THE PERIPHERAL NERVE

THE
PERIPHERAL NERVE

Edited by

D.N. LANDON

LONDON
CHAPMAN AND HALL

A Halsted Press Book
JOHN WILEY & SONS, INC., NEW YORK

First published 1976
by Chapman and Hall Ltd
11 New Fetter Lane, London EC4P 4EE
© *1976 Chapman and Hall Ltd*
Typeset by Preface Ltd
Salisbury, England
Printed and bound in the
United States of America

ISBN 0 412 11740 1

Distributed in the U.S.A.
by Halsted Press, a Division of
John Wiley and Sons, Inc., New York

CONTENTS

Contributors   *page* x
Preface   xi

1   THE MYELINATED NERVE FIBRE
    D. N. Landon and Susan Hall   1

    1.1   Introduction   1
    1.2   The axon   9
    1.3   The Schwann cell   13
    1.4   The node of Ranvier   27
    1.5   Axonal RNA   54
    1.6   The Schwann cell–axon relationship   58
    1.7   Intra-axonal transport systems   76
           References   90

2   THE UNMYELINATED NERVE FIBRE
    J. Ochoa   106

    2.1   Introduction   106
    2.2   Historical   107
    2.3   Fine structure   111
    2.4   Numbers and sizes of unmyelinated axons   130
    2.5   Growth of unmyelinated fibres   135
    2.6   Vulnerability of unmyelinated fibres and age changes   147
           References   150

3   THE PERINEURIUM AND CONNECTIVE TISSUE OF
    PERIPHERAL NERVE
    F. N. Low   159

    3.1   History of nerve sheaths   159
    3.2   General distribution   160
    3.3   Epineurium and endoneurium   161
    3.4   Perineurium   162

                                                                     v

3.5	Distal sheaths	168
3.6	Nerve root sheaths	173
3.7	Histogenesis of connective tissues	175
3.8	Blood supply of peripheral nerve	177
3.9	Barrier phenomena	178
3.10	Concluding remarks	179
	References	181

4 SENSORY GANGLIA
A. R. Lieberman 188

4.1	Introduction	188
4.2	General organization of sensory ganglia	189
4.3	Morphology and cytology of ganglion cells	198
4.4	Heterogeneity of neurons in sensory ganglia	218
4.5	Processes of sensory ganglion cells	225
4.6	The perineuronal satellite cell sheath	241
4,7	Development and differentiation of sensory ganglion cells	249
4.8	The trigeminal mesencephalic nucleus	253
4.9	Some functional considerations	256
	References	263

5 FUNCTIONAL ANATOMY OF THE ANTERIOR HORN MOTOR NEURON
S. Conradi 279

5.1	Introduction	279
5.2	Morphology of the motor neurons	280
5.3	Central connections of the motor neurons	296
5.4	Some aspects of the morphology of the motor neurons during development	312
5.5	Conclusion	319
	References	320

6 SPINAL AND CRANIAL NERVE ROOTS
H. J. Gamble 330

6.1	Introduction	330
6.2	Spinal nerve roots	331
6.3	Particular properties of cranial nerve roots	346
6.4	Degeneration and regeneration in nerve roots	349
	References	351

7   GANGLIA OF THE AUTONOMIC NERVOUS
    SYSTEM
    G. Gabella   355

    7.1   Sympathetic ganglia   355
    7.2   Sympathetic ganglia in amphibia   372
    7.3   The ciliary ganglion in mammals   376
    7.4   The ciliary ganglion in birds   379
    7.5   Intramural ganglia   382
          References   388

8   SENSORY TERMINALS OF PERIPHERAL NERVES
    L. H. Bannister   396

    8.1   Introduction   396
    8.2   Structure and functions of individual sensory endings 409
    8.3   Receptor arrays   446
          References   454

9   THE MOTOR END-PLATE: STRUCTURE
    Geraldine F. Gauthier   464

    9.1   General morphology of the motor end-plate   464
    9.2   Ultrastructure of the mammalian neuromuscular
          junction   465
    9.3   Ultrastructural and cytochemical manifestations of
          molecular configuration at the receptor site   478
    9.4   Recent functional interpretations of
          neuromuscular ultrastructure   481
    9.5   Summary and conclusion   487
          References   488

10 THE MOTOR END-PLATE: FUNCTION
    A. J. Buller   495

    10.1 Introduction   495
    10.2 Types of myoneural junctions   496
    10.3 Chemical transmission   498
    10.4 Transmitter release   500
    10.5 Post-synaptic events   506
    10.6 Non-transmitter action between nerve and muscle   508
    10.7 Summary and conclusions   509
          References   509

11 THE CHEMISTRY AND STRUCTURE OF MYELIN
     N. A. Gregson   512

     11.1   Introduction   512
     11.2   The composition of myelin   520
     11.3   Structural studies of myelin   533
     11.4   Short range interactions   542
     11.5   Modification of structure   544
     11.6   Myelin proteins and their properties   548
     11.7   Lipoprotein complexes isolated from myelin   562
     11.8   The synthesis and metabolism of myelin   565
     11.9   Abnormalities of myelin synthesis and metabolism
             in disease   577
     11.10   Current hypotheses of membrane structure and their
             relevance to myelin   585
             References   588

12 HISTOCHEMISTRY OF PERIPHERAL NERVES
     AND NERVE TERMINALS
     J. F. Hallpike   605

     12.1   Introduction   605
     12.2   The normal nerve   606
     12.3   **Wallerian degeneration**   628
     12.4   Demyelination   643
     12.5   Storage disorders   648
             References   652

13 PATHOLOGY OF THE PERIPHERAL NERVE
     G. Allt   666

     13.1   Introduction   666
     13.2   Experimental allergic neuritis – introduction   667
     13.3   Signs of EAN   667
     13.4   Histology of EAN   668
     13.5   Immune response in EAN   678
     13.6   EAN/EAE introduction processes and identity of the
             antigen   679
     13.7   Suppression of EAN   671
     13.8   Experimental diphtheritic neuropathy – introduction   682
     13.9   Signs of diphtheritic neuropathy   682
     13.10   Histology of diphtheritic neuropathy   683
     13.11   Effects of diphtheria toxin on cellular metabolism   695

13.12   Electrophysiological changes in EAN diphtheritic
        neuropathy   697
13.13   Wallerian degeneration and subsequent regeneration —
        introduction   701
13.14   Histology of Wallerian degeneration   703
13.15   Regeneration   716
13.16   Electrophysiological changes in Wallerian degeneration
        and subsequent regeneration   725
13.17   Conclusion   726
        References   728

14   ELECTROPHYSIOLOGICAL PROPERTIES OF
     PERIPHERAL NERVE
     J. J. B. Jack   740

14.1   Charge movements across the membrane   740
14.2   The spread of charge   779
14.3   Properties related to fibre size   795
14.4   Conclusion   806
        References   808

     Addenda   819

     Index   823

CONTRIBUTORS

G. Allt — Department of Anatomy, The Middlesex Hospital Medical School, Cleveland Street, London W1P 6DB.

L. H. Bannister — Department of Biology, Guy's Hospital Medical School, London Bridge SE1 9RT.

A. J. Buller — Department of Physiology, The Medical School, University Walk, Bristol ES8 1TD.

S. Conradi — Neurologiska Kliniken, Karolinska Sjuhuset, Fack, 1041 Stockholm 60, Sweden.

G. Gabella — Department of Anatomy and Embryology, University College, Gower Street, London WC1E 6BT.

H. J. Gamble — Anatomy Department, St. Thomas Hospital Medical School, London SE1 7RH.

Geraldine F. Gauthier — Wellesley College, Wellesley, Massachusetts 02181, U.S.A.

N. A. Gregson — Department of Anatomy, Guy's Hospital Medical School, London SE1 9RT.

Susan Hall — Department of Anatomy, Guy's Hospital Medical School, London SE1 9RT.

J. F. Hallpike — Wessex Neurological Centre, Southampton General Hospital, Tremona Road, Southampton SO9 4XY.

J. J. B. Jack — Physiology Laboratories, Parks Road, Oxford OX1 3PT.

D. N. Landon — Institute of Neurology, Queen Square, London WC1N 3BG.

A. R. Lieberman — Department of Anatomy and Embryology, University College, Gower Street, London WC1E 6BT.

F. N. Low — Department of Anatomy, University of North Dakota, Grand Forks, North Dakota 58201, U.S.A.

J. Ochoa — Division of Neurology, Dartmouth Medical School, Hanover, New Hampshire 03755, U.S.A.

PREFACE

"Our aim will be to make propositions about nerve-fibres which shall express as many aspects as possible of our experience of them, without allowing any to remain special or unrelated. We shall try to answer the question 'What is a nerve fibre?' in such a way as to relate the information about it to as wide a range of ideas as we can, and shall resolve not to be disquieted if the search leads us to some of the grandest questions of creation."

— J. Z. Young, from 'The History of the Shape of a Nerve Fibre' in *Essays on Growth and Form*, presented to D'Arcy Wentworth Thompson, 1945.

In the late 19th and early part of this century studies of the peripheral nerves and their distal terminations occupied a prominent place in accounts of the vertebrate nervous system, largely as a consequence of their accessibility for both microscopic examination and experimental manipulation. Thereafter the development of improved staining methods and electrophysiological techniques led to an increasing preoccupation with the integrative functions and internal connections of the central nervous system. Interest in the peripheral nervous system was renewed in the war, and early post-war, years as a result of concern for peripheral nerve injuries and their repair, and the structural bases responsible for the differing modalities of peripheral sensibility. However fashions change in biology, as in other fields of intellectual endeavour, and in many respects study of the peripheral nervous system has latterly become a poor relation to the more fashionable, and ostensibly more philosophically challenging, study of the structure and function of the central nervous system.

None-the-less the peripheral nervous system continues to offer many advantages to the experimenter concerned with the biology of nervous tissue and its functional behaviour, as well as the potential for greater and more immediate rewards in terms of the understanding and treatment of human pathology. Much has indeed been done in these fields within the last twenty years, but the information obtained is disseminated through a wide range of specialist publications and is not readily accessible to newcomers to the study of the nervous system, or to workers in other fields of biology and medicine. This book is intended to fulfill the need felt to exist at the time of its gestation for a concise yet well documented survey of present knowledge concerning the structure and function, and development and pathology of the mammalian peripheral nervous system.

The time has long since passed, however, when a genuinely comprehensive account of the peripheral nervous system could be contained within one volume, and emphasis has thus been placed upon recent advances in knowledge, particularly in the field of fine structure, and upon the nature of the biological interrelationships which exist between the neuron and it's supporting cells, end organs, and other surrounding tissues. Extensive references are provided to more detailed accounts of the individual topics discussed. Successive chapters deal with the myelinated and unmyelinated peripheral axons and their relationships to their satellite cells and connective tissue sheaths; with the cells of origin of such axons, both in the spinal cord and in the peripheral somatic and autonomic ganglia; and with their peripheral sensory and motor terminals. Further chapters are concerned with the structure and chemistry of myelin; with the histochemical reactions of peripheral nerves; with a review of the cytological phenomena associated with degeneration and regeneration in the peripheral nervous system; and with the physico-chemical processes underlying the initiation and conduction of the nerve impulse.

I am very grateful to the Medical Research Council and the Institute of Neurology, Queen Square, for the use of the research facilities needed for some of the work described in Chapter 1; to my wife Karen for her encouragement and support, and for much tedious typing; and to the contributors to this volume for the effort and care they have put into their individual chapters. I am sure that it is their hope, as much as it is mine, that this book may provide a useful foothold on the path towards a more complete understanding of the structure and function of the mammalian nervous system.

D.N.L.
July, 1975

1 THE MYELINATED NERVE FIBRE

D.N. Landon and Susan Hall

1.1 Introduction

The fundamental functional unit of the nervous system is the *neuron*, a remarkable cell which possesses the capacity to receive, conduct, process in the context of other incoming information, and subsequently transmit onwards, coded stimuli which converge upon it from a variety of central and peripheral sources, and is able to make functional contact with other neurons and with effector and receptor mechanisms via specialized sites of intercellular contact. The vertebrate neuron ·is a mononucleate, diploid cell which, for descriptive purposes, is usually subdivided into a cell body, the *soma* or *perikaryon*, and a population of fine cytoplasmic processes, collectively termed *neurites*, which are extensions of the soma into the surrounding tissues, and, like the soma, are covered with an excitable plasma membrane. By convention, a neurite that conveys information towards the soma is called a *dendrite*, and one that conveys information away from the soma, an *axon*. This division implies that conduction is unidirectional, as indeed is the case *in vivo*, although experimental studies have shown that axons can in fact conduct in either direction.

A neuron typically possesses but one axon, and a variable number of dendrites, arranged so as to form a *dendritic tree*, whose shape is often characteristic of the neuron. In some smaller neurons, the structure of the dendritic tree is relatively simple, but in the larger neurons, particularly in the higher centres, the dendrites branch more or less dichotomously many times, so that the resultant distribution of dendrites is an elaborate network in which the area of membrane surface available for the reception of stimuli is correspondingly increased, e.g., the cerebellar Purkinje cell. Although there is enormous variation in both the shape and dimensions of neurons in different loci, a morphological classification applicable to all vertebrate neurons is available, based upon the spatial relationships between a soma and its neurites: thus a neuron may be *unipolar* (e.g., dorsal root ganglion cells, granule cells of the olfactory bulb); *bipolar* (e.g., cells of the cochlear and vestibular ganglia), or, more commonly, *multipolar* (most of the cells of the central nervous system). In some rather rare instances the axon is absent – examples of such *anaxonic* neurons are the retinal bipolar cells and retinal amacrine cells.

Neurons may be located either wholly within the central nervous system, or, as in the case of cranial and sensory ganglia and dorsal root ganglion cells, cranial and spinal motor neurons and pre- and post-ganglionic autonomic neurons, their peripherally-directed axonal processes may lie wholly or partially within the peripheral nervous system, and are thus external to the pial envelope which covers the central nervous system.

An axon arises from its parent soma at the *axon hillock*, whence it continues into a short unmyelinated *initial segment* (see Chapter 5), distal to which it may extend for considerable distances before terminating in some specific site at the periphery. Though single throughout the initial segment and much of its subsequent course, an axon typically divides as it nears its termination, producing a terminal arborization of delicate *telodendria*. Between initial segment and terminal arborization, all axons are associated with a population of satellite cells; in the vertebrate central nervous system these are the *oligodendroglia*, and in the peripheral nervous system the *Schwann cells*.

1.1.1 The organization of a peripheral nerve trunk

In the peripheral nervous system, the functional unit constituted by an axon and its Schwann cells is termed a *peripheral nerve fibre*; and this unit may be further categorized as being either *non-myelinated* or *myelinated*, according to the nature of the structural relationship which obtains between the axon and its satellite. In the vertebrates, a major nerve trunk, e.g., one containing the nerve supply to part of a limb, is composed of many thousand non-myelinated and myelinated peripheral nerve fibres. In its proximal parts, where it is commonly incorporated in a limb plexus, it is a mixture of motor, sensory and post-ganglionic sympathetic fibres, having a plurisegmental derivation from the spinal cord. As the nerve trunk is traced distally, there is a gradual functional segregation of this initially heterogeneous population of fibres into bundles or *funiculi*, within which the majority of fibres are either motor or sensory. Repeated fasciculation (division of the funiculi), in conjunction with interchange of fibres between fascicles via numerous intraneural plexuses, continues the process of segregation according to destination, until ultimately small groups of fibres appear, each providing specific connections for a particular effector or receptor mechanism (see Sunderland, 1968).

A typical histological section through a peripheral nerve trunk would, therefore, contain numerous fibres, some emanating from anterior horn cells and conveying motor impulses to neuromuscular junctions, others the peripheral dendrites of dorsal root ganglia carrying pain, pressure, temperature and stretch impulses from either free endings in the skin or a number of specialized end-organs in skin, muscle, tendons, joints, connective tissue and bone. A more extensive functional classification of this spectrum of fibres has been derived from analyses of total fibre diameter and conduction velocity, parameters which show a direct proportional relationship in myelinated fibres (Hursh, 1939; Rushton, 1951). A fibre in any mixed peripheral nerve trunk may thus be

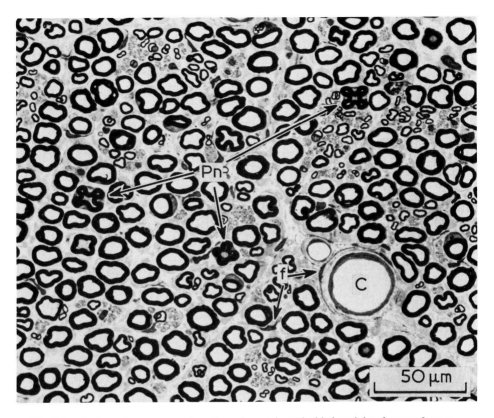

Fig. 1.1 A 1 μm transverse section through a resin embedded peripheral nerve from a baboon, stained with toluidine blue. Large and small diameter myelinated nerve fibres can be seen embedded in a matrix of longitudinally running collagen fibres. Also visible are endoneurial capillaries (C), fibroblasts (f), and crenated paranodal myelin sheaths (Pn).

allotted to one of three groups, A, B and C, originally defined by Erlanger and Gasser (1937), by comparing the shape of the compound action potential obtained from frog sciatic nerve with the fibre size histogram for that nerve. Group A comprises the largest fibres with the fastest conduction velocities, i.e., the myelinated somatic afferent and efferent fibres; group B contains the myelinated pre-ganglionic fibres of the autonomic nervous system, and group C is composed of the smallest-diameter, slowest-conducting, fibres, the unmyelinated visceral and somatic afferent fibres and the post-ganglionic autonomic efferents. Furthermore, as a result of numerous combined histological and electrophysiological studies of chronically de-afferented and de-efferented preparations, group A has been subdivided into groups I, II and III (all afferent fibres), and α, β and γ (all efferent fibres). In the following description of these subgroups, the values given in parentheses are respectively the diameter range and conduction velocity for the nerve fibres of the adult cat: it should be remembered however, that absolute values vary according to the species and the

3

site studied (see Boyd and Davey, 1968). Group I (10–20 μm, 50–100 m/sec) includes the primary sensory fibres from muscle spindles (Ia) and tendon organs (Ib); group II (5–15 μm, 20–70 m/sec) includes fibres from the secondary endings on the intrafusal muscle fibres within spindles and cutaneous afferent receptors; group III (1–7 μm, 5–30 m/sec) includes fibres which convey nociceptive impulses, afferent impulses from sensory plexuses in the walls of some blood vessels and from the follicles of fine 'down' hairs. In the efferent subdivision, α fibres (9–20 μm, 50–100 m/sec) are exclusively skeletomotor, β fibres (9–15 μm, 50–85 m/sec) are both skeletomotor and fusimotor, while γ fibres (4.5–8.5 μm, 20–40 m/sec) are exclusively fusimotor, both 'fast' and 'slow'.

Reference has already been made to the progressive ordering imposed upon an initially mixed population of fibres, by the process of fasciculation, and the question arises as to the means whereby fibres are retained within the appropriate bundle during their passage through the tissues to their termination. Some measure of mechanical restraint is undoubtedly provided by a system of three morphologically-distinct connective tissue sheaths, the *epineurium*, the *perineurium* and the *endoneurium*, which respectively surround a nerve trunk, its funiculi, and the individual fibres of which they are composed (see Chapter 3). Peripheral nerve fibres lie within the endoneurium, or endoneurial space, a loose collagenous matrix, which also contains occasional fibroblasts, mast cells and the intraneural capillary network. The perineurium, the layer intermediate between endoneurium and epineurium, is the most cellular of the three sheaths, being composed of a number of layers of characteristically flattened cells, each covered by a basal lamina and exhibiting evidence of considerable pinocytotic activity. As will be seen in a later chapter, many workers have demonstrated the effectiveness of the perineurium as a diffusion barrier responsible for the isolation of the peripheral nerve fibres it encloses from potentially noxious materials in the surrounding connective tissue spaces. The epineurium constitutes the adventitial coat of a nerve trunk, and consists of irregular, dense connective tissue, which is largely collagenous. These three components of the connective sheath of the peripheral nerve are described and discussed at length in Chapter 3.

1.1.2 *The basic organization of a myelinated peripheral nerve fibre*

In a normal mammalian myelinated peripheral nerve fibre, the Schwann cells, which are responsible for the elaboration and subsequent maintenance of the myelin sheath, are arranged in longitudinal sequence along the axonal surface, every Schwann cell territory defining the extent of an *internode*. In both immature and mature fibres, there is only one Schwann cell, and, hence, one Schwann cell nucleus, per internode, and when fibres branch this invariably occurs at a node. Internodal length is an easily measured dimensional parameter that is frequently employed in quantitative analyses of fibre populations, and it

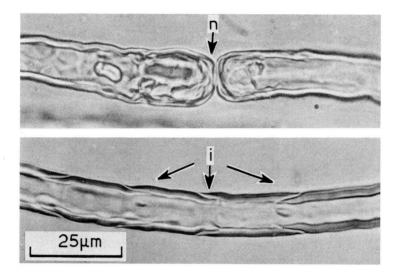

Fig. 1.2   Large myelinated nerve fibres from a mouse teased in saline, showing a node of Ranvier (n) with its paranodal bulbs, and a myelin sheath containing incisures of Schmidt–Lanterman (i).

bears a positive but variable correlation to external fibre diameter (e.g., Thomas and Young, 1949). In mammalian myelinated fibres, internodal length ranges from c. 300 μm in the smallest diameter fibres to c. 1500 μm in the largest (e.g., Vizoso and Young, 1948).

Every internode, irrespective of its length, and whether it is observed microscopically *in vivo* or *in vitro*, appears to be subdivided into a variable number of *cylindrico-conical segments* whose boundaries are delimited by a series of zones within the myelin sheath, the *incisures of Schmidt–Lanterman*. For over a century the latter were considered by the majority of histologists to be artefacts, but they are now known to be inclusions of Schwann cytoplasm within the myelin which pursue a spiral course across the sheath, and connect the external and internal layers of Schwann cell cytoplasm (Section 1.23). The cylindrico-conical segment becomes more apparent in the acute stage of Wallerian degeneration (Chapter 14), when it forms the basis of a primary degeneration ovoid; however, in the normal fibre, it has, as yet, no functional connotation, and thus remains merely a descriptive 'unit'.

The distribution of compact myelin and cytoplasm within a Schwann cell is such that an internode is organized internally into a series of concentric subcellular compartments which surround the axon, and insulate it, both morphologically and physiologically, from the endoneurium (Ranvier, 1878). The axon consists of a central core of cytoplasm or *axoplasm*, bounded by a continuous plasma membrane, the *axolemma*; this is surrounded in turn by a narrow peri-axonal space, the Schwann cell plasma membrane and a thin inner layer of Schwann cell cytoplasm, the numerous membranous lamellae of the

5

myelin sheath, an outer more extensive layer of Schwann cell cytoplasm, and finally a continuous Schwann cell plasma membrane and its basal lamina.

All internodes, with the obvious exception of the first and last along a fibre, are bounded proximally and distally by a *node of Ranvier*, a structure which appears by light microscopy to be narrow tranverse interruption seemingly separating neighbouring internodal segments (e.g., Ranvier, 1875; Hess and Young, 1952), and the region of the internode immediately adjacent to the nodal gap is accordingly termed the *paranode*. While the overall contour of an internode is usually envisaged to be that of a smooth-walled cylinder of more or less constant diameter, there is in fact considerable and consistent deviation from this shape in the region of the paranode and node of larger fibres, where the fibre first expands dramatically into a *paranodal bulb*, before narrowing at the nodal gap to a diameter which is considerably less than that of the internode Fig. 4. As will be seen later (Section 1.24), the paranodal bulb is a region at which there exist complex reciprocal alterations in the form and composition of both axon and Schwann cell (Williams and Landon, 1963; Berthold, 1968a). Unlike the incisure of Schmidt–Lanterman, which has been little investigated, and whose function is at present unknown, the nodal region has been the subject of numerous studies. The importance of the node in the propogation of the action potential has been recognized since the early 1940's (Tasaki and Takeuchi, 1941), and it is generally accepted that the nerve impulse is conducted along the fibre by saltation from node to node, and that this process involves rapid ionic fluxes across succesive nodal axon membranes (see Chapter 14).

1.1.3 *The development of ideas about the structure of the peripheral nerve fibre*

The process by which ideas are evaluated is a complex one, greatly influenced by previous experience, and therefore the ways in which our knowledge of the structure of the peripheral nerve fibre has developed will be briefly traced prior to describing current views concerning its morphology and functional activities.

The fibrous nature of the components of the peripheral nervous system has been recognized for almost two centuries, since the writings of Fontana (1781), who described in detail semi-transparent nervous cylinders within teased fibre bundles. During the first half of the last century, Remak described the unmyelinated nerve fibres which still bear his name, and recognized that the fibres of the organic (sympathetic) nervous system differed from those elsewhere in the body in that they lacked a white outer layer. Moreover, he was aware that within each nerve fibre in the peripheral nervous system, there was a thin-walled tube containing a flat ribbon (primitive Band), which corresponded to the whole grey fibre of the organic system, and he gave what is probably the first account of the maturation of peripheral nerve fibres (Remak, 1836, 1837).

During the nineteenth century, the shape of the peripheral nerve fibre, the nature of the myelin sheath, the physical consistency of the axon and the

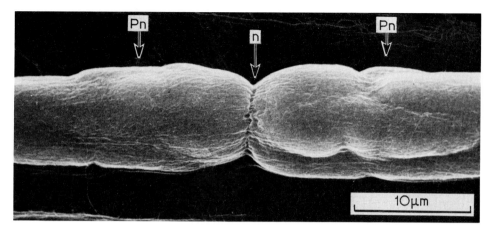

Fig. 1.3 Scanning electron micrograph of the nodal region of a 10 μm diameter myelinated fibre from the sciatic nerve of a rat. The structure of the node (n) is obscured by the overlying sheath of fine collagen fibrils (the sheath of Plenk and Laidlaw) and the Schwann cell basal lamina; (Pn) indicates the paranodal bulbs.

existence of anatomically-distinct regions within each fibre, in particular the nodes of Ranvier and the incisures of Schmidt—Lanterman, were examined by numerous workers, using a variety of complex histological techniques. For detailed accounts and contemporary critiques, the reader should consult the classic and extensive texts by Ranvier (1878), Gedoelst (1886) and Cajal (1928).

In retrospect, it is clear that many subsequent misconceptions concerning the significance of the structural features of peripheral nerve fibres were the inevitable consequences of first, an inadequate appreciation of the effects of excision and subsequent physico-chemical trauma on the excised fibre; second, an inappropriate choice of fixatives due to an ignorance of their chemistry and mode of action; and third, the almost complete absence of attempts to observe fibres *in vivo*. In an era in which the methods of investigation become ever more complex, these criticisms of empiricism remain sadly relevant. Interpretations of peripheral nerve fibre organization must therefore still be evaluated in an awareness of the paucity of information at present available concerning the nature and extent of alterations to the structure and dimensions of nerve fibres produced by preparative techniques (see Williams and Wendell-Smith, 1971).

The lipid/protein nature of the myelin sheath has been recognized for over a century. Ewald and Kühne (1874) wrote of a horny proteinaceous network in the myelin sheath of peripheral nerve fibres; Ranvier (1878) regarded myelin as being fluid, or nearly fluid, fat, and Gedoelst (1886) proposed that it consisted of lecithin and cerebrine; while the discovery of the birefringence of myelin is attributed to Ehrenberg (1849). Furthermore, in 1910, Nageotte, on the basis of preferential cleavage patterns produced by alcoholic extraction of lipid from myelin, described a system of repeating lipid and protein layers which bore a

7

superficial resemblance to modern interpretations of the organization of the myelin sheath.

During the 1930's Schmitt and his co-workers demonstrated both the radially positive intrinsic birefringence and the radially negative form birefringence of the sheath after lipid extraction (e.g., Schmitt, Bear and Palmer, 1935; Schmitt and Bear, 1937). On the basis of this work, together with the results of studies by Schmidt (e.g., Schmidt, 1936), a model of myelin was proposed in which radially disposed lipid and tangentially orientated protein moieties were arranged in alternating concentric laminae. Thus, the application of data integrated from the physical analytical techniques of X-ray diffraction and polarization optics, to a biological structure with an inherent geometrical regularity, enabled reasonably confident predictions to be made about sheath architecture over a decade before the publication of the earliest electron micrographs (Fernandez–Moran, 1950). The structure and chemistry of myelin are described in detail in Chapter 11.

Early attempts to describe the detailed morphology of the axon and Schwann cell, using light microscopy, or to determine their relationship to each other and to the myelin sheath, and the manner of myelinogenesis were less successful, although there were several investigations of the morphological changes which occur during maturation of the peripheral nerve fibre (e.g., Remak, 1836; Vignal, 1883; Westphal, 1894). Our present limited understanding of the mechanics of the formation of the myelin sheath owe much to the observations and deductions of Geren (1954), who described the wrapping of the elongated Schwann cell mesaxon around the axon in her classic 'jelly-roll' hypothesis. While it seems likely that this presents too simple a view of the processes involved, and that some appositional or interstitial growth must also occur (see p. 59, Section 1.6.1), an acceptance of Geren's proposals is implicit in most current interpretations of sheath morphology, and of the appearances of nerve fibres during remyelination.

In 1928, de Renyi defined the criteria necessary for the recognition of a 'normal, living' peripheral nerve fibre. It is clear in retrospect that these criteria were necessarily arbitrary, since they were based on studies of teased fibres; they were, however, of significance since their proposal indicated a recognition of the need for a definition of 'normality', and a determination to move away from the catalogues of often conflicting structural details described by the nineteenth century histologists. A protracted series of classic experimental observations on the nerve fibres of the living tadpole tail followed (Speidel, 1932, 1933, 1964), and the results of this work, and of the earlier observations by Harrison (1904) and by de Renyi, provided a frame of reference within which the results of conventional light microscopical histology could be assessed.

There have been surprisingly few attempts to compare the morphology of processed tissue with that of its living counterpart. In the peripheral nervous system, tissue density, thickness, and the experimental dislocation involved in the presentation of the field to the optical system, have precluded the

8

transillumination of substantially undisturbed mature mammalian nerve trunks; it is for these reasons that tissue culture has achieved such popularity. Tissue culture techniques in the nervous system have evolved from the hanging drop method introduced by Harrison (1904), into the more elaborate procedures developed by Murray and her co-workers over the last thirty years, capable of maintaining explanted embryonic and neo-natal tissues for considerable periods (Murray, 1965).

A technique has recently been developed for the observation of mature myelinated peripheral nerve fibres *in vivo*, using oblique incident illumination (Williams and Hall, 1970). Using this technique, some aspects of the *in vivo* structure of the peripheral nerve fibre have been described in the normal animal (Fig. 1.9) and during degeneration and demyelination (Williams and Hall, 1971a, b; Hall and Gregson, 1971).

1.2 The axon

The origins of the myelinated axons of the mammalian peripheral nervous system from their cell somata are described in detail in Chapters 5 and 6. These axons possess a diameter range of <1 μm to 10 or 15 μm: the extent to which an axon may taper along its length has not been systematically examined, nor have axonal diameters been systematically analysed in terms of their distribution within fibre populations. Most measurements of axon diameter have been directed toward evaluating its relationship to total fibre diameter (a ratio known as 'g'), because of its relevance to theories of saltatory conduction (Rushton, 1951; Hodgkin, 1971; Williams and Wendell-Smith, 1971). The internodal axon typically appears to be a smooth-walled cylinder, which becomes reciprocally indented at the outermost limits of the paranode, shaped by, or possibly shaping, the crenation of the myelin sheath in this region (Williams and Landon, 1963). At the node, in most myelinated fibres, the axon regains its cylindrical contour, but at the same time becomes dramatically constricted, so that its diameter is only $1/3 - 1/6$ of its internodal value (Landon and Williams, 1963; Berthold, 1968a and Section 1.5). Berthold (1968a) has described tortuous axonal projections which are given off from the paranodal/nodal axon of the largest myelinated fibres in the adult cat: their significance is unknown, although presumably they result in an increase in the surface area of contact between axon and Schwann cell. In small fibres, however, the nodal axon diameter appears to be larger than that of the internodal axon; according to Dun (1970), this may be predicted from an analysis of the relationship between fibre diameter and nodal diameter and length, using the transmission line theory.

An axon is composed of cytoplasm, the axoplasm, and is bounded by a continuous plasma membrane, the axolemma, which is separated from the Schwann cell plasma membrane along its internodal aspect by a $10 - 20$ nm peri-axonal space. Ultrastructurally, axoplasm consists of an electron-translucent

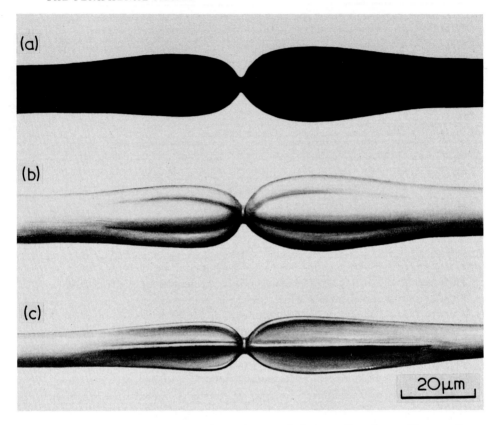

Fig. 1.4 An artist's impression of some features of a large myelinated nerve fibre near the node of Ranvier. (a) Silhouette of the paranodal bulbs showing their proximo-distal asymetry; (b) the surface contour of the bulbs; and (c) the surface contour of the subjacent axon with the myelin sheath removed. By courtesy of the editor of *Nature* (reproduced from Williams and Landon, 1963).

amorphous matrix, within which is found a characteristic population of organelles. In aldehyde-osmium fixed material, a fine granularity can usually be seen in the vicinity of the organelles, and immediately below the axolemma (this should not be confused with the denser undercoating of the nodal axolemma): this presumably reflects the deposition of stain on axoplasmic macro-molecules – the apparent clumping around the organelles is probably a fixation artefact.

The majority of axoplasmic organelles are either microtubules or neuro-filaments, normally aligned in parallel with the long axis of the fibre, although it is not unusual to find bundles of neurofilaments apparently cut obliquely in longitudinal sections. The microtubules are cylindrical, seemingly rigid struc-tures, 24 ± 2 nm in diameter, consisting of 12–13 slightly twisted rows of globular protein subunits, 4–5 nm in diameter. These subunits are a colchicine-binding protein, tubulin, having a molecular weight of c. 60 000

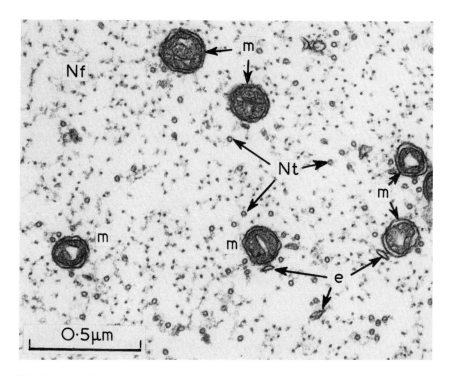

Fig. 1.5   An electron micrograph of a transverse section through the axoplasm of a large myelinated nerve fibre: (m) mitochondria; (e) smooth endoplasmic reticulum: (Nf) neurofilaments; and (Nt) neurotubules.

(Schmitt and Samson, 1968): the fact that tubulin binds colchicine has been exploited in numerous experimental investigations of axonal transport mechanisms (Section 1.86). In most tissues, including nerve, microtubules appear to be hollow following conventional preparative methods, but some axonal microtubules have a dense core – the significance of which is unknown. According to Weiss and Mayr (1971c) microtubules extend as single, continuous and undivided structures . . . 'from their roots in the neuronal soma through the length of the axon to its peripheral ending.' By counting microtubules in single branched axons (Aα and Ia fibres) innervating rat lumbrical muscles, they found that the combined total of numbers of tubules present in the distal branches equalled the number recorded in the proximal undivided stem, and they proposed that the microtubule grows exclusively from its base by accretion of subunits in the immediate vicinity of the nucleus, the coiling of the subunits seen in the mature microtubule being imposed by nuclear rotation (Weiss and Mayr, 1971c). Zenker and Hohberg (1973b) have recently confirmed that there is no change in the microtubule content of the axons of fibres immediately above and below the sites of fibre division. However their further finding that the mean density of microtubules is identical in the parent axon and its peripheral terminal branches indicates, when taken in conjunction with their earlier observation (Zenker and Hohberg, 1973a), that the sum of axonal cross sectional areas of all of the terminal branches of an Aα fibre exceeds the cross sectional area of their stem fibre by some eleven times, that many peripheral microtubules can have no direct continuity with the microtubules in the neuron soma. While the peripheral increase in the microtubule numbers could in theory represent the result of branching, this phenomenon has never been reported, and it appears probable that the additional microtubules are assembled locally, possibly from centrally synthesized molecules of tubulin monomer, in the numbers needed to match the peripheral increase in axoplasmic mass.

Neurofilaments are 8–9 nm diameter filaments, composed of globular subunits, frequently having small side-arms projecting from their surfaces (Wuerker, 1970). Satisfactory extraction and chemical and physical analyses of neurofilaments have not yet been acheived in the vertebrate nervous system, although such studies have been carried out on squid giant axons (Schmitt and Davison, 1961). There is much evidence to support the view that aggregations of neurofilaments provide the basis for the argentophilic fibrils seen by light miscroscopy using the reduced-silver methods of Cajal and Bielschowsky (Gray, 1970).

Other constituents of axoplasm include mitochondria – these are typically long and threadlike, at least two or three being seen within the internodal axoplasm in any transverse section – vesicles of varying shapes and sizes, and discontinuous membrane-bound profiles which are presumed to be agranular endoplasmic reticulum. Occasionally, ribosome-like particles, glycogen (especially within nodal axoplasm), multivesicular bodies, dense bodies and structures resembling the dense-cored vesicles typical of adrenergic axons are also visible.

It is of interest that since the biochemical demonstration of axonal RNA (Section 1.4), descriptions have appeared of axoplasmic ribosomes, or ribosome-like particles, in the initial segments of adult neurons (Peters, Proskauer and Kaiserman-Abramoff, 1968; Palay, Sotelo, Peters and Orkand, 1968), and in embryonic and foetal axons (e.g., Caley and Maxwell, 1968; Tennyson, 1969). Ribosomes have also been described recently in segments of foetal rabbit axon some distance (60 μm) from the perikaryon, in 'growth cones' (Tennyson, 1970), and in mature myelinated axons in the rat (Zelena, 1970). Such findings emphasize the tendency for the electron microscopist to concentrate on one particular aspect of a sample, and to ignore the morphology of adjacent areas; it is unlikely that the demonstration of axoplasmic ribosomes has resulted from any sudden improvement in technique, since the visualization of ribosomes, unlike that of microtubules, does not appear to be fixative-dependent.

It has been suggested that the axoplasm is organized internally into 'streets' within which the organelles become aligned in longitudinally-running columns – the mitochondria and vesicles lying in nose-to-tail fashion between bundles of microtubules and neurofilaments (e.g., Martinez and Friede, 1970a). There is little evidence however to support such precise compartmentalization in normal fibres; but in certain abnormal states, notably those following the induction of axonal swelling, longitudinal rows of mitochondria and degenerating organelles may be seen, separated by tangles of neurofilaments and degenerating microtubules (Martinez and Friede, 1970a, Hall, 1972). It may be well that this appearance is an expression of altered axonal flow characteristics, and the relevance of such morphological changes to the distribution of organelles within the axoplasm is doubtful. Some attempts have been made to analyse the distribution patterns of organelles within the axoplasm – but these are of limited value since it seems likely that while some bulk translocation of the axonal column does occur, the various organelles are transported at different rates, both as classes and as individuals (Section 1.83).

1.3 The Schwann cell

The Schwann cell is the neuronal satellite cell of the peripheral nervous system.

1.3.1 *Origin and development*

Some aspects of the early development of the Schwann cell, in particular its derivation, and its initial relationship to the whole peripheral nerve fibre bundle, remain unresolved. Since the classic series of experiments by Harrison (1904, 1924), a considerable body of experimental evidence has accumulated to support the view that the neural folds are the major source of the satellite cells of cranial and peripheral nerves (e.g., Yntema, 1937; Detwiler and Kehoe, 1939; Weston, 1963; Chibon, 1965; Johnston, 1966). At present, it is thought that the Schwann cell has a dual derivation, from both the neural crest and the neural tube: and while the relative contribution from either source to the emergent population of Schwann cells is not known, most evidence tends to indicate that the neural crest is the major cell donor (see Horstadius, 1950; Weston, 1970 and Chapter 10).

Do the Schwann cells influence the distribution patterns of the outgrowing peripheral nerve fibre bundles? Relatively little attention has been paid to this question, or to the related problem as to whether the Schwann cells are present *in situ* in the tissues before the appearance of the axons, largely because of the difficulty of identifying such undifferentiated cells as they migrate through the developing tissues. According to Harrison (1924), the relationship of sheath cells to motor nerve roots is initially variable in the frog, and Yntema (1943) found that the normal migration of motor fibres into the limb in *Ambystoma* failed to occur following the experimental removal of the (presumed) source of the sheath cells. Weston (1963) followed the migration of isotope labelled neural crest cells in the somitic mesenchyme of unlabelled hosts in the chick: labelled cells were observed lying along the ventral aspect of the neural tube at the time at which the first motor nerve fibres were emerging ... 'we only know that when nerve fibres can first be identified in radioautographic preparations, some labelled cells have already associated closely with them' (Weston, 1970). It is interesting that the relationship between labelled graft and developing fibre

13

bundles persisted even where the latter were abnormally sited in the embryo (Weston, 1963), suggesting a specific (and inductive?) response by the sheath cells to the presence of the axons.

Axons, 0.1—1.5 μm in diameter, grow out from the spinal cord in large bundles, within which they are in cell-to-cell contact in a manner similar to that found in the mature vertebrate olfactory nerve. A number of such bundles, collectively constituting the axonal complement of a definitive peripheral nerve trunk or funiculus, are initially surrounded by two cellular layers: an inner layer composed of the mesenchymal precursors of the connective tissue elements of the mature nerve, and an outer layer of migrating Schwann cells. These Schwann cells proliferate and, crossing the mesenchymal layer, invade the axonal groups — a process beginning on or before the 12th embryonic day in the rat (Diner, 1965) and mouse (Asbury, 1967), and in the 12th week *in utero* in the nerves of the brachial plexus and the sciatic nerves of the human foetus (Cravioto, 1965). The subsequent activities of the Schwann cells over a relatively short period (two weeks *in utero* in the human foetus), are important in establishing both the geometry and the physiological characteristics (in the sense of the distinction between future myelinated and non-myelinated fibres) of the mature nerve fibre bundle.

By 14 weeks *in utero* in man, the Schwann cells appear to be more or less uniformly distributed throughout the nerve, dissecting away groups of axons — foetal axons (Friede and Samorajski, 1968; Reier and Hughes, 1972) — from the main bundles by means of long exploratory cytoplasmic processes. Speidel (1964) has described primitive Schwann cells migrating proximo-distally along young unmyelinated fibres in amphibian larvae *in vivo*, the cells appearing to proceed by slow amoeboid movements, putting out fine pseudopodia. Initially, a number of axons are engulfed either singly or communally, within invaginations of each Schwann cell plasma membrane: according to Gamble (1966) and Dunn (1970), several hundred axons commonly share the same invagination at the earliest stages examined in the nerves of the human foetus. The largest axons tend to be arranged peripherally within the invaginated groups of axons, and on the basis of their subsequent developmental history, these have been identified as a recognizable population of *pro-myelin* fibres by some workers (Friede and Samorajski, 1968). As a result of repeated Schwann cell division, a situation is rapidly reached within the nerve bundle in which the majority of Schwann cells contain only one pro-myelin axon, i.e., the 1:1 relationship between axon and Schwann cell of the mature myelinated fibre has been established. The initiation of myelinogenesis, which has been suggested to be, at least in part, related to the attainment of a critical axon diameter (Friede and Somarajski, 1967, 1968 and Section 1.6.1, p. 63) is associated with both a cessation of Schwann cell proliferation and a period of Schwann cell hypertrophy. In an autoradiographic study, Asbury (1967) reported that by the 2nd post-natal day in the mouse, only one-quarter of the Schwann cells were still proliferating, a finding in accord with the rapid myelinogenesis taking place in the mouse at this time.

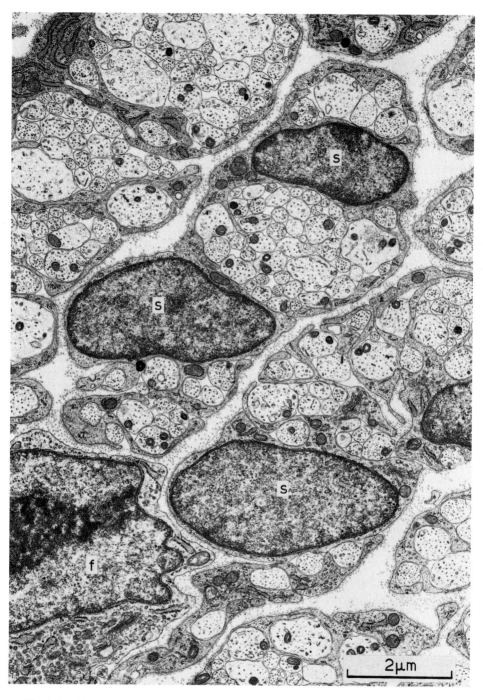

Fig. 1.6 Electron micrograph of a transverse section through the nerve to the medial gastrocnemius muscle of a neonatal rat. Three Schwann cell nuclei (s) and one fibroblast nucleus (f) are labelled. Numerous small axons of varying size are enclosed singly, or as groups, within extensions of Schwann cell cytoplasm.

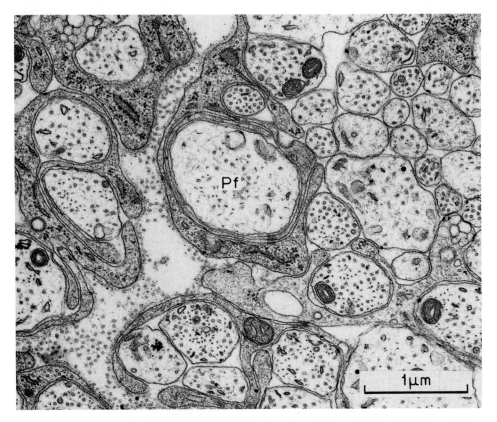

Fig. 1.7 A similar preparation to Fig. 1.6., showing a 'promyelin' fibre (Pf), segregated from an adjacent cluster of primitive unmyelinated axons by overlapping layers of Schwann cell cytoplasm. Earlier stages in the same process are visible around two fibres on the left.

1.3.2 *Morphology*

A Schwann cell is usually defined as a cell, within a peripheral nerve fibre trunk or bundle, enclosing an axon, or group of axons, and itself surrounded by a continuous basal lamina. Although in the normal nerve, no other cells are ever seen in such proximity to the axonal population, there are instances, as will be seen in a later chapter, in pathologically or experimentally altered nerve, when this is not the case, and an axon may become separated from its Schwann cell by an invading monocyte or small lymphocyte. Controversy has recently centred around the nature of certain axon-associated cells, lacking a basal lamina, at sites of active nerve regeneration (Morris, Hudson and Weddell, 1972). It seems unnecessary to invoke any special nomenclature to cover such cells however, and unless they can be shown to be of haematogenous origin, they should be considered to be Schwann cells, despite their (temporary?) lack of a basal lamina.

The life history of the Schwann cell is divisible into two distinct stages, a peri-natal migratory and proliferative phase, which is succeeded by the axon-associated, myelin-producing and -maintaining differentiated state: the mobility displayed by the Schwann cell during the former phase, and its relative quiescence during the latter, are reflected in the differing morphologies of the immature and mature Schwann cell.

The immature Schwann cell is initially a large rounded cell, with an oval nucleus possessing one, or sometimes two nucleoli. The cytoplasm is typically dense, containing numerous mitochondria, single ribosomes, polyribosomes and a few microtubules (Fig. 1.6). As the cells migrate, at first they assume a spindle shape, and subsequently become more irregular in outline with the production of shorter, thicker processes from nearer the main body of the cell (Cravioto, 1965). Frequent mitotic figures are seen at this and subsequent stages in the subdivision of the axon groups (Cravioto, 1965; Asbury, 1967; Dunn, 1970; Martin and Webster, 1973). The processes come to lie between the tightly-packed small diameter axons, which thus appear to be contained within deep invaginations of the Schwann cell plasma membrane (Webster, Martin and O'Connell, 1973).

Once a Schwann cell has achieved an appropriate quantitative relationship with an axon or group of axons, proliferation and migration cease: the proliferative and migratory potentials of the Schwann cell do not become apparent in the mature nerve except in response to an abnormal stimulus, e.g., the induction of axonal degeneration. In such cases, the Schwann cell is considered to exhibit signs of de-differentiation, in that it 'reverts' to its juvenile proliferative and migratory characteristics.

In developing myelinated and non-myelinated fibres, the Schwann cell presents an 'active' appearance, manifested by a relatively large volume of cytoplasm, rich in mitochondria, polyribosomes and granular endoplasmic reticulum, the moderately-dilated cisternae of which typically contain electron-dense material. Microfilaments and microtubules are particularly obvious, the latter lying in bundles parallel with the long axis (axes) of the invaginated axon (axons), and in the lips of the cytoplasm bounding the external mesaxon in myelinating fibres.

As the axons increase in diameter, and as the myelin sheath grows thicker, there is a gradual diminution in the apparent volume of the related Schwann cell cytoplasm, and Samorajski and Friede (1968) have found that in the sciatic and vagus nerves of the mouse the ratio of axoplasm to Schwann cell cytoplasm in a normal mature fibre increased in a curvilinear fashion with the increase in fibre size.

In electron micrographs of longitudinal sections of mature myelinated fibres, the Schwann cell cytoplasm is evident as a thin, often apparently discontinuous, pale strip lying external to the myelin sheath, and internal to the Schwann cell plasma membrane – this layer forms the outer compartment of Schwann cell cytoplasm. Only rarely is any Schwann cell cytoplasm observed internal to the myelin sheath in small mammals such as the mouse (Samorajski and Friede, 1968), but in larger mammals, e.g., the cat, the baboon and man, three or more longitudinally running bands of Schwann cytoplasm can usually be found within the myelin sheath of the larger fibres, indenting the external contour of the axon. However only at the paranodes, in the nodal gap fingers, throughout the spiral of the Schmidt—Lanterman incisures and in the perinuclear region, does any substantial volume of Schwann cell cytoplasm persist after myelination is completed. The distribution of the external compartment of the cytoplasm between these sites, i.e., over the major part of the uncomplicated internode, is apparently limited to narrow, longitudinally-disposed bands, linked at random by fine cross-bridges, thereby forming a diffuse network (e.g., Nemiloff, 1910; Nageotte, 1922; Cajal, 1928; Young, 1945; Berthold, 1968a; Samorajski and Friede, 1968), and is not, as has been proposed (Stoeckenius and Zeiger, 1956), a continuous sheet. There are undoubtedly inter- and intra-species and even inter-fibre differences in the arrangement described, but the basic plan appears to be common to the larger myelinated fibres of all vertebrates that have been examined. In such fibres, depending upon the physico-chemical conditions of fixation and subsequent preparation for electron microscopy, the external contour, indeed the whole thickness, of the myelin sheath may assume one of several forms in tranverse sections: it may be classically smooth and almost circular, or randomly-indented or even 'cog-wheel like' (the irregular pattern described by Berthold, 1968a). On aesthetic grounds, such indented sheaths are usually considered to be poorly fixed, and therefore fail to represent the 'true' shape of the fibre *in vivo*; a view disputed by Berthold (1968a). The Schwann cell cytoplasm is observed either lying in flattened, isolated demi-lunes around the circumference of the smooth sheaths, or occupying the troughs which are the inevitable accompaniment to the variously notched sheaths. In a brief ultrastructural analysis of the distribution of Schwann cell cytoplasm about the myelinated axon (other than at paranodes and nuclei), Samorajski and Friede (1968) found that 94% of the axons in the sciatic nerve of the mouse were covered by only two or three strands of cytoplasm, but they found that larger fibres may contain proportionately more strands, and multiple strands are evident in the photomicrographs of Berthold and Skoglund (1967).

The cytoplasm of the mature Schwann cell is less electron dense than that of the more immature 'active' cell, and in the narrow longitudinal processes running between paranodes and perinuclear region, it consists of a granular amorphous material containing an occasional microtubule or group of microfilaments, and more rarely a mitochondrion or dense body. In the paranodal region, however, the volume of cytoplasm increases considerably, filling the troughs created by the crenations of the paranodal sheath (Nageotte, 1922; Williams and Landon, 1963; Landon and Williams, 1963; Berthold and Skoglund, 1967) and characteristically, in the mature paranode, becomes rich in rod-shaped mitochondria, 0.3—4.0 μm long (Williams and Landon, 1963; Berthold and Skoglund, 1967, see Section 1.2.4 and Fig. 1.19). In a developmental study on the density

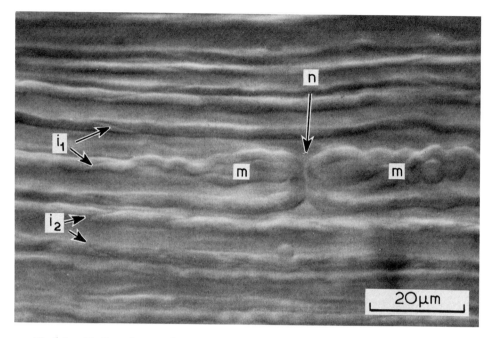

Fig. 1.8   Myelinated nerve fibres in the sciatic nerve of a mouse visualized by oblique incident illumination *in vivo*, and undisturbed. A node (n) is seen, together with several incisures of Schmidt–Lanterman (i). Note the folded and undulant outline of the myelin (m) over the paranodal bulbs.

of mitochondria in Schwann cell cytoplasm in ventral lumbar roots and peripheral nerve fibres of the cat, Berthold and Skoglund (1967) found an approximate ten-fold increase in the mean number of mitochondria per 100 square microns of paranodal Schwann cell cytoplasm with time, from birth up to at least one year, whereas the increase for internodal mitochodria was a third of this value. The distribution of Schwann cell cytoplasm may be inferred from the application of tinctorial histochemical methods designed to demonstrate the presence of characteristic (though by no means specific) mitochondrion-bound enzymes (Williams and Landon, 1965; Berthold and Skoglund, 1967). Light microscope evaluation of the activity pattern of $NADH_2$ — tetrazolium reductase in teased, fixed fibres of lumbar spinal roots and peripheral nerves in mature cats indicated a predominantly peri-nuclear and paranodal accumulation of formazan deposits, linked via delicate bands of activity (Berthold and Skoglund, 1967). Such a pattern correlates well with the known ultrastructural distribution of mitochondria within the Schwann cell cytoplasm of the mature internode and paranode.

In the study of the peripheral nerve, as of any other biological structure, the validity of attempts to extrapolate from the static microscope image to the *in vivo* state is always open to question. In the case of the distribution of Schwann cell cytoplasm around the internodal axon, it is clear that even if the tedious task of analysing semi-serial sections of a selected population of fibres were to be undertaken, the information thus obtained would be limited to a reasonably precise account of the morphological association between a small number of Schwann cells and their axons immediately prior to fixation/exicision (after due allowances have been made for the effects of these procedures). Furthermore, we do not know whether the Schwann cell is capable *in vivo* of altering its morphological relationship with the axon by re-arrangement of its cytoplasmic compartments.

At the node, the Schwann cell cytoplasm extends as a collar over and beyond the convex outer border of the terminating myelin sheath; from it protude a regular system of filament-containing finger-like processes. The latter are directed into the nodal space, interdigitating in the finely floccular gap substance with their counterparts from the collar of Schwann cell cytoplasm of the adjacent paranode. It seems that this part of the Schwann cell, at least, is capable of the rapid extension of exploratory processes into the endoneurium or along the adjacent axon, following alterations to the 'normal' environment of the fibre or to the 'normal' morphological association between Schwann cell/Schwann cell or Schwann cell and axon: examples of such processes are typically seen during incipient paranodal demyelination (e.g., Ballin and Thomas, 1969a).

The perinuclear Schwann cell cytoplasm contains numerous polyribosomes, microtubules, microfilaments, mitochondria and small dense bodies, a limited amount of granular endoplasmic reticulum, prominent Golgi vesicles and, less frequently, lysosomes and glycogen-like particles. A number of interesting perinuclear inclusion bodies have been described: while most are considered to be nothing more than preparative artefacts, there are two notable exceptions – Reich's π granules, and the corpuscles of Erzholz (see Cajal, 1928). Reich's π granules or 'protagon granules', are ellipsoidal structures $1-2\ \mu m$ long, composed of lamellae having an alternating 4 nm repeat of dark and light bands, separated by a finely granular matrix. In the peripheral nerve fibres of the rat and mouse, they are more numerous in developing and regenerating nerve than in normal, mature fibres, but similar lamellar bodies have been reported in the Schwann cytoplasm of myelinated fibres in apparently normal human cervical and lumbar dorsal roots (Gamble and Eames, 1966). The corpuscles of Erzholz, which are probably identical with the μ granules of Reich, have been described as spherical bodies $0.5-2.0\ \mu m$ in diameter, staining intensely with the Marchi method (Cajal, 1928). Ultrastructurally, they appear to be homogeneous lipid-like droplets (Babel, Bischoff and Spoendlin, 1970), and in view of their Marchi positive staining reaction, they almost certainly contain a considerable proportion of unsaturated cholesterol ester (Adams, 1962). It seems likely that the variety of other inclusion bodies observed are merely debris – expressions of the transient accumulation of the products of Schwann cell metabolism, perhaps as a result of myelin sheath remodelling. The fact that they are most frequently seen at times when the Schwann cell is engaged in myelin synthesis or regeneration would support this idea.

The Schwann cell nucleus is lozenge-shaped, heterochromatic, often mildly-indented and occupies a near mid-internodal position. *In vivo*, the presence of the nucleus may be inferred from a characteristic unilateral indentation of the myelin sheath, 6–8 μm long (Williams and Hall, 1970). Bremner and Smart (1965) analysed the position of the nucleus in relation to the mid-point of the internode in the phrenic nerves of adult rats, and found that only 12% of the Schwann nuclei lay at or within ±5 μm of the internodal midpoint, while 82% were displaced more than 5 μm distally, irrespective of the internodal length. It has been suggested that a distal displacement of the nucleus is indicative of an underlying continuous circulation of Schwann cell cytoplasm in a direction opposite to that of the proposed proximo-distal neuroplasmic flow, i.e., that the Schwann cell has the properties of an insulated counter-current exchange machine, the nucleus tending to move in the direction of flow, and the inner compartment of Schwann cell cytoplasm running counter to the direction of flow (Bremner and Smart, 1965). Interesting though this idea may be, it is not supported by any other morphological or physiological evidence, and indeed its credibility is weakened by the typical absence of any substantial inner compartments of Schwann cell cytoplasm. It appears more reasonable to consider nuclear displacement to be a not unexpected feature of a Schwann cell in which the distribution of cytoplasm about the axon has become polarized during, and as a consequence of, cellular maturation within a tissue environment that displays a diversity of growth patterns. A similar argument has been invoked to explain the asymmetry of the paranodal bulbs in peripheral nerve fibres (Williams and Kashef, 1968 and Section 1.40).

There have been various proposals that the Schwann cell cytoplasm actively participates in the production of the 'rippling' or 'wave-like' movements along the internode which have been observed *in vitro*, and particular emphasis has been placed upon the possible involvement of the Schmidt–Lanterman incisures in such activity (Robertson, 1958b; Singer, 1968). These movements are thought to occur either as expressions of mutual trophic/metabolic support between axon and Schwann cell, or, in a more popular view, as part of the mechanism underlying neuroplasmic flow (1.75). Although there is a considerable body of evidence, derived from tissue culture studies, of the existence of continuous, rhythmic low-amplitude alterations in contour along the internode, similar behaviour has not yet been observed *in vivo* (Williams and Hall, 1970, 1971a).

1.3.3 *The Schmidt–Lanterman incisure*

The significance of the finding of funnel shaped discontinuities in the internodal myelin sheath of normal nerve fibres has been disputed for more than a century. While many histologists dismissed these so-called incisures of Schmidt–Lanterman (Schmidt, 1874; Lanterman, 1877) as artefacts, the product of histological processing and post mortem change (e.g., Fuerst, 1897), Ranvier was satisfied from his studies of living frog nerves that these structures existed *in vivo*, and expressed his conviction that they represented slender protoplasmic connections between the Schwann cell cytoplasm within and outside the myelin sheath, effectively dividing it into a series of interlocking cylindro-conical segments (Ranvier, 1878). The early European workers succeeded in demonstrating a number of structural features of the incisure with relative consistency, the most commonly recognized being the 'spiral apparatus of Golgi—Rezzonico,' the 'plasmatic chambers', and the 'infundibular membrane' or 'cement' (Kühnt, 1876; Pertik, 1881; Golgi, 1881; Cajal, 1928). Despite Ranvier's observations, the pre-existence of these structures in the living nerve was doubted by many contemporary critics on the ground that complex and often capricious staining and fixation techniques were necessary for their demonstration; while others, such as Nageotte (1922), who accepted their reality *in vivo* disputed Ranvier's claim that they represented protoplasmic bridges penetrating the myelin sheath.

Although today we acknowledge that much of what is seen at the incisure in silver-impregnated or osmicated material is indeed artefactual, these appearances should not be dismissed lightly, since they are indicative of the underlying organization and structural lability of this region of the internode.

With the development and correlation of physical methods of analysing the myelin sheath, the Schmidt—Lanterman incisures were often assumed to be cracks in an otherwise regular protein-phospholipid array, produced in response to manipulative traumatization or to loss of 'turgor pressure' from the cell body after sectioning (Young, 1945). Undoubtedly, incisural widening, which is the consequence of alterations in the physico-chemical environment of the fibre such as are bound to occur *in vitro*, was persuasive evidence that the incisures were merely the commonest type of post mortem artefact (Bito, 1926).

In the early reports of electron microscope examination of peripheral nerve fibres, incisures were often categorized as artefactual, one of several types of shearing defects, resulting from slippage along preferential glide planes between adjacent lamellae (Robertson, 1958b), or they were assumed to be devoid of any internal structure, with individual myelin lamellae terminating on either side of the incisure (Gasser, 1952; Geren-Uzman and Noguiera-Graf, 1957). In retrospect, it is clear that most, if not all, 'cracks' within the normal internodal myelin sheath are attributable to inadequate control of fixation and subsequent processing, and bear little relation to the morphological state of the undisturbed fibre *in vivo*.

Observation of living, substantially undisturbed peripheral nerve fibres in the frog and adult mouse, has established the presence of Schmidt—Lanterman incisures as bilateral oblique dark lines of varying width, crossing the compact internodal myelin sheath, dividing every internode into cylindrico-conical segments of varying length (Ranvier, 1878; Hall and Williams, 1970). When freshly excised nerve fibres are teased gently apart in a pool of warmed isotonic saline, and examined with standard Köhler illumination, the incisures are again

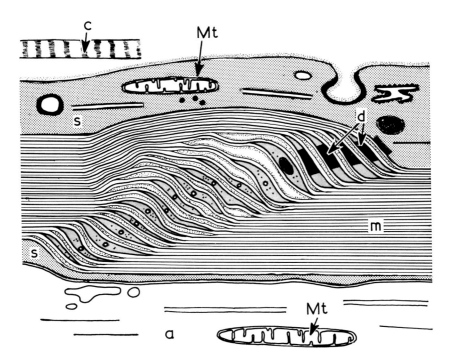

Fig. 1.9 A diagram showing the principal features of the structure of an incisure of Schmidt–Lanterman in a mature myelinated fibre. The incisure is shown in a moderately 'open' condition (see text). (a), axon; (c), endoneurial collagen; (d), desmosomes; (m), myelin sheath; (Mt), mitochondria; (s), Schwann cell cytoplasm. A continuous spiral of Schwann cell cytoplasm containing a single microtubule, dilates the dense 'period' line of each myelin lamella in turn. This process is accompanied by splitting of the adjacent 'intraperiod' lines to produce a coextensive spiral 'channel' connecting the extracellular space with the periaxonal space at the outer and inner mesaxons respectively. A series of 'desmosomes' (d) are present at the external end of the incisure. (Reproduced from Hall and Williams (1970), by courtesy of the editor of the *Journal of Cell Science*.)

apparent as discrete zones along the internode, and together with the nodes of Ranvier, constitute the only 'discontinuities' along the myelin sheath. However, whereas *in vivo*, the Schmidt–Lanterman incisures exhibit a narrow range of states, most appearing closed (i.e., as a thin dark line crossing the myelin sheath obliquely) and only a minority seeming to be moderately open (i.e., the midpoint width of the dark line being approximately twice that at its ends), *in vitro*, with time, all exhibit some degrees of widening, varying from a moderately open state, through further intermediate stages of widening, to irreversibly over-dilated zones in which discrete 'lamellae' can be seen crossing the incisural space (Hall and Williams, 1970). Concurrent, irreversible changes are seen in the nodal regions, involving retraction of paranodal myelin and collapse of paranodal contour, and the appearance of numerous pits, indicative of splits in the myelin sheath. These structural alterations – the response of the components of the unfixed nerve fibre to excision and removal from the body – at least in part

23

explain the consistently reproducible staining patterns reported by earlier workers. The osmotically induced widening of channels at the node and the incisure in continuity with the extracellular space, and the onset of autolytic degradation in the myelin sheath, allow access to structural components otherwise inaccessible to histological stains, thus permitting the demonstration of such features as the spiral apparatus of Golgi–Rezzonico (Fig. 1.4).

In the simplest, i.e., *in vivo* closed, condition of the Schmidt–Lanterman incisure in both immature and mature fibres the major dense line of the myelin sheath is split to enclose a characteristically granular spiral of Schwann cell cytoplasm (in a manner similar to that observed at the node), and it is the staining of this spiral that is responsible for the appearance of the spiral apparatus of Golgi–Rezzonico. In the mouse this helix of cytoplasm typically contains a single, central microtubule, c. 24 mm in diameter, increasing to two or three in the incisures of larger mammals. Unlike the longitudinal microtubules of the Schwann cell cytoplasm external to the myelin sheath, and those in the axoplasm, the incisural and paranodal microtubules run circumferentially. Although they seem to be a characteristic feature of the incisure, having been observed in peripheral nerve fibres in many species (e.g., Hall and Williams, 1970) and in fibres in rat spinal cord and rabbit medulla (Blakemore, 1969) their functional significance is uncertain. A great variety of speculative interpretations have appeared concerning the activity of the microtubules in the cells of other tissues, but it seems likely that in the incisure the microtubules are behaving as cytoskeletal elements (Porter, 1966), in some way related to the stabilization of the cytoplasmic spiral. Near the external surface of the incisure, stacks of desmosome-like thickenings are commonly found (Hall and Williams, 1970): similar structures have been described at the node of Ranvier (Harkin, 1964; Berthold, 1968a) and as isolated specializations of the external mesaxon in developing fibres in the rat, mouse and in the human foetal ulnar nerve (Gamble, 1966). As with the incisural microtubules, it is impossible to assign any specific function to these thickenings, other than by inference from the occurrence, and presumed function of similar structures (puncta adhaerens) in other tissues, and it has, accordingly, been tentatively suggested that they are concerned with maintaining the structural integrity of the spiral (Hall and Williams, 1970). Circumstantial evidence which may be cited in support of this suggestion is the observation that while dilatation of the incisure always spreads from its axonal aspect, the desmosome-like stacks are always confined to its outer half. The stacks are rarely bilateral however, and when examined in serial sections do not extend far into the mature incisure: they are much more evident in developing incisures.

Membrane-bound dense bodies and primary lysosomes have been reported as infrequent inclusions within the outer turns of the cytoplasmic spiral of the incisure (Hall and Williams, 1970); organelles of the size of mitochondria have also been observed within normal incisures, but there is some doubt as to their precise identity.

The intraperiod line of the myelin within the incisural region is double, the

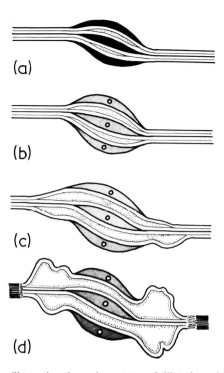

Fig. 1.10 A diagram illustrating the various states of dilatation which may be seen in an incisure. (a) the 'condensed' condition following prefixation immersion in hypertonic saline; (b) the normal 'closed' condition of the incisure seen at undisturbed incisures *in vivo*; (c) the moderately 'open' condition seen in incisures teased in isotonic saline, and also occasionally *in vivo*; and (d) an irreversibly widened incisure of the kind seen following mechanical trauma, or exposure to hypotonic solutions. (Reproduced from Hall and Williams (1970), by courtesy of the editor of the *Journal of Cell Science*.)

space between the two components containing an amorphous, moderately electron dense, material. This gap provides a potential channel of variable width in continuity with the extracellular space along the entire length of the cytoplasmic spiral, and has been shown to be accessible to lanthanum ions if these are added to the solution bathing the exterior of the fibre (Hall and Williams, 1971). It must be pointed out, however, that the commonly accepted view that lanthanum ions act simply as inert tracers delineating extensions of the extracellular space is a naïve one, since this ion is known to bind to the fixed anionic groups on membrane surfaces. Nevertheless the observed binding of lanthanum ions to the external surfaces of the components of the intraperiod lines suggests that at the incisure the constitution of the membranes differs from that obtaining elsewhere in the compact myelin, and it is possible that this is a region of increased hydration within the sheath. Rapid demyelination is initiated at the paranode and incisure after the intraneural injection of lysophosphatidyl choline (Hall and Gregson, 1971), and it was proposed that these sites are most vulnerable because they represent relatively large surface areas of the sheath membrane easily accessible to substances within the endoneurial fluid.

Dilatation of the incisures is a phenomenon which has been recognized since the earliest morphological descriptions: Stilling (1856) included drawings of swollen incisures in his work, some 20 years before the independent observations made by Schmidt (1874) and Lanterman (1877), but he paid them little attention since he believed them to be artefacts. Incisural dilatation has been considered to be a non-specific consequence of stretching and compression (Nageotte, 1922; Kimbarovskaya, 1953), electrical stimulation (Lázár and Maros, 1962), fibre aging (Lubińska, 1956), immersion in hypotonic solutions (Sotnikov, 1965; Hall and Williams, 1970) and a sensitive indicator of the onset of degenerative change (Williams and Hall, 1971b). It is probably the dilatation of unsuspected incisures that has been responsible for reports of sudden increases in their numbers per internode following traumatization (e.g., Webster, 1964b). Hall and Williams (1970) have demonstrated by immersing nerves in anisotonic saline solutions that incisural dilatation begins by widening of peri-incisural intraperiod lines, to produce intra-myelin spaces which become progressively confluent — the 'plasmatic chambers' of older descriptions. The cytoplasmic spiral remains intact at this stage and provides the morphological basis of the 'infundibular membrane'. Irreversible dilatation results from the disruptive effects of extensive separation at the peri-incisural intraperiod lines and the subsequent collapse of the membranes into a lamellar material with a 4 nm repeat within the spaces so formed.

The question of the biological significance of the incisure remains un-answered, and consequently invites speculation. A number of possible functions may be proposed from a consideration of its morphology and its relationship to the other components of the internode. Incisures may participate (i) in the transport of materials across the sheath; (ii) act as points for the initiation or augmentation of peristaltic waves (if any) along the sheath; (iii) or be foci for growth and remodelling of the sheath. The participation of incisures in any of these functions has yet to be convincingly demonstrated, but the first suggestion merits further investigation in view of the demonstrated continuity between endoneurium and peri-axonal space, and between the inner and outer compartments of the Schwann cell cytoplasm, via the incisural spiral.

The consistent, and approximately linear, relationship which exists between numbers of incisures, (the frequency of incisures increasing with increase in fibre diameter and myelin thickness, regardless of internodal length, Hiscoe, 1947), and the fact that incisures are present from the initiation of myelinogenesis both in developing and remyelinating fibres, imply that the incisure is an indispensable feature of all but the thinnest internodal myelin sheath. Perhaps the most definite evidence of the involvement of incisures in some aspects of internodal 'homeostasis' is that irreversible dilatation of the incisures, such as is seen after mechanical or chemical damage to the fibre, is always followed by breakdown of

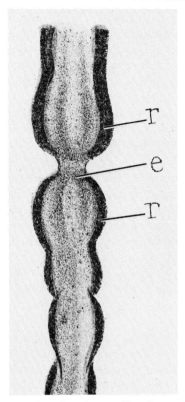

Fig. 1.11   The node of a teased osmicated nerve fibre from a frog: detail from plate I. of Ranvier (1878). (e) marks the nodal constriction, the *étranglement annulaire*, and (T) the terminal swellings of the myelin sheath, the *renflements terminaux*, which are shown to be asymmetrically dilated and longitudinally grooved. (Figure enlarged approximately 4 times the original lithograph.)

the cylindrico-conical segments into primary ovoids, and subsequent degeneration of the whole internodal myelin sheath (Williams and Hall, 1971b).

1.4 The node of Ranvier

Periodic annular constrictions of the external contour of peripheral myelinated nerve fibres, coinciding with interruptions to the myelin sheath, were first described by Ranvier in 1871. He observed that there was invariably only one Schwann cell nucleus between each pair of 'annular constrictions', or nodes, and this finding led him to propose that the interval between adjacent nodes represented the territory of a single Schwann cell. He was convinced moreover, that despite the interruption to the myelin sheath, the axis cylinder continued uninterrupted from segment to segment of the nerve tube, extending as an unbroken protoplasmic strand from its central origin to its peripheral termination. The myelin itself he regarded to be a liquid, or nearly liquid, fat droplet contained within the substance of the Schwann cell, concerned with both the mechanical protection of the axis cylinder, and with improving the impulse conduction capabilities of the nerve fibre by providing it with an electrically insulating layer; the 'annular constrictions' and Schmidt–Lanterman incisures serving to divide up the myelin tube and prevent its displacement by local mechanical forces or gravity (Ranvier, 1878). These conclusions were contested by a number of Ranvier's contemporaries and successors: Nageotte (1922), for example, held that the Schwann cell sheath was a continuous syncytium along the length of the nerve, and that the myelin sheath was an integral component of the axon (being formed by an elaborate arrangement of mitochondria at its surface), while a number of writers up to the time of von Muralt (1946) continued to maintain that the axon was interrupted by tranverse septa at the level of each node. Eventual vindication of the correctness of the majority of Ranvier's opinions awaited the advent of electron microscopy.

1.4.1 *Morphology of the nodes and paranodal bulbs*

(i) *Light microscopy*

Ranvier described the detailed appearance of the node both in the living frog, and in excised nerve fibres from a number of mammals, after a variety of different staining procedures. He observed that in nerves in which the myelin sheath had been stained with osmium tetroxide the ends of the 'nerve tube' on either side of the node were slightly swollen, often asymmetrically, and that on the surface of these terminal swellings there could be seen a series of bulging ribs or rounded lumps (Fig. 1.12), which augmented their capacity, and appeared to be pockets formed by the Schwann cell sheath to contain a greater quantity of myelin. On the nodal aspect of the swellings the myelin turned inwards towards the axis cylinder to provide the limits of a lucent biconcave meniscus traversed at the mid point of the node by a refractile band. From the examination of sectioned, and teased and stained preparations it could be seen that the axis cylinder underwent a 'biconical expansion' where it crossed the nodal meniscus, and was greatly narrowed in comparison to its internodal diameter to either side of the annular constriction, where it passed through the inturned ends of the myelin tube (Fig. 1.13).

Ranvier also observed that if unfixed nerves were immersed in dilute solutions of silver nitrate, and subsequently exposed to light, the position of every annular constriction was marked by the presence of a black or brown 'petite croix latine', the so-called 'cross of Ranvier'. He considered that the major part of the transverse bar of the cross was due to the presence of a ring of 'cement' substance around the nodal axon; the existence of similarly staining intercellular cement between the contiguous edges of pavement epithelial cells reinforcing his belief that the node represented the point of contact between adjacent Schwann cells. The vertical bar he believed represented the biconical nodal axon, together

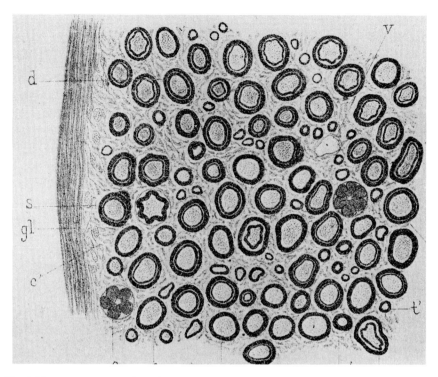

Fig. 1.12 Transverse section of part of an osmicated sciatic nerve of a dog: detail from Plate II of Ranvier (1878), enlarged × 2. Note the generally circular outline of the majority of both the large and small myelin sheaths, many of the larger having the double structure (d) indicative of a transverse section through an incisure; the interstitial connective tissue (c), and the enveloping perineurium, the *gaîne lammeleuse* (gl); note also the crenated outline, myelin pockets and reduced axon diameter of the three fibres sectioned through their paranodal regions, the external contour in each case being returned to a circle by a slender line.

with a variable proportion of the adjacent narrowed axon beneath the terminal swelling (Fig. 1.14); the longitudinal extent of the staining depending upon the duration of immersion of the fibres in silver nitrate. Ranvier demonstrated that these two components of the cross could be dissociated by the trauma inevitably associated with the process of teasing apart fibres for examination, the cement ring remaining at the point of apposition of the two terminal swellings, while the stained portion of the axon moved longitudinally to come to lie beneath one or other of the adjacent myelin segments (Fig. 1.14).

The node has continued to be the subject of histological interest during the century that has followed its original description, both in connection with studies of degeneration and regeneration in the peripheral nervous system (Nageotte, 1922; Cajal, 1928), and later with regard to its suggested role in the propagation of the saltatory nerve impulse (Lillie, 1925; Rushton, 1951; Hodgkin, 1971), but many of the details of its structure so vividly portrayed by

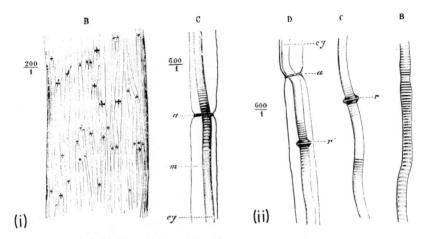

Fig. 1.13 The effects on peripheral nerve fibres of impregnation with dilute silver nitrate solutions. (i) 'B', is a small thoracic nerve from a mouse and shows numerous 'crosses of Ranvier'. 'C', is an individual silver impregnated node, the myelin (m) having been rendered transparent by immersion in glycerine, showing the 'cementing disc' at the node (a) and repeating transverse striations across the axis cylinder (cy), 'Frommann's lines'. (ii) 'D', illustrates the dissociation of the two components of the cross of Ranvier by mechanical trauma in a rabbit sciatic nerve fibre. The cementing disc remains at the original site of the node (a), while the nodal axon with its biconical expansion (r) has moved longitudinally beneath one of the adjacent myelin segments. 'C' and 'B' portray the appearances of 'Frommann's lines' on isolated axis cylinders from a rabbit sciatic nerve. (From text figures 5 and 6 of Ranvier (1878), slightly reduced from the original.)

Ranvier were subsequently overlooked, or dismissed as artefacts of preparation. Nemiloff (1910) described the staining of the nodal cement substance in unfixed nerves with methylene blue, the 'Nemiloff rings'; and Nageotte (1922), while differing from Ranvier on many points of interpretation of structure (v.s.) confirmed the latter's observation of the presence of strands of Schwann cell cytoplasm in the neighbourhood of the node corresponding to the grooves between the myelin ridges of the terminal swellings, and termed these strands the 'marginal protoplasmic network'. In addition Nageotte was able, with the aid of the same dichromate/acid fuchsin staining technique used to reveal the apparatus of Golgi–Rezzonico (q.v. p. 24), to demonstrate the existence of a new feature of the node which now bears his eponym the 'spiny bracelet of Nageotte'. This structure consists of a series of five or six circular crests decorated with curved spines, and surrounds the circumference of the narrowed portion of the axon where it passes through the inturned end of the myelin sheath, the spines penetrating the end of the sheath and following its curvature (Fig. 1.15). Nageotte considered that the spiny crests corresponded to circular streaks he had observed at the same location in living nerve fibres, and that they represented the insertion of the leaflets of myelin onto the axis cylinder.

Subsequent histological studies have added little of importance to these early descriptions, and the state of knowledge of the structure of the node, as

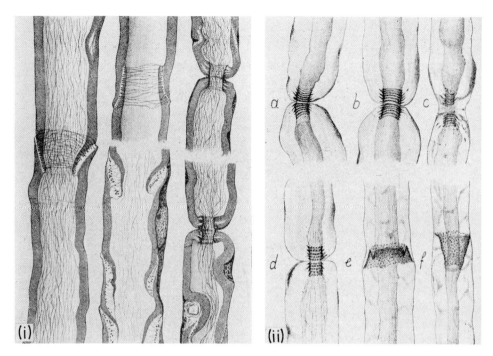

Fig. 1.14 (i) Myelinated fibres from the guinea pig, stained with potassium dichromate and acid fuchsin to demonstrate the spiral apparatus of Golgi-Rezzonico at the incisures. (ii) Fibres of the rabbit and guinea pig stained with the same technique, to show the 'spiny bracelet' (a,b,c and d) and two incisures (e and f). (Reproduced from Figures 24 and 25, Nageotte (1922), by courtesy of Alcan – Presses Universitaires de France: Paris.)

revealed by light microscopy, was reviewed by Hess and Young in 1952. They drew attention to a number of its features; these included the thickened corrugated myelin over the 'paranodal bulbs' extending back some 40 μm from the node, often in the form of a low spiral; the narrowing of the axon at the node, to at least a half of its internodal diameter in larger fibres; and the reduction in the length of exposed axon at the node in large fibres when compared to small ones, being reduced to as little as 0.5 μm in the largest fibres. They also confirmed that while the axoplasm of the node differed in its optical, staining, and therefore also presumably in its physical characteristics from that of the internode, no transverse boundary of the kinds suggested by Gedoelst (1886) and von Muralt (1946) could be detected across the nodal axon. Hess and Young considered that the 'spinous bracelet of Nageotte' represented a 'protein neurokeratin' component of the terminal portion of the myelin sheath, and that the 'cement disc' was a 'diaphragm' of 'scleroprotein material continuous with the neurilemma' having a radius of up to 5 μm in large fibres; its composition necessarily having some effect upon 'the passage of ions and other substances from the axon surface to the perinodal space'.

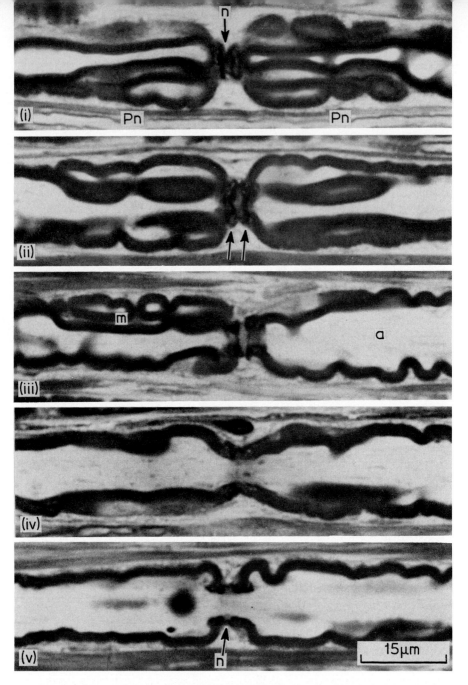

Fig. 1.15 A set of $1-2 \ \mu$m, resin embedded, longitudinal sections through different nodes in a limb nerve of a baboon: stained with toluidine blue. The series represents successively deeper levels of section through the node and paranodes of a typical large fibre, and illustrates normal appearances of the swollen paranodal bulbs with their undulating ridged and grooved myelin (m) (I–III) in such sections, and the narrowing of the axon (a) at the node and beneath the inturned ends of the myelin sheath (IV–V). The paired densities either side of the mid nodal point (arrows, II) represent artefactual distortion of the ends of the outermost myelin lamellae.

Hess and Young (1952) explored the familiar nodal staining effects of Methylene Blue and dilute silver nitrate solutions, appearances which they ascribed to 'the presence of active ionic interchanges perhaps with a high concentration of chloride and potassium ions', and suggested that since these materials stained the whole narrowed region of the axon, this, rather than the myelin-free area, constituted the effective nodal membrane. They confirmed the structural independence of the longitudinal and tranverse components of the 'Ranvier cross', by observing that pressure applied to the overlying coverslip caused their dissociation in the manner described by Ranvier. They also provided an explanation for the phenomenon known as 'Frommann's lines' (Frommann, 1861; Fig. 1.14), a series of transverse striations across the axon which appear following penetration of the node, or any point of damage along the fibre, by silver nitrate solutions; the separation of the lines increasing with increase in distance from the point of entry of the stain. Hess and Young proposed that this phenomenon was analogous to that described by Liesegang, in which periodic rings are produced in a gelatin gel by the diffusion into it of silver nitrate, and are thus the consequence of diffusion of an electrolyte into a colloid solution with which it reacts.

An additional feature of the paranodal bulbs, recognized by Ranvier but which has subsequently passed largely unremarked, is their longitudinal asymmetry, the proximal bulb at most nodes being larger than its more distal neighbour. This consistent polarization was observed by Lubińska (1954), and was explained in terms of the dynamics of axoplasmic flow by Lubinska and Lukaszewska (1956), who proposed that the constriction of the nodal axon led to a damming of axoplasmic material on the proximal side of each node, causing its distension. However, later observations on the morphology of nodes between normal internodes and regenerated intercalated segments, led Lubińska to doubt the correctness of this hypothesis (Lubińska, 1958).

Subsequent quantitative studies of paranodal asymmetry in normal nerves, and following regeneration in both mature and growing animals (Williams and Kashef, 1961; Williams and Landon, 1963; Williams and Kashef, 1968), have confirmed the validity of the quantitative observations of Lubińska and Lukaszewska (1956). Consistent proximo-distal polarization of the paranodes was found in mature limb nerves, and in regenerated nerves in which the regeneration had been accompanied by growth in limb length. Asymmetric paranodal bulbs without consistent polarization were found in normal dorsal and ventral root fibres, and symmetrical bulbs were seen in regenerated nerves in mature animals. The situation in the recurrent laryngeal nerve was of particular interest, since here the polarization of the paranodal bulbs maintained a consistent relationship to the cephalo-caudal axis of the body, the more cephalad of each pair being the larger, while reversing with respect to their relationship to the cell body; those on the recurved segment of the nerve showed no preferential polarization.

Williams and Kashef (1968) concluded that the asymmetry and polarization

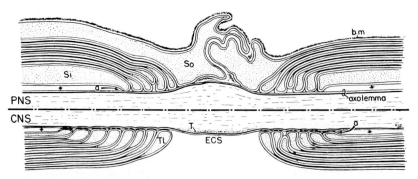

Fig. 1.16 A schematic representation of a longitudinal section through the region of the node of Ranvier of a small myelinated nerve fibre; the condition seen in the peripheral nervous system (above) is compared with that found in the central nervous system (below). The figure illustrates the serial attachment of the myelin 'pockets' adjacent to the node, a somewhat swollen nodal axon, and the presence of loosely interdigitating Schwann cell processes overlapping the nodal axolemma, in the former, and contrasts these features with the exposed nodal axolemma and the absence of a satellite cell compartment external to the myelin sheath seen in the latter. (Reproduced from Bunge (1968) by kind permission of the author and the editors of *Physiological Reviews*.)

While certain of the minor details of this drawing require modification in the light of more recent knowledge, e.g. it is now known that there is an interval between the terminal myelin 'pockets' and the juxtanodal axolemma, and that the intermittent densities of the outer leaflet of the axolemma beneath the zone of myelin termination, and the dense 'undercoating' beneath the nodal axolemma are both present at peripheral as well as at central nodes (see Fig. 1.32 and text), this figure provides a reasonably accurate representation of the anatomy of the node of a *small* peripheral myelinated nerve fibre. However it is not justifiable to extrapolate these appearances to the nodes of large peripheral fibres, in which the axon/Schwann cell relationships are both more complex and more ordered (see text and Fig. 1.19).

of the paranodal bulbs was unrelated to the position of the nerve cell body, and thus to the direction of flow of axoplasm, but could be correlated with differential growth and maturation gradients within the body segments through which any individual nerve passed. The considerable, and largely unidirectional, movements occurring between the growing elongating Schwann cell and its surrounding tissues during development were thought to lead to differences in the mechanical conditions operating at the 'advancing' and 'trailing' ends of the cell, and it was proposed that these differences could be responsible for the observed polarization of the paranodal bulbs. Furthermore it must be stressed that the paranodal bulbs are not simple fusiform swellings of the axon and myelin sheath, of a kind that might be expected to accompany the local accumulation of axoplasm consequent upon a partial block to axoplasmic flow (see Spencer, 1972), but involve elaborate and interrelated changes in the form and content of both the axon and Schwann cell (Figs. 1.16 and 1.19, and Section 1.4.2). The resulting 'paranodal apparatus' (Williams and Landon, 1963) has been suggested to reflect the presence of a highly ordered and functionally important interrelationship between the neuron and its satellite cells at the node (Landon and Williams, 1963).

(ii) Electron microscopy

The use of electron microscopy provided much new information concerning the structure of the nodes of amphibia and mammals (Gasser, 1952; Robertson, 1957a and b; 1959; Uzman and Villegas, 1960; Elfvin, 1961b; Sjöstrand, 1963). When examined in longitudinal section, the myelin lamellae were seen to end at either side of the node as a series of 'loops' produced by the presence of a small pocket of Schwann cell cytoplasm at the end of each major dense, or period, line, these 'pockets' representing sections through a continuous cytoplasmic spiral connecting the inner and outer compartments of the Schwann cell (Robertson, 1957a). Each loop appeared to make an oblique and close contact with the juxtanodal axolemma, the membranes being separated by a gap of no more than 2 nm. The Schwann cell sheath was found to be discontinuous at the node, as Ranvier had proposed, and the nodal gap, corresponding to the position of the cementing disc, contained irregular interdigitating finger-like projections from the ends of the Schwann cells, some of which made contact with the nodal axolemma (Robertson, 1957b; Uzman and Villegas, 1960). These microvillous processes were embedded in an amorphous matrix material, thought by Elfvin (1961b) to be an extension of the Schwann cell basal lamina, the only structure other than the axon having direct continuity across the nodal gap. The nodal axon itself was described as being somewhat swollen towards its mid-point, and to contain neurofilaments, vesicles and occasional dense bodies and mitochondria.

Such early accounts of nodal fine structure in general failed to mention any significant narrowing of the axon at the node when compared to its internodal diameter, or the presence of features comparable to the ridged and swollen terminal myelin segments, the 'paranodal bulbs', visible by light microscopy. Exceptions were the reports of Gasser (1952) and Hess and Lansing (1953), who described accumulations of Schwann cell cytoplasm rich in mitochondria adjacent to the node, in a position similar to that occupied by the 'marginal protoplasmic network' of Nageotte. For technical reasons these early electron microscopic descriptions dealt, in the main, with very limited samples of the smallest diameter myelinated fibres, and it has subsequently become apparent that, while accurate within their proper context, such descriptions have provided very misleading models of nodal ultrastructure when generalized to the much larger diameter fibres commonly studied by the light microscopist and the electrophysiologist. Subsequent improvements in electron microscopical techniques, and the extension of studies to large diameter myelinated fibres in a variety of mammals, including man, have yielded much new information concerning the fine structure of the nodal and paranodal regions (Williams and Landon, 1963, 1965; Landon and Williams, 1963; Berthold and Skoglund, 1967; Berthold, 1968b).

The myelin sheath of large nerve fibres (i.e., $>6\,\mu m$) has been found to undergo consistent changes in its form and dimensions as it passes through the region of the paranodal bulb, comparable to those previously observed by light

35

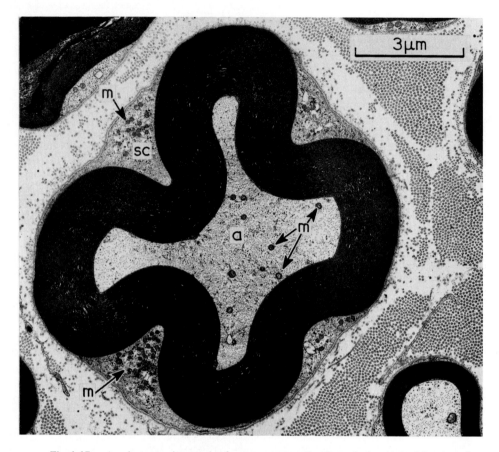

Fig. 1.17 An electron micrograph of a transverse section through the paranodal region of a medium sized (8–10 μm) myelinated fibre from the limb nerve of a baboon. The myelin sheath is folded into the form of a cross, the grooves on its external surface being filled with Schwann cell cytoplasm (sc) rich in mitochondria (m). The axoplasm (a), which contains relatively few mitochondria, fills the internal contour of the myelin sheath, adopting a fluted form similar to that depicted in Fig. 1.4.

microscopy (see p. 31). The sheath as a whole thickens due to an increase in radial spacing of its constituent lamellae from 11 nm to 13 nm in osmium fixed material, (Williams and Landon, 1963), and a concomitant increase in its circumference is accompanied by folding, to produce a series of longitudinal grooves and ridges, the number and dimensions of which increase in proportion to increase in internodal fibre diameter. The internal contour of the myelin sheath is completely filled by the underlying axon, which thus possesses reciprocal ridges and grooves on its external surface (Figs. 1.4 and 1.17). While there is little or no increase in the size of the internal compartment of the Schwann cell in this region, the grooves on the external surface of the paranodal myelin sheath are, on the contrary, filled by columns of Schwann cell

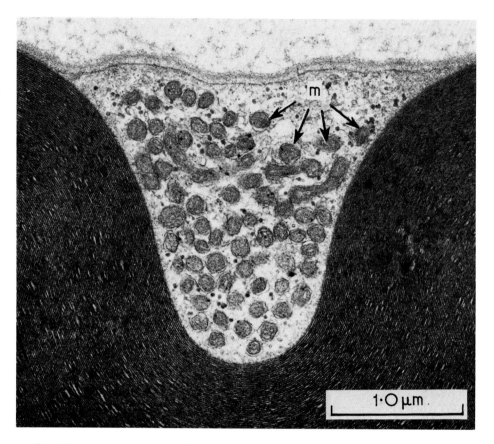

Fig. 1.18 A transverse section through one paranodal furrow of a large myelinated fibre from a baboon peripheral nerve; showing the large numbers of mitochondria (m) contained within the Schwann cell cytoplasm.

cytoplasm, and their presence, together with that of a thin veil of cytoplasm bridging the crests of the myelin ridges, returns the overall outline of the paranodal bulb to a circle. (Fig. 1.18). These local accumulations of Schwann cell cytoplasm external to the myelin sheath contain large aggregations of small rod shaped mitochondria, in concentrations ten to twenty fold greater than that found elsewhere along the internode, 100 or more being visible in a single cross section through a large (15 μm diameter) paranodal bulb (Williams and Landon, 1963). Other structures, apart from the external mesaxon, commonly found in the paranodal Schwann cell cytoplasm include small pieces of rough endoplasmic reticulum, occasional free ribosomes, glycogen granules and small (100 nm) dense granules, together with scattered filaments and occasional microtubules, the exact content depending upon the species examined.

Quantitative data concerning variation in a number of structural parameters at the node and paranodes, including change in the cross sectional areas of

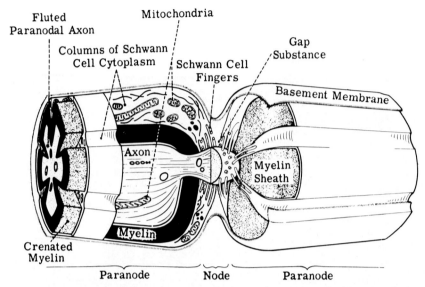

Fig. 1.19   A diagrammatic representation of the structure of a node of Ranvier of a large mammalian peripheral myelinated nerve fibre. (Reproduced by courtesy of the editors of *Gray's Anatomy* and J. and A. Churchill Limited, London.)

the axon and Schwann cell, and their content of mitochondria, have been obtained by Berthold (1968a) from serial tranverse sections through nodes of a small number of feline ventral root fibres. These agree in all essentials with results of earlier quantitative light microscope estimates of change in axon perimeter and cross sectional area, and electron microscope counts of mito-chondrial numbers in the axons and Schwann cells of large paranodes in limb nerves of the rabbit, mouse and rat (Williams and Landon, 1963). The large mitochondrial population of the paranodal Schwann cell cytoplasm can also be revealed by histochemical techniques for the demonstration of mitochondrial enzymes, such as succinic and lactate dehydrogenases (Williams and Landon, 1965) and NADH-tetrazolium reductase (Berthold and Skoglund, 1967).

As the immediate vicinity of the node is approached the ridges and grooves of the myelin sheath become shallower and disappear, the myelin lamellae finally curving inwards to run more or less radially towards their terminal pockets on the axon membrane; the smooth outward convexity of this terminal portion of the myelin sheath helping to further narrow the perinodal space. The juxtanodal flattening of the 'pleats' in the myelin sheath is accompanied by confluence of the columns of Schwann cell cytoplasm, to produce a continuous circum-ferential collar of cytoplasm immediately adjacent to the node. This collar contains only a few mitochondria, but often numerous small osmiophilic granules, and from it there arise two or more rows of regularly ordered microvillous, or 'finger-like', processes (Figs. 1.19, 1.20 and 1.21). The microvilli are directed radially inwards to end as a regularly spaced hexagonal array in close relationship to the nodal axolemma, and are embedded in an amorphous, moderately electron dense matrix, the 'gap substance', distinguishable as an entity from the continuous overlying Schwann cell basal lamina. The microvilli are similar in structure to those found on other cell types, have a diameter of 70–80 nm, and contain 4–6 fine internal filaments. While similar microvilli at the nodes of small (<5 μm diameter) fibres have been described to 'interdigitate',

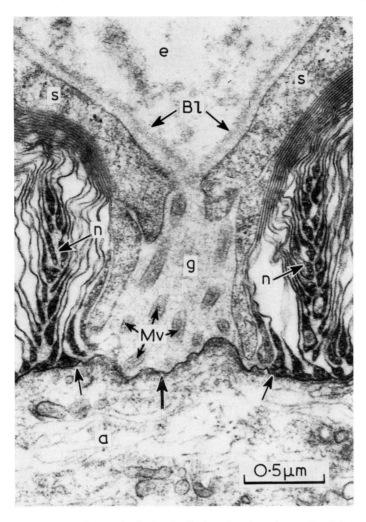

Fig. 1.20 Electron micrograph of a longitudinal section through one side of the node of a 10 μm fibre from a baboon limb nerve. The large arrow points to the nodal axolemma with its electron dense 'undercoat' which ceases at the point of attachment of the first myelin 'pocket' (small arrows). Note the continuity of the basal lamina (Bl) across the nodal gap. a – axoplasm; e – endoneurial space; g – gap substance; Mv – Schwann cell microvilli; n – myelin 'pocket' regressions of the 'spinous bracelet' of Nageotte; s – nodal collar of Schwann cell cytoplasm.

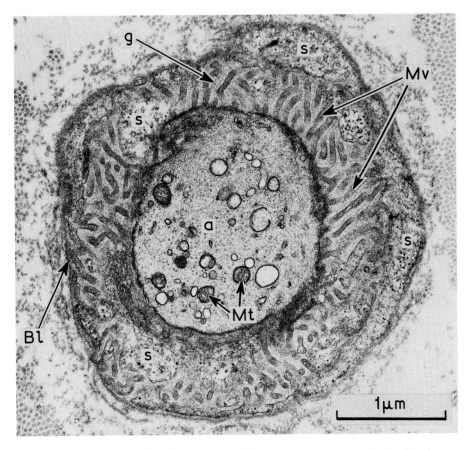

Fig. 1.21   Transverse section through a node of Ranvier. a – axoplasm; Bl – basal lamina; g – gap substance; Mt – mitochondria; Mv – radial Schwann cell microvilli.

and to be 'tangled' and 'irregular' (Robertson 1959, 1960), their arrangement at large nodes is highly ordered with a regular minimum separation of 70–80 nm (Figs. 1.20, 1.21, 1.22), their numbers, length and regularity increasing with increase in fibre size.

In large fibres, as in small, each myelin lamella appears, in longitudinal section, to end as a 'pocket' of Schwann cell cytoplasm by distension of the major dense or 'period' line, the 'pockets' representing sections through successive turns of a continuous cytoplasmic spiral connecting the inner and outer Schwann cell compartments (Robertson, 1957a, 1960). However in large fibres not all of the 'pockets' make contact with the axolemma, serial sets regressing in a stepwise fashion out into the substance of the terminal myelin sheath, to produce an image resembling an ear of corn (Fig. 1.20), the extracellular space between the 'pockets' often containing an amorphous material similar to the gap substance. Five or six of such regressions may occur along the region of myelin termination in a large fibre, and it is likely that they represent the structural basis for the 'spinous bracelet' of Nageotte. Those Schwann cell pockets that do reach the axon surface come into close contact with the axolemma, an apparent gap of only 2—3 nm intervening between the outer dense components of the opposed cell membranes. A series of inter-mittent increases in the electron density of the outer leaflet of the axolemma has been reported to occur at the region of myelin termination in some, but not all, fibres; first being seen at nodes in the central nervous system (Peters, 1966; Fig. 1.32) and later, as a less common occurrence, at the nodes of peripheral nerve fibres. These spots of increased density occur at a frequency such that three or four are present under each terminal 'pocket', and surface (i.e. paraxial) views reveal that they represent sections through a continuous shallow spiral of increased density in the outer leaflet of the axolemma. It has been suggested from 'tracer' studies using lanthanum salts that the space between adjacent turns of this spiral represents a low resistance pathway for the access of ions to the perinodal space (Hirano and Dembitzer, 1969). Such claims require to be treated with some reserve in view of the very high concentrations of lanthanum salts employed, and the known affinity of lanthanum ions for components of the cell surface coat. It is probable that, while no 'tight junctions' or other intercellular seals can be observed between the axon and Schwann cell membranes using the best modern techniques, the internodal axon is in fact effectively isolated from ionic events occurring at the node (an essential requirement of present views on saltatory conduction of the nerve impulse) by the high resistance to longitudinal ionic flux imposed by the length of the region of myelin termination, and the closeness of the apposition of its component 'pockets' to the axolemma. A detailed account of the freeze-etched appearances of the apposed cell membranes in this region has recently been published by Livingstone, Pfenninger, Moor and Akert (1973).

The terminal 'pockets' of the myelin sheath contain densely staining cyto-plasm, similar in consistency to that seen in the cytoplasmic spirals of the Schmidt—Lanterman incisures, and, like them, each pocket contains one or more microtubules. The transport functions ascribed to microtubules in the axon (Section 1.77) are obviously also relevant to the problems of intracellular communication presented by the extremely attenuated spiral pathway between the inner and outer Schwann cell compartments provided by the incisural cytoplasmic spirals and the myelin terminal 'pockets'. Microtubules have furthermore been ascribed functional roles in the morphogenesis of cells and cell organelles (Porter, 1966; McIntosh and Porter, 1967; Gibbons, Tilney and Porter, 1969), in addition to their well recognized functions in the mitotic spindle, and it is possible that their presence in the terminal myelin 'pockets' may indicate their having a similar role in the maintenance of the morphology of the region of myelin termination.

The reciprocal changes in the surface contour of the axon necessitated by the presence of the longitudinal folds in the paranodal myelin sheath have been

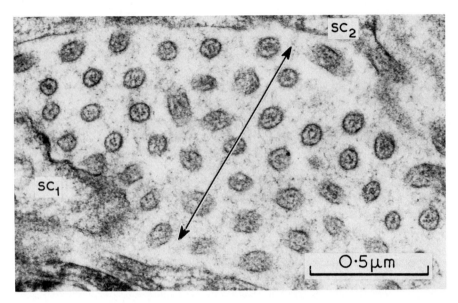

Fig. 1.22 Paraxial longitudinal section across the nodal gap of a large fibre. The radially directed Schwann cell microvilli (Mv) embedded in the amorphous gap substance (g) form a regular hexagonal array, and are sectioned transversely. Each has a central core of 4–6 fine filaments. The arrow indicates the longitudinal axis of the underlying axon and sc_1 and sc_2 the adjacent Schwann cells.

described earlier (Fig. 1.19). Measurements of large paranodes in limb nerves indicate that axonal perimeter, and thus axon surface area, significantly increases above its mean internodal value in both proximal and distal bulbs, although to a much greater extent in the former, while increase in the axonal cross-sectional area is restricted to the proximal bulb only (Williams and Landon, 1963). The axoplasm shows little change in its structure or content of organelles during its passage through the paranodal bulbs. The neurotubules tend to follow the line of the fibre axis, the recesses produced by the axonal ridges containing only neurofilaments and occasional embayed clusters of small mitochondria or aggregations of smooth membrane cisternae. Large threadlike mitochondria are a consistent feature of the paranodal axoplasm, as elsewhere along the internode, and while often being present in slightly greater numbers on the proximal side of the node, they in no way compare in frequency to those present in the adjacent Schwann cell cytoplasm external to the myelin sheath.

As the axon passes from the end of the paranodal bulb through the inturned end of the myelin sheath it regains a cylindrical contour, while its diameter is suddenly reduced to between $1/3$ and $1/6$ of its mean internodal value. This reduction in axon size is not accompanied by any appreciable change in the concentration of neurofilaments within the axoplasm, implying that many filaments end within the paranodal bulb. The neurotubules, on the other hand, are not reduced in number, and pass uninterrupted from one paranodal bulb to

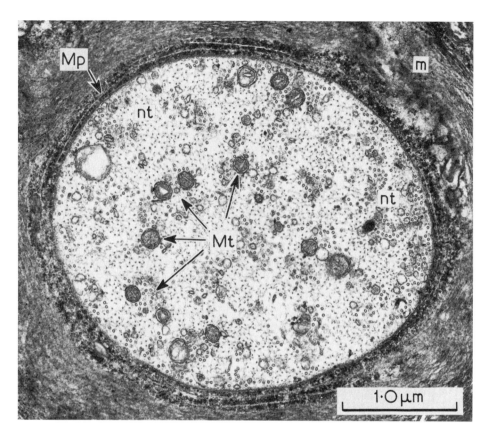

Fig. 1.23 Transverse section through a large myelinated fibre at the region of myelin termination. The axon diameter is reduced to between $\frac{1}{4}$ and $\frac{1}{5}$ th of its internodal value, and is surrounded by the myelin sheath (m) and terminal 'pockets' (Mp). While the lateral spacing of the neurofilaments is similar to that seen in the internode, the concentration of other organelles is increased. The most striking features are the pallisades of neurotubules (nt), both beneath the axolemma, and associated with the mitochondria (Mt) and vesicles.

the next; the compression of the internodal tubule population within a much smaller cross sectional area of axoplasm being associated, at least in the large nodes of larger mammals, with their aggregation into laterally aligned groups or 'ribbons' having a minimal separation of 30—35 nm (Fig. 1.24). These groups lack the cross-linkages of the fasciculated neurotubules characteristic of the initial segment of the axon (Palay, Sotelo, Peters and Orkand, 1968), and while some clusters lie near to the axon surface, others form pallisades around individual mitochondria or vesicles occasionally linked to them by dense cross-bridges (Raine, Ghetti and Shelanski, 1971) and thus provide morphological evidence for the suggested role of neurotubules in intra-axonal transport systems (Section 1.77; Fig. 1.34). An increase in the mitochondria and vesicle content is also apparent in the narrowed portion of the axon, but this is

43

possibly no more than another inevitable consequence of the reduction in axon cross-sectional area, and may have no particular metabolic significance.

The nodal axon is a barrel-shaped cylinder extending between the outermost attached 'pockets' of the two adjacent myelin sheaths. Its diameter increases at its mid point to rather more than that of the paranode in small fibres, and to between one quarter and one half of its mean internodal value in large fibres. Both the length of the exposed axon at the node, and its absolute diameter, increase with increasing fibre size, while the diameter of the nodal axon relative to its internodal value decreases with increase in fibre size. A precise knowledge of the area of physiologically active axon membrane at the node is of obvious importance to calculations concerning the changes in charge density and ionic flux associated with the propagation of the action potential. The values to be ascribed to this parameter, and how these may be affected by change in total fibre diameter, have been the subject of some controversy. While early estimates based on light and electron microscope studies of mammalian and frog nerves indicated that the area of exposed axon at the node remained approximately constant (Hess and Young, 1952), or even diminished (Robertson, 1959) with increase in fibre size, later electron microscope measurements showed that the axon surface area between the outermost 'pockets' of the myelin sheath increased significantly with increase in fibre size, being $3-5 \mu m^2$ and $15-25 \mu m^2$ is small and large feline ventral root fibres respectively (Berthold, 1968b); values in accord with those calculated from electrophysiological data. An unavoidable source of error affecting light microscopic estimates of the length of the nodal axon in large fibres is the difficulty of visualizing its longitudinal limits due to the outward convexity of the terminal swellings of the myelin sheath, as these further narrow the nodal gap to less than 50% of the length of the nodal axon visible in longitudinal sections.

On its external surface the nodal axolemma is related to a structural mosaic composed of the ends of the Schwann cell microvilli and the amorphous 'gap substance' which lies between them. No recognizable junctional complexes are visible between the ends of the microvilli and the nodal axon, but their adjacent membranes approach to within 2−5 nm of one another (Andersson−Cedergren and Karlsson, 1966; Berthold, 1968b), a considerably smaller gap than is normally seen between two apposed cell membranes. The internal aspect of the nodal axolemma is marked by the presence of an electron dense 'undercoating' of amorphous material some 25−30 nm thick (Fig. 1.20), an arrangement which is characteristic of the spike generating regions of both the initial axon segment and some sensory receptor terminals (see Chapter 4, p. 229). This density beneath the axon membrane is restricted to the nodal axolemma, ceasing abruptly at the point of attachment of the first myelin 'pockets' (Figs. 1.20 and 1.32), and on its deep surface it merges with a more diffuse increase in the density of the nodal and juxtanodal axoplasmic matrix. These regions of the axon are stained preferentially by the Hale colloidal iron technique (Abood and Abul Haj, 1956), and by cobalt hexamine (Langley, 1971; and Fig. 1.25(ii)), methods used for the histological detection of sulphated and nonsulphated mucopoly-saccharides (glycoaminoglycans) respectively, and it is probable that the increased density of the nodal axoplasmic matrix in conventional electron microscope preparations reflects the presence of such materials. Use of the Hale technique at the electron microscope level indicates that the sulphated mucopolysaccharides are present in highest concentrations both immediately beneath, and just outside the nodal axolemma, the former location coinciding with the position of the osmiophilic axolemmal 'undercoating' (Langley and Landon, 1967).

The organelle content of the nodal axoplasm differs little from that of the neighbouring juxtanodal regions. One to five, or occasionally more, mitochondria may be visible in a mid-nodal transverse section, depending upon the size of the fibre, and these are often situated towards its periphery. Local increases in the vesicle content of the axoplasm occur, frequently in the form of longitudinally aligned strings of round or ovoid vesicles having diameters ranging between 100–200 nm. Elements of the axonal 'smooth endoplasmic reticulum' (of which the chains of vesicles may be a distended component), lamellated autophagic vesicles, and dense lysosome-like granules of various sizes have also been described.

The identity and physicochemical properties of the gap substance, and the influence of the paranodal apparatus as a whole upon the impulse conducting properties of the node, are discussed in Section 1.4.3. A possible mechanical role for the gap substance, in accord with its older histological appellation of 'cementing disc', is suggested by observations that increase in length of peripheral nerve fibres when stretched is accommodated within the internodal segments, the dimensions of the nodes, the narrowest and ostensibly weakest portions of the fibres, remaining unchanged (Schneider, 1952; Kashef, 1966, and personal communication). However it is probably unjustified to ascribe all of this resistance to stretching shown by the node to the presence of the cementing disc, since the fine collagen fibrils of the endoneurial sheath of Plenk and Laidlaw provide a close knit continuous connective tissue tube spanning the nodal gap external to the basal lamina (Fig. 1.3); and by virtue of the presence of the paranodal bulbs this tube has a larger cross sectional area at the node and paranode than over the remainder of the internode.

1.4.2 *Development of the node and paranodal bulbs*

Numerous studies have been made of the development and differentiation of both Schwann cells and axons in growing peripheral nerves, and of the processes involved in myelination (see Sections 1.2.1, and 1.6.1), but only a few accounts have appeared concerning the morphogenesis of the nodes of Ranvier and paranodal regions of the nerve fibre, (Uzman and Nogueira–Graf, 1957; Berthold and Skoglund, 1967, 1968a and b; Berthold, 1968c; Allt, 1969a).

The positions of the future nodes are defined by the sites of contact between adjacent units of the Schwann cell column surrounding individual 'promyelin' nerve fibres, and are fixed at these particular positions by the onset of myelination. The subsequent increase in the length of the nerve, necessary to accommodate its dimensions to the postnatal growth of the parts within which it lies, is achieved by the increase in the length of the internodal segments of the axon and Schwann cells (Williams and Kashef, 1968; Schlaepfer and Myers, 1973), and nodal regions have little share in these growth processes. While the exposed length of axon at the node is said to be 'extensive' in the immature fibre (Allt, 1969a), it seldom measures more than 1.5 μm, a value differing little from that found at the nodes of mature large myelinated fibres, and the postmyelination increases in the diameter of the nodal and juxtanodal portions of the axon are seldom more than one quarter of those achieved elsewhere along its adjacent internodal segments. It thus appears appropriate to regard the narrowed axon of the nodal and juxtanodal regions of the larger mature myelinated axons (Section 1.4.1) to be the consequence of a local restriction of growth, itself in some way a result of the attachment of the spiral of Schwann cell membrane forming the end of the myelin sheath to the axon in this region, and not to be due to active constriction of the axon by the inturned end of the myelin sheath, as has been implied in some descriptions of nodal structure.

The timing of the onset and rate of progress of the processes of nodal morphogenesis varies between species, and with the position of the node along the cephalo-caudal and proximo-distal axes of the body. It is also related to future fibre size, and to variations in the functional demands made upon nerve fibres in different parts of the organism during the course of ontogenesis (Berthold, 1968c; Schwieler, 1968). In a growing 1–2 μm fibre, at the stage at which the first 4–6 compact myelin lamellae have been formed along the adjacent internodes, the future nodal axon is enveloped by overlapping or abutting 'cuffs' of Schwann cell cytoplasm. These cuffs are on the nodal side of the ends of a series of 'promyelin' lamellae, composed of several layers of uncompacted Schwann cell membranes and their contained cytoplasm, which surround the axon immediately adjacent to the node, true compact myelin only commencing some 5–10 μm from the mid-nodal point. The nodal axon is distinguishable even at this early stage by the presence of the characteristic, 30 nm thick, dense coat adherent to the inner surface of the axolemma (Berthold, 1968b); but the future 'nodal gap' is represented merely by a 20 nm interval between the opposed membranes of the 'cuffs' of Schwann cell cytoplasm, and a similar interval between these and the nodal axolemma. This perinodal cleft is continuous with a 10–30 nm gap between the axolemma and the ends of the uncompacted promyelin lamellae, which thus lack the close (1–2 nm) contact with the axon of the myelin 'pockets' of the mature node.

Subsequent increase in fibre diameter to 4–5 μm is accompanied by a number of interrelated changes in both the form and proportions of the structural components of the node and paranodal regions. The numbers of myelin lamellae rapidly increase (Section 1.6.1), and longitudinal spread of myelin compaction progressively reduces the extent of the zone of uncompacted 'promyelin' lamellae adjacent to the node. The 'promyelin' terminal pockets are initially obliquely inclined towards the axon, but with increase in numbers of lamellae their approach approximates to a right angle, thus deepening the nodal constriction. The nodal 'cuffs' of Schwann cell cytoplasm meanwhile diminish in size and withdraw from the nodal axolemma, to be replaced by an outgrowth of microvilli from their nodal surfaces. These microvilli are at first irregular in form and closely packed, and only later acquire their mature regularity and radial symmetry, with increase in fibre diameter above 6–7 μm (Berthold, 1968b; Allt, 1969a).

During the early stages of nodal development the Schwann cell cytoplasm in the paranodal regions is indistinguishable in its content of organelles from that surrounding the remainder of the internode, with the exception of that in the immediate neighbourhood of the nucleus, possessing filaments, microtubules, ribosomes (both free and attached to small rough endoplasmic reticular cisterns), small vesicles and occasional scattered mitochondria. Later growth in fibre diameter to ~4 μm, and the coincident changes in nodal morphology, including the appearance of the microvilli, are accompanied by a marked increase in the numbers of mitochondria present in the paranodal Schwann cell cytoplasm. A quantitative analysis of the occurrence of mitochondria per unit area of Schwann cell in the lumbar ventral root fibres of the cat, reveals a tenfold increase in the mitochondrial content of the paranodes between birth and 55 days of age (Berthold and Skoglund, 1967).

Concurrent but opposite changes affect the mitochondrial population of the axon, and the local accumulations of clusters of small mitochondria commonly seen at the nodes of fibres in the 1–2 μm diameter range, are no longer visible at the nodes of fibres of 4–5 μm diameter. Berthold (1968c) has suggested that the displacement of the predominant population from an intra to an extra-axonal position during development may represent a solution to the problem of maintaining a large enough energy supply system at the node to provide for the needs of the nodal axolemma, while avoiding its continual displacement by axoplasmic flow. This proposal provides a logistic explanation to support the earlier suggestions (Williams and Landon. 1963, 1964, 1965; Landon and Williams, 1963) that the great disproportion between the mitochondrial contents of the axon and the Schwann cell in the paranodal regions of the mature fibre (Section 1.4.1) might reflect a role for the Schwann cell in the supply of energy rich compounds for use at the nodal axon membrane, for example, in ionic pump mechanisms.

Increase in the paranodal mitochondrial population, and the development of the Schwann cell microvilli, are accompanied by the appearance of small vesicles containing a moderately electron dense granular material within the juxtanodal Schwann cell cytoplasm (Berthold, 1968c). This material may represent a precursor of the gap substance, which also makes its first appearance between the nodal Schwann cell microvilli at this stage of nodal morphogenesis. The concurrent development of the mature pattern of ridges and grooves of the paranodal myelin sheath may not always be the consequence of a simple progressive process of swelling and folding, superimposed upon the smooth, unswollen paranodes of the immature fibre of 2 μm diameter or less. Berthold and Skoglund (1968b) report the existence of an intermediate stage affecting cat ventral root fibres of between 3 and 4 μm diameter, during which slender filiform or fungiform outgrowths of the paranodal myelin sheath, containing either axoplasm or cytoplasm of the inner compartment of the Schwann cell, project out into the surrounding Schwann cell cytoplasm, to produce what they term a 'complex paranode'. With further growth in fibre diameter to 5–6 μm these processes become separated from their origins and are phagocytosed within the Schwann cell cytoplasm, to be replaced by the smooth or undulant myelin ridges, and intervening grooves filled by columns of mitochondria-rich Schwann cell cytoplasm, that characterize the mature 'paranodal apparatus'. 'Complex' paranodes have not yet been reported to occur in developing limb nerves, and the phenomenon may therefore be the product of developmental conditions specific to the nerve roots, possibly connected with the process, also peculiar to the ventral roots of kittens, by which whole Schwann cells supporting abnormally short myelin segments are eliminated from nerve fibres during development (Berthold and Skoglund, 1968a, b).

It is thus apparent that, in the nerve fibres most studied, i.e., the lumbar ventral root fibres of the cat and kitten (Berthold, 1968a, b, c; Berthold and Skoglund, 1967, 1968a, b), the node and paranodal apparatus have achieved something close to their mature morphology, albeit in miniature, by the stage of development at which the fibre has a mean internodal diameter of only 5 μm. Subsequent growth in internodal length and axon diameter involves only quantitative changes and remodelling, without further significant structural reorganization. Berthold and Skoglund (1967) have demonstrated that, in growing feline nerves, the time of appearance of the paranodal aggregations of mitochondria corresponds well with the attainment by the nerve of adult electrical properties with regard to absolute refactory period; and Schwieler (1968) has shown that the capabilities of nerves in the kitten to conduct continuously at high frequencies correlate better with the maturity of the pattern of NADH-Tetrazolium reductase activity at their nodes, than with their diameter. Such findings suggest that nodal maturity, which necessarily includes the aggregation of mitochondria at the paranodes, is a more important determinant of the impulse conducting properties of a nerve than absolute diameter. The implications of this proposal are considered further below (Section 1.4.3).

1.4.3 *The ionic environment of the node and nodal function*

Hess and Young (1952), in discussing their own, and previous observations (Ranvier, 1878; Macallum, 1905; Macallum and Menten, 1906; Nemiloff,

1908; Cajal, 1928) concerning the staining properties of the node of Ranvier, remarked that '. . . much remains obscure about the nature of the barrier around the fibre at the node', and that '. . . until the permeability properties of the cementing disc, perinodal space and outer endoneurium are known it cannot be assumed that at the node there is free diffusion between the axon surface and whatever tissue fluids constitute the external environment of the fibre'. These words of caution have passed unheeded by the majority of workers concerned with the electrophysiological studies of the role of the node in saltatory conduction of the nerve impulse (e.g., Tasaki, 1968; Hodgkin, 1971). Most theoretical calculations of charge density and ionic flux ignore the existence of the paranodal bulbs, and assume the node to be a straight sided cylinder, of length equal to he optically visible nodal gap in teased fibres, and in free commerce with an extracellular tissue fluid. As will have been seen from the description of nodal structure in Section 1.4.1, this 'ideal' node of the electrophysiologists bears little resemblance to the morphology of the nodes of the large myelinated peripheral nerve fibres usually employed in their experiments. An understanding of how this complex morphology is related to function, and specifically to ionic movements during the passage of the action potential, demands a detailed knowledge of the physico-chemical properties of the structural elements that constitute the environment of the nodal axolemma.

The black 'cross of Ranvier' produced at the node by immersion of nerve fibres in a dilute solution of silver nitrate and subsequent exposure to sunlight,

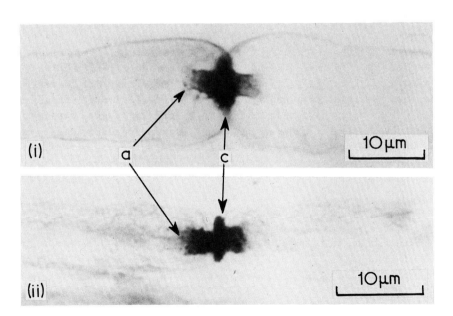

Fig. 1.24   The cross of Ranvier: nodes of rat sciatic nerves immersed in 0.1 m silver nitrate for short periods. (i) fixed in glutaraldehyde; (ii) unfixed. a – axon; c – cementing disc.

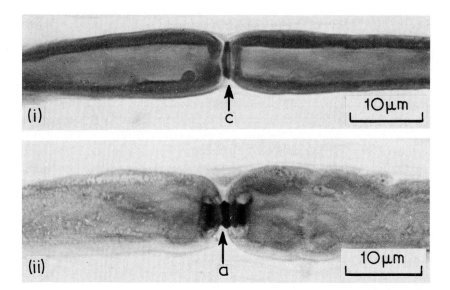

Fig. 1.25 (i) A teased osmicated myelinated nerve fibre; the cementing disc (c) at the node is stained with copper ferrocyanide (see text). (ii) A teased fibre fixed in glutaraldehyde and stained with cobalt hexamine followed by ammonium sulphide. The nodal axon (a) is stained, clearly demonstrating its biconical profile, but the cementing disc is unstained by this technique (see text). (Both preparations are reproduced by courtesy of Dr O. K. Langley and the editors of the *Histochemical Journal*.)

has been described earlier (Section 1.4.1 and Figs. 1.13 and 1.24), and the affinity of the region of the cementing disc for a wide variety of other metal salts has been demonstrated by several subsequent investigators, among whom were Macallum (1905), Macallum and Menten (1906), Herbst (1965) and Gerebtzoff and Mladenov (1967). An indication of the nature of the material responsible for this cation-binding capacity at the node was provided by Abood and Abul Haj (1956), who used the Hale colloidal iron stain to detect local concentrations of non-sulphated mucopolysaccharides at and around the nodes of peripheral nerve fibres. Subsequent fine structural studies of the Mowry modification of the Hale stain demonstrated the presence of material in a narrow zone spanning the nodal axolemma, which blocking reactions and enzyme digestion showed to be largely composed of sulphated mucopolysaccharides (Langley and Landon, 1967).

The known ion exchange properties of mucopolysaccharides have led to studies of cation binding and cation exchange at the nodes of Ranvier, using a variety of inorganic cations, and the organic polycation Alcian Blue (Landon and Langley, 1971; Langley, 1969, 1970, 1971). These studies have demonstrated the presence of a fixed anionic charge matrix surrounding the axon at the node, and fine structural studies of the distribution of the bound ions have localized this property to the nodal gap substance (Figs. 1.25 and 1.26). The strength of the bond between the cation and its binding site was found to increase with

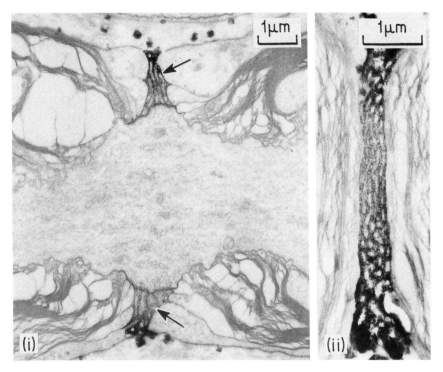

Fig. 1.26   Longitudinal sections through the nodes of rat sciatic nerve fibres demonstrating the binding of copper ions to the gap substance; identical preparations to that portrayed in Fig. 1.25(i). (i) An axial section in which a dense precipitate of copper ferrocyanide can be seen external to the axolemma between the Schwann cell microvilli (arrows). (ii) A paraxial section passing through the edge of the disc, the precipitate revealing the microvilli in negative contrast.

increasing valency, and to be inversely proportional to hydrated ionic radius; these properties, and the reversibility of the binding reaction, suggest that the cation-polyanion bond is an electrostatic one. While the sulphated material close to the nodal axolemma (see p. 45) must be expected to play a part in the observed ion binding reaction, the fine structural localization of the binding material, and its response to blocking reactions, enzyme digestion, and Alcian Blue staining at varying electrolyte concentrations, indicate that other polyanions, containing carboxyl, or a mixture of carboxyl and phosphate groups and thus unstained by the Hale method, are responsible for the majority of the ion binding effect (Landon and Langley, 1971; Langley, 1971). The extracellular cation binding material, although it is most conveniently studied in large fibres, is found around the nodes of peripheral nerve fibres of all diameters, the intensity and extent of the nodal staining being proportional to the electron optically visible quantity of gap substance. While this diminishes with decreasing fibre size, a proportionately higher concentration of sulphated mucopolysaccharides is found within the nodal axoplasm of small fibres. Material with similar staining and binding properties to the 'cementing disc' is found around the nodes of the larger myelinated fibres in the central nervous system, in a position corresponding to the amorphous electron dense perinodal matrix (Hildebrand, 1971; Hildebrand and Skoglund, 1971; Landon and Langley, unpublished observations.

The affinity of the nodal regions for metal ions has provided ground for criticism of the specificity of the localization of reaction products produced by histochemical methods claimed to demonstrate the presence of acetylcholin-esterase within the cementing disc (Gerebtzoff, 1962). While the specificity of the enzyme reaction itself is not in question, since it can be abolished by the use of appropriate enzyme inhibitors or exclusion of the specific substrate, acetylthiocholine, there exists a possibility that the products of acetylthio-choline hydrolysis may not be precipitated solely at the sites of acetylcholin-esterase activity. Copper ions in the incubation medium may be expected to accumulate within the ion binding matrix of the 'cementing disc', and will there be readily available to precipitate thiocholine diffusing from sites of enzyme activity elsewhere within the nodal complex (Zenker, 1964; Langley and Landon, 1969; Krammer and Lischka, 1973).

The physiological consequences of the presence of an ion binding matrix around the nodal axolemma are obviously very difficult to assess. While most of our knowledge of its properties is based upon studies of fixed material, and is thus inevitably incomplete, the physico-chemical constitution of the nodal gap sub-stance cannot simply be ignored in any serious analysis of the ionic mechanisms underlying nerve impluse transmission along peripheral myelinated nerve fibres.

Hodgkin (1951) has shown that small changes in sodium ion concentration external to nerve membranes, whilst they have little effect upon the resting potential, can greatly alter the magnitude and rate of rise of the action potential. The osmotic activity of counter cations within a polyanion domain is considerably lower than that of the same concentration of ions in simple solution (Salimen and Loumanmäki, 1963), and it is possible that the polyanionic matrix of the nodal gap substance has the capacity to concentrate and maintain a high, but osmotically, inactive, reservoir of sodium ions close to the nodal axolemma, available for transit across the axolemma during the passage of the action potential. The release of sodium ions from this reservoir in an osmotically active form may be triggered by the arrival within the matrix of inorganic (Tobias, 1964), or organic (Langley, 1970), counter cations withdrawn electronically from the membrane phase of the axon (Landon and Langley, 1971). The apparent contradiction between the observed extremely rapid responses of the electrical properties of nodes to changes in the concentration of external ions, (e.g., Vierhaus and Ulbricht, 1971), and the obvious structural impediments to the free diffusion of ions which have been described, can also be resolved by this proposal that the nodal gap substance acts as an ion-exchange 'buffer'. Access to the external aspect of the perinodal collar of Schwann cell microvilli and gap substance will be equivalent to direct access to the immediate vicinity of the nodal axolemma, and calculations of the effects of diffusion coefficients, convection factors and 'unstirred layers' are rendered largely irrelevant.

The presence of a polyanion matrix around the node may have the additional function of limiting diffusion away from the axon of the potassium ion that passes outwards through the axolemma during the passage of the nerve impulse, and thus hold it available for redistribution across the nodal axolemma during repolarization. Bennett (1963) has proposed that the 'glycocalyx' of striated muscle may have a similar function in limiting the loss of potassium ion from the immediate vicinity of the sarcolemma following the passage of a propogated action potential; and Seneviratne, Pieris and Weerasuriya (1972) have postulated that depression of nerve excitability by hypoxia may be due to efflux of potassium ion, and its accumulation immediately outside the axolemma as a consequence of the diffusion barrier presented by the materials in the nodal gap. Some of the properties of local anaesthetics may also be attributed to their interaction with the ion binding matrix at the node. These substances are organic bases that exist predominantly in the cationic form at physiological pH, and Langley (1973) has demonstrated that they bind to the nodal polyanions, and can be exchanged for metallic ions in fixed tissues, at concentrations that produce an electro-physiological effect on rat peripheral nerves *in vivo*. The pharmacological effects of local anaesthetics may therefore, in part at least, be related to a competitive interaction with sodium ion for the nodal binding sites, the consequent reduction in the concentration of sodium ion adjacent to the axolemma leading to a reduction in the amplitude of the action potential.

The perinodal gap substance has hitherto been discussed in isolation, and solely in terms of its properties as a passive ion binding matrix; it has been proposed, however, that the gap substance may form but a part of a functionally important unit, the 'paranodal apparatus', the other components of which are the mitochondria rich paranodal portions of the Schwann cell and the nodal microvilli (Williams and Landon, 1963; Landon and Langley, 1971). Earlier suggestions that this morphological complex could be responsible for the supply of energy-rich compounds to the nodal axolemma (Landon and Williams, 1963; Williams and Landon, 1963, 1964, 1965) have been referred to above (p. 47). The speculations of Berthold and Skoglund (1967) that the paranodal mitochondria might play a role in the maintenance of the ionic milieu of the node, based upon the known participation of mitochondria in the active transport of ions, and comparisons of the morphology of the nodal and paranodal portions of the Schwann cell with the structure of cells known to be concerned with the active transcellular movement of ions in other tissues, and with the cells of the salt secreting glands of marine vertebrates and the potassium secreting cells of the insect gut in particular, have led to the formulation of an alternative hypothesis concerning the function of the 'paranodal apparatus'.

Salt secreting cells characteristically contain large concentrations of mito-chondria close to their absorptive lateral and basal surfaces, and possess microvilli, or similar surface specializations, on their relatively small, apical secretory surfaces, often covered by a substantial coat of mucopoly-saccharide. It has been suggested (Landon and Langley, 1971) that the 'paranodal apparatus' of the Schwann cell may function in a similar manner to a salt secreting cell, and thus be concerned with the active accumulation of sodium ion in the region of the nodal gap; the mitochondria of the paranodal Schwann cell cytoplasm providing the energy necessary for the active translocation of sodium ion from the endoneurial matrix opposed to the outer surface of the Schwann cell, or from the periaxonal space via the Schmidt—Lanterman incisures, to the cells' microvillous apex at the node. Such a system of replenishment of the extracellular sodium ion adjacent to the node, while it might be of limited value to small, slowly conducting fibres, can be conceived to have considerable functional advantages for the larger diameter fibres responsible for conducting prolonged high frequency trains of impulses. It is in just such fibres that the 'paranodal apparatus' attains its greatest complexity and content of mito-chondria, and it will be recalled (p. 48) that it is the development of 'adult' paranodal morphology, rather than the achievement of any particular critical fibre diameter, that correlates best with the attainment of adult impulse conduction characteristics during ontogeny. While the assignment of such an active role in the control of the ionic environment of the node to the paranodal portions of the Schwann cell is at present pure speculation, supported by nothing more substantial than cytological analogy, it is important to emphasize that the functional behaviour of the nodal axon membrane cannot be considered in isolation from its natural morphological environment, and that knowledge of the properties of the node of Ranvier derived from electro-physiological studies relates to the properties of the node in its entirety, and not merely to those of the nodal axolemma.

1.5 Axonal RNA

The classic view of the distribution of RNA within the neuron, as inferred from semi-quantitative and qualitative light microscope observations of the arrangement of its presumed structural correlate, the basophilic Nissl material, was that RNA was confined to the somata and central segments of the dendrites. Such a view clearly implied the absence of any local protein synthesis by the axon. This distribution of RNA was apparently confirmed by the absence of axoplasmic ribosomes, and the failure of early ultra-violet microspectrophotometric methods to detect axonal RNA (Nurnberger, Engström and Lindström, 1952). However, with the development of more sensitive techniques, notably the direct microchemical analysis of Carnoy-fixed axons dissected free of myelin, and the unequivocal demonstration of small amounts of axonal RNA (0.02–0.07%) in the giant axon of the Mauthner neuron in the goldfish (Edström, Eichner and Edström, 1962), this view became untenable. It was shown that the RNA content of the axon exceeded that of the cell body by a factor of 4 in the specimens analyzed, even though the concentration of RNA (w/v) in the axon was about 1/20 that in the soma (Edström, 1964). RNA has also been shown to be present in axons from the lobster stretch receptor (0.06%) (Grampp and Edström, 1963); in the giant axon of the squid (0.02–0.03%) (Lasek, 1970) and crayfish abdominal cord (0.02%) (Andersson, Edström and Jarlstedt, 1970); and in the spinal accessory nerves of the cat (Koenig, 1965) and rabbit (Koenig, 1967a,b). In terms of concentration, the quantity of RNA in mammalian axons is an order of magnitude lower than that in the non-mammalian axons, i.e., 0.003 – 0.006%: Koenig (1970) has suggested however that concentration may not be a suitable parameter to examine in mammalian axons where the surface to volume ratio is high, since a significant proportion of their RNA may be associated with membranes, and with the axolemma in particular.

The source of this RNA is currently in dispute. The original assumption that the presence of axonal RNA was indicative of a centrifugal migration of somal RNA has been challenged by more recent experimental evidence which implies that some (perhaps all) axonal RNA is synthesized locally. There have been a number of studies, generally in piscine or avian retino-tectal systems, in which, following injection of labelled pre-cursors around the relevant perikarya, the intra-axonal migration patterns of labelled RNA and TCA-soluble nucleotide derivatives have been assessed biochemically and/or autoradiographically (e.g., Bray and Austin, 1968; Casola, Davis and Davis, 1969; Bondy, 1972; Wolburg, 1972; Ingoglia, Grafstein, McEwen and McQuarrie, 1973; Autilio-Gambetti, Gambetti and Shafer, 1973; Gambetti, Autilio-Gambetti, Shafer and Pfaff, 1973). The characteristic axonal distribution of radioactively-labelled RNA that is obtained by these methods is a gradient, in marked contrast to the sharply-defined peaks produced by distally-migrating proteins (see Section, 1.7.1 p. 78), and on the basis of this type of analysis, a range of intra-axonal velocities, both fast and slow, have been calculated for RNA. It appears that the rates reported reflect differences in the species and the age of experimental animal, the site of administration and the type of pre-cursor and, according to Bondy (1972), the duration of the phase of somal synthesis. Moreover, it is possible that the true levels of migrating RNA and TCA-soluble material are 'masked' by local synthesis of RNA, and it is this factor which has, until recently, been generally ignored.

There is now persuasive evidence available to support the concept of a local DNA-dependent synthesis of RNA; but the question of the site of synthesis, i.e., whether it is intra- or extra-axonal, remains unanswered. One of the more consistent findings in studies involving the use of radioactively-labelled pre-cursors has been the precocious intra-axonal appearance of labelled TCA-soluble material: and it has been inferred that at least some of the RNA subsequently detected in the axon has been synthesized locally from this population of pre-cursors. In support of this view, it has been shown that labelled pre-cursors are incorporated into axonal RNA *in vitro*, a process that is actinomycin D-sensitive, and that most of this labelled RNA is extra-mitochondrial (see Koenig, 1970). Autilio-Gambetti *et al.* (1973), using intra-ocular injections of ^{3}H-uridine to label RNA in the optic nerve of the rabbit, found that a $70 - 80\%$ reduction in the amount of detectable labelled RNA could be produced by the subsequent intra-cranial injection of actinomycin D: the intra-ocular injection of the latter, while severely inhibiting retinal RNA synthesis, had no effect on the incorporation of pre-cursors into RNA in the nerve.

Non-somal, extra-axonal synthesis of RNA implies satellite cell participation, but there is, unfortunately, little quantitative data available concerning the RNA content of satellite cells, primarily because of the technical difficulties inherent in obtaining pure samples. Edström and his co-workers have studied the local synthesis of RNA in Mauthner axons in the goldfish, by comparing the type of RNA obtained when axons are incubated with labelled pre-cursors *in situ* in the spinal cord with that obtained if the axons are dissected free from their glial covering before incubation (Edström, Edström and Hökfelt, 1969; Edström and Sjöstrand, 1969). It was found that whereas newly-synthesized RNA recovered from isolated axons was only 4S, that obtained from fibres incubated *in situ* was not only 4 S but also 16 S and 28–30 S (Edström *et al.*, 1969). The tentative interpretation of these findings was that the higher molecular weight RNA was derived from the satellite cell nuclei. In this context it is interesting that Peterson, Bray and Austin (1968) and Autilio-Gambetti *et al.* (1973), in light microscope autoradiographic analyses of the fate of injected radioactively-labelled RNA pre-cursors, have described the presence of silver grains not only within axons, but also within Schwann cells and glial 'spaces'. In a subsequent electron microscope autoradiographic study, Gambetti *et al.* (1973) found that following intra-ocular injection of ^{3}H-uridine in the rabbit, 74–83% of all the counted grains over the components of the optic nerve were extra-axonal, and that glial cell bodies were the most heavily labelled structures. In addition, the grain count over the axons was significantly higher than that expected as random scatter from myelin and glial processes: this labelled RNA was concentrated mainly around the periphery of the axon, and bore no obvious relation to the distribution of mitochondria.

The implications of the macromolecular transfer of material from axon to Schwann cell and *vice versa* are exciting, particularly in view of the recent reports of intercellular transfer of macromolecules in culture (Kolodny, 1971), and the demonstrated limited capacity of some axons to take up material by endocytosis (Section 1.63). However, these observations require corroboration from further ultrastructural, autoradiographical and biochemical investigations before they can be profitably discussed in greater detail.

1.5.1 *Axonal protein synthesis*

The neuron soma was believed, until recently, to be the exclusive source of axonal protein, and numerous studies over the past decade, in particular those involving autoradiography and liquid scintillation spectrography, have confirmed the somato-fugal, intra-axonal displacement of discrete bands of labelled protein. Most discussions of this phenomenon involve the tacit, and debatable, assumption that *all* protein reaches the periphery by this route, but as several workers have pointed out, the time taken for material to travel from soma to periphery (even at the fastest observed rates) seems inconsistent with the rapidity of neuronal responses to physiological stimuli. The idea that all axonal protein is soma-derived is open to question on a number of counts. First, it is possible that labelled material could leak into the blood stream at the injection site, and reach the periphery by an extra-axonal route, either in the blood stream, or in the endoneurial flow system described by Weiss, Wang, Taylor and Edds (1945); second, labelled pre-cursor may flow unincorporated along the axon to the periphery where protein synthesis occurs *in situ*; and third, protein may be synthesized locally along the axon from extra-axonal pre-cursors, and thus supplement the somal supply.

While there is evidence that leakage of material into the blood stream occurs in the optic tract of fishes (Rahmann, 1971), evidence for the flow of amino acids along the axon is equivocal; most workers have denied that it occurs (Bray and Austin, 1968; di Giamberardino, 1971), but Csanyi, Gervai and Lajtha (1973) have reported flow rates ranging from 5 to 110 mm/day for $L^{-14}C$ proline and D-glutamic acid in chick, rabbit and carp nerves.

There is now some experimental support for protein synthesis in the axon. The evidence includes the microchemical and autoradiographic demonstration of the incorporation of labelled amino acids into axonal protein *in vitro* (Edström, 1969); the demonstration of local ACHe synthesis (Koenig, 1967); the uptake of labelled amino acids into synaptosomal proteins *in vitro* (Morgan and Austin, 1968); and the demonstration of axonal RNA and local axonal RNA synthesis (Section 1.30). Furthermore, there have been a number of electron microscope autoradiographic studies in which labelled amino acids, after intraperitoneal administration, have been demonstrated in nerve bundles, localized over Schwann cells, myelin sheaths and axons (Singer and Salpeter, 1966; Singer, 1968; Freide and Samorajski, 1969): the interpretations placed upon these results are open to criticism however (Section 1.43). In spite of these findings, it must be pointed out that, in the systems which have been examined in most detail, i.e., invertebrate giant axons, axonal RNA is almost entirely 4S RNA containing functional tRNA (Lasek, Dabrowski and Nordlander, 1973), and there is little evidence of rRNA. Although it has been demonstrated that tRNA can be involved as an amino acid donor in reactions other than the mRNA-directed synthesis of polypeptides (e.g., Soffer, 1968), it remains difficult to reconcile the intra-axonal synthesis of protein with an almost total lack of high molecular weight axonal RNA.

1.6 The Schwann cell – axon relationship

The widespread adoption of the concept of a 'neuron-glia' unit, makes it pertinent to preface a consideration of the relationship this implies with the following question: are satellite cells necessary for the survival and adequate functioning of the neuron?

There are many sites in invertebrate central and peripheral nervous systems and in the vertebrate neuropil, at which small-diameter axons are either naked (Horridge, 1968), or are segregated within a satellite cell furrow into bundles in which the individual axons are not separated from their neighbours by tongues of satellite cell cytoplasm, but lie in direct cell-to-cell contact; e.g., in crustacea (Whitear, 1962), in octopus optic nerve (Dilly, Gray and Young, 1963; Robertson, 1964) and in the vertebrate olfactory nerve (Graziadei, 1966). Moreover, during the ontogeny of even the largest vertebrate myelinated nerve fibres, there is a period prior to myelinogenesis when there is little in the organization of bundles of fine axons and of the Schwann cells migrating in parallel with them, to suggest the complexity of the future association between these cell types (see Section 1.3.1 and Fig. 1.6). Axonal viability has been demonstrated experimentally in situations in which Schwann cell viability is less certain: axonal continuity, morphological integrity and, it is presumed, functional capacity, are all maintained during temporary alterations in the state of the Schwann cell, whether as a consequence of a primary demyelination (e.g., McDonald, 1967; Hall and Gregson, 1971), or a more complete interference with Schwann cell metabolism, leading to Schwann cell necrosis (e.g., Masurovsky, Bunge and Bunge, 1969). Even removal of most of the glial cytoplasm surrounding neurons in leech ganglia does not immediately impair neuronal activity (Kuffler and Potter, 1964). Large peripheral axons can survive for periods of at least one month *in vivo* with long stretches of their internodal surfaces devoid of all Schwann cell covering other than a collapsed basal lamina (Hall, unpublished observations), and naked, apparently viable, axons have recently been described within distemper plaques in the central nervous system, surviving three months after the development of the disease (Raine, 1972).

Axons can undoubtedly function in the absence of a satellite cell, or at least without sole claim to a satellite cell territory, but in all but the simplest nervous systems, some kind of satellite cell typically constitutes the most immediate cellular environment of the neuron. That there is a relationship between the neuron and its satellite cells, in terms of (i) the provision of specific metabolic support; (ii) interchange of various species of RNA and consequent genomic stimulation and modification; and (iii) an 'interlocking energetic system' (Hydén, 1967), is implicit in contemporary interpretations of integrated neuronal activity and the maintenance of homeostasis within the nervous system. Much of the evidence for this attractive concept of the 'neuron-glia unit' as the functional unit upon which the higher levels of organization of the nervous system are superimposed, is circumstantial however, and has been drawn largely from biochemical or autoradiographic analyses of experimentally-manipulated mammalian or non-mammalian tissue, 'neuronal-' or 'glial-enriched' fractionated material, and more recently, from the studies of individual cells isolated by micro-dissection, (see Johnston and Roots, 1972). Furthermore, although ideas of Schwann cell function are obviously coloured by the roles which have been proposed for glia (Bunge, 1968), it is uncertain to what extent we are justified in extrapolating conclusions based upon observations concerning the type of cellular organization existing in the central nervous system to that found in the peripheral nervous system.

In the vertebrate peripheral nervous system, the assumption that some functional reciprocity does exist seems warranted on morphological grounds (Section 1.2). In both non-myelinated and myelinated fibres, the Schwann cell defines the geometry of the peri-axonal space, by virtue of its monopoly of the outer surface of the axolemma, and the morphological relationship between Schwann cell and axolemma becomes more complex in the nodal region where the finger-like processes of adjacent Schwann cells interdigitate within the gap substance and abut upon the nodal axolemma (Landon and Williams, 1963 and Section 1.4.1).

The imputation of a metabolic or functional role to the interrelationship between the axon and its Schwann cells raises many questions. How accessible is the peri-axonal space to the general extracellular space? Does the Schwann cell modify the chemical and osmotic constitution of the peri-axonal space, and is the latter, as Lehninger (1968) has suggested, of the intercellular space between neurons and glia ... 'not merely a dilute aqueous solution of amorphous character, but very likely a structured matrix endowed with a number of interesting molecular properties.'

1.6.1 Myelination and axon-myelin relationships

The ontogenetic processes whereby the future myelinated nerve fibres are segregated during development from the outgrowing bundles of primitive unmyelinated axons, and thus achieve a one-to-one relationship with their own individual columns of Schwann cells, have been described earlier (Section 1.3.1, p. 14). The structural changes implicit in the subsequent acquisition of a myelin sheath by these fibres, and the factors which govern the adult relationships between axon calibre, myelin sheath thickness and inter-nodal length are also of considerable interest.

The mechanism proposed by Geren (1954) for the initiation of myelinogenesis in the chick, i.e., the rolling of the axon within a spiral of Schwann cell cytoplasm, with subsequent growth of the mesaxon and 'zippering' of the residual membrane spiral, was soon generally accepted to be valid for the myelinated fibres of other vertebrates (e.g., Robertson, 1960). However, when expressed in these simple terms the hypothesis clearly fails to provide an adequate description of the concurrent and interrelated changes in shape and dimensions which occur in a myelinating nerve fibre. Compact myelin is first seen when the axon is between 1 and 2 μm in diameter and the individual Schwann cells are only some 200–250 μm long. The subsequent increase in axon diameter with maturation, to between 10 and 15 μm in the largest mammalian myelinated fibres, necessitates adjustment of the already 'compacted' lamellar structure of the myelin to accommodate this change in axonal girth, while the growth in axon length which accompanies growth in the tissues surrounding the nerve, e.g., increase in limb length, requires a corresponding increase in the length of the Schwann cell column. Since the total numbers of Schwann cells along a nerve do not increase during normal myelination (Vizoso and Young, 1948), and may indeed slightly decrease (Berthold and Skoglund, 1968a), growth in length of the axon requires a four to six fold increase in the length of the individual Schwann cells, and therefore of their contained segments of myelin; i.e., from 250–300 μm to between 1000 and 1500 μm in large fibres.

Webster (1971) has recently described the fine structural details of the myelination process affecting a small number of fibres in a marginal bundle of the rat sciatic nerve. He found that the initial turns of the developing mesaxon spiral were highly variable with regard to both their direction and contour, frequently reversing. The spiral contained a larger number of turns at the level of the nucleus than towards the nodes, and whereas the external end of the mesaxon was in general, to be found within the same quadrant of the Schwann cell throughout its length, the inner, adaxonal, end of the mesaxon varied in its position around the circumference of the axon from point to point along the cell, in a manner which corresponded to the observed differences in the number of turns of the mesaxon spiral. Subsequent increase in the numbers of compact myelin lamellae was associated with increased regularity of form and loss of spiral reversals, and restriction of the Schwann cell cytoplasm to continuous longitudinal strips adjacent to the external mesaxon, and to narrow spirals at the Schmidt–Lanterman incisures and the nodes of Ranvier (Fig. 1.27). Measurements of the rate of addition of new myelin membrane showed that this increased rapidly during the growth of the first 4–6 layers (3–4 turns at 3 days, 17–28 turns at 7 days), and thereafter continued at a relatively constant level during the further enlargement of the compact myelin sheath, a somewhat similar acceleration of the increment of myelin membrane after the deposition of the first few turns was found by Friede and Samorajski (1968). Closely comparable morphological changes have been reported by Fraher (1973) in a study of the development of fibres in the anterior spinal roots of the rat (see also Martin and Webster (1973) and Webster, Martin and O'Connell, 1973).

The observed simultaneous increases in the internal circumference, thickness (numbers of lamellae) and the length of the myelin sheath during its development, have suggested to many observers both that the myelin lamellae are able to slip one upon another, and that new myelin constituents may be inserted into an already formed compact spiral, particularly during the processes of growth and remodelling. The familiar alternation of dense and pale lines in

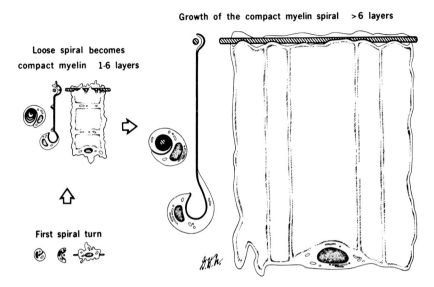

Growth of the compact myelin spiral > 6 layers

Loose spiral becomes
compact myelin 1-6 layers

First spiral turn

Fig. 1.27   A diagram of myelin formation in a Schwann cell showing how the position and relative size of the cytoplasmic interfaces of the myelin membrane change during growth of the myelin sheath. The appearance of the Schwann cell in transverse section is supplemented by transverse and *en face* views of the 'unrolled' cell, the three stages of growth being represented at the same magnification. (Reproduced from Webster (1971), by kind permission of the author and the editors of the *Journal of Cell Biology*.)

the electron microscope image of sectioned myelin has, in the past, fostered the impression gained from early biochemical studies (Davison, Dobbing, Morgan and Payling Wright, 1959) that this material is, *in vivo*, both structurally rigid and metabolically inert. It is now becoming apparent that myelin may, on the contrary, be a relatively labile material, the increase in the total area of the myelin lamellae which accompanies growth in axon length and diameter being achieved by the direct radial intercalation of new molecular constituents into the 'liquid crystal lattice' of the existing compact spiral. Such a process could account for the observed changes in the chemical composition of myelin during maturation (Banik and Davison, 1967; and Chapter 11).

The quantitative autoradiographic studies by Rawlins (1973) of the uptake of intra-peritoneally administered ^{3}H cholesterol into the myelin sheaths of suckling mice have recently demonstrated the rapidity with which sterols can be incorporated into, and can move through, juvenile compact myelin. Twenty minutes after injection the ^{3}H cholesterol was confined to the outer and inner edges of the myelin sheaths; at 1½ hours it occupied two corresponding but wider peripheral bands of myelin, and by 3 hours it was homogeneously distributed throughout the sheath. Both the Schwann cell cytoplasm and the axon were found to be labelled at all stages. The homogeneous distribution of the label across the thickness of the myelin 3 hours after injection indicates that, wherever it is first incorporated into the sheath, the cholesterol rapidly spreads or diffuses throughout its extent, and appears to be available for continuous exchanges between the Schwann cell cytoplasm, the myelin and the axoplasm, as well as for reutilization following myelin sheath degeneration (Rawlins, Villegas, Hedley-White and Uzman, 1972).

The possibility that the myelin lamellae may be able to slip over one another with relative ease *in vivo* provides one of the two basic assumptions upon which Friede (1972) has based his model of the process of myelin growth. The other is that the conversion of mesaxon into myelin is not simply a matter of compaction of the two cell membranes to produce a similar length or area of myelin leaflet, but that it involves a fundamental molecular rearrangement such that one unit of length of mesaxon gives rise to three units of myelin leaflet. The stimulus to myelin growth is postulated to be axon expansion rather than axon calibre *per se*, and the process is described as being a biphasic phenomenon in which elongation of the mesaxon induced by axon growth is followed by conversion to myelin, the consequent threefold increase in the circumferential dimension of the new myelin material driving additional turns onto the exterior of the spiral. In Friede's (1972) diagram the external mesaxon is shown to move while the inner, adaxonal mesaxon remains stationary. This may be unintentional, but in view of the absence of any convincing evidence that the Schwann cell nucleus rotates around the axon during myelination, even *in vitro*, and since the relatively elaborate specializations of the Schwann cell cytoplasm external to the myelin at the paranode (see p. 48) are present well before the fibres have achieved their adult dimensions (Berthold, 1968b), the more likely candidate for rotation is the inner adaxonal mesaxon. This suggestion is supported by Webster's (1971) description of the apparent mobility of the internal mesaxon during the early phase of myelination.

Whether or not slippage of the adjacent layers of the myelin does indeed occur, and whether this process, or the insertion of new material, or both, are responsible for the increase in the circumference of the growing myelin sheath, it is difficult to avoid the conclusion that the addition of new turns to the myelin spiral requires rotation of the whole myelin cylinder, together with its inner mesaxon. The motive force for such a rotation may be envisaged to be obtained from the insertion of new membrane components into the external surface membrane of the Schwann cell, either throughout its extent, or locally at the origin of the external mesaxon and at the incisures and nodes of Ranvier. The restraint imposed upon the longitudinal growth of the membrane by the juxtaposition of adjacent Schwann cells at the nodes would confine at least 98% of the resulting increase in myelin membrane area to the transverse dimension of the cell (see Williams and Wendell-Smith, 1971).

The most obvious structural impediment to this proposal is provided by the existence of the elaborate fluting of the paranodal myelin sheath which, as has been noted earlier (Berthold, 1968b), is well established early in myelination. However, here again one may be misled by the apparent solidity of the electron microscope image into attributing an unwarranted rigidity to the observed structure. The increased periodicity of the paranode myelin, from 11 to 13 nm in osmium fixed material (Williams and Landon, 1963) may indicate that it has a more hydrated structure than has the internode myelin, and the frequently observed spiral form of the paranodal ridges and furrows (Hess and Young, 1952; Williams and Landon, 1963; Berthold and Skoglund, 1967) may signal the direction of myelin sheath rotation, the movement of the paranode either lagging behind or running before that of the remainder of the myelin segment. The incisures of Schmidt–Lanterman, on the other hand, present no such obstacle to rotation, a strand of Schwann cell cytoplasm being merely wound in with the rotating myelin cylinder. Even the apparent attachment of the terminal myelin loops to the juxtanodal axon is less of a difficulty than it might at first appear since, even in the mature node of a large fibre, only a minority of the loops make contact with the axon, due to the existence of the 'spiny bracelets of Nageotte' (see p. 30). However, it is not the purpose of this account to provide a detailed justification of any particular putative mechanism of myelination, but rather to emphasize that all such theories are still, of necessity, expressed in very simple, indeed naive, mechanistic terms, an index of our present ignorance of the nature of the molecular events occurring during myelination, and of the biological drives responsible for its initiation and control.

In the past, extrapolations of data relating axon diameter to myelin sheath thickness have led to suggestions that the initiation of myelination is merely the consequence of an axon having attained a certain critical diameter (Duncan, 1934; Matthews, 1968). That this is unlikely to be true is indicated by both the appreciable overlap found between the size ranges of myelinated and unmyelinated fibres in adult animals and man (Friede and Samorajski, 1968; Ochoa amd Mair, 1969), and the evidence that the segregation of the developing 'promyelin' axons from their primitive unmyelinated neighbours occurs when they are of a size well within the range for that of the future mature unmyelinated fibre population. At present all that can be said with regard to the influence of axon size, as such, on myelination is that myelin is not found around axons of less than a certain critical size in any particular location; in the nerve roots for example, myelin is unlikely to be seen around axons of less than 3 μm in circumference (Fraher, 1972).

The observations that myelin increment proceeds *pari passu* with increase in axon diameter (Friede and Samorajski, 1968), and that the growth of axons can be directly correlated with increase in the volume of their cells of origin (Martinez and Friede, 1970b), have led Friede to propose that growth of the neuron is the major determinant of the progress and extend of myelination. He has sought evidence that this is the case from experiments, originally designed by Duncan (1948), in which the normal increase in axon girth with age in the distal part of a nerve trunk is delayed by the proximal application of a 'snug' ligature early in postnatal life (Friede, 1972). He found that growth of both axon diameter and myelin sheath thickness were retarded distal to the ligature, and that release of the nerve after 50 days resulted in accelerated axon growth and proportionately enhanced myelin formation in the distal portion of the nerve. Such experiments can be criticized on the grounds that pressure gradients may exist within the nerve, and that the constriction may not affect all of its cellular constituents, or indeed all axonal functions to an equal extent (see Section 1.7. p. 79). While the effect of a decrease in axon diameter cannot be unequivocally distinguished from the effects of a selective reduction in the supply of axonally derived myelin constituents for example, these experiments clearly demonstrate that the normal ratio of axon diameter to the diameter of the whole fibre (d/D, see p. 67) is maintained during the period of constriction. This finding carries the further, and unstated, implication that the myelin synthetic mechanism is able to respond separately and selectively to changes in either the radial of longitudinal dimensions of the axon. While the d/D ratio retained its normal value in the constricted fibres, the individual internodes must have continued to grow in length in direct proportion to the growth in length of the axon, itself keeping pace with the unimpeded growth of the limb within which it lay, while maintaining a constant myelin thickness. Evidence for the converse proposition, that normal growth of internodal length is necessary for the development of a normal thickness of myelin sheath, may be implicit in observations such as those of Schroder (1972) that in regenerated nerves (which have short internodes; see Chapter 14), the ratio of d/D is always increased: i.e., the myelin sheaths never regain their normal thickness in proportion to axon diameter. Similarly, the thin myelin sheaths found on the occasional, normally occurring, short internodes of large diameter fibres, such as the first internodal segment of the dorsal root ganglion neurons (see Chapter 7), may possibly have remained thin because these segments have failed to share in the process of lengthening with limb growth affecting the remainder of the fibre.

All attempts to induce myelination around inert artificial fibres have failed (see, for example, Field, Raine and Hughes, 1969), and one must conclude that myelination requires the active participation of both axon and Schwann cell, and that a direct relationship exists between axon growth, or some anabolic functions closely linked to growth, and myelin synthesis in peripheral nerve fibres, at least during their initial development. Similar considerations appear to apply to myelination in the central nervous system, and it has been claimed by Kornguth, Anderson and Scott (1966), that the onset of the period of rapid myelination in the rat spinal cord is associated with the synthesis, in the spinal cord and dorsal root ganglion neurons, of a specific basic protein antigenically similar to that found in adult rat myelin.

That under other circumstances changes in the diameter and length of the axon being remyelinated play little or no role as stimuli to successful myelin formation is indicated by the phenomenon of segmental remyelination. This process is a repair mechanism by which single segments of myelin, or short series of segments, lost from the axon as a consequence of either natural pathology, or experimental interference with agents such as lysophosphatidyl choline (Hall and Gregson, 1971; Hall, 1973) or diphtheria toxin (Allt, 1969b, 1972; and Chapter

13), are replaced by local Schwann cell proliferation and the subsequent formation of new myelin segments. While the new intercalated internodes are short, and the new myelin segments fail to achieve the adult d/D ratio of their normal neighbours on the same axon, substantial new myelin sheaths are formed in circumstances in which there are only minor changes in axon diameter and no increase in axon length (Hall, 1973). A comparable phenomenon has been observed in the central nervous system (Gledhill, Harrison and McDonald, 1973).

The quantitative relationships between axon diameter, myelin sheath thickness, total fibre diameter and internodal length have been much studied since the early part of this century (e.g, Donaldson and Hoke, 1905), on account of both the obvious and wide range of natural variation in these parameters, and their relevance to theories of the mechanism of nerve impulse conduction (Hodgin 1971, and Chapter 14). The problems inherent in obtaining accurate measurements from fresh or fixed, teased or sectioned, nerves have been explored by Wendell-Smith and Williams (1959) and Williams and Wendell-Smith (1960), and the possible influence of the errors introduced by such factors as fixation shrinkage, or the lens effect of myelin, upon the results of earlier studies of the dimensions of peripheral nerve fibres have been reviewed by Williams and Wendell-Smith (1971). They demonstrated that when appropriate correction factors were employed the relationship between axon diameter and myelin thickness (m) differed in the nerves to skin and to muscle, and was different yet again in the fibres of the nerve roots. They found that while the rate of increase of sheath thickness with increasing axon diameter was similar in skin and muscle nerves, the myelin sheath was always thicker in a muscle nerve for any given axon diameter (Fig. 1.28), and that, in contrast, the dorsal and ventral nerve

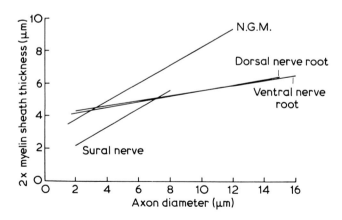

Fig. 1.28   Overall regression lines from pooled data for 4 specimens of the mature nerve to the medial gastrocnemius muscle; 4 specimens of the mature sural nerve; and 4 mature ventral and 2 mature dorsal spinal nerve roots; all from the rabbit. (Reproduced from Williams and Wendell-Smith (1971), by kind permission of the authors and the editor of the *Journal of Anatomy*.)

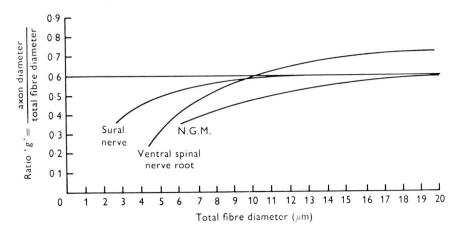

Fig. 1.29 Curves showing the relationship between the ratio 'g' (*d/D*) and total fibre diameter 'D' for fibres in the three nerves indicated in the rabbit. The curves are derived from the calculated regression lines of 2m and d given in Fig. 1.28. Note how the lines for the NGM and sural nerves flatten out at the theoretical optimum value of (g), i.e. 0.6. (Reproduced from Williams and Wendell-Smith (1971), by kind permission of the authors and the editor of the *Journal of Anatomy*.)

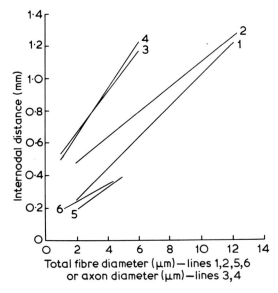

Fig. 1.30 Calculated regression lines for internodal length (l) on mean internodal fibre diameter (*D*) in rabbit nerve fibres; calculated for the mature NGM and sural cutaneous nerves for fibres in similar diameter groups (2–12 μm), lines 1 and 2; and for similar immature nerves at 2 weeks after birth, lines 5 and 6. Lines 3 and 4 refer to the same sample as lines 1 and 2 but in this case relate internodal distance (l) to axon diameter (*d*). (Reproduced from Williams and Wendell-Smith, (1971), by kind permission of the authors and the editor of the *Journal of Anatomy*.)

roots, which possess a much greater range of axon diameters, showed a much slower increase in sheath thickness with axon size.

Reference has been made earlier to the ratio relating axon diameter to total fibre diameter, d/D. This ratio has been held by Rushton (1951), Hodgkin (1971), and others to be an important determinant of internodal conduction time, their calculations indicating that the energetically most efficient value for d/D is 0.6. Williams and Wendell-Smith (1971) have shown that although earlier morphological estimates of this ratio based on fixed and stained histological preparations gave widely differing values, those obtained for the largest fibres in fresh frozen sections of the sural nerve and the nerve to the medial head of gastrocnemius in the rabbit were almost exactly 0.6, the predicted optimum. Smaller fibres in these nerves possessed smaller values for d/D, while the fibres of the ventral spinal root differed markedly from those in the two peripheral nerves, in that they gave progressively increasing values for d/D above 0.6 with increase in total fibre diameter above 10 μm (Fig. 1.29).

Internodal length has long been recognized to be related to fibre diameter, large diameter fibres having long internodes (Thomas and Young, 1949). The development of this relationship has been attributed to the early onset of myelination in the future large fibres, this event fixing the total number of Schwann cells along their length, so that subsequent growth in length of the fibre necessitated by the continued growth of the surrounding tissues is accommodated by elongation of this limited population of Schwann cells and their contained myelin segments. (Vizoso and Young, 1948; Schlaepfer and Myers, 1973).

Williams and Wendell-Smith (1971) have also examined the relationship between internodal length (l), fibre diameter and axonal diameter. They find that, in the rabbit, internodal length bears a closer relationship to axon diameter than to fibre diameter (Fig. 1.30), and that the growth patterns of the sural nerve and nerve to the medial gastrocnemius muscle indicate that the steady increment of new myelin lamellar material during growth proceeds at distinctly different rates in these two nerves (Fig. 1.31) Furthermore, while cessation of growth in sheath thickness in the sural nerve coincides with the end of growth in nerve length, both axon diameter and sheath thickness continue to increase in the nerve to the medial gastrocemius muscle for some time after the limb ceases to grow. Such observations as these underline the importance of specific local interactions between neurons and their satellite cells, related to their anatomical site and physiological functions, in determining such characteristics as myelin thickness and internodal length; in addition they emphasize the inadequacy of models of the myelination process that depend upon change in only one or two parameters (see p. 63) to explain the observed variety of morphological relationships between an axon and its Schwann cells in the peripheral nerve. Even where unanimity of opinion concerning the factors controlling specific aspects of differentiation appears to exist at present, this may merely be the consequence of restriction of experimental studies to too narrow a range of

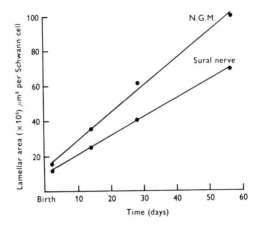

Fig. 1.31   Calculated regression lines of mean lamellar area per Schwann cell against time, for the largest fibre diameter group in the NGM and sural cutaneous nerves of the rabbit respectively. The two types of Schwann cell show constant but different rates of lamellar synthesis. (Reproduced from Williams and Wendell-Smith, (1971), by kind permission of the authors and the editor of the *Journal of Anatomy*.)

species. The observations of Jacobs and Cavanagh (1969) imply that the accepted correlation between internodal distance and limb growth cannot be extrapolated from mammals to birds; remyelination in the fowl, following either local demyelination or whole nerve degeneration and regeneration, being accompanied by a progressive increase in the length of the Schwann cells and their contained myelin segments with time, thus restoring the positive correlation between axon diameter and internodal length.

Despite what has been said above concerning the pitfalls inherent in too simplistic a view of the factors involved in ontogenesis, the combined results of observations on the normal growth of myelin, and of remyelination following segmental demyelination or whole nerve degeneration and regeneration, appear to point to the existence of a relationship between myelin sheath thickness and axon surface area. An 'axon-area' related stimulus to myelination would account for the observed greater effect of increase in axon diameter than axon length on myelin sheath thickness in any particular situation. Variation in the magnitude of the axonal stimulus, or variation in the competence of the Schwann cells at different locations to respond to identical stimuli, could provide the necessary dimension of freedom to account for the observed differences in the d/D ratios in skin and muscle nerves. The physiological advantages of d/D ratios tending towards a value of 0.6 may have ensured the natural selection of the appropriate balance between axon stimulus and Schwann cell response necessary to achieve this relationship where it would be of the greatest functional advantage, i.e., in the largest diameter limb nerves. Removal of the stimulus to myelin synthesis, or maintenance, by axon section or death permits the Schwann cell to rid itself of its now redundant organelle, the myelin, by the autophagic mechanisms characterizing the early phases of Wallerian degeneration (Chapter 13).

The experiments of Simpson and Young (1945) provided some evidence that Schwann cell populations at different anatomical sites may indeed differ in their ability to respond to the presence of axons by producing myelin. Outgrowing sprouts from the central ends of severed peripheral myelinated axons were caused to regrow into the Schwann tubes of a visceral autonomic nerve: while the splanchnic Schwann cells, which had formerly supported an almost wholly unmyelinated nerve fibre population, were able to make a few thin myelin sheaths around the ingrowing somatic axons, remyelination never approached the extent achieved when similar axons were allowed to regrow along their old peripheral (somatic) Schwann tubes.

It is probable that, while the stimuli leading to the formation of myelin around nerve fibres are 'simple', in the sense that they are common to all vertebrates, and involve fundamental interactions between two species of cell, the mechanisms by which the process of myelination is initiated and controlled are likely to prove to be exceedingly complex, the product of a long evolution of the relationship between the axon and its satellite cells.

1.6.2 *The peri-axonal space*

It is at present technically impossible to monitor the constitution of the narrow intercellular space between neurons and their satellite cells by direct sampling *in vivo*. Mathematical descriptions of ionic behaviour in the layer immediately external to he axolemma, either computed or derived from experimental observations, and the possible implications of such activity on neuron-neuron and neuron-glia interactions, relate almost entirely to the space around the neuron soma, or to the peri-axonal space of fibres of lower vertebrates or invertebrates (see Adelman and Palti, 1972).

It was widely assumed for many years that the intercellular cleft between satellite cell and neuron was of too small dimensions to allow the passage of materials or exchange of ions (e.g., Schmitt, 1958; Bunge, 1968), and that, as a consequence, some types of glia behaved as 'special compartments' providing an ionic environment functionally equivalent to that of the extracellular space surrounding other cells. This generalization now requires some modification, largely as a result of the development of techniques employing low molecular weight and colloidal substances as electron-opaque markers to follow the passage of materials across cellular barriers or through intracellular compartments. The apparent ease with which these substances enter intercellular clefts has been cited as strong evidence in support of the hypothesis that the perineuronal spaces are low-resistance pathways for the movement of water and solutes. 'Continuity' between extracellular space and Schwann cell-axon space, inferred from the presence of tracer in the latter following its introduction into the extracellular space, has been demonstrated using silver iodide in the crab (Baker,

1965); thorium dioxide in the squid (Villegas and Villegas, 1968); ferritin, in toad spinal ganglia, either in culture or *in vivo* (Rosenbluth and Wissig, 1964), in mouse neuropil (Brightman, 1965) and in non-myelinated fibre bundles in adult mouse sciatic nerve (Hall and Williams, 1971); horseradish peroxidase, in non-myelinated fibres in rat adrenal gland and in explanted mouse dorsal root ganglia (Holtzman and Peterson, 1969), in detached amphibian retinae (Lasansky and Wald, 1962), in mouse neuropil (Brightman and Reese, 1969), and in dissected walking limb nerves and around the giant axons of the circumoesophageal system in the lobster (Holtzman, Freeman and Kashner, 1970); and lanthanum in mouse neuropil (Brightman and Reese, 1969) and in myelinated nerve fibres in fresh and fixed rat forebrain (Hirano and Dembitzer, 1969).

There are, however, certain practical criteria which must be satisfied before a particular distribution of extracellular space can be established with confidence. Ideally, for a substance to behave as a genuine tracer, i.e., for it to delineate and not to 'stain', its distribution should not be affected by (i) preferential adsorption or chemical binding to cell surfaces, or (ii) lipid solubility within the tissue; (iii) it should not undergo alterations in molecular configuration as a result of (i) or (ii); (iv) it should not induce alterations in the molecular structure of the membranes with which it is in contact; (v) the method of its application should involve minimal alteration to physico-chemical parameters within the tissue; and (vi) it should be non-toxic, at least at the dose-levels employed.

Where tracers enter apparent spaces which have been demonstrated by other techniques, and whose frequency and location are independent of the method of fixation, it seems likely that they are utilizing normally patent anatomical channels. If, on the other hand, tracers are found free in damaged tissue, e.g., ferritin lying free within cytoplasm, it is probable that their presence is an artefact. Between these extreme conditions, there is an area fraught with problems of interpretation where, while the tissue appears undamaged, 'tracer' is found in situations which would not have been predicted from the known morphology of the tissue.

It is, therefore, an over-simplification to assume that solute or colloid diffusion within the peri-axonal space of loosely-ensheathed or non-myelinated axons is ever entirely free. Where the tracer has been administered either in conjunction with the fixative or to an excised sample, its presence in the peri-axonal space is of equivocal significance, and cannot be accepted as evidence of continuity between the extracellular space and the peri-axonal space *in vivo*. Even in those situations in which tracer has been administered *in vivo*, and in which there is minimal morphological alteration in the cell system, the presence of the introduced material within the periaxonal space does not necessarily imply complete freedom of access. Most workers assume that the satellite cell is active in influencing the composition of the peri-axonal space, and Bunge (1968) has suggested that satellite cells provide a cell gauntlet whereby . . . 'materials that might adversely affect axonal conduction are degraded either by the action of intercellular enzymes or by enzymes mounted on the membranes bounding the intercellular moat'.

Electrophysiological studies have revealed that diffusion of at least some ions is relatively limited, to the extent that the periaxonal space can be overloaded with them under conditions of experimental stress. In 1956, Frankenhauser and Hodgkin reported a now widely-recognized phenomenon, the apparent increase in K^+ concentration in the peri-axonal space of the giant axon of the squid during the repetitive conduction of nerve impulses: this accumulation was considered to be the result of the difference between K^+ transference numbers through the axolemma and the multicellular Schwann cell layer. Similar increases in the concentration of K^+ external to the axolemma have been computed during voltage clamp pulses in the same experimental system (Adelman and Palti, 1969). During repetitive firing, the K^+ concentration in the peri-axonal space is increased in non-myelinated mammalian nerve fibres (Ritchie and Straub, 1957), as well as in the central nervous systems of amphibia and the leech (Orkand, Nichols and Kuffler, 1966; Baylor and Nichols, 1969).

There is little doubt that there are changes in many membrane electrical parameters as a result of changes in the concentration of K^+ in the peri-axonal space of the systems examined, i.e., that neuronal activity, and possibly satellite cell activity, may be modulated by alterations in the ionic composition of these intercellular clefts. Electrophysiological evidence purporting to demonstrate the existence of some form of electrical coupling between the axon and the Schwann cell in the squid nerve fibre has recently been reported by Villegas (1972).

As the association between an axon and its satellite cell becomes more complex, there is a concomitant reduction in the area of axoplasm exposed to the bulk extracellular space. A relatively straightforward progression can be observed in phylogeny from the naked, non glial-associated axon through diverse types of invertebrate axonal sheaths (see Bunge, 1968; Gray, 1970), to the highly evolved 1:1 association between axon and Schwann cell found in the myelinated internode of the vertebrate peripheral nerve fibre. The systematic obliteration of the mesaxon is accompanied by a limitation of the points of continuity between peri-axonal space and endoneurium to tortuous and restricted inter- and intra-Schwann cell channels. It is usually assumed that the internodal peri-axonal space is isolated from the endoneurium by the close apposition of the innermost terminal loops of Schwann cell cytoplasm to the outer surface of the juxtanodal axolemma, e.g., ... 'there are no extracellular space channels between the axon membrane and the external medium in the internodal regions' (Aidley, 1971). An effective seal at this site is an essential premise for the theory of saltatory conduction (see Hodgkin, 1971), according to which, little of importance, in ionic terms, occurs in the internodal peri-axonal space during the propagation of the action potential except for a negligible capacitative leak through low-resistance regions of the sheath (possibly at the incisures).

In the myelinated nerve fibre, channels between the Schwann cells occur at the nodes of Ranvier. The existence of a channel open to the rapid flux of ions between the immediate nodal peri-axonal space and the endoneurium has been accepted for many years, and it has been calculated that in a large myelinated axon, 6×10^6 sodium ions enter each node per impulse (Hodgkin, 1971). Studies with electron dense materials such as ferritin (Hall and Williams, 1971), lanthanum (Hirano and Dembitzer, 1969; Hall and Williams, 1971), horseradish peroxidase (Hirano, Becker and Zimmerman, 1969) and microperoxidase (Feder, Reese and Brightman, 1969) have indicated that this channel may extend to include the peri-axonal space beneath the myelin loops.

In the absence of corroborative evidence derived from some other experimental source, it is difficult to know how much importance should be attached to these findings, which are subject to the difficulties of interpretation mentioned earlier. The apparent ease and rapidity with which tracers gain access to the peri-axonal space of the paranode/node complex may reflect a genuine communication between this space and general extracellular space; it could alternatively indicate the disruptive effects of these substances, or some specific reaction between the 'tracer' and components of the cell surfaces. The behaviour of ferritin at the node is particularly interesting in the light of the binding of a variety of metallic cations to the nodal gap substance (Langley and Landon, 1971; and Section 1.4.3, p. 50).

1.6.3 *Trophic support of the axon by the Schwann cell*

One of the more obvious roles which have been assigned to the Schwann cell is participation in local, i.e., non-somal, trophic support of the axon. Such a function implies the existence of an intermediate trans-myelin transport system: an idea which is by no means new (Kerr, 1904). This interesting problem has been investigated both with light and electron autoradiography, in general using parenterally administered labelled amino acids in amphibia (e.g., Singer and Salpeter, 1966; Singer, 1968). Studies with electron microscope autoradiography have revealed an apparently chronologically sequential transfer of labelled material from the endoneurium into the axon via the nucleus, cytoplasm and myelin sheath of the Schwann cell. While the published autoradiographs appear to give qualitative support to this hypothetical supplementary route into the axon via the Schwann cell, no attempt has yet been made to apply the available analytical techniques of circle analysis (Williams, 1969, 1973), or hypothetical grain distribution (Blackett and Parry, 1973) to the quantitative evaluation of this data. The inference that the presence of sparsely-distributed silver grains over such a complex multi-compartmental tissue system provides a definitive demonstration of a local Schwann cell-mediated uptake of material is therefore premature, but the uniform failure of these experiments to reveal any 'preferential localization' of label which might implicate a particular pathway, e.g., via paranode or incisure, may be of some significance.

There are at least three routes by which material may traverse the internodal myelin sheath: (i) by direct radial passage, penetrating successive myelin lamellae; (ii) along the intraperiod line to the peri-axonal space; (iii) along the

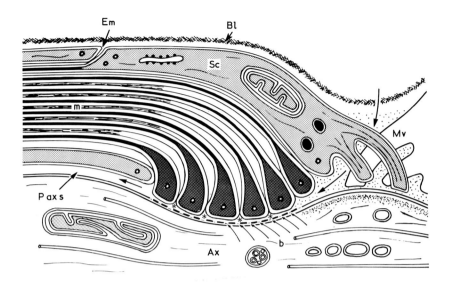

Fig. 1.32 A diagramatic representation of the membrane relationships existing between the axon and the end of one of its ensheathing Schwann cells at the node of Ranvier of a small myelinated nerve fibre. The radial dimension of the internodal periaxonal space, and the thickness and spacing of the components of the cell membranes have been exaggerated for clarity. The probable route by which materials gain access to the periaxonal space (P. ax s) is indicated by the 'heavy' arrows passing through the gap substance and under the myelin pockets at the node.

An alternative, spiral pathway suggested to be present at the node, between the dense bands in the outer leaflet of the axolemma (Hirano and Dembitzer, 1969), is indicated by a series of small curved arrows: a more plausible nodal extracellular spiral following the intervals between the adjacent myelin pockets is indicated by a series of asterisks. Ax — axon; b — spiral bands; Bl — basal lamina; Em — external mesaxon; Mv — Schwann cell microvilli; P ax S. — periaxonal space; Sc — Schwann cell cytoplasm.

major dense line to reach the adaxonal Schwann cytoplasm and subsequently enter the peri-axonal space. Routes (ii) and (iii) are of the order of at least $\times 10^6$ longer than that of direct nodal ingress, and can be of little significance in terms of rapid ionic fluxes. The major dense line is always single in normal tissue, except where it splits to enclose Schwann cell cytoplasm at the paranode and the incisure: there have been few references to breakdown of the major dense line even in pathological states, and in these cases, it occurs secondarily to the more common splitting of the intraperiod line.

A few workers have described a double intraperiod line after treatment with lanthanum (Revel and Hamilton, 1969), and after fixation in solutions containing digitonin 0.2% w/v (Napolitano and Scallen, 1969), but the chemistry involved in these reactions is complex and poorly understood, and their interpretation is at present difficult. In most studies of the normal myelin sheath the intraperiod line appears single, splitting only at the incisures and around the paranodal terminal loops. Unlike the major dense line, the intraperiod line displays great lability, being very rapidly affected by traumatization, whether this is osmotic, mechanical (Robertson, 1958a; Millington and Finean, 1961; Elfvin, 1961a), chemical (Aleu, Katzman and Terry, 1963; Scheinberg, Taylor, Herzog and Mandell, 1966) or pathological, particularly in association with Wallerian degeneration (Glimstedt and Wohlfart, 1960; Williams and Hall, 1971), experimental allergic encephalitis (Lampert, 1965), diphtheritic polyneuritis in peripheral nerve (Webster, 1964a) and lysophosphatidyl choline-induced demyelination (Hall and Gregson, 1971).

The ease with which the intraperiod line may be manipulated experimentally suggests that it is the site of considerable structural flexibility *in vivo*. The appearance of small intra-myelin space initiated by splits in the intraperiod line is an almost inescapable feature of electron micrographs of many 'normal' internodal sheaths, especially in the largest myelinated fibres, in conventinally-processed tissue. While such splits are usually dismissed as preparative artefacts, it cannot be denied that in some instances, splitting of the intraperiod line may indicate the presence of a dynamic process in which the intraperiod line continuously opens and closes *in vivo*, e.g., thus providing a relatively unimpeded, albeit tortuous, pathway for the trans-myelin passage of water and ions, or perhaps the motive force for the generation of a microperistaltic wave for the propulsion of the axonal column. Mugnaini and Schnapp (1974) have recently reported evidence from sectioned, and freeze fractured, central and peripheral myelin of the turtle, chick, and mammals, of the existence of a continuous tight junction or zonula occludens around the periphery of the myelin sheath; i.e., at the inner and outer mesaxons, and between the adjacent turns of the cytoplasmic spirals at the incisures and the paranodal 'pockets'. This junction is claimed to seal off an extracellular compartment between the paired intraperiod lines, 2.5 and 1.0 nm wide in peripheral and central myelin sheaths respectively, from the general extracellular space. They suggest that such a seal may limit extracellular diffusion, and thus enhances the insulative properties of the myelin sheath, and may in addition serve to sequester potential autoantigens from the immune system.

There is a possible precedent for the existence of extracellular space channels within the myelin sheaths elaborated by satellite cells. Using peroxidase, Holtzman *et al.* (1970) demonstrated a complex network of anastomosing tubules in the Schwann cell cytoplasm surrounding lobster walking limb axons, connecting the peri-axonal space with the medium external to the fibre. Similar systems have been described in other crustacean giant nerve fibres (Holtzman and Peterson, 1969), and it has been proposed that the large surface area of the anastomosing tubule systems would facilitate rapid ionic exchange between the Schwann cell and the external medium.

What is the fate of axon-destined material which has entered the peri-axonal space, either directly via the mesaxon, or following extrusion from the Schwann cell? The axolemma presents the final continuous, and presumably critical, barrier to this material. The rate and magnitude of the exchange of materials between the internodal axon and the narrow periaxonal space have

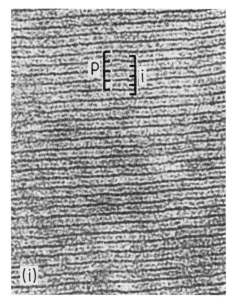 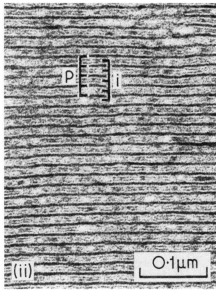

Fig. 1.33   Two examples of peripheral nerve myelin in transverse section, showing forms with single (i) and double (ii) intraperiod lines (see p. 74). p – period lines; i – intraperiod lines.

been little investigated for obvious reasons, and studies of transport across the axolemma have been largely concerned with the factors governing its exitability, and then usually in non mammalian nerves and without regard to the existence of its satellite cell sheath.

The large scale movements of ions across the axolemma following stimulation have been measured directly, using radio-isotopically labelled ions (e.g., Keynes, 1951), and over the last two decades, more accurate analyses of membrane conductance parameters have resulted from voltage clamp experiments (e.g, Hodgin and Huxley, 1952). Little is known, however, about the molecular basis of the permeability changes occurring in the axolemma during the propagation of the action potential (see Aidley, 1971).

It is possible that macromolecules enter the axon along its length by some form of endocytosis, thereby supplementing the supply of materials from the cell soma. There is morphological evidence of intensive pinocytotic activity at the growth cones of neurites in tissue culture (Hughes, 1953; Pomerat, Hendelman, Raiborn and Massey, 1967), and the formation of pinocytotic and coated vesicles at the surface of the neuron soma, along axons and at axon terminations both in normal tissues, and following the introduction of exogenous tracers, has been described by several authors. Waxman (1968) observed coated invaginations of the internodal axolemma in myelinated nerve fibres in mouse sciatic nerve, and suggested that they were involved in a micro-pinocytotic uptake of materials from the peri-axonal space. Similar coated axolemmal invaginations and pinocytotic vesicles have been seen along axons in mature non-myelinated nerve fibres in rat adrenal glands, and these have been implicated in the axonal uptake of peroxidase (Holtzman and Peterson, 1969). It has been suggested that, during the 'internalization' of fluid vacuoles observed at the periphery of growth cones, pinocytotic vesicles become continuous with the interconnected system of axonal agranular reticulum, and that subsequently fluid moves centripetally through the axon . . . 'within continuous channels of agranular reticulum . . . or as discontinuous cisternae that move independently'. (Tennyson, 1970).

Singer, Krishman and Fyfe (1972) proposed direct axonal commerce with the peri-axonal space via axolemmal 'pores' continuous with the agranular reticulum of the axon. There is no evidence to support this proposal: if transport is at an ionic level, i.e., if transient ion-specific 'tunnels' open within the axolemma, permitting the entry of ions into the axon, or, even if larger, less specific, pores exist, but open only randomly for very short time intervals, the structural changes involved would be almost impossible to detect with conventional observational techniques.

1.7 Intra-axonal transport systems

The existence of an elaborate system of cytoplasmic processes extending many centimetres from the neuron soma introduces special problems of intra-cellular communication and maintenance of structure which are not found in most other types of cell, the soma has long been recognized to be a trophic centre providing some, unspecified, support for its axon, a function demonstrable by the axonal degeneration which occurred distal to any interruption to its normal continuity with the soma (Cajal, 1928).

The proposition that material might be transported from the cell soma to the periphery down the axon was first suggested by Scott (1906). He found that after sectioning the dorsal roots in frogs close to their ganglia, and stimulating the central stump, the rate at which the reflex arc disappeared was a function of the frequency of stimulation, and proposed that the soma normally secreted some substance necessary for the functioning of the fibre, which passed down the nerve to its termination.

The concept of axonal flow was further developed by Weiss and his co-workers in the 1940's, in a classic series of experiments in which alterations in axonal morphology were produced by narrowing the total cross-section of a peripheral nerve fibre bundle by the application of a chronic circumferential constriction (Weiss and Hiscoe, 1948). The characteristic axonal adaptation to such a restriction was the appearance of a marked accumulation of material proximal to the obstruction, with a corresponding reduction in fibre diameter beneath and distal to the 'bottleneck'. That this axonal deformation was at least partially reversible was demonstrated by the redistribution of axonal material and partial redistension of the emaciated distal fibres upon release of the constriction. These responses were interpreted by Weiss to be the result of restricting a continuous somatofugal movement of the axonal matrix, together with at least part of its associated water. From an analysis of the mechanics of the damming process, it was proposed that axonal flow occurred as a non-Newtonian movement of a plastic semi-solid body: as will be seen, subsequent definitions were expanded to include intra-axonal transport rates a hundred times faster than this bulk axonal displacement. From the rate at which the pre-constriction dimensions of the distal fibres were regained after removal of the constriction, it was calculated that the rate of flow was of the order of 1–2 mm per day. Tentative, and as Weiss later conceded (Weiss, 1969), probably co-incidental, support for this value was provided by the calculation of the rate of protein de-amination in nerve fibres (Weiss and Hiscoe, 1948).

Spencer (1972), using an analogous experimental model to that employed by Weiss and Hiscoe, has recently shown that in a population of myelinated nerve fibres passing through an artificial constriction, only those members that had undergone degeneration and subsequent regeneration developed focal swellings proximal to the site of the ligature; accompanying undamaged fibres were not affected. He attributes the fact that axoplasmic 'damming' occurs solely in regenerating fibres to either a substantial increase in the net transport of axoplasm and its contained organelles in these fibres, as a consequence of distal regrowth, or to a change in the physical characteristics of their axoplasm, i.e., a change from 'gel' to 'sol', the 'gel' state of the axoplasm presumed to exist in the normal mature fibres being less conducive to local swelling.

The realization that some form of axonal flow was a consistent feature of the normal non-electric behaviour of the neuron was a significant event since it marked the beginning of a fundamental change in thinking about the nature of the neuron. Whereas the structure of the axon had previously been considered to be the passive substratum upon which the bio-electrical characteristics of the fibre were imposed, apparently incapable of growth or contractility after maturation, the demonstration of axoplasmic flow introduced a new dimension into interpretations of the possible inter-relationships of soma, axon, Schwann cell and myelin sheath.

1.7.1 *The rates of flow*

Definitive evidence supporting the occurrence of axonal flow has been provided by experimental studies using isotopically labelled tracer molecules. Early demonstrations of the transport of ^{32}P-orthophosphate (Ochs, Dalrymple and Richards, 1962), protein (Koenig, 1958) and phospholipid (Miani, 1962), confirmed the presence of a somatofugal transport of labelled compounds at a consistent flow rate of 1–3 mm per day. It was not until the introduction of tritiated marker molecules, and high resolution autoradiography, by Droz and Leblond (1963), that ideas concerning flow developed beyond the simple concept of a continuous bulk translocation of axoplasm, and the existence of a heterogeneity of flow rates was appreciated. The experimental approach most used has been to present a labelled protein pre-cursor to a population of nerve cells, either by a single pulse intravenous or intraperitoneal injection, or by a well-localized micro-injection near the neuron somata, and to measure the time-course of the movement of the incorporated label along the axon, or its speed of appearance at the nerve terminal.

In early studies using ^{32}P as pre-cursor, Ochs and his co-workers analyzed the outflow pattern of labelled material in ventral root fibres following injection near the motor neuron bodies of the lumbosacral spinal cord in the cat, and found a slow axoplasmic flow of 4—5 mm/day (Ochs *et al.* 1962; Ochs, 1966), a rate in reasonable agreement with the slow flow calculated by Weiss. Using ^{3}H-leucine as the labelled pre-cursor however, two slopes of activity were found in the ventral roots (Ochs, Johnson and Ng, 1967; Ochs, Sabri and Johnson, 1969), providing evidence not only of slow transport, but also of a more rapid component, visible as a crest of activity descending along the sciatic nerve at a rate of about 400 mm/day. A similar biphasic pattern of transport was reported in a study of sensory nerves by Lasek (1968).

These different rates of transport have been correlated with the ways in which labelled pre-cursor is handled by the soma. Using the blocking agents puromycin and cyclohexamide, Ochs and Ranish (1969) demonstrated that, whereas some of the labelled pre-cursor becomes involved in protein synthesis almost immediately after it has entered the soma, so that it is found in the axon within 30 minutes of its administration, a larger portion of the incorporated material enters an inaccessible compartment of the soma, from which it later emerges as a high molecular weight protein to be carried down the axon in the slow transport system. The Golgi apparatus has been cited as the 'gate' controlling the liberation of material from these somal compartments into the axon, on the basis of electron microscope autoradiographic studies (Droz, 1965; Ochs, Sabri and Ranish, 1970).

It is now generally accepted that intra-axonal transport occurs at a minimum of two velocities, the original slow neuroplasmic flow of 1—3 mm/day, and a much faster transport system operating against the background of that flow at daily rates of anything between 12—3000 mm/day (Grafstein, 1967; Lasek, 1968; Livett, Geffen and Austin, 1968; Karlsson and Sjöstrand, 1968; Ochs and Johnson, 1969; Barondes, 1969; Lasek, 1970; Dahlström, 1971).

The fast rate has been estimated in a number of ways: (i) from the rate of spread of radioactivity along a fibre (e.g., Ochs *et al.*, 1967); (ii) from the rate of accumulation of labelled material proximal to a constriction (e.g., Livett *et al.*, 1968) or at a synaptic terminal (Mc Ewen and Grafstein, 1968); (iii) from the rate of progress of a peak within the longitudinal distribution of radioactivity in a nerve (Karlsson and Sjöstrand, 1968).

Several workers have reported rates of flow which imply that the restriction to two categories is too rigid (Lux, Schubert, Kreutzberg and Globus, 1970; Karlsson and Sjöstrand, 1971; Schonbach and Cuénod, 1971). Karlsson and Sjöstrand (1971) have described at least four different phases of axonal transport in the retinal cells of the rabbit, viz., a fast phase (I) corresponding to the rapid component of axonal flow, calculated at 110–115 mm/day in the optic pathway (Karlsson and Sjöstrand, 1968); two intermediate phases, with rates of 40 mm/day (II) and 6–12 mm/day (III); and a classic slow phase of 2 mm/day (IV). Bradley, Murchison and Day (1971) have challenged even this demarcation, and have described a spectrum of velocities for axoplasmic flow in mouse sciatic nerve, claiming that there was no evidence from the velocity distribution histogram of a distinction into fast or slow transport components. In contrast to these findings, Ochs has recently determined the rate of fast axoplasmic transport in the motor and sensory sciatic nerve fibres of the monkey, dog, cat, rabbit, goat and rat: he found that in all fibres examined, the fast component of transport was in the range 390–420 mm/day, irrespective of fibre diameter, and suggested the existence of a single underlying mechanism (Ochs, 1972).

1.7.2 *Bidirectional flow*

Claims of the existence of bidirectional flow within normal nerve fibres have provided grounds for some controversy. Proponents of the occurrence of somato-petal flow point out that bidirectional streaming is a characteristic of almost all cultured cells, as well as of various protozoa and plant cells (see Lubińska, 1964). Furthermore, bidirectional migration of granules and 'mitochondria' have been observed in cultured axons (Pomerat et al., 1967); in exised, myelinated axons viewed with Normarski optics in the tadpole tail (Webster and Billings, 1972), *Xenopus* and rat sciatic nerves (Smith, 1971, 1972), chicken sural nerve (Kirkpatrick, Bray and Palmer, 1972), human sural nerve (Kirkpatrick and Stern, 1973); and in three species of amphibian embryos viewed with differential interference optics (Berlinrood, McGee-Russell and Allen, 1972). It should be remembered, however, that the behavioural characteristics displayed by excised mammalian nerve fibres or immature non-mammalian nerve fibres, whether *in situ* or *in vitro*, may not provide a strict parallel to the processes occurring in myelinated fibres *in vivo*.

Until recently, much of the evidence supporting bidirectional flow in nerve fibres was derived from the results of attempts at mechanical interference. After ligation or crush of a nerve fibre, whether myelinated or non-myelinated, a common finding is the temporary accumulation of material, particularly mitochondria and mitochondrial enzymes, on both the proximal and distal sides of the block (e.g., Kreutzberg and Wechsler, 1963; Lubińska, 1964; Zelená, 1969; Kapeller and Mayor, 1969a,b). In non-myelinated fibres there is, according to Kapeller and Mayor (1967), a differential displacement of axoplasmic organelles with respect to the site of the lesion, in that granular vesicles and some axoplasm continue proximo-distally to the nerve terminals, while mitochondria and some agranular vesicles move centripetally. These morphological findings have been supplemented by histochemical studies of the accumulation of enzymes such as acetylcholinesterase proximal and distal to similar lesions (see Lubińska, 1964; Lubińska, 1971; Lubińska and Niemierko, 1971).

While the findings from constriction experiments suggest that some movements in a proximal direction may occur, the experimental methods employed are open to question. The temporary accumulation of mitochondria and degenerating organelles distal to a lesion could simply be due to the non-specific displacement of axoplasm away from both sides of the lesion, or it could represent local synthesis as response to injury (e.g., Kapeller and Mayor, 1969a,b; Weiss and Mayr, 1971).

Some support for the concept of bidirectional flow does exist however which is not based on the effects of deliberate traumatization. Kristensson (1970) and Kristensson and Olsson (1971a, b and 1973) have demonstrated the selective accumulation of protein tracers such as albumin labelled with Evans blue and horseradish peroxidase, within appropriate spinal motor neurons after intradermal or intramuscular injection in suckling mice, and have further demonstrated that the apparent somatopetal movement of these markers is affected by ligation, temperature change and the intraneural injection of colchicine. Moreover, it has been thought for some time that certain viruses can be transported intra-axonally from the periphery to the neuron soma (e.g., Baringer and Griffith, 1970; Kristensson, Lycke and Sjöstrand, 1971).

The belief that the soma monitors and regulates the energetic state and metabolic requirements of its peripheral processes implies a feedback of information from the periphery to the soma: the existence of such an input has been inferred from the classic chromatolytic response of the soma to nerve section, in the same way that degeneration distal to a similar section is interpreted to indicate loss of the normal proximo-distal output of material. A number of hypotheses concerning the nature of this centrally-directed signal for chromatolysis have been proposed (see Cragg, 1970; Engh and Schofield, 1972), and several of these invoke the existence of a normal disto-proximal axoplasmic flow.

1.7.3 *The distribution of material between the flow systems*

Neuroplasmic flow is, by definition, assumed to involve most, if not all, of the axoplasmic constituents, conveying some of the particulate and most of the soluble proteins; it is thought that at least 80 per cent of the protein transported down the axon is carried in a soluble form (McEwen and Grafstein, 1968). Bray and Austin (1969) have reported 5–6 times more protein in the slow system than in the rapid flow. Fernandez, Huneeus and Davison (1970), demonstrated a complex population of proteins moving within the slow phase in studies on the crayfish cord, and analysis of this population by gel electrophoresis under conditions of denaturation revealed the presence of the microtubule protein. Extensive studies of the transport of soluble microtubular protein to the nerve endings have been carried out by Barondes and his co-workers (see Barondes,

1971): in essence, these experiments have involved the intracerebral injection of labelled pre-cursor, and the subsequent estimation of radioactivity in the synaptosome centrifuge fraction, which is interpreted to be due to the distal axonal transport of labelled protein synthesized in the soma. Barondes (1971) concluded that the overall rate of transport of microtubular soluble protein is similar to that of most of the other soluble proteins, i.e., it travels with the slow system. This finding is in agreement with the studies of the kinetics of colchicine, presumed to be bound to microtubules, in optic nerve axons (Grafstein, McEwen and Shelanski, 1970). Karlsson and Sjöstrand (1971) using ^{3}H-leucine and ^{14}C-leucine, demonstrated homogeneous labelling of the soluble proteins of the slow phase in the optic nerve and tract of the rabbit, and this was interpreted to indicate that, in this system at least, a particular class of proteins is limited to a specific phase.

Particulate matter, including some of the axoplasmic and somal organelles, neurotransmitters and metabolites is carried more rapidly. Attempts to categorize rates of rapid flow and associate them with specific subcellular components have relied largely on circumstantial evidence obtained either from the correlation of biochemical, autoradiographical and ultrastructural techniques (e.g. Karlsson and Sjöstrand, 1971; Elam, Neale and Agranoff, 1971), or by the semi-quantitative or qualitative assessment of histochemical or ultrastructural evidence of the accumulation of material proximal to an interruption in axonal continuity (e.g., Banks, Magnall and Mayor, 1969). After ultracentrifuge subfractionation of conventionally-prepared crude nuclear, mitochondrial and microsomal fractions of lateral geniculate body following the intra-ocular injection of ^{3}H-leucine, Karlsson and Sjöstrand (1971) found that the most rapidly-migrating material was associated with the lighter particulate fractions, whereas the mitochondria and lysosomes were conveyed at rates intermediate between the rapid and slow phases.

1.7.4 *Mitochondrial transport*

The mechanism and rate of movement of mitochondria have attracted much experimental attention, not surprisingly, since it seems reasonable to assume that such factors may be important in determining the intra-axonal distribution of these organelles necessary to maintain the various energy-requiring processes occurring along an axon. The kinetics of mitochondrial supply have been investigated by observing mitochondrial accumulation proximal to a ligation or section of a nerve bundle. The 'damming' of mitochondria under these conditions has been described ultrastructurally (Weiss and Pillai, 1965; Zelená, 1969), biochemically and histochemically (Freide, 1959; Kreutzberg and Wechsler, 1963; Barondes, 1969; Banks et al., 1969; Dahlström, Jonanson and Norberg, 1969) and has been analysed statistically by Scharf and Blume (1964). It is probable that the results of such experiments, like those designed to examine other facets of intra-axonal transport (Section 1.7.1), are influenced by the local axonal response to injury following the production of an abnormal state within the fibres (Kapeller and Mayor, 1969a,b): it has indeed been suggested that mitochondria converge upon a lesion as a result of ... 'local galvanotactic or electrophoretic displacement toward tissue debris at low pH.' (Weiss and Mayr, 1971.)

In some studies, it has been concluded that mitochondria are a component of the slow transport system, moving at 1—2 mm/day (e.g., Weiss and Pillai, 1965). In other experiments in which similar techniques have been used, more rapid rates have been reported. Banks *et al.* (1969) found a net somatofugal flow rate of 14 mm/day for mitochondria by measuring the rate of accumulation of cytochrome oxidase proximal to a ligation of the cat hypogastric nerve, and Elam *et al.* (1971), have reported the rapid axonal transport of mitochondria (or of proteins metabolically incorporated into mitochondria), in the goldfish visual system. Zelená (1968) and Zelená, Lubińska and Gutmann (1968) studied the accumulation of mitochondria at a nerve crush: they concluded that there was a rapid bidirectional movement of mitochondria (1.7.2).

Attempts have been made to determine mitochondrial flow rates in relatively undisturbed axons, thereby eliminating the effects of any local response to injury: the results, however, still indicate the existence of a variety of rates. Using ^{59}Fe as a marker for mitochondrial cytochromes, Jeffrey, James, Kidman, Richards and Austin (1972) found a slow-moving (1—4 mm/day), colchicine-sensitive peak of protein-bound ^{59}Fe in the sciatic nerve following injection of radioactive material into the ventral horn of the chicken spinal cord. Subsequent analysis of this material by subcellular fractionation revealed that the highest specific activity resided in the mitochondrial fraction. Cinemicrographic recordings of cultured axons, and observations of excised nerve fibres by No marski phase and dark field optics, have revealed numerous intra-axonal particles migrating rapidly, sometimes in a saltatory fashion, apparently both centripetally and centrifugally (Section 1.7.2). On the basis of their size it is often, and not unaturally, assumed, that some of these particles are mito-chondria: however, the unequivocal identification and categorization of particles at or near the limit of resolution of an optical system is difficult, and less satisfactory than the identification of a radioactively labelled subcellular fraction (e.g., Jeffrey *et al.*, 1972). Mitochondria are occasionally observed in close association with microtubules in the axoplasm in fixed fibres, and the relationship is sometimes so well ordered that, in transverse sections, the mitochondria appear to be surrounded by a regular pallisade of microtubules (Raine *et al.*, 1971, and Fig. 1.23). Several workers have indeed considered that the mitochondria are aligned by microtubules (Wuerker and Kirkpatrick, 1972; Hirano and Zimmerman, 1971). However, in our present state of knowledge, it would be unwise to read any great functional significance into this pattern.

A number of inferences may be drawn from the various studies outlined above concerning the intra-axonal transport of organelles. It appears probable that there may be species differences in mitochondrial flow rates; that mitochondria may flow at different rates in different nerves, or even within the same axon (e.g., Dahlström *et al.*, 1969); that different experimental procedures may preferentially emphasize different modes of flow; and that there may be local synthesis of organelles.

1.7.5 *Proposed mechanisms underlying neuroplasmic flow*

The physical mechanism mediating bulk axoplasmic displacement, the so-called neuroplasmic flow, remains uncertain. On theoretical mechanical grounds, and taking into consideration the rheological properties of axoplasm which the damming experiments were thought to reveal, Weiss proposed that the driving force was a slow somatofugal microperistaltic wave of small amplitude which travelled along the length of the fibre. Subsequent experimental attempts to test this hypothesis have primarily involved the long-term observation and direct recording by cinemicrography, of fibres *in vitro*, either in tissue culture systems (Murray and Herrmann, 1968; Singer and Bryant, 1969; Weiss, 1972), or *in vivo*, using oblique incident illumination (Williams and Hall, 1970, 1971) or Normarski phase contrast optics (Webster and Billings, 1972).

There is little doubt that local rythmic changes in contour are a consistent characteristic of fibres that have been excised and placed in a 'nutrient' medium, as well as in those maintained in a more permanent tissue culture environment. The results of extensive recordings may be summarized as follows: (a) pressure waves travel along the surface of the fibre and apparently involve both the sheath and the axolemma; (b) rhythmic movement continues in isolated fragments of nerve and in the walls of Wallerian degeneration-type ovoids; (c) the frequency of the surface wave has a constant time course of 17 mins/cycle; (d) damming of axonal contents occurs proximal to the more distal of two ligatures placed in tandem on a nerve, and at kinks in an excised fibre; and (e) peristaltic activity can start spontaneously in a previously inert fibre (for more detailed treatment of the results of cinemicrographic recording, refer to Weiss, 1972).

While the demonstration of a capacity for peristaltic behaviour *in vitro* is of interest, particularly in the light of reports of glial pulsatility in tissue culture (Pomerat *et al.*, 1967), it does not necessarily follow that similar behaviour occurs *in vivo*. It has been argued in favour of comparisons between the *in vitro* and *in vivo* situations that intracellular phenomena may be considered to operate, at least in part, independently of the establishment of intercellular connections and other more general external influences (Lubińska, 1964), and that extrapolations from the tissue culture situation to that obtaining in the living fibre might be expected to retain their validity. However, using direct observation of substantially undisturbed mature myelinated fibres *in vivo*,

Williams and Hall (1971) could find no evidence of pulsatility either in normal immature or mature fibres, or in degenerating fibres. Continuous viewing for periods up to 8 hours showed that there were no gross or relatively rapid changes in either internodal profile or in the state of paranodes or incisures, a period within which at least thirty 'cycles' should have occurred according to Weiss. It is interesting to note in this context, that Weiss reported inconclusive results when recording from small subcutaneous nerve bundles *in vivo* (Weiss, 1969).

Biondi, Levy and Weiss (1972) in an analysis of the rheological properties of axoplasm, concluded that ... 'this mechanism [of peristalsis] in mature nerve fibres is neither identical to, nor even rheologically comparable with, the mode of protrusion of filopodia from embryonic, regenerating or cultured cells or neurons ... the extremely high consistency, viscosity, and cohesiveness of the content of the mature nerve fibre contrasts so sharply with the cinemicrographically demonstrated high mobility of the substance of immature neuron sprouts that the physical requirements for orientated convection are radically different'. If such differences between immature and mature axoplasm exist *in vivo*, they could provide a partial explanation for the conflicting properties of the relatively reactive internode in culture and its static counterpart *in vivo*.

A recurring theme in the various reports of peristaltic activity in nerve fibres has been the apparent involvement of the Schmidt–Lanterman incisures in such dynamic behaviour. It has been suggested, for example, that incisures can move along the internode (Singer, 1968), and they have been implicated as foci for the initiation of rhythmicity. Beyond the observation that a small population of Schmidt–Lanterman incisures appear moderately open in a normal undisturbed population of fibres *in vivo*, there does not at present seem to be any evidence to support such ideas: the incisure always appears closed at the optical resolution achieved by the oblique incident light technique, and its dramatic, rapid, irreversible dilatation in response to traumatization is not associated with the development of peristalsis (Williams and Hall, 1971). It is possible that some form of a regular contraction-relaxation cycle could occur at a submicroscopic level of organization, e.g., within the myelin lamellae, with incisural participation within the limits of morphological reversibility, but at present this is mere speculation.

1.7.6 *Proposed mechanisms underlying rapid transport*

While it may appear that our knowledge of the dynamics of neuroplasmic flow is, by the kindest estimate, incomplete, we know even less about the mechanisms underlying fast intra-axonal transport: such evidence as is available is largely circumstantial and heavily dependent upon the production of abnormal states within the fibre. Davison (1970) has pointed out that it is possible that the entire range of velocities, including neuroplasmic flow, could be generated by a single process. The existence of a wide range of velocities within the collectively-grouped fast transport system implies either that they are mediated by a corresponding number of separate mechanisms, or that they share a common one which is sufficiently flexible to permit rates from 12–2000+ mm/day. It is impossible to discriminate between the fast and slow systems on the basis of sharply-defined differences between the substances they carry, since there may be local alterations in rate, in response to continuously varying environmental conditions and metabolic demands, which are not detectable by present experimental techniques. Mitochondria, for example, have been observed to move with high velocities for brief intervals of time, although it is generally considered that they are usually transported in the slow-moving axonal column (Burdwood, 1965; Kreutzberg, 1969). The amine storage granule is also apparently transported at differing rates, moving at 120–140 mm/day in cat sciatic and splenic nerve (Livett et al., 1968), and at 48–72 mm/day in rabbit sciatic nerves. Dahlström (1971) has pointed out that rates of transport for an organelle may differ within different neuron systems of the same species – the transport of nor-adrenaline granules in rat sciatic nerves having been shown to be 5–6 times faster than in the rat bulbo-spinal neurons, while the migration rates of ACHe and ChA in the rat vagus has been estimated to be three times faster than in the hypoglossal nerves (Frizell, Hasselgren and Sjöstrand, 1970).

Irrefutable evidence for the existence of at least two independent mechanisms for the somato-fugal movement of material would be obtained if it were possible to block one experimentally without inducing detectable changes in the kinetic characteristics of the other(s). The introduction of the drugs colchicine (and its derivatives) (Borisy and Taylor, 1967) and vinblastine (Weisenberg and Timasheff, 1969) appeared to provide such a method. Colchicine shows a strong, fairly specific binding affinity for tubulin, the protein subunit of microtubules, inducing microtubular depolymerization (Schmitt, 1968; Yamada, Spooner and Wessels, 1970), and vinblastine precipitates this protein, inducing the formation of paracrystalline arrays (Marantz, Ventilla and Shelanski, 1969; Berry and Shelanski, 1972). Initial experiments with colchicine indicated that it interfered with the fast component of flow (Dahlström, 1968; Kreutzberg, 1969), but it is now clear that with higher doses, the slow phase is also impaired: Karlsson and Sjöstrand (1971) found in rabbit optic nerve that whereas almost complete inhibition of the rapid phase occurred after the intra-ocular injection of 2.5 μg of colchicine 24 hours before the administration of ^{3}H-leucine, 10–25 μg were required to cause 85 per cent inhibition of the slow phase. James et al. (1970) reported that colchicine had a more pronounced blocking effect on the slow than on the rapid phases of flow in chicken sciatic nerve, and Fernandez et al. (1970) have found that slow transport ceases in crayfish cord at $3°–5°$C, a temperature range at which certain microtubules dissociate (e.g., Tilney and Porter, 1967): it is not certain, however, that all the tubules were destroyed in this preparation (Davison, 1970). The local administration of these agents results

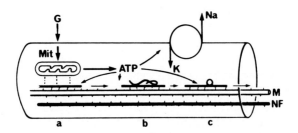

Fig. 1.34 A diagrammatic representation of the 'transport filament' hypothesis of Ochs (1974). Glucose (G) enters the fibre and after glycolysis and oxidative phosphorylation in the mitochondrion (Mit), the ATP produced supplies energy to the sodium pump, shown controlling the level of Na^+ and K^+ in the fibre, as well as to the 'transport filaments'. These are shown as short black bars to which various axonal components are bound for carriage down the fibre. At (a) mitochondria are temporarily attached (dashed lines) to both forward and retrograde moving transport filaments, to give rise to a fast to-and-fro movement with a net slow forward component. Soluble proteins (b) and particulate elements (c) are more firmly bound to the transport filaments. Cross bridges between the transport filaments and the microtubules (M) and/or the neurofilaments (NF) play a similar role in movement to that which has been proposed for the cross bridges between the actin and myosin filaments in the sliding filament hypothesis of muscular contraction. The energy required is supplied by ATP, and it is proposed that a wide range of cellular components may be carried at the same fast rate. (Reproduced from Ochs, (1974), by kind permission of the author and the editor of *The Peripheral Nervous System*, Plenum Press, New York.)

in changes in axonal ultrastructure consistent with an interruption to the normal somato-fugal movement of organelles, and a concomitant loss, and fibrillar disintegration, of the microtubules (Schlaepfer, 1971), and this leads to Wallerian-type degeneration.

Recent work by Ochs using the standard L7 ganglion-sciatic nerve preparation in the cat, has revealed that fast transport occurs independently of any somal propulsive force, that it is temperature and oxygen dependent, but independent of axon diameter and membrane polarization, and that the energetic supply mediating fast transport is present locally along the length of the axon. It was shown that *in vitro*, the mechanism of transport is dependent upon oxidative phosphorylation: while fast transport is maintained *in vitro* in the presence of oxygen, it is rapidly blocked by N_2, CN or DNP, and by short-term local anoxia produced by covering a length of nerve with petrolatum jelly to prevent entry of oxygen (Ochs, 1971, 1972). The obvious inference to be drawn from the action of DNP is that the maintenance of fast transport is ATP-dependent, as is the 'sodium pump'. According to Ochs (1972a,b), the ATP is required to activate cross-bridges between transported material and axonal microtubular subunits, in a manner analogous to that postulated to occur between the sliding filaments of muscle sarcomeres, and it is of interest that a major proportion of the ATP-ase present in the axon is of the Ca^{++}, Mg^{++} activated variety with similar properties to the actomoysin ATPase of muscle (Ochs, 1974).

1.7.7 *The postulated involvement of microtubules and neurofilaments*

In the absence of any convincing evidence supporting a specific structured-linked mechanism of axonal transport, it is not surprising that, at one time or another, most axoplasmic organelles have been assigned some transport function. Two obvious candidates for consideration are the microtubules and neurofilaments, although it often seems that they are chosen for no better reason than that they are consistently present in normal axoplasm, and, in the case of neurofilaments at least, lack any other proven function.

Microtubules have been observed in many cellular situations in which transport of some type is known to occur (see Jahn and Bovee, 1969). Several possible functions have been proposed for them: (i) that they may provide surfaces along which selected cell particles, e.g., chromosomes, melanin granules, are transported and orientated (Schmitt and Samson, 1968); (ii) that they may provide a cytoskeletal framework and be concerned with the maintenance of cellular asymmetry (Tilney, 1968); (iii) that they may be related to active cellular or subcellular motility – an idea which was initially supported by the apparent similarity between the amino acid compositions of actin and tubulin, before more recent work using peptide mapping showed that these two proteins are unrelated (Stephens and Linck, 1969).

Such a diversity of postulated activities is a consequence of the variety of subcellular sites at which microtubules are to be found, often in close association with particular organelles or particles, and it does not necessarily reflect actual physico-chemical differences between microtubular populations. However, in view of the reported differences in staining characteristics (Behnke and Zelander, 1967), and the protein heterogeneity of single microtubules (Bradley, 1973), it is probably unwise to extrapolate the behaviour of microtubules in one highly differentiated tissue to interpretations of their possible behaviour at another locus. This proviso is particularly pertinent to any speculations concerning microtubular contractility, a subject which has been raised earlier in discussions of the mechanics of axonal flow: it is unlikely that cytoplasmic movements similar to those brought about by the complex systems of microtubules in cilia, flagella and heliozoan axostyles, could be mediated by the single and apparently randomly located microtubules of the axoplasm. The surface chemistry of microtubules, and the fact that they selectively bind GTP, have been invoked in an ingenious mechanism for the rapid, directed conduction of some intra-axonal particles. Schmitt (1968) has suggested that specific, transitory binding occurs between the protein subunits of the microtubules and corresponding sites on selected axonal vesicles, the latter moving in a saltatory fashion along the microtubules in a GTP-dependent process not unlike the movement of ribosomes along mRNA during protein synthesis. In a somewhat similar vein, Ochs has advanced the hypothesis that lengths of protein 'transport' filament, to which are bound particulates, proteins and polypeptides, are continuously produced in the soma, and enter the axon to slide along the surface of the microtubules by means of ATP-activated cross-bridges (Section 1.7.6 and Fig. 1.34).

Cross-bridging between neighbouring microtubules has been reported at a number of sites at which they are arranged in closely-packed parallel bundles, e.g., in the initial segment of the axon (Palay *et al.*, 1968) and in the mitotic spindle (Hepler, McIntosh and Cleland, 1970), and it has been suggested that the bridges are 'mechanochemical' in nature, functioning so as to move substances attached to the microtubules, or to slide the individual microtubules past one another. The theories of both Schmitt and of Ochs embody the current trend in thought concerning the function of axonal microtubules, in that these are no longer considered to be part of the force-generating mechanism — this role being now ascribed to the side-arms. Although a regular arrangement of microtubules around axoplasmic organelles such as mitochondria may be seen occasionally in cross-sections of normal peripheral nerve fibres (Section 1.7.4), there have, as yet, been no reports of cross-bridging between these two components in the mammalian nervous system. Recently, however, Smith and his co-workers have described a close, and apparently transport related morphological association between microtubules and synaptic vesicles in the axons of the spinal cord of the lamprey, *Petromyzon marinus* (Smith, Järlfors and Beránek, 1970), the vesicles being attached to the microtubules by the cross-bridges (Smith, 1970).

The most widely cited, although still indirect, evidence that microtubules, themselves part of the slow-moving neuroplasmic flow system, may participate in the intra-axonal transport of material(s) comes from experiments with colchicine and the vinca alkaloids, vincristine and vinblastine (Section 1.7.6).

In the normal axon the neurofilaments are longitudinally arranged, are of indeterminate length, and have a strikingly regular lateral spacing (Section 1.2 and Fig. 1.5). It has been suggested that their arrangement represents a macrocrystalline lattice within the axoplasm, imposing a precise three-dimensional geometry upon the axonal matrix, thereby defining channels and surfaces through and along which transported materials may pass (Weiss, 1970). However no convincing evidence has yet been found to link neurofilaments to any known transport system. Some attempts have been made to interfere with neurofilament structure selectively, in much the same way that colchicine and the vinca alkaloids have been employed to produce microtubular disruption. The drug cytochalasin B is reported to affect contractile and motile systems in a variety of cells (e.g., Holtzer and Sanger, 1972), and it is apparently capable of disrupting neurofilaments in developing neurites (Yamada *et al.*, 1970). However, a recent study has indicated that while cytochalasin B produces a dose-related depression of fast transport in the rat optic nerve *in vitro*, there has as yet been no corroboration of these findings *in vivo* (Crooks and McClure, 1972). As with microtubules, there have been some suggestions that the neurofilaments effect the translocation of materials by sliding past one another (Lasek, 1970) and Wuerker and Palay (1969) have reported the presence of electron-dense fibrillar material, putative cross-bridges, linking neurofilaments in the anterior horn cells in the rat spinal cord.

Thus while a number of interesting hypotheses have been proposed concerning the possible roles of microtubules and neurofilaments in the alignment and transport of axoplasmic organelles, none can be considered to be more than hypotheses at the present time. Weiss and Mayr (1971a) have proposed that the neurofilaments are merely metastable vectors indicative of the presence of shear lines within the axonal matrix: it follows from this that their appearance in conventional, aldehyde-fixed tissue could bear little or no relation to their *in vivo* state.

1.7.8 *The fate of the transported material*

It is generally believed that each neuron soma continuously synthesises and delivers into its processes an heterogeneous population of macromolecules, soluble proteins and organelles, and that the components of this population are displaced centrifugally at varying rates, and probably by different mechanisms. However, in spite of numerous experimental studies particularly of the renewal of synaptic proteins (see Droz, 1973, for references), relatively little is known of the fate of this material.

A minor proportion of the slowly-moving axoplasmic mass is thought to be 'absorbed' in its passage along the axon, to be used in the maintenance of adequate intra-axonal levels of essential macromolecules, e.g., in the replacement of substances that have been catabolized *in situ*; in the provision of pre-cursors for the local synthesis of RNA and proteins (Sections 1.5 and 1.5.1), or in the renewal of the constituents of the axolemma. Furthermore it will be apparent from the foregoing sections that the neuron soma is unlikely to be the sole source of these metabolic materials, and that both the Schwann cells and peripheral terminals (e.g., Edstrom and Hanson, 1973) are potential contributors to an intra-axonal pool of metabolites.

While it has been suggested in the past that the slow-moving axonal proteins are excluded from the nerve endings (e.g., McEwen and Grafstein, 1968; Hendrickson, 1972) it is now generally considered that the bulk of both the fast and slow-moving compartments of the axonal column reach the axon termination. Recent experimental evidence indicates that the renewal of more than 98 per cent of the proteins and glycoproteins at the synapse is brought about by components which have been synthesized in the neuron soma and have subsequently migrated in the fast phase of axonal transport, many of them apparently within the smooth endoplasmic reticulum (Droz, Koenig and di Giamberardino, 1973). Several kinetic studies using high resolution auto-radiography and improved subcellular fractionation techniques have demonstrated the continuous turnover of proteins at nerve endings, at rates ranging from hours to weeks (Droz, 1973): these proteins are presumably destined for incorporation into the synaptic vesicles, and the axolemma and pre-synaptic plasma membranes. The contribution if any of the extracellular compartment to the local synthesis of protein within nerve endings is currently unknown.

From what is known of the transport of mitochondria it seems reasonable to assume that each axon terminal will contain the oldest members of the various populations of axoplasmic organelles: since these rapidly degenerate proximal to an experimental interruption to axonal flow, such as that produced by ligation, crush or the intraneural injection of cyanide (Hall, 1972), it is likely that a similar degeneration occurs within the natural interruption to flow constituted by the nerve terminal. Mitochondrial degeneration *in vivo*, as opposed to that produced artefactually during histological processing, has been reported within nerve endings ('mitochondrial graveyards') at neuromuscular junctions between motor nerve fibres and extra-ocular muscles in the rat (Weiss and Mayr, 1971). Hajós and Kerpel-Fronius (1973) have demonstrated histochemically that there are differences in cytochrome oxidase and succinic dehydrogenase activity in mitochondria from different intraneuronal sites, and they have correlated this evidence of a 'functional heterogeneity' of intraneuronal mitochondria with proximo-distal 'aging' of the migrating mitochondrial population. However, in spite of this apparent aging with distal migration, synaptic mitochondria retain their capacity to synthesize protein at nerve endings (e.g., Droz and Koenig, 1971; Gambetti, Autilio-Gambetti, Gonatas and Shafer, 1972; Ramirez, Levitan and Mushynski, 1972; Deanin and Gordon, 1973), and according to Gambetti *et al.* (1972) at least 20 per cent of the labelled amino acids incorporated locally into pre-synaptic endings *in vitro* could reflect mitochondrial activity.

References

Abood, L. G. and Abul-Haj, S. F. (1956) Histochemistry and characterization of hyaluronic acid in axons of peripheral nerve. *Journal of Neurochemistry,* 1, 119–125.

Adams, C. W. M. (1962) The histochemistry of the myelin sheath. In *Neurochemistry*, (eds.) Elliot, K. A. C., Page, I. H. and Quastel, J. H., pp. 85–112. C. C. Thomas: Springfield, Illinois.

Adelman, W. J. and Palti, Y. (1969) The influence of external potassium on the inactivation of sodium currents in the giant axon of the squid *Loligo Pealei. Journal of general Physiology,* 53, 685–703.

Adelman, W. J. and Palti, Y. (1972) The role of periaxonal and perineuronal spaces in modifying ionic flow across neural membranes. In *Current Topics in Membrane and Transport.* Vol. III. (eds.) Bronner, F. and Kleinzeller, A., pp. 199–235. Academic Press: New York.

Aidley, D. J. (1971) *The Physiology of Excitable Cells*. University Press: Cambridge.

Aleu, F. P. Katzman, R. and Terry, R. D. (1963) Fine structure and electrolyte analysis of cerebral edema induced by alkyl intoxication. *Journal of Neuropathology and experimental Neurology,* 22, 403–413.

Allt, G. (1969a) Ultrastructural features of the immature peripheral nerve. *Journal of Anatomy,* 105, 283–293.

Allt, G. (1969b) Repair of segmental demyelination in peripheral nerves: an electron microscope study. *Brain,* 92, 639–646.

Allt, G. (1972) An ultrastructural analysis of remyelination following segemental demyelination. *Acta Neuropathologica (Berlin),* 22, 333–344.

Andersson, E., Edström, A. and Jarlstedt, J. (1970) Properties of RNA from giant axons of the crayfish. *Acta physiologica scandinavica,* 78, 491–502.

Andersson-Cedergren, E. and Karlsson, U. (1966) Demyelination regions of nerve fibres in frog muscle spindles as studied by serial sections for electron microscopy. *Journal of Ultrastructure Research,* 14, 212–239.

Asbury, A. K. (1967) Schwann cell proliferation in developing mouse sciatic nerve. *Journal of Cell Biology,* 34, 735–743.

Autilio-Gambetti, L., Gambetti, P. and Shafer, B. (1973) RNA and axonal flow.

Biochemical and autoradiographic study in the rabbit optic system. *Brain Research*, **53**, 387–398.

Babel, J., Bischoff, A. and Spoendlin, H. (1970) *Ultrastructure of the Peripheral Nervous System and Sense Organs*. Churchill: London.

Baker, P. F. (1965) A method for the location of extracellular space in crab nerve. *Journal of Physiology, London*, **180**, 439–447.

Ballin, R. H. M. and Thomas, P. K. (1969a) Electron microscope observations on demyelination and remyelination in experimental allergic neuritis. 2. Remyelination. *Journal of the Neurological Sciences*, **8**, 225–237.

Ballin, R. H. M. and Thomas P. K. (1969b) Changes at the nodes of Ranvier during Wallerian Degeneration: an electron microscope study. *Acta Neuropathologica (Berlin)*, **14**, 237–249.

Banik, N. L. and Davison, A. N. (1967) Desmosterol in rat brain myelin. *Journal of Neurochemistry*, **14**, 594–596.

Banks, P., Magnall, D. and Mayor, D. (1969) The re-distribution of cytochrome oxidase, noradrenaline and adenosine triphosphate in adrenergic nerves constricted at two points. *Journal of Physiology, London*, **200**, 745–762.

Baringer, J. R. and Griffith, J. F.(1970) Experimental herpes simplex encephalitis: early neuropathologic changes. *Journal of Neuropathology and experimental Neurology*, **29**, 89–104.

Barondes, S. H. (1969) Axoplasmic transport. In *Handbook of Neurochemistry*, (ed.) Lajtha, A., Chapter 18, Vol. 2. Plenum Press: New York.

Barondes, S. H. (1971) Slow and rapid protein transport in brain. *Acta Neuropathologica*, Suppl. **5**, 97–103.

Baylor, D. A. and Nicholls, J. G. (1969) Changes in extracellular potassium concentration produced by neuronal activity in the central nervous system of the leech. *Journal of Physiology. London*, **203**, 555–569.

Behnke, O. and Zelander, T. (1967) Filamentous substructure of microtubules of the marginal bundle of mammalian blood platelets. *Journal of Ultrastructure Research*, **19**, 147–165.

Bennet, H. S. (1963) Morphological aspects of extracellular polysaccharides. *Journal of Histochemistry and Cytochemistry*. **11**, 14–23.

Berlinrood, M., McGee-Russell, S. M. and Allen, R. D. (1972) Patterns of particle movement in nerve fibres *in vitro* – an analysis by photokymography and microscopy. *Journal of Cell Science*, **11**, 875–886.

Berry, R. W. and Shelanski, M. L. (1972) Interactions of tubulin with vinblastine and guanosine triphosphate. *Journal of molecular Biology*, **71**, 71–80.

Berthold, C.-H. (1968a) Ultrastructure of the node-paranode region of mature feline ventral lumbar spinal-root fibres. *Acta Societatis Medicorum upsaliensis*, **73**, Suppl. 9, 37–78.

Berthold, C.-H (1968b) Ultrastructure of postnatally developing peripheral nodes of Ranvier. *Acta Societatis Medicorum upsaliensis*, **73**, Suppl. 9, 145–168.

Berthold, C.-H. (1968c) Ultrastructure of postnatally developing peripheral nodes of Ranvier. *Acta Societatis Medicorum upsaliensis*, **73**, 145–168.

Berthold, C.-H. and Skoglund, S. (1967) Histochemical and ultrastructural demonstration of mitochondria in the paranodal region of developing feline spinal roots and nerves. *Acta Societatis Medicorum upsaliensis*, **72**, 37–70.

Berthold, C.-H. and Skoglund, S. (1968a) Postnatal development of feline paranodal myelin-sheath segments. I. Light microscopy. *Acta Societatis Medicorum upsaliensis*, **73**, 113–126.

Berthold, C.-H. and Skoglund, S. (1968b) Postnatal development of feline paranodal myelin-sheath segments. II. Electron microscopy. *Acta Societatis Medicorum upsaliensis*, **73**, 127–144.

Biondi, R. J., Levy, M. J. and Weiss, P. A. (1972) An engineering study of the peristaltic drive of axonal flow. *Proceedings of the national Academy of Sciences*, **69**, 1732–1736.

Bito, F. (1926) Über eine Substanz welche die Schmidt–Lantermannschen einkerbungen Ausfullt. *Folia anatomica japonica*, **4**, 283–303.

Blackett, N. M. and Parry, D. M. (1973) A new method for analyzing electron microscope autoradiographs using hypothetical grain distributions. *Journal of Cell Biology*, **57**, 9–15.

Blakemore, W. F. (1969) Schmidt–Lanterman incisures in the central nervous system. *Journal of Ultrastructure Research*, **29**, 496–498.

Bondy, S. C. (1972) Axonal migration of various ribonucleic acid species along the optic tract of the chick. *Journal of Neurochemistry*, **19**, 1769–1776.

Borisy, G. G. and Taylor, E. W. (1967) The mechanism of action of colchicine. Binding of colchicine-^{3}H to cellular protein. *Journal of Cell Biology*, **34**, 525–533.

Boyd, I. A. and Davey, M. R. (1968) *Composition of Peripheral Nerves*. Livingstone: Edinburgh.

Bradley, M. O. (1973) Microfilaments and cytoplasmic streaming: inhibition of streaming with cytochalasin. *Journal of Cell Science*, **12**, 327–343.

Bradley, W. G., Murchison, D. and Day, M. J. (1971) The range of velocities of axoplasmic flow. A new approach and its application to mice with genetically inherited spinal muscular atrophy. *Brain Research*, **35**, 185–197.

Bray, J. J. and Austin, L. (1968) Flow of protein and ribonucleic acid in peripheral nerve. *Journal of Neurochemistry*, **15**, 731–740.

Bray, J. J. and Austin, L. (1969) Axoplasmic transport of ^{14}C protein at two rates in chicken sciatic nerve. *Brain Research*, **12**, 730–733.

Bremner, D. and Smart, I. (1965) The position of Schwann cell nuclei in relation to the internodal mid-point of myelinated nerve fibres. *Journal of Anatomy*, **99**, 194–195P.

Brightman, M. W. (1965) The distribution within the brain of ferritin injected into cerebrospinal fluid compartments. II Parenchymal distribution. *American Journal of Anatomy*, **117**, 193–220.

Brightman, M. W. and Reese, T. S. (1969) Junctions between intimately apposed cell membranes in the vertebrate brain. *Journal of Cell Biology*, **40**, 648–677.

Bunge, R. P. (1968) Glial cells and the central myelin sheath. *Physiological Reviews*, **48**, 197–251.

Burdwood, W. O. (1965) Rapid bidirectional particle movement in neurons. *Journal of Cell Biology*, **27**, 115A.

Cajal, S. R. y,(1909) *Histologie du système nerveux de l'homme et des vertébrés*. Maloine: Paris.

Cajal, S. R. y, (1928) *Degeneration and Regeneration of the Nervous System*. University Press: London.

Caley, D. W. and Maxwell, D. S. (1968) An electron microscopic study of neurons during postnatal development of the rat cerebral cortex. *Journal of Comparative Neurology*, **133**, 17–44.

Casola, L., Davis, G. A. and Davis, R. E. (1969) Evidence for RNA transport in rat optic nerve. *Journal of Neurochemistry*, **16**, 1037–1041.

Chambers, V. C. (1973) The use of ruthenium red in an electron microscope study of cytophagocytosis. *Journal of Cell Biology*, **57**, 874–878.

Chibon, P. (1965) Etude autoradiographique après marquage par la thymidine tritée des dérivés de la crête neurale troncale chez l'amphibian urodèle Pleurodeles (waltlii Micah). *Compte rendu hebdomadaire des séances de l'Académie des Sciences*, **261**, 5645–5648.

Cragg, B. G. (1970) What is the signal for chromatolysis? *Brain Research*, **23**, 1–21.

Cravioto, H. (1965) The role of Schwann cells during the development of human peripheral nerves. *Journal of Ultrastructure Research*, **12**, 634–651.

Crooks, R. F. and McClure, W. O. (1972) The effect of cytochalasin B on fast axoplasmic transport. *Brain Research*, **45**, 643–646.

Csanyi, V., Gervai, J. and Lajtha, A. (1973) Axoplasmic transport of free amino acids. *Brain Research*, **56**, 271–284.

Dahlström, A. (1968) Effect of colchicine on transport of amine storage granules in sympathetic nerves of rat. *European Journal of Pharmacology*, **5**, 11–113.

Dahlström, A. (1971) Axoplasmic transport (with particular respect to adrenergic neurons). *Philosophical Transactions of the Royal Society* B, **261**, 325–358.

Dahlström, A., Jonanson, J. and Norberg, K.-A. (1969) Monoamine oxidase activity in rat sciatic nerves after constriction. *European Journal of Pharmacology*, **6**, 248–254.

Davison, P. F. (1970) Microtubules and neurofilaments: possible implications in axoplasmic transport. *Advances in Biochemical Psychopharmacology*, **2**, 289–302.

Davison, A. N., Dobbing, J., Morgan, R. S. and Payling Wright, G. (1959) The persistance of 4-^{14}cholesterol in the mammalian central nervous system. *Lancet*, **I**, 658–660.

Deanin, G. G. and Gordon, M. W. (1973) Chloramphenicol- and cyclohexamide-sensitive protein synthetic systems in brain mitochondrial and nerve-ending preparations. *Journal of Neurochemistry*, **20**, 55–68.

de Renyi, J. (1928) The structure of cells in tissues as revealed by microdissection. II. The physical properties of the living axis cylinder in the myelinated nerve fibre of the frog. *Journal of Comparative Neurology*, **47**, 405–425.

Detwiler, S. R. and Kehoe, K. (1939) Further observations on the origin of the sheath cells of Schwann. *Journal of Experimental Zoology*, **81**, 415–435.

di Giamberardino, L. (1971) Independence of the rapid axonal transport of protein from the flow of free amino acids. *Acta Neuropathologica*, Suppl. 5, 132–135.

Dilly, P. N., Gray, E. G. and Young, J. Z. (1963) Electron microscopy of optic nerves and optic lobes of *Octopus* and *Eledone*. *Proceedings of the Royal Society*. B., **158**, 446–456.

Diner, O. (1965) Les cellules de Schwann en mitose et leur rapports avec les axones au cours du developpement du nerf sciatique chez le Rat. *Compte rendu hebdomadaire des séances de l'Académie des sciences*, **261**, 1731–1734.

Donaldson, H. H. and Hoke, G. W. (1905) The areas of the axis cylinder and medullary sheath as seen in cross sections of the spinal nerves of vertebrates. *Journal of Comparative Neurology*, **15**, 1–16.

Droz, B. (1965) Accumulation des protéines nouvellement synthétisées dans l'appareil de Golgi du neurone; étude radioautographique en microscopie electronique. *Compte rendu hebdomadaire des séances de l'Académie des sciences*, **260**, 320–322.

Droz, B. (1973) Renewal of synaptic proteins. *Brain Research*, **62**, 383–394.

Droz, B. and Koenig, H. L. (1971) Dynamic condition of protein in axons and axon terminals. *Acta Neuropathologica (Berlin)*. Suppl. 5, 109–118.

Droz, B., Koenig, H. L. and di Gianberardino, L. (1973) Axonal migration of protein and glycoprotein to nerve endings. I. Radioautographic analysis of the renewal of proteins in nerve endings of chicken ciliary ganglion after intracerebral injection of ^{3}H lysine. *Brain Research*, **60**, 93–127.

Droz, B. and Leblond, C. P. (1963) Axonal migration of proteins in the central nervous system and peripheral nerves as shown by radioautography. *Journal of Comparative Neurology*, **121**, 325–345.

Dun, F. T. (1970) The length and diameter of the node of Ranvier. *IEEE Transactions on Bio-Medical Engineering*, **17**, 21–24.

Duncan, D. (1934) A relation between axon diameter and myelination determined by measurement of myelinated spinal root fibres. *Journal of Comparative Neurology*, **60**, 437–471.

Duncan, D. (1948) Alterations in the Structure of nerves caused by restricting their growth with ligatures. *Journal of Neuropathology and Experimental Neurology*, **7**, 261–273.

Dunn, J. S. (1970) Developing myelin in human peripheral nerves. *Scottish Medical Journal*, **15**, 108–117.

DuShane, G. P. (1935) An experimental study of the origin of pigment cells in Amphibia. *Journal of Experimental Zoology*, **72**, 1–31.

Edström, A. (1964) The ribonucleic acid in the Mauthner neuron of the goldfish. *Journal of Neurochemistry*, **11**, 309–314.

Edström, A. (1969) Protein synthesis in the isolated Mauthner nerve fibre of goldfish. *Journal of Neurochemistry*, **16**, 67–81.

Edström, A., Edström, J. E. and Hökfelt, T. (1969) Sedimentation analysis of ribonucleic acid extracted from isolated Mauthner nerve fibre components. *Journal of Neurochemistry*, **16**, 53–66.

Edström, J. E., Eichner, D. and Edström A. (1962) The ribonucleic acid of axons and myelin sheaths from Mauthner axons. *Biochimica et biophysica acta*, **61**, 178–184.

Edström, A. and Hanson, M. (1973) Retrograde axonal transport of proteins *in vitro* in frog sciatic nerves. *Brain Research*, **61**, 311–320.

Edström, A. and Sjöstrand, J. (1969) Protein synthesis in the isolated Mauthner nerve fibre of goldfish. *Journal of Neurochemistry*, **16**, 67–82.

Ehrenberg (1849) Quoted by **Schmitt, F. O. and Geschwind, N.** (1957) The axon surface. *Progress in Biophysics and Biophysical Chemistry*, **8**, 166–215.

Elam, J. S., Neale, E. A. and Agranoff, B. W. (1971) Axonal transport in the goldfish visual system. *Acta Neuropathologica*, Suppl. 5, 257–266.

Elfvin, L. G. (1961a) Electron microscopic investigation of the plasma membrane and myelin sheath of autonomic nerve fibres in the cat. *Journal of Ultrastructure Research*, 5, 388–407.

Elfvin, L. G. (1961b) The ultrastructure of the nodes of Ranvier in cat sympathetic nerve fibres. *Journal of Ultrastructure Research*, 5, 374–387.

Engh, C. A. and Schofield, B. H. (1972) A review of the central response to peripheral nerve injury and its significance in nerve regeneration. *Journal of Neurosurgery*, 37, 195–203.

Erlanger, J. and Gasser, H. S. (1937) *Electrical Signs of Nervous Activity*. University of Pennsylvania Press: Philadelphia.

Ewald, A. and Kuhne, W. (1876) Die Verdaung als histologische Method. Ueber einen neuen Besdandtheil des Nerven-systems. *Verhandlungen des Naturhistorisch-medizinischen Vereins zu Heidelberg*, 1, 457.

Feder, N., Reese, T. S. and Brightman, M. W. (1969) Microperoxidase, a new tracer of low molecular weight. A study of the interstitial compartments of the mouse brain. *Journal of Cell Biology*, 43, 35–36A.

Fernandez, H. L., Huneeus, F. C. and Davison, P. F. (1970) Studies on the mechanism of axoplasmic transport in the crayfish cord. *Journal of Neurobiology*, 1, 395–409.

Field, E. J., Raine, C. S. and Hughes, D. (1969) Failure to induce myelin sheath formation around artificial fibres; with a note on the toxicity of polyester fibres for nervous tissue *in vitro*. *Journal of Neurological Sciences*, 8, 129–142.

Fernandez-Moran, H. (1950) Sheath and axon structures in the internode portion of vertebrate myelinated nerve fibres. An electron microscope study of rat and frog sciatic nerves. *Experimental Cell Research*, 1, 309–337.

Fontana, F. (1781) *Traite sur le venin de la vipère*. Florence.

Fraher, J. P. (1972) A quantitative study of anterior root fibres during early myelination. *Journal of Anatomy*, 112, 99–124.

Fraher, J. P. (1973) A quantitative study of anterior root fibres during early myelination. II. Longitudinal variation in sheath thickness and axon circumference. *Journal of Anatomy*, 115, 421–444.

Frankenhauser, B. and Hodgkin, A. L. (1956) The after-effects of impulses in the giant nerve fibres of *Loligo*. *Journal of Physiology, London*, 131, 341–376.

Friede, R. L. (1959) Transport of oxidative enzymes in nerve fibres; a histochemical investigation of the regenerative cycle in neurons. *Experimental Neurology*, 1, 441–466.

Friede, R. L. (1972) Control of myelin formation by axon calibre (with a model of the control mechanism). *Journal of Comparative Neurology*, 144, 233–252.

Friede, R. L. and Samorajski, T. (1967) Relation between the number of myelin lamellae and axon circumference in fibres of vagus and sciatic nerves of mice. *Journal of Comparative Neurology*, 130, 223–231.

Friede, R. L. and Samorajski, T. (1968) Myelin formation in the sciatic nerve of the rat. A quantitative electron microscopic, histochemical and radioautographic study. *Journal of Neuropathology and Experimental Neurology*, 27, 546–570.

Friede, R. L. and Samorajski, T. (1969) The clefts of Schmidt–Lanterman: a quantitative electron microscopic study of their structure in developing and adult sciatic nerves of the rat. *Anatomical Record*, 165, 89–101.

Frizell, M., Hasselgren, P. O. and Sjöstrand, J. (1970) Axoplasmic transport of acetylcholin-esterase and choline acetyl-transferase in the vagus and hypoglossal nerve of the rabbit. *Experimental Brain Research*, 10, 526–531.

Frommann, (1861) Zur Silberfärbung der Axencylinder. *Virchow's Archives*, 21, p. 151.

Fuerst, J. (1897) Ein Beitrag zur Kenntniss der Scheide der Nervenfasern. *Morphologisches Arbeiten (Schwalbe)*, 6.

Gambetti, P., Autilio-Gambetti, L. A., Gonatas, N. K. and Shafer, B. (1972) Protein synthesis in synaptosomal fractions. Ultrastructural radio-autographic study. *Journal of Cell Biology*, 52, 526–535.

Gambetti, P., Autilio-Gambetti, L., Shafer, B. and Pfaff, L. (1973) Quantitative autoradio-graphic study of labelled RNA in rabbit optic nerve after intraocular injection of ^{3}H uridine. *Journal of Cell Biology*, 59, 677–684.

Gamble, H. J. (1966) Further electron microscope studies of human foetal peripheral nerves. *Journal of Anatomy,* **100**, 487–502.

Gamble, H. J. and Eames, R. A. (1966) Electron microscopy of human spinal-nerve roots. *Archives of Neurology,* **14**, 50–53.

Gasser, H. S. (1952) Discussion in *The Hypothesis of Saltatory Conduction. Cold Spring Harbor Symposia on Quantitative Biology,* **17**, 32–36.

Gedoelst, L. (1886) Etude sur la constitution cellulaire de la fibre nerveuse. *La Cellule,* **3**, 114–226.

Gerebtzoff, M. A. (1962) Démonstration histochimique d'une activité de l'acétylinestérase au noeud de Ranvier. *Archives internationales de physiologie et de biochimie,* **70**, 418–420.

Gerebtzoff, M. A. and Mladenov, S. (1967) Affinity for metallic salts and acetylcholinesterase activity at Ranvier nodes. *Acta Histochemica (Jena),* **26**, 318–323.

Geren, B. B. (1954) The formation from the Schwann cell surface of myelin. *Experimental Cell Research,* **7**, 558–562.

Geren-Uzman, B. and Nogueira-Graf, G. (1957) Electron microscope studies of the formation of nodes of Ranvier in mouse sciatic nerves. *Journal of Biophysical and Biochemical Cytology,* **3**, 589–597.

Gibbons, J. R., Tilney, L. C. and Porter, K. R. (1969) Microtubules in the formation and development of the primary mesenchyme in *Arbacia punctulata:* I The distribution of microtubules. *Journal of Cell Biology,* **41**, 201–226.

Gledhill, R. F., Harrison, B. M. and McDonald, W. I. (1973) Pattern of remyelination in the C.N.S. *Nature,* **244**, 443–444.

Glimstedt, G. and Wohlfart, G. (1960–61) Electron microscopic observations on Wallerian degeneration in peripheral nerves. *Acta morphologica neerlando-scandinavica,* **3**, 135–146.

Golgi, C. (1881) Sulla struttura delle fibre nervose midollate periferiche e centrali. *Archivio per le scienze mediche,* **4**, 221–245.

Grafstein, B. (1967) Transport of protein by goldfish optic nerve fibres. *Science, New York,* **157**, 196–198.

Grafstein, B., McEwen, B. S. and Shelanski, M. L. (1970) Axonal transport of microtubule protein. *Nature, London,* **227**, 289–290.

Grampp, W. and Edström, J.-E. (1963) The effect of nervous activity on ribonucleic acid of the crustacean receptor neuron. *Journal of Neurochemistry,* **10**, 725–731.

Gray, E. G. (1970) The fine structure of nerve. *Comparative Biochemistry and Physiology,* **36**, 419–448.

Graziadei, P. (1966) Electron microscope observations of the olfactory mucosa of the mole. *Journal of Zoology,* **149**, 89–94.

Hajós, F. and Kerpel-Fronius, S. (1973) Comparative electron cytochemical studies of presynaptic and other neuronal mitochondria. *Brain Research,* **62**, 425–429.

Hall, S. M. (1972) The effects of injection of potassium cyanide into the sciatic nerve of the adult mouse: *in vivo* and electron microscopic studies. *Journal of Neurocytology,* **1**, 233–254.

Hall, S. M. (1973) Some aspects of remyelination after demyelination produced by the intraneural injection of lysophosphatidyl choline. *Journal of Cell Science,* **13**, 461–477.

Hall, S. M. and Gregson, N. A. (1971) The *in vivo* and ultrastructural effects of injection of lysophosphatidyl choline into myelinated peripheral nerve fibres of the adult mouse. *Journal of Cell Science,* **9**, 769–789.

Hall, S. M. and Williams, P. L. (1970) Studies on the 'incisures' of Schmidt and Lanterman. *Journal of Cell Science,* **6**, 767–792.

Hall, S. M. and Williams, P. L. (1971) The distribution of electron-dense tracers in peripheral nerve fibres. *Journal of Cell Science,* **8**, 541–555.

Harkin, J. C. (1964) A series of desmosomal attachments in the Schwann sheath of myelinated mammalian nerves. *Zeitschrift für Zellforschung und mikroskopische Anatomie,* **64**, 189–195.

Harrison, R. G. (1904) Neue Versuche und Beobachtungen über die Entwicklung der peripheren Nerven der Wirbeltiere. *Sitzungsberichte der Neiderrheinischen Gesellschaft Für Natur und Heilkunde zu Bonn*, 55–62.

Harrison, R. G. (1924) Neuroblast versus sheath cell in the development of peripheral nerves, *Journal of Comparative Neurology,* **37**, 124–205.

Hendrickson, A. E. (1972) Electron microscopic distribution of axoplasmic transport. *Journal of Comparative Neurology*, **44**, 381–397.

Hepler, P. K., McIntosh, J. R. and Cleland, S. (1970) Intermicrotubule bridges in mitotic spindle apparatus. *Journal of Cell Biology*, **45**, 438–444.

Herbst, F. (1965) Untersuchungen über Metallsalzreaktionen am der Ranvierschen schnaürringen. *Acta Histochemica (Jena)*, **22**, 223–233.

Hess, A. and Lansing, A. J. (1953) The fine structure of peripheral nerve fibres. *Anatomical Record*, **117**, 175–200.

Hess, A. and Young, J. Z. (1952) The nodes of Ranvier. *Proceedings of the Royal Society, London B*, 140, 301–320.

Hildebrand, C. (1971) Ultrastructural and light-microscopic studies of the nodal region in large myelinated fibres of the adult feline spinal cord white matter. *Acta Physiologica scandinavica*, Suppl., **364**, 43–80.

Hildebrand, C. and Skoglund, S. (1971) Histochemical studies of adult and developing feline spinal white matter. *Acta Physiologica scandinavica*, Suppl., **364**, 145–173.

Hirano A. and Dembitzer, H. M. (1969) The transverse bands as a means of access to the periaxonal space of the central myelinated nerve fibre. *Journal of Ultrastructure Research*, **28**, 141–149.

Hirano, A., Becker, N. H. and Zimmerman, H. M. (1969) Isolation of the periaxonal space of the central myelinated nerve fibre with regard to the diffusion of peroxidase. *Journal of Histochemistry and Cytochemistry*, **17**, 512–516.

Hirano, A. and Zimmerman, H. M. (1971) Some new pathological findings in the central myelinated axon. *Journal of Neuropathology and Experimental Neurology*, **30**, 325–336.

Hiscoe, H. B. (1947) Distribution of nodes and incisures in normal and regenerated nerve fibres. *Anatomical Record*, **99**, 447–476.

Hodgkin, A. L. (1951) The ionic basis of electrical activity in nerve and muscle. *Biological Review*, **26**, 339–409.

Hodgkin, A. L. (1971) *The Conduction of the Nervous Impulse*. University Press: Liverpool.

Hodgkin, A. L. and Huxley, A. F. (1952) Currents carried by sodium and potassium ions through the membrane of the giant axon of *Loligo. Journal of Physiology, London*, **116**, 449–472.

Holtzer, H. and Sanger, J. W. (1972) Cytochalasin B: microfilaments, cell movement, and what else? *Developmental Biology*, **27**, 444–446.

Holtzman, E. and Peterson, E. R. (1969) Uptake of protein by mammalian neurons. *Journal of Cell Biology*, **40**, 863–869.

Holtzman, E., Freeman, A. R. and Kashner, L. A. (1970) A cytochemical and electron microscope study of channels in the Schwann cells surrounding lobster giant axons. *Journal of Cell Biology*, **44**, 438–445.

Horridge, G. A. (1968) The origins of the nervous system. In *The Structure and Function of Nervous Tissue. I. Structure*, (ed.) Bourne, G. H., pp. 1–29. Academic Press: New York.

Hörstadius, S. (1950) *The Neural Crest.* Oxford University Press: London.

Hughes, A. (1953) The growth of embryonic neurites. A study on cultures of chick neural tissue. *Journal of Anatomy*, **87**, 150–162.

Hursh, J. B. (1939) Conduction velocity and diameter of nerve fibres. *American Journal of Physiology*, **127**, 131–139.

Hydén, H. (1967) Dynamic aspects of the neuron-glia relationship. In *The Neuron*. (ed.) Hydén, H., pp. 179–219. Elsevier: Amsterdam.

Ingoglia, N. A., Grafstein, B. M., McEwen, B. S. and McQuarrie, I. G. (1973) Axoplasmic transport of radioactivity in the goldfish optic system following intraocular injection of labelled RNA precursors. *Journal of Neurochemistry*, **20**, 1605–1616.

Jacobs, J. M. and Cavanagh, J. B. (1969) Species differences in internode formation following two types of peripheral nerve injury. *Journal of Anatomy*, **105**, 295–306.

Jahn, T. L. and Bovee, E. C. (1969) Protoplasmic movements within cells. *Physiological Reviews*, **49**, 793–862.

James, K. A. C., Bray, J. J., Morgan, I. G. and Austin, L. (1970) The effect of colchicine on the transport of axonal protein in the chicken. *Biochemical Journal*, **117**, 767–771.

Jeffrey, P, L., James, K. A. C., Kidman, A. D., Richards, A. M. and Austin, L. (1972) The flow of mitochondria in chicken sciatic nerve. *Journal of Neurobiology*, **3**, 199–208.

Johnston, M. C. (1966) A radioautographic study of the migration and fate of cranial neural crest cells in the chick embryo. *Anatomical Record,* 156, 143–155.

Johnston, P. V. and Roots, B. I. (1972) *Nerve Membranes.* Pergamon Press: Oxford.

Kapeller, K. and Mayor, D. (1967) The accumulation of mitochondria proximal to a constriction in sympathetic nerves. *Journal of Physiology, London,* 191. 70–71P.

Kapeller, K. and Mayor, D. (1969a) An electron microscopic study of the early changes proximal to a constriction in sympathetic nerves. *Proceedings of the Royal Society B,* 172, 39–51.

Kapeller, K. and Mayor, D. (1969b) An electron microscopic study of the early changes distal to a constriction in sympathetic nerves. *Proceedings of the Royal Society B,* 172, 53–63.

Karlsson, J.-O. and Sjöstrand, J. (1968) Transport of labelled proteins in the optic nerve and tract of the rabbit. *Brain Research,* 11, 431–439.

Karlsson, J.-O. and Sjöstrand, J. (1971) Axonal transport of proteins in the optic nerve and tract of the rabbit. *Acta Neuropathologica,* Suppl. 5, 207–215.

Kashef, R. (1966) *The node of Ranvier.* Ph.D. thesis. University of London.

Kerr, J. G. (1904) On some points in the early development of motor nerve trunks and myotomes in *Lepidosiren paradoxa* (Fitz.). *Transactions of the Royal Society of Edinburgh,* 41, 119–128.

Keynes, R. D. (1951) The ionic movements during nervous activity. *Journal of Physiology, London,* 114, 119–150.

Kimbarovskaya, E. M. (1953) Changes in peripheral nerve fibres resulting from stretching. Dissertation. Dnepropetrovsk.

Kirkpatrick, J. B., Bray, J. J. and Palmer, S. M. (1972) Visualization of axoplasmic flow *in vitro* by Nomarski microscopy: comparison to rapid flow of radioactive proteins. *Brain Research,* 43, 1–10.

Kirkpatrick, J. B. and Stern, L. Z. (1973) Axoplasmic flow in human sural nerve. *Archives of Neurology,* 28, 308–312.

Koenig, E. (1965) Synthetic mechanisms in the axon. II. RNA in myelin-free axons of the cat. *Journal of Neurochemistry,* 12, 357–361.

Koenig, E. (1967a) Synthetic mechanisms in the axon. III. Stimulation of acetylocholinesterase synthesis by actinomycin D in the hypoglossal nerve. *Journal of Neurochemistry,* 14, 429–435.

Koenig, E. (1967b) Synthetic mechanisms in the axon. IV. *In vitro* incorporation of ^{3}H-precursors into axonal protein and RNA. *Journal of Neurochemistry,* 14, 437–446.

Koenig, E. (1970) Membrane protein synthesizing machinery of the axon. *Advances in Biochemical Psychopharmacology,* 2, 303–315.

Koenig, H. (1958) An autoradiographic study of nucleic acid and protein turnover in the mammalian neuraxis. *Journal of Biophysical and Biochemical Cytology,* 4, 785–792.

Kolodny, G. M. (1971) Evidence for transfer of macromolecular RNA between mammalian cells in culture. *Experimental Cell Research,* 65, 313–324.

Kornthguth, S. E., Anderson, J. W. and Scott, G. (1966) Temporal relationship between myelinogenesis and the appearance of a basic protein in the spinal cord of the white rat. *Journal of Comparative Neurology,* 127, 1–18.

Krammer, E. B. and Lischka, M. F. (1973) Schwermetallaffine Strukturen des peripheren Nerven. I Potentieller Störfaktor beim cytochemischen AChE-Nachweis. *Histochemie,* 36, 269–282.

Kreutzberg, G. W. (1969) Neuronal dynamics and axonal flow. IV. Blockage of intra-axonal enzyme transport by colchicine. *Proceedings of the National Academy of Sciences of the United States of America,* 62, 722–728.

Kreutzberg, G. W. and Wechsler, W. (1963) Histochemische Untersuchungen oxydativer Enzyme am regenerierenden Nervus ischiadicus der Rattus. *Acta Neuropathologica (Berlin),* 2, 349–361.

Kristensson, K. (1970) Transport of fluorescent protein tracer in peripheral nerves. *Acta Neuropathologica, (Berlin),* 16, 293–300.

Kristensson, K., Lycke, E. and Sjöstrand, J. (1971) Spread of Herpes simplex virus in peripheral nerves. *Acta Neuropathologica (Berlin),* 17, 44–53.

Kristensson, K. and Olsson, Y. (1971a) Retrograde axonal transport of protein. *Brain Research,* 29, 363–365.

Kristensson, K. and Olsson, Y. (1971b) Uptake and retrograde axonal transport of peroxidase in hypoglossal neurons. Electron microscopical localization in the neuronal perikaryon. *Acta Neuropathologica (Berlin)*. **19**, 1–9.

Kristensson, K. and Olsson, T. (1973) Diffusion pathways and retrograde axonal transport of protein tracers in peripheral nerves. *Progress in Neurobiology*, **1**, 85–109.

Kuffler, S. W. and Potter, D. D. (1964) Glia in the leech central nervous system: physiological properties and neuron-glia relationship. *Journal of Neurophysiology*, **27**, 290–320.

Kühnt, J. H. (1876) Die peripherische markhaltige Nervenfaser. *Archiv für Mikroskopische Anatomie und Entwicklungsmechanik*, **13**, 427–464.

Lampert, P. W. (1965) The mechanism of demyelination in experimental allergic neuritis. Electron microscopic studies. *Laboratory Investigation*, **20**, 127–138.

Landon, D. N. and Langley, O. K. (1971) The local chemical environment of nodes of Ranvier: a study of cation binding. *Journal of Anatomy*, **108**, 419–432.

Landon, D. N. and Williams, P. L. (1963) Ultrastructure of the node of Ranvier. *Nature, London*, **199**, 575–577.

Langley, O. K. (1969) Ion exchange at the node of Ranvier. *Histochemical Journal*, **1**, 295–309.

Langley, O. K. (1970) The interaction between peripheral nerve polyanions and alcian blue. *Journal of Neurochemistry*, **17**, 1535–1541.

Langley, O. K. (1971) A comparison of the binding of Alcian Blue and inorganic cations to polyanions in peripheral nerve. *Histochemical Journal*, **3**, 251–260.

Langley, O. K. (1973) Local anaesthetics and nodal polyanions in peripheral nerve. *Histochemical Journal*, **5**, 79–86.

Langley, O. K. and Landon, D. N. (1967) A light and electron histochemical approach to the nodes of Ranvier and myelin of peripheral nerve fibres. *Journal of Histochemistry and Cytochemistry*, **15**, 722–731.

Langley, O. K. and Landon, D. N. (1969) Copper binding at nodes of Ranvier: a new electron histochemical technique for the demonstration of polyanions. *Journal of Histochemistry and Cytochemistry*, **17**, 66–69.

Lanterman, A. J. (1877) Ueber den feineren Bau der markhaltigen Nervenfasern. *Archiv für Mikroskopische Anatomie und Entwicklungsmechanik*, **13**, 1–8.

Lasansky, A. and Wald, F. (1962) The extracellular space in the toad retina as defined by the distribution of ferrocyanide. A light and electron microscope study. *Journal of Cell Biology*, **15**, 463–479.

Lasek. R. J. (1968) Axoplasmic transport in cat dorsal ganglion cells: as studied with L-leucine-H^3. *Brain Research*, **7**, 360–377.

Lasek, R. J. (1970) Protein transport in neurons. *International Review of Neurobiology*, **13**, 289–324.

Lasek, R. J., Dabrowski, C. and Nordlander, R. (1973) Analysis of axoplasmic RNA from invertebrate giant axons. *Nature, New Biology*, **244**, 162–165.

Lázár, L. and Maros, T. (1962) Beitrag zur funktionellen bedeutung der Schmidt–Lantermannschen–Einkerbungen. *Revue des Sciences Médicales*, **7**, 51–54.

Lehninger, A. L. (1968) The neuronal membrane. *Proceedings of the National Academy of Sciences of the United States of America*, **60**, 1069–1080.

Lillie, R. S. (1925) Factors affecting transmission and recovery in the passive iron nerve model. *Journal of General Physiology*, **7**, 473–507.

Livett, B. G., Geffen, L. B. and Austin, L. (1968) Proximodistal transport of [C-14] noradrenaline and protein in sympathetic nerves. *Journal of Neurochemistry*, **15**, 931–939.

Livingstone, R. B., Pfenninger, K., Moor, H. and Akert, K. (1973) Specialized paranodal and interparanodal glial-axonal functions in the peripheral and central nervous system: a freeze etching study. *Brain Research*, **58**, 1–24.

Lubińska, L. (1954) Form of myelinated nerve fibres. *Nature (London)*. **173**, 867.

Lubińska, L. (1956) The physical state of axoplasm in teased vertebrate nerve fibres. *Acta biologiae experimentalis*, **17**, 135–140.

Lubińska, L. (1958) Short internodes 'intercalated' in nerve fibres. *Acta biologiae experimentalis*, **18**, 117–136.

Lubińska, L. (1964) Axoplasmic streaming in regenerating and in normal nerve fibres. *Progress in Brain Research,* **13,** 56–66.
Lubińska, L. (1971) Acetylcholinesterase in mammalian peripheral nerves and characteristics of its migration. *Acta Neuropathologica,* Suppl. 5, 136–146.
Lubińska, L. and Lukaszewska, I. (1956) Shape of myelinated nerve fibres and proximo-distal flow of axoplasm. *Acta biologiae experimentalis,* 17, 115–133.
Lubińska, L. and Niemierko, S. (1971) Velocity and intensity of bi-directional migration of acetylcholinesterase in transected nerves. *Brain Research,* 27, 329–342.
Lux, H. D., Schubert, P., Kreutzberg, G. W. and Globus, A. (1970) Excitation and axonal flow: autoradiographic study on motoneurons intracellularly injected with a ³H- amino acid. *Experimental Brain Research,* 10, 197–204.
Macallum, A. B. (1905) On the distribution of potassium in animal and vegetable cells. *Journal of Physiology, London,* 32, 95–128.
Macallum. A. B. and Menten, M. L. (1906) On the distribution of chlorides in nerve cells and fibres. *Proceedings of the Royal Society of London, Series B,* 77, 165–193.
McDonald, W. I. (1967) Structural and functional changes in human and experimental neuropathy. In *Modern Trends in Neurology.* (ed.) Williams, D., pp. 145–164. Butterworths: London.
McEwen, B. and Grafstein, B. (1968) Fast and slow components in axonal transport of protein. *Journal of Cell Biology,* 38, 494–508.
McIntosh, J. R. and Porter, K. R. (1967) Microtubules in the spermatids of the domestic fowl. *Journal of Cell Biology,* 35, 153–173.
Marantz, R., Ventilla, M. and Shelanski, M. (1969) Vinblastine induced precipitation of microtubule protein. *Science, New York,* 165, 498–499.
Martin, J. R. and Webster, H. de F. (1973) Mitotic Schwann cells in developing nerve; their changes in shape, fine structure, and axon relationships. *Developmental Biology,* 32, 417–431.
Martinez, A. J. and Friede, R. L. (1970a) Accumulation of axoplasmic organelles in swollen nerve fibers. *Brain Research,* 19, 183–198.
Martinez, A. J. and Friede, R. L. (1970b) Changes in nerve cell bodies during the myelination of their axons. *Journal of Comparative Neurology,* 138, 329–338.
Masurovsky, E. B., Bunge, M. B. and Bunge, R. P. (1967) Cytological studies of organotypic cultures of rat dorsal root ganglia following X-irradiation *In vitro.* II. Changes in Schwann cells, myelin sheaths and nerve fibers. *Journal of Cell Biology,* 32, 497–518.
Matthews, M. A. (1968) An electron microscopic study of the relationship between axon diameter and the initiation of myelin production in the peripheral nervous system. *Anatomical Record,* 161, 337–352.
Miani, N. (1962) Evidence of a proximo-distal movement along the axon of phospholipid synthesised in the nerve-cell body. *Nature, London,* 193, 887–888.
Millington, P. and Finean, J. B. (1961) Electron microscope and X-ray diffraction studies of the effects of mercuric chloride on the structure of nerve myelin. *Journal of Ultrastructure Research,* 5, 470–484.
Morgan, I. G. and Austin, L. (1968) Synaptosomal protein synthesis in a cell-free system. *Journal of Neurochemistry,* 15, 41–51.
Morris, J. H., Hudson, A. R. and Weddell, G. (1972) A study of degeneration and regeneration in the rat sciatic nerve using electron microscopy. 2 The development of the 'regeneration unit'. *Zeitschrift für Zellforschung und mikroskopische Anatomie,* 124, 103–130.
Mugnaini, E. and Schnapp, B. (1974) The zonula occludens of the myelin sheath. *Journal of Cell Biology,* 63, 234a.
von Muralt, A. (1946) *Die Signalubermittling im Nerven.* Birkhauser: Basle.
Murray, M. (1965) Nervous tissues *in vitro.* In *Cells and Tissues in Culture,* (ed.) Willmer, E. N., pp. 373–455. Academic Press: New York.
Murray, M. and Herrmann, A. (1968) Passive movements of Schmidt–Lanterman clefts during continuous observation *in vitro. Journal of Cell Biology,* 38, 149–150P.
Nageotte, J. (1910) Note sur le mécanisme de la formation des réseaux artificiels dans la gaine de myéline. *Comptes rendus des séances de la Société de biologie,* 69, 628–631.

99

Nageotte, J. (1922) *L'organisation de la matière*. Felix Alcan: Paris.

Napolitano, L. M. and Scallen, T. J. (1969) Observations on the fine structure of peripheral nerve myelin. *Anatomical Record*, 163, 1–6.

Nemiloff, A. (1908) Einige Beobachtungen über den Bau des Nervengewebes bei Ganoiden und Knochen-fischen. II. Bau der Nervenfasern. *Archive für Mickroskopische Anatomie*, 72, 575–606.

Nemiloff, A. (1910) Über die Beziehung der sog. "Zellen der Schwannschen Scheide" zum Myelin in den Nervenfasern von Saugetieren. *Archiv für Mikroskopische und Entwicklungsmechanik*, 76, 329–348.

Nurnberger, J., Engström, A. and Lindström, b. (1952) Study of ventral horn cells of adult cat by two independent cytochemical microabsorption techniques. *Journal of Cellular and Comparative Physiology*, 39, 215–254.

Ochoa, J. and Mair, W. G. P. (1969) The normal sural nerve in man. I Ultrastructure and number of fibres and cells. *Acta Neuropathologica, Berlin*, 13, 197–216.

Ochs, S. (1966) Axoplasmic flow in neurons. In *Macromolecules and Behavior*, (ed.) Gaito, J., pp. 20–39. Appleton-Century-Crofts: New York.

Ochs, S. (1971) The dependence of fast transport in mammalian nerve fibers on metabolism. *Acta Neuropathologica*, Suppl. 5, 86–96.

Ochs, S. (1972a) Characteristics and a model for fast axoplasmic transport in nerve. *Journal of Neurobiology*, 2, 331–345.

Ochs, S. (1972b) Fast axoplasmic transport of materials in mammalian nerve and its integrative role. *Annals of the New York Academy of Sciences*, 193, 43–57.

Ochs, S. (1974) Axoplasmic Transport – Energy Metabolism and Mechanism. In *The Peripheral Nervous System*, (ed.) Hubbard J. I., Plenum Press: New York and London.

Ochs, S., Dalrymple, D. and Richards, G. (1962) Axoplasmic flow in ventral root nerve fibers of the cat. *Experimental Neurology*, 5, 349–363.

Ochs, S., Johnson, J. and Ng, M.-H. (1967) Protein incorporation and axoplasmic flow in motoneuron fibres following intra-cord injection of labelled leucine. *Journal of Neurochemistry*, 14, 317–331.

Ochs, S. and Johnson, J. (1969) Fast and slow phases of axoplasmic flow in ventral root nerve fibres. *Journal of Neurochemistry*, 16, 845–853.

Ochs, S. and Ranish, N. (1969) Characteristics of the fast transport system in mammalian nerve fibres. *Journal of Neurobiology*, 1, 247–261.

Ochs, S., Sabri, M. I. and Johnson, J. (1969) Fast transport system of materials in mammalian nerve fibres. *Science, New York*, 163, 686–687.

Ochs, S., Sabri, M. I. and Ranish, N. (1970) Somal site of synthesis of fast transported materials in mammalian nerve fibres. *Journal of Neurobiology*, 1, 329–344.

Orkand, R. K., Nicholls, J. G. and Kuffler, S. W. (1966) Effect of nerve impulses on the membrane potential of glial cells in the central nervous system of amphibia. *Journal of Neurophysiology*, 29, 788–806.

Palay, S. L., Sotelo, C., Peters, A. and Orkand, P. M. (1968) The axon hillock and the initial segment. *Journal of Cell Biology*, 38, 193–201.

Pertik, O. (1881) Untersuchungen über Nervenfasern. *Archiv für Mikroskopische Anatomie und Entwicklungsmechanik*, 18, 183–239.

Peters, A. (1966) The node of Ranvier in the central nervous system. *Quarterly Journal of experimental Physiology*, 51, 229–236.

Peters, A., Proskauer, C. C. and Kaiserman-Abramof, I. R. (1968) The small pyramidal neuron of the rat cerebral cortex. The axon hillock and the initial segment. *Journal of Cell Biology*, 39, 604–619.

Peterson, J. A., Bray, J. J. and Austin, L. (1968) An autoradiographic study of the flow of protein and RNA along peripheral nerve *Journal of Neurochemistry*, 15, 741–745.

Pomerat, C. M., Hendelman, W. J., Raiborn, C. W. Jr. and Massey, J. F. (1967) Dynamic activities of nervous tissue *in vitro*. In *The Neuron*. (ed.) Hydén, H., pp. 119–178. Elsevier: Amsterdam.

Porter, K. R. (1966) Cytoplasmic microtubules and their functions. In *Principles of Biomolecular Organisation*, (ed.) Wolstenholme, G. E. W. and O'Connor, M., pp. 308–356. Churchill: London.

Rahmann, H. (1971) Different modes of substance flow in the optic tract. *Acta Neuropathologica (Berlin)*, Suppl. 5, 162–170.

Raine, C. S. (1972) Viral infections of nervous tissue and their relevance to multiple sclerosis. In *Multiple Sclerosis, Immunology, Virology and Ultrastructure*, (eds.) Wolfgram, F., Ellison, G. W., Stevens, J. G. and Andrews, J. M., pp. 91–118. Academic Press: New York.

Raine, C., Ghetti, B. and Shelanski, M. (1971) On the association between microtubules and mitochondria within axons. *Brain Research*, **34**, 389–393.

Ramirez, G., Levitan, I. B. and Mushynski, W. E. (1972) Highly purified synaptosomal membranes from rat brain; incorporation of amino acids into membrane proteins *in vitro*. *Journal of Biological Chemistry*, **247**, 5382–5390.

Ranvier, L. A. (1871) Contributions à l'histologie et à la physiologie des nerfs périphérique. *Comptes rendus hebdominal seances d'Academie des Sciences, Paris*, **73**, 1168–1171.

Ranvier, L. A. (1875) *Traite technique d'histologie*. Savy: Paris.

Ranvier, M. L. (1878) *Leçons sur l'histologie du systeme nerveux*. Savy: Paris.

Raven, C. P. (1936) Zur entwicklung der Ganglienleiste; über die Differenzierung des Rumpfganglienleisten-materials. *Archiv für Entwicklungsmechanik der Organismen*, **134**, 122–146.

Rawlins, F. A. (1973) A time sequence autoradiographic study of the *in vivo* incorporation of [1, 2 ^{3}H] cholesterol in peripheral nerve myelin. *Journal of Cell Biology*, **58**, 42–53.

Rawlins, F. A., Villegas, G. M., Hedley-Whyte, E. T. and Usman, B. G. (1972) Fine structural localization of cholesterol-1, 2 -^{3}H in degenerating and regenerating mouse sciatic nerve. *Journal of Cell Biology*, **52**, 615–625.

Reier, P. J. and Hughes, A. F. (1972) An effect of neonatal radiothyroidectomy upon non-myelinated axons and associated Schwann cells during maturation of the mouse sciatic nerve. *Brain Research*, **41**, 263–282.

Remak, R. (1836) Vorläufige Mittheilung microskopischer Beobachtungen über den innern Bau der Cerebro-spinal-nerven und über die Entwickelung ihrer Formelemente. *Muller's Archiv für Anatomie und Physiologie*, 145–161.

Remak, R. (1837) Weitere mikroscopische Beobachtungen über die Primitivfasern des Nervensystems der Wirbelthiere. *Froriep's neue Notizen aus dem Gebiete der Natur – und Heilkunde*, 36–41.

Revel, J. P. and Hamilton, D. W. (1969) The double nature of the intermediate dense line in peripheral nerve myelin. *Anatomical Record*, **163**, 7–16.

Ritchie, J. M. and Straub, R. W. (1957) The hyperpolarisation which follows activity in mammalian non-medullated fibres. *Journal of Physiology, London*, **136**, 80–97.

Robertson, J. D. (1957a) The ultrastructure of the myelin sheath near nodes of Ranvier. *Journal of Physiology, London*, **135**, 56p.

Robertson, J. D. (1957b) The ultrastructure of nodes of Ranvier in frog nerve fibres. *Journal of Physiology, London*, **137**, 8p.

Robertson, J. D. (1958a) Structural alterations in nerve fibres produced by hypotonic and hypertonic solutions. *Journal of Biophysical and Biochemical Cytology*, **4**, 349–364.

Robertson, J. D. (1958b) The ultrastructure of Schmidt–Lanterman clefts and related shearing defects of the myelin sheath. *Journal of Biophysical and Biochemical Cytology*, **4**, 39–46.

Robertson, J. D. (1959) Preliminary observations on the ultrastructure of nodes of Ranvier. *Zeitschrift fur Zellforschstellung und mikroscopische Anatomie*, **50**, 553–560.

Robertson, J. D. (1960) The molecular structure and contact relationships of cell membranes. *Progress in Biophysics*, **10**, 343–418.

Robertson, J. D. (1964) Unit membranes: a review with recent new studies of experimental alterations and a new subunit structure in synaptic membranes. In *Cellular Membranes in Development*, (ed.) Locke, M., pp. 1–81. Academic Press: New York.

Rosenbluth, J. and Wissig, S. L. (1964) The distribution of exogenous ferritin in toad spinal ganglia and the mechanism of its uptake by neurons. *Journal of Cell Biology*, **23**, 307–325.

Rushton, W. A. H. (1951) A theory of the effects of fibre size in medullated nerve. *Journal of Physiology, London*, **115**, 101–122.

Salimen, S. and Loumanmäki, K. (1963) The binding of sodium and potassium ions by Heparin. *Biochimica et biophysica acta*, **69**, 533–537.

Samorajski, T. and Friede, R. L. (1968) Size-dependent distribution of axoplasm, Schwann cell cytoplasm and mitochondria in the perpheral nerve fiber of the mouse. *Anatomical Record,* 161, 281–292.

Scharf, J.-H. and Blume, R. (1964) Uber die Abhängigkeit der axonalen Mitochondrienzahl vom Kaliber der segmentierten Nervenfaser auf Grund einer Regressionanalyse. *Journal für Hirnforschung.* 6, 361–376.

Scheinberg L. C., Taylor, J. M., Herzog I. and Mandell S. (1966) Optic and peripheral nerve response to triethyltin intoxication in the rabbit: biochemical and ultrastructural studies. *Journal of Neuropathology and Experimental Neurology* 25, 202–213

Schlaepfer, W. W. (1971) Vincristine-induced axonal alterations in rat peripheral nerve. *Journal of Neuropathology and Experimental Neurology,* 30, 488–505.

Schlaepfer, W. W. and Myers, F. K. (1973) Relationship of myelin internode elongation and growth in the rat sural nerve. *Journal of Comparative Neurology,* 147, 255–266.

Schmidt, H. D. (1874) On the construction of the dark or double-bordered nerve fibre. *Monthly Microscopical Journal (London),* 11, 200–221.

Schmidt, W. J. (1936) Doppelbrechung und Feinbau der Markscheide der Nervenfasern. *Zeitschrift für Zellforschung und mikroskopische Anatomie,* 23, 657–676.

Schmitt, F. O. (1958) Axon-satellite cell relationships in peripheral nerve fibers. *Experimental Cell Research,* Suppl. 5, 33–57.

Schmitt, F. O., Bear, R. S. and Palmer G. L. (1935) X-ray diffraction studies on nerve *Radiology,* 25, 131–151.

Schmitt, F. O. and Bear, R. S. (1937) The optical properties of vetebrate nerve axons as related to fiber size. *Journal of Cellular and Comparative Physiology,* 9, 261–273.

Schmitt, F. O. and Davison, P. F. (1961) Biologie moleculaire des neurofilaments. In *Actualités Neurophysiologiques,* Série 3, (ed.) Monnier, A. M., Masson: Paris.

Schmitt, F. O. and Samson, F. E. (1968) Neuronal fibrous proteins. *Neurosciences Research Program Bulletin,* 6, 113–219.

Scheider, D. (1952) Die Dehnbarkeit der markhaltigen Nervanfaser des Froches. In *Abhängigkeit von funktion und struktur. Zeitschrift fur Naturforschung,* 7b, 38–48.

Schmitt F. O. (1968) Fibrous proteins – neuronal organelles. *Proceedings of the National Academy of Sciences of the United States of America,* 60, 1092–1101

Schonbach, J. and Cuénod, M. (1971) Axoplasmic streaming and proteins in the retino-tectal neurons of the pigeon. *Acta Neuropathologica* Suppl, 5, 153–161.

Schroder, J. M. (1972) Altered ratio between axon diameter and myelin sheath thickness in regenerated nerve fibres. *Brain Research,* 45, 49–65.

Schwieler, G. H. (1968) Respiratory regulation during postnatal development in cats and rabbits and some of its morphological substrate. *Acta Physiologica scandinavica* Suppl. 304.

Scott, F. H. (1906) On the relation of nerve cells to fatigue of their nerve fibres. *Journal of Physiology, London,* 34, 145–162.

Seneviratne, K. N., Peiris, O. A. and Weerasuriya, A. (1972) Effects of hyperkalaemia on the excitability of peripheral nerve. *Journal of Neurology, Neurosurgery and Psychiatry,* 35, 149–155.

Simpson, S. A. and Young, J. Z. (1954) Regeneration of fibre diameter after cross-unions of visceral and somatic nerves. *Journal of Anatomy,* 79, 48–65.

Singer, M. (1968) Penetration of labelled amino acids into the peripheral nerve fiber from surrounding body fluids. In *Growth of the Nervous System,* (eds.) Wolstenholme, G. E. W. and O'Connor, M., pp. 200–215. Churchill: London.

Singer, M. and Salpeter, M. M. (1966) The transport of ^{3}H-l histidine through the Schwann and myelin sheath into the axon, including a re-evaluation of myelin function. *Journal of Morphology,* 120, 281–315.

Singer, M. and Bryant, S. V. (1969) Movements in the myelin Schwann sheath of the vertebrate axon. *Nature, London,* 221, 1148–1150.

Singer, M., Krishman, N. and Fyfe, D. A. (1972) Penetration of ruthenium red into peripheral nerve fibers. *Anatomical Record,* 173, 375–390.

Sjöstrand, F. S. (1963) The structure and formation of the myelin sheath. In *Mechanisms of Demyelination,* pp. 1–43, McGraw-Hill Book Company: New York.

Smith, D. S. (1970) Bridges between vesicles and axoplasmic microtubules. *Journal of Cell Biology,* 47, 195–196A.

Smith, D. S., Järlfors, U. and Beránek, R. (1970) The origin of synaptic axoplasm in the lamprey (*Petromyzon marinus*) central nervous system. *Journal of Cell Biology*, **46**, 199–219.

Smith, R. S. (1971) Centripetal movement of particles in myelinated axons. *Cytobios*, **3**, 259–262.

Smith, R. S. (1972) Detection of organelles in myelinated nerve fibers by dark-field microscopy. *Canadian Journal of Physiology and Pharmacology*, **50**, 467–469.

Soffer, R. L. (1968) The arginine transfer reaction. *Biochimica et biophysica acta*, **155**, 228–240.

Sotnikov, O. S. (1965) Structure of Schmidt–Lanterman incisures. *Federation Proceedings. Federation of American Societies for Experimental Biology*, **25**, T 204–210.

Speidel, C. C. (1932) Studies of living nerves. I. The movements of individual sheath cells and nerve sprouts correlated with the process of myelin sheath formation in amphibian larvae. *Journal of Experimental Zoology*, **61**, 279–332.

Speidel, C. C. (1933) Studies of living nerves. II. Activities of amoeboid growth cones, sheath cells and myelin segments, as revealed by prolonged observation of individual nerve fibres in frog tadpoles. *American Journal of Anatomy*, **52**, 1–79.

Speidel, C. C. (1964) In vivo studies of myelinated nerve fibers. *International Review of Cytology*, **16**, 173–231.

Spencer P. S. (1972) Reappraisal of the model for 'Bulk Axoplasmic Flow'. *Nature New Biology, London* **240**, 283–285

Stephens, R. E. and Linck, R. W. (1969) Comparison of muscle actin and ciliary microtubule protein in the mollusk *Pecten irradians*. *Journal of Molecular Biology*, **40**, 497–501.

Stilling, B. (1856) *Uber den Bau der Nerven-primitivfasern und der Nervenzelle*. Frankfurt.

Stoeckenius, W. and Zeiger, K. (1956) Morphologie der segmentierten Nervenfaser. *Ergebnisse der Anatomie und Entwicklungsgeschichte*, **35**, 420–534.

Sunderland, S. (1968) *Nerves and Nerve Injuries*. Livingstone: Edinburgh.

Tasaki, I. and Takeuchi, T. (1941) Der am Ranvierschen Knoten entstehende Aktionsstrom und seine Bedeutung für die Erregungsleitung. *Pflüger's Archiv für die gesamte Physiologie des Menschen und der Tiere*, **244**, 696–711.

Tasaki, I. (1968) 'Nerve excitation – a macromolecular approach'. C. C. Thomas: Springfield, Illinois.

Tennyson, V. M. (1969) The fine structure of the developing nervous system. In *Developmental Neurobiology*, (ed.) Himwich W., pt 2 Chapter 3. C. C. Thomas: Springfield, Illinois.

Tennyson, V. M. (1970) The fine structure of the axon and growth cone of the dorsal root neuroblast of the rabbit embryo. *Journal of Cell Biology*, **44**, 62–79.

Thomas, P. K. and Young, J. Z. (1949) Internodal lengths in the nerves of fishes. *Journal of Anatomy*, **83**, 336–350.

Tilney, L. G. (1968) The assembly of microtubules and their role in the development of cell form. *Developmental Biology Supplement*, **2**.

Tilney, L. G. and Porter K. R. (1967) Studies on the microtubules in Heliozoa II. The effect of low temperature on these structures in the formation and maintenance of the axopodia *Journal of Cell Biology* **34**, 327–343.

Tobias, J. M. (1964) A chemically specified mechanism underlying excitation in nerves. A hypothesis. *Nature, London*. **203**, 13–17.

Uzman, B. G. and Villegas, G. M. (1960) A comparison of nodes of Ranvier in sciatic nerves with node-like structures in optic nerves of the mouse. *Journal of Biophysical and Biochemical cytology*, **7**, 761–762.

Vierhaus, J. and Ulbricht, W. (1971) Effect of a sudden change in sodium concentration on repetitively evoked action potentials of single nodes of Ranvier. *Pflügers' Archives*, **326**, 76–87.

Vignal, W. (1883) Mémoire sur le développement des tubes nerveux chez les embryons de mammifères. *Archives de physiologie*, **15**, 513–534.

Villegas, G. M. and Villegas, R. (1968) Ultrastructural studies of the squid nerve fibers. *Journal of General Physiology*, **51**, 44–60S.

Villegas, J. (1972) Axon-Schwann cell interaction in the squid nerve fibre. *Journal of Physiology, London*, **225**, 275–296.

Vizoso, A. D. and Young, J. Z. (1948) Internode length and fibre diameter in developing and regenerating nerves. *Journal of Anatomy*, 82, 110–134.

Waxman, S. G. (1968) Micropinocytotic invaginations in the axolemma of peripheral nerves. *Zeitschrift für Zellforschung und mikroskopische Anatomie*, 86, 571–574.

Webster, H. de F. (1964a) Some ultrastructural features of segmental demyelination and myelin regeneration in peripheral nerve. *Progress in Brain Research*, 13, 151–174.

Webster, H. de F. (1964b) The relationship between Schmidt–Lanterman incisures and myelin segmentation during Wallerian degeneration. *Annals of the New York Academy of Sciences*, 122, 29–38.

Webster, H. de F. (1971) The geometry of peripheral myelin sheaths during their formation and growth in rat sciatic nerves. *Journal of Cell Biology*, 48, 348–367.

Webster, H. de F. and Billings, S. M. (1972) Myelinated nerve fibers in *Xenopus* tadpoles: *in vivo* observations and fine structure. *Journal of Neuropathology and Experimental Neurology*, 31, 102–112.

Webster, H. de F., Martin, J. R. and O'Connell, M. F. (1973) The relationships between interphase Schwann cells and axons before myelination: a quantitative electron microscope study. *Developmental Biology*, 32, 401–416.

Weisenberg, R. G. and Timasheff, S. N. (1970) Aggregation of microtubule subunit protein. Effect of divalent cations, colchicine and vinblastine. *Biochemistry*, 9, 4110–4116.

Weiss, P. A. (1969) Neuronal dynamics. *Neurosciences Research Program Bulletin*, 5, 371–400.

Weiss, P. A. (1970) Neuronal dynamics and neuroplasmic flow. In *Neurosciences Review, a Second Study Program*, (eds.) Schmitt, F. O., Quarton, G. C., Melnechuck, T. and Adelman, G., pp. 840–850. Rockefeller Press: New York.

Weiss, P. A. (1972) Neuronal dynamics and axonal flow: axonal peristalsis. *Proceedings of the National Academy of Sciences*, 69, 1309–1312.

Weiss, P., Wang, H., Taylor, A. C. and Edds, M. V. (1945) Proximo-distal fluid convection in the endoneurial spaces of peripheral nerves, demonstrated by colored and radioactive (isotope) tracers. *American Journal of Physiology*, 143, 521–540.

Weiss, P. A. and Hiscoe, H. B. (1948) Experiments in the mechanism of nerve growth. *Experimental Zoology*, 107, 315–395.

Weiss, P. A. and Pillai, A. (1965) Convection and fate of mitochondria in nerve fibers: axonal flow as vehicle. *Proceedings of the National Academy of Sciences*, 54, 48–56.

Weiss, P. A. and Mayr, R. (1971a) Organelles in neuroplasmic ('axonal') flow: neurofilaments. *Proceedings of the National Academy of Sciences of the United States of America*. 68, 846–850.

Weiss, P. A. and Mayr, R. (1971b) Neuronal organelles in neuroplasmic ('axonal') flow. I. Mitochondria. *Acta Neuropathologica*, Suppl. 5, 187–197.

Weiss, P. A. and Mayr, R. (1971c) Neuronal organelles in neuroplasmic ('axonal') flow. II. Neurotubules. *Acta Neuropathologica (Berlin)*, Suppl. 5, 198–206.

Wendell-Smith C. P. and Williams, P. L. (1959) The use of teased preparations and frozen sections in quantitative studies of mammalian peripheral nerve *Quarterly Journal of Microscopical Science*. 100. 499–508.

Weston, J. A. (1963) A radioautographic analysis of the migration and localisation of trunk neural crest cells in the chick. *Developmental Biology*, 6, 279–310.

Weston, J. A. (1970) The migration and differentiation of neural crest cells. *Advances in Morphogenesis*, 8, 41–114.

Westphal, A. (1894) Die elektrischen Erregbarkeitsver-hältnisse des periphererishcen Nervensystems des Menschen in jugendlichem Zustand und ihre Bezieungen zu den anatomischen Bau desslben. *Archiv für Psychiatrie und Nervenkrankheiten*, 26, 1–98.

Whitear, M. (1962) The fine structure of crustacean proprioceptors. I. The chordotonal organs in the legs of the shore crab *Carcinus maenas*. *Philosophical Transactions of the Royal Society B.*, 245, 291–325.

Williams, M. A. (1969) The assessment of electron microscopic autoradiographs. *Advances in Optical and Electron Microscopy*, 3, 219–272.

Williams, M. A. (1973) Electron microscopic autoradiography: its application to protein biosynthesis. In *Techniques in Protein Biosynthesis*, (eds.) Campbell, P. N. and Sargent, J. R., Vol. 3, pp. 126–190. Academic Press: New York.

Williams, P. L. and Hall, S. M. (1970) *In vivo* observations on mature myelinated nerve fibres of the mouse. *Journal of Anatomy*, 107, 31–38.

Williams, P. L. and Hall, S. M. (1971a) Prolonged *in vivo* observations of normal peripheral nerve fibres and their acute reactions to crush and deliberate trauma. *Journal of Anatomy*, 108, 397–408.

Williams, P. L. and Hall, S. M. (1971b) Chronic Wallerian degeneration – an *in vivo* and ultrastructural study. *Journal of Anatomy*, 109, 487–503.

Williams, P. L. and Kashef, R. (1961) Asymmetry of the node of Ranvier in mammals – an experimental study. *Journal of Anatomy*, 95, 610.

Williams, P. L. and Kashef, R. (1968) Asymmetry of the node of Ranvier. *Journal of Cell Science*, 3, 341–356.

Williams, P. L. and Landon, D. N. (1963) Paranodal apparatus of peripheral nerve fibres of mammals. *Nature, London*, 198, 670–673.

Williams, P. L. and Landon, D. N. (1964) The energy source of the nerve fibre. *New Scientist*, 21, 166–169.

Williams, P. L. and Landon, D. N. (1965) 'The node of Ranvier'. *Journal of Anatomy*, 100, 437.

Williams, P. L. and Wendell-Smith, C. P. (1960) The use of fixed and stained sections in quantitative studies of peripheral nerve. *Quarterly Journal of Microscopical Science*, 101, 43–54.

Williams, P. L. and Wendell-Smith, C. P. (1971) Some additional parametric variations between peripheral nerve fibre populations. *Journal of Anatomy*, 109, 505–526.

Wolburg, H. (1972) Intraaxonaler Transport von Ethidium-Bromid-sensitiven RNS- und niedermolekularen 3H-Uridin-Verbindungen im Tractus opticus von Teleosteern. *Experimental Brain Research*, 15, 348–363.

Wuerker, R. B. (1970) Neurofilaments and glial filaments. *Tissue and Cell*, 2, 1–9.

Wuerker, R. B. and Kirkpatrick, J. B. (1972) Neuronal microtubules, neurofilaments and microfilaments. *International Review of Cytology*, 33, 45–75.

Wuerker, R. B. and Palay, S. L. (1969) Neurofilaments and microtubules in anterior horn cells of the rat. *Tissue and Cell*, 1, 387–402.

Yamada, K. M., Spooner, B. S. and Wessels, N. K. (1970) Axon growth: roles of microfilaments and microtubules. *Proceedings of the National Academy of Sciences*, 66, 1206–1212.

Yntema, C. L. (1937) Experimental study of origin of cells which constitute seventh and eighth cranial ganglia and nerves in the embryo of *Ambystoma punctatum*. *Journal of Experimental Zoology*, 75, 75–101.

Yntema, C. L. (1943) Deficient efferent innervation of the extremities following removal of the neural crest in *Amblystoma*. *Journal of Experimental Zoology*, 94, 319–343.

Young, J. Z. (1945) The history of the shape of a nerve fibre. In *Essays on Growth and Form*, (eds.) Clark, W. E. L. and Medawar, P. B., pp. 41–93. Clarendon Press: Oxford.

Zelená, J. (1968) Bidirectional movements of mitochondria along axons of an isolated nerve segment. *Zeitschrift für Zellforschung und mikroskopische Anatomie*, 92, 186–196.

Zelená, J. (1969) Bidirectional shift of mitochondria in axons after injury. In *Cellular Dynamics of the Neuron*, (ed.) Barondes, S. H., Vol. 8, pp. 73–94. Academic Press: New York.

Zelená, J. (1970) Ribosome-like particles in myelinated axons of the rat. *Brain Research*, 24, 359–363.

Zelená, J., Lubińska, L. and Gutmann, E. (1968) Accumulation of organelles at the ends of interrupted axons. *Zeitschrift für Zellforschung und mikroskopische Anatomie*, 91, 186–196.

Zenker, W. (1964) Über die Anfärbung der Ranvierschen Schnürringe beim Koelle Verfahren zum Histochemischen Nachweis der Cholinesterase. *Acta Histochem (Jena)*, 19, 67–72.

Zenker, W. and Hohberg, E. (1973) A–α-Motorische Nervenfasen: Axonquerschnittsfläche von Stammfaser und Endästen. *Zeitschrift für Anatomie und Entwicklungsgeschichte*, 139, 163–172.

Zenker, W. and Hohberg, E. (1973b) A-α-nerve fibre: number of neurotubules in the stem fibre and in the terminal branches. *Journal of Neurocytology*, 2, 143–148.

2 THE UNMYELINATED NERVE FIBRE

J. Ochoa

2.1 Introduction

An unmyelinated nerve fibre is composed of a bundle of small axons covered by a chain of satellite cells. Remak, in 1838, was the first to recognize that this class of nerve fibre differed in structure from those at that time called 'tubuli primitivi'. Subsequent improvements in histological techniques, and the cumulative observations of many subsequent workers have since contributed to define the essential anatomical distinctions between myelinated fibres ('tubuli primitivi') and unmyelinated fibres (Remak fibres), as well as a number of their electro-physiological properties.

The axons of unmyelinated fibres are extremely slender neuronal processes, barely visible in the light microscope, and for this reason the structure of unmyelinated fibres was ill-defined prior to the early 1950s, and some controversy arose concerning the possible existence of a tenuous myelin sheath surrounding unmyelinated axons. It is clear today that in most peripheral nerves there exist large numbers of mature, small calibre nerve fibres whose axons are completely and permanently devoid of myelin, and the presence or absence of myelin continues to be the most widely used criterion for the sub-classification of nerve fibres. One must be careful not to overestimate the significance of this criterion, however, since it is based upon a subsidiary feature of the nerve fibres concerned. Indeed, axons devoid of myelin do not form a homogeneous group: there are the true unmyelinated fibres (Remak fibres) which even in the mature state are normally devoid of myelin, and also myelinated axons which may temporarily lack myelin due to immaturity or disease. Another reason to regard myelin as a subsidiary feature of nerve fibres is the fact that to some extent the onset, degree and rate of myelination are dependent on axonal calibre (Duncan, 1934; Friede and Samorajski, 1968; Matthews, 1968; Friede, 1972), and that below a certain size limit, growing axons fail to become myelinated. From such evidence Duncan (1934) argued that unmyelinated axons are devoid of myelin because they do not reach the critical calibre for myelination. It appears, however, that such extrapolation to unmyelinated axons of the properties of immature axons awaiting myelination is without justification since we now know that in a mature nerve unmyelinated axons may greatly exceed the supposed 'critical diameter' necessary for myelination (Ochoa and Mair,

1969a; Ochoa, 1971). Furthermore, Duncan's argument involves the unlikely assumption that, as regard their trophic influences upon the Schwann cells, the neurons which give rise to myelinated and unmyelinated axons have a similar potential. On the contrary the evidence available supports the concept that myelinated and unmyelinated neurons constitute distinct groups in that they subserve specific functional modalities, and possess specific metabolic characteristics in so far as these can be deduced from their preferential involvement in certain pathological processes. Thus, it seems unreasonable to regard unmyelinated axons as being devoid of myelin simply because they are of small calibre; it appears more likely that this absence can be attributed to an intrinsic difference from those axons endowed with the property of stimulating the Schwann cells to form myelin.

Peripheral unmyelinated fibres may therefore be defined as those peripheral nerve elements formed by the axons of small neurons (and their accompanying satellite cells) which even in their mature state are normally of small calibre and lack myelin. They may also be referred to as non-medullated fibres, Remak fibres or C-fibres.

2.2 Historical

Although terms 'unmyelinated' or 'non-myelinated' imply the recognition of the substance called myelin, unmyelinated fibres were known as 'fibrae organicae' long before the myelin sheath was identified as a distinct entity. The discovery of unmyelinated fibres is credited to Robert Remak, who published in Berlin in 1838 a remarkable monograph, written in Latin, describing aspects of the structure of the nervous system as gross as the anatomy of the spinal cord and as subtle as his 'fibrae organicae'. Remak's discovery was the more remarkable when it is realized that he was using very primitive microscopes and a limited repertoire of histological techniques. Remak used nerves from animals and from man, which he simply teased apart in water. He described 'fibrae organicae' in somatic and in autonomic nerves but his best illustrations represent fibres from autonomic sympathetic trunks (Fig. 2.1a). In the figure reproduced here, Remak refers explicitly to nucleated corpuscles present in association with the fibres, but the significance of such corpuscles was not grasped by Remak at that time, and, it was Theodor Schwann, one of the pioneers of the cell theory, who fully described the satellite cells of peripheral nerve fibres in his famous monograph published only a year after Remak's. It is interesting, however, that the chance of having described these satellite cells governed Schwann's attitude to theories of the origin of nerve fibres, and he subsequently neglected the axon and pioneered the erroneous cell-chain theory of development of nerve fibres.

The discoverer of unmyelinated fibres was also the discoverer of the axis cylinder in myelinated fibres (Remak, 1837), but Remak failed to describe axons in his unmyelinated fibres and the credit for this is reserved for Tuckett (1895). A feature of unmyelinated fibres which was emphasized by Remak was

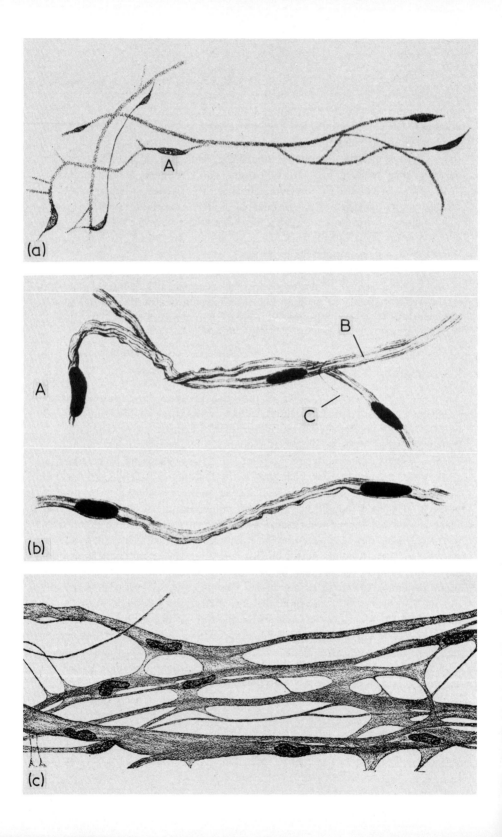

(a)

(b)

(c)

A

B

C

A

their occurrence in practically all nerves . . . 'provided you are skillful enough to prepare the nerves and acquainted with their features' . . . but a number of authors contemporaneous with Remak were convinced he had mistaken connective fibres for nerves.

In 1895 Tuckett published a definitive account of work done in Cambridge which established the basic structure of unmyelinated fibres. By combining microdissection of fresh sympathetic and olfactory nerves with subsequent staining, Tuckett demonstrated that unmyelinated fibres are made of cores surrounded by cellular sheaths (Fig. 2.1b). He insisted that the sheath cells are an intimate component of the fibres and that the cores are processes of neurons which carry the nervous impulse. Tuckett also described some of the degenerative and and regenerative changes seen in unmyelinated fibres following nerve transection.

Another crucial contribution to the study of unmyelinated fibres was made by Walter Ranson (1911) when he modified Cajal's silver stain and applied it to peripheral nerves. Ranson's pyridine-silver technique exposed the unmyelinated axons to microscopic examination better than any previous method (Figs. 2.2a and 2.2b) and initiated an era of counts of unmyelinated axons. Although unmyelinated fibres had been seen in somatic nerves before, Ranson can be regarded as the effective discoverer of somatic unmyelinated fibres. He first remarked upon their abundance in somatic nerves in man and animals (Ranson, 1911), and he demonstrated that the majority of them take origin in the small neurons of the dorsal root ganglia (Ranson, 1911, 1912a). He subsequently traced their centrally directed branches, via the dorsal root, into the medial part of the Lissauer's tract of the spinal cord (Ranson, 1913, 1914), and he attributed to unmyelinated fibres a role in the conduction of impulses related to pain (Ranson, 1915). When Bishop, Heinbecker and O'Leary (1933) contested Ranson's view that the vast majority of unmyelinated axons in somatic nerves are afferent, Ranson, Droegemueller, Davenport and Fisher (1935) produced further convincing evidence to vindicate their own views, today universally accepted.

Nageotte, one of the most perceptive masters of neuro-histology, took a special interest in unmyelinated fibres. He examined them with the advantages of the use of twentieth century light microscopes and his own method of dissociation of the nerve with weak acid solutions following fixation with alcohol. Like Ranvier (1878), Nageotte (1922) noted that unmyelinated fibres

---

Fig. 2.1a   Fibrae organicae from the sympathetic nerve of a man, enlarged about 150 times. A − nodule with a nucleolus. (Reproduced from Remak, (1838), Fig. 3.)

b Fibres of Remak from the carotid canal of a rabbit: teased in aqueous humour, fixed in 1% osmic acid. Grubler's hematoxylin and eosin in glycerine. These fibres, being somewhat flattened through teasing and crushing, show how the sheath breaks into fibrils: A − nucleus; B − core of the fibre; C − sheath. (Reproduced from Tuckett, (1895), *Journal of Physiology,* **19**, Fig. 6.)

c Unmyelinated fibres from the cervical sympathetic of the cat. (Reproduced from Nageotte, (1922), Fig. 41.)

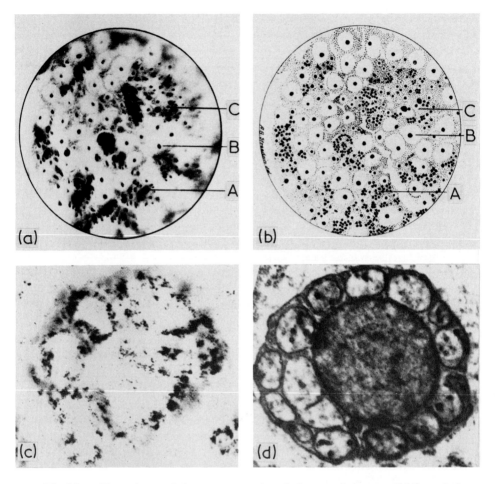

Fig. 2.2a Photomicrograph from a cross section of a human sciatic nerve. Cajal's method. A – non-medullated fibres; B – large medullated fibres; C – small medullated fibres. (Reproduced from Ranson, (1911), *American Journal of Physiology*, **12**, Fig. 7.)

b From a transverse section of a human sciatic nerve. Cajal's method. A – non-medullated fibres; B – large medullated fibres; C – small medullated fibre. (Reproduced from Ranson, (1911), *American Journal of Physiology*, **12**, Fig. 1.)

c Electron microscope picture of C fibres in the saphenous nerve of the cat, stained with silver by the Ranson method. Note the silver precipitation about the fibres. To derive the better known light pictures with this stain, it should be borne in mind that in sections 10 to 20 times as thick (1 to 2 μm) the granules about the fibres would form a continuous ring. Without special precautions in microphotography the rings are caused to appear as solid black dots as the result of light diffraction (Gasser, 1950). (Reproduced from Gasser, (1955), *Journal of General Physiology*, **38**, Fig. 3.)

d Schwann cell sheath containing C fibres in the hypogastric nerve of the cat. (Reproduced from Gasser, (1955), *Journal of General Physiology*, **38**, Fig. 4.)

are arranged in anastomosing fibrous systems, but he improved upon Ranvier's description in his emphasis that only the satellite cells branch and reunite and that axons do not anastomose within the plexus (Fig. 2.1c); he further stressed that each of the anastomosing 'fibres' contains several axons. A feature of unmyelinated fibres which light microscopists, including Nageotte, and early electron-microscopists failed to describe correctly was the fact that their component satellite cells do not form a syncytium, and it is now clear that while these cells are certainly very closely apposed, they retain their individual identity.

Weddell has long been interested in unmyelinated fibres, with particular regard to their relationship to sensation, and his work on unmyelinated fibres has, therefore, been concerned with somatic unmyelinated fibres. The bulk of Weddell's work was carried out before the routine use of electron microscopy in anatomy, but he and his associates wrote extensively concerning degeneration and regeneration of unmyelinated fibres in the skin (Weddell and Glees, 1941; Weddell, Guttmann and Gutmann, 1941; Weddell, 1942). The contributions of Weddell and his school to knowledge of the regeneration of unmyelinated fibres, together with the work of de Castro, are reviewed in Section 2.5.3 of this chapter.

Gasser, an outstanding physiologist, was the first to describe some of the features of unmyelinated fibres visible with electron microscopy (Gasser, 1952, 1955). He had earlier examined the unmyelinated fibres by light microscopy using both fixed nerves stained with silver, and fresh nerves examined using phase contrast optics (Gasser, 1950), but he realized that any new information would come from the use of the electron microscope. From his early observations, it became clear that it is the axonal membranes which bind silver (Figs. 2.2c and 2.2d) and Gasser was able to count unmyelinated axons with greater confidence than had been hitherto possible in light microscope silver preparations. The relatively crude techniques available to electron microscopists in the early fifties were the cause of some misconceptions, particularly with regard to the possible syncytial nature of the Schwann cells and the apparent intracytoplasmatic position of the axons within them. In the mid-fifties, shortly after Geren (1954) published her fundamental paper on the basic fine structural relations of axon and Schwann cell in developing nerves, Gasser (1955) revised his previous opinions and demonstrated that unmyelinated axons are extra cellular and that his 'mesaxon' is a reflected double layer of Schwann cell plasma membrane. This work, together with that of Hess (1956) proved a turning point in our knowledge of the structure of unmyelinated fibres.

2.3 Fine structure

2.3.1 *The Axon*

Axons consist of cell cytoplasm, the axoplasm, contained within a cell membrane, the axolemma. Formed elements such as neurofilaments, microtubules, mitochondria, and very sparse smooth endoplasmic reticulum are

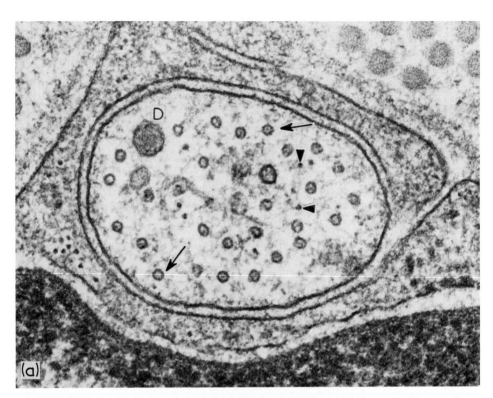

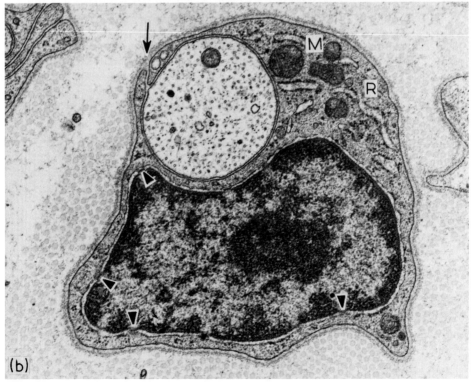

present in the axoplasm of any type of mature or developing axon (Figs. 2.3a, 2.3c and 2.5a). Even before the introduction of aldehyde fixatives for electron microscopy by Sabatini, Bensch and Barnett (1963), microtubules had been described in unmyelinated axons in the cornea of the mouse fixed with osmium tetroxide by Whitear (1960), where she called them 'tubules'. In similarly fixed axons from the cat splenic nerve, Elfvin (1961) described neurotubules as 'thick filaments'. The use of glutaraldehyde fixation as a routine procedure resulted in preservation of microtubules in the cytoplasm of many cells, and in particular in the mitotic spindle, cilia and flagella. The morphology of the fibrous organelles of protein composition such as microtubules and neurofilaments, has been studied extensively in recent years (Palay, McGee-Russell, Gordon and Grillo, 1962; Porter, 1966; Wuerker and Kirkpatrick, 1972) and their participation in the mechanisms for transport of particles within the cytoplasm is receiving increasing acceptance (Schmitt, 1968) (cf.Chapter 1). Microfilaments, even finer than neurofilaments and claimed to be the basis of certain cell movements, may also occur within cell processes (Wessells, Spooner, Ash, Bradley, Luduena, Taylor, Wrenn and Yamada, 1971); in axons such microfilaments are present in growth cones, and it has been shown that their reversible disintegration results in reversible arrest of cone movement (Yamada, Spooner and Wessells, 1971).

Axonal mitochondria are long and have a consistent longitudinal arrangement within the axon. In the sural nerve in man, Dyck and Lambert (1969) have reported the occurrence of 0–4 mitochondria per ultrathin cross section of unmyelinated axons and in the medial popliteal nerve of the baboon mitochondria occur at an average density of one per unmyelinated axon cross section (Fowler and Ochoa, 1975): a similar incidence is found in the majority of laboratory animals. Samorajski and Friede (1968) counted mitochondria per unit cross-sectional area of axon and Schwann cell in myelinated and unmyelinated fibres from sciatic and vagus nerves in adult mice. They found that mitochondrial density in the axoplasm decreased with increasing fibre size, while increasing in the Schwann cell cytoplasm, and they discussed the possible metabolic implications of these findings.

Granular or dense cored vesicles are a prominent feature of some autonomic axons, particularly towards their distal endings; they range in size from 30 nm to 120 nm and have been found to be best preserved by fixation in 3% buffered potassium permanganate (Richardson, 1966). Dense cored vesicles are also seen sparsely scattered along the course of most unmyelinated axons in nerves known to contain both autonomic and somatic fibres (Fig. 2.3a), suggesting that they

---

Fig. 2.3a   Unmyelinated axon from the sural nerve of a child aged 9. The axon contains neurofilaments (arrow heads) and microtubules (arrows). A dense core vesicle (D) is also present. Glutaraldehyde immersion-fixation; osmium tetroxide. (x 104 000.)
b Schwann cell nucleus indented by unmyelinated axon of rounded cross section. Source as in Fig. 2.3a. Note nuclear pores (arrow heads), the mesaxon (arrow), mitochondria (M), and granular endoplasmic reticulum (R) in the Schwann cell. Glutaraldehyde immersion-fixation; osmium tetroxide. (x 24 500.)

113

may also be a normal constituent of somatic unmyelinated axons. Similar granular vesicles occur amongst agranular vesicles in some sensory nerve endings (Banker and Girvin, 1971; Landon, 1972) and in the growth cones of developing and regenerating myelinated and unmyelinated axons. However, following the demonstration of catecholamines in the sediment of granules recovered after ultracentrifugation of homogenized autonomic nerves by von Euler and Hillarp (1956), convincing evidence was produced using electron microscopic autoradiography that dense cored vesicles are the organelles which bind labelled noradrenaline (Wolfe, Potter, Richardson and Axelrod, 1962). While it has been observed that the larger vesicles are not exclusively located in adrenergic endings they nevertheless also appear to bind labelled noradrenaline (Taxi and Sotelo, 1972). The chemical content of dense cored vesicles in axons other than those of autonomic adrenergic neurons remains to be determined.

Dense cored vesicles have been used as natural submicroscopic markers for the indirect assessment of axoplasmic transport in autonomic unmyelinated axons. Dahlström and Fuxe (1964) showed, by means of the fluorescence method of Falck (1962), that catecholamines rapidly accumulate above a local constriction in adrenergic axons; they predicted that this was probably the result of damming up of storage granules manufactured in the neuron cell bodies and transported distally. This hypothesis was subsequently tested by Kapeller and Mayor (1967) using electron microscopy, who confirmed that the material accumulating in the axon under these circumstances consists of dense cored vesicles. It is also possible however that local synthesis could be responsible for the phenomenon, especially in view of the finding of some accumulation of catecholamines distal to the constriction. Actual movement of catecholamines along the nerve was then proved by Livett, Geffen and Austin (1968), who demonstrated the distal displacement of a peak of radioactive noradrenaline between autonomic ganglion cells and the site of nerve constriction. The intra-axonal localization of the tracer was subsequently demonstrated using electron microscopic autoradiography by Geffen, Descarries and Droz (1971).

Like somatic motor nerve fibres, cholinergic autonomic fibres are commonly identified ultrastructurally by the presence of agranular 'synaptic' vesicles in their endings (de Robertis and Bennett, 1955). Such vesicles, however, are not normally seen along the course of axons away from the nerve endings. Cholinergic unmyelinated axons bind methylene blue near their endings, both intravitally and supravitally, whereas adrenergic axons do not (Ehinger, Sporrong and Stenevi, 1967; Richardson, 1968), but the physical basis for this staining specificity, and its possible connection with the presence of acetycholine, has not been determined.

In addition to adrenergic and cholinergic unmyelinated axons, other types can be distinguished on the basis of the contents of their terminals. The use of false neuro-transmitters (e.g. 5 hydroxydopa) and studies of the ultrastructural features of their contained vesicles have enabled Baumgarten, Holstein and Owman (1970) to identify what they term 'p-type fibres' in the Auerbach's plexuses of mammals and man. Such axons contain large granular vesicles (85–150 nm) resembling neurosecretory granules and these, like the granules of endocrine cells, contain a polypeptide substance.

2.3.2 *The Schwann cell*

Satellite cells associated with unmyelinated axons and those associated with myelinated axons have a common embryological origin. The potential ability of satellite cells associated with unmyelinated axons to myelinate has been established from observations on their behaviour in living nerves (Speidel, 1932), and from the results of experiments in which myelinated and unmyelinated nerves were cross-anastomosed (Simpson and Young, 1945; Hillarp and Olivercrona, 1946). It is not surprising, therefore, that there are many structural features shared in common between cells associated with the two types of axon, and also with those associated with fetal axons. For this reason, and because Schwann first described these cells in Remak fibres as well as in developing and mature myelinated nerves, the satellite cells of peripheral nerve fibres of any kind are commonly referred to as 'Schwann cells'. While some authors prefer to call satellite cells of unmyelinated axons 'Remak cells', this has not yet been sanctioned by usage, nor, as was noted earlier, did Remak provide a clear description of these cells.

The nuclei of satellite cells associated with unmyelinated axons are elongated and smooth in contour, aligned longitudinally like a series of bacilli (Figs. 2.1b and 2.5a), and possess one or more nucleoli. They have a reciprocal and variable spatial relationship to their neighbouring axons, which either indent the nucleus or themselves become flattened. In material fixed in glutaraldehyde, the nuclear chromatin tends to accumulate near the surface as an homogeneous stratum fenestrated at the nuclear pores (Fig. 2.3b); but as in other cell types the exact distribution of the chromatin is fixative dependent (Ericsson, Saladino and Trump, 1965). Mitoses are not normally observed in the satellite cells of unmyelinated fibres in the mature animal.

The cytoplasm of the satellite cells contains a variety of organelles in the perinuclear region (Figs. 2.4a–d and 2.5a), while elsewhere in the cytoplasm only occasional filaments, microtubules and sparse mitochondria can be seen in ultrathin sections (Fig. 2.6a). It may, therefore, on occasion be impossible to distinguish between an axon and a Schwann cell process on the grounds of their cytoplasmic features alone, although sometimes such a distinction is facilitated by the more homogeneous density of the Schwann cell cytoplasm matrix (Fig. 2.14c). Elements of the Golgi complex are consistently found near the nucleus of Schwann cells of unmyelinated fibres and were first observed by Cajal (1928, see his Fig. 5) with the help of a special method of silver impregnation. Two centrioles, arranged at right angles, also occur near the nucleus; one of these is usually parallel to the long axis of the cell, so its transverse diameter is frequently seen in cross sections of the Schwann cells (Fig. 2.4a). Rough

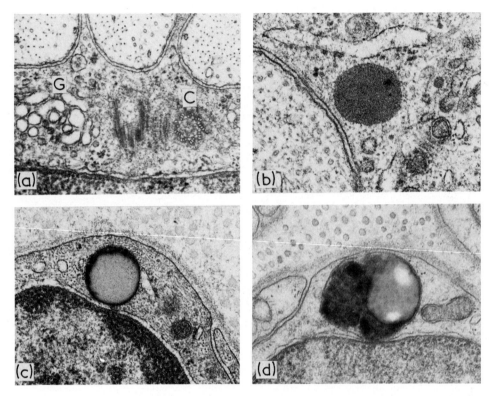

Fig. 2.4a Golgi apparatus (G) and centrioles (C) in Schwann cell of unmyelinated fibre. Cat spinal nerve root. Glutaraldehyde perfusion-fixation followed by osmium tetroxide perfusion fixation. (x 33 500.)
b Membrane bound dense body in the perinuclear cytoplasm of an unmyelinated fibre. Sural nerve from child aged 9. Glutaraldehyde immersion fixation; osmium tetroxide. (x 39 200.)
c Partially extracted osmiophilic droplet (probably lipid), in the perinuclear cytoplasm of unmyelinated fibre. Source and preparation as in Fig. 2.4b (x 32 500.)
d Lysosome in the perinuclear cytoplasm of unmyelinated fibre. From the sural nerve of a man aged 59. Osmium tetroxide immersion fixation. (x 34 000.)

endoplasmic reticulum also occurs, mainly in the perinuclear cytoplasm, together with dense bodies and lipid inclusions. 'Pi' granules are not a feature of the Schwann cells associated with unmyelinated axons, although they are a prominent feature of those of myelinated fibres (cf. Chapter 1.). By contrast, globular inclusions with a content of varying electron density classifiable within the general category of lysosomes, may be prominent within Schwann cells of unmyelinated fibres (Fig. 2.4d), and these appear to increase with age in man (Sharma and Thomas, 1975). Dense bodies similar in appearance to those illustrated in Fig. 2.4b were shown by Weller and Herzog (1970) to have positive acid phosphatase reactions in the Schwann cells of unmyelinated fibres in human nerves.

Whereas the cytoplasm of Schwann cells associated with unmyelinated axons is

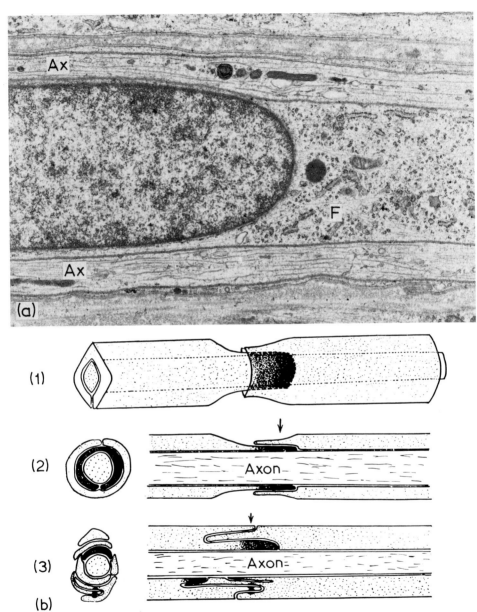

Fig. 2.5a Nuclear region of unmyelinated fibre, from the medial popliteal nerve of baboon, cut longitudinally. Note filaments (F) and ribosomes in Schwann cell cytoplasm and two parallel axons (Ax) near the surface. Glutaraldehyde perfusion-fixation; osmium tetroxide. (x 14 300.)

b Line drawings to show simple ensheathing by part of one Schwann cell of part of the next at a junctional zone (in 1 and 2), and (in 3) interdigitation of one cell with the next, along unmyelinated axons. (Reproduced from Eames and Gamble, (1970), *Journal of Anatomy*, **106**, Fig. 5.)

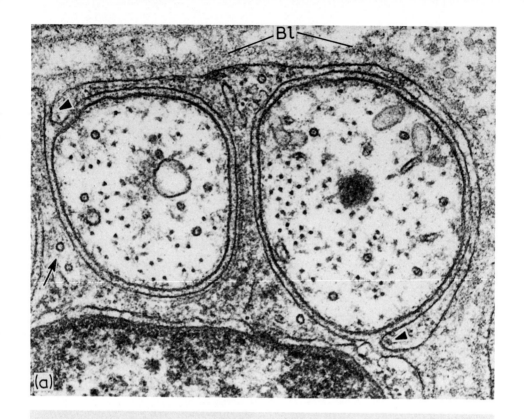

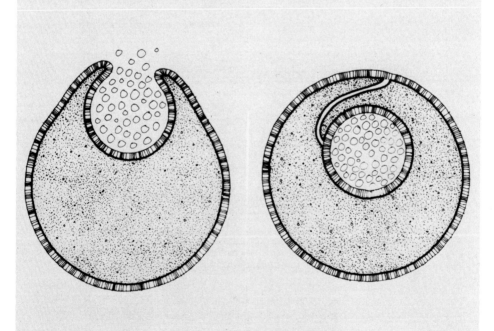

quite electronlucent, an increase in the density has been reported in some of the cell processes that interlock with those of adjacent cells in the chain at their points of contact (Eames and Gamble, 1970) (Fig. 2.5b). Electrondense Schwann cell cytoplasm may occur in other situations than at the cell junctions, and may indeed be quite a striking feature, particularly in nerves primarily fixed with glutaraldehyde, but superficially similar dark appearances may also follow the deliberate use of hypertonic solutions to soak nerves prior to fixation with osmium tetroxide (Elfvin, 1962) (Fig. 2.11f). We have examined a substantial number of nerve biopsies taken from patients suffering from various kinds of peripheral neuropathy, and also from human volunteers without obvious abnormalities of their peripheral nerves, and have only seen such dark Schwann cell processes in nerve fascicles fixed with glutaraldehyde, and taken from a small proportion of the patients suffering from peripheral neuropathies. We have seldom seen such cells in normal or traumatized medial popliteal nerves from anesthetized adult baboons, perfusion-fixed with glutaraldehyde (Fowler and Ochoa, (1975). Carlsen, Knappeis and Schmalbruch (1969) interpreted similar dark profiles observed in nerves from five patients suffering from peripheral neuropathies and fixed with 'isotonic' glutaraldehyde, to be necrotic Schwann cell processes. Appenzeller and Kornfeld (1972) also attributed an abnormal significance to similar dark cell processes in nerves, primarily fixed with glutaraldehyde, taken from two young female patients suffering from cogenital indifference to pain, and proposed the name 'mosaic Schwann cells' to describe them. Morris, Hudson and Weddell (1972) have also remarked upon the presence of a small percentage of 'dark staining' Schwann cells in normal rat sciatic nerves, and in their Fig. 3 they illustrate one such cell cut through the nuclear region and associated with normal axons. In sections from well fixed normal nerves to the internal anal sphincter of rhesus monkeys, Baumgarten, Holstein and Stelzner (1973) have shown light and dark Schwann cell processes, sometimes intermingled in single bundles of unmyelinated fibres. The exact significance of these dark Schwann cells is not at present apparent, but while the phenomenon may be fixation dependent it would seem that such appearances need not necessarily be either artefactual or abnormal; it is possible that the increased electron density may reflect a transient alteration in the functional activity of the Schwann cell.

Fig. 2.6a Two unmyelinated axons totally enveloped by Schwann cell tongues (arrow heads) which define short 'mesaxons'. The cell surface is invested by basal lamina (Bl). Note the gap of regular width between the osmiophilic layer of plasma membranes of axon and Schwann cell. Note also microtubules in Schwann cell cytoplasm (arrow). Source, as in Fig. 2.4a (×78 000.)
b Schematic representation of collagen pockets; open on the left and on the right enclosed by further over growth of all tongues to form a cleft. (Reproduced by courtesy of Mr. L. Moraleda).

2.3.3 *Longitudinal arrangement of the Schwann cells in unmyelinated fibres*

Until relatively recently it was believed that the Schwann cells of unmyelinated fibres formed a syncytium, and it was only in 1958 that Elfvin demonstrated the consecutive nuclei in unmyelinated fibres to belong to individual cells. It was not until very recently however that the actual junction zone between consecutive Schwann cells was specifically studied by Eames and Gamble (1970), who described these junctions in unmyelinated fibres from human nerves, from reconstructions of their fine anatomy seen in electron micrographs of longitudinal and transverse sections (Fig. 2.5b). From their observations it appears that (at least in cutaneous nerves in man) the surface of unmyelinated axons is never wholly devoid of Schwann cell coverage and thus exposed to the endoneurial space since at the cell junctions the processes of adjacent satellite cells interlock. These junctions being rather inconspicuous, measurement of the lengths of Schwann cells associated with unmyelinated axons cannot be made as accurately as in myelinated fibres, where the nodes of Ranvier conveniently mark the edges of adjacent Schwann cell territories. Nevertheless, Peyronnard, Aguayo and Bray (1973) and Peyronnard, Terry and Aguayo (1975), have produced estimates of internuclear distances in unmyelinated fibres from developing, adult and regenerating nerves, and these provide an indirect means of estimating Schwann cell lengths, and therefore, a potential method of assessing the condition of unmyelinated fibres in mature nerves. De la Motte (1972) has claimed that the calibre of unmyelinated axons tend to narrow roughly midway between consecutive cell nuclei and has speculated as to whether this may be related in some way to the site of the junctions between the satellite cells.

2.3.4 *Surface relations between Schwann cell, axon and endoneurial elements*

The plasma membranes of Schwann cells and axons have no distinctive ultrastructural peculiarities that can be resolved by current techniques. Specific molecular features of the cell membranes of unmyelinated fibres, probably relevant to their ability to handle ions, appear to be reflected in the manner in which conduction of the nervous impulse in these fibres is affected by Δ^9 Tetrahydrocannabinol (Byck and Ritchie, 1973), and also the way in which these fibres and other cells bind tetrodotoxin (Colquhoun, Henderson and Ritchie, 1972). It is to be hoped that improvements in microscopical techniques will eventually open to the human eye other aspects of the cell's structure and function concerning which today we can experience only a remote flavour through biochemistry. Some other indications of the existence of special molecular features in the Schwann cell plasma membrane may be gained from its consistent association with a basal lamina, and its apparent affinity for the axonal surface membranes. The interface between the apposed axon and Schwann cell plasma membranes is seen in tissue sections as a gap of very regular width (10–15 nm) when the tissues have been prepared for electron microscopy in the conventional manner (Figs. 2.3a and 2.6a). This finding does not however mean that there is an empty space separating the adjacent membranes, and that they are not actually in contact. It so happens that routine preparatory techniques reveal only the inner part of the plasma membrane, and the apparent 'gap' contains an 'intercellular substance' corresponding to the outer components of the apposed membranes, and these can be revealed by special techniques (cf. Chapter 1). In addition, discretely localized phosphatases and esterases have been demonstrated at both the Schwann cell-axon interfaces and the mesaxons of unmyelinated fibres, by the use of electron histochemistry (Novikoff, Quintana, Villaverde and Forschirm, 1966). Indirect evidence of uptake of substances from the intercellular gap into axon and Schwann cell is provided by the occasional visualization of coated pits, suggesting that micropinocytosis is occurring at the plasma membranes on both sides of the gap (Figs. 2.7a and 2.7b). A similar mechanism would appear to be the chief source of synaptic vesicle formation at the presynaptic terminal axonal membrane in the central nervous system (Turner and Harris, 1973), and at motor end plates (Heuser and Reese, 1973).

The amount of axonal surface which is enclosed by the adjacent Schwann cell processes varies greatly. Unmyelinated axons may be in contact with other neighbouring axons, and in such cases only a sector of the axonal surface may attain contact with the Schwann cell. Sometimes there is no apparent obstacle to the Schwann cell encircling the axon and yet part of the axonal surface may be covered only by basement membrane. Often however, the whole perimeter of the axon is encircled by a Schwann cell, the apposed surfaces of the superficial process forming a membrane-bounded cleft, the mesaxon. The length of the mesaxon obviously depends on the extent to which the apposed tongues overlap. Spiral formation by further growth of the Schwann cell processes, as seen in the early stages of myelination, does not occur to any extent in relation to unmyelinated axons. By contrast, up to three turns may occur around discrete bundles of collagen fibrils adjacent to unmyelinated fibres, implying that unmyelinated axons may actually inhibit further spiral growth of the Schwann cell processes associated with them.

Bundles of collagen fibrils, with or without an intervening cushion of basal lamina are often encircled by processes from Schwann cells of unmyelinated fibres (Figs. 2.6b and 2.7b), and possible mechanisms by which the cell tongues may encircle collagen bundles were illustrated in Fig. 19 by Ochoa and Vial (1967). These interesting formations are what Gamble (1964), and Gamble and Eames (1964) have called 'collagen pockets', and they regarded them to be the result of the active engulfment by Schwann cells of pre-existing collagen. It has been found that in the sural nerve of the human fetus such collagen pockets have not appeared by the eighteenth week of life (Ochoa, 1971). When they are formed is not known, but pockets certainly occur in the nerves of young human adults and in several laboratory animals, in which they are also exclusively associated with unmyelinated fibres. Collagen pockets may be quite numerous in

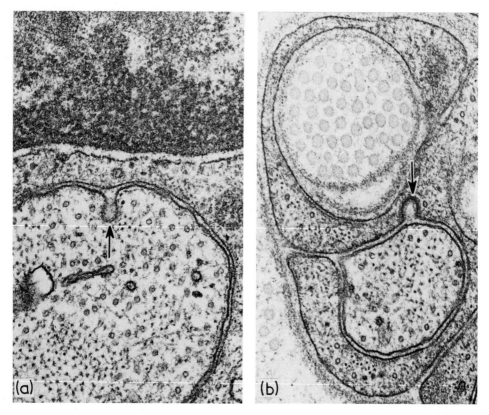

Fig. 2.7a Uptake vesicle (arrowed) in unmyelinated axon, open to the intercellular gap. (x 36 000.)
b Uptake vesicle (arrowed) in Schwann cell, open to the intercellular gap. Note collagen pocket. x 42 000. Fig. 2.7a and b, are taken from the sural nerve of a child aged 9. Glutaraldehyde immersion-fixation, osmium tetroxide.

Fig. 2.8a Some of the developing axons devoid of myelin are still in contact with their fellows; others are held individually by Schwann cell processes. From the sural nerve of a human fetus 18 weeks of age. Glutaraldehyde immersion-fixation; osmium tetroxide (x 9800.)
b Unmyelinated axons just separated from each other by slender Schwann cell septa. The 'fibre' is made of two compact subunits. Medial popliteal nerve of baboon. Glutaraldehyde perfusion-fixation; osmium tetroxide. (x 10 100.)
c Unmyelinated axons well separated from each other. Many are contained in separate Schwann cell processes. From the sural nerve of a boy aged 15. Osmium tetroxide immersion fixation. (x 7200.) Reproduced from Ochoa and Mair, (1969), *Acta Neuropathologica,* **13**, Fig. 6. (Courtesy of Springer Verlag, Berlin-Heidelberg-New York.)
d A well defined unit limited by a common basement membrane, made of Schwann cell subunits of complementary shapes. The collagen fibrils found within the complex are thinner than those found outside. These are the features of regenerated clusters containing axons before myelination. From the sural nerve of a patient suffering from diabetic neuropathy. Osmium tetroxide immersion-fixation. (x 5400.)

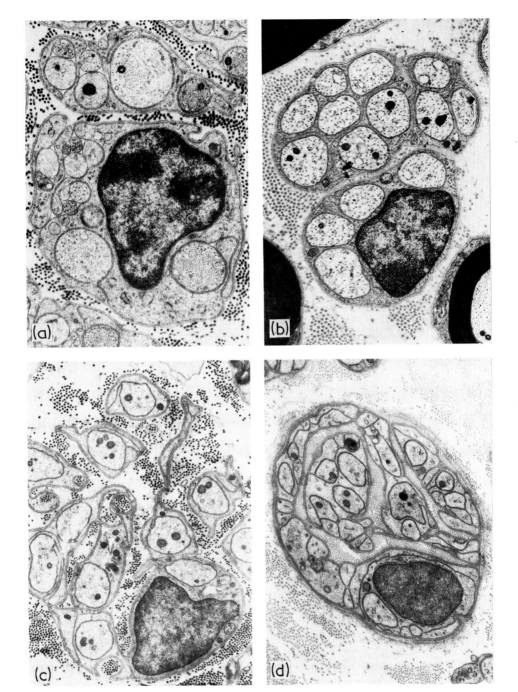

some neuropathies, and this finding has been taken to indicate that newly formed collagen comes to occupy the place of unmyelinated axons after these have degenerated (Thomas, 1973).

2.3.5 *The pattern of axons in unmyelinated fibres*

In peripheral nerves early in development, large numbers of small axons are found lying in close contact with one another. Subsquently the bundles of axons become progressively subdivided through the intervention of the processes of the proliferating Schwann cells (Fig.2.8a). In mature nerves several unmyelinated axons invariably continue to share a common Schwann cell, but the specific pattern of enclosure varies in different species, and in different nerves in the same species. In rare instances, the pattern in mature nerves resembles the fetal arrangement: several unmyelinated axons crowd together in contact with one another, being enclosed as a group by the encircling Schwann cell processes. Olfactory nerves provide the classic example of such an arrangement. In autonomic nerves and in deeply situated somatic nerves, unmyelinated axons are more elaborately enwrapped by Schwann cell processes: axons here are separated from one another by slender tongues, and yet the multiaxonal fibre remains a well-defined compact columnar unit (Fig. 2.8b). An extreme example of the differentiation of unmyelinated fibres occurs in cutaneous nerves in man (Fig. 2.8c); here each unmyelinated axon is again enwrapped individually but the Schwann cells branch into bundles of small processes each enclosing one or two axons which run separately, to reunite only near the nuclear region of the next Schwann cell in the chain. This arrangement, as opposed to the more simple patterns previously described, may be envisaged to serve the purpose of preventing electrical interaction between axons. This relatively elaborate pattern was first noticed by Gamble and Eames (1964) in cutaneous nerves in man, and its characteristic appearance is clearly distinguishable in cross sections from that of units of regenerating axons prior to myelination (Fig. 2.8d). The use of montages of electron micrographs, covering relatively large cross sectional areas of abnormal human cutaneous nerves, greatly assists the recognition of the characteristic patterns of genuine unmyelinated fibres as distinct from clusters of regenerated axons awaiting myelination. This technique permits differential counts of axons devoid of myelin, and prevents evidence of loss of unmyelinated axons from being masked by a contaminating population of regenerating axons (Fig. 2.12c) (Ochoa and Mair, 1969b; Ochoa, 1970a; Ochoa, 1970b).

2.3.6 *The course of unmyelinated axons in the Schwann cell columns*
It is of some theoretical importance to know whether axons which are close neighbours at one point along the nerve fibre continue to be so at other levels, since this anatomical feature is relevant to the possibility of the cross excitation of a resting axon by an adjacent active axon. Katz and Schmitt (1940) were

concerned with this problem in regard to myelinated fibres. On the basis of the estimated spike duration of the action potentials, and the length of the regions of active ionic inflow along unmyelinated axons, Gasser (1955) deduced a minimum length of parallel contact beyond which cross excitation between neighbouring unmyelinated axons could be anticipated. Gasser made unsuccessful attempts to follow the course of unmyelinated axons in teased preparations and in electron micrographs of longitudinal sections of nerves, and he finally turned to reconstructions of unmyelinated fibres from electronmicrographs of consecutive cross sections. Gasser was able in this way to trace the course of fifty odd axons over 500 μm of fibre in the saphenous nerve of the cat and observed that the composition of an individual bundle changed continuously. He came to the conclusion that axons ran in close association for only short distances, and that electrical interaction sufficient to result in cross excitation was unlikely to occur within bundles of unmyelinated axons under normal circumstances. Aguayo and Bray (1975), who have also made elegant three-dimensional reconstructions of unmyelinated fibres from the cervical sympathetic nerve of the rat (Fig. 2.9), similarly emphasize that axons constantly interchange between the anastomosing systems of fibres.

As has been mentioned earlier, electrical interaction is perhaps even more unlikely in cutaneous nerves in man, where unmyelinated axons are often held individually within the processes of branched Schwann cells, and it is of interest that the results of intraneural recordings from single C-fibre units within a cutaneous nerve in human subjects appear to support the view that there is no electrical interaction between such units (Torebjörk and Hallin, 1970).

The question of whether the unmyelinated axons themselves normally branch within the nerve trunks after the stage of their initial development remains an open one. Ranson et al. (1935) commented that unmyelinated axons probably dichotomize and that this would provide an explanation for the greater abundance of axons in peripheral nerves than in their corresponding roots, as had been reported by Davenport and Bothe (1934). However, speculations based solely upon light microscopic counts of axons impregnated with silver are open to question, especially in view of the fact that unmyelinated axons are more closely packed in the roots than in nerve trunks. A direct demonstration of branching of unmyelinated axons by electron microscopy, or alternatively, a demonstration of a significant increase in the number of axons over a long stretch of unbranched nerve, based on electron microscope counts, is still awaited.

Unmyelinated axons undoubtedly branch near their terminals and evidence that this occurs is available from a variety of sources. In so far as sensory unmyelinated axons are concerned there is electrophysiological evidence of branching of unmyelinated fibres in the skin of man, a single C-unit being activated by cutaneous stimulation from more than one site (Hallin and Torebjörk, 1970). Likewise the phenomenon of the 'Axon reflex', observed to follow the application of mustard oil to the conjunctival sac, intradermal

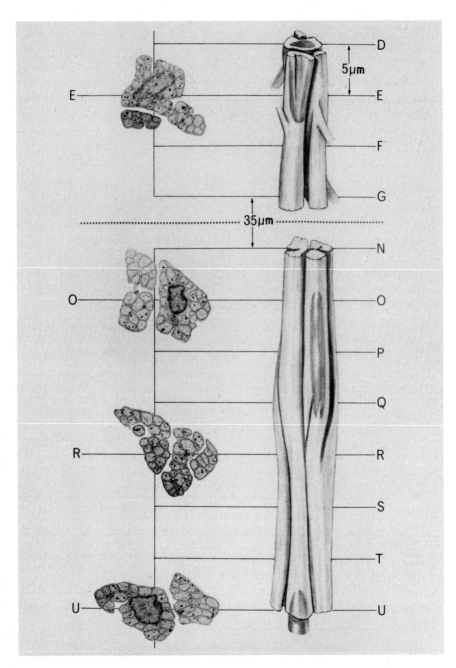

Fig. 2.9 Three-dimensional reconstruction of unmyelinated fibres from a normal rat cervical sympathetic trunk based upon electron micrographs of serial transverse sections (D to U) cut at 5 µm intervals. Four of the electron micrographs are reproduced. The arrangement of axons within Schwann cell units varies from level to level due to branching and fusion of adjacent units. Schwann cell nuclei are present at levels D, O and U. (Reproduced by courtesy of Drs A. J. Aguayo and G. M. Bray, 1974).

injection of histamine or local irritation of the skin by other means (Bruce, 1910; Lewis, 1927), implies connection of individual pain fibres with both the epithelium and a blood vessel (Celander and Folkow, 1953), and necessitates terminal branching of the sensory unmyelinated fibres. Extensive morphological studies of the distribution of unmyelinated fibres in the skin (Weddell, 1941; Weddell, Pallie and Palmer, 1954; Weddell, 1966) using methylene blue intravital staining have not conclusively established the existence of terminal axonal branching, both because of the difficulty in distinguishing true branching from simple separation of overriding axons in a bundle when seen under the light microscope, and because the terminal arborizations of myelinated axons are also unmyelinated and may intermingle with the true unmyelinated terminals. Electron microscopic studies of the innervation of skin have not yet provided us with convincing illustrations of branching of unmyelinated axons but Cauna (1968) states that '. . . non-myelinated fibres divide regularly and the fibre sets gradually split into smaller units. Single (axonal) branches leave such sets to continue their progress within their own Schwann cell covering, and to divide again'. Branching of terminal Schwann cells of unmyelinated fibres to accommodate the multiple small terminal axons in the 'penicillate endings' of the human skin has been illustrated in detail by Cauna (1973).

It is probable that autonomic unmyelinated terminals also dichotomize and observations of axon reflex phenomena involving autonomic effectors support this possibility (Lewis and Marvin, 1927; Bickford, 1938; Coon and Rothman, 1939, 1940; Wada, Aoki and Koyama, 1958).

2.3.7 *Distribution of unmyelinated fibres within the nerve trunks*

In nerves containing both myelinated and unmyelinated fibres, a statement which applies to most somatic nerves, unmyelinated fibres are usually found over the whole cross sectional area of the nerve fascicle (Figs. 2.2a and 2.2b). However, in any particular quadrant it will be found that unmyelinated fibres are not evenly distributed; several multiaxonal fibres usually occurring in groups separated from similar groups by appreciable distances, and small myelinated fibres are often mixed with the groups of unmyelinated fibres (Fig. 2.10a). The association of small myelinated fibres and unmyelinated fibres in some species is sufficiently consistent to enable one to trace the sites at which unmyelinated fibres are abundant in light microscope preparation stained for myelin. This close association between small myelinated and unmyelinated fibres in mature nerves is presumably a consequence of the way in which nerve fibres differentiate during development. Mature large diameter fibres are those which have myelinated first (Boughton, 1906) and hence are the first to be segregated from the primitive bundles of axons devoid of myelin. Unmyelinated fibres are presumably the direct descendants of such stem bundles and may, therefore, be expected to retain a close spatial relationship with the last

127

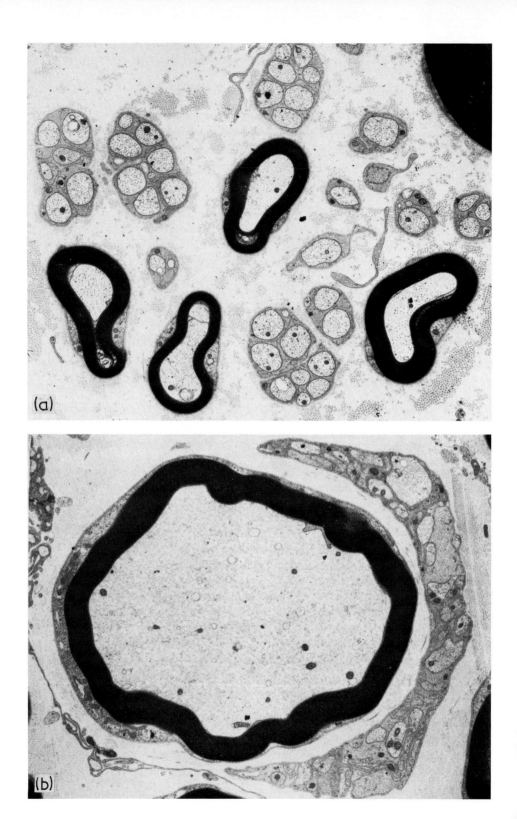

myelinated fibres to be segregated from the bundles, i.e. the small myelinated fibres.

Under some special circumstances unmyelinated and myelinated fibres may acquire new spatial inter-relationships. Regenerated unmyelinated fibres may elect to regrow along pre-existing myelinated fibres, rather than along their previous pathway. This phenomenon probably occurs more frequently than is generally realized, but may be to some extent obscured by the presence within the nerve of unmyelinated regenerating branches from myelinated fibres superficially similar to genuine unmyelinated axons. A happy anatomical circumstance permitted Evans and Murray (1954) to describe this curious phenomenon in the vagus nerve, which divides into a purely myelinated branch, the recurrent laryngeal, and a largely unmyelinated branch, the abdominal vagus. Following a crush in the neck, regenerating autonomic unmyelinated fibres, destined for the stomach, became misdirected into the recurrent laryngeal nerve. Division of the vagus nerve proximal to the nodose ganglion after regeneration demonstrated that the new population of unmyelinated axons in the recurrent laryngeal were not branches of myelinated fibres, since the former persisted whereas all the myelinated fibres degenerated. These exciting experiments were studied by light microscopy but the conclusions have been confirmed subsequently using electron microscopy, and there remains no doubt that genuine unmyelinated fibres can be found in the recurrent laryngeal branch arranged in close relation to myelinated fibres, just outside their basal laminae (King and Thomas, 1971), (Fig. 2.10b). Impressed by the paucity of unmyelinated fibres in neuropathies associated with 'onion bulb' formations and by the resemblance of the outermost components of the whorls of 'onion bulbs' to partially denervated unmyelinated fibres, we concluded that unmyelinated fibres contribute to these formations, and speculated whether a similar tropism to that resulting in the Evans and Murray phenomenon might operate in these neuropathies (Ochoa and Mair, 1969b; Ochoa, 1970b, 1970c).

2.3.8 *Deviations from the natural structure of unmyelinated fibres, caused by preparative procedures*

No one has yet observed normal unfixed unmyelinated fibres at a sufficiently high resolution to permit any final conclusions concerning either the shape or the volume of the axons and the Schwann cell processes. Procedures that are generally thought to preserve the shape of tissues and cells with maximal fidelity, such as freeze-etching, usually result in images of unmyelinated axons

---

Fig. 2.10a   Small myelinated fibres intermingled with groups of unmyelinated fibres: a characteristic association. From the middle popliteal nerve of baboon. Glutaraldehyde perfusion-fixation, osmium tetroxide. (x 6700.)
b Regenerated unmyelinated fibres, misdirected into a nerve not normally containing unmyelinated fibres, are arranged around a myelinated fibre. (x 6340.) (Reproduced by courtesy of Drs Rosalind King and P. K. Thomas.)

which are regularly round or oval in cross section (see illustrations in articles by Bischoff, 1970, and by Devine, Simpson and Bertaud, 1971).

The shape, volume and composition of living structures are greatly changed in the course of preparation for electron microscopy. These changes occur chiefly at the stage of fixation, different fixatives preferentially preserving some subcellular components at the expense of others. The final appearance following primary fixation with osmium may be quite different from that which follows the use of glutaraldehyde, especially in respect to cell volume and the structure of the unit membranes and microtubules (cf. Figs. 2.6a and 2.15b). Osmolarity is one of the most important variables of the fixative and may greatly influence such features of the preparation as volume and shape, and the effect on unmyelinated fibres of changes in the osmolarity of the fixative was the specific subject of a study by Elfvin (1962). By treating nerves with solutions of different compositions before and during fixation, Elfvin provoked changes in the shape and volume of axonal and Schwann cell processes, involving both swelling and shrinkage. In the situation in which nerves were exposed to distilled water prior to fixation, there was shrinkage of the axons, while the Schwann cells became swollen (Fig. 2.11). A valuable survey of the chemical and morphological changes caused by fixatives in general are given in a review by Hopwood (1969). Besides changes in structure of the tissues caused by the fixative itself, changes may occur due to metabolic derangement immediately prior to fixation. Interference with the blood supply to the nerve, possibly caused by haemostatic manoeuvres during biopsy, may result in mitochondrial disruption, indistinguishable from early post mortem changes in axons and Schwann cells. Other rapid, and possibly reversible changes in volume are known to occur in unmyelinated axons subjected to metabolic stress (Mire, Hendelman and Bunge, 1970). Finally, it cannot be emphasized too strongly that changes in shape and volume which may at first sight appear to be a genuine consequence of cell damage, may equally be the result of fixation or preparation, and such changes obviously affect the validity of axonal measurements.

2.4 Numbers and sizes of unmyelinated axons

Unmyelinated fibres are the most numerous components of mixed nerves, autonomic nerves and cutaneous nerves; but counting and measuring their axons with confidence requires much labour and the use of the electron microscope. The need to discern whether a rounded profile is an axon or a collagen pocket or a Schwann cell process arises continuously, and this requires some deliberation and experience. Even when it is quite clear that a given profile is an axon, it is possible to mistake the node of a small myelinated fibre for an unmyelinated axon, and in nerves containing regenerating myelinated fibres it may be difficult to distinguish genuine unmyelinated axons from axon sprouts that will in time become myelinated. The need to recognize and discount such small and as yet unmyelinated regenerating axons is mandatory if one is to obtain unbiased

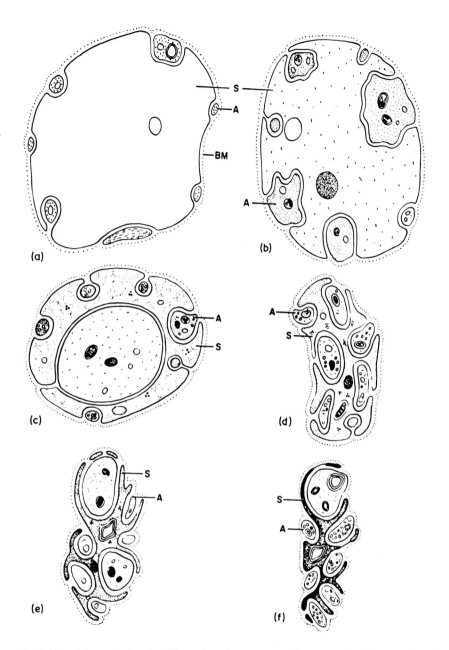

Fig. 2.11 Schematic drawing illustrating the structure of cross-sectioned unmyelinated nerve fibres which have been exposed to hypotonic or hypertonic milieu for 2 hours before fixation with osmium tetroxide. The soaking fluids were in (a) distilled water; (b) Tyrode's solution without NaCl; (c) NaCl Tyrode; (d) 2 NaCl Tyrode; (e) 5 NaCl Tyrode; (f) 10 NaCl Tyrode. A – axon; S – Schwann cell; B – basement membrane. (Reproduced from Elfvin, (1962), *Journal of Ultrastructure Research,* 7, Fig. 19.)

estimates of the numbers of unmyelinated fibres in cases of peripheral neuropathy, where such contamination is to be expected (Fig. 2.12c). In some species, unfortunately, such distinctions cannot be made with confidence.

Interest in the numbers of unmyelinated axons in peripheral nerves and nerve roots started with the work of Ranson and his associates (1935), who initiated systematic counts of axons from animals and man stained with silver, using the light microscope. Ranson and his colleagues reported that amongst somatic peripheral nerves, cutaneous nerves were those which contained the highest numbers of unmyelinated axons. Anyone familiar both with silver staining techniques and with electron microscopy might have predicted that counts of unmyelinated axons stained with silver would underestimate their true numbers (see Fig. 2.2c). However, the differential estimates of Ranson *et al.* (1935) in cutaneous nerves in man are close to those calculated using electron microscopy by Ochoa and Mair (1969a) in the sural nerve in man. Such surprising agreement is perhaps explicable by the peculiarity of the cutaneous nerves in man described in a previous section, by which the axons are held independently by branched Schwann cells and can be distinguished individually even when only roughly outlined by the silver deposits. From the data put forward by Ranson *et al.* (1935) and by Ochoa and Mair (1969a), unmyelinated axons outnumber myelinated axons in cutaneous nerves in man by the ratio of 3 or 4 to 1. In the rat, Landon and Preston (1963), using electron microscopy, found that unmyelinated axons predominated in the ratio of 4:1 in the saphenous nerve, whereas in the nerve to the medial head of the gastrocnemius muscle, myelinated and unmyelinated axons were equally represented.

One of the most thorough quantitative studies of the numbers and calibres of unmyelinated axons on record was carried out by Gasser (1950) using silver impregnation techniques. Gasser analysed the optical problems involved in the measurements of enlarged photomicrographs and also made the necessary corrections for tissue shrinkage. He proposed a size range of 0.4–1.25 μm for unmyelinated axons in the saphenous nerve of the cat and published the first histogram of unmyelinated axon diameters, which had an unimodal distribution. A few years later, Gasser reported a size range of 0.25–1.4 μm for unmyelinated axons in the sural nerve of the cat based on electron microscopy; this size distribution was also unimodal (Gasser, 1955).

The fibre size spectrum of myelinated fibres is known to vary intra-specifically, and it would be reasonable to expect a fair degree of variation of unmyelinated axon diameter in individuals of the same species and age group. This variation is perhaps reflected in the lack of agreement between the various reports of unmyelinated axonal size, in any given species. However, many of the differences between published reports are probably due to change in volume and shape during the preparation of the nerves for microscopy and are most pronounced when tissue prepared by different methods is compared. If such comparisons are restricted to quantitative studies based on electron microscopy of cutaneous nerves in adult man, the extreme values reported for unmyelinated

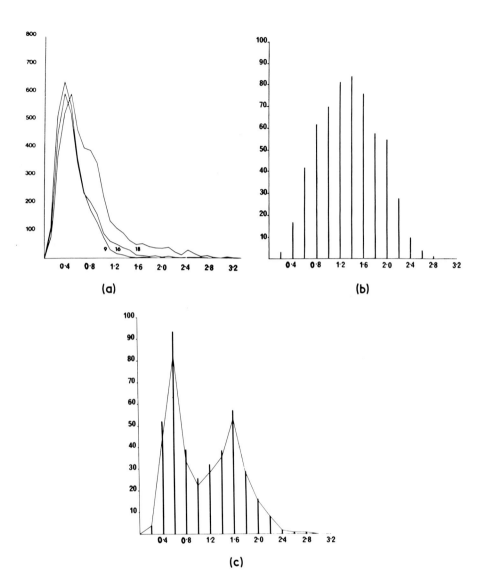

Fig. 2.12a Contours of histograms of diameters of developing axons in sural nerves from three human fetuses aged 9, 16 and 18 weeks. (Reproduced from Ochoa, (1971), *Journal of Anatomy,* 108, Fig. 4.)
b A unimodal histogram of diameters of unmyelinated axons in the sural nerve from a young normal adult. Reproduced from Ochoa and Mair, (1969), *Acta Neuropathologica,* 13, Fig. 7b, (by courtesy of Springer Verlag, Berlin-Heidelberg-New York).
c Bimodal histogram of diameters of unmyelinated axons in the sural nerve of a patient suffering from neuropathy due to isoniazid. Note that the additional population of minute axons nearly coincides in size range with that of fetal axons (in Fig. 2.12a). Axons devoid of myelin other than genuine unmyelinated axons have been discounted and their contribution separated above the continuous line. (Reproduced from Ochoa, (1970), *Brain,* 93, Fig. 4.)

fibre diameters from pooled data are 0.2–3.5 μm. Values from specific reports have been 0.5–3.5 μm (Weller, 1967); 0.2–3 μm (Ochoa and Mair, 1969a); 0.3–1.5 μm (Dyck and Lambert, 1969); 0.2–2–2 μm (Dyck, Lambert and Nichols, 1971). Which of these values best approaches the *in vivo* state is unknown, but for practical purposes this is unimportant.

The question of the size range and frequency distribution of unmyelinated axon diameters, in normal and abnormal nerves, is still a matter of debate but has some significance in pathological diagnosis. It was noted in early counts of unmyelinated axons in normal and abnormal nerves that the usual diameter distribution is unimodal (Ochoa and Mair, 1969a) (Fig. 2.12b), whereas in abnormal nerves there is an increase in the proportion of the small diameter axons (Ochoa and Mair 1969b; Ochoa 1970a) (Fig. 2.12c). Bray, Peyronnard and Aguayo (1972b) have also illustrated a change from an unimodal to a bimodal histogram in partially degenerated autonomic nerves of the rabbit. As discussed in another section (Section 2.5.3), we regarded the small axons responsible for the bimodality to be regenerating sprouts and we regard evidence of regeneration of unmyelinated axons to be a useful criterion for the recognition of previous damage to unmyelinated fibres. Other workers in the field have reported unimodal histograms in normal cutaneous nerves (Aguayo, Nair and Bray, 1971; Carlsen and Knappeis, 1973), but Dyck, Lambert and Nichols (1971) report having found bimodal size distributions in the sural nerves of some young persons. Unmyelinated fibres in animal material fixed by aldehyde perfusion also usually show a unimodal size distribution (see Fig. 2.14a) (Marotte, 1972; Bray *et al.*, 1972b; Dyck and Hopkins, 1972; Aguayo and Bray, 1975; Fowler and Ochoa, 1975).

When it comes to estimates of the numbers of unmyelinated axons in nerves, problems arise which relate to the technical difficulties inherent in attempts to achieve total counts in the whole nerve, and the limited significance of numbers per unit area. The limitations to the latter approach depend to some extent on the patchy distribution of unmyelinated fibres in the nerves, but more importantly concern the variable volume changes caused by different preparation procedures. For the practical purposes of pathological diagnosis we find that the detection of the presence of Schwann cell bands devoid of axons (Figs. 2.15a and b) is a straightforward exercise and is as reliable an indication of a loss of axons as is the more time-consuming demonstration of an absolute loss of axons by counting their numbers (Ochoa, 1970c).

In summarizing the essential points concerning counts and measurements of unmyelinated axons in normal adult nerves using electron microscopy, it is possible to state that their mean diameter is smaller in small than in large animals and also smaller in autonomic than in somatic nerves; that the smallest axons of all have a diameter in the region of 0.2 μm, while the largest can be at least as large as the smallest myelinated axons; and that normal unmyelinated axons usually have a unimodal distribution in size-frequency histograms, and major deviations from this unimodal distribution indicate abnormality.

2.5 Growth of unmyelinated fibres

2.5.1 *Elongation, orientation and differentiation of developing axons*

The axons of peripheral unmyelinated fibres are the outgrowths of small neurons of the sensory ganglia and from autonomic neurons of the sympathetic chain and parasympathetic ganglia. Unmyelinated fibres are also found in the ventral roots (Coggeshall, Coulter and Willis, 1973); their cells of origin are probably situated in the dorsal root ganglia. Knowledge concerning the process of elongation of developing unmyelinated fibres and of their orientation towards their end organs, as distinct from the similar processes undergone by myelinated fibres, is limited. In most sensory and mixed nerves, an understanding of these phenomena is limited by the difficulties in distinguishing true unmyelinated fibres from the unmyelinated precursors of myelinated fibres. However, there is no indication that the course of events differs significantly in the two types of fibre, and such brief accounts of the early development of peripheral sympathetic nerves as have been published suggest that similar growth mechanisms occur in the two types of fibre. Cajal (1905a) for example referred to developing sympathetic nerves in mammals as consisting at an early stage of 'naked Remak axons with no interstitial cells', and he also described frequent branching of these neuronal outgrowths and the presence of 'growth cones'.

Amongst the most informative contributions to the subject of growth of developing axons were those derived from studies of living nerves by Harrison (1924) and by Speidel (1932, 1933, 1935). In his classic series of reports on microscopic observations of living nerves of amphibian larvae, Speidel illustrated a number of fascinating dynamic aspects of the behaviour of axons, Schwann cells and interstitial tissues, and the process of axonal elongation and the activities of the Schwann cells of 'myelin emergent' and 'non-myelin emergent' sprouts were described in detail. With regard to the behaviour of the axonal outgrowths themselves, he found that they appeared to have a common repertoire of reactions: elongation, amoeboid movements of the growth cones, the production of branches, interaction with neighbouring fibres and cells, all occurred in a similar fashion in both 'myelin emergent' and 'non-myelin emergent' axons, although the rate of elongation was faster in 'non-myelin emergent' sprouts, and, as Speidel commented, a number of the so-called 'non-myelin emergent' sprouts must have been immature genuine unmyelinated fibres. As to the behaviour of the 'sheath cells', Speidel insisted that cells related to 'non-myelin emergent' sprouts could migrate freely towards other fibres and could engage in myelin formation, whereas cells connected with myelinated fibres could not migrate. If these observations are applicable to other species, they are the most direct proof of the existence of a single type of Schwann cell for myelinated and unmyelinated fibres, and they endorse the view that myelination is controlled by the particular properties of the axon. Webster and Billings (1972) have recently observed developing nerves *in vivo* using a differential interference microscope, and have been able to trace mitochondrial movements and to prepare samples of selected areas of nerve for electron microscopy.

An aspect of the problem of growth which remains almost totally obscure is the mechanism of guidance of growing axons towards their peripheral endings. In the case of regenerating axons within nerve trunks, their course towards the periphery is largely determined by pre-existing columns of Schwann cells (Cajal, 1905b; Ranson, 1912b) but even in this undoubtedly over-simplified model there may be selectivity, as for instance in insects (Pearson and Bradley, 1972), where fast and slow motor neurons are claimed to appropriately reinnervate fast and slow muscle after nerve transection. In the case of developing axons in the embryo it must be remembered that, initially, axons grow towards the periphery in the absence of satellite cells: these appear at a later stage and migrate along the bundles of axons (Harrison, 1924). This represents a basic difference between development and regeneration to which little attention is usually paid.

The nature of the process that determines the course of pioneer axons during development, and their orientation towards their end organs has interested many biologists in the past. Theories *en vogue* in earlier decades of this century have included chemotaxis (Cajal, 1892); the influence of electrical fields, so-called galvanotropism (Käppers, 1971), the influence of rapidly growing neighbouring peripheral organs (Detwiler, 1936, quoted by Weiss, 1955); and stereotropism (Lewis and Lewis, 1912; Speidel, 1933; Weiss, 1941). Paul Weiss (1955) has reviewed this topic and has argued convincingly against a role for 'galvanotropism' and 'chemotaxis', and in favour of local physical phenomena which he termed 'contact guidance'. Dunn (1971) in recent years has analysed the processes involved in the orientation of axon outgrowths in tissue culture of chicken dorsal root ganglia, and has reached the conclusion that the axonal behaviour can best be explained by 'contact inhibition', a phenomenon initially described by Loeb (1921) from observations of the movement of amoebocytes *in vitro*. Dunn has used time-lapse cine-microphotography to document the realignment of the path of the growing tip of an axon when it makes contact with a neighbour and has confirmed the earlier observations of Nakajima (1965). Growth in a more or less straight line would, according to Dunn (1971) be the course least likely to be obstructed by other cells. It is possible that similar inhibitory mechanisms contribute to the definition of the terminal territories innervated by any given neural unit: excessive extension by branching might normally be curtailed by the presence of neighbour neurites.

There has recently been remarkable progress in the field of study concerned with the growth and differentiation of neurons, and in particular of those giving rise to unmyelinated axons. The early experiments of Rita Levi-Montalcini in collaboration with Cohen opened up a new era in the study of the biology of the neuron, as they led to the discovery and subsequent identification of a powerful protein agent that promotes growth of embryonic sympathetic and sensory nerve cells, later called 'Nerve Growth Factor'. Levi-Montalcini and

Cohen first detected this factor in mouse sarcomata, then in snake venom, and subsequently found it in large amounts in the submaxillary salivary gland of the male mouse (Levi-Montalcini and Booker, 1960a; Cohen, 1960). The preparation of a nerve growth factor anti-serum (Cohen, 1960) and its experimental use in newborn animals resulted in dramatic destruction of sympathetic neurons (Levi-Montalcini and Booker, 1960b) and hence of unmyelinated fibres in cervical sympathetic nerves (Aguayo, Martin and Bray, 1972). With these findings in mind Aguayo *et al.* (1971) have proposed that familial disorders in which development of sympathetic and sensory unmyelinated fibres appear to be selectively arrested, such as Familial Dysautonomia (Riley-Day Syndrome), may be due to some abnormal process involving nerve growth factor. It is also interesting that systemic administration to newborn animals of adrenergic blocking agents, such as 6-hydroxydopamine (Thoenen and Tranzer, 1968; Angeletti and Levi-Montalcini, 1972) may also result in selective degeneration of catecholamine containing sympathetic neurons, but in this instance there is sparing of sensory neurons, as also of parasympathetic neurons. More recently selective degeneration of central serotonin containing neurons and their axons has been induced by 5–6 dihydroxytryptamine (Baumgarten, Björklund, Holstein and Nobin, 1972; Daly, Fuxe and Jonsson, 1973). Much remains to be discovered about the mechanisms that bring about neuronal degeneration following the administration of neurotransmitter blocking agents.

2.5.2 *Quantitative studies and the fine structure of developing axons*

At an early stage of development, all axons in both autonomic and somatic nerves are uniformly narrow and devoid of myelin. When Schwann cells join the developing nerve trunks, they embrace bundles of axons each of which continues for some time to lie in contact with several of its fellows (Fig. 2.8a). The processes by which some of these axons become segregated from neighbours and myelinate are described in Chapter 6 (p. 333). The remaining axons, i.e. those that will not myelinate, also increase their diameter to a limited extent, but they retain many features of their undifferentiated precursors, such as the sharing of the same Schwann cell by several axons and the absence of myelin sheaths: these axons will constitute the unmyelinated axons of mature somatic and autonomic nerves (Peters and Muir, 1959; Cravioto, 1965; Gamble, 1966; Allt, 1969; Ochoa, 1971; Webster, 1971; Aguayo and Bray, 1975).

It is impossible to tell in an early developing axon-Schwann cell bundle to which category any particular axon belongs, because of their structural uniformity. In the sural nerve of the human fetus, for example, the smallest axons between the fetal ages of 9–18 weeks are of the order of 0.1 μm in diameter, but with advancing maturation bimodality becomes evident (Fig. 2.12a), probably due to the faster rate of growth of a second population with initially closely similar dimensions (Ochoa, 1971). When as a result of further maturation the populations of myelinated fibres become distinguishable from the unmyelinated population, the latter continues to have a unimodal distribution both in somatic and autonomic nerves in man (Ochoa and Mair, 1969a; Sharma and Thomas, 1975) and in several animal species (Gasser, 1950; 1955; Marotte, 1972; Dyck and Hopkins, 1972; Aguayo and Bray, 1975; Fowler and Ochoa, 1975).

In developing autonomic nerves, such as the sympathetic trunk of the rat, the smallest axons present just before birth have a diameter of the order of 0.3 μm. With further maturation the axons increase in size, the total number of Schwann cells also increasing, so that as in somatic nerves the number of axons contained within each Schwann cell unit progressively falls with time (Aguayo and Bray, 1975). Despite this increase in number of Schwann cells, elongation of the unmyelinated axons with growth is accompanied by progressive longitudinal separation of Schwann cells, whose territories must therefore extend to continue to provide coverage for their contained axons. This effect, which has its counter part in the increase in internodal length of myelinated fibres with growth, has been demonstrated in unmyelinated fibres of the sympathetic trunk in the rat (Peyronnard, Terry and Aguayo, 1975) by the finding of an increase in Schwann cell internuclear distance with maturation.

The conduction velocities of unmyelinated fibres in the cervical sympathetic trunk of growing rats has been shown by Hopkins and Lambert (1973) to increase, from half of their normal adult values to adult values, between the tenth and the fifty-eighth day after birth. They attribute the observed increase in conduction velocity to the expected increase in axonal diameter over that period.

Developing axons contain neurofilaments, microtubules, smooth endoplasmic reticulum and mitochondria suspended in an amorphous matrix, but the axonal processes of very small diameter are barely able to accommodate a mito-chondrion. In developing autonomic nerves (Pick, Gerdin and Delemos, 1964; Aguayo and Bray, 1975), and also in developing mixed nerves, some axons in the sections can be seen to contain the dense cored granules usually considered to contain catecholamines. Occasional developing axons may be cut through swollen portions which contain abundant vesicles, mitochondria, endoplasmic reticulum and lamellated bodies. These have been interpreted to be evidence of spontaneous degeneration (Reier and Hughes, 1972), but growth cones consisting of the dilated portions at the tips of growing axons (Cajal, 1892; Harrison, 1907; Speidel, 1933) also contain a variety of submicroscopic organelles. Although some useful criteria have been recommended to aid the fine structural distinction between regenerating and degenerating axons, that depend upon their subcellular contents as seen in ultrathin sections (Lampert, 1967), only limited reliance can be placed upon such recommendations since it has been shown that within the tips of growing axons there may occur marked longitudinal stratification of organelles (Ochoa and Morgan-Hughes, 1974), the cytoplasmic contents in cross sections having quite different appearances at the different levels of section through the axon tip. Evidence is available that would appear to support either of these interpretations. On one hand it is known that, during certain stages of development, the number of peripheral neurons increase. This event has been documented quantitatively in dorsal root ganglia from the human fetus (McKinnis, 1935), and from the chicken embryo (Hamburger and Levi-Montalcini, 1949), and would be in keeping with the finding of axonal tips within developing nerves. On the other hand, there is also evidence of degeneration of neurons in developing dorsal root ganglia of the chicken embryo (Hamburger and Levi-Montalcini, 1949), and a clear fall in the total number of axons during post-natal development of autonomic nerves in rat (Aguayo, Terry and Bray, 1973), and in the ventral roots of developing tadpoles (Prestige and Wilson, 1972). It seems clear that during development the two processes of new growth and limited degeneration occur *pari passu*, and that at different times and in different body segments one or the other predominates. This balance appears to be at least partially controlled by the properties of the corresponding peripheral end organs (Hamburger and Levi-Montalcini, 1949).

There has been justified interest in recent years in studying the fine structure and dynamics of growth cones in central and peripheral neurons. Our understanding of the motile processes of growth cones was significantly increased when a network of peculiar microfilaments 5 nm in diameter, half the size of neurofilaments and similar in appearance to those of the contractile ring of cleaving eggs and dividing cells (Schroeder, 1968; 1973), was demonstrated beneath the plasma membrane in growth cones of axons of dorsal root ganglion neurons undergoing elongation *in vitro* (Yamada, Spooner and Wessells, 1970, 1971). They were found to disappear following administration of cytochalasin B, a substance which is capable of arresting some forms of cytokinesis, including movement of growth cones, without apparently affecting protein synthesis or axonal transport (Yamada *et al.*, 1971; Wessells *et al.*, 1971).

There appear to be some subtle differences in the reported ultrastructural features of growth cones from various types of neurons. Whether these are real differences related to neuronal type or the result of different techniques of preparation or culture (or even of planes of section) on essentially similar structures is however unknown. The particular ultrastructural features of growth cones of sensory unmyelinated fibres during development have not been determined but those of sympathetic neurons in tissue culture have been elegantly illustrated by Bunge (1973).

2.5.3 *Regeneration of unmyelinated fibres*

While the amount of information available concerning regeneration of myelinated fibres far outweighs that available on the regeneration of unmyelinated fibres, it would nevertheless be a mistake to underestimate the value of early light microscope observations and what they teach about such regenerative processes. When Cajal (1905b, p. 205) wrote that 'growth, branching and orientation of regenerated nerve fibres is governed by the attractive action of chemotactic substances produced by the cells of Schwann', and later '. . . such influence, analogous to the one we proposed many years ago to explain the phenomenon of growth and connection of embryonic nerve fibres . . .' he was not referring exclusively to myelinated fibres but to nerve fibres of all types. Despite the fact that his silver technique was not ideally suited to explore unmyelinated fibres, and the difficulties inherent in attempts to distinguish between the types of regenerated fibre in the distal stump of an interrupted nerve, Cajal (1905b, p. 160) described many interesting changes in the unmyelinated fibres of the proximal stumps of transected nerves. These included the branching of unmyelinated axons in the proximal stump, their minute growth cones, the orientation of most sprouts towards the scar, and the recurrent course taken by a minority. Another phenomenon described by Cajal (1905b) and illustrated in his Fig. 13e, is the association of regenerated sprouts of unmyelinated fibres with a surviving myelinated fibre which thus becomes surrounded by unmyelinated branches. This may be a prominent, though unremarked, example of the tropism by which unmyelinated become associated with myelinated fibres (see Section 2.3.7).

Walter Ranson (1912b) contributed valuable data, seldom quoted today, concerning the degeneration and regeneration of unmyelinated fibres in the sciatic nerve of the dog following nerve transection. The use of his pyridine-silver method (a modification of Cajal's method) enabled Ranson to produce a lucid report of continuing authority, all the more so when it is remembered that, at that time, the polygenistic theory of theory of axonal regeneration still retained many adherents. Together with a detailed description of degenerative changes in the distal stump, he described retrograde changes affecting unmyelinated axons for a short distance proximal to the lesion. He found that by the fourteenth day following transection, when unmyelinated fibres just proximal to the scar still showed signs of traumatic degeneration, numerous new axons had been produced from unmyelinated fibres higher up in the proximal stump. Because of the compact grouping of the regenerated axons, Ranson was not able to witness the actual sites of axon branching, but this could be presumed from the great increase in the total number of axons present. While it was not possible to distinguish the unmyelinated from the future myelinated sprouts within the scar, this could be achieved in the proximal stump by virtue of the higher level at which sprouting occurred in unmyelinated fibres (Ranson, 1912b). Sprouts with growth cones then penetrated the distal stump (guided by 'stereotropism' and 'chemotaxis') and many appeared to invade appropriate slender protoplasmic bands that Ranson believed he could distinguish from the larger bands of Büngner corresponding to the pre-existing myelinated fibres.

Studies of degeneration, and more particularly of regeneration, of unmyelinated fibres, are bound to be more informative when performed on autonomic rather than on somatic nerves, since the possibility of confusion caused by the presence of unmyelinated sprouts of myelinated axons is minimized. The monumental work by Fernando de Castro, from Madrid, who by 1930 had published the results of experiments on the sympathetic nerves of 160 cats and 9 dogs, probably constitutes the most comprehensive document available on this subject. Although little credit is given to de Castro's contribution today, its scope has yet to be matched by electron microscopic studies of greater resolution, but necessarily more limited perspective based on ultrathin tissue sections. Some earlier studies by Langley (1897) and by Tsukagushi (1916), although less extensive than de Castro's, also deserve attention. De Castro clearly illustrated and minutely described regeneration of unmyelinated fibres in pre- and post-ganglionic sympathetic nerves. He found that the processes of collateral branching and terminal growth started in the proximal stump between 50–60 hours after injury in post-ganglionic fibres and a little earlier in the pre-ganglionic fibres (Fig. 2.13), but the very rapid regeneration, reported by Cajal (1950b) in the sciatic nerve, was not observed by de Castro. Some axonal outgrowths followed a recurrent path but the majority invaded the scar and elongated in close association with pre-existing Schwann cell columns. The regenerated fibres did not necessarily grow into their corresponding old tubes in the distal stump, and de Castro attributed some of the functional anomalies which may occur after regeneration of autonomic nerves to this mismatching. Chromatolytic changes in the nerve cell body during the course of regeneration of sympathetic nerves were also described in this report.

An issue which is dealt with only superficially in the reports cited above concerns the orientation of regenerating unmyelinated axons with relation to the Schwann cell columns of the distal stump. It is probable that after being crushed, providing that the Schwann cell sheath (basal lamina) retains its continuity, each axonal sprout enters its corresponding old Schwann tube. After nerve transection, however, regenerating fibres are not necessarily directed toward their own particular columns of Schwann cells and endings, and it appears that each regenerating neuron may eventually make contact with a larger periphery than normal as a result of intrafascicular axonal branching (de Castro, 1930; Murray and Thompson, 1957). Another difficult question which has received little attention is whether, after transection of nerves containing a mixed population of myelinated and unmyelinated fibres, the regenerated axons grow specifically into Schwann cell columns of the appropriate type and achieve appropriate peripheral connections. We do know that when given no other choice, for example after cross-union of myelinated and unmyelinated nerves (Simpson and Young, 1945), regenerating axons invade the wrong type of Schwann cell band, and that bands formerly belonging to unmyelinated fibres can be induced to myelinate their new axons. We also know that regenerating unmyelinated fibres may follow the course of myelinated fibres and become misdirected into a myelinated branch of a nerve rather than follow their previous course into an unmyelinated nerve. As mentioned earlier, this rare phenomenon was described by Evans and Murray by light microscopy in 1955 in a series of convincing experiments on the recurrent laryngeal nerve and their observations have recently been corroborated by King and Thomas (1971) using electron

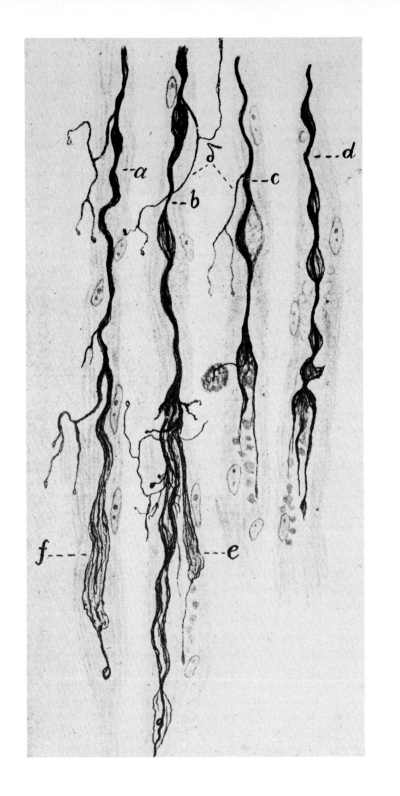

microscopy. A probable isolated example of such tropism is illustrated in Fig. 13e of Cajal (1950b). How frequently these departures from normal behaviour are found in regenerating nerves is hard to tell, but it might be profitable for physiologists to reflect upon how such anomalous regenerations might affect the interpretation of their physiological experiments.

Another intriguing facet of axon regeneration, well described for unmyelinated fibres, is the growth of collateral branches from intact axons following the loss of others within sympathetic nerve trunks (Murray and Thompson, 1957), and the analogous process of the growth of branches, particularly from intact unmyelinated fibres, into denervated areas of the skin originally supplied by other nerves (Speidel, 1933; Weddell and Glees, 1941; Weddell et al., 1941). The latter process was suggested to provide an explanation (Weddell et al., 1941) for the progressive shrinkage in the area of loss of pain sensation and autonomic function earlier than could be explained by direct regeneration from the proximal stump of a divided nerve (Pollock, 1920). Such phenomena presumably indicate the existence of a dormant potential for growth in nerve cells, normally suppressed in a subtle equilibrium about which we know very little. A further interesting aspect of the regeneration of unmyelinated fibres in the skin, recently revealed by electron microscopy, concerns the reinnervation of skin grafts (Orgel, Aguayo and Williams, 1972). These authors observed that scrotal skin transplanted to the ear of the rabbit was rapidly reinnervated by unmyelinated and myelinated axons. Quantitative electron microscopy showed a marked numerical imbalance in favour of the unmyelinated axons, many of which were of very small diameter and it was their opinion that such an imbalance could result in distorted sensation.

Apart from occasional isolated observations, and some reports on counts of unmyelinated axons, the contribution of electron microscopy of tissue sections to the study of regeneration of unmyelinated fibres has been scanty. To date we have not been shown the sites of emergence of axonal branches, the structural features of regenerating growth cones at various levels of section, evidence of recurrent axons, etc. Unfortunately light microscopy does not adequately resolve the finer unmyelinated fibres, and electron microscope studies other than those based on the use of serial sections, lack sufficient perspective. Electron microscopy of single isolated unmyelinated fibres awaits further technical developments; one may hope that it may prove as useful as the recent studies of single myelinated fibres (Spencer and Thomas, 1970; Dyck and Lais, 1970; Ochoa, 1972). Such technical limitations have led to past claims concerning

---

Fig. 2.13   Onset of the regenerative process in some axons of the central stump of the internal carotid nerve, 60 hours after section (cat). c, d, live axons showing hypertrophy and their connection with the necrosed segment (below); a, b, other axons in state of 'turguescence divisoire'; f, e, newly formed terminal expansions; δ, newly produced collaterals. Cajal's method-pyridine. (Reproduced from de Castro, (1930), *Travaux du Laboratoire des Recherches Biologiques de Madrid*, **26**, Fig. 33.)

unmyelinated axons to be called in question, since these have been largely based upon electron microscopy of random ultrathin sections, and it is true for example that there is no definite proof that the miniature profiles, rounded or oval in cross section, having a primitive or embryonic type of relationship to Schwann cells, which several authors have taken to be regenerating axons (Ochoa and Mair, 1969b; Ochoa, 1970a; Ochoa, 1970b; Bray *et al.*, 1972b; Orgel, *et al.*, 1972; Aguayo and Bray, 1975) are indeed axons and not proliferating Schwann cell processes. Dyck and Hopkins (1972), for instance, experienced some difficulty in identifying profiles seen in transverse sections of regenerating rat cervical sympathetic trunk. However, in the sural nerve in man, reasonable confidence in their correct identification as axons has been gained from several lines of indirect evidence: (a) the processes identified as regenerating axons are of the same order of size as developing axons (Figs. 2.12a and c); (b) they are of similar size and bear a similar topological relationship to Schwann cells as do the terminal axonal branches in the skin (Cauna, 1968, 1973); (c) Schwann cell processes (in the sural nerve in man) tend to be plate-like rather than rounded or oval in cross section. Although this issue is not yet settled, the author considers that in so far as cutaneous nerves in man are concerned, unmyelinated axonal sprouts can be identified with reasonable confidence. It is a different matter to regard such small rounded profiles in abnormal nerves as pieces of axons undergoing fragmentation, a view proposed in a pioneer electron microscopic study of autonomic nerve degeneration (Taxi, 1959). With increasing experience, most investigators would today agree that these are not the appearances to be expected in degeneration, and in view of the fast rate of regrowth of unmyelinated axons, the majority would probably consider that such rounded profiles represent regenerating axon sprouts.

Before quantitative electron microscopy of unmyelinated axons became a commonplace procedure for experimental animal material, Ochoa and Mair (1969b) and Ochoa (1970a) postulated that the presence of an additional population of (presumed) axons in partially damaged human nerves was evidence of regeneration, and emphasized the value of an acquired bimodality in the fibre-size spectrum of unmyelinated axons as an indication of previous damage to unmyelinated axons (Fig. 2.12c). This proposition has been questioned by Dyck *et al.* (1971a) on the grounds of their having found equivocal histograms of unmyelinated axon size in some of their normal control material. In view of the limited number of normal human control specimens available, one does not know whether to attribute these differences to differences of methodology, unsuspected pathology or to true intraspecific variation. It appears to us significant, however, that in perfusion-fixed material from baboon sciatic nerves, the histograms of unmyelinated axons were found to be consistently unimodal in normal nerves, whereas those from animals previously subjected to local nerve injury were often bimodal (Fowler and Ochoa, 1975) (Fig. 2.14a), while similar bimodal histograms following sympathetic trunk injury in the rat have been published by Bray *et al.* (1972b). A significant exception to the usual occurrence

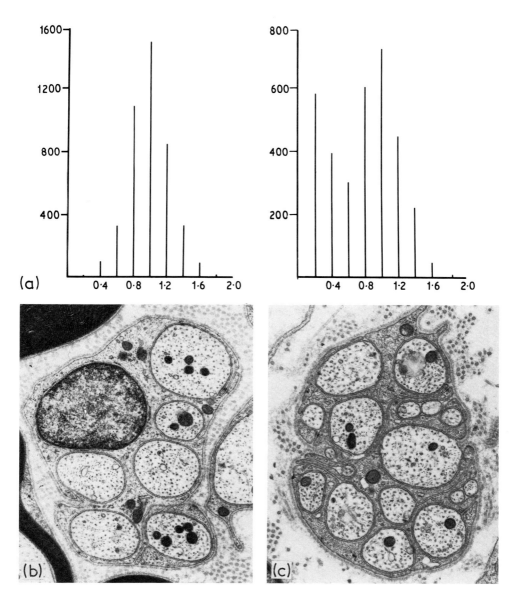

Fig. 2.14a   Left: Pooled histogram of diameters of over 4000 unmyelinated axons from fifteen samples of six medial popliteal nerves from normal adult baboons. Right: Pooled bimodal histogram of diameters of over 4000 unmyelinated axons from eleven samples of two medial popliteal nerves from two baboons. Partial injury was inflicted months previously by relatively severe local compression with a pneumatic cuff inflated around the knee. (Modified from Fowler and Ochoa (1975).)

b Representative sample of axons contributing to the histogram on the left. (x 14 000.)

c Axons contributing to the histogram on the right: an additional population of minute axons, which give rise to bimodality, is obvious. (x 16 200.)

of axonal sprouts in partially damaged nerves is seen following administration of nerve growth factor antiserum to newborn animals. This procedure causes loss of a substantial percentage of unmyelinated axons and their parent cell bodies, and also appears to prevent collateral axon sprouting (Aguayo et al., 1972). The duration of these inhibitory effects has been tested in separate experiments and it was found that the normal ability of the neurons in question to sprout following axonal interruption was unaffected in adult rats that had received nerve growth factor antiserum neonatally (Bray, Aguayo and Martin, 1972).

The fate of a proportion of the excess axonal sprouts formed following nerve injury appears to be eventual resorption. This was directly observed and explicitly described by Weddell (1942) in his study of regeneration of nerve fibres in the skin, and also deduced by inference from axonal counts in regenerating autonomic nerves by Dyck and Hopkins (1972). It was suggested by Ochoa (1970a), that failure to attain peripheral connection was perhaps one of the factors which inhibited the maturation of the regenerated population of miniature unmyelinated axons, a well established phenomenon with myelinated fibres (Weiss and Taylor, 1944; Weiss, Edds and Cavanaugh, 1945; Sanders and Young, 1945; Evans and Murray, 1956). It has been recently shown that experimental blockade of the longitudinal growth of regenerating autonomic nerve fibres also results in arrested maturation of unmyelinated axons in the rabbit (Aguayo, Peyronnard and Bray, 1973).

In nerves containing myelinated and unmyelinated fibres there may occur, following various kinds of injury, miniature regenerating axons devoid of myelin, as outgrowths from either type of fibre. As has been mentioned earlier (Section 2.3.4), in human cutaneous nerves the genuine unmyelinated fibres can be clearly distinguished from axon sprouts awaiting myelination (Figs. 2.8c and d). Estimates of the relative proportions of the two classes of unmyelinated axon can, therefore, be made with reasonable confidence (Fig. 2.12c). It is unfortunately not possible to apply the same criteria to deep nerves or to cutaneous nerves in other species, where unmyelinated fibres may have a less characteristic arrangement. It can be presumed that in mixed nerves containing sprouts awaiting myelination there is no way to distinguish between the contributions of the two kinds of axon devoid of myelin to a compound nerve action potential, where both would crowd within the C elevation since they conduct at similar velocities (Berry, Grundfest and Hinsey, 1944; Sanders and Whitteridge, 1946).

Like developing axons, regenerating unmyelinated axons conduct nervous impulses before attaining their mature size. Murray and Thompson (1957) demonstrated the occurrence and functional activity of collateral sprouts in the sympathetic nervous system of the cat, and Hopkins and Lambert (1972a) have shown an increase in the conduction velocity of regenerated unmyelinated axons with time, following a crush of the cervical sympathetic trunk in the rat. The latter also showed that the presence of the superior cervical ganglion was necessary for the recovery of the compound nerve action potential, and suggested that the formation of an effective synaptic connection was a prerequisite for the return of conduction velocity to normal values in regenerating axons.

2.6 Vulnerability of unmyelinated fibres and age changes

Following axonal division, unmyelinated fibres distal to the cut degenerate. Ranson (1912b) paid special attention to this process, as did de Castro (1930), and in recent years electron microscopists have described some of the fine structural changes involved (Roth and Richardson, 1969; Berger, 1971; Dyck and Hopkins, 1972; Bray *et al.*, 1972b; Thomas and King, 1974). One somewhat unexpected finding was that of Cajal (1928), who believed that a crush injury to nerves of mixed fibre types may selectively spare some unmyelinated fibres. This is not entirely surprising, however, since as a rule such fibres escape injury following milder forms of acute local compression (Ochoa, Fowler and Gilliatt, 1972; Fowler and Ochoa, 1975). Such relative resistance of unmyelinated fibres to mechanical manoeuvres which induce displacement of axoplasm in their myelinated neighbours, in no way conflicts with their greater physiological sensitivity to mechanical stimuli (Lindquist, Nilsson and Skoglund, 1973).

The selective sparing of unmyelinated fibres sometimes seen in peripheral nerve disorders, may of course be due to factors other than their small dimensions. Particular molecular or metabolic interactions must be decisive in determining the specificity of the damage seen in those axonal neuropathies in which large diameter fibres are predominantly affected. Some kind of molecular specificity probably also explains the exclusive or predominant involvement of somatic and autonomic unmyelinated fibres (or their cell bodies) in amyloid neuropathy (Dyck and Lambert, 1969), the neuropathy of Familial Dysautonomia (Aguayo *et al.*, 1971), and the effects of nerve growth factor antiserum during development. Further molecular or metabolic differentiation appears to determine the selectivity in disorders which discriminate between autonomic and somatic unmyelinated fibres. An example of an almost pure primary autonomic degeneration leading to orthostatic hypotension was described by Shy and Drager (1960), and it was later confirmed by Johnson, Lee, Oppenheimer and Spalding (1966) that the disorder is the consequence of degeneration of the intermediolateral column cells in the thoraco-lumbar spinal cord, but they failed to confirm Shy and Drager's observation that there were also changes in the neurons of the sympathetic ganglia (for a review, see Bannister, 1971). Specific antigenic properties of sympathetic neurons appear to determine the extent of the lesions in an allergic autonomic neuropathy in the rabbit (Appenzeller, Arnason and Adams, 1965), and the existence of special metabolic features may explain the specific damage to adrenergic neurons induced by adrenergic blocking agents. Whether these experimentally produced pathologies bear any relationship to rare forms of acute autonomic neuropathy in man

(Thomashefsky, Horwitz and Feingold, 1972) is not known. Examples of degeneration affecting predominantly the sensory unmyelinated and small myelinated neurons are found in some forms of insensitivity to pain (Appenzeller and Kornfeld, 1972), and in Tangier disease (Kocen, King, Thomas and Haas, 1973).

Some potentially toxic therapeutic agents, like isoniazid, have been shown by electron microscopy to damage peripheral unmyelinated fibres (as well as myelinated fibres) both in animals (Schröder, 1970), and in man (Ochoa, 1970a). However, studies of nerve conduction in animals intoxicated with isoniazid and with acrylamide (Hopkins and Lambert, 1972b), have led to this evidence being questioned. The persistence of C potentials, in the presence of reduced A components, which correspond to the large myelinated fibres, led Hopkins and Lambert to conclude that unmyelinated fibres were selectively spared in somatic nerves, as they appeared to be in autonomic nerves. Since in partially damaged nerves containing mixed fibre types there may be regeneration *pari passu* with degeneration despite continued administration of some toxic substances (Cavanagh, 1967; Ochoa, 1970a; Morgan-Hughes *et al.*, 1974), and unmyelinated sprouts from myelinated fibres may be expected to contribute to the C elevation of the compound nerve action potential, it is possible that the C elevations in Hopkins and Lambert's somatic nerves were of heterogenous origin. We would therefore agree that '. . . it is not possible in a mixed nerve to study the changes in conduction velocity of unmyelinated fibres . . .' (Hopkins and Lambert, 1972a). The same bias may well operate in the hypertrophic neuropathy of Dejerine-Sottas, a disorder in which we firmly believe unmyelinated (as well as myelinated) axons to be affected (Ochoa, 1970c), and thus differ from Dyck, Ellefson, Lais, Smith, Taylor and Van Dyke (1970) who maintained that the unmyelinated fibres are spared. The possibility that nerve fibres other than genuine unmyelinated fibres may contribute to the apparently normal C elevation of the sural nerve action potential, in patients suffering from that disorder was, however, recognized by Dyck, Lambert, Sanders and O'Brien (1971b).

Ochoa and Mair (1969b) concluded, from an examination of unmyelinated fibres in sural nerves of seven healthy persons aged between 15 and 59 years of age, that with ageing there was increasing evidence of morphological changes involving both degeneration and regeneration. On the basis of these findings, criteria were enunciated for the electron microscopic evaluation of partially

---

Fig. 2.15a   Only one unmyelinated axon (A) survives in this conglomerate of denervated, budded Schwann cell bands of the unmyelinated type. From the sural nerve of a man aged 59. Osmium tetroxide immersion fixation. (x 14 700). Reproduced from Ochoa and Mair, (1969), *Acta Neuropathologica*, **13**, Fig. 6b, (courtesy of Springer Verlag, Berlin-Heidelberg-New York.)
b Denervated Schwann cell band of unmyelinated type made of four flattened processes unusually twisted like a spiral galaxy. From the sural nerve of a patient suffering from neuropathy due to isoniazid intoxication. Osmium tetroxide immersion-fixation. (x 53 500). (Reproduced from Ochoa and Vial, (1967), *Journal of Anatomy*, **102**, Fig. 16.)

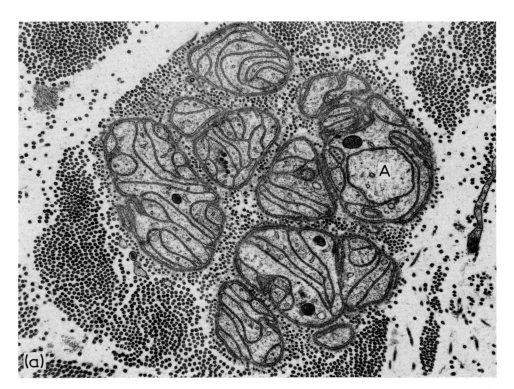

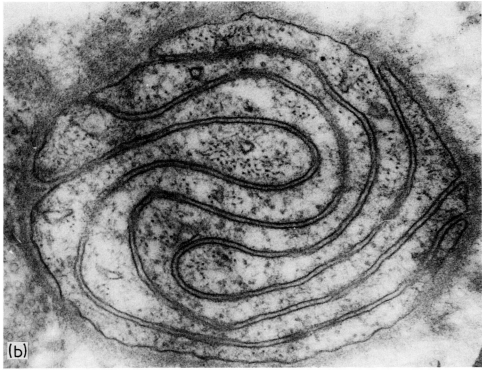

damaged nerves, including the recognition of recent degeneration of fibres, of attempts at regeneration, and the presence of denervated Schwann cell bands. Confidence in these criteria was enhanced when a similar, though exaggerated, picture was found in a study of material from a number of neuropathies (Ochoa, 1970a). Behse, Buchthal, Carlsen and Knappeis (1973) have not been able to confirm the existence of age changes in sural nerves in man, but their nerves were taken from a less exposed site in the leg than were our own. This negative finding raises the question of whether the changes which Ochoa and Mair (1969b) described, might have resulted from minor local trauma, rather than from nerve cell degeneration. Support for this possibility is provided by the apparent absence of axonal degeneration with ageing in the abdominal vagus in man reported by Sharma and Thomas (1975), who nevertheless noted the presence of abundant Schwann cell bands devoid of axons in every instance, and a marked increase in the number of collagen pockets with ageing. On the other hand, Pick (1970) illustrates fibres from the lumbar sympathetic trunk of three men aged 52, 54 and 57 that show both denervation and probably also active degeneration (see Figs. 5.47d and 5.50 in Pick, 1970). It must remain an open question as to whether or not the changes seen in the sural nerve of man with increasing age are caused by minor local trauma, but one can be confident that Schwann cell bands devoid of axons, and composed of flattened processes, are abnormal and indicate axonal loss (Fig. 2.15a). One can equally be confident that excess numbers of miniature axons represent attempts at regeneration, and are also therefore abnormal (Fig. 2.14c).

At the end of this review, the reader may well feel that the balance of its contents is far from optimal. To some extent this may be an expression of the author's personal bias, but it may also be a reflection of the paucity of our current knowledge; much remains to be discovered about dynamic aspects of unmyelinated fibres, even at the simplest morphological levels. As a supplement to this study, the reader is invited to enjoy the farsightedness and style of the erudite writings of Ranson, De Castro and Gasser alluded to above, and to follow in those of Aguayo and Bray accounts of many fascinating contemporary experiments.

References

Aguayo, A. J., Nair, C. P. V. and Bray, G. M. (1971) Peripheral nerve abnormalities in the Riley-Day Syndrome. *Archives of Neurology,* **24**, 106–116.

Aguayo, A. J., Martin, J. B. and Bray, G. M. (1972) Effects of nerve growth factor antiserum on peripheral unmyelinated nerve fibres. *Acta Neuropathologica (Berlin),* **20**, 288–298.

Aguayo, A. J. and Bray, G. M. (1975) Experimental pathology of unmyelinated nerve fibers. In *Peripheral Neuropathy,* (ed.) Dyck, P. J., Thomas. P. K. and Lambert, E. H. Saunders: Philadelphia.

Aguayo, A. J., Terry, L. C. and Bray, G. M. (1973) Spontaneous loss of axons in sympathetic unmyelinated nerve fibers of the rat during development. *Brain Research,* **54**, 360–364.

Aguayo, A. J., Peyronnard, J. M. and Bray, G. M. (1973) A quantitative ultrastructural study of regeneration from isolated proximal stumps of transected unmyelinated nerves. *Journal of Neuropathology and Experimental Neurology*, **32**, 256–270.

Allt, G. (1969) Ultrastructural features of the immature peripheral nerve. *Journal of Anatomy*, **105**, 283–293.

Angeletti, P. U. and Levi-Montalcini, Rita (1972) Growth inhibition of sympathetic cells by some adrenergic blocking agents. *Proceedings of the National Academy of Sciences, Washington*, **69**, 86–88.

Appenzeller, O., Arnason, B. G. and Adams, R. D. (1965) Experimental autonomic neuropathy: An immunologically induced disorder of reflex vasomotor function. *Journal of Neurology, Neurosurgery and Psychiatry*, **28**, 510–515.

Appenzeller, O. and Kornfeld, M. (1972) Indifference to pain: A chronic peripheral neuropathy with mosaic Schwann cells. *Archives of Neurology*, **27**, 322–339.

Banker, Betty Q. and Girvin, J. P. (1971) The ultrastructural features of the mammalian muscle spindle. *Journal of Neuropathology and Experimental Neurology*, **30**, 155–195.

Bannister, R. G. (1971) Degeneration of the autonomic nervous system. *Lancet*, 175–179.

Baumgarten, H. G., Holstein, A. F. and Owman, Ch. (1970) Auerbach's plexus of mammals and man: electron microscopic identification of three different types of neuronal processes in myenteric ganglia of the large intestine from Rhesus monkeys, guinea-pigs and man. *Zeitschrift für Zellforschung und mikroskopische anatomie*, **106**, 376–397.

Baumgarten, H. G., Björklund, A., Holstein, A. F. and Nobin, A. (1972) Chemical degeneration of indolamine axons in rat brain by 5,6-dihydroxytryptamine. *Zeitschrift für Zellforschung und mikroskopische anatomie*, **129**, 256–271.

Baumgarten, H. G., Holstein, A. F. and Stelzner, F. (1973) Nervous elements in the human colon of Hirschsprung's disease. *Virchows Archiv für pathologische Anatomie*, **358**, 113–136.

Behse, F., Buchthal, F., Carlsen, F. and Knappeis, G. G. (1973) Personal Communication.

Berger, B. (1971) Etude ultrastructurale de la dégénérescence Wallerienne experimentale d'un nerf entièrement amyélinique: le nerf olfactif. 1. Modifications axonales. *Journal of Ultrastructure Research*, **37**, 105–118.

Berry, C. M., Grundfest, H. and Hinsey, J. C. (1944) The electrical activity of regenerating nerves in the cat. *Journal of Neurophysiology*, **7** 103–115.

Bickford, R. G. (1938) The mechanism of local sweating in response to faradism. *Clinical Science*, **3**, 337–341.

Bischoff, A. (1970) In *Ultrastructure of the peripheral nervous system and sense organs* (ed.) Babel, J., Bischoff, A. and Spoendlin, H. J. and A. Churchill: London.

Bishop, G. H., Heinbecker, P. and O'Leary, J. L. (1933) The function of the non-myelinated fibers of the dorsal roots. *American Journal of Physiology*. **106**, 647–669.

Boughton, T. H. (1906) The increase in the number and size of the medullated fibers in the oculomotor nerve of the white rat and of the cat at different ages. *Journal of Comparative Neurology and Psychology*, **16**, 153–165.

Bray, G. M., Aguayo, A. J. and Martin, J. B. (1972a) Effects of crush injury on cervical sympathetic trunks in rats treated neonatally with nerve growth factor antiserum (AS-NGF). *Clinical Research*, **10**, 948.

Bray, G. M., Peyronnard, J. M. and Aguayo, A. J. (1972b) Reactions of unmyelinated nerve fibers to injury. An ultrastructural study. *Brain Research*, **42**, 297–309.

Bruce, A. N. (1910) Uber die Beziehung der sensiblen Nervenendigungen zum Entzundungsvorgang. *Archiv für experimentelle Pathologie und Pharmakologie*, **63**, 424–433.

Bunge, Mary B. (1973) Fine structure of nerve fibers and growth cones of isolated sympathetic neurons in culture. *Journal of Cell Biology*, **56**, 713–735.

Byck, R. and Ritchie, J. M. (1973) Tetrahydrocannabinol: Effects on mammalian nonmyelinated nerve fibers. *Science*, **180**, 84–85.

Cajal, S. R. (1892) La rétine des vértebrés. *La cellule*. **9**, 119.

Cajal, S. R. (1905a) Génesis de las fibras nerviosas del embrión. *Trabajos del Laboratorio de investigaciones biologicas de la Universidad de Madrid*, **4**, 227–294.

Cajal, S. R. (1905b) Mecanismo de la regeneración de los nervios. *Trabajos del Laboratorio de investigaciones biologicas de la Universidad de Madrid*, **4** 119–210.

Cajal, S. R. (1928) *Degeneration and Regeneration of the Nervous System,* Vol. 1, Oxford University Press.

Carlsen, F., Knappeis, G. G. and Schmalbruch, H. (1969) Schwann cell 'necrosis' in unmyelinated nerve fibres of patients with polyneuropathy. *Virchows Archiv für pathologische Anatomie,* 348, 306–308.

Carlsen, F. and Knappeis, G. G. (1973) personal communication.

Castro, F. de (1930) Recherches sur la dégénération et la régénération du système nerveux sympathique. Quelques observations sur la constitution des synapses dans les ganglions. *Trabajos del Laboratorio de investigaciones biologicas de la Universidad de Madrid,* 26, 357–456.

Cauna, N. (1968) Light and electron microscopal structure of sensory end-organs in human skin. In *The Skin Senses, Proceedings of the First International Symposium on the skin senses.* (ed.) Kenshalo, D. R. , C. C. Thomas, Springfield: Illinois.

Cauna, N. (1973) The free penicillate nerve endings of the human hairy skin. *Journal of Anatomy,* 115, 277–288.

Cavanagh, J. B. (1967) On the pattern of change in peripheral nerves produced by isoniazid intoxication in rats. *Journal of Neurology, Neurosurgery and Psychiatry,* 30, 26–33.

Celander, O. and Folkow, B. (1953) The nature and the distribution of afferent fibres provided with the axon reflex arrangement. *Acta physiologica scandinavica,* 29, 359–376.

Coggeshall, R. E., Coulter, J. D., and Willis, W. D. (1973) Unmyelinated fibers in the ventral root. *Brain Research,* 57, 229–233.

Cohen, S. (1960) Purification of a nerve growth promoting protein from the mouse salivary gland and its cytotoxic antiserum. *Proceedings of the National Academy of Sciences, Washington,* 46, 302–311.

Colquhoun, D., Henderson, R. and Ritchie, J. M. (1972) The binding of labelled tetrodotoxin to non-myelinated nerve fibres. *Journal of Physiology,* 227, 95–126.

Coon, J. M. and Rothman, S. (1939) The nature of the sweat response to drugs with nicotine-like action. *Proceedings of the Society of Experimental Biology and Medicine,* 42, 231–233.

Coon, J. M. and Rothman, S. (1940) The nature of the pilomotor response to acetylcholine; some observations on the pharmacodynamics of the skin. *Journal of Pharmacology and Experimental Therapy,* 68, 301–311.

Cravioto, H. (1965) The role of Schwann cells in the development of human peripheral nerves. An electron microscopic study. *Journal of Ultrastructure Research,* 12, 634–651.

Dahlström, A. and Fuxe, K. (1964) A method for the demonstration of adrenergic nerve fibres in peripheral nerves. *Zeitschrift für Zellforschung und mikroskipische Anatomie,* 62, 602–607.

Daly, J., Fuxe, K. and Jonsson, G. (1973) Effects of intracerebral injections of 5,6-dihydroxytryptamine on central monoamine neurons: Evidence for selective degeneration of central 5-hydroxytryptamine neurons. *Brain Research,* 49, 476–482.

Davenport, H. A. and Bothe, R. T. (1934) Cells and fibers in spinal nerves. *Journal of Comparative Neurology,* 59, 167–174.

De la Motte, D. (1973) personal communication.

Devine, C. E., Simpson, F. O. and Bertaud (1971) Freeze-etch studies on the innervation of mesenteric arteries and vas deferens. *Journal of Cell Science,* 9, 411–425.

Duncan, D. (1934) A relation between axone diameter and myelination determined by measurement of myelinated spinal root fibers. *Journal of Comparative Neurology,* 60, 437–471.

Dunn, G. A. (1971) Mutual contact inhibition of extension of chick sensory nerve fibres in vitro. *Journal of Comparative Neurology,* 143, 491–508.

Dyck, P. J. and Lambert, E. H. (1969) Dissociated sensation in amyloidosis. *Archives of Neurology,* 20, 490–507.

Dyck, P. J., Ellefson, R. D., Lais, A. C., Smith, R. C., Taylor, W. F. and Van Dyke, R. A. (1970) Histologic and lipid studies of sural nerves in inherited hypertrophic neuropathy: preliminary report of a lipid abnormality in nerve and liver in Dejerine-Sottas disease. *Mayo Clinic Proceedings,* 45, 286–327.

Dyck, P. J. and Lais, A. C. (1970) Electron microscopy of teased nerve fibres: method permitting examination of repeating structures of same fibre. *Brain Research*, **23**, 418–424.

Dyck, P. J., Lambert, E. H. and Nichols, Penny C. (1971a). Quantitative measurement of sensation related to compound action potential and number and sizes of myelinated and unmyelinated fibers of sural nerve in health, Friedreich's ataxia, hereditary sensory neuropathy and tabes dorsalis. *Handbook of Electroencephalography and Clinical Neurophysiology*, **9**, 83–118.

Dyck, P. J., Lambert, E. H. and Sanders, K. and O'Brien, P. C. (1971b) Severe hypomyelination and marked abnormality of conduction in Dejerine-Sottas hypertrophic neuropathy: myelin thickness and compound action potential of sural nerve *in vitro. Mayo Clinic Proceedings*, **46**, 432–436.

Dyck, P. J. and Hopkins, A. P. (1972) Electron microscopic observations on degeneration and regeneration of unmyelinated fibres. *Brain*, **95**, 223–234.

Eames, Rosemary A. and Gamble, H. J. (1970) Schwann cell relationships in normal human cutaneous nerves. *Journal of Anatomy*, **106**, 417–435.

Ehinger, B., Sporrong, B. and Stenevi, U. (1967) Combining the catecholamine fluorescence and methylene blue staining methods for demonstrating nerve fibres. *Life Sciences*, **6**, 1973–1974. Great Britain: Pergamon Press Ltd.

Elfvin, L.-G. (1958) The ultrastructure of unmyelinated fibers in the splenic nerve of the cat. *Journal of Ultrastructure Research*, **1**, 428–454.

Elfvin, L.-G. (1961) Electron-microscopic investigation of filament structures in unmyelinated fibers of cat splenic nerve. *Journal of Ultrastructure Research*, **5**, 51–64.

Elfvin, L.-G. (1962) Electron microscopic studies on the effect of anisotonic solutions on the structure of unmyelinated splenic nerve fibers of the cat. *Journal of Ultrastructure Research*, **7**, 1–38.

Ericsson, J. L. E., Saladino, A. J. and Trump, B. F. (1965) Electron microscopic observations of the influence of different fixatives on the appearance of cellular ultrastructure. *Zeitschrift für Zellforschung und mikroskopische Anatomie*, **66**, 161–181.

von Euler, U. S. and Hillarp, N. A. (1956) Evidence for the presence of Noradrenaline in submicroscopic structures of adrenergic axons. *Nature*, **177**, 44–45.

Evans, D. H. L. and Murray, J. G. (1954) Regeneration of non-medullated nerve fibres. *Journal of Anatomy*, **88**, 465–480.

Evans, D. H. L. and Murray, J. G. (1956) A study of regeneration in a motor nerve with a unimodal fiber diameter distribution. *Anatomical Record*, **126**, 311–333.

Falck, B. (1962) Observations on the possibilities of the cellular localization of monoamine by a fluorescence method. *Acta Physiologica Scandinavica*, **56**, *Supplement*, **197**, 1–26.

Fowler, T. J. and Ochoa, J. (1975) Electron microscopic observations and measurements of unmyelinated fibres in normal and injured peripheral nerves in the baboon. *Neuropathology and Applied Neurobiology*, **1**, 247–265.

Friede, R. L. and Samorajski, T. (1968) Myelin formation in the sciatic nerve of the rat. A quantitative electron microscope, histochemical and radioautographic study. *Journal of Neuropathology and Experimental Neurology*, **27**, 546–570.

Friede, R. L. (1972) Control of myelin formation by axon caliber (with a model of the control Mechanism). *Journal of Comparative Neurology*, **144**, 233–252.

Gamble, H. J. (1964) Comparative electron-microscopic observations on the connective tissues of a peripheral nerve and a spinal nerve root in the rat. *Journal of Anatomy*, **98**, 17–25.

Gamble, H. J. (1966) Further electron microscope studies of human foetal peripheral nerves. *Journal of Anatomy*, **100**, 487–502.

Gamble, H. J. and Eames, Rosemary A. (1964) An electron microscope study of the connective tissues of human peripheral nerve. *Journal of Anatomy*, **98**, 655–663.

Gasser, H. S. (1950) Unmedullated fibers originating in dorsal root ganglia. *Journal of General Physiology*, **33**, 651–690.

Gasser, H. S. (1952) In discussion of 'The hypothesis of saltatory conduction' *Symposium on Quantitative Biology, Cold Spring Harbour*, **17**, 32.

Gasser, H. S. (1955) Properties of dorsal root unmedullated fibers on the two sides of the ganglion. *Journal of General Physiology*, **38**, 709–728.

Geffen, L. B., Descarries, L. and Droz, B. (1971) Intraaxonal migration of (^{3}H) norepinephrine injected into the caeliac ganglion of cats: radioautographic study of the proximal segment of constructed splenic nerves. *Brain Research,* **35**, 315–318.

Geren, Betty B. (1954) The formation from the Schwann cell surface of myelin in the peripheral nerves of chick embryos. *Experimental Cell Research,* **7**, 558–562.

Hallin, R. G. and Torebjörk, H. E. (1971) Afferent and Efferent C Units Recorded from human skin nerves in situ. *Acta Societatis medicorum upsaliensis,* **72**, 277–281.

Hamburger, V. and Levi-Montalcini, Rita (1949) Proliferation, differentiation and degeneration in the spinal ganglia of the chick embryo under normal and experimental conditions. *Journal of Experimental Zoology,* **111**, 457–501.

Harrison, Ross G. (1907) Observations on the living developing nerve fiber. *Anatomical Record,* **1**, 116–118.

Harrison, Ross G. (1924) Neuroblast versus sheath cell in the development of peripheral nerves. *Journal of Comparative Neurology,* **37**, 123–197.

Hess, A. (1956) The fine structure and morphological organisation of non-myelinated nerve fibres. *Proceedings of the Royal Society (Series B),* **144**, 496–506.

Heuser, J. E. and Reese, T. S. (1973) Evidence for recycling of synaptic vesicle membrane during transmitter release at the frog neuromuscular junction. *Journal of Cell Biology,* **57**, 315–344.

Hillarp, N. and Olivecrona, H. (1946) The role played by the axon and the Schwann cells in the degree of myelination of the peripheral nerve fibre. *Acta Anatomica,* **2**, 17–32.

Hopkins, A. P. and Lambert, E. H. (1972a) Conduction in regenerating unmyelinated fibres. *Brain,* **95**, 213–222.

Hopkins, A. P. and Lambert, E. H. (1972b) Conduction in unmyelinated fibres in experimental neuropathy. *Journal of Neurology, Neurosurgery and Phychiatry,* **35**, 163–169.

Hopkins, A. P. and Lambert, E. H. (1973) Age changes in conduction velocity of unmyelinated fibers. *Journal of Comparative Neurology,* **147**, 547–552.

Hopwood, D. (1969) Fixatives and fixation: a review. *Histochemical Journal,* **1**, 323–360.

Johnson, R. H., Lee, G. deJ., Oppenheimer, D. R. and Spalding, J. M. K. (1966) Autonomic failure with orthostatic hypotension due to intermediolateral column degeneration. *Quarterly Journal of Medicine,* **35**, 276–292.

Kapeller, K. and Mayor, D. (1967) The accumulation of noradrenaline in constructed sympathetic nerve as studied by fluorescence and electron microscopy. *Proceedings of the Royal Society (Series B),* **167**, 282–292.

Käppers, C. U. A. (1917) Further contribution on neurobiotaxis. *Journal of Comparative Neurology,* **27**, 261–298.

Katz, B. and Schmitt, O. (1940) Electric interaction between two adjacent nerve fibres. *Journal of Physiology,* **97**, 471–488.

King, R. H. M. and Thomas, P. K. (1971) Electron microscope observations on aberrant regeneration of unmyelinated axons in the vagus nerve of the rabbit. *Acta Neuropathologica,* **18**, 150–159.

Kocen, R. S., King, Rosalind, Thomas, P. K. and Haas, L. (1973) Nerve biopsy findings in two cases of Tangier disease. *Acta Neuropathologica,* in press.

Lampert, P. W. (1967) A comparative electron microscopic study of reactive degenerating, regenerating, and dystrophic axons. *Journal of Neuropathology and Experimental Neurology,* **26**, 345–368.

Langley, J. N (1897) On the regeneration of pre-ganglionic and post-ganglionic visceral nerve fibres. *Journal of Physiology,* **22**, 215–230.

Landon, D. N. (1972) The fine structure of the equatorial regions of developing muscle spindles in the rat. *Journal of Neurocytology,* **1**, 189–210.

Landon, D. N. and Preston, G. M. (1963) Unpublished observations.

Levi-Montalcini, Rita and Booker, Barbara (1960a) Excessive growth of the sympathetic ganglia evoked by a protein isolated from mouse salivary glands. *Proceedings of the National Academy of Sciences, Washington,* **46**, 373–384.

Levi-Montalcini, Rita and Booker, Barbara (1960b) Destruction of the sympathetic ganglia in mammals by an antiserum to a nerve-growth protein. *Proceedings of the National Academy of Sciences, Washington,* **46**, 384–391.

Lewis W. H. and Lewis, M. R. (1912) The cultivation of sympathetic nerves from the intestine of chick embryos in saline solutions. *Anatomical Record,* **6**, 7–32.

Lewis, T. (1927) *The blood vessels of the human skin and their responses.* Shaw: London.

Lewis, T. and Marvin, H. M. (1927) Observations upon a pilomotor reaction in response to Faradism. *Journal of Physiology,* 64, 87–106.

Lindquist, C., Nilsson, B. Y. and Skoglund, C. R. (1973) Observations on the mechanical sensitivity of sympathetic and other types of small-diameter nerve fibers. *Brain Research,* 49, 432–435.

Livett, B. G., Geffen, L. B. and Austin, L. (1968) Proximo-distal transport of (^{14}C) noradrenaline and protein in sympathetic nerves. *Journal of Neurochemistry,* 15, 931–939.

Loeb, L. (1921) Ameboid movement, tissue formation and consistency of protoplasm. *American Journal of Physiology,* 56, 140–167.

Marotte, L. R. (1972) personal communication.

Matthews, M. A. (1968) An electron microscopic study of the relationship between axon diameter and the initiation of myelin production in the peripheral nervous system. *Anatomical Record,* 161, 337–352.

McKinnis, Mary E. (1936) The number of ganglion cells in the dorsal root ganglia of the second and third cervical nerves in human foetuses of various ages. *Anatomical Record,* 65, 255–259.

Mire, J. J., Hendelman, W. J. and Bunge, R. P. (1970) Observations on a transient phase of focal swelling in degenerating unmyelinated nerve fibres. *Journal of Cell Biology,* 45, 9–22.

Morgan-Hughes, J. A., Sinclair, Sally and Durston, J. H. J. (1974) The pattern of peripheral nerve regeneration induced by crush in rats with severe acrylamide neuropathy. *Brain,* 97, 215–232.

Morris, J. H., Hudson, A. R. and Weddell, G. (1972) A study of degeneration and regeneration in the divided rat sciatic nerve based on electron microscopy. I. The traumatic degeneration of myelin in the proximal stump of the divided nerve. *Zeitschrift für Zellforschung und mikroskopische Anatomie,* 124, 76–102.

Murray, J. G. and Thompson, J. W. (1957) The occurrence and function of collateral sprouting in the sympathetic nervous system of the cat. *Journal of Physiology,* 135, 133–162.

Nakajima, S. (1965) Selectivity in fasciculation of nerve fibres in vitro. *Journal of Comparative Neurology,* 125, 193–205.

Nageotte, J. (1922) *L'Organisation de la matière dans ses rapports avec la vie.* (ed.) Alcan, F., Paris.

Novikoff, A. B., Quintana, N., Villaverde, H. and Forschirm, Regina (1966) Nucleoside phosphatase and cholinesterase activities in dorsal root ganglia and peripheral nerve. *Journal of Cell Biology,* 29, 525–545.

Ochoa, J. (1970a) isoniazid neuropathy in man: Quantitative electron microscope study. *Brain,* 93, , 831–850.

Ochoa, J. (1970b) Electron microscope observations on unmyelinated fibres in normal and pathological human nerves. *Proceedings of the VI International Congress of Neuropathology.* Masson: Paris.

Ochoa, J. (1970c) The structure of developing and adult sural nerve in man and the changes which occur in some diseases. A light and electron microscopic study. *University of London, PhD. Thesis.*

Ochoa, J. (1971) The sural nerve of the human foetus: electron microscope observations and counts of axons. *Journal of Anatomy,* 108, 231–245.

Ochoa, J. (1972) Ultrathin longitudinal sections of single myelinated fibres for electron microscopy. *Journal of neurological Sciences,* 17, 103–106.

Ochoa, J. and Vial, D. (1967) Behaviour of peripheral nerve structures in chronic neuropathies with special reference to the Schwann cell. *Journal of Anatomy,* 102, 95–111.

Ochoa, J. and Mair, W. G. P. (1969a) The normal sural nerve in man. I. Ultrastructure and numbers of fibres and cells. *Acta Neuropathologica,* 13, 197–216.

Ochoa, J. and Mair, W. G. P. (1969b) The normal sural nerve in man. II. Changes in the axons and Schwann cells due to ageing. *Acta Neuropathologica,* 13, 217–239.

Ochoa, J., Fowler, T. J. and Gilliatt, R. W. (1972) Anatomical changes in peripheral nerves compressed by a pneumatic tourniquet. *Journal of Anatomy,* 113, 433–455.

Ochoa, J. and Morgan-Hughes, J. A. (1974) The tips of myelinated axons in a neuropathy of the dying-back type: single fibre electron microscopic study. To be published.

Orgel, M., Aguayo, A. and Williams, H. B. (1972) Sensory nerve regeneration: an experimental study of skin grafts in the rabbit. *Journal of Anatomy*, 111, 121–135.

Palay, S. L., McGee-Russell, S. M., Gordon, S. and Grillo, Mary A. (1962) Fixation of neural tissues for electron microscopy by perfusion with solutions of osmium tetroxide. *Journal of Cell Biology*, 12, 385–410.

Pearson, K. G. and Bradley, A. B. (1972) Specific regeneration of excitatory motoneurons to leg muscles in the cockroach. *Brain Research*, 47, 492–496.

Peters, A. and Muir, A. R. (1959) The relationship between axons and Schwann cells during development of peripheral nerves in the rat. *Quarterly Journal of Experimental Physiology*, 44, 117–130.

Peyronnard, J. M., Aguayo, A. J. and Bray, G. M. (1973) Schwann cell internuclear distances in normal and regenerating unmyelinated nerve fibres. *Archives of Neurology*, 29, 56–59.

Peyronnard, J. M., Terry, L. C. and Aguayo, A. J. (1975) Schwann cell internuclear distances in developing unmyelinated nerve fibers. *Archives of Neurology*, 32, 36–38.

Pick, J. (1970) The histology and fine structure of autonomic nerves. In *The Autonomic Nervous System* (ed.) Lippincott, J. B. Philadelphia.

Pick, J., Gerdin, C. and Delemos, C. (1964) An electron microscopical study of developing sympathetic neurons in man. *Zeitschrift für Zellforschung und mikroskopische Anatomie*, 62, 402–415.

Pollock, L. J. (1920) Nerve overlap as related to the relatively early return of pain sense following injury to the peripheral nerves. *Journal of Comparative Neurology*, 32, 357–378.

Porter, K. R. (1966) Cytoplasmic microtubules and their functions. In *Ciba Foundation Symposium on Principles of Biomolecular organisation.* (ed.) Wolstenholme, G. E. W. and O'Conor, M. Little and Brown: Boston.

Prestige, M. C. and Wilson, Margaret A. (1972) Loss of axons from ventral roots during development. *Brain Research*, 41, 467–470.

Ranson, S. W. (1911) Non-medullated nerve fibres in the spinal nerves. *American Journal of Anatomy*, 12, 67–87.

Ranson, S. W. (1912a) The structure of the spinal ganglia and of the spinal nerves. *Journal of Comparative Neurology*, 22, 159–175.

Ranson, S. W. (1912b) Degeneration and regeneration of nerve fibers. *Journal of Comparative Neurology*, 22, 487–545.

Ranson, S. W. (1913) The course within the spinal cord of the non-medullated fibers of the dorsal roots: a study of Lissauer's tract in the cat. 23, 259–281.

Ranson, S. W. (1914) An experimental study of Lissauer's tract and the dorsal roots. *Journal of Comparative Neurology*, 24, 531–545.

Ranson, S. W. (1915) Unmyelinated nerve-fibers as conductors of protopathic sensation. *Brain*, 38, 381–389.

Ranson, S. W., Droegemueller, W. H.. Davenport, H. K. and Fisher, C. (1935) Number, size and myelination of the sensory fibers in the cerebrospinal nerves. Research Publications. *Association for Research in Nervous and Mental Diseases*, 15, 3–34.

Ranvier, M. L. (1878) *Lecons sur l'Histologie due Système Nerveux.* F. Savy: Paris.

Reier, P. J. and Hughes, A. (1972) Evidence for spontaneous axon degeneration during peripheral nerve maturation. *American Journal of Anatomy*, 135, 147–155.

Remak, R. (1837) Weitere microscopische Beobachtungen über die Primitivfasern des Nervensystems der Wirbelthiere. *Frorieps neue notizen aud dem gebiete der Natur und heilkunde*, 3, 35–42.

Remak, R.. (1838) *Observationes anatomicae et microscopicae de systematis nervosi structura.* Berlin.

Richardson, K. C. (1966) Electron microscopic identification of autonomic nerve endings. *Nature*, 210, 756.

Richardson, K. C. (1968) Cholinergic and adrenergic axons in methylene blue-stained rat iris: an electromicroscopical study. *Life Sciences*, 7, 599–604.

DeRobertis, E. D. P. and Bennett, H. S. (1955) Some features of the sub-microscopic morphology of synapses in frog and earthworm. *Journal of Biophysical and Biochemical Cytology,* 1, 47–58.

Roth, C. D. and Richardson, C. (1969) Electron microscopical studies on axonal degeneration in the rat iris following ganglionectomy. *American Journal of Anatomy,* 124, 341–360.

Sabatini, D. D., Bensch K. and Barnett, R. J. (1963) Cytochemistry and electron microscopy. The preservation of cellular ultrastructure and enzymatic activity by aldehyde fixation. *Journal of Cell Biology,* 17, 19–58.

Samorajski, T. and Friede, R. L.(1968) Size-dependent distribution of axoplasm, Schwann cell cytoplasm, and mitochondria in the peripheral nerve fibers of mouse. *Anatomical Record,* 161, 281–292.

Sanders, F. K. and Young, J. Z. (1945) Effect of peripheral connexion on the diameter of nerve fibers. *Nature, London,* 155, 237–238.

Sanders, F. K. and Whitteridge, D. (1946) Conduction velocity and myelin thickness in regenerating nerve fibres. *Journal of Physiology (London),* 105, 152–174.

Schmitt, F. O. (1968) Fibrous proteins-neuronal organelles. *Proceedings of the National Academy of Sciences, Washington,* 60, 1092–1101.

Schröder, J. M. (1970) Die Feinstruktur marklöser (Remakscher) Nervenfasern bei der Isoniazid-Neuropathie. *Acta Neuropathologica (Berlin),* 15, 156–175.

Schroeder, T. E. (1968) Cytokinesis: filaments in the cleavage furrow. *Experimental Cell Research,* 53, 272–318.

Schroeder, T. E. (1973) Actin in dividing cells: contractile ring filaments bind heavy meromyosin. *Proceedings of the National Academy of Sciences of the U.S.A.,* 70, 1688–1692.

Schwann, T. (1839) *Mikroskopische Untersuchungen über die Uebereinstimmung in der Struktur und dem Wachstum der Tiere und Pflanzen.* Sander: Berlin.

Sharma, A. K. and Thomas, P. K. (1975) Quantitative studies on age changes in unmyelinated fibres in the vagus nerve in man. *Proceedings of the Giessen Symposium on Neuromuscular Diseases,* (eds.) Kunze, K. and Desmedt, J. E., Karger: Basel.

Shy, G. M. and Drager, G. A (1960) A neurological syndrome associated with orthostatic hypotension. *Archives of Neurology,* 2, 42–57.

Simpson, S. A. and Young, J. Z. (1945) Regeneration of fibre diameter after cross-unions of visceral and somatic nerves. *Journal of Anatomy,* 79, 48–65.

Speidel, C. C. (1932) Studies of living nerves. I. The movements of individual sheath cells and nerve sprouts correlated with the process of myelin-sheath formation in amphibian larvae. *Journal of Experimental Zoology,* 61, 279–331.

Speidel, C. C. (1933) Studies of living nerves. II. Activities of ameboid growth cones, sheath cells, and myelin segments, as revealed by prolonged observation of individual nerve fibers in frog tadpoles. *American Journal of Anatomy,* 52, 1–79.

Speidel, C. C. (1935) Studies of living nerves. IV. Growth, regeneration, and myelination of peripheral nerves in salamanders. *Biological Bulletin,* 68, 140–161.

Spencer, P. S. and Thomas, P. K. (1970) The examination of isolated nerve fibres by light and electron microscopy, with observation on demyelination proximal to neuromas. *Acta Neuropathologica (Berlin),* 16, 177–186.

Taxi, J. (1959) Etude au microscope électronique de la dégénérescence wallerienne des fibres nerveuses amyéliniques. *Comptes Rendus Academie des Sciences,* 248, 2796–2798.

Taxi, J. and Sotelo, C. (1972) Le Probléme de la migration des catécholamines dans les neurones sympathiques. *Revue Neurologique, Paris,* 127, 23–36.

Thoenen, H. and Tranzer, J. P. (1968) Chemical Sympathectomy by selective destruction of adrenergic nerve endings with 6-Hydroxydopamine. *Archiv fur Pharmakologie und experimentelle Pathologie,* 261, 271–288.

Thomas, P. K. (1973) The ultrastructural pathology of unmyelinated nerve fibres. *New Developments in Electromyography and Clinical Neurophysiology.* (ed.) Desmedt, J. E. Vol. 2 pp. 227–239. Karger: Basel.

Thomas, P. K. and King, R. M. H. (1974) The degeneration of unmyelinated axons following nerve section. *Journal of Neurocytology,* 3, 497–512.

Thomashefsky, A. J., Horwitz, S. J. and Feingold, M. H. (1972) Acute autonomic neuropathy. *Neurology, 22,* 251—255.

Torebjörk, H. E. and Hallin, R. G. (1970) C-fibre units recorded from human sensory nerve fascicles *in situ. Acta Societatis medicorum upsaliensis, 75,* 81—84.

Tsukaguchi, R. (1916) On the regeneration of the cervical sympathetic after section. *Journal of Experimental Physiology, 9,* 281—327.

Tuckett, I. L. (1895) On the structure and degeneration of non-medullated nerve fibres. *Journal of Physiology, 19,* 267—311.

Turner, P. T. and Harris, A. B. (1973) Ultrastructure of synaptic vesicle formation in cerebral cortex. *Nature, 242,* 57—58.

Wada, M., Aoki, T. and Koyama, W. (1958) The axon reflex sweating produced by potassium and sodium cyanides. *Experientia, 14,* 102—103.

Webster, H. deF. (1971) The geometry of peripheral myelin sheaths during their formation and growth in rat sciatic nerves. *Journal of Cell Biology, 48,* 348—367.

Webster, H. deF. and Billings, Susan M. (1972) Myelinated nerve fibers in *Xenopus* tadpoles: *in vivo* observations and fine structure. *Journal of Neuropathology and Experimental Neurology, 31,* 102—112.

Weddell, G. (1941) The pattern of cutaneous innervation in relation to cutaneous sensibility. *Journal of Anatomy, 75,* 346—367.

Weddell, G. (1942) Axonal regeneration in cutaneous nerve plexuses. *Journal of Anatomy, 77,* 49—62.

Weddell, G. (1966) The relationship between pain sensibility and peripheral nerve fibers. *Pain — Henry Ford Hospital International Symposium,* (eds.) Knighton, R. S. and Dumke, P. R., Little, Brown and Co: Boston.

Weddell, G. and Glees, P. (1941) The early stages in the degeneration of cutaneous nerve fibres. *Journal of Anatomy, 76,* 65—93.

Weddell, G., Guttmann, L. and Gutman, E. (1941) The local extension of nerve fibres into denervated areas of skin. *Journal of Neurology and Psychiatry, 4,* 206—225.

Weddell, G., Pallie, W. and Palmer, E. (1954) The morphology of peripheral nerve terminations in the skin. *Quarterly Journal of Microscopical Science, 95,* 483—501.

Weiss, P. (1941) Nerve patterns: the mechanics of nerve growth. *Growth, Third Growth Symposium, 5,* 163—203.

Weiss, P. (1955) *Nervous system (Neurogenesis) in Analysis of Development,* ed. Willier, B. H., Weiss, P. A. and Hamburger, V. Section VII, 346—401.

Weiss, P. and Taylor, A. C. (1944) Further experimental evidence against 'neurotropism' in nerve regeneration. *Journal of Experimental Zoology, 95,* 233—257.

Weiss, P., Edds, M. V. and Cavanaugh, M. (1945) The effect of terminal connections on the caliber of nerve fibers. *Anatomical Records, 92,* 215—233.

Weller, R. O (1967) An electron microscopic study of hypertrophic neuropathy of Dejerine and Sottas. *Journal of Neurology, Neurosurgery and Psychiatry, 30,* 111—125.

Weller, R. O. and Herzog, I. (1970) Schwann cell lysosomes in hypertrophic neuropathy and in normal human nerves. *Brain, 93,* 347—356.

Wessells, N. K., Spooner, B. S., Ash, J. F., Bradley, M. O., Luduena, M. A., Taylor, E. L., Wrenn, J. T. and Yamada, K. M. (1971) Microfilaments in cellular and developmental processes. *Science, 171,* 135—143.

Whitear, M. (1960) An electron microscope study of the cornea in mice, with special reference to the innervation. *Journal of Anatomy, 94,* 388—408.

Wolfe, D. E., Potter, L. T., Richardson, K. C. and Axelrod, J. (1962) Localising tritiated norepinephrine in sympathetic axons by electron microscopic autoradiography. *Science,* 138, 440—442.

Wuerker, R. B. and Kirkpatrick, J. B (1972) Neuronal microtubules, neurofilaments, and microfilaments. *International Review of Cytology,* No. 33, 45—75.

Yamada, K. M., Spooner, B. S. and Wessells, N. K. (1970) Axon growth: Roles of microfilaments and microtubules. *Proceedings of the National Academy of Sciences, 66,* 1206—1212.

Yamada, K. M., Spooner, B. S. and Wessells, N. K. (1971) Ultrastructure and function of growth cones and axons of cultured cells. *Journal of Cell Biology, 49,* 614—635.

3 THE PERINEURIUM AND CONNECTIVE TISSUE OF PERIPHERAL NERVE

F.N. Low

3.1 History of nerve sheaths

Knowledge of the histological organization of tissues ensheathing peripheral nerve dates from the classic contributions of Key and Retzius (1873, 1876). These authors recognized three connective tissue sheaths which they called by names that are still in general use (Fig. 3.1). The outermost sheath, the epineurium, constituted the connective tissue that surrounded the entire nerve and blended insensibly with the connective tissue of nearby parts. The middle sheath, the perineurium, was made up of more compact cellular layers concentrically arranged and was also interpreted as connective tissue. The perinuerium enclosed individual fascicles of longitudinally running nerve fibres. The innermost sheath, the endoneurium, was simply the connective tissue that surrounded Schwann cells and their enclosed nerve fibers within a single fascicle.

The second comprehensive study of nerve sheaths was offered by Ranvier (1875, 1882) who used different terminology. The outermost sheath was the perifascicular fibrous tissue. The middle sheath was the 'gaine lamelleuse'. This was often translated as the 'lamellated sheath of Ranvier' since concentric layers of cells were its most conspicuous feature. The innermost sheath in Ranvier's terminology became the intrafascicular fibrous tissue.

Both of these early investigations recognized three connective tissue sheaths around peripheral nerve. Later, certain subdivisions of these sheaths were discovered through the independent investigations of Plenk (1927) and Laidlaw (1929, 1930). Both of these workers studied the argyrophilic properties of peripheral nerve. They described a closely fitting web of argyrophilic fibres surrounding individual nerve fibres (see Nageotte, 1930); This 'inner' portion of the endoneurium became the 'sheath of Plenk and Laidlaw', and the latter investigator likened this sheath to the Fibrillenscheide of Key and Retzius or the intrafascicular connective tissue of Ranvier. The outer portion of the endoneurium, according to Gray (1970), corresponds to he sheath of Key and Retzius which he states was sometimes called the sheath of Henle (1841). However, Nageotte (1930) considered only the perineurium of the far periphery, where it was very thin, to be the sheath of Henle. Whatever may be the preferred terminology, it became evident that silvering techniques revealed a compact sheath of reticular fibres in the endoneurium close to individual nerve fibres.

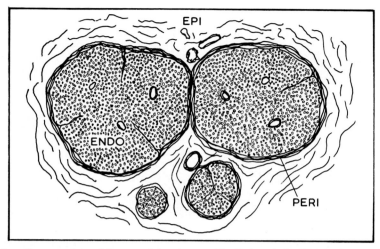

Fig. 3.1   *Cross section of large peripheral nerve*   The Epineurium (EPI) is the connective tissue that forms the outermost of the peripheral nerve sheaths. The endoneurium (ENDO) is the connective tissue that surrounds the longitudinally running neurites and their Schwann cells. The perineurium (PERI) consists of flattened layers of cells and intervening connective tissue. It effectively seals off the endoneurium from the epineurium.

This contrasted with less compactly arranged connective tissue elements elsewhere in the endoneurium. More detailed accounts of the light microscopic era of investigation have been given in the reviews of Nageotte (1930), Causey (1960) and Gray (1970).

3.2 General distribution

The pattern described above, that of three concentric sheaths for peripheral nerves, is remarkably constant throughout the entire body. In a comprehensive review of the thickness of perineurium in relation to nerve size Sunderland and Bradley (1952) make no mention of lack of this sheath. It routinely persists in small motor nerves (Burkel, 1966, 1967, 1970) and in cutaneous nerves (Glees, 1943). However, exceptions to the presence of perineurium do occur in the acoustic nerve (Ross and Burkel, 1970), and in larger mixed nerves of the dental pulp (Stockinger, 1965). Olfactory nerves traversing the subarachnoid space are covered only by a single cellular layer (pia-arachnoid) instead of the multilayered root sheath present in spinal nerves (Low, unpublished observations), the deeper layers of the latter being analogous to the deeper layers of perineurium. The autonomic nervous system possesses sheaths with essentially the same organization as those of the somatic nerves, and Wilson and Silva (1965) have described perineurium of the phrenic nerve in some detail. Around ganglia, both spinal (Andres, 1961) and autonomic (Barton and Causey, 1958; Lieberman, 1968), the perineurium of connecting nerve branches. In ganglia the flattened·capsule cells that surround individual neurons are homologous, and continuous with, the Schwann cells that enclose their axons; they are therefore surrounded by the endoneurium. When nerves are very small both endoneurium and perineurium tend to become indistinguishable from neighbouring connective tissue. However, for the sake of consistent terminology it is best to adhere to the terms endoneurium and epineurium wherever a perineurial sheath separates the two parts of the connective tissue space.

3.3 Epineurium and endoneurium

Electron microscopy affords deeper insight into the significance of peripheral nerve sheaths (Babel, Bischoff and Spoendlin, 1970). The morphology of the epineurium and endoneurium is readily understood by direct observation, and they are clearly composed of similar connective tissue elements to those encountered all through the organism. The extracellular elements are chiefly unit collagenous fibrils which vary in diameter from 30 to 200 nm in various parts of the body (Porter, 1966). These conspicuous fibrils are now recognized to make up the substructure of both collagen fibres, where they are large, and reticular fibres where they are somewhat smaller. In the epineurium, where most of them contribute to collagen fibres, their diameters vary from 60 to 110 nm (Gamble and Eames, 1964a). The collagen fibrils of the perineurium run circumferentially around the nerve trunk and are thus at right angles to both the regular longitudinally arranged endoneurial fibres, and the somewhat less regular and larger, longitudinal and spiral fibrils of the epineurium. In the endoneurium, where the majority make up the reticular fibres of the sheath of Plenk and Laidlaw, they vary from 30 to 65 nm in diameter (Thomas, 1963). Elastic fibres with their associated microfibrils are routinely found in the epineurium but are rare in the endoneurium. Microfibrils (Low, 1962; Haust, 1965), as everywhere else in the body, tend to aggregate near to the surface of basement membranes.

Cellular populations differ in the epineurium and endoneurium. In the epineurium fibroblasts, macrophages and mast cells are present in numbers and distribution that suggest no differences from loose connective tissue in general. In the endoneurium, where Schwann cells and endothelial cells of blood vessels account for most of the population, fibroblasts make up only 4% of the total cell population (Causey and Barton, 1959). Some of the cells counted as fibroblasts may be macrophages but no one seems to have offered definite identification of this cell type in the endoneurial tissue space. At best macrophages are very rare in the endoneurium. Mast cells have been reported by several authors (Gamble, and Goldby, 1961; Gamble, 1964; Olsson, 1965, 1968; Enerbäck, Olsson, and Sourander, 1965).

The connective tissue of normal and degenerated human peripheral nerves was scrutinized by Gamble and Eames (1964b) who pointed out that endoneurial collagen in the human does not form sheaths as in the rabbit and cat. However, all evidence indicates that both epineurium and endoneurium are connective tissues. The restricted cell population of endoneurium is notable, that this may be in some measure due to certain peculiar features of the perineurium will become evident in following paragraphs.

3.4 Perineurium

The fine structure of perineurium presents a unique interpretative problem (Fig. 3.2). Although its extracellular parts are clearly connective tissue, its cellular organization is not comparable to that of any other tissue in the body. It is, therefore, necessary to examine basic patterns of histological fine structure that are recurrent throughout the body in order to provide some background against which to evaluate the perineurium. At the risk of lengthy digression from the primary subject matter of this chapter, sections on boundary (basement) membranes and connective tissue space are offered below as these subjects have a direct bearing on the histological organization of the perineurium. The same

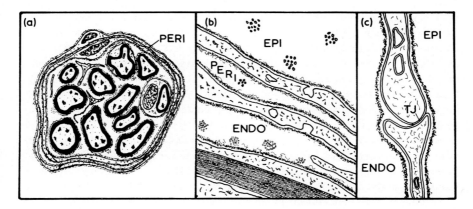

Fig. 3.2   *Fine structure of perineurium*   (Drawn from Burkel, 1967)
a *Cross section of small nerve with bilayered perineurium*   The perineurial layers completely surround the endoneurium which contains eleven neurites and their Schwann cells. The latter are separated from the endoneurial connective tissue space by boundary membranes.
b *Detail of bilayered perineurium*   This drawing represents a cross-section of a portion of a peripheral nerve. Both surfaces of each layer of perineurial cells are covered by boundary membranes. Between each cellular layer lies a variable amount of connective tissue space which may contain unit collagenous fibrils and other extracellular components of the connective tissues. The unit collagenous fibrils, whose size differs notably between endoneurium and epineurium, run predominantly in a direction longitudinal to the course of the nerve. This arrangement characterizes peripheral nerves in general.
c *Tight junction between perineurial cells*   A pentalaminar junction (TJ), which involves fusion of the outer (dense) layer of the plasmalemma of each cell, seals off the neighbouring portions of the connective tissue space from each other. Where only one perineurial layer is present, as illustrated above, this 'tight' junction (TJ) separates epineurium from endoneurium. Wherever more than one perineurial layer is present tight junctions characterize the deepest layer, the one lying next to the endoneurium.

may be said of the fine structural organization of epitheia, an account of which will be presented later, in logical order.

3.4.1 *Boundary (basement) membranes*

Basement membranes were first described by Bowman (Todd and Bowman, 1845) who recognized a difference in the connective tissue substrate immediately underlying epithelia and, for about a century, basement membranes were considered to be exclusively subepithelial. They were described as being present or absent depending upon the ability of the techniques then in use to demonstrate them. A notable change in our concept of basement membranes came about with the demonstration by Gersh and Catchpole in 1949 of periodic acid-Schiff (PAS) positive areas not only underneath all epithelia, but separating all non-connective tissue cells and fat from bordering connective tissue space. These PAS positive layers were all called basement membranes. As electron microscopic techniques improved following the introduction of polyester and Epoxy embedments in the late 1950s, a set of much thinner structures (25–50 nm) were consistently observed in the same histological locations (Fig. 3.3), and by association the term basement membrane was carried over into electron microscopy.

It soon became evident that the connective tissue space at the level of fine structure contained fibrous extracellular connective tissue (elastic fibres, unit collagenous fibrils and microfibrils) in company with connective tissue cells, all of which except fat cells were free in the sense that they were not covered by basement membranes. All other cells were separated from the connective tissue space by such membranes and these thus formed the boundaries of the space (Fig. 3.3). To leave the connective tissue space any particle would, with very few exceptions (lymphatic capillaries blood vascular sinusoids, Majno, 1965), have to pass through such a membrane. Hence the term 'boundary membrane' was suggested in place of the less accurate 'basement membrane' of former use (Low 1961, 1964; Battig and Low, 1961; Deane, 1964; Low and Burkel 1965), since these membranes limit or bound the connective tissue space. The term boundary membrane also referred this structure to the space occupied by the connective tissues, of which these membranes are now regarded to be a part.

3.4.2 *Connective tissue space*

The term boundary membrane proves useful in understanding new areas in fine structure because of the somewhat surprising extent of the connective tissue space itself. A small amount of this space persists between the boundary membranes of capillaries and parenchymal cells in almost all parts of the body (Fig. 3.3). Indeed, the connective tissue space is obliterated between blood vessels and parenchyma in only five known areas; the capillary network of the brain (Peters, Palay and Webster, 1970), between the glomerular capillaries and

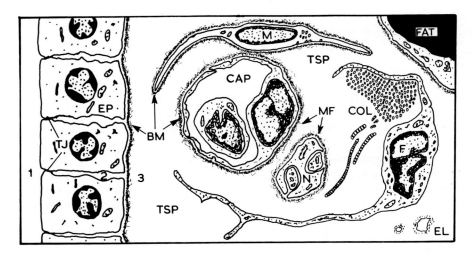

Fig. 3.3 *Boundary membrane histology* Boundary membranes (BM) separate non-connective tissues and fat from the connective tissue space (TSP). Included among the non-connective tissues are epithelium (EP) (including endothelium (CAP) and mesothelium), muscle (M) and peripheral nerve (N), whose Schwann cells and perineurial cells fall into this category. The connective tissues, both cellular (F) and extracellular occupy the continuous connective tissue space without intervening boundary membranes. Fibrillar components recognizable in fine structure include elastic fibres (EL), unit collagenous fibrils (COL) and microfibrils (MF). The fine structural organization of epithelia creates three separate spaces; the space outside the free surface of the epithelium (1, far left above), the intercellular space of the epithelium (2) and the connective tissue space (3, TSP). Spaces 1 and 2 are separated by tight junctions (TJ) and 2 and 3 by a boundary membrane (BM).

Bowman's capsule of the kidney corpuscle (Roth and Greep, 1966), the alveolar walls of the lung (Low, 1961), the stria vascularis of the cochlear duct (Smith, 1957; Hinojosa and Rodriguez-Echandia, 1966) and in certain portions of the chorioallantoic placenta (Jollie, 1964; Carlson and Ollerich, 1969). Elsewhere the connective tissue space persists, suggesting a remarkable continuity. In fact, actual geometric compartmentation of the connective tissue space apparently occurs only in the alveolar walls of the lung, where the rich network of anastomosing capillaries press closely against the alveolar epithelium and divide the connective tissue space into small compartments (Weibel, 1963). An appreciation of the implications of this continuity for the total organism may be obtained by contemplating the situation that is obvious in the early embryo before organogenesis has become established (Low, 1964). All of the labyrinthine, intrusive growths of later development fail to obliterate the connective tissue space between the boundary membranes of non-connective tissue cells (except in the five cases cited), and succeed in true geometric compartmentation of this space only in the lung. The situation now recognizable in fine structure is essentially a recapitulation of the frequently repeated maximum of the early histologists: 'The connective tissues are continuous throughout the body'.

3.4.3 *Basic concepts*

Certain basic ideas may be derived from the foregoing considerations. (i) When cells are associated with boundary membranes they are not connective tissue cells. (ii) The connective tissue space is enclosed by and contains cells covered by boundary membranes which mark off its limits. (iii) The connective tissue space is a continuum throughout the body. With these principles in mind, the fine structure of the perineurium may be critically examined.

The number of concentric cellular layers of perineurium may be as great as ten (Gray, 1970) or even twelve (Lieberman, 1968). This number diminishes in linear relationship to the diameter of the nerve (Sunderland and Bradley, 1952) until a single layer is left (Burkel, 1967; Fig. 3.2), the thinnest layers being beyond the limit of resolution of the light microscope. Boundary membranes cover both surfaces of perineurial cells. Outer cellular layers of cells are separated by layers of connective tissue space of variable thickness, these layers tending to be thinner toward the inner aspect of the perineurium. Unit collagenous fibrils in these areas measure 40 to 80 nm in diameter (Gamble and Eames, 1964a), and are thus larger than those of the endoneurium (30 to 65 nm) and smaller than those of the epineurium (60 to 110 nm). Ocasional fibroblasts are present and may be recognized by their lack of boundary membranes. Mast cells have also been reported (Gamble and Goldby, 1961; Olsson, 1968).

Diffusion barrier The innermost layer of perineurial cells forms a complete sleeve around the endoneurium and its contained nerve fibres (Fig. 3.2), the individual endoneurial cells being connected by tight junctions (Burkel, 1967; Thomas and Jones, 1967; Gray, 1970). Experimental work confirms the barrier function of this innermost layer of perineurial cells since it is impermeable to ferritin (Waggener, Bunn, and Beggs, 1965), to small molecule proteins such as horseradish peroxidase (Klemm, 1970), and to exogenous proteins (Olsson and Reese, 1969). Even a molecule as small as $FeCl_3$, although it penetrates deeply into the perineurium in three minutes, takes three hours to reach the endoneurium (Röhlich and Knoop, 1961). The passage of $AgNO_3$ through the perineurium is also slow (Krnjević, 1954). This anatomical and experimental evidence has direct bearing on the question of where the physiological diffusion barrier known to exist in peripheral nerve is located. Its site still seems to be in dispute despite the concrete fine structural evidence cited above. Counter opinion centres about the connective tissue of the epineurium as the effective barrier (Feng and Liu, 1949; Crescitelli, 1951; Causey and Palmer, 1953; Lehmann, 1953), but much of the evidence favouring the epineurium depends on de-sheathing techniques, and in most cases the nature of the remaining coverings of the nerve was not determined. Recent reviews, however (Sunderland, 1965; Lieberman, 1968; Gray, 1970), favour the perineurial site. It seems only reasonable to accept the evidence of tight junctions in the basal layer of perineurial cells and the impermeability or delaying action of this layer on molecular tracers. One may reasonably conclude then, that the innermost layer of perineurial cells is the site of the diffusion barrier long known to physiologists and neurologists. In insects tight junctions form a similar barrier around the central nervous system (Lane and Treherne, 1972).

Some insight into the terminology applied to the perineurium over the years is of interest at this point. This is necessary since certain interpretations of perineurium, now more or less established, are inconsistent with known principles of modern histology. The original interpretation of perineurial cells as flattened fibroblasts must be questioned because of the presence of boundary membranes wherever these cells border on the connective tissue space. Conversely, one may say that, if they are fibroblasts, they represent the only aggregation of such cells anywhere in the body in which the individual cells are separated from the connective tissue space by boundary membranes. Among these cells, the more compactly organized layer is on record under no less than eight different names (Lieberman, 1968); endothelium (Key and Retzius, 1876), mesothelium (Sunderland, 1965), epithelium (Krnjević, 1954), perineural epithelium (Shanthaveerappa or Shantha and Bourne, 1962–1968; Shantha-veerappa, Hope and Bourne, 1963), perilemma (Röhlich and Weiss, 1955), neurothelium (Lehmann, 1957), perineurothelium (Cravioto, 1966a) and *stratum internum perineurii* (Clara and Özer, 1959). These names represent the choice of individual investigators, being largely descriptive according to preference. However, those implying an epithelial organization are open to question for the reasons explained below.

3.4.4 *Epithelium in fine structure*

The fine structure and function of epithelia are clearly set forth in a series of studies by Farquhar and Palade (1963, 1964, 1965, 1966). These workers demonstrate in epithelia a set of cell junctions, notably those now called tight junctions or 'occluding zonules'. These attach the distal margins of epithelial cells to each other in a manner that seals the space outside the free surface of the epithelium (Hay, 1973) from the intercellular space of the epithelium itself (Fig. 3.3). The latter extends everywhere throughout the epithelium, wherever contiguous cells are not attached to each other by cell junctions, and is always separated from the connective tissue space by a boundary membrane. Thus, in confirmation of Ussing's (1960) electrochemical studies, Farquhar and Palade show that the basic organization of epithelium creates three spaces: first, the space outside the free surface; second, the intercellular space and third, the connective tissue space on the deep side of the boundary membrane (Fig. 3.3). This work is principally derived from intestinal epithelium and frog skin but the pattern established is now considered to be applicable to all epithelia, including endothelium (Majno, 1965) and mesothelium. 'Leaky' epithelia do occur wherever the junctions near the free surface are not tight (Majno, 1965) but the basic organization of the epithelium does not vary.

These criteria for fine structural organization of epithelium make it clear that the histology of perineurium cannot be reconciled with an epithelium in the sense interpreted by Krnjević (1954) and others, notably Shanthaveerappa or Shantha and Bourne (1962–1968) and Shanthaveerappa, Hope and Bourne (1963). *Both* surfaces of perineurial cells possess boundary membranes; They face the connective tissue space, and no 'free surface' is present. The interlaminar spaces in perineurium are typical parts of the connective tissue space and contain unit collagenous fibrils, a circumstance never encountered in the intercellular space of epithelia. Moreover, the resistance of many epithelia to penetration by tracer substances contrasts with the ready penetration of tracers into areas such as the surface of the brain that are covered only by pial connective tissue cells with fenestrations (Waggener, 1964; Brightman, 1965). While the basal layer of perineurium with its tight junctions resembles the junctional organization of many epithelia, the total organization of perineurium belies this interpretation.

Identity of perineurium   The elimination of the cells of both connective tissue and epithelium as tissues to which perineurium might belong poses a problem of identification. Among the fundamental tissues of the body only muscle and nervous tissue are left. Although it is tempting to immediately discard muscle as a possible contender, contractile properties based on fine structure in perineurium have been claimed by Ross and Reith (1969), and this may be related to the slow proximo-distal flow of fluid in the endoneurium described by Weiss (1943) and Weiss, Wang, Taylor and Edds (1945). However, none of the other characteristics of perineurium suggest muscle. Furthermore, the elimination of connective tissue derivation for perineurial cells does not meet with universal acclaim. Thomas and Jones (1967) report that regenerating perineurium is at first devoid of boundary membranes, and acquires them only as a secondary event. In addition fetal perineurial cells, and mesodermally derived tissues such as muscle and endothelium, acquire boundary membranes only slowly in normal development (Low, 1967). It should be clear from these conflicting considerations that a definitive identification of perineurium in terms of recognized basic histological tissues is not feasible. Perhaps the least objectionable interpretation of the status of perineurial cells is to class them frankly with the auxiliary non-conductive nervous tissues, most closely akin to Schwann cells. This classification stands up well when boundary membrane relationships and intracellular organelles are compared, the two being indistinguishable except for their gross cellular outlines (Cravioto, 1966b). Perineurial cells, like Schwann cells, possess a wrap-around tendency, differing from Schwann cells only in that they enclose whole fascicles of nerves and endoneurium rather than individual axons. Of all possible identities that can be assigned to perineurial cells on the basis of their fine structure, the role of modified Schwann cells seems to be the most appropriate.

The isolation of the endoneurial tissue space by the tight junctions of the basal layer of perineurial cells, while functionally effective, is not structurally complete. Burkel (1967) points out that individual sheaths of perineurium accompany blood vessels close to where these pierce the perineurium to enter the endoneurium. Just outside the perineurium even a reticular fibre may have a sheath of perineurium around it. Both of these situations reflect the tendency of perineurial cells, frequently noted in Schwann cells elsewhere, to wrap around any longitudinal structure close to them. The portion of the connective tissue space thus enclosed would, in the case of the blood vessel at least, be continuous with the endoneurial connective tissue space and would represent an inter-ruption to the continuity of the perineurium. Burkel (1967) indicates that the number of perineurial layers of cells may decrease by termination of the innermost one along the course of the nerve, or by the fact that nerve branches are accompanied by the innermost layer of perineurium when they depart from the parent nerve. Apparently these discontinuities of the perineurial sheath are minor ones since they do not appear to interfere with the functional isolation of the endoneurial connective tissue space.

3.5 Distal sheaths

The peripheral termination of the perineurium is comparable to an open-ended sleeve (Burkel, 1967). This occurs some distance from the myoneural end-plate (Fig. 3.4) and allows unbroken continuity between the epineurial and endoneurial portions of the connective tissue space (Burkel, 1970). Substantially the same thing is illustrated by Robertson (1956, 1960) in much earlier studies of the myoneural junction. Robertson observed, before the days of recognized tissue patterns in fine structure, the terminal open end of the perineurial sleeve and unfortunately labelled it 'endoneurial sheath cells'. In the myoneural junction, the Schwann cell enveloping the terminating axon may either accompany it to the margin of the muscle cell or terminate a very short distance from it. This seems to be the situation in peripheral terminations of nerve fibres in general, wherever structurally specialized nerve endings are not present. The open ended perineurium is always separated by some connective tissue space from the Schwann cell which encloses the axon. Both of these are covered by boundary membranes. It appears from evidence incidentally gleaned that the Schwann cell enclosing the near-terminal axon may do one of three things: (1) it may end short of the nerve ending so that the axon is naked for a short distance, (2) it may leave the axon as described above as the latter makes contact with its destination and course for some distance on the surface of the 'receiving' cell (Robertson, 1960), or (3) the Schwann cell may accompany the axon for some distance as it enters the intercellular space of an epithelium or epithelioid structure such as an islet of Langerhans (Winborn, 1963). Whatever may be their situation, the perineurial cells always remain separated from the Schwann cells enclosing axons by at least a small interval of connective tissue space. The peripheral open-endedness of perineurium is apparently of functional signifi-cance since this is the area where toxins can most easily enter the endoneurial connective tissue space (Fedinec, 1958). In the following section on differently

168

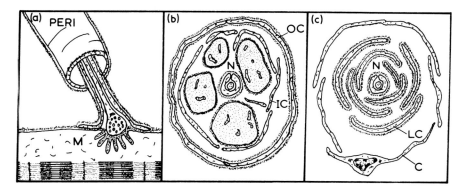

Fig. 3.4a *Motor end plate* The perineurium (PERI) terminates as an open-ended sleeve. At this point the epineurial and endoneurial portions of the connective tissue space are freely continuous with each other. The neurite with its Schwann cell is covered by a boundary membrane which becomes continuous with the boundary membrane of the muscle cell (M).

b *Muscle spindle, tendon spindle, Pacinian corpuscle* A common basic organization is shared by these three types of nerve endings. An outer capsule (OC) is made up of flattened cells covered by boundary membranes. This capsule is perineurial. Within it an inner capsule (IC) contains cells without boundary membranes. These are of endoneurial identity. Other structures such as intrafusal fibers (muscle spindle) and collagen fibers (tendon spindle) may occupy the greater part of the endoneurial area. In the Pacinian corpuscle the greater part of this area is occupied by cells of the inner capsule. Also in this area is found the neurite (N), single or branched, with its Schwann cell and boundary membrane.

c *Meissner's corpuscle, genital corpuscle and others* In these types of ending the centrally located neurite is surrounded by laminar (or lamellar) cells that are covered on both surfaces by boundary membranes. These cells represent the perineurial component of the peripheral nerve sheath. Farther from the neurite are capsular cells. These are connective tissue cells that possess·no boundary membranes. They are essentially epineurial in position. The endoneurium in these endings is greatly reduced and without cellular representation. The neurite (N) is centrally located.

structured nerve endings it will be shown that, whatever their complexity, the composition of these endings may be interpreted in terms of epineurium perineurium and endoneurium.

3.5.1 *Motor end plates*

Motor end plates have come to occupy a prominent place in the literature of fine structure, but only their sheath characteristics will be considered here. The first full scale article throwing light on the sheaths near end plates was offered by Robertson in 1956, who later published a more extensive report in 1960. This early work concentrated chiefly on the relationship of the axon to the muscle cell, with only incidental attention to peripheral nerve sheaths, and the cells of the latter, in reality perineurial, were first interpreted to be endoneurial. Later Burkel (1966, 1967), concentrating on the perineurium, demonstrated its open endedness close to muscle cells and made clear that the endoneurial and epineurial portions of the connective tissue space were continuous with each other at this point (Burkel, 1970; Fig. 3.4). The sheaths of peripheral nerve thus present a very simple structural organization in the neighbourhood of the motor end plate.

3.5.2 *Muscle spindles*

Muscle spindles have been described in fine structure by a number of authors (Merrillees, 1960; Uehara and Hama, 1965; Karlsson and Anderson-Cedergren, 1966, 1971; Matthews, 1971; Santini and Ibata, 1971). The intrafusal fibres of the spindle with their sensory or motor endings are surrounded by a more or less complete inner capsule of cells having thinly attenuated cytoplasm and incomplete or absent boundary membranes. Outside this is an outer capsule, often some distance from the inner one, which differs from it in being covered by boundary membranes. The outer sheath may be equated with the perineurium and the inner with connective tissue cells (fibroblasts) whose location is essentially endoneurial (Fig. 3.4b). The nerve terminations and the intrafusal fibres present no peculiar features. They, too are located in the endoneurium. Continuity of the outer capsule with the perineurium is at present only a presumption, as is whether or not the outer capsule itself is open ended at its peripheral termination within the muscle, but if it is indeed perineurium, this would be the expected situation.

3.5.3 *Golgi tendon organs*

The fine structure of Golgi tendon organs has also been described (Merrillees, 1962; Bridgeman, 1968; Schoultz and Swett, 1971, 1972). They possess an organization remarkably similar to that of muscle spindles (Fig. 3.4b). A well defined capsule several cell layers thick encloses the luminal space of the organ, and the capsule cells are demonstrably continuous with the perineurium of the entering nerve. They are covered on both surfaces with boundary membranes and there is some tendency toward fenestration. The luminal space thus enclosed contains longitudinally running collagen fibres intimately associated with Schwann cells; these fibres are best interpreted as homologues of the intrafusal fibres of the muscle spindle. Also present in the luminal space are partitions consisting of cellular elements differing distinctly from the capsule cells, and these Schoulz and Swett (1972) designate septal cells. The capsule cells of Golgi tendon organs are perineurial and correspond to the outer capsule of muscle spindles. The septal cells are connective tissue and correspond to the inner capsule. The luminal space enclosed by the capsule of the tendon organ essentially corresponds to the endoneurial connective tissue space.

3.5.4 *Pacinian corpuscles*

The Pacinian corpuscle represents the most complex and highly developed of the sensory nerve endings. Nevertheless it illustrates a basic principle of fine structural organization in peripheral nerve endings. The perineurium of its nerve is known to be continuous with the outermost sheath of the corpuscle (Denny-Brown, 1946). The same circumstance is emphasized by Shantha-veerappa and Bourne (1963). Transmission electron microscopic studies show that the outer cellular layers of the corpuscle possess boundary membranes. These may clearly be interpreted to be perineurium that is continuous with the portion of the perineurium sheathing the nerve fibres just proximal to the corpuscle. Deeper within the corpuscle there are many concentric layers of cells closely packed together around the nerve fibers (Nishi, Oura and Pallie, 1969, 1970; Spencer and Schaumberg, 1973). In this area the connective tissue space is compressed into very thin laminae and a very considerable amount of cloudy or fluffy material is present. However, after reviewing micrographs from an earlier study (Pease and Quilliam, 1957; reported in Pease and Pallie, 1959) to determine the presence or absence of boundary membranes, Pease reports that boundary membranes can readily be recognized in the outer portions of the corpuscle but not in the core. He prefers to interpret the core cells as perineurial despite their lack of boundary membrane investment. The more recent work of Spencer and Schaumberg (1973) shows some boundary membranes around the inner core cells where these cells do not abut directly against each other. In the light of comparison with the somewhat simpler organization of other nerve endings, the core cells of the Pacinian corpuscle may be interpreted as connective tissue cells in a position that is essentially endoneurial (between perineurium and a centrally located axon). This affords a direct comparison between the simply organized muscle and tendon spindles with their outer (perineurial) and inner (endoneurial) capsules and the vastly more complex Pacinian corpuscle. In all three perineurium surrounds an endoneurial aggregation of variable cellular density (Fig. 3.4b).

3.5.5 *Meissner's, genital and other corpuscles*

The remainder of structurally organized nerve endings may conveniently be grouped together since, as Patrizi and Munger (1965) point out, they are modulations on a common organizational theme (Fig. 3.4.3). A number of the better known ones have been the subject of scrutiny at the level of fine structure: Meissner's corpuscles (Cauna and Ross, 1960) digital tactile corpuscles (Pease and Pallie, 1959), genital corpuscles (Patrizi and Munger, 1965; Polacek and Malinowsky, 1971), Herbst and Grandry corpuscles (Munger, 1965) and miscellaneous cutaneous endings (Munger, 1965; Suzuki and Kurosumi, 1972). In an extensive study of genital corpuscles in the rat penis Patrizi and Munger

(1965) reported capsular cells resembling fibroblasts without boundary membranes and laminar cells with boundary membranes. The latter are interpreted to be modified Schwann cells. Capsular cells delineate the margins of the corpuscle and the laminar cells are deposited in regular register around the central neurite. Cauna and Ross (1960) describe essentially the same situation in Meissner's corpuscles of the human finger-tip. Laminar cells dominate the area around the neurite while capsular cells are found in the periphery. Boundary membranes are not described but the intercellular substance seems, in their micrographs, to be organized as boundary membranes around the deeply located laminar cells. Pease and Pallie (1959) interpret the cells enclosing the nerve terminals to be extensions of the perineurium, and these, with their conspicuous boundary membranes correspond to the laminar cells of Patrizi and Munger (1965) and Cauna and Ross (1960). More peripherally placed are connective tissue cells that correspond to the capsular cells of these authors. The laminar cells then may be interpreted to be perineurial and the capsular cells to be epineurial. Other less detailed accounts of the fine structure of nerve endings do not appear to conflict with the pattern described above.

Summary of nerve endings A comprehensive interpretation of fine structure in nerve endings can easily be formulated (Fig. 3.4), despite the fact that muscle and tendon spindles and Pacinian corpuscles possess an outer lamination of cells covered by boundary membranes, while just the reverse situation occurs in other endings, notably Meissner's tactile corpuscle, genital corpuscles and the like. However, when one recalls the nature of the sheaths prevailing along the greater part of the course of peripheral nerve, i.e. perineurium with a connective sheath on each side, it can be seen that all nerve endings have a basic structural organization that is essentially an expression of the organization of the sheaths common to all peripheral nerve. A basic interpretation may therefore proceed along the following lines.

First it is necessary to accept the concept that perineurium continues uninterruptedly into the structural organization of nerve endings, a circumstance perhaps best illustrated in the Pacinian corpuscle, and then to remember that the endoneurium between perineurium and the Schwann cell-enclosed neurites and the epineurium outside the perineurium are both connective tissue. The sheaths of nerve endings may therefore consist of either perineurium coupled with an overgrowth of the endoneurium between it and the neurite (muscle spindle, Golgi tendon organ, Pacinian corpuscle), or of perineurium rather closer than usual to the neurite with epineurial connective tissue for an outer capsule (Meissner's tactile corpuscle, genital corpuscles and others). The fine structure and identity of the cellular and interstitial layers involved in many structurally organized nerve endings have not yet been recorded but enough evidence has now accumulated to warrant the prediction that the fine structural organization of all nerve endings will be amenable to interpretation in terms of the recognized basic sheaths of peripheral nerve; endoneurium, perineurium and epineurium.

3.6 Nerve root sheaths

The central termination of the perineurial sleeve has received less attention, but four papers from this author's laboratory have touched on this general area (McCabe and Low, 1969; Haller and Low, 1971; Himango and Low, 1971; Haller, Haller and Low, 1972).

3.6.1 *The subarachnoid angle*

Where the dorsal and ventral roots of a peripheral nerve enter the subarachnoid space, the epineurium becomes continuous with the dura mater. The endoneurium continues uninterruptedly and without change along the nerve root to the central nervous system where it terminates against the boundary membrane of the brain or spinal cord (Tarlov, 1937). The perineurium, however, undergoes radical change when it reaches the subarachnoid angle (McCabe and Low, 1969; Fig. 3.5). Although lamination is frequently hard to follow here, it appears

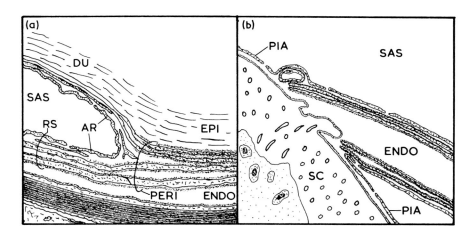

Fig. 3.5 *Central termination of perineurium*
a *Subarachnoid angle* In this diagram four layers of perineurial cells (PERI), all possessing boundary membranes, pass between the epineurium (EPI) and the endoneurium (ENDO). As the subarachnoid space (SAS) is approached the outer layers separate from the inner ones, loose their boundary membranes, acquire lucent cytoplasm and course between dura (DU) and arachnoid (AR). The lower layers continue centrally as the deep layers of the root sheath (RS), whose superficial layer is formed by the arachnoid. A longitudinally running myelin sheath occupies the lower portion of the diagram. (McCabe and Low, 1969).
b *Attachment of nerve root to spinal cord* (SC) The outer layer of the root sheath is continuous with the pia mater (PIA). The inner layers (central continuations of perineurial layers) end as an open cylinder just short of the surface of the central nervous system. There the endoneurial connective tissue space (ENDO) becomes continuous with the pial connective tissue space. The latter communicates with the subarachnoid space (SAS) through fenestrations in the cellular pia. Nerve fibres in the endoneurium are not represented. (Haller, Haller and Low, 1972).

that the outer layers of the perineurium separate from the inner ones and extend for some distance between the dura mater and the arachnoid membrane. This layer of cells is separated from the arachnoid by an extracellular dense line of irregular thickness (Himango and Low, 1971; Morse and Low, 1972). In this location the cytoplasm of the cells becomes lucent, so strikingly so that this area was mistaken in light microscopy for a space and was named the 'subdural' space. Although no 'open' space is present at the electron microscopic level, there should be no doubt that a physical weakness exists here. Resistance to fluid pressure appears to be low with the result that subdural haemorrhages settle in this area.

3.6.2 *On the root sheath*

The deeper layers of the perineurium pass the subarachnoid angle without essential change and, continuing along the nerve root as it crosses the subarachnoid space, make up the deeper layers of the root sheath (Haller and Low, 1971). The more superficial layers of the root sheath are continuations of the pia or arachnoid according to location and may be designated pia-arachnoid. The deepest layer of the root sheath is very closely knit and apparently possesses tight junctions as in the same layer of the perineurium along the more peripheral extent of the nerve. The boundary membrane separating the basal layer of this portion of the perineurium (root sheath; Haller and Low, 1971) is complete. In between the individual layers in the root sheath the boundary membranes are intermittent, but there are connective tissue fibrils present just as in the more peripheral perineurium. In this respect the perineurium of the root sheath appears to provide less insulation between the endoneurium and the subarachnoid space than elsewhere in peripheral nerve since the pia-arachnoid covering which forms the outer layer of the root sheath is fenestrated. However, the closely-knit continuity of the basal layer of the root sheath with its continuous boundary membrane may be adequate isolation in the more protected environment of the spinal canal and the surrounding cerebro-spinal fluid, and may be functionally comparable to the more complete structural isolation of epineurium from endoneurium farther out in the more peripheral course of the nerve.

3.6.3 *At the central nervous system*

The central termination of the nerve root, where it attaches to the central nervous system is an area of particular interest which has been described for the spinal cord (Haller, Haller and Low, 1972; Fig. 3.5). Here the outer layer of the root sheath becomes continuous with pia mater covering the spinal cord, while the inner layers of the root sheath, actually prolongations of the deep layers of perineurium, are open-ended at the point of attachment of nerve root and spinal cord Here the endoneurial connective tissue space becomes continuous with the pial connective tissue space. Since the cellular pial covering of the central nervous system is fenestrated there is direct continuity between the endoneurial connective tissue space and the cerebrospinal fluid. The central termination of the perineurial sleeve is thus effectively open-ended. The subarachnoid space, because of (1) the non-epithelial nature of its linings, (2) fenestrations connecting it with the surrounding areas of connective tissue space, and (3) presence of occasional connective tissue fibrils within it, is best interpreted as a cleared out portion of the connective tissue space (Frederickson and Haller, 1971), the same connective tissue space which extends uninterruptedly throughout the entire body (Low, 1964; Frederickson and Low, 1969).

3.7 Histogenesis of connective tissues

Since connective tissue makes up the greater part of peripheral nerve sheaths any interpretation of the function and significance of these sheaths should be cognizant of modern concepts of connective tissue histogenesis, and should emphasize contributions to such concepts that have derived from fine structural studies. Although the position of the fibroblast as the chief source of extracellular connective tissue fibrils is unassailable, an interesting body of evidence is emerging that points to the production of connective tissue fibrils by cells other than fibroblasts. This concept seems worthy of brief review.

In the chick the earliest expression of extracellular connective tissue is found in a primitive boundary membrane which underlies the epiblast at the time of laying (Low, 1967). During the first 24 hours of incubation this epithelial boundary membrane becomes complete and is then essentially identical to the boundary membranes of adult tissue. These membranes consist of a layer of conspicuous fuzzy material which is supported by a network of extremely fine fibrils that are much more difficult to demonstrate. These primary fibrils (Low, 1968) appear to be permanent constituents of the boundary membranes around the endothelium of capillaries (Palade, 1961; Majno, 1965). Thus if one is willing to accept the idea that ontogeny recapitulates phylogeny, boundary membranes and primary fibrils may be regarded as the phylogenetic forerunners of the extracellular connective tissues.

At the beginning of the second day of incubation in the chick, microfibrils (Low, 1962, 1968) begin to appear. The earliest visible as distinct structural entities apparently arise from the edge of the ectodermal boundary membrane that faces towards the future connective tissue space. This apparent 'delamination' is soon followed during the third day by an intense growth of microfibrils in the connective tissue space around the notochord (Duncan, 1957; Jurand, 1962; Low, 1968). Perinotochordal microfibrils have been studied enzymatically and it has been shown that the smaller ones are susceptible to enzymes that attack mucopolysaccharides while the larger ones (20 nm) are destroyed by the action of collagenase (Frederickson and Low, 1971). The former finding is in keeping with the mucopolysaccharide-rich environment in which perinoto-chordal microfibrils develop (O'Connell and Low, 1970). As fibrillogenesis continues, cells that have migrated from the break-up of the sclerotome of the somite take their place in the perinotochordal area (Hay, 1968; Olson and Low, 1971). These are the first cells anywhere in the embryo that have reached a stage of differentiation that merits their being called fibroblasts. The most significant aspect of the earliest synthesis of extracellular connective tissues relevant to the present discussion is the fact that extensive fibrillogenesis occurs before identifiable fibroblasts have become differentiated anywhere in the organism.

This synthesis of extracellular connective tissues in the absence of fibroblasts naturally arouses curiosity as to what kinds of cells can perform the complex synthesis leading to collagen fibre formation. Collagen synthesis has been reported in the chick cornea by Trelstad, and by Trelstad and Coulombre (Trelstad, 1969, 1971; Trelstad and Coulombre, 1971), in neuroepithelium by Cohen and Hay (1971) and in the chick notochord by Carlson (1973), and Carlson and Evans (1973). Each set of investigations supports the conclusions that the epithelium of the cornea, neural tube and notochord can produce collagen, a potentiality once exclusively reserved for the fibroblast. In later stages of development, the growing aorta presents a pattern of growth in fine structure that indicates non-fibroblastic synthesis of other extracellular connec-tive tissue components (Karrer, 1960; Ross and Bornstein, 1971; Newman and Low, 1973). The connective tissue space in the aortic wall contains microfibrils, elastic fibres and unit collagenous fibrils which, taken together, represent the three basic fibrillar elements of the extracellular connective tissues (Newman and Low, 1973). The same structural situation is reported by Pease and Molinari (1960) and by Pease and Paule (1960). The only cell type present is the myoblast (during development) or the smooth muscle cell (in mature tissue); fibroblasts are absent. The ability of the smooth muscle cell to synthesize connective tissue proteins (Ross and Klebanoff, 1971) and elastic fibres (Ross, 1971) stands conclusively demonstrated, and the non-fibroblastic origin of connective tissue fibrils in large arteries can no longer be doubted.

It seems reasonable to suppose that such synthetic properties of non-connective tissue cells may be retained, as a poorly recognized competence by adult cells that possess boundary membranes. Primary fibrils can be demon-strated in adult boundary membranes where connective tissue surrounds surfaces that are heavily invested with a tangle of microfibrils. Larger unit collagenous fibrils are usually found nearby, as are occasional processes of fibroblasts. By analogy with the condition in the embryo one may reasonably suspect that cells in the adult organism possessing boundary membranes are able to undertake extracellular fibrillogenesis through the microfibril stage, thus providing a source of microfibrils to which fibroblasts might supply additional tropocollagen. The ultimate result of such a process would be the production of extracellular fibrils of larger diameter with axial periodicity.

176

3.7.1 *Schwann cells and collagen*

The idea that Schwann cells can synthesize small unit collagenous fibrils receives strong support from an experimental study by Nathaniel and Pease (1963). In nerve fibres regenerating after crush injury the cytoplasmic component is reduced so that the boundary membrane separates from the Schwann cell plasmalemma, sometimes becoming convoluted but not discontinuous. A new boundary membrane forms in close association with the shrunken parent cell. Small unit collagenous fibrils of the size usually found in the endoneurium appear between the two boundary membranes. Observations leading to similar conclusions may be found in the publications of Nathaniel (1962) and Thomas (1964a,b). The production of collagen by Schwann cells has not been unsuspected even in light microscopic literature. Murray and Stout (1942) in an *in vitro* study of Schwann cells (although their transplants were contaminated with fibroblasts) note that reticulin fibres developed in areas occupied only by Schwann cells. Lyons and Woodhall (1949), in reviewing the situation relative to peripheral nerve injuries, suggested that zones of influence in connective tissue formation are so vague that it is difficult to tell where the fibroblast leaves off and the Schwann cell begins.

The possibilities for connective tissue formation in peripheral nerve is very great since both Schwann cells and connective tissue cells are present in abundance. Indeed, the only tissue components not suspected of participating in collagen formation are the axons themselves, and even these possess well known regenerative powers when located in the central stump. It is therefore not surprising, when one considers that all of the cells present are capable of new growth, that in studies of peripheral nerve pathology one is presented with such a confusing and highly variable tangle of cellular and extracellular components, at least two major cell types, fibroblasts and Schwann cells, being capable of both mitosis and extensive extracellular fibrillogenesis. It is beyond the scope of this contribution to analyse the pathology of peripheral nerve, and the reader is referred to classic sources in this field (Foot, 1940; Penfield, 1932), however, it is hoped that the principles expounded here may be useful in classifying tumours of peripheral nerve.

3.8 Blood supply of peripheral nerve

The blood supply of peripheral nerve is well documented in the literature of light microscopy, the chief contributions to which are reviewed by Adams (1942). Other, more recent studies (Adams, 1943; Tobin, 1943; Sunderland, 1945a,c) have confirmed a generally recognized pattern. The source of supply is from regional arteries which enter the epineurium, where they ramify and branch, and a similar arrangement is found in ganglia (Bergmann and Alexander, 1941). Although very little detailed information has been offered concerning the size of vessels in the endoneurium it has been stated that precapillary vessels penetrate the perineurium (Sunderland, 1945b), and it has been shown that the passage of these small vessels through the perineurium is very oblique (Gunderson and Low, 1968). The endoneurial vascular plexus itself consists largely or exclusively of capillaries (Waksman, 1961). The vessels leaving the endoneurium are apparently still capillaries, or at most the very smallest venules, and it seems reasonable to interpret the endoneurial circulation in terms of a capillary network. This circumstance assumes importance in the light of recent work on vascular permeability.

The effect and site of action of histamine and serotonin, both known to produce vascular leakage, was the subject of searching work performed by investigators from Harvard Medical School in Boston and the Rockefeller Institute in New York City (Majno and Palade, 1961; Majno, Palade and Schoefl, 1961). Their rather surprising results, obtained with tracer substances, make it clear that capillaries are not the primary vessels responsible for the increased vascular permeability. All detectable leakage occurred from the venules, from the smallest, post-capillary vessels of 6 to 7 μm in diameter to venules of moderate size, about 70 to 80 μm in diameter; the leakage stopped abruptly where these larger vessels join still larger veins. Venules 20 to 30 μm in diameter were the most sensitive to substances tending to cause leakage (Majno *et al.* 1961).

This evidence strongly suggests that vascular permeability to solutes of large molecular weight is reduced to a minimum in the endoneurium through the absence of veins. This situation contrasts with that found in other loose connective tissues, i.e. those that possess 'normal' venous plexuses. The significance of the non-permeable character of the endoneurial vasculature is emphasized in the work of Olsson and Reese (1969) who found the endoneurium of mouse sciatic nerve to be inaccessible to exogenous proteins. According to these investigators, flourescent albumen or horseradish peroxidase injected into the blood stream cannot find its way into the endoneurium, and they attributed this finding to the presence of tight junctions in the capillary network. The endoneurial vasculature is interpreted by these authors to constitute as effective a barrier to the entry of exogenous proteins as the barrier in the perineurium. Thus, evidence of a very special, insulated environment for the endoneurium may be attributed as much to the retention of large molecules by its vascular system as to the diffusion barrier present in the perineurium. In both areas the 'sealing-off' effect of tight intercellular junctions appears to be the reason for the prevailing isolation.

3.9 Barrier phenomena

The tight junctions present in both perineurium (Burkel, 1967: Thomas and Jones, 1967: Gray, 1970 and others) and endoneurial capillaries (Olsson and Reese, 1969) are capable of isolating the tissue spaces on the two sides of their cells from one another (Farquhar and Palade, 1963). This type of barrier is effective against colloidal lanthanum and phosphotungstate, both of which can penetrate interstices 2 nm wide in gap junctions (Goodenough and Revel, 1970). The efficiency of this junctional system as a barrier could be affected by three factors: (1) pinocytosis across perineurial and endoneurial cells, (2) transport phenomena across the plasmalemmae of the same cells and (3) structural deficiencies in the perineurial encasement.

Pinocytosis is common in both perineurium (Cravioto, 1966b; Burkel, 1967) and endothelium (Bruns and Palade, 1968a; Palade and Bruns, 1968). This form of 'transport in quanta' (Palade, 1960, 1961; Bruns and Palade, 1968b) might overcome the barrier function of the tight junctions were it not for the boundary membranes of perineurium and endothelium. These structures serve as macromolecular filters (Palade, 1961; Palade and Bruns, 1964; Majno, 1965; Bruns and Palade, 1968b) which retard or completely block particulate material transported across cytoplasmic layers by pinocytosis. Transport activity across the plasmalemmae is concerned principally with small molecules and ions and represents, for the most part, an active transport system (Danielli, 1973). Such a system could presumably circumvent the barrier effects of both tight junctions and boundary membranes. It is, however, unlikely that there is much transmembrane transport activity in the structurally unspecialized perineurium and endothelium since conspicuous morphological modifications are usually present wherever this activity is high, as in the kidney tubules and their associated counter-current capillary system (Bulger, 1973).

Structural deficiencies in the perineurial encasement appear to provide the most likely source of observed inefficiencies in the barrier function of some parts of the perineurium. These occur at the central end of the perineurial sleeve (Haller, Haller and Low, 1972), at its peripheral end (Burkel, 1967), and along the course of the peripheral nerve at the points of entry and exit of blood vessels and reticular fibres (Burkel, 1967). The central end of the perineurial sleeve is in a very protected position and the passage of blood vessels through the perineurial layers is very oblique (Gunderson and Low, 1968). Both of these circumstances would tend to oppose any reduction in the effectiveness of the isolation barrier provided by the perineurial sleeve that might result from free flow of materials along the endoneurial connective tissue space. Indeed, the open peripheral end of the perineurial sleeve appears to be the chief location at which failure of isolation produces noticeable results and such effects occur principally in the neighbourhood of the motor end plate (Fedinec, 1958).

3.10 Concluding remarks

Peripheral nerve sheaths may be summarized as consisting of two connective tissue sheaths, an outer (epineurium) and an inner (endoneurium), having a sheath of modified Schwann cells (perineurium) between them. The perineurium constitutes a diffusion barrier which produces an environment in the endoneurial connective tissue space that differs from that in the external epineurial connective tissue space. The blood vascular system of endoneurium likewise constitutes an effective diffusion barrier between the blood and the endoneurial connective tissue space. Both ends of the perineurial sleeve are effectively open-ended. This is especially true near motor end plates, where epineurial and endoneurial connective tissue space communicate freely. Structurally organized nerve endings are essentially peripheral extensions of these three sheaths. Some speculations may be offered concerning this basic structural pattern.

The structural and physiological organization of peripheral nerve sheaths emphasizes a single outstanding feature; the effective physiological isolation of the endoneurium from the remainder of the connective tissue space (Shantha and Bourne, 1968). Although the perineurial sleeve is open-ended, it is effectively closed to surrounding tissues along most of the course of the peripheral nerve. This is clearly illustrated by the part played by nerve trunks as pathways in infection (Wright, 1953), the entry of toxins and other foreign material being achieved through the open-ended perineurial sleeve, especially in situations like the motor end plate where there is no complex, structurally organized nerve ending to prevent free entry. In the case of nerve endings with a highly ordered structure, such as the Pacinian corpuscle, neither experimental studies nor clinical evidence implicates these endings in the entry of latent infections that travel along the nerve trunks. Thus a complex nerve ending apparently produces an effective closure of the perineurial tube. Fedinec (1958), in his study of the passage of tetanus toxin, notes that entry into the nerve sheaths is most effectively achieved when the toxin is inserted into muscle, and least when injected into the blood stream. This finding fits well with the existence of open-ended perineurium near motor end plates and the tight junctions in endoneurial capillaries. Once inside the endoneurial connective tissue space foreign proteins are 'protected' by the absence or paucity of macrophages and by the sealing effect of tight junctions of both perineurium and endoneurial capillaries. The situation pertaining when toxins in the endoneurium arrive at the proximal end of the nerve roots in the subarachnoid space is, however, still a puzzle. The central nervous system itself is usually attacked in these circumstances and to do this the boundary membrane of the central nervous system must be penetrated (see Chapter 6). One wonders why this did not occur at the Schwann cell boundary membranes along the course of the nerve.

However many questions may remain unanswered concerning the sheaths of peripheral nerve it is now clear that their fine structural organization and basic histological patterns are similar to those that characterize the remainder of the organism, and their unique physiological peculiarities are traceable to the special positioning of fine structural characteristics that are commonly found elsewhere throughout the organism.

Acknowledgements

The author's laboratory is supported by a grant from the United States Public Health Service, NS 09363 from the Institute of Neurological Diseases and Stroke.

References

Adams. W. E. (1942) The blood supply of nerves. I. Historical review. *Journal of Anatomy, (London)*, 76, 323–341.

Adams, W. E. (1943) The blood supply of nerves. II. The effects of exclusion of its regional sources of supply on the sciatic nerve of the rabbit. *Journal of Anatomy*, 75, 243–250.

Andres, K. H. (1961) Untersuchungen über den Feinbau von Spinalganglien. *Zeitschrift für Zellforschung und mikroskopische Anatomie*, 55, 1–48.

Babel, J., Bischoff, A. and Spoendlin, H. (1970) *Ultrastructure of the Peripheral Nervous System and Sense Organs* (ed.) Bischoff, A. C. V. Mosby Co., St. Louis, Missouri.

Barton, A. A. and Causey, G. (1958) Electron microscopic study of the superior cervical ganglion. *Journal of Anatomy, (London)*, 92, 399–407.

Battig, C. G. and Low, F. N. (1961) The ultrastructure of human cardiac muscle and its associated tissue space. *American Journal of Anatomy*, 108, 199–230.

Bergmann, L. and Alexander, L. (1941) Vascular supply of the spinal ganglia. *Archives of Neurology and Psychiatry, (Chicago)*, 46, 761–782.

Bridgman, C. F. (1968) The structure of tendon organs in the cat: a proposed mechanism for responding to muscle tension. *Anatomical Record*, 162, 209–220.

Brightman, M. W. (1965) The distribution within the brain of ferritin injected into cerebrospinal fluid compartments. II. Parenchymal distribution. *American Journal of Anatomy*, 117, 193–219.

Bruns, R. R. and Palade, G. E (1968a) Studies on blood capillaries. I. General organization of blood capillaries in muscle. *Journal of Cell Biology*, 37, 244–276.

Bruns, R. R. and Palade, G. E. (1968b) Studies on blood capillaries. II. Transport of ferritin molecules across the wall of muscle capillaries. *Journal of Cell Biology*, 37, 277–299.

Bulger, R. E. (1973) The urinary system. In *Histology*, 3rd edn. (ed.) Greep, R. O., pp. 713–760. McGraw-Hill: New York.

Burkel, W. E (1966) Perineurium, endoneurium and tissue space in peripheral nerves. *Anatomical Record*, 154, 325 (Abstract).

Burkel, W. E. (1967) The histological fine structure of perineurium. *Anatomical Record*, 158, 177–190.

Burkel, W. E. (1970) Continuity of epineurium and endoneurium at terminations of perineural sheaths. *Anatomical Record*, 166 285 (Abstract).

Carlson, E. C. (1973) Intercellular connective tissue fibrils in the notochordal epithelium of the early chick embryo. *American Journal of Anatomy*, 136, 77–90.

Carlson, E. C. and Evans, D. K. (1973) Ultrastructural evidence for the production of extracellular connective tissue fibrils by isolated chick notochord *in vitro*. *Anatomical Record*, 175, 284 (Abstract).

Carlson, E. C. and Ollerich, D. A. (1969) Intranuclear tubules in trophoblast III of rat and mouse chorioallantoic placenta. *Journal of Ultrastructure Research*, 28, 150–160.

Cauna, N. and Ross, L. L. (1960) The fine structure of Meissner's touch corpuscles of human fingers. *Journal of Biophysical and Biochemical Cytology*, 8, 467–482.

Causey, G. (1960) *The Cell of Schwann*. E. and S. Livingstone, Ltd., London.

Causey, G. and Barton, A. A. (1959) The cellular content of the endoneurium of peripheral nerve. *Brain*, 82, 594–598.

Causey, G. and Palmer, E. (1953) The epineural sheath of a nerve as a barrier to the diffusion of phosphate ions. *Journal of Anatomy, (London)*, 87, 30–36.

Clara, M. and Özer, N. (1959) Untersuchungen über die songenannte Nervenschiede. *Acta neurovegetativa, (Wien)*, 20, 1–18.

Cohen, A. M. and Hay, E. D (1971) Secretion of collagen by embryonic neuroepithelium at the time of spinal cord-somite interation. *Developmental Biology*, **26**, 578–605.

Cravioto, H. (1966a) The mesenchymal components of peripheral nerves. An electron microscopic study. *Journal of Neuropathology and Experimental Neurology*, **25**, 157.

Cravioto, H. (1966b) The perineurium as a diffusion barrier–ultrastructural correlates. *Bulletin of the Los Angeles Neurological Society*, **31**, 196–208.

Crescitelli, F. (1951) Nerve sheath as a barrier to the action of certain substances. *American Journal of Physiology*, **166**, 229–250.

Danielli, J. F. (1973) The bilayer hypothesis of membrane structure. *Hospital Practice*, **8**, 63–71.

Deane, H. W. (1964) Some electron microscopic observations on the lamina propria of the gut, with comments on the close association of macrophages, plasma cells and eosinophils. *Anatomical Record*, **149**, 453–473.

Denny-Brown, D. (1946) Importance of neural fibroblasts in the regeneration of nerve. *Archives of Neurology and Psychiatry*, (*Chicago*), **55**, 171–215.

Duncan, D. (1957) Electron microscope study of the embryonic neural tube and notochord. *Texas Reports of Biology and Medicine*, **15**, 367–377.

Enerbäck, L., Olsson, Y. and Sourander, P. (1965) Mast cells in normal and sectioned peripheral nerve. *Zeitshrift für Zellforschung und mikroskopische Anatomie*, **66**, 596–608.

Farquhar, M. G. and Palade, G. E. (1963) Junctional complexes in various epithelia. *Journal of Cell Biology*, **17**, 375–412.

Farquhar, M. G. and Palade, G. E. (1964) Functional organization of amphibian skin. *Proceedings of the National Academy of Sciences of the United States of America*, **51**, 569–577.

Farquhar, M. G. and Palade, G. E. (1965) Cell junctions in amphibian skin. *Journal of Cell Biology*, **26**, 263–291.

Farquhar, M. G. and Palade, G. E. (1966) Adenosine triphosphatase localization in amphibian epidermis. *Journal of Cell Biology*, **30**, 359–379.

Farquhar, M., Wissig, S. L. and Palade, G. E. (1961) Glomerular permeability. I. Ferritin transfer across the normal glomerular capillary wall. *The Journal of Experimental Medicine*, **113**, 47–66.

Fedinec, A. A. (1958) The role of the peripheral nerve barrier in the passage of tetanus toxin in the rat. *Anatomical Record*, **130**, 299 (Abstract).

Feng, T. P. and Liu, Y. M. (1949) The connective tissue sheath of nerve as an effective diffusion barrier. *Journal of Cellular and Comparative Physiology*, **34**, 1–16.

Foot, N. C (1940) Histology of tumors of the peripheral nerves. *Archives of Pathology and Laboratory Medicine*, **30**, 772–805.

Frederickson, R. G. and Haller, F. R. (1971) The subarachnoid space interpreted as a special portion of the connective tissue space. *Proceedings of the North Dakota Academy of Science*, **XXIV**: 142–159.

Frederickson, R. G. and Low, F. N. (1969) Blood vessels and tissue space associated with the brain of the rat. *American Journal of Anatomy*, **125**. 123–146.

Frederickson, R. G. and Low, F. N. (1971) The fine structure of perinotochordal microfibrils in control and enzyme-treated chick embryos. *American Journal of Anatomy*, **130**, 349–376.

Gamble, H. J (1964) Comparative electron-microscopic observations on the connective tissues of a peripheral nerve and a spinal nerve root in the rat. *Journal of Anatomy*, (*London*), **98**, 17–25.

Gamble, H. J. and Breathnach, A. S. (1965) An electron microscope study of human foetal peripheral nerves. *Journal of Anatomy*, (*London*), **99**, 573–584.

Gamble, H. J. and Eames, R. A. (1964a) Electron microscopy of the connective tissues of normal and degenerated human peripheral nerves. *Journal of Anatomy*, (*London*), **98**, 478 (Abstract).

Gamble, H. J. and Eames, R. A. (1964b) An electron microscope study of the connective tissues of human peripheral nerve. *Journal of Anatomy*, (*London*), **98**, 655–663.

Gamble, H. J. and Goldby, S. (1961) Mast cells in peripheral nerve trunks. *Nature*, (*London*), **189**, 766–767.

Gersh, I. and Catchpole, H. R. (1949) The organization of ground substance and basement membrane and its significance in tissue injury, disease and growth. *American Journal of Anatomy,* 85, 457–521.

Glees, P. (1943) Observations on the structure of the connective tissue sheaths of cutaneous nerves. *Journal of Anatomy, (London),* 77, 153–159.

Goodenough, D. A. and Revel, J. P. (1970) A fine structural analysis of intercellular junctions in the mouse liver. *Journal of Cell Biology,* 45, 272–290.

Gray, E. G. (1970) The fine structure of nerve. *Comparative Biochemistry and Physiology,* 36, 419–448.

Gunderson, L. L. and Low, F. N. (1968) Perineurium and connective tissues of peripheral nerve. *American Journal of Veterinary Research,* 29, 455–461.

Haller, F. R., Haller, A. C. and Low, F. N. (1972) The fine structure of cellular layers and connective tissue space at spinal nerve root attachments. *American Journal of Anatomy,* 133, 109–124.

Haller, F. R. and Low, F. N. (1971) The fine structure of the peripheral nerve root sheath in the subarachnoid space in the rat and other laboratory animals. *American Journal of Anatomy,* 131, 1–20.

Haust, M. D. (1965) Fine fibrils of extracellular space (microfibrils): Their structure and role in connective tissue organization. *American Journal of Pathology,* 47, 1113–1137.

Hay, E. D. (1968) Organization and fine structure of epithelium and mesenchyme in the developing chick embryo. In *Epithelial-mesenchymal Interactions.* (ed.) Fleischmajer, R. and Billingham, R., pp. 31–55. The Williams and Wilkins Co. Baltimore.

Hay, E. D. (1973) Epithelium. In *Histology,* 3rd edition, (ed.) Greep, R. O. and Weiss, L., pp. 107–138, McGraw-Hill: New York.

Henle, H. (1841) *Allgemeine Anatomie.* Leipzig.

Himango, W. A. and Low, F. N. (1971) The fine structure of a lateral recess of the subarachnoid space in the rat. *Anatomical Record,* 171, 1–20.

Hinojosa, R. and Rodriguez-Echandia, E. L. (1966) The fine structure of the stria vascularis of the cat inner ear. *American Journal of Anatomy.* 118, 631–664.

Jollie, W. P. (1964) Fine structural changes in the placental labyrinth of the rat with increasing gestational age. *Journal of Ultrastructure Research,* 10, 27–47.

Jurand, A. (1962) Autoradiographic studies of the notochord in chick embryos. *Journal of Embryology and Experimental Morphology,* 10, 602–621.

Karlsson, U. and Andersson-Cedergren, E. (1966) Motor myoneural junctions on frog intrafusal muscle fibers. *Journal of Ultrastructure Research,* 14, 191–211.

Karlsson, U. and Andersson-Cedergren, E. (1971) Satellite cells of the frog muscle spindle as revealed by electron microscopy. *Journal of Ultrastructure Research,* 34, 426–438.

Karrer, H. E (1960) Electron microscope study of developing chick embryo aorta. *Journal of Ultrastructure Research,* 4, 420–454.

Key, A. and Retzius, G. (1873) Studien in der Anatomie des Nervensystems. *Archiv für mikroskopische Anatomie (und Entwicklungsmechanik),* 9, 308–386.

Key, A. and Retzius, G. (1876) *Studien in der Anatomie des Nervensystems und des Bindegewebes.* Samson and Wallin: Stockholm.

Klemm, H. (1970) Das Perineurium als Diffusions-barriere gegenuber Peroxydase bei epi-und endonneuraler Application. *Zeitschrift Für Zellforschung und mikroskopische Anatomie,* 108, 431–445.

Krnjević, K. (1954) The connective tissue of the frog sciatic nerve. *Quarterly Journal of Experimental Physiology and Cognate Medical Sciences,* 39, 55–72.

Laidlaw, G. F. (1929) Silver staining of the skin and of its tumors. *American Journal of Pathology,* 5,, 239–248.

Lane, N. J. and Treherne, J. E. (1972) Studies on perineurial junctional complexes and the sites of uptake of microperoxidase and lanthanum in the cockroach central nervous system. *Tissue and Cell,* 4, 427–436.

Lehmann, H. J. (1953) The epineurium as a diffusion barrier. *Nature, (London),* 172, 1045–1046.

Lehmann, H. J. (1957) Über Struktur und Funktion der perineuralen Diffusion Barrier. *Zeitschrift für Zellforschung und mikroskopische Anatomie,* 46, 232–241.

Lieberman, A. R. (1968) The connective tissue elements of the mammalian nodose ganglion. *Zeitschrift für Zellforschung und mikroskopische Anatomie,* 89, 95–111.

Low, F. N. (1961) The extracellular portion of the human blood-air barrier and its relation to tissue space. *Anatomical Record,* **139**, 105–124.

Low, F. N. (1962) Microfibrils: fine filamentous components of the tissue space. *Anatomical Record,* **142**, 131–138.

Low, F. N. (1964) A boundary membrane concept of ultrastructure applicable to the total organism. *Proceedings of the 3rd European Regional Conference on Electron Microscopy,* Prague, pp. 115–116.

Low, F. N. (1967) Developing boundary (basement) membranes in the chick embryo. *Anatomical Record,* **159**, 231–238.

Low, F. N. (1968) Extracellular connective tissue fibrils in the chick embryo. *Anatomical Record,* **160**, 93–108.

Low, F. N. and Burkel, W. E. (1965) A boundary membrane concept of ultrastructural morphology. *Anatomical Record,* **151**, 489–490.

Lyons, W. R. and Woodhall, B. (1949) *Atlas of Peripheral Nerve Injuries.* W. B. Saunders Co., Philadelphia.

McCabe, J. S. and Low, F. N. (1969) The subarachnoid angle: an area of transition in peripheral nerve. *Anatomical Record,* **164**, 15–34.

Majno, G. (1965) Ultrastructure of the vascular membrane. *Handbook of Physiology,* **3**, 2293–2375.

Majno, G. and Palade, G. E. (1961) Studies on inflammation: I. The effect of histamine and serotonin on vascular permeability: An electron microscopic study. *Journal of Biophysical and Biochemical Cytology,* **11**, 571–605.

Majno, G., Palade, G. E. and Schoefl, G. I. (1961) Studies on inflammation. II. The site of action of histamine and serotonin along the vascular tree: A topographic study. *Journal of Biophysical and Biochemical Cytology,* **11**, 607–626.

Matthews, P. B. (1971) Recent advances in the understanding of the muscle spindle. *Scientific Basis of Medicine,* 99–128.

Merrillees, N. C. R (1960) The fine structure of muscle spindles in the lumbrical muscles of the rat. *Journal of Biophysical and Biochemical Cytology,* **7**, 725–740.

Merrillees, N. C. R (1962) Some observations on the fine structure of a Golgi tendon organ of a rat.. In *Symposium on Muscle Receptors* (ed.) Barker, D., pp. 199–206. Hong Kong University Press: Hong Kong.

Morse, D. E. and Low, F. N. (1972) The fine structure of a pia mater in the rat. *American Journal of Anatomy,* **133**, 349–368.

Munger, B. L. (1965) The intraepidermal innervation of the snout skin of the opossum. A light and electron microscope study, with observations on the nature of Merkel's *Tastzellen. Journal of Cell Biology,* **26**, 79–97.

Munger, B. L. (1966) The ultrastructure of Herbst and Grandry corpuscles. *Anatomical Record,* **154**, 391–392 (Abstract).

Munger, B. L. (1971) In *Handbook of Sensory Physiology,* (ed.) Loewenstein, W. R., Vol. 1, Chapter 17, pp. 523–556. Springer: Berlin.

Murray, M. R. and Stout, A. P. (1942) Characteristics of human Schwann cells *in vitro. Anatomical Record,* 275–294.

Nageotte, J. (1930) Sheaths of the peripheral nerves. In *Cytology and Cellular Pathology of the Nervous System.* (ed.) Penfield, W. Paul B. Hoeber, Inc.: New York.

Nathaniel, E. J. H. (1962) Collagen formation by Schwann cells in regenerating dorsal roots of rats. *Anatomical Record,* **142**, 262 (Abstract).

Nathaniel, E. J. H. and Pease, D. C. (1963) Collagen and basement membrane formation by Schwann cells during nerve regeneration. *Journal of Ultrastructure Research,* **9**, 550–560.

Newman, T. L. and Low, F. N. (1973) The effect of enzymes on extracellular connective tissue components in the developing chick aorta. *American Journal of Anatomy,* (in press).

Nishi, K., Oura, C. and Pallie, W. (1969) Fine structure of Pacinian corpuscles in the mesentery of the cat. *Journal of Cell Biology,* **43**, 539–552.

Nishi, K., Oura, C. and Pallie, W. (1970) Ultrastructure of the mature Pacinian corpuscle in the mesentery of the cat. *Journal of Anatomy,* **106**, 208 (Abstract).

O'Connell, J. J. and Low, F. N. (1970) A histochemical and fine structural study of early extracellular connective tissue in the chick embryo. *Anatomical Record,* **167**, 425–438.

Olson, M. D. and Low, F. N. (1971) The fine structure of developing cartilage in the chick embryo. *American Journal of Anatomy,* 131, 197–216.

Olsson, Y. (1965) Storage of monoamines in mast cells of normal and sectioned peripheral nerve. *Zeitschrift für Zellforschung und mikroskopische Anatomie,* 68, 255–265.

Olsson, Y. (1968) Mast cells in the nervous system. *International Review of Cytology,* 24, 27–79.

Olsson, Y. and Reese, T. S. (1969) Inaccessibility of the endoneurium of mouse sciatic nerve to exogenous proteins. *Anatomical Record,* 163, 318–319 (Abstract).

Palade, G. E. (1960) Transport in quanta across the endothelium of blood capillaries. *Anatomical Record,* 136, 254 (Abstract).

Palade, G. E. (1961) Blood capillaries of the heart and other organs. *Circulation,* XXIV, 368–384.

Palade, G. E. and Bruns, R. R. (1964) Structure and function in normal muscle capillaries. In *Small Blood Vessel Involvement in Diabetes Mellitus. The American Institute of Biological Sciences,* pp. 39–49.

Palade, G. E. and Bruns, R. R. (1968) Structural modulations of plasmalemmal vesicles. *Journal of Cell Biology,* 37, 633–649.

Patrizi, G. and Munger, B. L. (1965) The cytology of encapsulated nerve endings in the rat penis. *Journal of Ultrastructure Research,* 13, 500–515.

Pease, D. C. and Molinari, S. (1960) Electron microscopy of muscular arteries; pial vessels of the cat and monkey. *Journal of Ultrastructure Research,* 3, 447–468.

Pease, D. C. and Pallie, W. (1959) Electron microscopy of digital tactile corpuscles and small cutaneous nerves. *Journal of Ultrastructure Research,* 2, 352–365.

Pease, D. C. and Paule, W. J. (1960) Electron microscopy of elastic arteries; the thoracic aorta of the rat. *Journal of Ultrastructure Research,* 3, 469–483.

Pease, D. C. and Quilliam, T. A. (1959) Electron microscopy of the Pacinian corpuscle. *Journal of Biophysical and Biochemical Cytology,* 3, 331–342.

Penfield, W. (1932) Tumors of the sheaths of the nervous system. In *Cytology and Cellular Pathology of the Nervous System,* Vol. 3, pp. 955–990.

Peters, A., Palay, S. L. and Webster, H. de F. (1970) *The Fine Structure of the Nervous System.* Harper Medical Division, Harper and Row: New York

Plenk, H. (1927) Über argyrophile Fasern (Gitterfasern) und ihre Bildungszellen. *Ergebnisse der Anatomie und Entwicklungsgeschichte,* 27, 302–412.

Poláček, P. and Malinovský, L. (1971) Die Ultrastruktur der Genitalkörperchen in den Clitoris. *Zeitschrift für mikroskopisch-anatomische Forschung. Abt. 2, Jahrbuch für Morphologie und mikroskopische Anatomie,* 84, 293–310.

Porter, K. R. (1966) *Mesenchyma and connective tissue.* In *Histology* (ed.) Greep, R. O. Chapter 4, pp. 99–133.

Ranvier, L. (1875) *Traité technique d'Histologie.* Paris.

Ranvier, L. (1882) Des modifications de structure qu'eprouvent les tube nerveux en passant des racines dans la moelle épinière. Comptes rendus de l'Académie de Science, 95, 1069.

Robertson, J. D. (1956) The ultrastructure of a reptilian myoneural junction. *Journal of Biophysical and Biochemical Cytology,* 2, 381–402.

Robertson, J. D. (1960) Electron microscopy of the motor end plate and the neuromuscular spindle. *American Journal of Physical Medicine,* 39, 1–43.

Röhlich, P. and Knoop, A. (1961) Elektronenmikroskopische Untersuchungen an den Hullen des N. Ischiadicus der Ratte. *Zeitschrift für Zellforschung und mikroskopische Anatomie,* 53, 299–312.

Röhlich, P. and Weiss, M. (1955) Studies on the histology and permeability of the peripheral nervous barrier. *Acta morphologica Academiae Scientiarum Hungaricae,* 5, 335–347.

Ross, Michael H. and Reith, E. J. (1969) Perineurium: evidence for contractile elements. *Science,* 165, 604–606.

Ross, Muriel D. and Burkel, W. E. (1970) Electron microscopic observations of the nucleus, glial dome and meninges of the rat acoustic nerve. *American Journal of Anatomy,* 130, 73–92.

Ross, R. (1971) The smooth muscle cell. II. Growth of smooth muscle in culture and formation of elastic fibers. *Journal of Cell Biology,* 50, 172–186.

Ross, R. and Bornstein, P. (1971) Elastic fibers in the body. *Scientific American,* 224, 44–52.

Ross, R. and Klebanoff, S. J. (1971) The smooth muscle cell. II. *In vivo* synthesis of connective tissue proteins. *Journal of Cell Biology,* **50**, 159–171.

Roth, W. D. and Greep, R. O. (1966) In *Histology,* 2nd Ed. (ed.) Greep, R. O., pp. 595–630. McGraw-Hill: New York.

Santini, M. and Ibata, Y. (1971) The fine structure of thin unmyelinated axons within muscle spindles. *Brain Research,* **33**, 289–302.

Schoultz, T. W. and Swett, J. E. (1971) Fine structure of Golgi tendon organs in the cat. *Physiologist,* **14**, 226 (Abstract).

Schoultz, T. W. and Swett, J. E. (1972) The fine structure of the Golgi tendon organ. *Journal of Neurocytology* **1**, 1–26.

Shantha, T. R. and Bourne, G. H. (1968) The perineural epithelium – a new concept. In *The Structure and Function of Nervous Tissue,* **1**, 379–459 (ed.) Bourne, G. H. Academic Press: New York.

Shanthaveerappa, T. R. and Bourne, G. H. (1962) The 'perineural epithelium', a metabolically active, continuous protoplasmic cell barrier surrounding peripheral nerve fasciculi. *Journal of Anatomy, (London),* **96**, 527–537.

Shanthaveerappa, T. R. and Bourne, G. H. (1962) A perineural epithelium. *Journal of Cell Biology,* **14**, 343–346.

Shanthaveerappa, T. R. and Bourne, G. H. (1963a) New observations on the structure of the Pacinian corpuscle and its relation to the perineural epithelium of peripheral nerves. *American Journal of Anatomy,* **112**, 97–109.

Shanthaveerappa, T. R. and Bourne, G. H. (1963b) Demonstration of perineural epithelium in vagus nerves. *Acta anatomica,* **52**, 95–100.

Shanthaveerappa, T. R. and Bourne, G. H. (1963c) Demonstration of perineural epithelium in whale and shark peripheral nerves. *Nature,* **197**, 702–703.

Shanthaveerappa, T. R. and Bourne, G. H. (1963c) The perineural epithelium: nature and significance. *Nature,* **199**, 577–579.

Shanthaveerappa, T. R. and Bourne, G. H. (1964) The perineural epithelium of sympathetic nerves and ganglion and its relation to the pia-arachnoid mater of the central nervous system and perineural epithelium of peripheral nerves. *Zeitschrift für Zellforschung und mikroskopische Anatomie,* **61**, 742–753.

Shanthaveerappa, T. R. and Bourne, G. H. (1965) Histological and histochemical studies of the choroid of the eye and its relations to the pia-arachnoid mater of the central nervous system and perineural epithelium of the peripheral nervous system. *Acta anatomica, (Basel),* **61**, 379–398.

Shanthaveerappa, T. R. and Bourne, G. H. (1966) Perineural epithelium: a new concept of its role in the integrity of the peripheral nervous system. *Science,* **154**, 1464–1467.

Shanthaveerappa, T. R., Hope, J. and Bourne, G. H. (1963) Electron microscope demonstration of the perineural epithelium in rat peripheral nerve. *Acta anatomica,* **52**, 193–201.

Smith, C. A. (1957) Structure of the stria vascularis and the spiral prominence. *Annals of Otology, Rhinology and Laryngology,* **66**, 521–536.

Stockinger, L. (1965) Nervenabschnitte ohne Perineurium. *Acta anatomica,* **60**, 244–252.

Spencer, R. S. and Schaumberg, H. H. (1973) An Ultrastructural Study of the Inner Core of the Pacinian Corpuscle. *Journal of Neurocytology,* **2**, 217–235.

Sunderland, S. (1945a) The intraneural topography of the radial, median and ulnar nerves. *Brain,* **68**, 243–299.

Sunderland, S. (1945b) Blood supply of the nerves of the upper limb in man. *Archives of Neurology and Psychiatry,* **53**, 91–115.

Sunderland, S. (1945c) Blood supply of peripheral nerves: practical considerations. *Archives of Neurology and Psychiatry,* **54**, 280–282.

Sunderland, S. (1965) The connective tissues of peripheral nerves. *Brain,* **88**, 841–854.

Sunderland, S. and Bradley, K. C. (1952) The perineurium of peripheral nerves. *Anatomical Record,* **113**, 125–141.

Suzuki, H. and Kurosumi, K. (1971) Fine structure of the cutaneous nerve endings in the mole snout. *Archivum histologicum Japonicum,* **34**, 35–50.

Tarlov, I. M. (1937) Structure of the nerve root. Nature of the junction between the central and the peripheral nervous systems. *Archives of Neurology and Psychiatry,* **37**, 556–583.

Thomas, P. K. (1963) The connective tissue of peripheral nerve: an electron microscopic study. *Journal of Anatomy, (London)*, 97, 35–44.

Thomas, P. K. (1964a) The deposition of collagen in relation to Schwann cell basement membrane during peripheral nerve regeneration. *Journal of Cell Biology*, 23, 375–382.

Thomas, P. K. (1964b) Changes in the endoneurial sheaths of peripheral myelinated nerve during Wallerian degeneration. *Journal of Anatomy, (London)* 98, 175–182.

Thomas, P. K. and Jones, D. G. (1967) The cellular response to nerve injury. 2. Regeneration of the perineurium after nerve section. *Journal of Anatomy*, 101, 45–55.

Tobin, C. E. (1943) Injection method to demonstrate blood supply of nerves. *Anatomical Record*, 87, 341–344.

Todd, R. B. and Bowman, W. (1845) *The Physiological Anatomy and Physiology of Man.* John W. Parker: London.

Trelstad, R. L. (1969) The role of the Golgi apparatus in collagen excretion by the chick corneal epithelium. *Journal of Cell Biology*, 43, 147a.

Trelstad, R. L. (1971) Vacuoles in the embryonic chick corneal epithelium, an epithelium which produces collagen. *Journal of Cell Biology*, 48, 689–694.

Trelstad, R. L. and Coulombre, A. J. (1971) Morphogenesis of the collagenous stroma in the chick cornea. *Journal of Cell Biology*, 50, 840–858.

Uehara, Y. and Hama, K. (1965) Some observations on the fine structure of the frog muscle spindle. (I) On the sensory terminals and motor endings of the muscle spindle. *Journal of Electron Microscopy, (Japan)*, 14, 34–42.

Ussing, H. H. (1960) The frog skin potential. *Journal of General Physiology*, 43, 135.

Waggener, J. D (1964) Electron microscopic studies of brain barrier mechanisms. *Journal of Neuropathology and Experimental Neurology*, 23, 174.

Waggener, J. D., Bunn. S. M. and Beggs, J. (1965) The diffusion of ferritin within the peripheral nerve sheath: an electron microscopy study. *Journal of Neuropathology and Experimental Neurology*, 24, 430–443.

Waksman, B. H. (1961) Experimental study of diphtheric polyneuritis in the rabbit and guinea pig. III. The blood-nerve barrier in the rabbit. *Journal of Neuropathology and Experimental Neurology*, 20, 35–77.

Weibel, E. R. (1963) *Morphometry of the human lung.* Springer: Berlin.

Weiss, P. (1943) Endoneurial edema in constricted nerve. *Anatomical Record*, 86, 491–522.

Weiss, P., Wang, H., Taylor, A. C. and Edds, V. (1945) Proximo-distal fluid convection in the endoneurial spaces of peripheral nerves, demonstrated by colored and radioactive (isotype) tracers. *American Journal of Physiology*, 143, 521–540.

Wilson, A. S. and Silva, D. G. (1965) Ultrastructure of the phrenic nerve. *Nature*, 208, 707–708.

Winborn, W. B. (1963) Light and electron microscopy of the islets of Langerhans of the Saimiri monkey pancreas. *Anatomical Record*, 147, 65–94.

Wright, G. P. (1953) Nerve trunks as pathways in infection. *Proceedings of the Royal Society of Medicine*, 46, 319–330.

SENSORY GANGLIA

A.R. Lieberman

4.1 Introduction

With the exception of the primary sensory neurons of the visual and olfactory systems, and the unusual collection of nerve cells constituting the mesencephalic nucleus of the trigeminal nerve (see Section 4.8), the cell bodies of adult vertebrate primary sensory neurons lie outside the central nervous system in ganglia intercalated along the course of the segmental dorsal roots and those cranial nerves with a sensory component.

The dorsal root ganglia and cranial sensory ganglia are collectively referred to as cerebrospinal, craniospinal or sensory ganglia. Each ganglion houses the perikarya of a variable number of ganglion cells, together with the proximal portions of their axons, the associated satellite and Schwann cell sheaths, and the usual connective tissue elements of the peripheral nervous system.

Over the last 100 years the cerebrospinal ganglia of virtually every vertebrate group have been subjected to exhaustive light microscopic scrutiny by many investigators using most of the available neurohistological techniques. Many comprehensive treatises on the microscopic anatomy and comparative anatomy of cerebrospinal ganglia resulted from these investigations (e.g. Van Gehuchten, 1892a, b; Hatai, 1901; Dogiel, 1908; Levi, 1908; Cajal, 1909; Marinesco, 1909; De Castro, 1932; Scharf, 1958). In surveying this vast and detailed literature, one is struck by the feeling that the efforts expended on the structural analysis of cerebrospinal ganglia were out of proportion to the insights acquired, and were to some extent the consequence of the relative accessibility of the ganglia.

Much additional information has accumulated in recent years, particularly as a result of ultrastructural studies on the normal fine structure, development, pathology and injury responses of the cells in sensory ganglia. It must be acknowledged, however, that cerebrospinal ganglia are intrinsically less interesting from the point of view of sensory information processing than the sensory centres of the brain and spinal cord, and, again by comparison with the central nervous system, display a relatively uniform and simple organization.

In this chapter, a survey of the organization of the ganglia and of the morphology and cytology of the ganglion cells and their satellite cells will be given, together with comments on other topics of current interest. Only selected reference will be made to the extremely extensive literature on sensory ganglia and no attempt has been made to include a comprehensive bibliography. In many cases the references given to support particular points may be the more recent of a very large number of relevant papers, or may be reviews rather than primary sources. It is hoped that the marginal loss of historical perspective that this approach entails will not be too significant. If such a loss is felt, however, it may be effectively remedied by consulting the writings of Van Gehuchten (1892a, b), Levi (1908), Ranson (1906, 1908), Cajal (1909), Marinesco (1909), De Castro (1932) and Scharf (1958), in which the antecedent literature is reviewed comprehensively.

4.2 General organization of sensory ganglia

The sensory ganglia comprise ovoid or fusiform swellings of the dorsal roots and the sensory cranial nerves. In spinal ganglia the neuronal perikarya are usually grouped together around or lateral to the bundles of root fibres: in some spinal ganglia, particularly of lower vertebrates, the cell bodies are concentrated as a cortex and the axial region of the ganglion contains the root fibres and rather few ganglion cell bodies. Some cranial sensory ganglia are eccentrically situated with respect to their nerve: most of the ganglion cells of the rabbit nodose ganglion for example, are grouped to one side of the sensory and other fibre bundles of the vagus nerve.

The basic tissue units of the ganglia, distinct both at the light and electron microscope levels, comprise individual ganglion cells, a variable extent of the initial portion of the axon (the only long process to which the cells give rise), and a capsule of satellite cells enclosed within a continuous basal lamina (Figs. 4.1, 4.2, 4.11–4.15).

4.2.1 *Ganglionic capsule and connective tissue*

The ganglia are surrounded by a multilamellate perineurial sheath and a fibrous outer epineurium. Since the ganglionic sheaths do not differ in any fundamental respects from those of peripheral nerve trunks (Lieberman, 1968a) and because peripheral nerve sheaths are described in detail elsewhere (Low, Chapter 3) the ganglionic capsule will not be considered further here.

The ganglion cell—satellite cell complexes and the intraganglionic fibre bundles lie within a highly vascularized connective tissue compartment, the endo-neurium, limited by the perineurium of the capsule and to some extent compartmentalized by fine trabeculae of perineurial cells extending from the innermost aspect of the capsule (Lieberman, 1968a).

Within the endoneurial compartment, collagen fibrils are the predominant extracellular formed element, for the most part displaying the staining characteristics of reticulin (Laidlaw, 1930). Elastic fibres do not normally occur within the endoneurium, but microfibrils (Haust, 1965) are relatively common

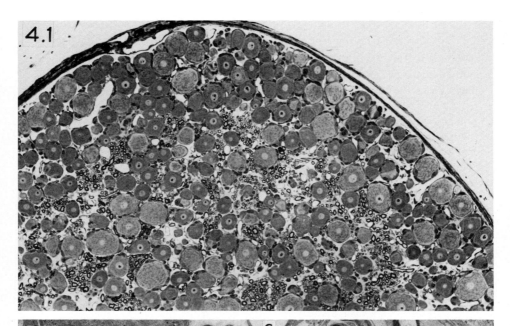

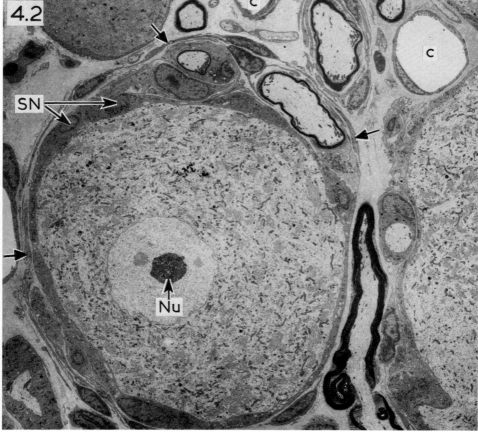

(Lieberman, 1968a). Occasionally small bundles of microfibrils are found in association with an amorphous material (Fig. 4.3) an appearance reminiscent of immature elastic fibres (Greenlee, Ross and Hartman, 1966). The reticular fibres may be disposed as incomplete sheaths around some of the neuron-satellite cell complexes, around the nerve fibres (particularly the large myelinated fibres) and around the blood vessels (Lieberman, 1968a). These fibrous sheaths are usually distinct in reticular fibre preparations (Laidlaw, 1930; De Castro, 1932; Scharf, 1958) and in scanning electron micrographs (Fig. 4.4, 4.5), but are less clearly defined in transmission electron micrographs.

In the older literature, and in some major reference works of the last 15 years, a second capsule of mesodermal elements, cellular as well as fibrous, has been described around the ganglion cell—satellite cell complexes (Cajal, 1909, 1928; De Castro, 1932; Scharf, 1958). Cajal (1909) described this outer capsule as lined on its inside by a continuous layer of flattened 'endothelial' cells. More recent electron microscope studies have failed to confirm the presence of a second complete cellular investment. However, attenuated cell processes are sometimes seen incompletely encircling a ganglion cell—satellite cell complex or an axon (Fig. 4.2). These processes are covered on both surfaces by basal lamina and are probably of satellite cell origin: some of the processes can be traced from perineuronal satellite cells, others from cell bodies resembling satellite cells in their ultrastructural appearance, but which are apparently lying free in the endoneurial space (Jacobs, unpublished observations). In addition, fibroblast processes occasionally appear partially to surround ganglion cell—satellite cell complexes.

Mast cells, which are common components of the connective tissues of vertebrate peripheral nerve trunks, but which are not normally found in dorsal or ventral roots, *are* components of the connective tissues of sensory ganglia (Olsson, 1968b). There are, however, some interesting site and species

---

Fig. 4.1   Survey light micrograph of the cortical region of a cervical dorsal root ganglion of a rabbit. One μm plastic section stained with toluidine blue. The cells are most closely packed beneath the capsule (at top) and the number of myelinated fibres increases more centrally (towards bottom). The wide range of perikaryal diameters, the intermingling of cells of different size and the rich capillary bed are all evident. ($\times$ 128: Reproduced by courtesy of J. M. Jacobs.)

Fig. 4.2   Medium-sized pale neuron sectioned at mid-nucleolar level in a survey electron micrograph of rat cervical ganglion. Parts of the perikarya of a small dark neuron (top left) and of a large pale neuron (right), with an emerging axonal process, are also seen. The neurons are completely enclosed within a capsule of satellite cell cytoplasm (nuclei at SN), which is more electron dense than the neuronal cytoplasm. The ganglion cell-satellite cell complex at the centre is further partially surrounded by the processes of flattened cells (arrows), which also enclose two of three thinly myelinated axons (at centre, top). The latter are proximal segments of the myelinated portion of probably a single stem process (see Section 4.5.2). The longitudinally sectioned myelinated fibre between the two pale cells displays thicker myelin on one side of the node than on the other and is therefore almost certainly a myelinated stem process (see section 4.5.2 and Figs. 4.29 and 4.29a). c — capillaries; Nu — nucleolus ($\times$ approx. 1500: Reproduced by courtesy of J. M. Jacobs.)

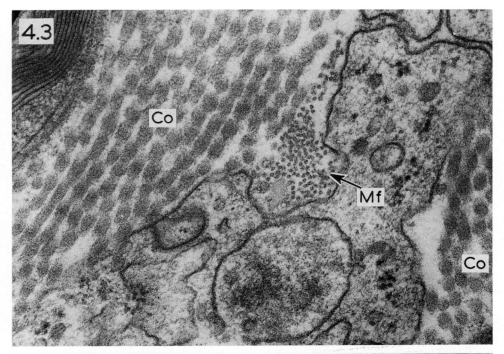

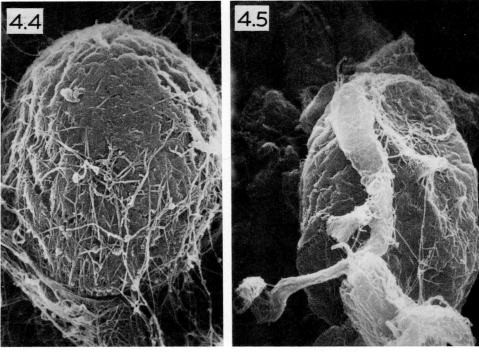

differences. For example, mast cells are present in the capsule of rat spinal and cranial ganglia (Olsson, 1968b), but do not occur within the endoneurium (Olsson, 1968b), or are extremely rare therein (Friede and Johnstone, 1967).

The endoneurium of the nodose ganglion in the rat (and also in the rabbit and guinea pig) is similarly devoid of mast cells (Lieberman, 1968a), whereas the trigeminal ganglion in the same species contains numerous mast cells (Mazza and Dixon, 1972). The specific role or roles of mast cells in sensory ganglia and the significance of the variations in their distribution have yet to be established.

4.2.2 Blood vessels

General features

Sensory ganglia are considerably more densely vascularized than are the nerve roots and peripheral nerves (Adams, 1942), or sympathetic ganglia (Szabó and Bölönyi, 1955). The intraganglionic blood vessels are predominantly capillaries, but precapillary arterioles and venules are also present (Bergmann and Alexander, 1941). Arterioles are relatively sparse and are concentrated beneath the capsule of the ganglion. Intraganglionic vessels originate from vessels that penetrate the capsule of the ganglion from an arterial plexus situated within, and superficial to, the capsule of the ganglion, and drain into a similar periganglionic venous plexus (Bergmann and Alexander, 1941; Adams, 1942; Brierley, 1955). As they pentrate the ganglion from the capsule, some vessels carry a 'sleeve' of perineurium with them for a variable distance into the ganglion (Lieberman, 1968a). The intraganglionic capillaries show considerable variation in overall diameter and endothelial cell width: some capillaries have conspicuously large lumina but relatively thin walls (Lieberman, 1968a). Very large focal dilatations of the intraganglionic capillaries ('ampullar dilatations'), particularly in the cell-rich zones, have been described in some studies (Bergmann and Alexander, 1941; Szabó and Bölönyi, 1955; Andres, 1961; Waksman, 1961). Bergmann and Alexander (1941) found such dilatations to be particularly characteristic of human dorsal root ganglia, and like Gardner (1940), found them to be increasingly prominent with age.

The intraganglionic capillary plexus is particularly rich in the cortical zones of the ganglion where cell bodies are most concentrated (Bergmann and Alexander,

---

Fig. 4.3 Microfibrils (Mf) in a depression at the surface of an endoneurial cell, and collagen fibrils (Co), in the endoneurium of the guinea pig nodose ganglion. (x 104 000: Reproduced from Lieberman, 1968a, by courtesy of Springer Verlag.)

Figs. 4.4 and 4.5 Scanning electron micrographs of critical point-dried cells teased from rat lumbar dorsal root ganglia. Fig. 4.4 was teased before fixation and Fig. 4.5 after fixation. The endoneurial collagen fibres condensed around the ganglion cell-satellite cell complex are particularly prominent in Fig. 4.4. In Fig. 4.5 the stem process of the axon emerges from the one pole of the cell (at top). (Fig. 4.4 x 6000; Fig. 4.5 x 3400: Reproduced by courtesy of D. N. Landon.)

1941), and it has been suggested that each ganglion cell is surrounded by a capillary loop or a more extensive network (Bergmann and Alexander, 1941; Brierley, 1955). One consequence of the less dense vascularization of the central zone of the ganglion is that cells close to the centre of ganglia are more susceptible to the effects of vascular occlusion than those situated in the cortex (Viraswami, 1965). Capillaries deeply invaginated into ganglion cell bodies have also been described in several species, including man (Scharf, 1958).

Ultrastructure

Although ultrastructural data is rather scanty, it would appear that, for the most part, intraganglionic capillaries are of the continuous, unfenestrated variety (Andres, 1961; Lieberman, 1968a). The endothelial cells, in addition to the usual organelles, are richly endowed with micropinocytotic vesicles, are linked by *occludens* junctions (see below) and sometimes display endothelial 'flaps' close to the interendothelial cell junctions. The capillaries are enclosed within a basal lamina that is sometimes split to accommodate a pericyte, and a distinct condensation of reticular fibres around the capillaries is evident in reticular fibre preparations (e.g. Laidlaw, 1930) but is less obvious in electron micrographs (Lieberman, 1968a). Although extensive ultrastructural studies of rabbit, rat and guinea pig nodose ganglia revealed only one or two examples of fenestrated endothelial cells (Lieberman, unpublished observations) and in spite of the fact that fenestrations have not been described or illustrated in most other studies of sensory ganglia (e.g. Andres, 1961; Dixon, 1963; Schlaepfer, 1971), Olsson (1971) has described the common occurrence of fenestrated capillaries (and of 'open' interendothelial cell junctions) in the dorsal root ganglia of the rhesus monkey, and Jacobs (unpublished observations) has observed occasional examples in rat sensory ganglia (Fig. 4.8). In addition, Gabbiani and Majno (1969), Arvidsson, Kristensson and Olsson (1973) and Gabbiani, Badonnel, Mathewson and Ryan (1974) have commented on the constant and normal presence of endothelial microvilli extending into the capillary lumen in the rat and rabbit trigeminal ganglia. There would thus appear to be distinct species and site variations in the ultrastructure of intraganglionic capillaries.

Vascular permeability in sensory ganglia

In some species at least, peripheral and cranial nerve trunks (and, to a lesser extent, roots also) maintain a blood-nerve barrier to certain molecules of a rather similar nature to the blood-brain barrier. Thus, in rats and mice, following the intravenous injection of protein tracers such as Evans blue albumin, fluorescein—labelled albumin, or horseradish peroxidase, the endoneurium remains free of tracer although the epineurial connective tissue and the outer perineurium display evidence of extensive extravasation of the labelled protein (Olsson, 1968a, 1972). The barrier is apparently maintained by the endothelial cells of the endoneurial capillaries, and by the innermost lamellae of the perineurium (Olsson and Reese, 1971; Kristensson and Olsson, 1973). The latter are linked by extensive continuous tight junctions (Reale, Luciano and Spitznas, 1975) and act as a very effective barrier to the diffusion of many different ions and molecules out of or into the endoneurium (Olsson and Reese, 1971; Low, Chapter 3), and the endoneurial capillaries, unlike those of the perineurium and epineurium (which are freely permeable) do not allow the passage of tracer between endothelial cells or transport it across the vessel wall in vesicles or other membrane bounded systems (Olsson and Reese, 1971). However, the endoneurial vessels of both spinal and cranial sensory ganglia, in all species so far studied *are* permeable to these same protein tracers (Waksman, 1961; Olsson, 1968a; Olsson, Kristensson and Klatzo, 1971; Arvidsson et al., 1973), especially those vessels in the cell-rich areas of the ganglia (Arvidsson et al., 1973). This phenomenon is illustrated in Fig. 4.6 (from unpublished work of Jacobs) in which the endoneurial compartment is massively labelled with horseradish peroxidase 5 minutes after intravenous injection of the tracer. The presence in routine electron micrographs (after aldehyde perfusion or immersion fixation) of patchily distributed moderately electron-dense material within the endo- neurial spaces resembling precipitated protein (Figs. 4.2, 4.12, 4.30) suggests that components of the plasma (perhaps serum proteins) probably leak out in considerable quantities under normal conditions. Curiously the vessels of the trigeminal ganglion appear to be rather less permeable to tracers than those of the spinal ganglia of the same animal (Arvidsson et al., 1973). Endoneurial vessels within the nerve roots are also relatively permeable, but become less so with increasing distance from the ganglion (Olsson, 1968a, 1972). Permeability of ganglionic vessels to protein tracers is even more marked during acute cadmium intoxication (Schlaepfer, 1971) in which the primary toxic effect appears to be on the endothelial cells and the integrity of their intercellular junctions (Gabbiani, 1966; Schlaepfer, 1971; Gabbiani et al., 1974).

The structural basis or bases for the differences in vascular permeability considered above (i.e. between the endoneurial vessels of different sensory ganglia in one species; between the endoneurial vessels of ganglia, nerve roots and nerve trunks; between endoneurial vessels in different species; and between endoneurial vessels on the one hand and perineurial and epineurial vessels on the other hand) remain to be conclusively established. The presence of fenestrated endoneurial vessels in sites characterized by relatively high vascular permeability suggests an obvious correlation, but, although Olsson and Reese (1971) report the presence of a few fenestrated capillaries in the epineurium of mouse sciatic nerve, most reports do not suggest that perineurial and epineurial vessels are fenestrated, and it is unlikely that differences in the distribution of fenestrated capillaries account for general permeability differences. It may be that the differences in vascular permeability reside predominantly in differences in the extent, activity, and selectivity of transendothelial transport systems or in differences in the degree of 'tightness' of interendothelial cell junctions, or in a

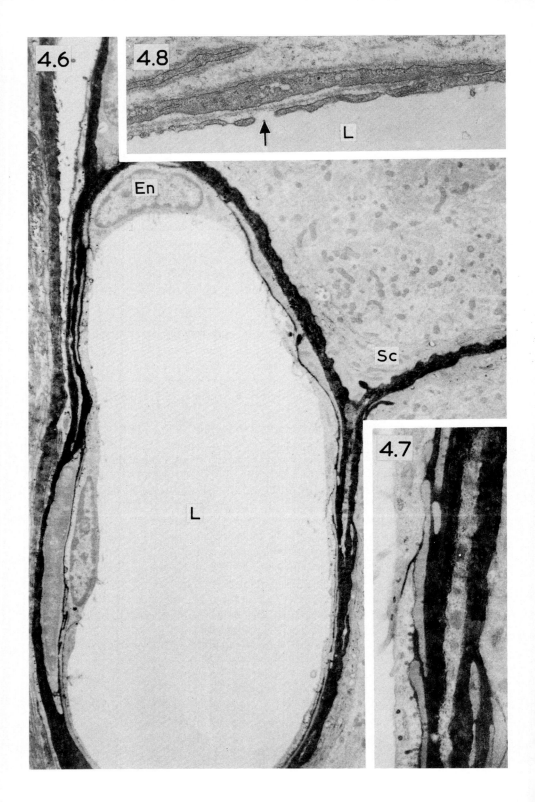

combination of these two factors. There are indications that regulation of the transendothelial cell route is likely to be important so far as the escape of protein is concerned. After intravenous injection of horseradish peroxidase, the tracer does not penetrate between endothelial cells to reach the endoneurium of rat sensory ganglia, but is found within endothelial microvesicles (Figs. 4.6, 4.7; Jacobs, unpublished observations). Furthermore, even very small protein molecules pass across 'leaky' muscle capillaries within vesicles (Simionescu, Simionescu and Palade, 1973) or through transient open channels formed by fused chains of such vesicles (Simionescu, Simionescu and Palade, 1975), rather than between the endothelial cells. On the other hand, Karnovsky (1968) has found that horseradish peroxidase escapes from muscle capillaries *between* endothelial cells, and Olsson and Reese (1971) have shown the same tracer passing from the lumina of epineurial and perineurial vessels between endothelial cells. Further ultrastructural tracer experiments and freeze fracture studies may help to decide the relative importance of these two routes of egress.

There is every reason to believe that the fact that serum proteins, and presumably other molecules, are able to pass from the circulation into the endoneurium of sensory ganglia is of both physiological and pathological significance, and may well be related to the special sensitivity of sensory ganglia to toxic agents such as cadmium (Gabbiani, 1966) and to certain neurological disorders in which ganglia rather than roots or nerves are primarily affected. Furthermore, species differences in the permeability of intraganglionic vessels may underlie differences in susceptibility to, among other conditions, experimental allergic neuritis and diphtheritic neuropathy (e.g. Waksman, 1961; Olsson, 1968a; Arvidsson *et al.*, 1973).

The permeability of intraganglionic capillaries to serum proteins also raises interesting questions about the disposal route of the leaked proteins, since there are no lymphatics within the ganglionic endoneurium (Ranvier, 1878; Lieberman, 1968a). Under normal conditions there is a constant proximo-distal flow of endoneurial fluid within peripheral nerves (Weiss, Wang, Taylor and

---

Fig. 4.6   Blood vessel (venule) situated immediately beneath the capsule of a rat lumbar ganglion. The tissue was fixed 5 minutes after intravenous injection of horseradish peroxidase. Electron dense reaction product fills the endoneurial space, and is also present between the cells forming the wall of the blood vessel, between satellite cells and between the satellite cells and the surface of the neurons. L – lumen; En – endothelial cell nucleus; Sc – satellite cell (x 5000: Reproduced by courtesy of J. M. Jacobs.)

Fig. 4.7   Enlargement of part of the wall of the blood vessel in Fig. 4.6. Reaction product can be seen in the endoneurial space, between the cells constituting the wall of the vessel (but not between the apical portions of the endothelial cells in the region of the junctional complex), and in numerous micropinocytotic vesicles, especially at the abluminal aspect of the endothelial cells. (x 19 500).

Fig. 4.8   Fenestrated, thin-walled capillary in rat cervical ganglion. One of the endothelial fenestrae lacks a pore diaphragm (arrow). L – lumen (x 26 000: Reproduced by courtesy of J. M. Jacobs.)

Edds, 1945; Mellick and Cavanagh, 1967) and it is possible that the leaked proteins are transported distally as components of the endoneurial fluid, to be released ultimately into extraneural connective tissue spaces at the open 'ends' of the perineurial sheaths (see Low, Chapter 3). Another possibility is that proteins are taken up by perineurial cells and transported from the endoneurial compartment to the epineurium, in which there are known to be lymphatics (Olsson, 1972). Allt (1972) has proposed that just such a mechanism of transperineurial bulk protein transport might operate in experimental allergic neuritis to dispose of serum proteins which leak into the endoneurium in particularly large quantities in this condition (see also Hall, 1972). There is also some evidence that lipid materials may be removed from the endoneurial compartment of peripheral nerves by a comparable process (see Williams and Hall, 1971). Finally, it may be that some leaked proteins are taken up by endothelial cells and returned to the circulation across the walls of the blood vessels. However, recent tracer experiments using intravenously injected horse-radish peroxidase indicate that within two hours, most of the leaked peroxidase in the endoneurial compartment of rat sensory ganglia, is taken up by macrophages: no evidence was found for a transperineurial route of disposal (Jacobs, unpublished observations).

4.3 Morphology and cytology of ganglion cells

4.3.1 *Size and number of ganglion cells*

Sensory ganglion cells vary enormously in size, both between different ganglia and within individual ganglia (Figs. 4.1, 4.11). Bühler (1898) gives a diameter range of from $10\mu m$ for the smallest cells of small vertebrates to $120\mu m$ for the largest spinal ganglion cells of man. In most ganglia the range of diameters is smaller: the cells of the lumbar ganglia in adult rats, for example, range from $20-50\mu m$ (Hatai, 1901), $10-80\mu m$ (Cavanaugh, 1951) or $18-75\mu m$ (Andres, 1961). In the first sacral ganglion of adult humans, however, almost the full range of diameters ($15-110\mu m$) is represented (Ohta, Offord and Dyck, 1974). Most of the cells are spheroidal, with round or oval profiles in section: some of the smaller cells appear to be ellipsoidal, and the smaller cells commonly appear angular in sections (e.g. Hatai, 1901; Scharf, 1958; Bunge, Bunge, Peterson and Murray, 1967), although less commonly so in well-fixed, plastic-embedded material.

Notwithstanding the transient differences between the ventrolateral and dorsomedial cell groups during early development (Section 7.3), and reports that small cells are more numerous at the centre and large cells at the periphery of developing human spinal ganglia (McKinnis, 1936), it would appear that in the spinal ganglia of adult mammals, cells of all sizes are distributed randomly. In the spinal ganglia of lower vertebrates, however, small cells may be particularly numerous in the zone surrounding the central axis of sensory root fibres (e.g. Berthold, 1966).

There is a postive correlation between cell size and axonal diameter: this relationship is soundly based on qualitative histological observations of normal adult ganglia (e.g. Cajal, 1909; Marinesco, 1909), on quantitative histological studies demonstrating an approximately parallel increase in cell and axonal diameter during the extended period of postnatal growth in rats (Donaldson and Nagasaka, 1918), and on quantitative histological studies establishing a selective loss of small diameter axons concomitant with the loss of small cells in certain pathological states (Ohnishi and Dyck, 1974). This correlation is also supported by physiological observations (e.g. Svaetichin, 1951). There is also a positive relationship between ganglion cell size and body size, the largest neurons occurring in the ganglia of the large mammals (Levi, 1908; Marinesco, 1909). The positive relationship between cell body size and the size of the peripheral territory innervated — originally propounded by Levi (1906, 1908), is amply confirmed by many studies demonstrating an increase in cell body size when the peripheral field of innervation is increased, either during normal postnatal growth (Donaldson and Nagasaka, 1918; Ohta *et al.*, 1974) or under experimental conditions (see Pannese, 1963 for review and references).

The continued growth of spinal ganglion cells as the size and surface area of the body increases is a striking illustration of this relationship. In man, for example, spinal ganglion cells continue to enlarge and the profile of perikaryal diameters progressively changes up to about 12 years, at which age the adult condition is reached (Ohta *et al.*, 1974). In rats, which continue to grow throughout life, perikaryal diameter increases in proportion to the increase in body surface area over at least the first year of life (Donaldson and Nagasaka, 1918), although Lawson Caddy and Biscoe (1974), measuring from electron micrographs, found no increase in the mean diameter of rat lumbar spinal ganglion cells after the 100th day.

The number of cells per ganglion varies enormously from the few hundred in the spinal ganglia of lower vertebrates to scores of thousands in the corresponding human ganglia. The numbers in individual ganglia also vary and marked differences in cell number between corresponding ganglia or groups of ganglia on opposite sides of the body have been described (DeLorenzi, 1937). As might be expected, thoracic ganglia contain significantly fewer cells than cervical or lumbar ganglia. Rat cervical ganglia contain about 11 000 cells whereas thoracic ganglia contain approximately 7000 cells (Hatai, 1902): in the cat, ganglia $T_3 - L_3$ contain 8–12 000 cells whereas ganglia $C_2 - T_1$ contain 18–33 000 cells (Holmes and Davenport, 1940).

The maximum number of cells in human S1 ganglia is reached by 3 years. It has been reported that signs of ganglion cell death appear with increasing frequency in ganglia from older people (Scharf and Blumenthal, 1967), and some counts have indicated a loss of cells with age (Gardner, 1940). Other studies, however, have not provided evidence for a significant decrease with age in numbers of sensory ganglion cells (e.g. Hatai, 1902, rat spinal ganglia; Ohta *et al.*, 1974, human S1 ganglion).

4.3.2 *Nucleus*

General features

The nuclei of sensory ganglion cells are large in relation to perikaryal volume, particularly in the small cells (Hydén, 1943): cell size and nuclear size are positively correlated but the relationship is not rectilinear (Hatai, 1907).

The nuclei normally occupy a central position in the cell body: they are generally spherical, with a smooth outline and few indentations (Fig. 4.1). In a small proportion of ganglion cells, nuclei are eccentrically situated: the proportion of such cells is larger in some ganglia and species than others (see, for example, Pannese, Bianchi, Calligaris, Ventura and Weibel, 1972). Binucleate neurons can occur but are extremely rare.

Apart from the nucleolus, the nucleolus associated chromatin and the sex chromatin (in the females of some species), the nucleus shows minimal staining with Nissl and conventional nuclear dyes, and by electron microscopy displays an evenly dispersed, unclumped chromatin pattern, quite unlike that of the satellite cells, Schwann cells and the various other non-neuronal nuclei of the ganglia, all of which have prominent heterochromatin aggregations, particularly at the nuclear margin (Fig. 4.2). Scattered singly among the finely dispersed chromatin particles, or clustered (often close to the nucleolus) are larger particles (range 25—40 nm), the perichromatin and interchromatin granules.

Intranuclear bodies

Spherical inclusion bodies ranging from less than 0.5μm to about 1μm in diameter are occasionally seen by electron microscopy in the nuclei of sensory ganglion cells (Moses, Beaver and Ganote, 1965, monkey trigeminal ganglion; Beaver, Moses and Ganote, 1965, human trigeminal ganglion; Figs. 4.9a–c rabbit nodose ganglion). They appear to lie relatively close to the nuclear periphery and sometimes also close to the nucleolus (Figs. 4.9a, b). Their morphology is somewhat variable but they most commonly exhibit an external or capsular element 50—100 nm wide, in which concentrically arranged filaments can usually be resolved (Figs. 4.9a–c), enclosing a central region containing electron dense granular material similar to chromatin granules or to nucleolar component granules (Figs. 4.9a, b). More rarely tubular or vesicular elements may occur within the nuclear bodies (Fig. 4.9c). Similar bodies have been described in other neurons, including sympathetic ganglion cells in dogs (Ishikawa, 1964), rats and rabbits (Lieberman, unpublished observations) and birds (Masurovsky, Benitez, Kim and Murray, 1970), and in a variety of other cell types, both normal and pathological (references in Popoff and Stewart, 1968; Dupuy-Coin and

Bouteille, 1972, 1975). There is some evidence that the granular internal components may contain RNA and derive from the nucleolus (Dupuy-Coin and Bouteille, 1972). There are also indications that the bodies contain protein (the capsular filaments, for example, are digested by pronase) and may be sites in which proteins, newly synthesized by nucleus or cytoplasm, accumulate (Dupuy-Coin and Bouteille, 1975).

Nucleolus

Most nuclei contain only a single spherical nucleolus, some 2–4μm in diameter (Figs. 4.1, 4.2). The nucleolus is normally centrally situated, but may sometimes lie very close to the nuclear periphery. Since the nucleus is also centrally situated, most nucleoli lie close to the centre of the cell body. Pannese *et al.* (1972), however, found consistent differences between species in the degree of nucleolar eccentricity in thoracic spinal ganglion cells: in rabbits more than 90 per cent of the nucleoli fall within a contour representing the cell outline reduced to 1/3 of its size (i.e. within approximately 1/3 of a radius from the cell centre), whereas less than 50 per cent of nucleoli lie within the central zone in guinea pigs, about 60 per cent in the rat, and nearly 80 per cent in the cat.

There is a close and direct relationship between nucleolar size (and nucleolar RNA content) and cytoplasmic RNA content (Hydén, 1960). In cells with two or more nucleoli, the individual nucleoli are relatively small, and the total nucleolar volume in such cells is probably not greater than in cells of comparable size with only a single nucleolus. The nucleoli display the prominent nucleolonemal organization characteristic of neuronal nucleoli (Figs. 4.2, 4.9a) and have been subjected to detailed ultrastructural and cytochemical analysis (e.g. Izard and Bernhard, 1962; Marinozzi, 1964; Hardin, Spicer and Greene, 1969). Occasionally, intranucleolar bodies resembling the nucleololus of monkey cerebellar neurons (see Dutta, Siegesmund and Fox, 1963) occur in sensory ganglion cells (Fig. 4.10, rat nodose ganglion, Lieberman, 1968b; see also Moses *et al.*, 1965 and Beaver *et al.*, 1965, monkey and human trigeminal ganglion cells).

4.3.3 *Cytoplasmic organization*

The pioneer studies of Palay and Palade (1955) and a considerable number of subsequent observations have made familiar the ultrastructural features of cytoplasmic organelles in these cells (Peters, Palay and Webster, 1970). For this reason only selected aspects of certain organelles will be stressed in this section.

Nissl substance, granular endoplasmic reticulum and ribosomes

Cells of all sizes are rich in Nissl substance, which may be distributed in a variety of patterns. In some cells it may occur as fine dust-like particles evenly

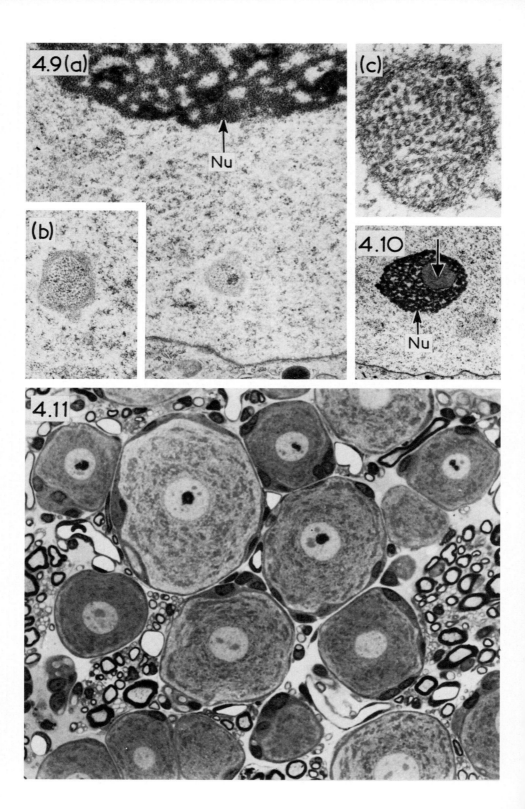

distributed throughout the cytoplasm, or it may comprise a virtually homogeneous mass in which distinct Nissl bodies are not obvious. In the majority, however, and certainly in all of the larger cells, discrete Nissl bodies of variable size are present, separated by diffusely basiphil or non-basiphil areas. In such cells the Nissl bodies may be distributed evenly throughout the cytoplasm or may be concentrated at the periphery or around the nucleus.

So diverse are the Nissl distribution patterns that numerous attempts have been made to classify sensory ganglion cells in terms of these differences. Histologists such as Cajal, Nissl, Dogiel, Cox, Van Gehuchten and Lugaro, and many others besides, produced classifications of varying complexity (see Orr and Rows, 1901; Marinesco, 1909, and Clark, 1926, for comprehensive reviews). Most of these classifications were esoteric, few show more than a superficial correspondence one with another and none are now of any great importance; (although in the future, when we have a greater understanding of subtle variations in the metabolic activities of different cells, such differences may acquire some significance). One common theme, however, does run through most of these classifications and that is the difference – first remarked upon on the basis of *intra vitam* methylene blue and metallic impregnation methods – between *large clear* cells and *small obscure* cells (Dogiel, 1908; Cajal, 1909). This subdivision of the neurons of sensory ganglia will be considered in more detail in Section 4.4.1.

At the ultrastructural level, Nissl substance is represented by granular endoplasmic reticulum and associated free ribosomes. The organization of the reticulum is somewhat variable, but the pattern throughout any one cell tends to be similar. At one extreme is an arrangement of the reticulum as extensive flattened sacs, usually stacked in parallel to form straight or curved arrays with minimal interconnection between adjacent sacs (e.g. Fig. 4.13). At the other extreme the granular reticulum comprises much shorter, less flattened sacs or cisterns, usually randomly arranged with respect to one another and commonly branched and anastomosing. Both varieties may be arranged in focal concentrations, or may be diffusely distributed throughout the cytoplasm. Cell size-related differences in the organization of granular endoplasmic reticulum will be considered in Section 4.4.1.

Fig. 4.9 Nuclear bodies in nodose ganglion neurons of guinea pig (Fig. 4.9a) and rabbit (Figs. 4.9b,c). The 'capsular' component of the bodies apparently contains circumferentially arranged filaments enclosing a core in which electron dense granules (Figs. 4.9a,b) or rarely, vesicular or tubular elements (Fig. 4.9c) are contained. Nu – nucleolus. (Figs. 4.9a,b × 20 000; Fig. 4.9c × 70 000.)

Fig. 4.10 Intranucleolar body (nucleololus, arrowed) in a rat nodose ganglion cell. Nu – nucleolus. (× 4000.)

Fig. 4.11 Light and dark cells in a toluidine blue-stained 1 μm plastic section of rabbit cervical dorsal root ganglion. (× 640: Reproduced by courtesy of J. M. Jacobs.)

As is the case in most other neurons, the granular reticulum, no matter how arranged, is always associated with large numbers of free ribosomes, which lie between and surround the endoplasmic elements. The free ribosomes are considerably more numerous than membrane-attached ribosomes (by a factor of at least 4:1 and perhaps as much as 20:1). As is the case for the membrane-attached ribosomes when seen *en face*, the free ribosomes all appear to be in polyribosomal arrays, the most common form of which is a 5 or 6 ribosome rosette (Palay and Palade, 1955).

Golgi apparatus and GERL

The Golgi apparatus is particularly prominent in sensory ganglion cells. When examined by light microscopy in metal-impregnated tissue, or after the histochemical reaction for nucleoside diphosphatase (NDPase) or thiamine pyrophosphatase (TPPase), the Golgi apparatus in most neurons appears to comprise a complex network of interconnected sheet-like and tubular elements surrounding the nucleus (Figs. 4.16, 4.17). The precise pattern varies from cell to cell and a considerable range of appearances is depicted in Fig. 4.16. Detailed descriptions of the light microscopically visualized apparatus have been given by, among others, Penfield (1920), Sosa and De Zorilla (1966) and Lieberman (1968b, 1969b) in metallic impregnations, and by Shanthaveerappa and Bourne (1965), Holtzman, Novikoff and Villaverde (1967) and Novikoff (1967a) in histochemical preparations. In general, the Golgi apparatus revealed by the two techniques appears similar, but the histochemically visualized reticulum appears to be slightly more complex, with a greater variety of positively-stained elements than is the case in osmium or silver-impregnated specimens.

By electron microscopy, in conventional thin sections, elements of the Golgi apparatus appear as discrete units ('dictyosomes'), each composed of a stack of flattened cisterns or saccules associated with numerous vesicles and with other tubular and cisternal elements of the smooth endoplasmic reticulum (Palay and Palade, 1955; Novikoff, 1967a; Lieberman, 1968b, 1969b; Peters *et al.*, 1970; Peach, 1972a; Fig. 4.18).

Fig. 4.12 Survey electron micrograph of rat cervical ganglion showing a small dark cell (at centre) and parts of a similar cell (bottom) and of two large pale cells (right and left). The stem process of the small dark cell emerges from the perikaryon (at A1) and curves around the parent cell (A2 and A3). F — nucleus of endoneurial fibroblast; SN — satellite cell nucleus. (x approx. 2600: Reproduced by courtesy of J. M. Jacobs.)

Figs. 4.13—4.15 Illustrate the principal cytoplasmic characteristics of small dark and large light cells and are taken from Jacobs *et al.* (1975a) (Reproduced by courtesy of the authors and Blackwell Scientific Publications Ltd.) In each case the survey electron micrograph inset is at (x 1300) and the main figure at (x 15 000.)
(4.13) Small dark cell from rat trigeminal ganglion. The cell contains an abundant, highly organized granular reticulum.

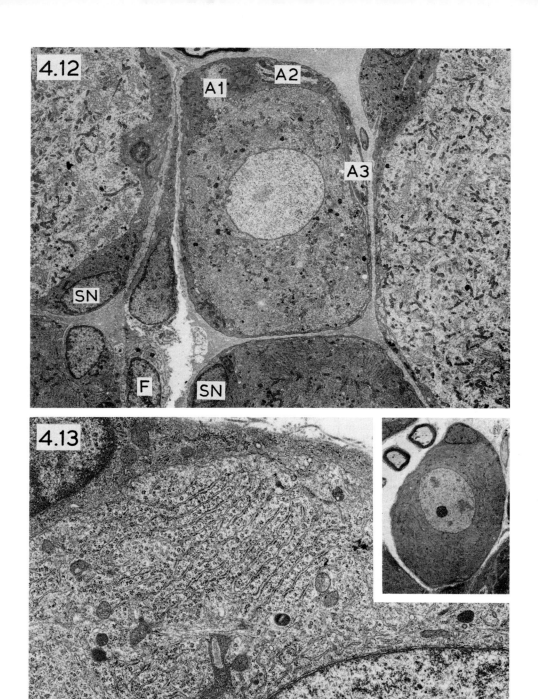

Certain enzymes (including NDPase and TPPase) and some glycoproteins increase in concentration or are only detectable at the inner ('mature') face of the stacks (Novikoff, 1967a; Novikoff, Novikoff, Quintana and Hauw, 1971; Rambourg, Marraud and Chrétien, 1973; Rambourg, Clermont and Marraud, 1974). The NDPase and TPPase-containing element consists of a hexagonal array of interconnected tubules, and is best seen in cytochemically reacted semi-thin sections (0.5μm) viewed *en face* in the electron microscope (Novikoff *et al.*, 1971). The study of such sections and reconstructions from serial thin sections lead to the conclusion that the NDP/TPPase positive inner element of the individual dictyosomes forms a continuum throughout the cell and thus accounts for the reticulum seen in histochemical preparations by light microscopy (Novikoff *et al.*, 1971).

Lying within the concavity of the mature face of the Golgi apparatus, and immediately adjacent to the NDP/TPPase-positive innermost element, is the GERL (Golgi-associated smooth Endoplasmic Reticulum with associated Lyso-somes; Novikoff, 1967a) which consists of a series of flattened cisterns and tubules connected to one another, and also to nearby elements of the granular endoplasmic reticulum, by narrow tubules (Fig. 4.18). The GERL complex is completely NDP/TPPase negative, but is strongly positive for acid phosphatase (Novikoff, 1967a; Novikoff *et al.*, 1971) and for this and other reasons Novikoff *et al.* (1971) consider that GERL is a distinct organelle system, rather than a component of the Golgi apparatus. The GERL appears to be involved in the formation of dense body lysosomes and acid hydrolase-containing coated vesicles (Holtzman *et al.*, 1967) from both its cisternal and tubular components (Novikoff *et al.*, 1971) (Fig. 18a), and it is reasonable to assume that newly synthesized acid hydrolases reach the GERL complex via its continuities with the granular endoplasmic reticulum, within which they are in all probability synthesized.

The outermost (generally convex) 'forming' face of the Golgi stacks apparently consists of a fenestrated, relatively wide cistern in most electron micrographs (Fig. 4.18). Continuities between this element and the granular endoplasmic reticulum can sometimes be traced in thin sections. This outermost component of the Golgi apparatus alone — for reasons that are completely unknown at present — is selectively 'stained' by prolonged osmication (Novikoff *et al.*, 1971; Rambourg *et al.*, 1973, 1974). Such preparations, especially when viewed as stereopairs of sections in the 0.5—7μm range photographed in the high voltage electron microscope (Rambourg *et al.*, 1973, 1974), show that the outermost element of the forming face of individual dictyosomes comprises a polygonal network of tubules (the primary network) interconnected to form a

---

(4.14) Large pale cell of the A1 variety from rat trigeminal ganglion. The clumps of granular reticulum are separated by narrow bundles of neurofilaments.
(4.15) ,Large pale cell of the A2 variety from rat cervical ganglion. The small clumps of granular reticulum are separated by prominent bundles of neurofilaments.

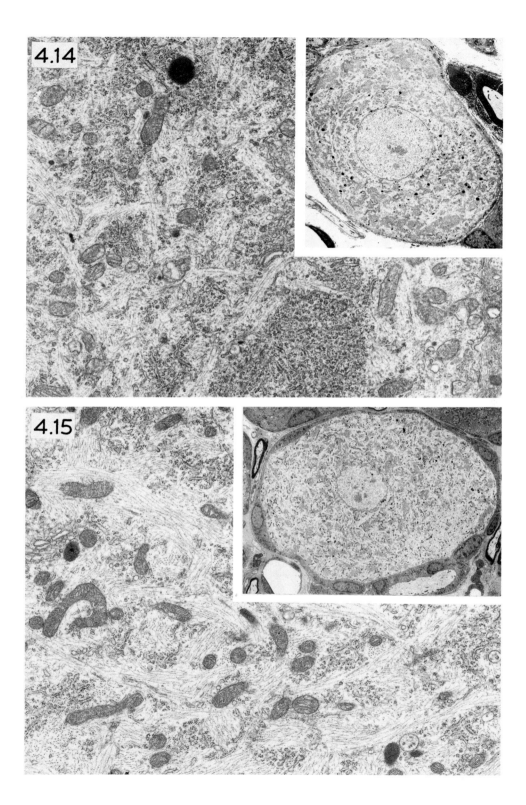

continuous reticulum surrounding the nucleus (the secondary network) and thus corresponding to the light-microscopically visualized Golgi apparatus seen in osmium-impregnated tissue (Novikoff *et al.*, 1971; Rambourg *et al.*, 1974).

It is therefore clear that the Golgi apparatus of light microscopy corresponds to one of two approximately coextensive, but structurally, chemically and functionally distinct, membrane systems: the osmiophilic, interconnected outermost elements of the forming face of the dictyosomes and the NDP/TPPase positive, interconnected inner elements of the mature face of the dictyosomes. The other cisterns of the dictyosomes (generally 2–6) are commonly fenestrated and are sandwiched between these two systems as disc-like stacks, but are probably not interconnected from one dictyosome to another. Furthermore, because the cisterns of GERL are interconnected by tubules, the GERL itself constitutes a third distinct endocellular reticulum, approximately coextensive with the Golgi apparatus of light microscopy: the many reports of acid phosphatase reaction product distributed in a reticular form (e.g. Kokko, 1965; Kalina and Bubis, 1968) are thus explained. It remains to be established which part or parts of the Golgi/GERL complexes are impregnated with the silver techniques. Novikoff (1967a) has suggested that the Da Fano silver technique impregnates the GERL in sensory ganglion cells because his preparations showed a reticulum only in small neurons (which have a complex GERL), whereas in the larger neurons only a granular, lysosome-like impregnation was produced: it is probable, however, that the large cells had not been successfully impregnated (see Figs. 4.16 and 4.17 and Lieberman, 1969a, b).

The functions of the Golgi apparatus and of the GERL are only partially understood. Autoradiographic studies have established that, as in other neurons and other cell types, the Golgi apparatus of the sensory ganglion cell is involved in the sequestration of newly synthesized proteins (Droz, 1965) and is the site of carbohydrate synthesis (Droz, 1967b) and presumably also of glycoprotein assembly. The presence of nucleoside phosphatase in the innermost element of the Golgi apparatus (see above) may indicate that glycosyl transferases are located at this level and suggests that glycoprotein synthesis occurs in or close to the innermost element of the Golgi apparatus (Novikoff *et al.*, 1971).

Not all newly synthesized protein passes through the Golgi apparatus. Many of the proteins migrating along the axon bypass the Golgi apparatus (Droz, 1967a) and newly synthesized acid hydrolases may pass through only the GERL on their way to lysosomal bodies (see below).

For extensive discussions of the functions of the Golgi apparatus and GERL see Novikoff (1967a, b), Novikoff *et al.* (1971) and Holtzman *et al.* (1973).

Modifications of the endoplasmic reticulum

Lamellar bodies. Modifications of the endoplasmic reticulum consisting of stacks of (or in rare cases, individual) agranular cisternae with compressed and almost obliterated lumina, spaced evenly and in parallel, and associated with an amorphous or 'fluffy' electron dense intercisternal material, have been described in sensory ganglion cells (Rosenbluth, 1962a, b; Lieberman, 1968b; Krajci, 1972). The possible significance of these lamellar bodies, which are continuous with unmodified elements of the granular reticulum is unknown, and the possibility that they and similar lamellar bodies are fixation-dependent artefacts has not, as yet, been adequately evaluated.

Subsurface cisterns. Both compressed and less flattened subsurface cisterns are common in sensory ganglion cells (Fig. 4.35) (Rosenbluth, 1962a, b, 1963; Lieberman, 1968b; Krajci, 1972). They are also prominent in sensory ganglion cells maintained *in vitro* (Bunge *et al.*, 1967). The outer surface of the subsurface cistern maintains a constant separation of 10–15 nm from the neuronal plasmalemma and faithfully follows its every undulation. Subsurface cisterns, particularly the non-compressed variety, may bear ribosomes on their cytoplasmic surface and both varieties are commonly in continuity with granular endoplasmic reticulum and may show a positive reaction within their lumina for acetyl cholinesterase (Brzin, Tennyson and Duffy, 1966). Although they most commonly occur singly, a stack of cisterns resembling the lamellar bodies described above may occasionally occur in a subsurface position (Rosenbluth, 1962a; Krajci, 1972).

In chick embryo dorsal root ganglia at about 5–7 days, coextensive confronting subsurface cisterns are commonly observed beneath the plasma membranes of contiguous neuroblasts (Pannese, 1968; Weis, 1968). As the neuroblasts become encapsulated by satellite cells (see Section 4.7.4), the confronting cisterns disappear: Weis (1968) has speculated that these transient junctional specializations may be involved in contact inhibition of neuroblast migration (see also Section 4.7.3).

The structural variations in subsurface cisterns of many different classes of adult nerve cell have recently been reviewed by Le Beux (1972b), who also offers some speculations concerning the possible physiological significance of the subsurface cistern.

Glycogen-membrane arrays. Glycogen granules are only occasionally seen in the perikarya of adult mammalian sensory ganglion cells although they may be abundant in the corresponding cells of lower vertebrates (Berthold, 1966). Stacks of parallel smooth surfaced cisterns associated with glycogen aligned in a single row of evenly spaced particles between each pair of cisterns have been observed in sensory ganglion cells in a variety of sites and species and following different methods of fixation (Bunge *et al.*, 1967; Lieberman, 1968b; Pannese, 1969b; Fig. 4.20a). Occasionally one or a small stack of these glycogen-membrane arrays may lie in a subsurface position (Fig. 4.20b).

Lysosomes

A variety of familiar cytoplasmic constituents contain acid hydrolases, and can therefore be classified as lysosomes (Novikoff, 1967a, b). The family of lysosomes

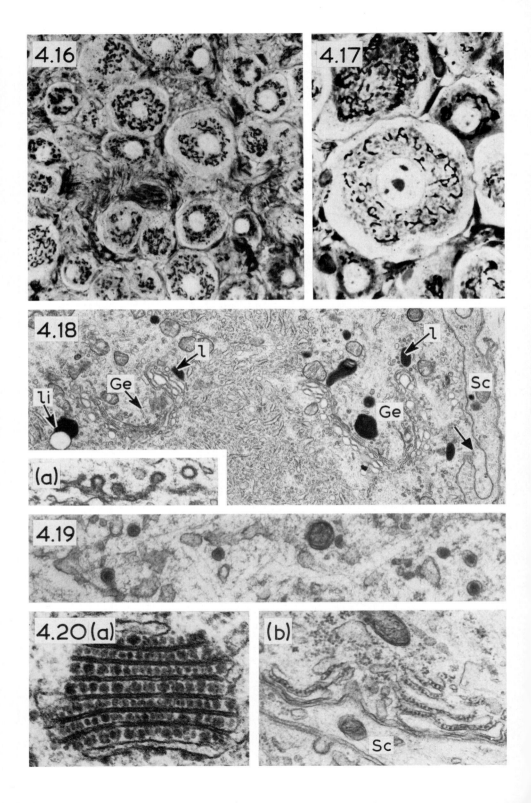

includes the prominent and numerous 'dense bodies' (Figs. 4.18, 4.22a), multi-vesicular bodies (Fig. 4.21), autophagic vacuoles (which are uncommon), coated (or alveolate) vesicles, generally from 40—100 nm diameter which may lie both close to the plasma membrane (Fig. 4.36), and close to and often apparently budding from the elements of the Golgi apparatus and GERL (Fig. 4.18a), smooth surfaced vesicles associated with the Golgi apparatus and GERL, the GERL itself (Fig. 4.18 and see above), and lipofuscin bodies (Figs. 4.18, 4.21).

The dense bodies comprise a heterogeneous population: most are ovoid or spherical and they range from less than 0.2μm to over 1μm in diameter. All are limited by a single unit membrane. Many dense body lysosomes, particularly the smaller ones, have a matrix of moderate electron density comprised of a fine granular, homogeneously distributed material. Others, particularly the larger lysosomes, contain scattered larger electron dense granules, and whorls or stacks of membrane-like material. The size, heterogeneity and internal complexity of the dense body lysosomes increase with age or after a regenerative response to injury of the peripherally directed cell process (Lieberman, 1971).

The small cells of sensory ganglia apparently contain a higher concentration of dense body lysosomes than the larger cells, and acid hydrolase activity evaluated at the light microscope level is markedly greater in the small cells (Kokko, 1965; Novikoff, 1967a, b; Peach, 1972b). This feature appears to be correlated with a more prominent Golgi apparatus and GERL in the small cells (Novikoff, 1967a). The difference between large and small cells with respect to acid hydrolase activity appears to be qualitative as well as quantitative. Knyihár (1971) reports that although cells of all sizes in rat dorsal root ganglia show acid phosphatase activity, the small cells alone contain a fluoride-resistant (and

---

Fig. 4.16   Golgi apparatus of rabbit nodose ganglion neurons shown by the Da Fano silver impregnation technique. (x 400. Reproduced from Lieberman, 1969b, by courtesy of the Cambridge University Press.)

Fig. 4.17   Golgi apparatus (Da Fano technique) and Nissl substance (haematoxylin counterstain) in rabbit nodose ganglion cells. (x 800. Reproduced from Lieberman, 1971, by courtesy of Academic Press.)

Fig. 4.18   Two elements of the Golgi apparatus in an electron micrograph of a rabbit nodose ganglion cell. Note the distended, fenestrated outer cisternae of the forming face and the elements of GERL (Ge) at the mature face. Lipofuscin (li), smaller lysosome-like dense bodies (l), the satellite cell (Sc) and a paraphyte (arrowed) are also seen. (x 12 500.)

Fig. 4.18a   Mature face of Golgi apparatus in a rabbit nodose ganglion neuron. Coated vesicles associated with a tubule or cistern of GERL are prominent. (x 40 000.)

Fig. 4.19   Dense-cored vesicles in peripheral cytoplasm of rabbit nodose ganglion neuron. (x 40 000.)

Fig. 4.20   Glycogen-membrane complexes in cat cervical dorsal root ganglion (Fig. 4.20a) and in a subsurface position in a rabbit nodose neuron (Fig. 4.20b). Sc — satellite cell. (Fig. 4.20a x 86 000; Fig. 4.20b x 40 000: Reproduced by courtesy of D. N. Landon.)

perhaps non-lysosomal) isoenzyme. This fluoride-resistant acid phosphatase is transported cellulifugally along the dorsal roots, since it is present in the synaptic endings of these cells in the dorsal horn (Knyihár, László and Tornyos, 1974; Coimbra, Sodré-Borges and Magalhães, 1974), accumulates on the ganglionic side of a ligature tied along the central dorsal root (Knyihár, 1971) and rapidly disappears from the terminal distribution field in the dorsal horn following section of the central dorsal root or ganglionectomy (Knyihár, 1971; Knyihár et al., 1974; Coimbra et al., 1974).

There is considerable evidence, though as yet inconclusive, that acid hydrolases synthesized in the granular endoplasmic reticulum are concentrated and packaged into primary lysosomes within the GERL complex (see reviews in Novikoff, 1967b; Novikoff et al., 1971; Holtzman et al., 1973). Both coated vesicles and small dense body lysosomes are probably included in the population of primary lysosomes (Novikoff et al.,1971). The larger dense bodies, especially those with internal differentiations are probably secondary lysosomes (Novikoff, 1967b; see also Sekhon and Maxwell, 1974). A discussion of the role of lysosomes in sensory ganglion cells is beyond the scope of this chapter: the subject is dealt with in considerable detail by Novikoff, 1967b and Novikoff et al., 1971).

Pigment granules

Two classes of pigment are accumulated within sensory ganglion cells: a brown pigment which is a form of melanin (neuromelanin) and the yellow (to pale brown) pigment, lipofuscin. The melanin-like pigment occurs only rarely, most notably in primate trigeminal ganglion cells (De Castro, 1932), and in mesencephalic neurons (Hinrichsen and Larramendi, 1970), but lipofuscin is extremely common.

Lipofuscin pigment granules ('Abnutzungspigment') are PAS-postive, stain with Sudan Black B, are autofluorescent and, of course, are acid hydrolase-positive, although rather weakly so (Kokko, 1965; Novikoff, 1967b). It is generally accepted that lipofuscin granules are a class of lysosomal residual body: they appear to develop from dense body lysosomes by the progressive accumulation within the latter of the indigestible remnants of autophagic and/or heterophagic activity and by pigment deposition (Novikoff, 1967b; Sekhon and Maxwell, 1974).

A few lipofuscin granules are present in the ganglion cells of young animals, but the size and complexity of the individual granules and the size of the accumulations of lipofuscin granules all increase with age (Moses et al., 1965; Samorajski, Ordy and Rady-Reimer, 1968; Glees and Gopinath, 1973). A minority of ganglion cells in young adult animals contains conspicuous clusters of lipofuscin (Jacobs, unpublished observations), and in older animals many cells contain large numbers of granules sometimes clustered in a crescent-shaped mass at one pole of the nucleus: in some cells the entire cytoplasm appears to be packed with granules (e.g. Gardner, 1940). In fact, the accumulation of lipofuscin with age is a general phenomenon in vertebrate neurons, and is perhaps the most consistent and reliable ultrastructural correlate of cellular ageing in the neuron (see Sekhon and Maxwell, 1974).

The granules themselves are rather polymorphic: they are generally $1-3$ μm or more in diameter, are commonly lobulated, are limited by a single unit membrane, and display a wide spectrum of internal differentiations, the most prominent of which are extremely electron dense granules of a range of sizes, straight or curved linear arrays of membrane-like material, and one or more peripherally located lipid globules or vacuoles (Fig.4.21). Detailed descriptions of the lipofuscin granules* in sensory ganglion cells are given by Samorajski et al. (1965, 1968); Beaver et al. (1965); Moses et al. (1965); Pineda, Maxwell and Kruger (1967); Hasan and Glees (1972) and Glees and Gopinath (1973).

Melanin-like pigment also accumulates with increasing age in some ganglion cells (De Castro, 1932; Beaver et al., 1965). At the ultrastructural level, however, melanin and lipofuscin-containing pigment bodies are indistinguishable in these cells (Beaver et al., 1965), a finding that accords well with the demonstration that the neuromelanin granules of locus coeruleus and substantia nigra neurons do not resemble cutaneous melanin, but are very similar to mature lipofuscin granules (Moses, Ganote, Beaver and Schuffman, 1966; Hirosawa, 1968). It would seem possible, therefore, that some lipofuscin bodies become melanized in the sensory ganglion cells of older animals.

Other cytoplasmic organelles

Microtubules and filaments. Both filaments and tubules are abundant in the perikarya of sensory ganglion cells, disposed either singly (and apparently in random orientation) or in bundles (Figs. 4.14, 4.15, 4.21). Bundles of filaments are particularly numerous in large pale cells (Section 4.4.1) and form prominent roads ('plasmastrassen', Andres, 1961), between aggregates of granular endoplasmic reticulum and other cytoplasmic organelles (Fig. 4.15). Filaments and tubules are occasionally concentrated in the immediately perinuclear zone, in which, apart from mitochondria and free polyribosome clusters, they constitute the principal cytoplasmic component. The larger bundles of filaments correspond to the neurofibrils of light microscopy.

*Since the only valid criterion for identifying a cytoplasmic inclusion as liposfuscin is the presence in it of the pigment, it is by no means certain that all inclusions identified as lipofuscin bodies on histochemical or ultrastructural grounds do in fact contain pigment. As pigment accumulates in neurons, coarse electron dense granules appear within presumptive lipofuscin bodies (see Sekhon and Maxwell, 1974) but the distinction between large dense body lysosomes and lipofuscin granules is a somewhat arbitrary one at the electron microscope level. Most authors designate large irregularly shaped electron dense bodies with complex differentiations of the matrix (and particularly with lipid vacuoles) as lipofuscin bodies.

213

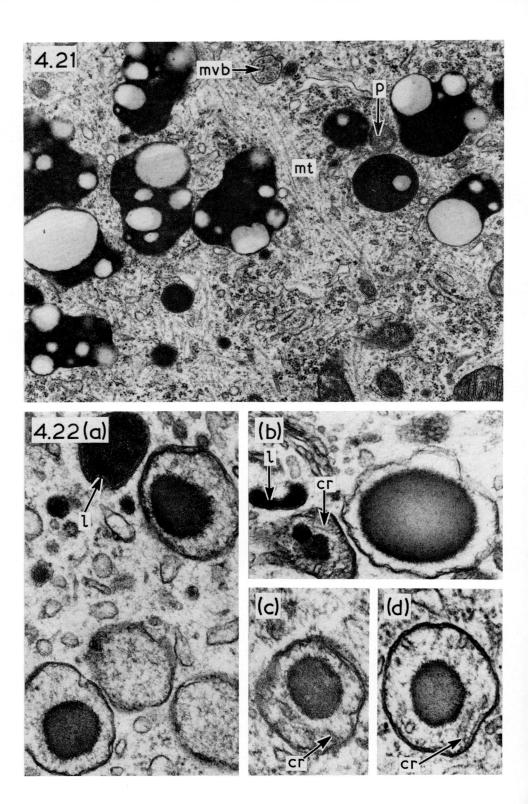

Mitochondria. The perikaryal mitochondria form an apparently homogeneous population. Most appear to be thread-like and branched, with a diameter of 0.2–0.4 μm (apparently unrelated to cell size) and have prominent cristae oriented for the most part perpendicular to the long axis of the mitochondrion.

Matrix granules of the type common in non-neuronal cells, especially in epithelial cells with ion-transporting functions, that probably represent storage sites for divalent cations (Peachey, 1964) are not normally present in these mitochondria (though see Bunge *et al.*, 1967). There are, however, several descriptions of distinctive matrix granules in the mitochondria of some ganglion cells (Moses *et al.*, 1965, mammalian trigeminal ganglia; Lieberman, 1968b, rat and rabbit nodose ganglia; Glees and Gopinath, 1973, spinal ganglia). The mitochondria studied by Lieberman (1968b) contained either one to several small granules only a few nanometres in diameter, or a single large granule (0.5 to 1 μm or more in diameter) with a characteristically 'frayed' border (Fig. 4.22). The granules were homogeneous in texture, electron-dense (though sometimes less so at their centres) and filled the entire mitochondrial matrix so that the mitochondria were only recognizable as such by their double membranes and the remnants of cristae. There was morphological evidence (apparent in most cells with 'mature' intra-mitochondrial granules) of a developmental progression from mitochondria of essentially normal appearance to the abnormal mitochondria containing a single large granule (Fig. 4.22). These mitochondrial inclusions were found in only some animals, but were always present in many cells: they were therefore interpreted to be of pathological significance (Lieberman, 1968b). Glees and Gopinath (1973), however, have placed an entirely different interpretation upon the similar inclusions observed in their material: they consider them as lipofuscin precursors, which they believe, contrary to most opinions, to be derived from mitochondria rather than lysosomes (see above).

Dense-cored vesicles. Smooth surfaced vesicles, from 50 to 150 nm in diameter with homogeneous electron dense cores are surprisingly common in sensory ganglion cells (Moses *et al.*, 1965; Lieberman, 1968b; Fig. 4.19). Some of the dense cores appear to be in tubules of smooth endoplasmic reticulum rather than in vesicles. Although many of the dense-cored vesicles resemble amine-storage granules, sensory ganglion cells do not display specific fluorescence and probably do not contain catecholamines.

Recently, Peach and Koch (1974) have described somewhat similar electron dense inclusions in mouse trigeminal ganglion cells. Comparable inclusions were

---

Fig. 4.21 Collection of complex lipofuscin granules in trigeminal ganglion cell of adult cat. Microtubules (mt), a multivesicular body (mvb) and a possible peroxisome (p) are also illustrated. (x 32 500. Reproduced by courtesy of D. N. Landon.)

Fig. 4.22 Intramitochondrial inclusions in rabbit (Figs. 4.22a-c) and rat (Fig. 4.22d) nodose neurons. (1 – lysosome-like dense body; cr – remains of mitochondrial cristae). (Fig. 22a x 60 000; Fig. 22b x 51 000; Figs. 4.22c,d x 80 000.)

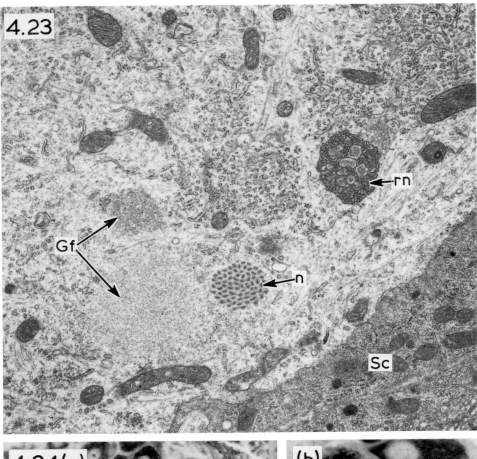

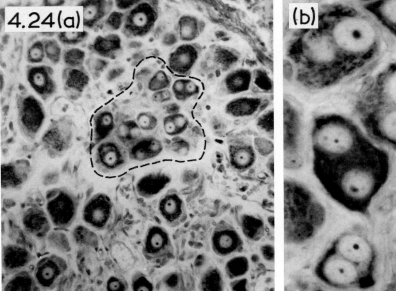

not found in rat trigeminal ganglion cells and Peach and Koch (1974) have interpreted them as viral inclusions because of their similarity to type A virus particles.

Peroxisomes. Peroxidase-containing bodies about 0.2 μm in diameter are present in sensory ganglion cells, but are not numerous and are considerably less conspicuous than in the perineuronal satellite cells (Citkowitz and Holtzman, 1973; Holtzman *et al.*, 1973; and see Section 4.6.1). Their significance is presently unknown.

Nematosomes and other granular/filamentous bodies. Nematosomes ('thread-like bodies'), originally identified as cytoplasmic components of sympathetic ganglion cells (Grillo, 1970), also occur in rat trigeminal and spinal ganglion cells (Peach, 1972c; Jacobs, Carmichael and Cavanagh, 1975a). The nematosomes are non membrane-bound approximately spherical inclusions about 1 μm in diameter, comprised of numerous interwoven threads of electron-dense material (Fig. 4.23 from unpublished work of Jacobs). The individual threads or strands are about 40 nm thick, have a filamentous substructure and are concentrated at the periphery of the large cells (Peach, 1972c). More than one nematosome may be present in a single cell. Peach (1972c) has drawn attention to the resemblance of nematosomes to, and suggested the possibility that they may be derived from, the paranucleolar body and/or the accessory body of Cajal, and according to Grillo (1970), who suggests a derivation from the nucleolus, nematosomes contain RNA as well as non-histone protein.

Other types of non-membrane-bound cytoplasmic body occur in sensory ganglion cells. The type most frequently seen is an approximately spherical body, generally less than 1 μm in diameter, comprised of granules 60–170Å in diameter which may be tightly or loosely packed and may be associated with filaments: these bodies are referred to here as granular/filamentous bodies (Rosenbluth, 1962a; Lieberman, 1968b; Le Beux, 1972a; Krajci, 1972; Fig. 4.23). They resemble bodies described in neurons of the central nervous system (e.g. Karlsson, 1966; Kishi, 1972): similar bodies also occur in non-neural cells. Kishi (1972) considered that bodies of this type resembled nucleoli, but cytochemical examination of the bodies has revealed the presence of protein but not of RNA. A possible variation of this type of body is a larger mass of loosely-packed finely granular and filamentous material within which are

Fig. 4.23 Non-membrane-bound cytoplasmic inclusions in rat cervical ganglion cell. Simple granular-filamentous bodies (Gf), a nematosome (n) and a reticular nematosome (rn) all lie close to one another at the periphery of a large pale cell. Sc – satellite cell. (x 17 500. Reproduced by courtesy of J. M. Jacobs.)

Fig. 4.24 Cluster of binucleate multipolar neurons (outlined in Fig. 4.24a) situated close to the superior pole of a rabbit nodose ganglion. The neurons are clearly different from the surrounding sensory ganglion cells, and the staining properties of the endoneurium also differ in the two regions. The cells, seen at higher magnification in a serial section in Fig. 4.24b, closely resemble rabbit sympathetic neurons. (Fig. 4.24a x 250; Fig. 4.24b x 800; cresyl violet stain.)

217

contained small clumps of more closely aggregated granules (Jacobs *et al.*, 1975a).

Another, quite different non membrane-bound body also present in sensory ganglion cells consists of filaments forming a wide-meshed network, and a core, or several cores of filaments that closely resemble ordinary neurofilaments (Fig. 4.23 from unpublished work of Jacobs). These bodies, which have been described in rat lateral vestibular neurons by Sotelo and Palay (1968) (who termed them fibrillary inclusions), and in neurons of the rat and cat substantia nigra by Le Beux (1972a) (who termed them reticular nematosomes), have been seen in rabbit nodose neurons (Lieberman, unpublished observations) and in rat sensory ganglion cells (Jacobs *et al.*, 1975a; Jacobs, Cavanagh and Carmichael, 1975b). Simple granular/filamentous bodies, nematosomes, and reticular nematosomes have been found in close association with one another in rat sensory ganglion cells (Jacobs *et al.* 1975a; and see Fig. 4.23). The functions of these different types of non-membrane-bound electron dense body are not yet known.

Special features of the axon hillock region

Sensory ganglion cells do not possess a prominent axon hillock (see Section 4.5.2) but there is normally a Nissl-free cytoplasmic zone close to the origin of the axon. In most cells this zone is cone-like, with its base extending into the cytoplasm, sometimes quite deeply, and its apex at the root of the axon. At the electron microscope level the axon hillock region is characterized by a small number of free ribosomes, sparsely distributed endoplasmic reticulum having extensively degranulated membranes, an absence of elements of the Golgi apparatus, and the orientation towards the axon of filaments and microtubules (Jacobs *et al.*, 1975b). Cisterns of the granular endoplasmic reticulum abutting this region also commonly show signs of degranulation (Jacobs *et al.*, 1975b) and the presence of this rather extensive volume of 'physiologically chromatolyzed' cytoplasm (see Fig. 4.30), is a factor of significance in experimental and pathological studies of sensory ganglion cells at the electron microscopic level.

4.4 Heterogeneity of neurons in sensory ganglia

4.4.1 *'Light' cells and 'dark' cells*

Although there appears to be no conclusive evidence for a distinct bimodal size distribution of sensory ganglion cells (e.g. Hatai, 1907), it is generally considered that these neurons may be divided into two classes in both cranial and spinal ganglia: large light cells (A cells) and small dark cells (B cells) (Scharf, 1958; Andres, 1961). The relative proportions of the two classes differ from ganglion to ganglion and according to certain variables in the preparative techniques (see below); for example, roughly 50 per cent of the cells in rat spinal ganglia fall into the category of small dark cells (e.g. Clark, 1926; Andres, 1961), and 62 per cent in the chicken trigeminal ganglion (Gaik, 1973). The small dark cells display a more intense basiphilia and are also more argyrophilic and osmiophilic than the large pale cells: for these reasons they have been referred to as *cellules obscures, pyknomorphic cells* and *chromophilic cells* (see Van Gehuchten, 1897; Hatai, 1907; Marinesco, 1909).

There is good evidence that at least some types of dark cell are avoidable artefacts (Cammermeyer, 1962) and that the nature of the fixative, and certain other variables in the preparation of tissue for histological study have a profound influence on the frequency with which dark cells are observed (e.g. Fisher and Ranson, 1934; Bacsich and Wyburn, 1953; Cammermeyer, 1962). It is therefore probable that at least some dark cells, especially those described in earlier studies of sensory ganglia, are shrunken and hyperchromic cells, and the basis for the light cell-dark cell classification, which was originally made in material sub-optimally fixed by current standards, has as a result been called into question on numerous occasions (see for example Kokko, 1965; Pineda *et al.*, 1967).

The bulk of the available evidence, however, does suggest that there are unshrunken small cells in well-fixed material with developmental, histochemical and ultrastructural features that distinguish them from the large pale cells. This evidence lends considerable support to the notion that sensory ganglion cells can be meaningfully subdivided into 'large pale' and 'small dark' classes, but it is as yet far from clear in what respects the differences are functionally significant (see p. 221).

Many authors have found consistent ultrastructural differences between the large light cells and the small dark cells (Hossack and Wyburn, 1954; Dawson, Hossack and Wyburn, 1955; Hess, 1955; Andres, 1961; Moses *et al.*, 1965; Berthold, 1966; Novikoff, 1967a, b; Peach, 1972a; Lawson *et al.*, 1974; Jacobs *et al.*, 1975a). The principal ultrastructural differences between the two classes relate to the arrangement and relative amount of granular endoplasmic reticulum and ribosomes. In the small dark cells, granular endoplasmic reticulum and ribosomes are highly concentrated, and discrete, small aggregates of granular reticulum are relatively rare. Such cells often display a highly organized lamellar granular endoplasmic reticulum, with long parallel cisterns extending in an almost uninterrupted ring around the cell, often located peripherally and enclosing a cytocentrum in which free polyribosomes are numerous (Fig. 4.13). In the large light cells, on the other hand, the granular endoplasmic reticulum is composed of discrete clumps (Figs. 4.14, 4.15). Furthermore, the large light cells contain a relatively high proportion of neurofilaments and these, together with microtubules, tend to run in prominent bundles between the aggregates of granular endoplasmic reticulum (Peach, 1972a; Lawson *et al.*, 1974; Jacobs *et al.*, 1975a). According to Jacobs *et al.* (1975a) the large light cells may be further subdivided on the basis of their neurofilament content into A_1 cells (Fig. 4.14) with relatively fewer neurofilaments than A_2 cells, in which the granular endoplasmic aggregates are small and the neurofilamentous 'roads' between them particularly prominent (Fig. 4.15). The A_1 and A_2 cells probably represent the extremes of a continuous spectrum in Nissl body size and neurofilament content in class A cells (Jacobs, personal communication). [Because of the similarity between the highly filamentous A_2 cells and some cells undergoing a retrograde perikaryal response to axotomy (Lieberman, 1971), the fact that such cells are normally present in sensory ganglia is of considerable relevance to the interpretation of experimental and pathological observations on sensory ganglia]. There are other ultrastructural differences between light and dark cells: the Golgi apparatus, GERL and lysosomal bodies (see appropriate parts of Section 4.3.3) all appear to be more highly developed in the small cells than in the large cells. A variety of histochemical differences, some of which are closely related to the ultrastructural differences, have also been described (e.g. Tewari and Bourne, 1962; Kokko, 1965; Matsuura, 1967; Kalina and Bubis, 1968, 1969; Knyihár, 1971; Robain and Jardin, 1972; Peach, 1972b). Of special interest is the finding that fluoride-resistant acid phosphatase is restricted to the small cells of rat spinal ganglia (Knyihár, 1971), while in frog spinal ganglia a characteristic distinguishing feature of the small cells is their high glycogen content (Berthold, 1966).

Differences between light and dark cells are also apparent prenatally in mammals (Tennyson, 1965, 1970; Lawson et al., 1974), and before hatching in birds (Gaik, 1973). The recent H^3 thymidine autoradiographic studies of Lawson et al. (1974) indicate that the large light cells are formed approximately one day earlier than the small dark cells (day 12 vs. day 13) in rat lumbar spinal ganglia. Future light and dark cells can also be distinguished in prenatal spinal ganglia of the rabbit on the basis of differences in the amount and distribution of granular endoplasmic reticulum in their cell bodies (Tennyson, 1965), and in the organelle content of the proximal portions of their processes (Tennyson, 1970). Although differences between light and dark cells are not very marked at birth in rat dorsal root ganglia (Kalina and Wolman, 1970; Yamadori, 1970; Lawson et al., 1974), and could not be detected in prenatal mouse trigeminal ganglia by Peach (1973), the two classes become progressively more distinct over the first few postnatal days. At the ultrastructural level of examination, this differentiation is associated with an enormous increase in the neurofilament content of the light cells (Yamadori, 1970). Some of the histochemical differences between the light and dark cells of the adult also become apparent during this period, and Kalina and Wolman (1970) who studied the differentiation of rat spinal and trigeminal ganglia during the first few postnatal weeks, have provided particularly dramatic descriptions of the progressive histochemical differentiation of large light and small dark cells.

Further observations favouring the existence of distinct classes of cell are the anatomical evidence indicating that the small cells give rise to unmyelinated axons and the large cells myelinated axons (e.g. Svaetichin, 1951; Ohnishi and Dyck, 1974; reviewed by Scharf, 1958; see Section 4.5.2), the different distribution of large and small cells in some ganglia (e.g. frog spinal ganglia; Berthold, 1966) and the presence of light and dark cells in long-term organotypic cultures of rat spinal ganglia (Bunge *et al.*, 1967).

The functional differences between light and dark cells, if any, are still obscure. It has been suggested that cells of different types subserve different functional modalities (see reviews by Clark, 1926; Scharf, 1958; Crosby, Humphrey and Lauer, 1962; Robain and Jardin, 1972), and in particular that the dark cells are visceral afferent neurons (e.g Crosby *et al.*, 1962).

There is, however, only a very limited amount of evidence to support this contention. If small dark cells were associated with visceral afferent functions, one might expect them to be particularly numerous in ganglia such as the nodose ganglion of the vagus nerve: although De Castro (1932) did indeed consider that the nodose ganglion contained cells that are among the smallest in the cerebrospinal ganglia, other observations do not support this general proposition (Clark, 1926; Lieberman, 1968b). Recently, Knyihár (1971) and Gobel (1974) have suggested that the small dark cells of the spinal and trigeminal ganglia are specifically nociceptive, and there is clinical and quantitative histological evidence to support this contention (see Ohnishi and Dyck, 1974). Another suggestion, that the small cells are cholinergic (Giacobini, 1959; Kokko, 1965; Kalina and Bubis, 1969), appears to be less well founded as it is based upon the particularly high concentration of acetylcholine esterase found in the small cells (Giacobini, 1959; Kokko, 1965; Kalina and Bubis, 1969; Kalina and Wolman, 1970), and not upon the demonstration of either choline acetylase within, or of acetylcholine release from their central terminals. Nevertheless, consistent differences in the content of cholinesterase, acid phosphatases (e.g. Kokko, 1965; Kalina and Bubis, 1968; Knyihár, 1971), and other enzymes (see especially Robain and Jardin, 1972) all suggest that there may be significant metabolic differences between the large and small cells. However, there appears to be little evidence for, and much against, the proposal of Tewari and Bourne (1962), that dark cells are in the active stage, and light cells in the quiescent stage of an oscillatory functional cycle.

In the eighth nerve ganglia of mammals there are distinct ganglion cell subtypes, distinguished on the basis of perikaryal morphology, size, and the characteristics of their satellite cells. The details of these differences and their possible functional significance are discussed by Rosenbluth (1962a) and others (see Adamo and Daigneault, 1973; Perkins, 1973).

4.4.2 'Atypical' cells, 'pericellular terminal arborizations', 'receptor apparatus' and 'synapses' in sensory ganglia

Up to this point the neuronal population of sensory ganglia has been treated as if it were homogeneous, i.e. a single population of primary sensory neurons. Having discussed the problem of light and dark cells, and the question of structural and functional subdivisions within this population, reports of the occurrence within sensory ganglia of nerve cells significantly different in morphology and function from the primary sensory neurons will now be considered.

'Atypical' cells

In most of the early histological studies of sensory ganglia 'atypical' ganglion cells were described and various interpretations were placed upon their significance (e.g. Dogiel, 1896, 1897, 1908; Cajal, 1907, 1909; Levi, 1908; Marinesco, 1909; De Castro, 1932; Blair, Bacsich and Davies, 1935; Scharf, 1958; Fernandez, 1966). Although a variety of such atypical cells has been described (and many classes or subclasses of atypical cell were considered to exist by some observers), in essence the atypical cells usually described were unipolar cells, having in addition a number of short dendrite-like processes originating from the cell body and initial tract of the axon: less commonly, they were described as being frank multipolar cells. Cajal (1907) and many others originally accepted that the processes of such cells were functional dendrites and that they represented the sites of synaptic contact with the fine pericellular nests of fibres described by Dogiel (1896) and Cajal (1906, 1909) around some cells in sensory ganglia (see below). Kiss (1932), in work which is now largely discredited (see Fisher and Ranson, 1934), went so far as to interpret multipolar cells in sensory ganglia, particularly in the vagal and other cranial ganglia, as sympathetic neurons and to call into question the existence of a cranial parasympathetic system. But even before Kiss's work, and long before it was established by electron microscopy that synapses do not occur in sensory ganglia (see below), the studies of degeneration and regeneration conducted by Cajal (1928) and others, and those of Nageotte (1906, 1907) on tabetic human ganglia and transplanted rabbit spinal ganglia, led to a change of opinion, and Cajal (1928) came to hold the view that the multipolar cell types were 'structures of a pathological and more or less ephemeral character'. Nageotte (1906, 1907) proposed that the short processes of the atypical cells (processes which he designated as *paraphytes* to distinguish them from processes making functional contact with other neurons — *orthophytes*) developed as the result of attempts by a cell to compensate for adverse conditions. The sprouting of paraphytes from the soma and initial axon was seen by Nageotte primarily as an injury response and he even suggested that such regenerative attempts ('collateral regeneration') might sometimes lead to the establishment of an orthophyte. However, a determined attempt to verify Nageotte's conclusions directly, by assessing the frequency of atypical cells in cat spinal ganglia at various intervals after sectioning the sciatic nerve or dorsal roots (Barris, 1934) revealed no increase: Barris was able to find an increase in atypical cells only after directly incising and traumatizing the ganglia.

How then are the paraphytes and atypical cells to be interpreted? Of great relevance are the findings that atypical cells may be present in preparations of foetal and neonatal ganglia (see Barris, 1934), and that atypical cells are seen less commonly in well-fixed, minimally shrunken preparations in normal, pathological and experimental animals of all ages, than in poor preparations in which cell shrinkage is marked. Most of the illustrations of 'dendrites' and of multipolar neurons suggest very strongly that the cells in question have undergone severe shrinkage and/or distortion, and a comparison of the paraphytes in such illustrations with the non-synaptic perikaryal evaginations demonstrated by electron microscopy (Section 4.6.2) suggests a close correspondence between the two, particularly if allowance is made for cell shrinkage and artefactual elongation of the paraphytes in the light microscope preparations (Pannese, 1960; Pineda et al., 1967; Section 4.6.2).

Ectopic autonomic neurons

Figs. 4.24a, b which show a cluster of undistorted multipolar cells in serial sections of the rabbit nodose ganglion (from unpublished work of Lieberman) represent quite a different phenomenon. The cells of the cluster, which lie close to the superior pole of the ganglion, are very similar to sympathetic ganglion cells. This similarity is reinforced by the binucleate nature of many of the cells, since rabbit superior cervical ganglion cells are also commonly binucleate (unpublished personal observations; Gabella, Chapter 5). These cells are therefore interpreted to be ectopic sympathetic ganglion cells within the nodose ganglion. Such conspicuous clusters of sympathetic neurons in the rabbit nodose ganglion are very rare: but in view of the very close developmental and anatomical relationship between the vagus nerve and the cervical sympathetic system, they do not represent a surprising anomaly and might be expected to occur occasionally in other sensory ganglia as well.

Pericellular arborizations

The pericellular nests of Dogiel (1896) and Cajal (1906, 1909) were described by both as similar to those found in association with autonomic ganglion cells. Interestingly enough, Van Gehuchten (1892a, b) in his studies of cranial and spinal ganglia, emphasized that fine intraganglionic nerve fibres were never disposed in the pericellular configuration characteristic of preganglionic fibres in sympathetic ganglia. In this case, he was perhaps the more reliable observer, for Cajal (1928) later came to regard the pericellular fibres as manifestations of much the same phenomenon as the paraphytes. Originally, however, Cajal (1909) considered the pericellular nests to be the terminal arborizations of sympathetic fibres of extrinsic origin. Dogiel, on the other hand, inclined to the view that they comprised the receptor apparatus (sensory 'terminals') of other cells within the ganglion and his interpretations have been reinforced by a series of subsequent studies, chiefly by Eastern European workers (see Milokhin and Reshetnikov, 1972, for references).

The observations and interpretations of Cajal have also been supported by more recent studies, notably the fluorescence histochemical observations of Owman and Santini (1966) and Santini (1966) who have described pericellular skeins of adrenergic fibres around a few cells in cat cerebrospinal ganglia, and found these to be reduced in number following sympathectomy. Lukáš, Čech and Buriánek (1970) have made similar observations on the rabbit trigeminal ganglion, and offer the suggestion that the adrenergic fibres may innervate parasympathetic neurons scattered among the sensory ganglion cells. Furthermore, there have been over the years many physiological studies, the results of which have been taken to imply the presence of autonomic ganglion cells in sensory ganglia (e.g. Bayliss, 1901; Kuré, Saégusa, Kawaguchi and Shiraishi, 1930; Mathews, 1934). Recently Uemura, Fletcher, Dirks and Bradley (1973) and Uemura, Fletcher and Bradley (1974) have found degenerating vesicle-containing terminals in the wall of the bladder after removal of sacral or lumbar dorsal root ganglia, and they have interpreted their findings to indicate the presence of postganglionic autonomic neurons in the excised ganglia.

It cannot be emphasized too strongly, however, that in the 20 years or so during which sensory ganglia have been subjected to electron microscope study, no multipolar neurons, no convincing afferent or efferent nerve endings, and no synaptic contacts between an axon terminal and a ganglion cell body or process have as yet been demonstrated. Milokhin and Reshetnikov (1972) have published electron micrographs which purport to show receptor nerve endings and a specialized 'synapse' between such endings and a ganglion cell in rat dorsal root ganglia, but the micrographs are poor and their interpretations unacceptable since their 'nerve endings' appear to be paraphytes (or in some cases, perhaps, satellite cell processes). It is true that under the abnormal conditions of dissociated cell cultures, chick dorsal root ganglion cells grown *in vitro*, have been shown to develop rare interneuronal synaptic contacts (Miller, Varon, Kruger, Coates and Orkand, 1970; Lodin, Faltin, Booker, Hartman and Sensenbrenner, 1973), but under the more 'normal' conditions of explant cultures, synapse formation does not occur even after many months in culture (Bunge *et al.*, 1967; Bird, personal communication). Thus, in spite of the vast volume of anatomical and physiological literature in which it is assumed, or in which indirect evidence has been obtained and interpreted to indicate that autonomic ganglion cells are *normally* present in sensory ganglia (cf. p. 223), or that the sensory ganglion themselves are innervated by receptor terminals of other sensory neurons, or by efferent, autonomic endings, it should be remembered that the best available anatomical and physiological evidence lends no support whatever to such assumptions.

4.4.3 *Chromaffin-like cells*

There is no doubt, however, about the presence within certain sensory ganglia, notably the nodose ganglion of the vagus nerve, of clusters of small cells that obviously differ from the sensory ganglion cells. These cells, which do not resemble the autonomic neurons described above, but show some morphological similarities to adrenal medullary cells and to the principal cells of the carotid body, fall within the general class of cells designated as *paraganglia* (Goormaghtigh, 1936; Coupland, 1965). In fact, paraganglia are found not only within the nodose ganglion (Goormaghtigh, 1936, mouse; Muratori, 1932, birds; Grillo, Jacobs and Comroe, 1974, cat), but all along the course of the vagus nerve and its branches (vagal paraganglia) in mice (Goormaghtigh, 1936), hamsters (Chen and Yates, 1970) and probably other mammals as well.

Very recently these cells have been studied in some detail by Grillo *et al.* (1974) in the cat nodose ganglion, using fluorescence histochemistry and electron microscopy. These authors have established very close similarities between the paraganglion-like cells of the nodose ganglion and the granular cells or SIF cells (Small Intensely Fluorescent cells) which occur in certain mammalian sympathetic ganglia, notably the rat superior cervical ganglion (reviewed by Gabella, Chapter 5). Like the SIF cells of sympathetic ganglia, these cells contain catecholamines stored in large dense cored vesicles, lie immediately adjacent to fenestrated capillaries and receive synaptic contacts of unknown origin upon their perikarya. From physiological and pharmacological evidence presented by Jacobs and Comroe (1971) and by others, it would appear that the SIF cells of the cat nodose ganglion are of physiological importance and are probably involved in producing the reflex apnoea, bradycardia, hypertension and vasodilation in the limb vessels, that follows injection of 5-hydroxy-tryptamine or phenyldiguanide when the carotid sinus nerve has been sectioned. Much remains to be learnt about these cells however (whence, for example, do they derive their afferents?; do they give rise to efferent synapses?; do they secrete catecholamine into the associated capillaries?; do they have a functional relationship with the sensory ganglion cells?). It is not surprising that so little is known about them when it is remembered that the SIF cells of the superior cervical ganglion have been subjected to very detailed anatomical scrutiny and occur in an autonomic ganglion which has been well studied by physiologists, and yet remain enigmatic cells whose precise relationship to the preganglionic fibres and to the sympathetic ganglion cells is unclear and whose physiological significance is unknown.

4.5 Processes of sensory ganglion cells

4.5.1 *General features and terminology*

Kolliker (1844) studying frog dorsal root ganglia, is generally credited with having been the first to recognize the unipolar character of sensory ganglion cells. There ensued, however, a period of considerable uncertainty concerning the nature of the processes of sensory ganglion cells, as a result of the demonstration by many workers that fish spinal ganglion cells were bipolar, a condition more in keeping with what was known concerning impulse conduction in neurons at that time. It was not until later, following further comparative anatomical studies (see for example Chase, 1909), the influential histogenetic studies of His (1886), and the decisive developmental studies of Cajal and others (see Section 4.7) that it became clear that the bipolar organization characteristic of adult fish cerebrospinal ganglion cells, in general gives way to the unipolar condition in higher vertebrates.

Ranvier (1875), Key and Retzius (1876) and Retzius (1880) were chiefly responsible for establishing the relationship between the single process of the ganglion cells and the dorsal root fibres. They demonstrated the origin of the latter from a bifurcation of the initial process of the ganglion cells into centrally and peripherally directed branches and it was shown soon after that the central processes enter and terminate within the spinal cord.

Various studies, especially those of Van Gehuchten (1892a, b) confirmed the essential similarity of spinal ganglia and cranial sensory ganglia, with the exception of the spiral and vestibular ganglia, within which the bipolar condition of the neuron is retained (see Section 4.6.5).

The single principal process to which each perikaryon gives rise, is here referred to as the *stem process* or *initial tract of the axon*. On leaving the cell body the stem process often pursues a tortuous course in the vicinity of the cell body. The T or Y-shaped bifurcation occurs at a variable distance from the cell body, commonly close to or within the axial fibre region.

Both the peripherally directed and the centrally directed processes, and the stem process that connects them with the cell body, are structurally axons and all three may be myelinated. It is quite common, however, to find the peripheral process referred to as a dendrite and the stem process as a 'dendro-axonal process' (e.g. Warwick and Williams, 1973). The designation of the peripheral process of sensory ganglion cells as a dendrite was made by many early histologists. Van Gehuchten (1892b) and Cajal (1909) in particular championed this point of view, which was based largely on the fact that the direction of impulse conduction in the peripheral process is towards rather than away from the cell body, and to a lesser extent upon developmental and phylogenetic considerations. More than 10 years ago, Bodian (1962) discussed this anomaly and pointed out that the position of the cell body is irrelevant in terms of the 'dynamic polarization' of the cell. Bodian proposed that the 'dendritic zones' of neurons are those regions in which responses are generated – whether by transducer or synaptic activity – and that the receptor terminals, and they alone, represent the dendritic zone of the sensory ganglion cell. Viewed in this light, the functional objection ceases to have any validity.

There are, it is true, significant differences in development, biochemistry, axoplasmic flow characteristics and fine structure, between central and peripheral processes, and these differences will be considered in Section 4.5.5. But despite these differences, and allowing for the possibility that the unusual features of the vertebrate primary sensory neuron reflect a phylogenetic trend for the progressive displacement of sensory neuron perikarya from a superficial position in the body, in which location their receptor terminals arise directly from the soma, to a more protected paravertebral position, there is still no reason why the term dendrite should be applied to the peripheral process of a sensory ganglion cell.

4.5.2 *The initial tract of the axon (stem process) and the axonal glomerulus*

The intial tract of the axon or stem process is defined here as the portion of the axon extending from the cell body to the bifurcation into centrally and peripherally directed processes. Thus, the stem process includes both the glomerular portion of the axon and the portion distal to the glomerulus (in the case of cells with axonal glomeruli: see below), and includes both the unmyelinated and myelinated portions of those stem processes which are myelinated along their distal extent. At its origin, the stem process is small (generally less than 3 μm in diameter in small mammals) and leaves the perikaryon rather abruptly, commonly at an acute angle. A multiple derivation of the axon from a series of short roots that originate independently from the soma and unite to form the axon within the confines of the satellite cell capsule has been described in many studies employing the metal impregnation and methylene blue techniques (see especially Dogiel, 1908 and Levi, 1908): but an artefactual basis for such observations cannot be excluded (see Section 4.4.2).

The diameter of the stem process may increase at some distance from the cell body (Pineda *et al.*, 1967; Spencer, Raine and Wiśniewski, 1973) and the unmyelinated part of the stem process is usually considerably larger than unmyelinated axons of peripheral nervous tissue, and is endowed with a more complex satellite cell sheath (see Section 4.6.3). Very large stem processes, with diameters of up to 15 μm were observed by Spencer *et al.* (1973) in adult cat and monkey dorsal root ganglia.

Fine structure of the proximal portion of the stem process

With the electron microscope the initial portion of the stem process shows several distinctive features (those of the axon hillock region of the cell body are considered in Section 4.3.3). Microtubules and microfilaments funnel into it from the perikaryon, as do mitochondria and smooth endoplasmic reticulum, and lysosome-like dense bodies are commonly concentrated in this region. Prominent aggregates of granular endoplasmic reticulum do not generally extend into the axon from the perikaryon, but ribosomes and even small granular endoplasmic aggregates occur in the unmyelinated and myelinated portions of the stem process of rat dorsal root ganglia (Zelená, 1970, 1972; Spencer *et al.*, 1973), and are certainly more prominent in the proximal portion of the stem

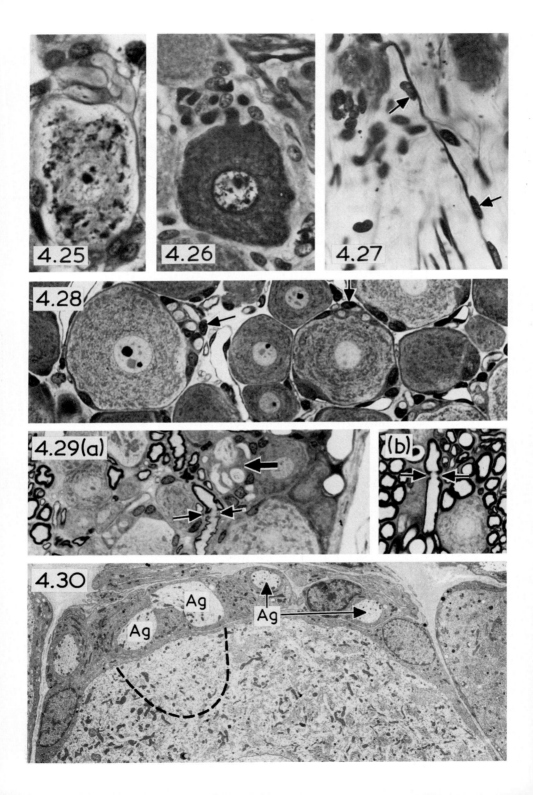

process following lesions of the peripheral axon than under normal conditions (Lieberman, 1968b).

Zelená (1971), and more recently Peach (1975), have described fascicles of microtubules within the initial portion of the stem process of some rat spinal ganglion and mouse trigeminal ganglion cells and apparent microtubule fascicles have also been observed in the processes of chick spinal ganglion cells grown *in vitro* (Fig. 4.32; unpublished work of Bird), and in Fig. 4.31, pairs of linked microtubules (arrows) are indicated in the stem process of a cat trigeminal ganglion cell, which also displays an indistinct undercoating. But these are isolated observations and in the vast majority of studies of sensory ganglion cells, both *in vivo* and *in vitro*, neither fasciculated microtubules nor an electron dense sub-axolemmal coating, have been described in this region. In vertebrate multipolar neurons, fasciculated microtubules and an axolemmal undercoating are characteristic of the axonal initial segment (Peters *et al.*, 1970), the region in which the final ionic events leading to the initiation of a propagated action potential are known to occur. The absence of the morphological specializations of the initial segment at the origin of the stem process of the sensory ganglion cell (in which region action potentials are not normally generated), supports the suggestion that the fasciculated microtubules and undercoating are concerned with action potential initiation and propagation. It is interesting, incidentally, that although an undercoating is present in the receptor terminals of at least some primary sensory neurons (mechanoreceptors: Hashimoto, 1973; Spencer

---

Fig. 4.25   Axonal glomerulus of a large cell in rabbit nodose ganglion. (Haematoxylin and eosin; x 1000.)

Fig. 4.26   Origin of the axon and the axonal glomerulus of a rabbit nodose neuron. (Bodian silver method; x 800.)

Fig. 4.27   Origin of an axon from a small neuron in rabbit nodose ganglion. This axon does not display an axonal glomerulus. Schwann cell nuclei associated with the axon are arrowed. (Bodian silver method; x 625.)

Fig. 4.28   Axonal glomeruli (arrows) of a large and of a medium sized neuron in a rabbit cervical dorsal root ganglion. (One μm toluidine-blue stained section; x 512. Reproduced by courtesy of J. M. Jacobs.)

Figs. 4.29a and 4.29b   Longitudinally sectioned myelinated stem processes in one μm toluidine blue-stained sections of rat lumbar ganglion (Fig. 4.29a) and rat trigeminal ganglion (Fig. 4.29b). In both micrographs the myelin of the internode above the arrows marking the node of Ranvier is thicker than that of the other internode. The thinly myelinated internode is situated closer to the origin of the axon than the more thickly myelinated internode. Fig. 29a also shows the profiles of an unmyelinated stem process comprising a glomerulus (block arrow): the parent cell can not be identified in this section. (x 512: Reproduced by courtesy of J. M. Jacobs.)

Fig. 4.30   Survey electron micrograph of the axon hillock region (dotted line) and part of the axonal glomerulus (Ag) of a rat cervical ganglion cell. The origin of the axon from the cell body is not seen in this micrograph. (x 2200: Reproduced by courtesy of J. M. Jacobs.)

and Schaumberg, 1973), and at the first heminode at which the myelin sheath is acquired, there has been to date no description of fasciculated microtubules in the action potential generating region of the peripheral process of the primary sensory neuron (see, for example, Andres and Düring, 1973; Bannister, Chapter 6).

The surface of the initial portion of the stem process is not always smooth. In many light microscopic studies employing the methylene blue technique (see especially Huber, 1896; Dogiel, 1908), and metallic impregnation methods (e.g Levi, 1908; Huber and Guild, 1913), protrusions of variable shape, length and complexity, often ending in an expanded 'end-bulb' have been described, extending from the intracapsular portion of the initial axon and invaginating the satellite cells in precisely the same fashion as the many evaginations of the cell body (Section 4.6.2). The extensive literature on these structures has recently been reviewed by Kohno and Nakayama (1973) who have studied them with the electron microscope in the dorsal root ganglia of an amphibian (Rana), in which class they are particularly well-developed and were originally described by Huber (1896 – 'axon collaterals of Huber'). Kohno and Nakayama (1973) found the axon collaterals of Huber to contain longitudinally aligned filaments, mitochondria and vesicles, with prominent whorls of filaments in the terminal expansions. Comparable evaginations have also been examined by electron microscopy in the craniospinal ganglia of various mammals (e.g. Pineda *et al.*, 1967; Lieberman, 1968b; Fig. 31), where they appear to be less well-developed than in the frog spinal ganglia. The term *axonal paraphytes* for these structures will be adopted here. The axonal paraphytes of mammalian ganglia display a morphology very similar to that of the inital tract of the axon from which they arise (Fig. 4.31). Their significance and the significance of the more complex axon collaterals of Huber, remain unknown.

The axonal glomerulus

The convolutions of the stem process in the vicinity of the parent cell body, which are sometimes concentrated close to the point of emergence of the axon and sometimes spread over the entire surface of the cell, were called *glomeruli* by Cajal (1909). Although the glomeruli are best seen in methylene blue preparations (e.g. Dogiel, 1908; Cajal, 1907, 1909), and in metallic impregnation preparations (Fig. 4.26) they can also be demonstrated with considerable clarity in Nissl preparations (Fig. 4.25), in semithin plastic sections (Figs. 4.28, 4.29; see Pineda *et al.*, 1967; Spencer *et al.*, 1973) and in electron micrographs (Fig. 4.30).

Since preparations in which glomeruli are demonstrated to the greatest advantage are the least suitable for quantitation, it is difficult to determine the proportion of cells with axonal glomeruli and the relationship between cell size and glomerular complexity. It is clear, however, that not all ganglion cell axons give rise to glomeruli (Figs. 4.27, 4.33), and that glomeruli vary enormously in complexity: they are, for example, far more conspicuous in mammalian than in frog ganglia (Svaetichin, 1951; Scharf, 1958), but less well-developed in the spinal ganglia of the rat than in the ganglia of other mammals (Andres, 1961), especially carnivores, whose ganglion cells apparently give rise to the most highly developed glomeruli (Chase, 1909). Large cells give rise to more prominent glomeruli than do smaller cells (Van Gehuchten, 1897; Cajal, 1907; Pannese, 1960; Andres, 1961; Fernandez, 1966; Pineda et al., 1967; Spencer et al., 1973), and according to Ha (1970) very few small cells in cat dorsal root ganglia have glomeruli. But even large cells are sometimes without an axonal glomerulus (De Castro, 1932). Furthermore, observations on rabbit and rat sensory ganglia (Lieberman, 1968b) and many published micrographs and drawings (e.g. Levi, 1908; Chase, 1909; Truex, 1939; Scharf, 1958) suggest that it is not uncommon for the initial axon of a ganglion cell to bifurcate very close to its origin, the central and peripheral processes diverging from a very short unmyelinated stem process (e.g. Fig. 33).

Glomeruli are not present or are only poorly developed at birth in mammals, and are formed during the first few postnatal weeks (Cajal, 1909; Pannese, 1960). In dogs and cats, for example, the first loops and convolutions do not appear until 8 days after birth and the adult pattern is established after about 1 month. It is interesting and may well prove significant that even in the most mature and well-myelinated long-term organotypic cultures of dorsal root ganglia *in vitro*, the ganglion cells do not develop axonal glomeruli (Bunge et al., 1967; Bird, personal communication).

The myelinated portion of the stem process

At a variable distance from its origin, but commonly immediately after it emerges from the glomerulus, the stem process of the larger ganglion cells acquires a myelin sheath, the sheath beginning at a heminode, where periaxonal satellite cells of the unmyelinated stem process give way to a Schwann cell. The myelinated portion of the stem process axon may comprise only one or may include several internodal segments. In frogs, for example, the distance from the origin of the axon to the bifurcation is of the order of $100-400 \mu m$, and 3 or 4 internodal segments may precede the bifurcation (Svaetichin, 1951). In mammals, this distance may be much greater in the case of the largest cells, and it has long been appreciated that the myelin of this segment is thinner than the myelin of the fibres in the dorsal roots (Rexed and Sourander, 1949).

Recently Spencer et al. (1973) have shown that in this region of relatively thin myelin in mammalian dorsal root ganglia, the usual relationships between axonal diameter and myelin sheath thickness and between fibre diameter and internodal length (see, for example, Friede and Samorajski, 1968 and Chapter 1) are not followed. It is clear from the data of Svaetichin (1951) that a similar situation obtains along the stem process of frog dorsal root ganglion cells. In mammals, successive internodes en route to the axonal bifurcation have

231

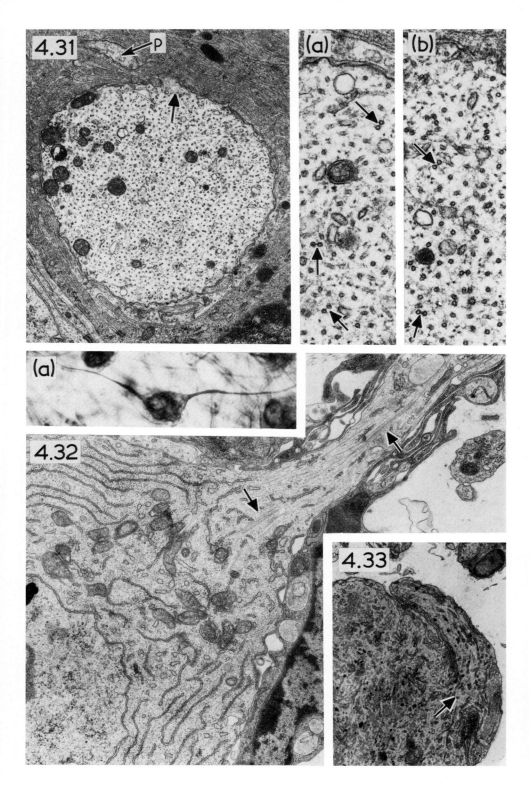

progressively thicker myelin sheaths (Figs. 4.2, 4.29, 4.29a), but the centrally and peripherally directed fibres beyond the bifurcation adhere to the usual axon: sheath diameter relationship of peripheral nerve fibres. As Spencer *et al.* (1973) point out, this finding has interesting implications in relation to current concepts concerning the factors initiating and controlling myelination in the peripheral nervous system (see also Chapter 1).

According to Cajal (1907, 1909), the glomerular portion of the axon is never myelinated, although Dogiel (1897) did claim to have observed myelinated glomerular axons and Pineda *et al.* (1967) have described the formation of loose myelin around the distal part of some glomerular axons in the trigeminal ganglion. Since the first part of the myelinated portion of the stem process may remain in the vicinity of the parent cell body, and in electron micrographs (e.g. Fig. 4.2) is sometimes seen to be partially included (with the parent cell body) in a discontinuous, but occasionally distinct 'second capsule' of flattened cells (see Section 4.2.1), a case could be made for including this part of the stem process also, as a component of the axonal glomerulus.

The significance of the axonal glomerulus, of the differences between the properties of cells with complex glomeruli and of those without extensive glomeruli, and of the unusual pattern of myelination of the stem process are, for the moment, obscure and remain matters for speculation and perhaps experimental investigation.

4.5.3 *Structural features of the stem process branch point*

Myelinated stem processes bifurcate at a node of Ranvier and give rise to a single peripheral process and a single central process, both of which are also myelinated (Dale, 1900; Rexed and Sourander, 1949). The axon is normally constricted at the node (Ranson, 1912; Ranson and Davenport, 1931; Ha, 1970). The ultrastructural and general histochemical features of this node are identical to

---

Fig. 4.31   Transversely sectioned unmyelinated stem process of a neuron from adult cat trigeminal ganglion. Note the complex arrangement of the periaxonal satellite cells and the axonal paraphyte (P) which originates from the axon at the arrow. Figs. 4.31a and b are high power micrographs of parts of the same axon illustrating pairs of microtubules apparently linked by cross bridges (arrows). The axolemma appears to be associated with a poorly defined undercoating. (Fig. 4.31 x 14 000; Figs. 4.31a,b x 40 000: Reproduced by courtesy of D. N. Landon.)

Fig. 4.32   Process arising from the cell body of a dorsal root ganglion cell in a 41 day dissociated cell culture of 12 day chick embryo. Apparent microtubule fascicles are arrowed. The cell body and process are invested in satellite cell processes. It is not certain whether this is a bipolar or unipolar cell: at this stage both varieties are present and Fig. 4.32a shows a typical bipolar sensory ganglion cell from a similar culture. (Fig. 4.32 x 15 000; Fig. 4.32a x 192: Reproduced by courtesy of M. Bird.)

Fig. 4.33   Rabbit nodose ganglion neuron showing bifurcation of a stem process immediately distal to its origin from the cell body (arrow). (x approx. 3000.)

those of nodes in other parts of the peripheral nervous system (Ha, 1970; Gerebtzoff, 1971). In silver preparations, neurofibrils pass from the stem process into the central and peripheral branches, but not between the central and peripheral branches (e.g. Truex, 1939). The same finding with respect to filaments and microtubules has been made by electron microscopy (Ha, 1970).

Much less is known about the branch point of unmyelinated stem processes. In silver preparations the branch point has always been identified as a bifurcation, characterized, in contrast to the myelinated branch point, by a distinctive triangular expansion (Ranson, 1912; Ranson and Davenport, 1931; Ha, 1970). The branch point of unmyelinated stem processes has yet to be described by electron microscopy. Further consideration will be given in Section 4.5.6 to the question of whether all unmyelinated stem processes branch in a simple dichotomous fashion.

4.5.4 *Size difference between the centrally and peripherally directed branches*

It is widely, and often uncritically, accepted that the peripherally directed branch is always thicker than the corresponding centrally directed branch. That this is sometimes the case is unquestionably true (see the illustrations in almost any account of sensory ganglia based on the methylene blue or metal impregnation techniques): but, whether in fact a size disparity is a *consistent* feature of the bifurcation is called into question by numerous studies. Dale (1900) made careful measurements of osmicated nerve roots and trunks in cat and rat, and could find no consistent differences in the myelinated fibre diameter spectra proximal and distal to the ganglia. The findings of Rexed and Sourander (1949) were similar: they found an identical myelinated fibre diameter spectrum on either side of the dorsal root ganglion in human and feline lumbo-sacral roots. They also found an identical spectrum close to the central pole of the ganglion and close to the spinal cord in cats, indicating a constant diameter along the dorsal roots, although in the human material some evidence was found for a thickening of small myelinated central fibres as they approached the cord.

So it would appear that, for mammalian spinal ganglion cells at least, the size disparity must be a feature of the smaller cells with unmyelinated axons. There is much evidence to support this contention. Ranson and Davenport (1931) observed a size disparity only in the case of small cells with unmyelinated processes in their silver preparations, and Ha (1970) has confirmed these observations using the Golgi method and electron microscopy. Furthermore, ultrastructural studies of the unmyelinated axons central and peripheral to sensory ganglia have shown a marked reduction in the mean diameter and in the range of diameters on the central side and have provided an explanation for observed differences in the conduction velocities of C-fibres on the two sides of the ganglion (Gasser, 1950, 1955; Mei, Boyer and Condamin, 1971).

It must be acknowledged, however, that in some sites, centrally directed myelinated axons as well as unmyelinated axons may be smaller than their peripheral counterparts. Mei *et al.* (1971), for example, present persuasive quantitative ultrastructural evidence for a general decrease in the diameters of myelinated (as well as of unmyelinated) axons from below to above the nodose ganglion in cats and it is of considerable interest to note that Van Gehuchten (1892a, b) stressed that the difference in thickness between centrally directed and peripherally directed processes was more marked in the mammalian nodose ganglion (cat, dog, and man) than in any of the many other sites he studied and that this observation was supported by later studies of Ranson, Foley and Alpert (1933).

It has been claimed, not only for nodose ganglion cells (Mei *et al.*, 1971) but also for spinal ganglion cells (Ha, 1970), that some cells give rise to an unmyelinated central process and to a myelinated peripheral process. The evidence in the case of the nodose ganglion is strong and is based on measurements and counts showing a reduction in the number of myelinated fibres central to the ganglion: Ha's evidence is principally from measurements of axonal diameter in Golgi preparations, in which the difference between central and peripheral axon diameter was so great for some cells (0.3 μm vs. 1.8 μm) that Ha (1970) considered such cells must have a myelinated peripheral process. In an unillustrated abstract, Ha (1969) also reports the observation of such a bifurcation by electron microscopy. It would, however, be relatively easy to interpret the heminode at the commencement of the myelin sheath (see Section 4.5.2) as part of an unequal bifurcation and the author does not describe the characteristics of the stem process at the bifurcation in question. Because of this, and because Golgi-impregnated material is not ideal for measurements of axonal diameter, and in view of the existence of evidence of a very small disparity in the number of myelinated axons central and peripheral to spinal ganglia (Dale, 1900; Rexed and Sourander, 1949), it is probable that unequal branching of this type is uncommon in mammalian spinal ganglia.

4.5.5 *Developmental, ultrastructural and axoplasmic flow differences between central and peripheral processes*

Although it was stressed above (Section 4.5.1) that both centrally and peripherally directed processes are axons, there are a number of well-established differences between them. These differences almost certainly reflect the different structural and functional properties of the peripheral receptor terminals and the central synaptic endings (with respect, for example, to requirements for transmitter metabolism or for trophic interactions) and perhaps also the rather large differences in the total axoplasmic volume of the two branches in some cells.

Differences in the central and peripheral process can be detected both *in vivo* and *in vitro* at early developmental stages. The peripherally growing process of

235

the bipolar neuroblast is thicker and more precocious in its elongation than the centrally directed process (Pannese, 1974). In developing rabbit dorsal root ganglia, one process of the bipolar neuroblast (the presumed future peripheral process) was found consistently to contain more granular endoplasmic reticulum than the other process (Tennyson 1965). Zelená (1972) occasionally observed ribosomes in the peripheral process, but never in the central process of adult rat spinal ganglion cells, a possible reflection of this developmental difference.

Another ultrastructural difference observed in developing neurons – the presence of a greater number of microtubules in the peripherally directed, and of filaments in the centrally directed process of chick embryo spinal ganglion cells *in vitro* (Barasa, Maccotta and Filgamo, 1970) – also appears to be reflected in the fine structure of the mature neuron. Quantitative ultrastructural studies of spinal roots and nerves by Smith (1973) in *Xenopus* and by Zenker, Mayr and Gruber (1973, 1975) in the rat, reveal consistently lower microtubule densities in the myelinated fibres of the dorsal root fibres proximal to the ganglion than in those distal to the ganglion. According to Smith (1973) filament density in proximal dorsal root axons (circa 120 filaments per μm^2) is approximately the same as that in distal dorsal root axons (and is also the same as that in ventral root fibres), whereas microtubule density in the proximal root axons is about 2 microtubules per μm^2 compared to 15 microtubules per μm^2 in the distal root axons, and the microtubules at this level (and in the ventral root axons) are closely associated with mitochondria. The differences between proximal and distal dorsal root fibres found by Zenker *et al.* (1975) for the rat are less dramatic but consistently in the same direction (approximately 26 microtubules per μm^2 vs. 34 microtubules per μm^2 for small axons and 13 vs. 17 per μm^2 for large axons), and like Smith (1973), Zenker *et al.* (1973) find a paucity of smooth endoplasmic elements in the central dorsal root axons.

The most significant aspect of these ultrastructural findings is that they correlate closely with differences in the axoplasmic flow characteristics and patterns of intra-axonal organelle movement in the two processes. Proteins synthesized in the cell bodies of the ganglionic neurons are transported somatofugally at various rates along both processes (Droz, 1965; Lasek, 1968). The rate of fast transport is identical along the central and peripheral processes (about 16 mm/h or 400 mm/day), the characteristic fast transport rate for a variety of neurons (Lasek, 1970b; Ochs, 1972). However, the net somatofugal flow along the central process is considerably less than the flow along the peripheral process, both in adult cat (Lasek, 1968) and in the kitten (Lasek, 1970a): approximately 50 per cent less protein passes centrally from the dorsal root ganglion than peripherally (Anderson and McClure, 1973).

Of considerable significance is the demonstration by Anderson and McClure (1973) of qualitative differences between the centrally and peripherally transported proteins: electrophoretic analysis of radioactively labelled proteins in the axons of the dorsal columns and of the sciatic nerve following H^3-leucine injection into cat L7 spinal ganglion revealed two peaks, corresponding to proteins of molecular weight 100 000 and 18 000 in the sciatic axons and a single major peak, corresponding to a molecular weight of 65 000 in the proteins extracted from the dorsal column axons. The functional significance of these differences is impossible to assess while the precise differences between centrally and peripherally transported proteins are unknown. It is, however, reasonable to speculate, as Anderson and McClure (1973) have done, that proteins transported centrally may be associated with transmitter functions at the spinal cord and brain stem synaptic endings, whereas those transported peripherally may be associated with sensory transduction. Or perhaps the peripherally transported proteins are associated with some aspects of the trophic relationship between the peripheral sensory ending and related cells.

There is additional evidence that the sensory ganglion cell is able selectively to direct somatofugally transported molecules into the central and peripheral processes. The concentration of glutamate in the central portion of the dorsal roots is high and is equivalent to the concentration in the dorsal root ganglia, but is much lower in the peripheral portion of the dorsal root or cutaneous nerve (Duggan and Johnston, 1970; Johnson and Aprison,1970). Similar findings have been made with respect to substance P (Takahashi and Otsuka, 1975). In these cases the functional significance of the difference is immediately apparent, for both glutamate and substance P are considered to be possible transmitters at the central terminals of the primary sensory neuron (see Section 4.9.3).

Recently the movement of intra-axonal organelles has been compared in myelinated fibres of the proximal and distal dorsal roots (and of the ventral roots and spinal nerves) of frogs and mammals, using Nomarski or dark-field light microscopic techniques (Smith, 1972, 1973; Cooper and Smith, 1974). In both processes, saltatory movement of small particles (0.2–0.5 μm diameter), most of which are almost certainly mitochondria or large vesicles of smooth endoplasmic reticulum, occurs in both directions along definite intra-axonal 'tracks'. Surprisingly enough, the particles move predominantly somatopetally (i.e. towards the dorsal root ganglion) both in the proximal and distal dorsal root (Smith, 1972; Cooper and Smith, 1974): 10–15 times as many particles pass towards the cell bodies as away from them and many of the particles moving towards the cell body are larger than those passing somatofugally. Most of the particles travel at about the same net velocity as the 'fast' axoplasmic flow system (e.g. Lasek, 1970b; Ochs, 1972), i.e. at approximately 1 μm per second, usually slightly faster in the somatofugal than in the somatopetal direction (Cooper and Smith, 1974).

Although the difference between somatofugal and somatopetal movement is seen on both sides of the ganglion, the number of particles moving in the axons of the proximal dorsal root is far fewer than in the distal root fibres (or in the ventral root or spinal nerve fibres). This 'sluggishness', Smith (1973) correlates with the low microtubule density, absence of microtubule-mitochondrial associations and paucity of smooth endoplasmic reticulum in the central axons.

4.5.6 *Some numerical considerations*

Ratio of myelinated to unmyelinated central processes

There is, in general, a considerable excess of ganglion cells over myelinated axons in the corresponding roots (Bühler, 1898; Hatai, 1902; Ranson, 1908; Ranson and Davenport, 1931; Duncan and Keyser, 1938). The difference is generally assumed to represent the number of cells giving rise to unmyelinated axons. The best available estimates and counts suggest that the number of unmyelinated central processes is significantly greater than the number of myelinated processes at most spinal levels. Duncan and Keyser (1938) using silver impregnation found a very constant 72 per cent of unmyelinated axons in the central dorsal roots at thoracic levels in the adult cat. This figure was endorsed by Holmes and Davenport (1940). More recent counts, employing electron microscopy to identify and enumerate unmyelinated axons, have yielded rather similar proportions of unmyelinated axons in dorsal roots of the rat (82 per cent unmyelinated axons in T8, Nunnemacher and Sutherland, 1969; twice as many unmyelinated as myelinated axons, Steer, 1971), and in the dorsal root of the seventh spinal nerve in the frog (just below 70 per cent, Sutherland and Nunnemacher, 1974). At other spinal levels in the cat, the percentage of unmyelinated dorsal root axons is generally lower (approximately 60 per cent at lumbo-sacral levels; just over 50 per cent in C_2) and in C_1 all but about 6.5 per cent of the dorsal root axons are myelinated (Duncan and Keyser, 1938). In the sensory root of the baboon trigeminal nerve, analysed by electron microscopy, the unmyelinated axons account for only 40 per cent of the total (Young and King, 1973).

Is there a 1:1:1 ratio between the number of ganglion cells, the number of central and the number of peripheral root axons?

A most important numerical consideration, to which a number of workers have addressed their attention over the years, is whether the total number of centrally directed axons corresponds to the number of ganglion cells. Less attention has been paid to the equally interesting and closely related question of whether the number of peripherally directed axons also corresponds to these totals. In many early studies a considerable excess of cells over total dorsal root axons was found (Hatai, 1902; Davenport and Ranson, 1931; Barnes, 1935; see review in Barnes and Davenport, 1937). Almost certainly these results were due to incomplete visualization of unmyelinated axons. Duncan and Keyser (1936, 1938) and Holmes and Davenport (1940) both working with adult cat spinal roots and Foley and Dubois (1937) working with cat vagus nerve are among those whose cell and fibre counts show a close correspondence between the number of ganglion cells and the number of centrally directed axons. Duncan and Keyser (1938) and

Holmes and Davenport (1940) carried out particularly careful counts and found a 1:1 correspondence at every spinal level, with a slight excess in favour of cells at most levels (Duncan and Keyser, 1938). A further indication that the ratio of central axons to ganglion cells is 1:1 is given by a comparison of electron microscope-based total axon counts of rat T_8 dorsal root (8 000 axons; Nunnemacher and Sutherland, 1969) with the cell counts of Hatai (1902) for rat spinal ganglia T_4 (7406) and L_2 (8315).

Clearly the data summarized above favour the existence of a 1:1 ratio between the number of ganglion cell bodies and of central processes. But how reliable are they? Much of the data are indirect and/or based on light microscopic studies of reduced silver preparations in which it is assumed that all of the axons are stained and independently resolved. Electron microscopy has shown that the diameter of many unmyelinated axons is close to the resolving power of the light microscope, and Gasser (1955) working with cat lumbo-sacral dorsal roots found that a substantial proportion of the axons was less than 0.2 μm in diameter. Thus, light microscope counts may underestimate the true number by a variable amount. The dramatic increase in the percentage of unmyelinated ventral root axons determined by electron microscopy (nearly 30 per cent; Coggeshall, Coulter and Willis, 1974) over the figures for the same roots and species based on light microscopy (consistently less than 10 per cent; Holmes and Davenport, 1940) bears eloquent testimony to this possibility. However, the error will depend upon the quality of the silver impregnation, the diameter spectrum of the population of unmyelinated axons and the optical properties of the imaging system used. Gasser (1955) concluded that the total number of centrally directed axons was greatly in excess of the number of dorsal root ganglion cells, and that multiple branching of unmyelinated axons must occur, with more branches directed centrally than peripherally. Just such a pattern of branching was occasionally observed by Dogiel (1897, 1908) in methylene blue preparations (see especially Fig. 4b in Dogiel, 1897). A survey of the literature, however, suggests that the light microscopic counts of dorsal root unmyelinated axons may not be as seriously underestimated as Gasser (1955) and others have assumed. Many authors, it is true, have concluded that groups of unmyelinated axons (especially the several axons grouped together as a single unmyelinated fibre), rather than individual unmyelinated axons, are commonly impregnated as a unit with the reduced silver methods (see, for example, Gasser, 1955; Egar and Singer, 1971). However, the illustrations in some of the key papers show preparations of high quality, in which axons well under 0.5 μm in diameter are clearly defined and individually resolved within the Remak cells of single unmyelinated fibres (see especially Duncan and Keyser, 1936 and Chapter 2). The rather close correspondence between the unmyelinated axon proportions of cat dorsal roots given by Duncan and Keyser (1938) and the figures based on electron microscopy (Nunnemacher and Sutherland, 1969; Sutherland and Nunnemacher, 1974) also suggest that most of the unmyelinated axons can be resolved, and it is possible that Gasser's figures for the diameters of cat dorsal root unmyelinated axons may have been too small, perhaps because of shrinkage problems. There does not appear to have been a more recent quantitative ultrastructural study in which the diameter spectrum of unmyelinated dorsal root axons has been analyzed, but other studies of dorsal and cranial sensory root axons in a variety of species suggest that comparatively few of the axons lie below the resolving power of the light microscope. For example, Gamble and Eames (1966) give the size range of human unmyelinated lumbar dorsal root axons as 0.4 to 1.6 μm; Young and King (1973) found a spectrum of 0.3 to 2.3 μm in the baboon trigeminal sensory root; the mean diameter of unmyelinated axons in the supranodose vagus of the cat is 0.8 μm (Mei *et al.*, 1971); Steer (1971) gives 0.2–0.8 μm as the range for unmyelinated axons very close to the cord in rat dorsal roots; and although the ranges are not given, all of the unmyelinated axons from the dorsal roots of frogs illustrated by Pick, Gerdin and De Lemos (1963) are within the resolving power of light microscopy. It is also tempting to put forward the existence of the 1:1 ratio as evidence that the best light microscope counts are accurate, but this involves an essentially circular argument.

There is a final relevant consideration. Nearly 30 per cent of ventral root axons in all vertebrate species so far studied are unmyelinated (Coggeshall *et al.*, 1974, 1975). The extremely careful studies of Coggeshall *et al.* (1974) have established that most of these axons are afferent and there is good physiological evidence that most of these ventral root afferents have peripheral receptive fields. The unmyelinated axons in cat sacral ventral roots are predominantly visceral afferents, with receptive fields in perirectal tissue, the wall of the bladder, the urethra and the vagina, and are activated by stimuli such as distension of the rectum, bladder or vagina (Clifton, Vance, Applebaum, Coggeshall and Willis, 1974) [Other authors recording from ventral root afferents at other levels and in other species, and chiefly it would seem, from myelinated afferents, have found receptive fields in skin, muscle and joints (Dimsdale and Kemp, 1966; Kato and Tanji, 1971) so that representations of most or all of the modality classes of dorsal root afferents may also be found in ventral roots].

It has been suggested that the sensory ventral root fibres derive from aberrant sensory ganglion cells that histological study shows are common constituents of ventral roots (Windle, 1931; Dimsdale and Kemp, 1966; Webber and Wemett, 1966; Kato and Hirata, 1968; Stacey, 1969). However, Coggeshall *et al.* (1974) found that most of the unmyelinated axons in the ventral roots of the cat disappeared following removal of the corresponding dorsal root ganglion. Although this finding is not in line with those of Dimsdale and Kemp (1966), who found that afferent activity in rat ventral root was not abolished by removal of the L_4 dorsal root ganglion 5 days earlier, it suggests that in cat at least, there are cells in the dorsal root ganglion with a central process that leaves the ganglion in the distal dorsal root and enters the central nervous system via the corresponding (or an adjacent) ventral root. The presence of significant numbers of such cells in the dorsal root ganglia would not be compatible with a 1:1 ratio between cells and axons in the dorsal root.

In conclusion, the evidence is, on balance, against the existence of a 1:1:1 relationship for all cells and root axons in the sensory ganglia, although this relationship almost certainly holds for the larger cells with myelinated processes and probably also for a majority of the remaining cells with unmyelinated processes. Other cells may give rise to more than a single central and/or peripheral process, either by further intraganglionic branching distal to the first branch point or by multiple branching at the first branch point. The cell-fibre relationship is further complicated by the probable presence in most ganglia of some cells with both (or all) processes leaving the ganglion on the peripheral side.

Finally, it is noteworthy that fine nerve bundles commonly interconnect the ganglia and roots of adjacent segments: careful dissections in the rat by Jacob and Weddell (1975) revealed many connections, particularly in the lumbar and sacral regions, between adjacent dorsal root ganglia, between ganglia and adjacent dorsal roots, between ganglia and adjacent ventral roots (perhaps the pathway for some of the ventral root afferents: see above) and between adjacent dorsal roots. The connecting bundles when examined by light and electron microscopy were found to contain both myelinated and unmyelinated fibres and from 6 per cent to as much as 28 per cent of the total number of myelinated fibres in a dorsal root were found to be contributed by the 'connectives'. The existence of such fine, intersegmental connections (and they are not confined to the rat lumbo-sacral region but are common at all spinal levels in monkeys and in man; see Jacob and Weddell, 1975, for references) enormously complicates attempts to obtain reliable quantitative data on the problem of cell: fibre ratios in the dorsal roots and ganglia.

4.6 The perineuronal satellite cell sheath

Each neuronal perikaryon is contained within a capsule of several flattened cells. Although the term *satellite cell* introduced by Cajal (1899; see Cajal, 1909) is the most widely used for these cells, they are also referred to under a bewildering variety of synonyms (see Pannese, 1960), among them *amphicytes, capsular cells* and *perisomatic gliocytes*. The perineuronal satellite cells display many close similarities, both morphological and functional, to the cells that ensheath the initial, unmyelinated portion of the ganglion cell axon (see Section 4.6.3) and to the Schwann cells of peripheral nerve fibres; probably all are variants of a single cell type with a common embryological origin from the neural crest (Yntema, 1937; though see Weston, 1970).

4.6.1 *Morphology and cytology of satellite cells*

The satellite cells are somewhat polymorphic: a few are stellate, some are polygonal with short processes and many are fusiform (Pannese, 1960). Their flattened cell bodies and narrow, laminar processes are interlocked, and embrace and envelop the neuronal perikaryon.

The cytological features of satellite cells have been established in a number of electron microscope studies (e.g. Hess, 1955; Wyburn, 1958; Pannese, 1960; Rosenbluth, 1963; Bunge *et al.*, 1967; Pineda *et al.*, 1967). Their nuclei are elongated and often slightly curved to conform with the contour of the neuron. Commonly, the perinuclear region bulges inwards and indents the neuron (Figs. 4.11, 4.12). The chromatin pattern resembles that of Schwann cells with prominent aggregates around most of the nuclear periphery. Under normal conditions the satellite cell nuclei do not display prominent nucleoli.

The cytoplasmic organelles of the satellite cells are concentrated in the perinuclear region (Fig. 4.34). Under normal conditions these comprise a relatively sparse granular endoplasmic reticulum, a modestly developed Golgi apparatus, mitochondria, microtubules and filaments, lysosome-like dense bodies, multivesicular bodies, coated vesicles and occasionally glycogen granules, centrioles and cilia. In older animals, lipofuscin granules are commonly clustered in this region (e.g. Moses *et al.*,1965). Further from the nucleus, the narrow cytoplasmic laminae normally contain no granular reticulum or elements of the Golgi apparatus: the most conspicuous organelles in these cell extensions are microtubules and filaments, tubular and vesicular elements of the smooth endoplasmic reticulum, and occasional mitochondria.

Recently a distinctive new class of cytoplasmic organelle, the peroxisome (or microperoxisome), which contains peroxidase and probably other enzymes, has been identified and characterized by light and electron microscopy in the satellite cells (and also in the Schwann cells) of rat dorsal root ganglia (Citkowitz and Holtzman, 1973; Holtzman *et al.*, 1973). Peroxisomes (identified following incubation with substrate under appropriate conditions) occur both in the satellite cell processes and in the perinuclear cytoplasm (where they are extremely numerous) as membrane-bound bodies approximately 0.2 μm in diameter. In non-incubated material the peroxisomes display a moderately electron-dense 'fluffy' matrix, and resemble the peroxisomes of other tissues, although they do not contain the nucleoids characteristic of hepatic peroxisomes in most species. The peroxisomes are closely associated with smooth endoplasmic reticulum and occasionally show a 'tail' suggestive of a derivation from the smooth reticulum (Citkowitz and Holtzman, 1973). The functions of peroxisomes in satellite cells are unknown: like peroxisomes in other tissues they may be involved in carbohydrate, lipid or coenzyme metabolism, but Citkowitz and Holtzman (1973) suggest that they may play a more specific role in sensory ganglion satellite cells, perhaps in the breakdown of materials taken up from the extracellular space. One possibility – that they are involved in the degradation of amino acid transmitters – is compatible with the demonstration that these cells have a high affinity uptake system for glutamate (Schon and Kelly, 1974) a possible contender for the role of dorsal root ganglion cell transmitter (see Section 4.11).

An important contribution of ultrastructural studies has been to define more precisely than was possible by light microscopy, the relationships between individual satellite cells, between the satellite cells and the neuron, and between the neuron-satellite cell complex and the endoneurial compartment.

The extent of interdigitation between contiguous satellite cells is even more extensive and striking than is suggested by the form of these cells in light microscope preparations. Although in some places the sheath is composed of only a single cellular lamina, most of the surface of the ganglion cells, particularly of the larger cells, is related to a multilamellate sheath of extensively interdigitated satellite cell processes. The number of satellite cell processes comprising the sheath and the thickness of the sheath both tend to increase close to the root of the axon. Interdigitation appears to be somewhat less extensive in lower vertebrates than in mammals (Pannese, 1964).

The satellite cells are separated from one another (and from the surface of the ganglion cells), by a narrow intercellular space of less than 20 nm. In places, the intercellular space between adjacent satellite cell processes is narrowed even further by the formation of what appear from thin-section criteria to be gap junctions (Figs. 4.35, 4.37) (see also Pannese, 1969a). The extracellular spaces between satellite cell processes and between the latter and the neuronal surface are, however, freely permeable to molecules of relatively large molecular weight (Rosenbluth and Wissig, 1964). Adjacent satellite cell laminae are also occasionally linked by small adhesion plaques or maculae adhaerentes.

The outer surface of the satellite cell, or in the case of a multilamellate sheath, the free surface of the outermost satellite cell lamina, is generally smooth (though see Section 4.2.1), and abuts a continuous basal lamina some 20–30 nm thick, which separates the neuron-satellite cell complex from the endoneurial compartment. Adjacent neurons, sharing a common satellite cell over an extensive area of contiguity and not separated by basal laminae are, however, occasionally observed (Lieberman, 1968b).

Suggestions that the satellite cell sheath might be commonly absent (e.g. Truex, 1939), syncytial (Ortiz-Picón, 1955), incomplete or even in cytoplasmic continuity with the neuron (references in Pannese, 1960), have been contraverted by electron microscopy (e.g. Hess, 1955; Wyburn, 1958; Pannese, 1960). It is, however, understandable that such misconceptions should have developed since the satellite cell capsule is occasionally too thin to be resolved adequately by light microscopy (Pannese, 1960, 1964).

4.6.2 *The satellite cell-neuronal interface*

The interface between the ganglion cell and the satellite cells is seldom smooth in adult animals. It is complicated by invaginations and evaginations of the neuronal surface, which are followed by the surface of the (innermost) satellite cells. In osmium-immersion-fixed ganglia the interdigitated plasma membranes may break down into chains of vesicles: the artefactual nature of this vesiculation was clearly demonstrated by Rosenbluth (1963), and later confirmed by Moses *et al.* (1965). The most conspicuous and extensive surface irregularities comprise irregular villiform and lamelliform evaginations of the neuron into the satellite cell sheath (Pannese, 1960; Rosenbluth, 1963) (Figs. 4.18, 4.34–4.36). Pineda *et al.* (1967) found such evaginations to be more extensive in monkey than in cat trigeminal ganglion and to be most prominent in large cells and close to the origin of the axon. Invagination of the neuronal perikaryon by satellite cell processes also occurs, but much less commonly, and the invaginations do not penetrate deeply into the ganglion cell body.

Surface irregularities at the neuron-satellite cell interface are not present at birth in mammals, but develop in the early postnatal period (Pannese, 1960, 1969a, 1974; Yamadori, 1970); they also become apparent in long-term cultures of dorsal root ganglia grown *in vitro* as the cultures mature (Bunge *et al.*, 1967). They increase the true surface area of the neuron (and of the neuron-satellite cell interface) by a considerable amount, but the functional significance of this amplification is presently unclear: Gray (1969) has hypothesized that the surface evaginations are comparable to the trophospongium* of invertebrate neurons and represent an alternate means whereby the surface area available for metabolic exchange can be increased in an otherwise adendritic cell body (see also Section 4.6.4 below).

The neuronal evaginations, particularly the larger ones, exaggerated by neuronal shrinkage and other artefacts of histological processing, are almost certainly the ultrastructural counterparts of the processes described by many early neurohistologists ('intracapsular unmyelinated fibres', 'subcapsular dendrites'; 'accessory processes'; see for example Dogiel, 1908; Levi, 1908; Chase, 1909; Cajal, 1909) and named paraphytes by Nageotte (1906) (see also Section 4.4.2).

Adhaerens-like junctions are occasionally observed between the neuronal plasma membrane and the adneuronal surface membrane of a satellite cell (Pannese, 1969a, 1974; Adamo and Daigneault, 1972), but gap junctions have never been described at this interface.

4.6.3 *The periaxonal satellite cells*

Satellite cells related to the proximal portion of the stem process (periaxonal satellite cells of Pannese, 1960) display a few ultrastructural differences from the

---

*In invertebrates, many large unipolar neurons are deeply invaginated by an extensive system of branching glial and connective tissue septa (e.g. Gray, 1969). These invaginations are referred to as 'trophospongium' and as the name implies are generally thought to have a trophic function. In a series of studies at the turn of this century, Holmgren (1900, 1901, 1902, 1904), described an extensive system of intracytoplasmic spaces and canals in dorsal root ganglion and other nerve cells, in vertebrates, as well as in a variety of invertebrate neurons. These canals were initially considered to be intracellular lymph channels (continuous with a supposed system of pericellular lymph vessels) but were later described as trophospongium (Holmgren, 1904; Marinesco, 1909). Since vertebrate neurons do not, in fact, show glial and connective tissue invaginations comparable with the invertebrate trophospongium, it is possible that Holmgren's observations were due at least in part to visualization of the negative image of the Golgi apparatus or the interstices of the metallophil reticulum (see Section 4.3.3). However, it is possible that some of the large dorsal root ganglion cells of *Lophius* included in the material studied by Holmgren (1904) do display deeper invaginations of their cell bodies by satellite cells than is the case for spinal ganglion cells in higher vertebrates.

satellite cells related to the cell body. Pineda *et al.* (1967) found their cytoplasm to be consistently more electron dense than that of perisomatic satellite cells and precisely the same observation was made by Yamadori (1970) in newborn rat spinal ganglia. Furthermore, they commonly contain considerable numbers of microtubules and filaments (Jacobs, unpublished observations; Peach, 1975) and the presence of microtubules may well be related to the most conspicuous feature of these cells, their striking tendency to spiral around the axon ('espirocitos'). Pannese (1960) has maintained that perisomatic and periaxonal satellite cells are always distinct elements with an abrupt transition at the root of the axon. In electron microscope studies of rabbit and rat nodose ganglion, however, satellite cells shared between the cell body and the emerging axon were commonly encountered (Lieberman, 1968b) and the basal lamina continues without interruption from the perisomatic to the periaxonal satellite cells; these morphological features constitute a further argument in favour of the essential similarity and common origin of the satellite cells of ganglion cell perikarya, and of their stem processes and the Schwann cells of peripheral nerves and roots (see Section 4.7.4).

4.6.4 *Quantitative relationships between satellite cells and neurons*

Microscopic inspection of sensory ganglia readily shows that the number of satellite cell nuclei per ganglion cell, and the thickness of the satellite cell sheath, are both greater around large than around small neurons and, according to De Castro (1932), greater in the case of cells with a complex axonal glomerulus (see Section 4.5.2) than in the case of cells of comparable size without an axonal glomerulus. In a series of interesting studies the linearity of these relationships has been established quantitatively in adult vertebrates under normal conditions, in developing ganglia, and under conditions resulting in chages of ganglion cell volume and surface area (Pannese, 1960, 1964, 1969a; Pannese *et al.*, 1972; Pannese, Ventura and Bianchi, 1975; Humbertson, Zimmerman and Leedy, 1969; Zimmerman, Karsh and Humbertson, 1971). Thus, for example, Pannese (1960), estimated (using light microscopy) that each satellite cell of both small and large ganglion cells in both newborn and adult animals (rats) corresponds to about 400 μm^2 of perikaryal surface (ignoring the considerable amplification of the latter by surface evaginations in the adult animal – see below), and to 2 000–2 500 μm^3 of perikaryal volume in the adult rat.

In the most recent of these studies, in which ultrastructural stereological methods were applied, it was shown that the volume of the satellite cell sheath is directly proportional both to the volume of the associated ganglion cell, and also (because of the considerable increase in perikaryal surface area due to the numerous perikaryal evaginations) to the surface area of the ganglion cell, in the dorsal root ganglia of adult rabbits and cats (Pannese *et al.*, 1972), and reptiles (Pannese *et al.*, 1975). A curious sidelight of these studies was the finding that for a given perikaryal volume or surface area, the satellite cell volume was always greater in cats than in rabbits, and substantially smaller in reptiles than in mammals.

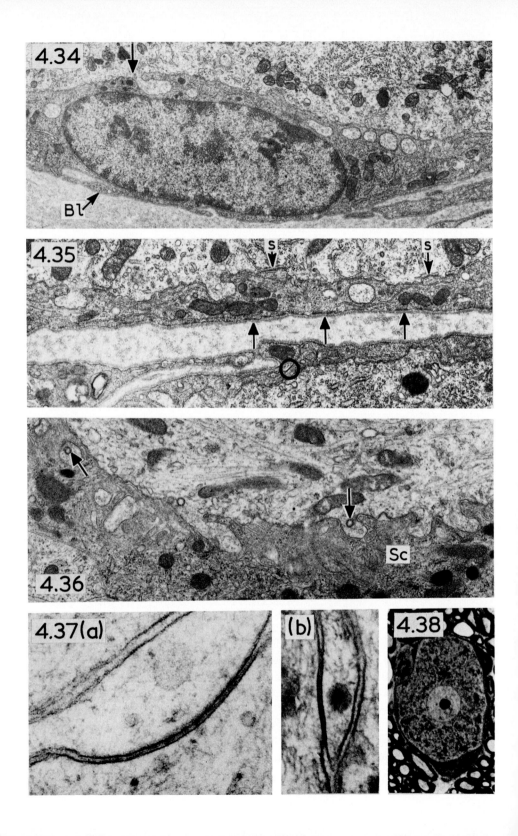

4.34

Bl

4.35

s   s

O

4.36

Sc

4.37(a)

(b)

4.38

The functional significance of this quantitative balance between neuronal perikarya and their satellite cell sheath is not clear. Developmental studies show that the satellite cells increase in number as the ganglion cell perikarya increase in size (Pannese, 1960, 1969a, 1974). Studies on axotomized neurons show a hypertrophy and hyperplasia of satellite cells soon after axotomy (Pannese, 1964; Humbertson *et al.*, 1969) at a time when dramatic metabolic changes are occurring in the neurons (Lieberman, 1971) and when cell swelling commonly occurs. But whether the maintenance of this satellite sheath-neuron relationship is related to the long-standing but still experimentally unvalidated hypothesis that satellite cells provide trophic support to the neurons they surround (Pannese, 1960, 1964), or to a requirement for regulating the passage of materials between neurons and blood vessels via the intercellular clefts of the sheath (see Pannese, 1960 and Pannese *et al.*, 1972), or to other factors, remains to be established. It has been claimed that dissociated chick spinal ganglion cells are able to survive, undergo differentiation and produce electrically active processes in the apparent absence of satellite or Schwann cells (Scott, Engelbert and Fisher, 1969; Okun, 1972) and that heart fibroblasts promote chick embryo spinal ganglion cell differentiation *in vitro* as effectively as satellite cells (Ludueña, 1973). If valid these observations would raise interesting questions about the roles of satellite cells in the normal development and metabolic maintenance of neurons. Others, however, have found that the survival and differentiation of sensory ganglion cells *in vitro* depends upon their association with satellite cells (e.g. Shimizu, 1965b). Furthermore, electron microscopy was

---

Fig. 4.34 Perinuclear region of a satellite cell; rat cervical dorsal root ganglion. A series of paraphytes, including one in continuity with the perikaryon (arrow) are apparent. Bl − basal lamina of satellite cell. (x 9000. Reproduced by courtesy of J. M. Jacobs.)

Fig. 4.35 Satellite cell sheaths and peripheral cytoplasm of two adjacent ganglion cells in rat cervical spinal ganglion. Subsurface cisterns (s), hemidesmosome-like specializations abutting the basal lamina (arrows) and what appears to be a close membrane apposition between the plasma membranes of contiguous satellite cells (circled) are indicated. (x 9000: Reproduced by courtesy of J. M. Jacobs.)

Fig. 4.36 Neuron-satellite cell interface in adult cat trigeminal ganglion. Paraphytes and coated vesicles, some of them closely associated with the paraphytes (arrows) are prominent. The presence of coated veiscles budding from (or possibly fusing with) the neuronal plasmalemma and free in the peripheral cytoplasm is a characteristic feature of sensory ganglion cell. Sc − satellite cell. (x 16 000: Reproduced by courtesy of D. N. Landon.)

Figs. 4.37a and **4.37b** Close membrane appositions, probably gap junctions, between satellite cell processes in rabbit nodose ganglion. (Fig. 4.37a x 80 000; Fig. 4.37b x 120 000.)

Fig. 4.38 Satellite cell undergoing mitosis in normal rat spinal ganglion. (Toluidine blue-stained one μm section; x 512: Reproduced by courtesy of J. M. Jacobs.)

not employed by Scott *et al.* (1969), Okun (1972) or Ludueña (1973) to confirm the complete absence of satellite cell processes from around the neurons. Bird (personal communication) has monitored events by electron microscopy in previously dissociated cell cultures of embryonic mouse and chick dorsal root ganglia, and has found that the surviving and differentiating neurons are *always* associated with satellite cell processes (e.g. Fig. 4.32).

4.6.5 *Myelinated ganglion cells*

In the ganglia of the eighth cranial nerve, a majority of the neuronal cell bodies, virtually all of which are bipolar cells, possess myelin sheaths. Myelinated perikarya are a consistent and striking feature of the vestibular and spiral ganglia in all vertebrate species and are also occasionally observed in the spinal ganglia of teleost fishes (Scharf, 1958).

The myelin around the vestibular and spiral ganglion cells may be loose, semi-compact or compact (in which case it is indistinguishable from that formed around adjacent nerve fibres) or a mixture of all three (Rosenbluth and Palay, 1961; Rosenbluth, 1962a; Nishimura, Kon, Awataguchi, Ishida and Yamamoto, 1965; Adamo and Daigneault, 1973). Some cells have only 1 or 2 myelin lamellae, but in the goldfish up to 90 lamellae have been counted (Rosenbluth and Palay, 1961). In mammals, maxima of 20 and 25 compacted lamellae have been counted in the rat (Rosenbluth, 1962a) and in the cat (Adamo and Daigneault, 1973). The individual lamellae in regions of loose or semi-compact myelin may be linked across the thickness of the sheath by a stack of adhaerens-like junctions (Rosenbluth, 1962a; Adamo and Daigneault, 1972, 1973). The myelin sheath around the cell body invariably continues along the two processes issuing from it, and terminates at nodes of Ranvier situated approximately equidistant from the perikaryon. The perikaryon plus the proximal portions of the two processes thus constitute a specialized myelinated internodal segment along the path of the auditory and vestibular nerve fibres, a path in which rapid and controlled conduction velocities are of critical functional significance. The probable importance of myelinated perikarya in determining the conduction properties of specific classes of fibre is emphasized by electrophysiological observations that suggest the existence of heterogeneity in the discharge and conduction properties of auditory fibres, and that the more heavily myelinated cells in the mammalian spiral ganglion are related to inner hair cells, whereas the minority population of unmyelinated neurons is connected to the outer hair cells (see Adamo and Daigneault, 1973, for references).

However, it is not only in the context of the electrophysiological properties of afferent nerve fibres that the myelinated perikarya of the eighth nerve ganglia are of interest. They are also important in at least two other respects: (1) in relation to considerations concerning the mechanisms of myelination, and (2) in relation to the debate on the functions of perineuronal satellite cells, with particular regard to hypotheses concerning metabolic interactions between neurons and glia.

(1) Electron microscope studies show that myelination of ganglion cell perikarya must involve mechanisms which differ fundamentally, in at least some respects, from the mechanisms operating during normal myelinogenesis of peripheral nerve. Thus, more than one satellite cell is involved in the myelination of the internodal segment containing the perikaryon (Rosenbluth and Palay, 1961; Rosenbluth, 1962a; Nishimura et al., 1965), and furthermore, one satellite cell may contribute to the sheaths of adjacent ganglion cells (Adamo and Daigneault, 1973). Finally, the perikaryal sheaths are commonly extremely irregular, with interruptions in the lamellae and a variety of departures from the normal arrangement seen in myelinated peripheral fibres: these irregularities are discussed in great detail by Rosenbluth (1962a). As Rosenbluth points out, a simple helical wrapping mechanism involving a single myelinogenic cell could not have produced the patterns seen in adult sheaths and studies on developing ganglia would be of great value in elucidating the myelinogenic mechanisms. In explant cultures of 12–15 day chick embryo stato-acoustic ganglia, the cell bodies acquire myelin sheaths, but at a much slower rate than normal (Shimizu, 1965a): such a system offers considerable advantages for ultrastructural analyses of perikaryal myelinogenesis.

(2) In regard to the question of possible metabolic interactions between myelinated neuronal perikarya and their satellites, it is difficult to envisage how a perikaryon surrounded by compact myelin, which is usually considered to be relatively inert and inpenetrable, could receive the metabolic support it is commonly supposed to do (e.g. Pannese, 1960). It is equally difficult to see how the fine control of diffusion to and from the neuronal perikaryon could be exerted through the intercellular clefts of the myelin sheath, as postulated by Pannese (1960) and Pannese et al. (1972) for spinal ganglia.

4.7 Development and differentiation of sensory ganglion cells

4.7.1 Embryological origins

The neurons of the spinal ganglia, like those of the autonomic ganglia and a variety of other adult cell types, derive from the neural crest. Those cells of the neural crest that migrate to a dorsolateral position along the neural tube and subsequently become arranged into clusters related to (and dependent for their formation upon the presence of) individual somites, constitute the rudiments of the sensory ganglia (Hörstadius, 1950; Weston, 1970; Pannese, 1974).

The embryological origins of the cranial sensory ganglia are more complex and not as yet fully understood. Although there is some evidence that neural crest is not involved in their formation in amphibia, most of the evidence available suggests that the cranial neural crest does contribute to the formation of the cranial sensory ganglia in conjunction with placodal ectoderm (Weston, 1970;

Johnston and Hazelton, 1972). Thus, the ganglion cells of the root or upper ganglia of the facial nerve, glossopharyngeal nerve, and vagus (jugular ganglion) are apparently derived predominantly from cranial neural crest (although the jugular ganglion may also receive cells from the trunk crest), whereas the neurons of the trunk or inferior ganglia of the facial nerve (geniculate ganglion), the glossopharyngeal nerve (petrosal ganglion) and the vagus (nodose ganglion) are derived predominantly from the ectodermal placodes, which also give rise to the neurons of the vestibulo-acoustic nerve ganglia. The trigeminal ganglion is thought to receive contributions both from cranial neural crest and placodal ectoderm (Johnston and Hazelton, 1972). In the chick, the neural crest apparently gives rise to the larger, more argyrophilic cells and the trigeminal placode to the smaller cells of the ganglion (Hamburger, 1961). Furthermore, Hamburger (1961) found that extirpation of the placode resulted in a deficiency of large cells and exteroceptive fibres and proposed that the small cells of this ganglion are predominantly proprioceptive. Whether the neural crest-derived neurons and the placodal ectoderm-derived neurons are indeed structurally and functionally differentiated as proposed by Hamburger (1961) has been questioned by Weston (1970). Weston has emphasized how difficult it is at present to make definitive statements about the origins of the cranial sensory ganglion cells on the basis of the ablation and labelling techniques currently employed. Cells originating in the neural crest, for example, may well contribute to the formation of the placodes as a result of the complex morphogenetic movements that occur during early embryogenesis, or as a result of early migrations, or the placodes may be induced by underlying neural crest, thus invalidating many of the conclusions drawn from ablation experiments.

4.7.2 *Cell turnover and the control of cell number in developing sensory ganglia*

The patterns of cell proliferation, of differentiation and histogenetic degeneration, and the relative contributions of intrinsic and extrinsic factors in determining the final cell number in sensory ganglia are of enormous interest, but are beyond the scope of this chapter. Most of the relevant data on the latter point derive from studies of sensory ganglia in birds and amphibians, in which experimental access to the embryo for the purpose of increasing or decreasing the peripheral innervation territory at various developmental stages, is relatively simple, and in which the numbers of ganglion cells are relatively small (see for example Hamburger and Levi-Montalcini, 1949; Mitolo, Selvaggi and Selvaggi, 1965). The literature on the control of cell number in avian and amphibian sensory ganglia has been reviewed by several authors, including Hughes (1968), Jacobson (1970) and Prestige (1970), and Pannese (1974) has provided a beautifully illustrated and thorough account of cell death during the development of chick dorsal root ganglia. A recent quantitative study of spinal ganglion development in a marsupial (Hughes, 1973) has paved the way for similar studies in at least this order of mammals, since dramatic changes in cell numbers occur after birth in the pouch-young (Hughes, 1973) which are considerably more accessible to experimental manipulation than the embryos of eutherian (placental) mammals.

4.7.3 *Differentiation of ganglion cells*

The ganglionic rudiments possess an epithelium-like structure initially, comprised of a basement lamina-enclosed group of closely packed mitotic cells separated by approximately 20 nm intercellular spaces, and are devoid of the blood vessels and the connective tissue elements which make their appearance only later in development (Pannese, 1974). Subsequent cell proliferation, and the incorporation of additional migrating neural crest cells, lead to rapid enlargement of the ganglionic rudiment. Cells in the ventrolateral portion of the ganglion show a more rapid differentiation than cells in the dorsomedial portion, particularly in birds (Hamburger and Levi-Montalcini, 1949; Gaik, 1973; Pannese, 1974), but later (towards the end of incubation in birds) differences between the ventrolateral and dorsomedial cells are no longer detectable. In rat lumbar dorsal root ganglia the final divisions of nearly all the neuroblasts occur on days 11–15 of gestation, with most of the future large light cells (see Section 4.4.1) being generated on day 12 and most of the small dark cells on day 13 (Lawson *et al.*, 1974).

The small undifferentiated cells, whose cytoplasm is characterized by abundant free polysomes but few other organelles, commonly have several small irregular processes, but these disappear during mitosis. The first stage of differentiation of the post-mitotic neuroblast also involves the disappearance of these processes, elongation of the neuroblast along the ganglionic axis and the outgrowth of one process from each of the two poles of the cell. The process that extends towards the periphery is commonly thicker than that growing towards the central nervous system, and grows at a faster rate (Pannese, 1974). (See also Section 4.5.5). Because developing sensory ganglion cells pass through this distinctive bipolar phase (see Fig. 4.32a), and for additional phylogenetic and comparative anatomical reasons (see Section 4.5.1) the mature ganglion cell is sometimes, but unnecessarily, referred to as a pseudounipolar cell.

The neural crest cells, and the mitotic neuroblasts to which they give rise, are small cells (8–12 μm in diameter in developing rat spinal ganglia; Lawson *et al.*, 1974). Following the final cell division, the postmitotic neuroblasts enlarge dramatically. According to Sobkowicz, Hartmann, Monzain and Desnoyers (1973) the cells show a rather constant, very rapid rate of size increase from the 11th embryonic to the 11th postnatal day (over which period their volume increases nearly 25-fold), after which they continue to enlarge only very slowly. An interesting observation of Lawson *et al.* (1974) slightly at variance with the findings of Sobkowicz *et al.* (1973), although also made in rat spinal ganglia, was that the 'growth spurt' started only 3 days or so *after* the formation of the majority of the cells – i.e. at embryonic day 15. The increase in cell body size during the early part of this period of growth is eccentric, and the bipolar neuroblast acquires a bell-shaped perikaryon with the polar processes aligned along the 'rim' of the bell. This stage occurs as early as 5 days in the chick (Pannese, 1974) and 15 days in the rabbit (Tennyson, 1965). Subsequently, the perikaryon 'pulls away' from the rim of the bell and moves closer to the ganglionic periphery: as this occurs the cytoplasmic 'neck' connecting the perikaryon with the bases of the processes narrows and elongates to give rise to the initial portion of the axon (the 'connecting piece' of Cajal, 1907). This differential growth leads to the establishment of the T-junction of the differentiated neuron at the point at which the initial axon bifurcates into peripheral and central processes (Tennyson, 1965, 1970; Pannese, 1974). It is perhaps worth emphasizing that the remodelling mechanism leading to the establishment of a monopolar neuron does not entail fusion of the proximal portions of the two original processes. Although clearly refuted by Cajal's and subsequent observations (e.g. Tennyson, 1965) accounts of such a fusion of processes are still to be found in some standard texts of recent years.

Concurrent with the phase of cellular remodelling leading to the acquisition of the unipolar form, granular reticulum proliferates and Nissl bodies become apparent, the Golgi apparatus forms and acquires its adult configuration, microtubules and filaments become more numerous, and an enormous increase occurs in the number of mitochondria (Pannese, 1974). Between the 11th day of gestation and birth the RNA content per neuron increases almost six fold in rat spinal ganglia (Sobkowicz *et al.*, 1973). A further five-fold increase in RNA content occurs over the first 11 postnatal days and thereafter there is a slow increase to the adult level of about 1250 pg per cell (Sobkowicz *et al.*, 1973). Detailed accounts of nuclear and cytoplasmic differentiation and of the genesis of organelles are to be found in the papers of Hydén (1943), Tennyson (1965, 1970) Pannese (1968, 1974), and Sobkowicz *et al.* (1973), and various aspects of the histochemical maturation of sensory ganglion cells are considered by Sarrat (1970), Tennyson and Brzin (1970), Giacobini, Marchisio, Giacobini and Koslow (1970) and Pannese (1974) (see also Section 4.4.1). It is interesting to note that, although many signs of chemodifferentiation of sensory ganglia cells become apparent soon after the final neuroblast division (Sarrat, 1970; Pannese, 1974), mitotic neuroblasts synthesize acetylcholinesterase and therefore display at least some chemodifferentiation at a very early developmental stage (Tennyson and Brzin, 1970; Pannese, 1974).

Throughout the early stages of development and differentiation, until, in fact, the ganglion cells become invested in their satellite cell capsules (see below) adjacent cells are commonly observed to be linked by adhesion plaques, and by gap junctions (Pannese, 1974). The presence of the latter is likely to be of considerable developmental significance (see for example, Bennett, 1973).

4.7.4 *Origin and development of satellite cells*

It is probable that the satellite and Schwann cells of the cerebrospinal ganglia arise from the neural crest (and placodal ectoderm) (Pannese, 1974). This would make the situation in the sensory ganglia comparable to that in the central nervous system, where both neurons and macroglia originate from neural ectoderm. There is, however, some experimental evidence indicating that some satellite and Schwann cells may derive from the neural tube (see Weston, 1970).

The satellite cells make their appearance in the ganglion rudiments after the neuroblasts (Levi, 1908; Pannese, 1974), but an intimate neuron-satellite cell relationship is established very early in development (Peach, 1973; Pannese, 1974). The satellite cells are initially stellate, with processes related to more than one neuroblast, but subsequently they tend to assume a simpler shape (see Section 4.6.1), perhaps as a result of process retraction (Pannese, 1969a), and become related to only one neuron. As is the case for developing ganglion cells (see above) satellite cells may be linked by gap junctions both during the early stages (i.e. before a relationship with a single neuron has been established) and later in development, when the junctions are between adjacent cells of the same perineuronal capsule (Pannese, 1974).

The satellite cells retain their mitotic capability as they differentiate, and, as the ganglion cells to which they are related enlarge, the number of satellite cells undergoes a proportional increase. In the early postnatal period, during which considerable enlargement of ganglion cell bodies occurs (see Section 4.3.1), mitotic satellite cells are consistently observed (Skoglund, 1967; 1-25 day old kittens). A small but consistent proportion of satellite cells is labelled by tritiated thymidine in adult rodents: Friede and Johnstone (1967) found 16 labelled satellite cells per 100 ganglion cells in adult rats and Smith and Adrian (1972) found that approximately 0.5 per cent of perineuronal satellite cells were labelled under similar conditions in adult mice (see also Fig. 4.38). In adult cats, however, Skoglund (1967) found no evidence for mitotic activity. Further aspects of the relationships between satellite cells and the neurons they invest are considered in Section 4.6.

4.8 The trigeminal mesencephalic nucleus

An anomaly among nuclei of the central nervous system, the mesencephalic nucleus of the trigeminal nerve, is a column of primary sensory neurons situated within the rostral pons and the entire caudo-rostral extent of the mid-brain. There is experimental evidence (Weston, 1970) that the neurons comprising this nucleus migrate into the brain from the neural crest and this developmental history, when taken in conjunction with the known anatomy and physiology of these cells (see below), makes it reasonable to consider this nucleus to be a homologue of the cranio-spinal sensory ganglia.

The peripheral processes of most of the mesencephalic neurons leave the brain stem in the ipsilateral mandibular division of the trigeminal nerve, and there is both anatomical and physiological evidence that they innervate the spindles and tendon organs of the masticatory muscles. Thus, chromatolysis or perikaryal degeneration occurs after lesions of the mandibular nerve (e.g. Bortolami, Callegari and Lucchi, 1972; Imamoto, 1972a, b) and the intracranial axons and cell bodies of these cells can be filled with cobalt by iontophoresis of cobaltous ions into the cut end of the trigeminal nerve (Prior and Fuller, 1973). Physiological evidence for the proprioceptive nature of the information carried by these axons is equally convincing (e.g. Corbin and Harrison, 1940; Jerge, 1963; Dale Smith, 1969). There is further, less complete evidence, that mesencephalic trigeminal neurons also provide a proprioceptive innervation to other muscles (facial, lingual, laryngeal, extraocular), to articular tissues of the tempero-mandibular joint, and to periodontal tissue (Dale Smith and Marcarian, 1968; Dault and Dale Smith, 1969; Darian-Smith, 1973; Warwick and Williams, 1973; Alvarado-Mallart et al., 1975).

The destination of the centrally directed processes of the mesencephalic neurons has long been a subject of controversy. It would appear, however, that for the most part they terminate in the cerebellar cortex, reaching the latter by way of the superior cerebellar peduncle (Brodal and Saugstad, 1965; Cupédo, 1970; a conclusion criticized by Hinrichsen and Larramendi, 1969). Collaterals to the trigeminal motor nucleus (Bortolami et al., 1972) and to other brain stem nuclei have also been described.

The cell bodies of mesencephalic trigeminal neurons are very similar in histological appearance to cranio-spinal ganglion cells. Most appear to be large, spherical, unipolar cells (Cajal, 1909; Corbin and Harrison, 1940; Dault and Dale Smith, 1969; Hinrichsen and Larramendi, 1969), but Cajal (1909) and others (e.g. Dault and Dale Smith, 1969; Bortolami et al., 1972) have reported the presence of a minority of small multipolar cells within the nucleus. In vitro, mesencephalic neurons resemble sensory ganglion cells grown under similar conditions, and most of the cells are unipolar, some bipolar and a few tripolar (Hild, 1966).

By electron microscopy, mesencephalic neurons have an initial axon segment similar to that of sensory ganglion cells (Hinrichsen and Larramendi, 1970; Alley, 1973) — i.e. free of synaptic contacts and without a sub-axolemmal undercoating or fasciculated microtubules (Section 4.5.2). The axon hillock region also resembles that of sensory ganglion cells in being almost Nissl-free (Brodal and Saugstad, 1965) and at the ultrastructural level containing few ribosomes (Alley, 1973).

In spite of the structural, functional and embryological affinities between these neurons and sensory ganglion cells, there are other equally striking and in some ways more interesting differences. Perhaps the most fundamental difference is that, unlike the sensory ganglion cell bodies which are completely ensheathed by satellite cells and devoid of synaptic contacts, mesencephalic neurons are set in a sea of complex neuropil (Imamoto and Shimizu, 1970) and are only partially enclosed by glial (astrocytic) processes so that the somal surface comes into direct contact with neuropil elements, particularly with sparse axon terminals that establish axo-somatic synapses (Hinrichsen and Larramendi, 1968, 1970; Imamoto and Shimizu, 1970; Bortolami *et al.*, 1972; Alley, 1973). Nothing is yet known about the physiological significance or sources of these endings. The mesencephalic neurons give rise to numerous short spines and crests. While Imamoto and Shimizu (1970) found rare synaptic contacts on such evaginations, most appear to be devoid of synaptic contacts (Hinrichsen and Larramendi, 1970; Alley, 1973) and in this respect are more akin to paraphytes (see Section 4.6.2) than to the usual postsynaptic spines of neurons in the central nervous system.

The clustering of mesencephalic neurons into small groups of cells, originally commented upon by Cajal (1909; see also Hinrichsen and Larramendi, 1969), and also observable *in vitro* (Hild, 1957), represents another interesting peculiarity of the trigeminal neurons. Ultrastructural studies have shown that extensive areas of direct plasmalemmal contact occur between neurons within such clusters, and that the interface is characterized by a series of closely spaced adhaerens-like maculae (Hinrichsen and Larramendi, 1968, 1970; Imamoto and Shimizu, 1970) and by areas of close membrane apposition resembling gap junctions (Hinrichsen and Larramendi, 1968, 1970). Evidence of electrotonic coupling between the neurons within a cluster (Baker and Llinás, 1971) suggests that the cells of a cluster may function as a unit, with ionic coupling between them mediated by the gap junctions.

There are other striking differences between mesencephalic neurons and sensory ganglion cells revealed by their different responses to axonal injury. In the first place, mesencephalic neurons of both fully grown mammals (Cupédo, 1970) and birds (Bortolami, Veggetti and Ciampoli, 1969; Bortolami *et al.*, 1972) appear to be unusually sensitive to lesions of their peripheral processes, and undergo degeneration following lesions that would certainly not produce such a severe response in sensory ganglion cells subjected to interruption of their peripheral processes at comparable distances from the perikarya and in animals of similar age (Lieberman, 1971, 1974).

Even more striking is the difference between sensory ganglion cells and trigeminal mesencephalic cells in response to interruption of their centrally directed processes. The former show little histological or ultrastructural evidence of an injury response to lesions of their central axons, even when the latter are cut quite close to the cell bodies, and in spite of the fact that the interrupted axons show active regenerative growth and a perikaryal metabolic response (Section 4.9.4). Mesencephalic neurons, on the other hand, show marked perikaryal changes following damage to their central axons, particularly when the injury is close to the cell bodies, changes that closely resemble those induced by lesions of their peripheral processes (Brodal and Saugstad, 1965; Bortolami *et al.*, 1972).

255

4.9 Some functional considerations

4.9.1 *Electrophysiological properties of sensory ganglion cells*

Under physiological conditions, action potentials in sensory ganglion cells are initiated at or close to the receptor terminals. Because of the off-stream position of the perikaryon in relation to the impulse traffic 'through-route', ganglion cell perikarya play a far less dominant role in the electrophysiological activities of the cell than is the case in multipolar neurons. Indeed, as long ago as 1899, Steinach maintained that the ganglion cell bodies themselves were of no significance, save in the trophic sense, to the normal physiological activities of cell. He based his conclusions on experiments in which reflex activity dependent upon certain dorsal roots in the frog, could still be elicited 1 and 2 days after the blood supply to the ganglia of these roots had been cut off. Although Steinach's experiments do not really provide adequate proof of the irrelevance of the cell bodies, the facts that the perikaryon and initial axon of the ganglion cell are devoid of synaptic contacts (Section 4.4.2) and are not normally action potential-generating regions, strengthen the notion that these parts of the cell are of limited significance in determining the pattern of afferent activity conveyed along the processes of the sensory ganglion cell to the central nervous system.

From the electrophysiological point of view, the interesting parts of the sensory ganglion cell are thus the terminal portions of the peripheral process, and the synaptic endings of the central process. In many ways, the anatomy and physiology of the spinal cord and brain stem nuclei in which the sensory ganglion cells terminate represent the most important aspects of the sensory ganglion cell, for it is in these regions that activity in second order neurons is generated and reflex activity controlled. Furthermore, it is the first level at which peripherally generated afferent activity in sensory nerve fibres comes under central control, and the only level at which the sensory ganglion cell can be influenced by other neurons, including other sensory ganglion cells. It would not be appropriate to discuss here the synaptic circuitry in which the central terminals of sensory ganglion cells participate or the physiology of spinal cord and brain stem primary afferent-receiving nuclei; excellent reviews and bibliographies are to be found in Wall (1973) (dorsal horn); Norton (1973) (dorsal column nuclei) and Darian Smith (1973) (trigeminal complex).

It should not be thought, however, that the perikaryon and initial part of the axon are completely silent. The cells maintain a resting membrane potential of 20–90 mV (references in Scott *et al.*, 1969), and although action potentials are not normally initiated at the level of the cell body, microelectrode studies of intact, freshly isolated and cultured ganglion cells show that the soma is always invaded by the action potential passing along its processes (amphibian dorsal root ganglia – Svaetichin, 1951; Dun, 1955; Ito, 1959; Ito and Saiga, 1959: mammalian dorsal root ganglia – Sato and Austin, 1961; Letbetter and Willis, 1969: chick dorsal root ganglia in explant cultures – Crain, 1956: chick dorsal root ganglia in dissociation cultures – Scott *et al.*, 1969; Varon and Raiborn, 1971). Conduction along the glomerular segment of the initial axon is slow, however, and the central terminals of at least those ganglion cells with large diameter myelinated axons are depolarized before the soma (Darian-Smith, 1973). Svaetichin (1951) also showed minor but consistent differences between the electrophysiological properties of small cells connected with unmyelinated axons and those of large cells with myelinated axons.

More interesting is the fact that a certain amount of evidence has accumulated from microelectrode studies to indicate that the intra-ganglionic portions of the sensory ganglion cell may not be completely irrelevant in determining the sequencing and pattern of peripherally generated impulses. In the first place, there is a passive influence in the form of a delay in the transmission of impulses through the ganglion. The question of a delay at the level of the ganglion was a controversial one for many years, but re-examination of the question by Dun (1955) demonstrated a consistent delay in transmission through frog dorsal root ganglia for both orthodromic and antidromic impulses. The delay almost certainly arises at the junction between the peripheral and central axons and the stem process (see Section 4.5.3).

Secondly, and of much greater significance, are recent studies of spinal ganglion cells by Tagini and Camino (1973) and of cat and rabbit spinal ganglion cells by Kirk (1974), which have revealed hitherto unsuspected active properties of the ganglion cells under special conditions. Tagini and Camino (1973) found that when large cells with myelinated processes were repeatedly activated and fatigued by electrical stimulation of the peripheral nerve, an action potential was sometimes generated by or close to the cell body following the electrically induced spike: the second action potential always travelled antidromically from the ganglion to the periphery. An additional curious finding in this study was that the second action potential does not propagate into the central process (i.e. towards the spinal cord in the orthodromic direction). Tagini and Camino (1973) suggest that this is because the latter is generally thinner and thus less excitable, but the anatomical evidence does not support this assumption (see Section 4.5.4).

Kirk (1974) was able to record regularly occurring spontaneous impulses from dorsal rootlets of rabbit and cat spinal ganglia isolated from the periphery by transection of the spinal nerve. These action potentials were found to propagate centrally from the ganglion towards the cord, but not peripherally from the ganglion towards the cut nerve. This strange phenomenon could be detected only one day or more after isolation of the ganglion from the periphery and primarily involved ganglion cells of small diameter with myelinated fibres.

Neither these studies, nor those showing spontaneous discharges of spinal ganglion cells maintained *in vitro* (e.g. Peacock, Nelson and Goldstone, 1973; but cf. Crain, 1956; Varon and Raiborn, 1971) offer any clue as to whether impulse generation by ganglion cell perikarya can occur, and if so what its function may be, under normal physiological conditions. But perhaps that is not the point: it may be that the capacity to generate action potentials at the level of the cell body develops only under abnormal conditions such as excessive stimulation or peripheral nerve section, and may in some as yet obscure fashion serve to mitigate the effects of the consequent hyper or hypo-activity.

4.9.2 *Somatotopic organization within sensory ganglia*

Ganglion cells innervating a common peripheral territory are grouped close to one another within the ganglion and the central processes of such cells remain adjacent to one another as they approach the cord or brain stem. In some cases at least, adjacent peripheral territories are innervated by adjacent groups of ganglion cells. The evidence for this somatotopic pattern of organization is extensive. Section of different branches of the vagus and trigeminal nerves, for example, results in retrograde changes (chromatolysis; see Section 4.9.4) in different groups of adjacent cells within the nodose ganglion (Molhant, 1913; Lieberman, 1968a, b) and the trigeminal ganglion (Allen, 1924; Mazza and Dixon, 1972). Molhant (1913) showed that in the rabbit nodose ganglion, cells innervating the heart and larynx are located close to the superior pole, those innervating the lungs in the middle and lower portions of the external border, cells innervating the stomach at the centre of the ganglion, and cells innervating the oesophagus and trachea in a diffuse zone extending from close to the superior pole to the centre of the ganglion. Major cell groups contributing peripheral processes to only one branch of a nerve may even show anatomically well-defined borders: the cells in the superior pole of the rabbit nodose ganglion, whose peripheral processes enter the superior laryngeal nerve, may be separated by a perineurial partition from the other cells of the ganglion (Lieberman, 1968a, b). Mazza and Dixon (1972) who cut the inferior alveolar, mental, infraorbital, external or superior labial nerves in young rats and mapped the chromatolytic cell groups in serial sections of the trigeminal ganglion, found a somatotopic organization similar to that found by Allen (1924) in cats, using the same approach. External nasal cells were located at the medial border of the ophthalmic-maxillary part of the ganglion and superior labial cells along its lateral border, with some degree of overlap ventrally: inferior alveolar cells were found to be closely packed into a lateral protuberance at the base of the mandibular division of the ganglion, with mental nerve cell bodies lying dorsal to them.

More recently, new anatomical techniques have become available for studying this aspect of sensory ganglion organization. One of these, autoradiography of roots and nerves following localized microinjection of labelled amino-acid into the ganglion, has already been used effectively by Burton and McFarlane (1973). They injected ^{3}H proline into different sectors of the cat L7 spinal ganglion and correlated the position of the cell bodies exposed to the tracer with the distribution of labelled central processes in the dorsal rootlets. Burton and McFarlane (1973) found that the rostral rootlets carry the central processes of cells located laterally in the ganglion, with the central processes of those cells lying most proximally (i.e. closest to the spinal cord) occupying the most rostral rootlet(s); the caudal rootlets carry the central processes of cells in the medial part of the ganglion, the central processes of the cells situated most distally occupying the most caudal rootlet(s). It is also possible to use this technique to trace the distribution of the peripheral processes of small groups of cells (e.g. Fink, Kish and Byers, 1975).

Of even greater potential value is the horseradish peroxidase technique: recent studies have shown that sensory ganglion cell perikarya can be labelled after injection of the horseradish peroxidase close to the receptor terminals of, or at the site of injury of their peripheral axons (Furstman Saporta and Kruger, 1975; Luiten, 1975; Kristensson and Olsson, 1975), and it also appears to be possible to label and identify the central axons of cells whose peripheral axons or receptor terminals have taken up the tracer (Furstman et al., 1975). It is therefore now possible to carry out detailed high resolution mapping studies using the horseradish peroxidase technique by labelling individual or very small groups of receptor terminals: Furstman et al. (1975), for example, were able to label a compact group of 5 or fewer cells at the periphery of the trigeminal ganglion following injection of the tracer into the pulp cavity of a single incisor tooth.

Finally, Stoeckel, Schwab and Thoenen (1975) have shown that it is also possible to use radioactively labelled nerve growth factor to localize the perikarya of ganglion cells into whose peripheral terminal field the nerve growth factor has been injected. These authors found that nerve growth factor injected into the forepaw of young or adult rats ascends the sensory axons at about 13 mm/h and accumulates in the large cell bodies of the cervical ganglia on the injected side.

There is also extensive physiological evidence for somatotopy based on recording evoked activity in single ganglion cells (or very small groups of cells) following physiological or electrical stimulation of the peripheral receptors or the peripheral or central axons in specific nerve branches or central rootlets. Mei (1964, 1970) working with the cat nodose ganglion has found a pattern of somatotopic organization corresponding rather well with that shown by the less refined anatomical analysis of the corresponding ganglion in the rabbit by Molhant (1913). Similar physiological studies have revealed the somatotopic organization of the trigeminal ganglion of several different species (Kerr and Lysak, 1964; Beaudreau and Jerge, 1968; Darian-Smith, 1973).

Burton and McFarlane (1973) also used physiological methods in their study of the L7 spinal ganglion of the cat. Antidromic activation of ganglion cells by stimulation of individual dorsal rootlets confirmed the relationship between the position of the cell and the rootlet carrying its central process found in the anatomical study (see above). These authors also mapped the receptive fields of the ganglion cells: electrode penetrations passing from one side of the ganglion to the other reveal a pattern of shifting overlap in the receptive fields of the cells encountered, (from preaxial to postaxial leg in the case of a lateral to medial penetration), whereas a penetration along the proximo-distal (longitudinal) axis reveals cells with non-overlapping receptive fields confined for the most part to the same small area of the hind limb.

The significance of the somatotopic organization of sensory ganglia is not entirely clear. For discussion of this topic, for comments on the intraganglionic distribution of cells related to different modalities, and for references, see Mei (1970), Darian-Smith (1973) and Burton and McFarlane (1973).

4.9.3 *Sensory ganglion cell transmitter(s)*

There are currently two principal candidates for the role of transmitter at the central terminals of sensory ganglion cells; L-glutamate and substance P. Glutamate exerts a powerful depolarizing effect on spinal cord and brain stem neurons (Johnson, 1972; Curtis and Johnston, 1974) and is the only excitatory amino acid present in high concentration both in the central portion of the dorsal root and in the dorsal root ganglia, but in low concentration in the peripheral dorsal root (Duggan and Johnston, 1970; Johnson and Aprison, 1970). Substance P, a polypeptide (undecapeptide) is some 200 times more potent than L-glutamate in depolarizing frog and rat motor neurons, is present in high concentration in the central dorsal roots of a variety of species and in even higher concentration (by a factor of about x 50) in the region of the dorsal horn of the cat spinal cord in which the central terminals are known to be concentrated; after section or ligation of the central dorsal root (cat; roots $L_5 - S_1$), the concentration of substance P falls dramatically in the dorsal horn and substance P accumulates on the ganglionic side of the lesion (Takahashi and Otsuka, 1975). Takahashi and Otsuka (1975) also report that glutamate levels do not fall in the dorsal horn after dorsal rhizotomy and that glutamate does not accumulate on the ganglionic side of a central dorsal root lesion.

Recent studies by Schon and Kelly (1974) showing uptake of H^3 glutamate into the perineuronal satellite cells and not into the neurons of cat dorsal root ganglia, also raise some doubts about glutamate as the transmitter of sensory ganglion cells. A possible explanation considered by Schon and Kelly (1974) for the failure of the cells to take up a presumed transmitter was that all of the available glutamate is sequestered by the satellite cells before it can reach the ganglion cells: a similar explanation has been offered for the failure of cerebellar Purkyně cells to show uptake of exogenous GABA (γ aminobutyric acid) under most conditions, although their transmitter is almost certainly GABA (Curtis and Johnston, 1974). One reason for doubting this explanation is that GABA, which is not a transmitter candidate for the sensory ganglion cells, is taken up just as avidly as glutamate by the satellite cells of isolated dorsal root ganglia (Schon and Kelly, 1974), and yet cat nodose and spinal ganglion cells show marked depolarizing responses to GABA (DeGroat, 1972; De Groat, Lalley and Saum, 1972) which suggests that the high affinity uptake system of the satellite cells does not prevent the GABA, and by inference, glutamate from reaching the surface of the neurons.

[The responsiveness of the sensory ganglion cells to GABA is also interesting in another respect as there is evidence that GABA is the transmitter responsible for depolarizing the terminals of sensory ganglion cells in the spinal cord and brain stem (Curtis and Johnston, 1974). The presence of GABA receptors on the ganglion cell bodies, though somewhat surprising in view of the absence of presynaptic terminals at this locus, can be taken as supporting evidence for GABA as the transmitter mediating presynaptic inhibition at the central terminals of the ganglion cells].

On balance, the case for substance P as the transmitter of lumbosacral dorsal root ganglion cells, appears to be stronger than that for glutamate, at least in the cat. But, it may be that both of these substances, and possibly others may act as transmitters in different sensory ganglion cells: more work is obviously needed.

4.9.4 *Regenerative capacities and injury responses of sensory ganglion cells*

Sensory ganglion cells display an impressive regenerative capability: vigorous axonal regrowth follows interruption of the peripheral process, and of the central process within the dorsal root or cranial sensory root. Regeneration of the peripheral process may lead to reinnervation of the denervated periphery, and in some cases to functional recovery. A discussion of the factors determining the rate and extent of regeneration, maturation and recovery of sensation would be beyond the scope of this chapter (see Young, 1942; Guth, 1956; Lieberman, 1974; Thomas, 1974).

Regenerating central dorsal or cranial sensory root fibres grow at approximately the same rate as regenerating peripheral fibres (Cajal, 1928; Moyer, Kimmel and Winborne, 1953; Carlsson and Thulin, 1967). Furthermore, although the regenerating axons do not normally enter the spinal cord or brain stem, their regenerative growth is vigorous and can be sustained by providing them with an artificially extended path along which to grow (see Lieberman, 1971).

In view of the many similarities between central and peripheral processes and the comparable regenerative growth they display after injury, it might be expected that the perikaryal responses associated with the injury and regenerative phase would be similar after lesions of either process. However it has been known for nearly 100 years that the ganglion cell perikarya show no or only very slight morphological evidence of an injury response after lesions of their centrally directed axons, whereas a series of distinctive perikaryal alterations is elicited by peripheral axon injury.

Among the changes induced in and around the cell bodies of sensory ganglion cells following injury of their peripheral processes, the most conspicuous are *chromatolysis*, which consists of a breakdown of large Nissl bodies and a loss of Nissl substance from the central portion of the cell, and displacement of the nucleus from its usual position at or close to the cell centre, towards the cell periphery. Other changes include nucleolar enlargement, an increase in neuro-filaments, proliferation and enlargement of lysosomes, cell swelling (in some cases at least), and hypertrophy and hyperplasia of the perineuronal satellite cells. The significance of these changes and the principal metabolic responses of the cell body to axonal injury are best known, not from studies on sensory ganglion cells, but from studies on mammalian cranio-spinal motor neurons.

In rat hypoglossal neurons the initial response to axonal injury is a change in the nuclear DNA (indicated by an increased capacity of the latter to bind Actinomycin D; Watson, 1974a) associated with a burst of nuclear RNA synthesis, the time of onset and duration of which are determined by the distance from the cell body of the site of injury (Watson, 1968). The increase in nuclear RNA synthesis is associated with an increase in nucleolar RNA content (and hence size), with an increase in the rate of transfer of newly-synthesized RNA from nucleus to cytoplasm (Watson, 1965), with an increase in cytoplasmic RNA content, and following closely on the latter, an increase in cytoplasmic protein synthesis and protein content (Watson, 1968). The cytoplasmic RNA content increases in proportion to the length of the period of enhanced nuclear RNA synthesis and is thus determined by the site of the injury since the period of increased synthesis is shorter and the increase in cytoplasmic RNA correspondingly less with lesions close to the cell body (Watson, 1968). Chromatolysis – an apparent reduction in cytoplasmic basiphil material (i.e. RNA) – is therefore in effect an optical illusion, brought about by changes in the distribution, in the regional concentration and (because of cell swelling) in the net cytoplasmic concentration of RNA. The more 'severe' chromatolysis seen with more proximal lesions reflects the lesser increase in cytoplasmic RNA under these conditions (Watson, 1968).

The various metabolic and morphological changes in axotomized neurons are certainly related in part to the regenerative growth of the interrupted axon, but also reflect to some extent a fall in the demand for the provision of certain materials to the nerve endings, and relate to changes in the surface properties of the injured neuron and in its relationships with presynaptic boutons and postsynaptic elements (Lieberman, 1971; Watson, 1974b; Grafstein, 1975).

The metabolic responses of sensory ganglion cells to interruption of their peripherally directed processes have not been studied so intensively. Because most of the morphological and histochemical changes in sensory ganglion cells after such an injury are very similar to those seen in motor neurons after axotomy, it is reasonable to suppose that the metabolic changes are also similar: preliminary studies of nucleolar and cytoplasmic RNA content and of cytoplasmic protein content in rat cervical dorsal root ganglion cells after section of their peripheral processes, strongly indicate that this is so (Watson, 1973).

Following injury of the central processes of sensory ganglion cells along the dorsal (or cranial sensory) roots or intraspinally, changes in the cell bodies are difficult to detect or are minimal when viewed by either by light or electron microscopy: this is the case even when the central processes are grown along an artificially extended pathway, or after repeated crush injuries, after very long post-operative survival periods, or in very young animals (Lieberman, 1969a, 1971; though c.f. Nathaniel and Nathaniel, 1973). In spite of this apparent unresponsiveness, some metabolic responses to central axotomy are to be expected (Lieberman, 1971), and Watson (1973) has reported small increases in nucleolar and cytoplasmic RNA content in rat spinal ganglion cells following division of the dorsal root. Of great additional interest was the demonstration by Watson in the same study, of a more marked metabolic response after division of *adjacent* dorsal roots: this finding suggests that the intraspinal sprouting of the uninjured dorsal root fibres that occurs as a result of the degeneration of neighbouring terminals acts as a more poweful stimulus to the cell body than a direct injury to the central axon.

It is therefore clear that the perikarya of sensory ganglion cells are affected by lesions of their central processes, that changes in the cell's RNA and protein metabolism may occur in the absence of detectable chromatolysis and that although this may not be reflected in the morphology of the cells, the response is qualitatively, if not quantitatively comparable both to that elicited by peripheral axon section and to that seen in axotomized motor neurons. The reason for the apparent differences in the responsiveness of the ganglion cells to central and peripheral axonal lesions is still not fully understood and is discussed by Lieberman (1969a, 1971), by Cragg (1970) and by Grafstein (1975).

Acknowledgements

I am extremely grateful to Dr. Jean Jacobs (Institute of Neurology) for her comments and criticisms on parts of the manuscript and for allowing me to cite her unpublished findings and to use so much of her material in the illustrations. I am also grateful to Dr. Margaret Bird (University College London) for discussion and for the loan of micrographs and to Dr. David Landon, for comments on the manuscript, for the loan of micrographs and for unfailingly courteous and helpful editorial guidance.

I am also indebted to Miss Ann Harris for outstanding secretarial help and to Miss Julie Barron and Mrs. Hilary Samson for printing the illustrations.

References

Adamo, N. J. and Daigneault, E. A. (1972) Desmosome-like junctions in the spiral ganglia of cats. *American Journal of Anatomy*, 135, 141–146.

Adamo, N. J. and Daigneault, E. A. (1973) Ultrastructural features of neurons and nerve fibres in the spiral ganglia of cats. *Journal of Neurocytology*, 2, 91–103.

Adams, W. E. (1942) The blood supply of nerves. I. Historical review. *Journal of Anatomy (London)*, 76, 323–341.

Allen, W. F. (1924) Localization in the ganglion semilunare of the cat. *Journal of Comparative Neurology*, 38, 1–25.

Alley, K. E. (1973) Quantitative analysis of the synaptogenic period in the trigeminal mesencephalic nucleus. *Anatomical Record*, 177, 49–60.

Allt, G. (1972) Involvement of the perineurium in experimental allergic neuritis: electron microscopic observations. *Acta neuropathologica (Berlin)*, **20**, 139–149.

Alvarado-Mallart, R. M., Batini, C., Buisseret, C., Gueritaud, J. P. and Horcholle-Bossavit, G. (1975) Mesencephalic projections of the rectus lateralis muscle afferents in the cat. *Archives Italiennes de Biologie*, **113**, 1–20.

Anderson, L. E. and McClure, W. O. (1973) Differential transport of protein in axons: comparison between the sciatic nerve and dorsal columns of cats. *Proceedings of the National Academy of Science, U.S.A.*, **70**, 1521–1525.

Andres, K. H. (1961) Untersuchungen über den Feinbau von Spinalganglien. *Zeitschrift für Zellforschung und mikroskopische Anatomie*, **55**, 1–48.

Andres, K. H. and Düring M. v. (1973) Morphology of cutaneous receptors. In *Handbook of Sensory Physiology* (ed.) Iggo, A., Vol. 11, Somatosensory System, Springer Verlag: Berlin-Heidelberg-New York

Arvidsson, B., Kristensson, K. and Olsson, Y. (1973) Vascular permeability to fluorescent protein tracer in trigeminal nerve and gasserian ganglion. *Acta neuropathologica (Berlin)*, **26**, 199–205.

Bacsich, P. and Wyburn, G. M. (1953) Formalin-sensitive cells in spinal ganglia. *Quarterly Journal of Microscopical Science*, **94**, 89–92.

Baker, R. and Llinás, R. (1971) Electrotonic coupling between neurons in the rat mesencephalic nucleus. *Journal of Physiology (London)*, **212**, 45–63.

Barasa, A, Maccotta, V. and Filogamo, G. (1970) Étude au microscope electronique des prolongement peripherique et central des cellules de ganglions spinaux d'embryons de poulet cultivés *in vitro*. *Bulletin de l'Association des Anatomistes*, 55° Congrès (Nancy), *115–122*.

Barnes, J. F. (1935) Cell to fiber ratios in the upper thoracic nerves of cat. *Anatomical Record*, **61**, Suppl. p. 3.

Barnes, J. F. and Davenport, H. A. (1937) Cells and fibers in spinal nerves. 3. Is a 1:1 ratio in the dorsal root the rule? *Journal of Comparative Neurology*, **66**, 419–469.

Barris, R. W. (1934) The frequency of atypical neurones in the spinal ganglia under normal conditions and after lesions of the roots, nerves or ganglia. *Journal of Comparative Neurology*, **59**, 325–339.

Bayliss, W. U. (1901) On the origin from the spinal cord of the vasodilator fibres of the hind-limb and on the nature of these fibres. *Journal of Physiology (London)*, **26**, 173–209.

Beaudreau, D. E. and Jerge, C. R. (1968) Somatotopic representation in the Gasserian ganglion of tactile peripheral fields in the cat. *Archives of Oral Biology*, **13**, 247–256.

Beaver, D. L., Moses, H. L. and Ganote, C. E. (1965) Electron microscopy of the trigeminal ganglion. II. Autopsy study of human ganglia. *Archives of Pathology*, **79**, 557–570.

Bennett, M. V. L. (1973) Function of electrotonic junctions in embryonic and adult tissues. *Federation Proceedings*, **32**, 65–75.

Berthold, C.-H. (1966) Ultrastructural appearance of glycogen in the B-neurons of the lumbar spinal ganglia of the frog. *Journal of Ultrastructure Research*, **14**, 254–267.

Bergmann, L. and Alexander, L. (1941) Vascular supply of the spinal ganglia. *Archives of Neurology and Psychiatry (Chicago)*, **46**, 761–782.

Blair, D. M., Bacsich, P. and Davies, F. (1936) The nerve cells in the spinal ganglia. *Journal of Anatomy, (London)*, **70**, 1–9.

Bodian, D. (1962) The generalized vertebrate neuron. *Science*, **137**, 323–326.

Bortolami, R., Callegari, E. and Lucchi, M. L. (1972) Anatomical relationship between mesencephalic trigeminal nucleus and cerebellum in the duck. *Brain Research*, **47**, 317–329.

Bortolami, R., Veggetti, A. and Ciampoli, A. (1969) Electron microscopic observations on the mesencephalic trigeminal nucleus (MTN) of duck. *Journal of Submicroscopic Cytology*, **1**, 235–245.

Brierley, J. B. (1955) The sensory ganglia: recent anatomical, physiological and pathological contributions. *Acta psychiatrica scandinavica*, **30**, 553–576.

Brodal, A. and Saugstad, L. F. (1965) Retrograde cellular changes in the mesencephalic trigeminal nucleus in the cat following cerebellar lesions. *Acta morphologica neerlando – scandinavica*, **6**, 147–159.

Brzin, M., Tennyson, V. M. and Duffy, P. E. (1966) Acetylcholinesterase in frog sympathetic and dorsal root ganglia: a study by electron microscope cytochemistry and microgasometric analysis with the magnetic diver. *Journal of Cell Biology*, 31, 215–242.

Bühler, A. (1898) Untersuchungen über den Bau der Nervenzellen. *Verhandlungen der Physikalisch-medizinischen Gesselschaft zu Würzburg*, 31, N.F. No. 8.

Bunge, M. B., Bunge, R. P., Peterson, E. P. and Murray, M. R. (1967) A light and electron microscope study of long term organized cultures of rat dorsal root ganglia. *Journal of Cell Biology*, 32, 439–466.

Burton, H. and McFarlane, J. J. (1973) The organization of the seventh lumbar spinal ganglion of the cat. *Journal of Comparative Neurology*, 149, 215–232.

Cajal, S. R. y (1907) Die Struktur des sensiblen Ganglien des Menschen und der Tiere *Ergebnisse der Anatomie und Entwicklungsgeschichte* 16, 177–215.

Cajal, S. R. y (1909) Histologie du système nerveux de l'homme et des vertébrés Vol. 1 French translation by Azouley, L. C.S.I.C. Madrid 1952.

Cajal, S. R. y (1928) *Degeneration and regeneration of the nervous system*. Vol. 1, ed. and translator May, R. M. Oxford University Press: London.

Cammermeyer, J. (1962) An evaluation of the significance of the 'dark' neuron. *Ergebnisse der Anatomie und Entwicklungsgeschichte*, 36, 1–61.

Carlsson, C.-A. and Thulin, C.-A. (1967) Regeneration of feline dorsal roots. *Experientia (Basel)*, 23, 125–126.

Cavanaugh, M. W. (1951) Quantitative effects of the peripheral innervation area on nerves and spinal ganglion cells. *Journal of Comparative Neurology*, 94, 181–219.

Chase, M. R. (1909) A histological study of sensory ganglia. *Anatomical Record*, 3, 121–140.

Chen, I-Li, and Yates, R. D. (1970) Ultrastructural studies of vagal paraganglia in Syrian hamsters. *Zeitschrift für Zellforschung und mikroskopische Anatomie*, 108, 309–323.

Citkowitz, E. and Holtzman, E. (1973) Peroxisomes in dorsal root ganglia. *Journal of Histochemistry and Cytochemistry*, 21, 34–41.

Clark, S. L. (1926). Nissl granules of primary afferent neurones. *Journal of Comparative Neurology*, 41, 423–451.

Clifton, G. L., Vance, W. H., Applebaum, R. E., Coggeshall, R. E. and Willis, W. D. (1974) Responses of unmyelinated afferents in the mammalian ventral root. *Brain Research*, 82, 163–167.

Coggeshall, R. E., Coulter, J. D. and Willis, W. D. (1974) Unmyelinated axons in the ventral roots of the cat lumbosacral enlargement. *Journal of Comparative Neurology*, 153, 39–58.

Coimbra, A., Sodré-Borges, B. P. and Magalhães, M. M. (1974) The substantia gelatinosa Rolandi of the rat. Fine structure, cytochemistry (acid phosphatase) and changes after dorsal root section. *Journal of Neurocytology*, 3, 199–217.

Cooper, P. D. and Smith, R. S. (1974) The movement of optically detectable organelles in myelinated axons of *Xenopus laevis*. *Journal of Physiology (London)*, 242, 77–97.

Corbin, K. B. and Harrison, F. (1940) Function of mesencephalic root of fifth cranial nerve. *Journal of Neurophysiology*, 3, 423–435.

Coupland, R. E. (1965) *The natural history of the chromaffin cell*. Longman Green and Co., Ltd.: London.

Cragg, B. G. (1970) What is the signal for chromatolysis? *Brain Research*, 23, 1–21.

Crain, S. M. (1956) Resting and action potentials of cultured chick embryo spinal ganglion cells. *Journal of Comparative Neurology*, 3, 423–435.

Crosby, E. C., Humphrey, T. and Lauer, E. W. (1962) *Correlative Anatomy of the Nervous System*, Macmillan: New York.

Cupédo, R. N. J. (1970) Indirect wallerian degeneration of afferents from the masticatory muscles. *Acta morphologica neerlando – scandinavica*, 8, 101–118.

Curtis, D. R. and Johnston, G. A. R. (1974) Amino acid transmitters in the mammalian central nervous system. *Ergebnisse der Physiologie*, 69, 97–188.

Dale, H. H. (1900) On some numerical comparisons of the centripetal and centrifugal medullated nerve fibres arising in the spinal ganglia of the mammal. *Journal of Physiology (London)*, 25, 196–206.

Dale Smith, R. (1969) Location of the neurons innervating tendon spindles of masticator muscles. *Experimental Neurology*, 25, 646–654.

Dale Smith, R. and Marcarian, H. Q. (1968) Centripetal localization of tooth and tongue tension receptors. *Journal of Dental Research*, 47, 616–621.

Darian-Smith, I. (1973) The trigeminal system. In *Handbook of Sensory Physiology Vol. II Somatosensory System*, (ed.) Iggo, A. pp. 271–314. Springer-Verlag: Berlin-Heidelberg-New York.

Dault, S. H. and Dale Smith, R. (1969) A quantitative study of the nucleus of the mesencephalic tract of the trigeminal nerve of the cat. *Anatomical Record*, 165, 79–88.

Davenport, H. A. and Ranson, S. W. (1931) Ratios of cells to fibers and of myelinated to unmyelinated fibers in spinal nerve roots. *American Journal of Anatomy*, 49, 193–207.

Dawson, I. M., Hossack, J. and Wyburn, G. M. (1955) Observations on the Nissl's substance, cytoplasmic filaments and the nuclear membrane of spinal ganglion cells. *Proceedings of the Royal Society of London, (Series B)*, 144, 132–142.

De Castro, F. (1932) Sensory ganglia of the cranial and spinal nerves. Normal and pathological. In: *Cytology and Cellular Pathology of the Nervous System.* (ed.) Penfield, W. Vol. 1 pp. 93–143. Hoeber: New York.

De Groat, W. C. (1972) GABA-depolarization of a sensory ganglion: antagonism by picrotoxin and bicuculline. *Brain Research*, 38, 429–432.

De Groat, W. C., Lalley, P. M. and Saum, W. R. (1972) Depolarization of dorsal root ganglia in the cat by GABA and related amino acids: antagonism by picrotoxin and bicuculline. *Brain Research*, 44, 273–277.

DeLorenzi, E. (1937) Bilateral inequality in the number of sensory neurons in the trunk of vertebrates. *Journal of Comparative Neurology*, 66, 301–306.

Dimsdale, J. A. and Kemp, J. M. (1966) Afferent fibres in the ventral nerve roots in the rat. *Journal of Physiology (London)*, 187, 25–26.

Dixon, A. D. (1963) Fine structure of nerve-cell bodies and satellite cells in the trigeminal ganglion. *Journal of Dental Research*, 42, 990–999.

Dogiel, A. S. (1896) Der Bau der Spinalganglien bei den Säugetieren. *Anatomischer Anzeiger*, 12, 140–152.

Dogiel, A. S. (1897) Zur Frage über den feineren Bau der Spinalganglien und deren Zellen bei Säugetieren. *Internationale Monatschrift für Anatomie und Physiologie*, 14, 73–116.

Dogiel, A. S. (1908) *Der Bau der Spinalganglien des Menschen und der Säugetiere.* Gustav Fisher: Jena.

Donaldson, H. H. and Nagasaka, G. (1918) On the increase in the diameters of nerve cell bodies and of the fibers arising from them during the later phases of growth (albino rat) *Journal of Comparative Neurology*, 29, 529–552.

Droz, B. (1965) Fate of newly synthesized proteins in neurons In: *The use of radioautography in investigating protein synthesis* (eds.) Leblond, C. P. and Warren K. B., pp. 159–175. Academic Press: New York and London.

Droz, B.(1967a) Synthèse et transfert des protéins cellulaires dans les neurones ganglionnaires. Etude radioautographique quantitative en microscopie électronique. *Journal de Microscopie*, 6, 201–228.

Droz, B. (1967b) L'appareil de Golgi comme site d'incorporation du Galactose-[3] H dans les neurons ganglionnaires spinaux chez le rat. *Journal de Microscopie*, 6, 419–424.

Duggan, A. W. and Johnston, G. A. R. (1970) Glutamate and related amino acids in cat spinal roots, dorsal root ganglia and peripheral nerves. *Journal of Neurochemistry*, 17, 1205–1208.

Dun, F. T. (1955) The delay and blockage of sensory impulses in the dorsal root ganglion. *Journal of Physiology (London)*, 127, 252–264.

Duncan, D. and Keyser, L. L. (1936) Some determinations of the ratio of nerve fibers to nerve cells in the thoracic dorsal roots and ganglia of the cat. *Journal of Comparative Neurology*, 64, 303–311.

Duncan, D. and Keyser, L. L. (1938) Further determinations of the numbers of fibers and cells in the dorsal roots and ganglia of the cat. *Journal of Comparative Neurology*, 68, 479–490.

Dupuy-Coin, A. M. and Bouteille, M. (1972) Developmental pathway of granular and beaded nuclear bodies from nucleoli. *Journal of Ultrastructure Research*, 40, 55–67.

Dupuy-Coin, A. M. and Bouteille, M. (1975) Protein renewal in nuclear bodies as studied by quantitative ultrastructural autoradiography. *Experimental Cell Research*, 90, 111–118.

Dutta, C. R., Siegesmund, K. A. and Fox, C. A. (1963) Light and electron microscopic observations of an intranucleolar body in nerve cells. *Journal of Ultrastructure Research,* 8, 452–551.

Egar, M. and Singer, M. (1971) A quantitative electron microscopic analysis of peripheral nerve in the urodele amphibian in relation to limb regenerative capacity. *Journal of Morphology,* 133, 387–398.

Fernandez, J. (1966) Etude histologique du ganglion de Gasser. Types de neurones et leur fréquence. *Acta neurovegetativa,* 29, 297–322.

Fink, B. R., Kish, S. J. and Byers, M. R. (1975) Rapid axonal transport in trigeminal nerve of rat. *Brain Research,* 90, 85–95.

Fisher, C. and Ranson, S. W. (1934) On the so-called sympathetic cells in the spinal ganglia. *Journal of Anatomy (London),* 68, 1–10.

Foley, J. O. and Dubois, F. S. (1937) Quantitative studies of the vagus nerve in the cat. I. The ratio of sensory to motor fibers. *Journal of Comparative Neurology,* 67, 49–68.

Friede, R. L. and Johnstone, M. A. (1967) Responses of thymidine labeling of nuclei in gray matter and nerve following sciatic transection. *Acta neuropathologica (Berlin),* 7, 218–231.

Friede, R. L. and Samorajski, T. (1968) Myelin formation in the sciatic nerve of the rat. *Journal of Neuropathology and Experimental Neurology,* 27, 546–570.

Furstman, L., Saporta, S. and Kruger, L. (1975) Retrograde axonal transport of horseradish peroxidase in sensory nerves and ganglion cells of the rat. *Brain Research,* 84, 320–324.

Gabbiani, G. (1966) Action of cadmium chloride on sensory ganglia. *Experientia (Basel),* 22, 261.

Gabbiani, G. and Majno, G. (1969) Endothelial microvilli in the vessels of the rat gasserian ganglion and testis. *Zeitschrift für Zellforschung und mikroskopische Anatomie,* 97, 111–117.

Gabbiani, G., Badonnel, M.-C., Mathewson, S. M. and Ryan, G. B. (1974) Acute cadmium intoxication: early selective lesions of endothelial clefts. *Laboratory Investigation,* 30, 686–695.

Gaik, G. C. (1973) A morphological analysis of the neurons in the developing and adult chicken trigeminal ganglion. *Anatomical Record,* 175, 326 (abstract).

Gamble, H. J. and Eames, R. A. (1966) Electron microscopy of human spinal-nerve roots. *Archives of Neurology,* 14, 50–53.

Gardner, E. (1940) Decrease in human neurons with age. *Anatomical Record,* 77, 529–536.

Gasser, H. S. (1950) Unmedullated fibers originating in dorsal root ganglia. *Journal of General Physiology,* 33, 651–690.

Gasser, H. S. (1955) Properties of dorsal root unmedullated fibers on the two sides of the ganglion. *Journal of General Physiology,* 38, 709–728.

Gerebtzoff, M. A. (1971) Analyse histochimique des structures nodales a la bifurcation axonale dans le ganglion spinal. *Comptes rendus des séances de la Société de Biologie,* 165, 198.

Giacobini, E. (1959) Quantitative determination of cholinesterase in individual spinal ganglion cells. *Acta physiologica scandinavica,* 45, 238–254.

Giacobini, G., Marchisio, P. C., Giacobini, E. and Koslow, S. H. (1970) Developmental changes of cholinesterases and monoamine oxidase in chick embryo spinal and sympathetic ganglia. *Journal of Neurochemistry,* 17, 1177–1185.

Glees, P. and Gopinath, G. (1973) Age changes in the centrally and peripherally located sensory neurons in rat. *Zeitschrift für Zellforschung und mikroskopische Anatomie,* 141, 285–298.

Gobel, S. (1974) Synaptic organization of the substantia gelatinosa glomeruli in the spinal trigeminal nucleus of the adult cat. *Journal of Neurocytology,* 3, 219–243.

Goormaghtigh, N. (1936) On the existence of abdominal vagal paraganglia in the adult mouse. *Journal of Anatomy (London),* 71, 77–90.

Grafstein, B. (1975) The nerve cell body's response to axotomy. *Experimental Neurology* (in press).

Gray, E. G. (1969) Electron microscopy of the glio-vascular organization of the brain of *Octopus. Philosophical Transactions of the Royal Society of London (Series B),* 255, 13–32.

267

Greenlee, T. K. Jr., Ross, R. and Hartman, J. L. (1966) The fine structure of elastic fibers. *Journal of Cell Biology,* **30,** 59–71.

Grillo, M. A. (1970) Cytoplasmic inclusions resembling nucleoli in sympathetic neurons of adult rats. *Journal of Cell Biology,* **45,** 100–117.

Grillo, M. A., Jacobs, L. and Comroe, J. H. Jr. (1974) A combined fluorescence histochemical and electron microscopic method for studying special monoamine-containing cells (SIF cells). *Journal of Comparative Neurology,* **153,** 1–14.

Guth, L. (1956) Regeneration in the mammalian peripheral nervous system. *Physiological Reviews,* **36,** 441–478.

Ha, H. (1969) Fine structure of spinal ganglia of the cat. *Anatomical Record,* **163,** 192–3 (abstract).

Ha, H. (1970) Axonal bifurcation in the dorsal root ganglion of the cat: a light and electron microscopic study. *Journal of Comparative Neurology,* **140,** 227–240.

Hall, S. M. (1972) The effects of injection of potassium cyanide into the sciatic nerve of the adult mouse: *in vivo* and electron microscopic studies. *Journal of Neurocytology,* **1,** 233–254.

Hamburger, V. (1961) Experimental analysis of the dual origin of the trigeminal ganglion in the chick embryo. *Journal of Experimental Zoology,* **147,** 91–123.

Hamburger, V. and Levi-Montalcini, R. (1949) Proliferation, differentiation and degeneration in the spinal ganglia of the chick embryo under normal and experimental conditions. *Journal of Experimental Zoology,* **111,** 457–501.

Hardin, J. H., Spicer, S. S. and Greene, W. B. (1969) The paranucleolar structure, accessory body of Cajal, sex chromatin, and related structures in nuclei of rat trigeminal neurons: a cytochemical and ultrastructural study. *Anatomical Record,* **164,** 403–432.

Hasan, M. and Glees, P. (1972) Electron microscopical appearance of neuronal lipofuscin using different preparative techniques including freeze-etching. *Experimental Gerontology,* **7,** 345–351.

Hashimoto, K. (1973) Fine structure of perifollicular nerve endings in human hair. *Journal of Investigative Dermatology,* **59,** 432–441.

Hatai, S. (1901) The finer structure of the spinal ganglion cells in the white rat. *Journal of Comparative Neurology,* **11,** 1–24.

Hatai, S. (1902) Number and size of the spinal ganglion cells and dorsal root fibers in the white rat at different ages. *Journal of Comparative Neurology,* **12,** 107–124.

Hatai, S. (1907) A study of the diameters of the cells and nuclei in the second cervical spinal ganglion of the adult albino rat. *Journal of Comparative Neurology,* **17,** 469–491.

Haust, M. D. (1965) Fine fibrils of extracellular space (microfibrils): their structure and role in connective tissue organization. *American Journal of Pathology,* **47** 1113–1137.

Hess, A. (1955) The fine structure of young and old spinal ganglia. *Anatomical Record,* **123,** 399–424.

Hild, W. (1957) Observations on neurons and neuroglia from the area of the mesencephalic fifth nucleus of the cat *in vitro. Zeitschrift für Zellforschung und mikroskopische Anatomie,* **47,** 127–146.

Hild, W. (1966) Cell types and neuronal connections in cultures of mammalian central nervous tissue. *Zeitschrift für Zellforschung und mikroskopische Anatomie,* **69,** 155–188.

Hinrichsen, C. F. L. and Larramendi, L. M. H. (1968) Synapses and cluster formation of the mouse mesencephalic fifth nucleus. *Brain Research,* **7,** 296–299.

Hinrichsen, C. F. L. and Larramendi, L. M. H. (1969) Features of trigeminal mesencephalic nucleus structure and organization. I. Light microscopy. *American Journal of Anatomy,* **126,** 497–506.

Hinrichsen, C. F. L. and Larramendi, L. M. H. (1970) The trigeminal mesencephalic nucleus. II. Electron microscopy. *American Journal of Anatomy,* **127,** 303–320.

Hirosawa, K. (1968) Electron microscopic studies on pigment granules in the substantia nigra and locus coeruleus of the Japanese monkey *(Macaca fuscata yakui). Zeitschrift für Zellforschung und mikroskopische Anatomie,* **88,** 187–203.

His, N. (1886) Zur Geschichte des menschlichen Rückenmarkes und der Nerven-wurzeln. *Abhandlungen der Sächsischen Akademie der Wissenschaften. (Leipzig),* **13,** 479–513.

Holmes, F. W. and Davenport, H. A. (1940) Cells and fibers in spinal nerves. IV. The number of neurites in dorsal and ventral roots of the cat. *Journal of Comparative Neurology*, 73, 1–5.

Holmgren, E. (1900) Weitere Mitteilungen über die "Saftkanälchen" der Nervenzellen. *Anatomischer Anzeiger*, 18, 290–296.

Holmgren, E. (1901) Beiträge zur Morphologie der Zelle. 1. Nervenzellen *Anatomischer Anzeiger*, 18, 267–325.

Holmgren, E. (1902) Einige Worte über das "Trophospongium" verschiedener Zellarten. *Anatomischer Anzeiger*, 20, 433–440.

Holmgren, E. (1904) *Über die Trophospongien der Nervenzellen.* Anatomischer Anzeiger, 24, 225–244.

Holtzman, E., Novikoff, A. B. and Villaverde, H. (1967) Lysosomes and GERL in normal and chromatolytic neurons of the rat ganglion nodosum. *Journal of Cell Biology*, 33, 419–436.

Holtzman, E., Teichberg, S., Abrahams, S. J., Citkowitz, E., Crain, S. M., Kawai, N., and Peterson, E. R. (1973) Notes on synaptic vesicles and related structures, endoplasmic reticulum, and peroxisomes in nervous tissue and the adrenal medulla. *Journal of Histochemistry and Cytochemistry*, 21, 349–385.

Hörstadius, S. (1950) *The Neural Crest.* Oxford University Press: London and New York.

Hossack, J. and Wyburn, G. M. (1954) Electron microscopic studies of spinal ganglion cells. *Proceedings of the Royal Society of London, Series B*, 65, 239–250.

Huber, G. C. (1896) The spinal ganglia of amphibia. *Anatomischer Anzeiger*, 12, 417–425.

Huber, G. C. and Guild, S. R. (1913) Observations on the histogenesis of protoplasmic processes and of collaterals, terminating in end bulbs, of the neurones of peripheral sensory ganglia. *Anatomical Record*, 7, 331–353.

Hughes, A. (1968) *Aspects of neural ontogeny.* Logos Press,

Hughes, A. (1973) The development of dorsal root ganglia and ventral horns in the opossum. A quantitative study. *Journal of Embryology and Experimental Morphology*, 30, 359–376.

Humbertson, A. Jr., Zimmerman, E. and Leedy, M. (1969) A chronological study of mitotic activity in satellite cell hyperplasia associated with chromatolytic neurons. *Zeitschrift für Zellforschung und mikroskopische Anatomie*, 100, 507–515.

Hydén, H. (1943) Protein metabolism in the nerve cell during growth and function. *Acta physiologica scandinavica*, Supplement 17, 1–136.

Hydén, H. (1960) The neuron. In *The Cell.* (eds.) Brachet, J. and Mirsky, A. E. Vol. IV. pp. 215–223. Academic Press: New York and London.

Imamoto, K. (1972a) Histochemical changes in the mesencephalic nucleus and motor nucleus following neurotomy of the third division of the trigeminal nerve. *Archivum histologicum japonicum*, 34, 19–33.

Imamoto, K. (1972b) Electron microscopic observations in the trigeminal mesencephalic nucleus following neurotomy of the third division of the trigeminal nerve. *Archivum histologicum japonicum*, 34, 361–374.

Imamoto, K. and Shimizu, N. (1970) Fine structure of the mesencephalic nucleus of the trigeminal nerve in the rat. *Archivum histologicum japonicum*, 32, 51–67.

Ishikawa, H. (1964) Peculiar intranuclear structures in sympathetic ganglion cells of a dog. *Zeitschrift für Zellforschung und mikroskopische Anatomie*, 62, 822–828.

Ito, M. (1959) An analysis of potentials recorded intracellularly from the spinal ganglion cell. *Japanese Journal of Physiology*, 9, 20–32.

Ito, M. and Saiga, M. (1959) The mode of impulse conduction through the spinal ganglion. *Japanese Journal of Physiology*, 9, 33–42.

Izard, J. and Bernhard, W. (1962) Analyse ultrastructurale de l'argentophilie du nucléole. *Journal de Microscopie*, 1, 421–434.

Jacob, M. and Weddell, G. (1975) Neural intersegmental connection in the spinal root and ganglion region of the rat. *Journal of Comparative Neurology*, 161, 115–124.

Jacobs, J. M., Carmichael, N. and Cavanagh, J. B. (1975a) Ultrastructural changes in the dorsal root and trigeminal ganglia of rats poisoned with methyl mercury. *Neuropathology and Applied Neurobiology*, 1, 1–19.

Jacobs, J. M., Cavanagh, J. B. and Carmichael, N. (1975b) The effect of chronic dosing with mercuric chloride on dorsal root and trigeminal ganglia of rats. *Neuropathology and Applied Neurobiology* (in press).

Jacobs, L. and Comroe, J. H. Jr. (1971) Reflex apnea, bradycardia and hypotension produced by serotonin and phenyldiguanide acting on the nodose ganglia of the cat. *Circulation Research,* **29**, 145–155.

Jacobson, M. (1970) *Developmental neurobiology.* Holt Rinehart and Winston, New York.

Jerge, C. R. (1963) Organization and function of the trigeminal mesencephalic nucleus. *Journal of Neurophysiology,* **26**, 379–392.

Johnson, J. L. (1972) Glutamic acid as a synaptic transmitter in the nervous system. A review. *Brain Research,* **37**, 1–19.

Johnson, J. L. and Aprison, M. H. (1970) The distribution of glutamic acid, a transmitter candidate, and other amino acids in the dorsal sensory neuron of the cat. *Brain Research,* **24**, 285–292.

Johnston, M. C. and Hazelton, R. D. (1972) Embryonic origins of facial structures related to oral sensory and motor functions. Chapter 4. In *Oral Sensation and Perception.* (ed.) Bosma, J. F. Charles C. Thomas: Springfield, Illinois.

Kalina, M. and Bubis, J. J. (1968) Histochemical studies on the distribution of acid phosphatases in neurones of sensory ganglia; light and electron microscopy. *Histochemie,* **14**, 103–112.

Kalina, M. and Bubis, J. J. (1969) Ultrastructural localization of acetylcholine esterase in neurones of rat trigeminal ganglia. *Experientia (Basel)* **25**, 388–389.

Kalina, M. and Wolman, M. (1970) Correlative histochemical and morphological study on the maturation of sensory ganglion cells in the rat. *Histochemie,* **22**, 100–108.

Karlsson, U. (1966) Three-dimensional studies of neurons in the lateral geniculate nucleus of the rat. I. Organelle organization in the perikaryon and its proximal branches. *Journal of Ultrastructure Research,* **16**, 429–481.

Karnovsky, M. J. (1968) The ultrastructural basis of transcapillary exchanges. *Journal of General Physiology,* **52**, 64s–95s.

Kato, M. and Hirata, Y. (1968) Sensory neurons in the spinal ventral roots of the cat. *Brain Research,* **7**, 479–482.

Kato, M. and Tanji, J. (1971) Physiological properties of sensory fibers in the spinal ventral roots in the cat. *Japanese Journal of Physiology,* **21**, 71–77.

Kerr, F. W. L. and Lysak, W. R. (1964) Somatotopic organization of trigeminal-ganglion neurones. *Archives of Neurology,* **11**, 593–602.

Key, A. and Retzius, G. (1876) Studien in der Anatomie des Nervensystems und des Bindegewebes, Part 2. Samson and Wallin: Stockholm.

Kirk, E. J. (1974) Impulses in dorsal spinal nerve rootlets in cats and rabbits arising from dorsal root ganglia isolated from the periphery. *Journal of Comparative Neurology,* **155**, 165–176.

Kishi, K. (1972) Fine structural and cytochemical observations on cytoplasmic nucleoluslike bodies in nerve cells of rat medulla oblongata. *Zeitschrift für Zellforschung und mikroskopische Anatomie,* **132**, 523–532.

Kiss, F. (1932) Sympathetic elements in the cranial and spinal ganglia. *Journal of Anatomy (London),* **66**, 488–498.

Knyihár, E. (1971) Fluoride-resistant acid phosphatase system of nociceptive dorsal root afferents. *Experientia (Basel),* **27**, 1205–1207.

Knyihár, E., László, I. and Tornyos, S. (1974) Fine structure and fluoride resistant acid phosphatase activity of electron dense sinusoid terminals in the substantia gelatinosa Rolandi of the rat after dorsal root transection. *Experimental Brain Research,* **19**, 529–544.

Kohno, K. and Nakayama, Y. (1973) Fine structure of the axon collaterals of Huber in frog spinal ganglia. *Journal of Neurocytology,* **2**, 383–391.

Kokko, A. (1965) Histochemical and cytophotometric observations on esterases in the spinal ganglion of the rat. *Acta physiologica scandinavica,* **66**, *Suppl.* 261.

Kölliker, A. von (1844) cited by Scharf (1958).

Krajči, D. (1972) Ultrastructure of the spinal ganglia in adult cat. I. Cytoplasm of perikarya. *Acta Universitatis Palackianae Olomucensis, Facultatis Medicae,* **61**, 45–64.

Kristensson, K. and Olsson, Y. (1973) Diffusion pathways and retrograde axonal transport of protein tracers in peripheral nerves. In: *Progress in Neurobiology* Vol 1, part 2 (eds.) Kerkut, G. A. and Phillis, J. W. Pergamon Press: Oxford and New York, pp. 85–109.

Kristensson, K. and Olsson, Y. (1975) Retrograde transport of horseradish peroxidase in transected axons. II. Relations between the rate of transfer from the injury to the perikaryon and the onset of chromatolysis. *Journal of Neurocytology,* 4, 653–661.

Kuré, K. G., Saégusa, G-I, Kawaguchi, K. and Shiraishi, K. (1930) On the parasympathetic (spinal parasympathetic) fibres in the dorsal roots, and their cells of origin in the spinal cord. *Quarterly Journal of Experimental Physiology,* 20, 51–66.

Laidlaw, G. F. (1930) Silver staining of the endoneurial fibers of the cerebrospinal nerves. *American Journal of Pathology,* 6, 435–444.

Lasek, R. J. (1968) Axoplasmic transport in cat dorsal root ganglion cells: as studied with [^{3}H]-L-leucine. *Brain Research* 7, 360–377.

Lasek, R. J. (1970a) Axonal transport of proteins in dorsal root ganglion cells of the growing cat: a comparison of growing and mature neurons. *Brain Research,* 20, 121–126.

Lasek, R. J. (1970b) Protein transport in neurons. *International Review of Neurobiology,* 23, 289–324.

Lawson, S. N., Caddy, K. W. T. and Biscoe, T. J. (1974) Development of rat dorsal root ganglion neurones. Studies of cell birthdays and changes in mean cell diameter. *Cell and Tissue Research,* 153, 399–413.

Le Beux, Y. J. (1972a) An ultrastructural study of a cytoplasmic filamentous body, termed nematosome, in the neurons of the rat and cat substantia nigra. *Zeitschrift für Zellforschung und mikroskopische Anatomie,* 133, 289–325.

Le Beux, Y. J. (1972b) Subsurface cisterns and lamellar bodies: particular forms of the endoplasmic reticulum in the neurons. *Zeitschrift für Zellforschung und mikroskopische Anatomie,* 133, 327–352.

Letbetter, W. D. and Willis, W. D. Jr. (1969) Electrophysiological characteristics of cat dorsal root ganglion cells. *The Physiologist,* 12, 283.

Levi, G. (1906) Studi sulla grandezza delle cellule. I. Ricerche comparative sulla grandezza delle cellule dei mammiferi. *Archivio italiano di Anatomia e di Embriologia,* 5, 291–358.

Levi, G. (1908) I ganglî cerebrospinali. Studi di Istologia comparata e di Istogenesi. *Archivio italiano di Anatomia e di Embriologia* 7, (Supplement), 1–392.

Lieberman, A. R. (1968a) The connective tissue elements of the mammalian nodose ganglion. *Zeitschrift für Zellforschung und mikroskopische Anatomie,* 89, 95–111.

Lieberman, A. R. (1968b) An investigation by light and electron microscopy of chromatolytic and other phenomena induced in mammalian nerve cells by experimental lesions. *Ph.D. Thesis,* University of London.

Lieberman, A. R. (1969a) Absence of ultrastructural changes in ganglionic neurons after supranodose vagotomy. *Journal of Anatomy (London),* 104, 49–54.

Lieberman, A. R. (1969b) Light- and electron-microscope observations on the Golgi apparatus of normal and axotomized primary sensory neurons. *Journal of Anatomy (London),* 104, 309–325.

Lieberman, A. R. (1971) The axon reaction. A review of the principal features of perikaryal responses to axon injury. *International Review of Neurobiology,* 14, 49–124.

Lieberman, A. R. (1974) Some factors affecting retrograde neuronal responses to axonal lesions. In *Essays on the Nervous System,* eds. Bellairs, R. and Gray, E. G. pp. 71–105. Clarendon Press: Oxford.

Lodin, Z., Faltin, J., Booher, J., Hartman, J. and Sensenbrenner, M. (1973) Formation of intercellular contacts in cultures of dissociated neurons from embryonic chicken dorsal root ganglia. *Neurobiology,* 3, 376–390.

Luduena, M. A. (1973) Nerve cell differentiation *in vitro. Developmental Biology,* 33, 268–284.

Luiten, P. G. M. (1975) The horseradish peroxidase technique applied to the teleostean nervous system. *Brain Research,* 89, 181–186.

Lukáš, Z., Čech, S. and Buriánek, P. (1970) Cholinesterase and biogenic monoamines in ganglion semilunare (Gasseri). *Histochemie,* 22, 163–168.

McKinniss, M. E. (1936) The number of ganglion cells in the dorsal root ganglia of the second and third cervical nerves in human fetuses of various ages. *Anatomical Record,* 65, 255–259.

Marinesco, G. (1909) *La cellule nerveuse.* Doin et fils: Paris.

Marinozzi, V. (1964) Cytochimie ultrastructurale du nucléole – RNA et protéines intra-nucléolaires. *Journal of Ultrastructure Research,* 10, 433–456.

Masurovsky, E. B., Benitez, H. H., Kim, S. U. and Murray, M R. (1970) Origin, development and nature of intranuclear rodlets and associated bodies in chicken sympathetic neurons. *Journal of Cell Biology*, 44, 172–191.

Mathews, B. M. C. (1934) Impulses leaving the spinal cord by dorsal nerve roots. *Journal of Physiology (London)*, 81, 29–31P.

Matsuura, H. (1967) Histochemical observation of bovine spinal ganglia. *Histochemie*, 11, 152–160.

Mazza, J. P. and Dixon, A. D. (1972) A histological study of chromatolytic cell groups in the trigeminal ganglion of the rat. *Archives of Oral Biology*, 17, 377–387.

Mei, N. (1964) Mise en évidence d'une somatotopie au niveau du ganglion plexiforme du chat. *Comptes rendus des séances de la Societé de Biologie*, 158, 2363–2367.

Mei, N. (1970) Disposition anatomique et propriétés électrophysiologiques des neurones sensitifs vagaux chez le chat. *Experimental Brain Research*, 11, 465–479.

Mei, N., Boyer, A. and Condamin, M. (1971) Etude comparée des deux prolongements de la cellule sensitive vagale. *Comptes rendus des séances de la Société de Biologie*, 165, 2371–2374.

Mellick, R. and Cavanagh, J. B. (1967) Longitudinal movement of radioiodinated albumin within extravascular spaces of peripheral nerves following three systems of experimental trauma. *Journal of Neurology, Neurosurgery and Psychiatry*, 30, 458–463.

Miller, R., Varon, S., Kruger, L., Coates, P. W. and Orkand, P. M. (1970) Formation of synaptic contacts on dissociated chick embryo sensory ganglion cells *in vitro*. *Brain Research*, 24, 356–358.

Milokhin, A. A. and Reshetnikov, S. S. (1972) Morphology of receptor innervation of spinal ganglia. *Neuroscience and Behavioural Physiology*, 5, 59–69 (translated from *Arkhiv Anatomii, Gistologii i Embriologii*, 60, 93–103 1971).

Mitolo, V., Selvaggi, F. and Selvaggi, L. (1965) Influences of the extent of the peripheral field of innervation on the volume of spinal ganglia and on the number of their nerve cells in chick embryos. *Acta Embryologiae et Morphologiae Experimentalis*, 8, 150–169.

Molhant, M. (1913) Le nerf vague. Etude anatomique et expérimentale. III. Les ganglions périphériques du vague. *Névraxe*, 15, 521–579.

Moses, H. L., Beaver, D. L. and Ganote, C. E. (1965) Electron microscopy of the trigeminal ganglion. I. Comparative ultrastructure. *Archives of Pathology*, 79, 541–556.

Moses, H. L., Ganote, C. E., Beaver, D. L. and Schuffman, S. S. (1966) Light and electron microscopic studies of pigment in human and rhesus monkey substantia nigra and locus coeruleus. *Anatomical Record*, 155, 167–184.

Moyer, E. K., Kimmel, D. L. and Winborne, L. W. (1953) Regeneration of sensory spinal nerve roots in young and senile rats. *Journal of Comparative Neurology*, 98, 283–300.

Muratori, G. (1932) Contributo all'innervazione del tessuto paragangliare annesso al sistema del vago (glomo carotico, paragangli estravagali ed intravagali) e all'innervazione del seno carotideo. *Anatomischer Anzeiger*, 75, 115–123.

Nageotte, J. (1906) Régéneration collatérale de fibres nerveuses terminées par des massues de croissance, à l'état pathologique et à l'état normal; lésions tabétiques des racines médullaires. *Nouvelle Iconographie de la Salpêtrière*, 19, 217–238.

Nageotte, J. (1907) Recherches expérimentales sur la morphologie des cellules et des fibres des ganglions rachidiens. *Revue Neurologique*, 15, 357–368.

Nathaniel, E. J. H. and Nathaniel, D. R. (1973) Electron microscopic studies of spinal ganglion cells following crushing of dorsal roots in adult rat. *Journal of Ultrastructure Research*, 45, 168–182.

Nishimura, T., Kon, I., Awataguchi, S., Ishida, M. and Yamamoto, N. (1965) Submicroscopic studies on the spiral ganglion in guinea pigs. *Hirosaki Medical Journal*, 17, 1–19.

Norton, A. C. (1973) The dorsal column system of the spinal cord: its anatomy, physiology, phylogeny, and sensory function. *Brain Information Service Updated Review*, (1973 update by Kruger, L.).

Novikoff, A. B. (1967a) Enzyme localization and ultrastructure of neurons. In *The Neuron*, ed. Hydén, H. Chapter 6. Elsevier Publishing Company: Amsterdam, London and New York, pp. 255–318.

Novikoff, A. B. (1967b) Lysosomes in nerve cells. In *The Neuron*, ed. Hydén, H. Chapter 7. Elsevier Publishing Company: Amsterdam, London and New York, pp. 319–377.

Novikoff, P. M., Novikoff, A. B., Quintana, N. and Hauw, J-J. (1971) Golgi apparatus,

GERL, and lysosomes of neurons in rat dorsal root ganglia studied by thick section and thin section cytochemistry. *Journal of Cell Biology*, 50, 859–886.

Nunnemacher, R. F. and Sutherland, R. M. (1969) Fibers in the rat's eighth thoracic nerve. *American Zoologist*, 9, 1150.

Ochs, S. (1972) Fast transport of materials in mammalian nerve fibers. *Science*, 176, 252–260.

Ohnishi, A. and Dyck, P. J. (1974) Loss of small peripheral sensory neurons in Fabry disease. *Archives of Neurology*, 31, 120–127.

Ohta, M., Offord, K. and Dyck, P. J. (1974) Morphometric evaluation of first sacral ganglia of man. *Journal of the Neurological Sciences*, 22, 73–82.

Okun, L. M. (1972) Isolated dorsal root ganglion neurons in culture: cytological maturation and extension of electrically active processes. *Journal of Neurobiology*, 3, 111–151.

Olsson, Y. (1968a) Topographical differences in the vascular permeability of the peripheral nervous system. *Acta neuropathologica (Berlin)*, 10, 26–33.

Olsson, Y. (1968b) Mast cells in the nervous system. *International Review of Cytology*, 24, 27–70.

Olsson, Y. (1971) Studies on vascular permeability in peripheral nerves: IV. Distribution of intravenously injected protein tracers in the peripheral nervous system of various species. *Acta neuropathologica (Berlin)*, 17, 114–126.

Olsson, Y. (1972) The involvement of vasa nervorum in diseases of peripheral nerves. In: *Handbook of Clinical Neurology* Vol. 12 (eds.). Vinken P. J. and Bruyn, G. W. North-Holland, Amsterdam, pp. 644–664.

Olsson, Y., Kristensson, K. and Klatzo, I. (1971) Permeability of blood vessels and connective tissue sheaths in the peripheral nervous system to exogenous proteins. *Acta neuropathologica (Berlin)*, Suppl. V, 61–69.

Olsson Y. and Reese. T. S. (1971) Permeability of vasa nervorum and perineurium in mouse sciatic nerve studied by fluorescence and electron microscopy. *Journal of Neuropathology and Experimental Neurology*, 30, 105–119.

Orr, D. and Rows, R. G. (1901) The nerve-cells of the human posterior root ganglia and their changes in general paralysis of the insane. *Brain*, 24, 286–309.

Ortiz-Picón, J. M. (1955) The neuroglia of the sensory ganglia. *Anatomical Record*, 121, 513–529.

Owman, C. and Santini, M. (1966) Adrenergic nerves in spinal ganglia of the cat. *Acta physiologica scandinavica*, 68, 127–128.

Palay, S. L. and Palade, G. E. (1955) The fine structure of neurons. *Journal of Biophysical and Biochemical Cytology*, 1, 69–88.

Pannese, E. (1960) Observations on the morphology, submicroscopic structure and biological properties of satellite cells (S.C.) in sensory ganglia of mammals. *Zeitschrift für Zellforschung und mikroskopische Anatomie*, 52, 567–597.

Pannese, E. (1963) Investigations on the ultrastructural changes of the spinal ganglion neurons in the course of axon regeneration and cell hypertrophy. II. Changes during cell hypertrophy and comparison between the ultrastructure of nerve cells of the same type under different functional conditions. *Zeitschrift für Zellforschung und mikroskopische Anatomie*, 61, 561–586.

Pannese, E. (1964) Number and structure of perisomatic satellite cells of spinal ganglia under normal conditions or during axon regeneration and neuronal hypertrophy. *Zeitschrift für Zellforschung und mikroskopische Anatomie*, 63, 568–592.

Pannese, E. (1968) Developmental changes of the endoplasmic reticulum and ribosomes in nerve cells of the spinal ganglia of the domestic fowl. *Journal of Comparative Neurology*, 132, 331–364.

Pannese, E. (1969a) Electron microscopical study on the development of the satellite cell sheath in spinal ganglia. *Journal of Comparative Neurology*, 135, 381–422.

Pannese, E. (1969b) Unusual membrane-particle complexes within nerve cells of the spinal ganglia. *Journal of Ultrastructural Research*, 29, 334–342.

Pannese, E. (1974) The histogenesis of the spinal ganglia. *Advances in Anatomy and Cell Biology*, 47, part 5, 1–97.

Pannese, E., Bianchi, R., Calligaris, B., Ventura, R. and Weibel, E. R. (1972) Quantitative relationships between nerve and satellite cells in spinal ganglia. An electron microscopical study. 1. Mammals. *Brain Research*, 46, 215–234.

Pannese, E., Ventura, R. and Bianchi, R. (1975) Quantitative relationships between nerve and satellite cells in spinal ganglia: an electron microscopical study. II. Reptiles. *Journal of Comparative Neurology*, **160**, 463–476.

Peach, R. (1972a) Fine structural features of light and dark cells in the trigeminal ganglion of the rat. *Journal of Neurocytology*, **1**, 151–160.

Peach, R. (1972b) Acid phosphatase distribution in the trigeminal ganglion of the rat. *Anatomical Record*, **174**, 239–250.

Peach, R. (1972c) Nematosomes in the rat trigeminal ganglion. *Journal of Cell Biology*, **55**, 718–721.

Peach, R. (1973) Cellular differentiation in the mouse trigeminal ganglion. *Anatomical Record*, **175**, 408–409 (abstract).

Peach, R. (1975) Tubules and filaments in satellite cells and axons of sensory neurons. *American Journal of Anatomy*, **142**, 385–390.

Peach, R. and Koch, W. E. (1974) A cytoplasmic inclusion in mouse trigeminal neurons. *American Journal of Anatomy*, **140**, 439–444.

Peachey, L. (1964) Electron microscopic observations on the accumulation of divalent cations in intramitochondrial granules. *Journal of Cell Biology*, **20**, 95–111.

Peacock, J. A., Nelson, P. G. and Goldstone, M. W. (1973) Electrophysiologic study of cultured neurons dissociated from spinal cords and dorsal root ganglia of fetal mice. *Developmental Biology*, **30**, 137–152.

Penfield, W. G. (1920) Alterations of the Golgi apparatus in nerve cells. *Brain*, **43**, 290–305.

Perkins, R. E. (1973) Innervation patterns in cochleas of cat and rat: study with rapid Golgi techniques. *Anatomical Record*, **175**, 410 (abstract).

Peters, A., Palay, S. L. and Webster, H. deF. (1970) *The fine structure of the nervous system: The cells and their processes.* Harper and Row: New York and London.

Pick, J., Gerdin, C. and De Lemos, C. (1963) On the ultrastructure of spinal nerve roots in the frog *(Rana pipiens). Anatomical Record*, **146**, 61–84.

Pineda, A, Maxwell, D. S. and Kruger, L. (1967) The fine structure of neurons and satellite cells in the trigeminal ganglion of cat and monkey. *American Journal of Anatomy*, **121**, 461–488.

Popoff, N. and Stewart, S. (1968) The fine structure of nuclear inclusions in the brain of experimental golden hamsters. *Journal of Ultrastructure Research*, **23**, 347–361.

Prestige, M. C. (1970) Differentiation, degeneration and the role of the periphery: quantitative considerations. In: *The Neurosciences: Second Study Program* (ed.) Schmitt, F. O. p. 73–82. Rockefeller University Press: New York, N.Y.

Prior, D. J. and Fuller, P. M. (1973) The use of a cobalt iontophoresis technique for identification of the mesencephalic trigeminal nucleus. *Brain Research*, **64**, 472–475.

Rambourg, A., Clermont, Y. and Marraud, A. (1974) Three-dimensional structure of the osmium-impregnated Golgi apparatus as seen in the high voltage electron microscope. *American Journal of Anatomy*, **140**, 27–46.

Rambourg, A., Marraud, A. and Chrétien, M. (1973) Tri-dimensional structure of the forming face of the Golgi apparatus as seen in the high voltage electron microscope after osmium impregnation of the small nerve cells in the semilunar ganglion of the trigeminal nerve. *Journal of Microscopy*, **97**, 49–57.

Ranson, S. W. (1906) Some new facts touching upon the architecture of the spinal ganglion in Mammals. *American Journal of Anatomy*, **5**, Suppl. 13.

Ranson, S. W. (1908) The architectural relations of the afferent elements entering into the formation of the spinal nerves. *Journal of Comparative Neurology*, **18**, 101–119.

Ranson, S. W. (1912) The structure of the spinal ganglia and of the spinal nerves. *Journal of Comparative Neurology*, **22**, 159–175.

Ranson, S. W. and Davenport, H. K. (1931) Sensory unmyelinated fibres in the spinal nerves. *American Journal of Anatomy*, **48**, 331–353.

Ranson S. W., Foley J. O. and Alpert, C. D. (1933) Observations on the structure of the vagus nerve. *American Journal of Anatomy*, **53**, 289–315.

Ranvier, L. (1875) Des tubes nerveux en T et de leurs relations avec les cellules ganglionaires – *Comptes rendus de l'Academie des sciences (Paris)*, **81**, 1274–1276.

Ranvier, L. (1878) *Leçons sur l'histologie du système nerveux.* F. Savy: Paris.

Reale, E., Luciano, L. and Spitznas, M. (1975) Freeze-fracture faces of the perineurial sheath of the rabbit sciatic nerve. *Journal of Neurocytology*, **4**, 261–270.

Retzius, G. (1880) Untersuchungen über die Nervenzellen der cerebrospinalen Ganglien und der übrigen peripherischen Kopfganglien mit besonderer Berücksichtgung auf die Zellnausläufer. *Archiv für Anatomie und Entwichlungsgeschichte*, 369–402. 402.

Rexed, B. and Sourander, P. (1949) The caliber of central and peripheral neurites of spinal ganglion cells and variations in fiber size at different levels of dorsal spinal roots. *Journal of Comparative Neurology*, **91**, 297–306.

Robain, O. and Jardin, L. (1972) Histoenzymologie du ganglion spinal du lapin. *Journal of the neurological Sciences*, **17**, 419–433.

Rosenbluth, J. (1962a) The fine structure of acoustic ganglia in the rat. *Journal of Cell Biology*, **12**, 329–359.

Rosenbluth, J. (1962b) Subsurface cisterns and their relationship to the neuronal plasma membrane. *Journal of Cell Biology*, **13**, 405–421.

Rosenbluth, J. (1963) Contrast between osmium-fixed and permanganate-fixed toad spinal ganglia. *Journal of Cell Biology*, **16**, 143–157.

Rosenbluth, J. and Palay, S. L. (1961) The fine structure of nerve cell bodies and their myelin sheaths in the eighth nerve ganglion of the goldfish. *Journal of Biophysical and Biochemical Cytology*, **9**, 853–877.

Rosenbluth, J. and Wissig, S. L. (1964) The distribution of exogenous ferritin in toad spinal ganglia and the mechanism of its uptake by neurons. *Journal of Cell Biology*, **23**, 307–325.

Samorajski, T., Ordy, J. M. and Keefe, J. R. (1965) The fine structure of lipofuscin age pigment in the nervous system of aged mice. *Journal of Cell Biology*, **26**, 779–795.

Samorajski, T., Ordy, J. M. and Rady-Reimer, P. (1968) Lipofuscin pigment accumulation in the nervous system of ageing mice. *Anatomical Record*, **160**, 555–574.

Santini, M. (1966) Adrenergic fibres in the feline Gasserian ganglia. *Life Sciences*, **5**, 283–287.

Sarrat, R. (1970) Zur Chemodifferenzierung des Rückenmarks und der Spinalganglien der Ratte. *Histochemie*, **24**, 202–213.

Sato, M. and Austin, G. (1961) Intracellular potentials of mammalian dorsal root ganglion cells. *Journal of Neurophysiology*, **24**, 569–582.

Scharf, J.-H. (1958) Sensible ganglien. *Handbuch der mikroskopischen Anatomie des Menschen*, Bd. IV/3. Nervensystem III, Springer: Berlin-Göttingen-Heidelberg.

Scharf, J.-H. and Blumenthal, H.-J. (1967) Neuere Aspekte zur Altersabhängigen Involution des sensiblen peripheren Nervensystems. *Zeitschrift für Zellforschung und mikroskopischen Anatomie*, **78**, 280–302.

Schlaepfer, W. W. (1971) Sequential study of endothelial changes in acute cadmium intoxication. *Laboratory Investigation*, **25**, 556–564.

Schon, F. and Kelly, J. S. (1974) Autoradiographic localisation of [³H]GABA and [³H]Glutamate over satellite glial cells. *Brain Research*, **66**, 275–288.

Scott, B. S., Engelbert, V. E. and Fisher, K. C. (1969) Morphological and electrophysiological characteristics of dissociated chick embryonic spinal ganglion cells in culture. *Experimental Neurology*, **23**, 230–248.

Sekhon, S. S. and Maxwell, D. S. (1974) Ultrastructural changes in neurons of the spinal anterior horn of ageing mice with particular reference to the accumulation of lipofuscin pigment. *Journal of Neurocytology*, **3**, 59–72.

Shanthaveerappa, T. R. and Bourne, G. H. (1965) The thiamine pyrophosphatase technique as an indicator of the morphology of the Golgi apparatus in the neurons. *Acta histochemica*, **22**, 155–178.

Shimizu, Y. (1965a) Note on myelin formation around the stato-acoustic ganglion cells cultivated *in vitro*. *Acta anatomica nipponica* **40**, 133–139.

Shimizu, Y. (1965b) The satellite cells in cultures of dissociated spinal ganglia. *Zeitschrift für Zellforschung und mikroskopische Anatomie*, **67**, 185–195.

Simionescu, N., Simionescu, M. and Palade, G. E. (1973) Permeability of muscle capillaries to exogenous myoglobin. *Journal of Cell Biology*, **57**, 424–452.

Simionescu, N., Simionescu, M. and Palade, G. E. (1975) Permeability of muscle capillaries to small heme-peptides. Evidence for the existence of patent transendothelial channels. *Journal of Cell Biology*, **64**, 586–607.

Skoglund, S. (1967) On the possible postnatal formation of new nerve fibres in the dorsal roots from new nerve cells in the ganglia. *Acta Societatis medicorum upsaliensis,* **72**, 25–29.

Smith, M. L. Jr., and Adrian, E. K. Jr. (1972) On the presence of mononuclear leucocytes in dorsal root ganglia following transection of the sciatic nerve. *Anatomical Record,* **172**, 581–588.

Smith, R. S. (1972) Detection of organelles in myelinated nerve fibers by dark-field microscopy. *Canadian Journal of Physiology and Pharmacology,* **50**, 467–469.

Smith, R. S. (1973) Microtubule and neurofilament densities in amphibian spinal root nerve fibres: relationship to axoplasmic transport. *Canadian Journal of Physiology and Pharmacology,* **51**, 798–806.

Sobkowicz, H. M. Hartmann, H. A., Monzain, R. and Desnoyers, R. (1973) Growth, differentiation and ribonucleic acid content of the fetal rat spinal ganglion cells in culture. *Journal of Comparative Neurology,* **148**, 249–283.

Sosa, J. M. and De Zorilla, B. (1966) Spinal ganglion cytological response to axon and to dendrite sectioning. *Acta anatomica,* **65**, 236–255.

Sotelo, C. and Palay, S. L. (1968) The fine structure of the lateral vestibular nucleus in the rat. I. Neurons and Neuroglial cells, *Journal of Cell Biology,* **36**, 151–179.

Spencer, P. S., Raine, C. S. and Wisniewski, H. (1973) Axon diameter and myelin thickness – unusual relationships in dorsal root ganglia. *Anatomical Record,* **176**, 225–244.

Spencer, P. S. and Schaumburg, H. H. (1973) An ultrastructural study of the inner core of the Pacinian corpuscle. *Journal of Neurocytology,* **2**, 217–235.

Stacey, M. J. (1969) Free nerve endings in skeletal muscle of the cat. *Journal of Anatomy (London),* **105**, 231–254.

Steer, J. M. (1971) Some observations on the fine structure of rat dorsal spinal nerve roots. *Journal of Anatomy (London),* **109**, 467–485.

Steinach, E. (1899) Über die centripetale Erregungsleitung im Bereiche des Spinalganglions. *Pflügers Archiv,* **78**, 291–314.

Stoeckel, K., Schwab, M. and Thoenen, H. (1975) Specificity of retrograde transport of nerve growth factor (NGF) in sensory neurons: a biochemical and morphological study. *Brain Research,* **89**, 1–14.

Sutherland, R. M. and Nunnemacher, R. F. (1974) Fibers in the ventral spinal nerves of the frog. *Journal of Comparative Neurology,* **156**, 39–48.

Svaetichin, G. (1951) Electrophysiological investigations on single ganglion cells. *Acta physiologica scandinavica,* **24**, Suppl. 86.

Szabó, Z and Bölönyi, F. (1955) Blood supply of the ganglia. *Acta morphologica Academiae scientiarum hungaricae,* **5**, 165–170.

Tagini, G. and Camino, E. (1973) T-shaped cells of dorsal ganglia can influence the pattern of afferent discharge. *Pflügers Archiv,* **344**, 339–347.

Takahashi, T. and Otsuka, M. (1975) Regional distribution of substance P in the spinal cord and nerve roots of the cat and the effect of dorsal root section. *Brain Research,* **87**, 1–11.

Tennyson, V. M. (1965) Electron microscopic study of the developing neuroblast of the dorsal root ganglion of the rabbit embryo. *Journal of Comparative Neurology,* **124**, 267–318.

Tennyson, V. M. (1970) The fine structure of the axon and growth cone of the dorsal root neuroblast of the rabbit embryo. *Journal of Cell Biology,* **44**, 62–79.

Tennyson, V. M. and Brzin, M. (1970) The appearance of acetylcholinesterase in the dorsal root neuroblast of the rabbit embryo. *Journal of Cell Biology,* **46**, 64–80.

Tewari, H. B. and Bourne, G. H. (1962) Histochemical evidence of metabolic cycles in spinal ganglion cells of rat. *Journal of Histochemistry and Cytochemistry,* **10**, 42–64.

Thomas, P. K. (1974) Peripheral nerve injury. In *Essays on the Nervous system,* (eds.) Bellairs, R. and Gray, E. G. pp. 44–70. Clarendon Press: Oxford.

Truex, R. C. (1939) Observations on the chicken Gasserian ganglion with special reference to the bipolar neurons. *Journal of Comparative Neurology,* **71**, 473–486.

Uemura, E., Fletcher, T. F., Dirks V. A. and Bradley, W. E. (1973) Distribution of sacral afferent axons in cat urinary bladder. *American Journal of Anatomy,* **136**, 305–314.

Uemura, E., Fletcher, T. F., and Bradley, W. E. (1974) Distribution of lumbar afferent axons in muscle coat of cat urinary bladder. *American Journal of Anatomy,* **139,** 389–398.

Van Gehuchten, A. (1892a) Contribution à l'étude de ganglions cerebrospinaux. *La Cellule,* **8,** 209–231.

Van Gehuchten, A. (1892b) Nouvelles recherches sur les ganglions cerebrospinaux. *La Cellule,* **8,** 233–254.

Van Gehuchten, A. (1897) L'anatomie fine de la cellule nerveuse. *Neurologisches Zentralblatt,* **16,** 905–911.

Varon, S. and Raiborn, C. (1971) Excitability and conduction in neurons of dissociated ganglionic cell cultures. *Brain Research,* **30,** 83–98.

Viraswami, V. (1965) The effect of vascular occlusion on the chromatolytic cycle in the spinal ganglia of the rabbit. *Acta anatomica,* **62,** 528–538.

Waksman, B. H. (1961) Experimental study of diphtheritic polyneuritis in the rabbit and guinea-pig. III. The blood-nerve barrier in the rabbit. *Journal of Neuropathology and Experimental Neurology,* **20,** 35–77.

Wall, P. D. (1973) Dorsal horn electrophysiology. In *Handbook of Sensory Physiology Volume II Somatosensory Systems,* (ed) Iggo, A. Springer-Verlag: Berlin-Heidelberg New York. pp. 253–270.

Warwick, R. and Williams, P. L. (1973) Gray's Anatomy 35th Edition, Longman: London.

Watson, W. E. (1965) An autoradiographic study of the incorporation of nucleic acid precursors by neurons and glia during nerve regeneration. *Journal of Physiology, (London),* **180,** 741–753.

Watson, W. E. (1968) Observations of the nucleolar and total cell body nucleic acid of injured nerve cells. *Journal of Physiology (London),* **196,** 655–676.

Watson, W. E. (1973) Some responses of neurones of dorsal root ganglia to axotomy. *Journal of Physiology (London),* **231,** 41–42P.

Watson, W. E. (1974a) The binding of actinomycin D to the nuclei of axotomised neurones. *Brain Research,* **65,** 317–322.

Watson, W. E. (1974b) Cellular responses to axotomy and to related procedures. *British Medical Bulletin,* **30,** 112–115.

Webber, R. H. and Wemett, A. (1966) Distribution of fibers from nerve cell bodies in ventral roots of spinal nerves. *Acta anatomica,* **65,** 579–583.

Weis, P. (1968) Confronting subsurface cisternae in chick embryo spinal ganglia. *Journal of Cell Biology,* **39,** 485–488.

Weiss, P., Wang, H., Taylor, A. C., Edds, Mac V., Jr. (1945) Proximodistal connection in the endoneurial spaces of peripheral nerves demonstrated by colored and radioactive (isotope) tracers. *American Journal of Physiology,* **143,** 521–540.

Weston, J. A. (1970) The migration and differentiation of neural crest cells. *Advances in Morphogenesis,* **8,** 41–114.

Williams, P. L. and Hall, S. M. (1971) Chronic Wallerian degeneration – an *in vivo* and ultrastructural study. *Journal of Anatomy (London),* **109,** 487–503.

Windle, W. F. (1931) Neurons of the sensory type in the ventral roots of man and of other mammals. *Archives of Neurology and Psychiatry (Chicago),* **26,** 791–800.

Wyburn, G. M. (1958) The capsule of spinal ganglion cells. *Journal of Anatomy (London),* **92,** 528–533.

Yamadori, T. (1970) A light and electron microscopic study on the postnatal development of spinal ganglia in rats. *Acta anatomica nipponica,* **45,** 191–205.

Yntema, C. L. (1937) An experimental study of the origin of the cells which constitute the VIIth and VIIIth cranial ganglia and nerves in the embryo of *Amblystoma punctatum. Journal of Experimental Zoology,* **75,** 75–101.

Young, R. F. and King, R. B. (1973) Fiber spectrum of the trigeminal sensory root of the baboon determined by electron microscopy. *Journal of Neurosurgery,* **38,** 65–72.

Young, J. Z. (1942). The functional repair of nervous tissue. *Physiological Reviews,* **22,** 318–374.

Zelená, J. (1970) Ribosome-like particles in myelinated axons of the rat. *Brain Research,* **24,** 359–363.

Zelená, J. (1971) Neurofilaments and microtubules in sensory neurons after peripheral nerve section. *Zeitschrift für Zellforschung und Mikroskopische Anatomie,* **117,** 191–211.

Zelená, J. (1972) Ribosomes in myelinated axons of dorsal root ganglia. *Zeitschrift für Zellforschung und mikroskopische Anatomie,* **124**, 217–229.

Zenker, W., Mayr, R. and Gruber, H. (1973) Axoplasmic organelles: quantitative differences between ventral and dorsal root fibres of the rat. *Experientia (Basel),* **29**, 77–78.

Zenker, W., Mayr, R. and Gruber, H. (1975) Neurotubules: different densities in peripheral motor and sensory nerve fibres. *Experientia (Basel),* **31**, 318–320.

Zimmerman, E., Karsh, D. and Humbertson, A. Jr. (1971) Initiating factors in perineuronal cell hyperplasia associated with chromatolytic neurons. *Zeitschrift für Zellforschung und mikroskopische Anatomie,* **114**, 73–82.

5 FUNCTIONAL ANATOMY OF THE ANTERIOR HORN MOTOR NEURON

S. Conradi

5.1 Introduction

The nerve impulses governing the activity of most skeletal muscles reach those muscles through the axons of the spinal motor neurons. Although the functional demands on the various motor axons associated with the transmission of nerve impulses are essentially similar, the pattern of neural control of different muscle fibres varies considerably. These variations are accomplished by differences in the central connections of the various motor neurons, each motor neuron bearing several thousand synapses on the cell body and dendrites. Besides being the site of impulse-origin, the central part of the motor neuron also influences growth and metabolism of the motor axon. The central and peripheral parts of the motor neuron are thus functionally closely interrelated.

Since the electrical activity of the spinal motor neurons is made manifest as muscle contractions, (which are easy to record), the functional properties of these cells were studied early and the study of the motor neuron still occupies a central position in neurophysiology. The spinal cord of the cat is thus a standard site for neurophysiological studies and most of our knowledge of motor control has been derived from this preparation, while the complex central connections of the motor neuron have been looked upon as a model of neuronal circuitry in general. Sherrington's concepts of excitation and inhibition were formulated after experiments upon cat spinal motor neurons, and studies on these cells using intracellular microelectrodes have provided further information concerning not only the physiology of motor control (see e.g. Granit, 1970), but also the basic physiological properties of nerve cells and synapses (Eccles, 1957, 1964).

Due to their size and accessibility, the spinal motor neurons are also well suited to studies by methods other than those of the physiologist, and the extent of our knowledge of these cells permits useful correlations to be made between disciplines; in the context of the motor neuron as a model system, such correlations may be of general value. The morphology of the large ventral horn motor neurons has been the object of many studies and is proportionately well understood. Electron microscopy has also rendered the synapses of the motor neurons accessible to morphological studies, but the great complexity of the synaptic connections still provides a formidable obstacle to attempts to reveal even the most simple patterns of the structural basis of neuronal circuitry. Some help has been derived from the occurrence of several distinct morphological types of synapses on the motor neurons and there is reason to believe that such morphological typing has a functional significance. In addition physiological studies on the motor neurons employing the intracellular microelectrode technique allow predictions to be made as to the localization on the cell surface of some of the active synapses, assisting comparisons with morphological data.

Rather than aiming at presenting a complete review of the vast field of knowledge concerning the structure of the motor neurons, the present article is intended to give some basic information concerning their morphology, and this will then be discussed with emphasis upon those aspects which appear to have the greatest functional significance; and as it is hoped will become apparent, many questions concerning the function of the motor neuron have important morphological implications. The following aspects of motor neuron structure appear to be of particular interest in this respect at the present time:

(a) The morphological definition of the motor neurons. Criteria are required for delimiting them from other neurons in the ventral horn and for distinguishing between the two main types described by the physiologists, i.e. alpha and gamma motor neurons.

(b) The dimensions and cell geometry of the motor neurons. These data need to be correlated with physiological measurements of their electrical properties, particularly since it has been argued (Henneman, Somjen and Carpenter, 1965), that motor neuron excitability varies with cell size.

(c) The morphology of the motor neurons in various functional states; for example following damage to the axon or under other pathological conditions.

(d) The synaptology of the motor neurons. Due to the central role played by the synapses in the impulse generating activity of the motor neuron, questions concerning the structure, origin and distribution of the various synapses on the cell surface are of major interest, and will be thoroughly discussed.

(e) Morphological aspects of the development of the motor neurons will also be dealt with, although present knowledge in this field is somewhat sparse. Correlations between morphology and function may be especially rewarding when made at stages when new functional abilities are added, and may provide information relevant to the situation in the adult.

5.2 Morphology of the motor neurons

5.2.1 *The large cells of the ventral horn*

A population of large multipolar neurons containing abundant Nissl substance, and having cell bodies of between 30–60 μm diameter, occupies the ventral and lateral parts of the ventral horn of the spinal cord. Several thick and branching dendrites are sent out in different directions from each of these neurons, and the thick, heavily myelinated axons enter the ventral spinal root after a short course through the ventral horn, during which one or more branches may leave each axon. The cells were recognized by the early light-microscopists (Deiters, 1865) (Fig. 5.1), but at that time, due to a lack of suitable staining methods, it was no more than an assumption that these cells were the sole source of the ventral root fibres. The possibility could not then, for example, be excluded that part of the ventral root fibres emanated from the descending tracts in the white substance of the cord. Not until Golgi and Ramon y Cajal introduced staining methods allowing impregnation of whole neurons (Fig. 5.2), could the course of the axons of these cells be ascertained. In recent experiments with intracellular injection of fluorescent dye, or radioactive material, through microelectrodes (Barrett and Graubard, 1970; Lux, Schubert and Kreutzberg, 1970) (Fig. 5.3), the location of individual motor neurons among these cells has been visualized in a new way.

The cell bodies of the large neurons are intermingled with smaller neurons, forming fields within the ventral horn with a characteristic cytoarchitecture, the lamina IX of Rexed (1952) (Fig. 5 4). The cell bodies of these large cells are spheroid or slightly ovoid, as judged from observations on serial sections (Barr, 1939) or on isolated neurons (Chu, 1954). According to some authors (Lhermitte and Kraus; 1925, Weil, 1927), the cell bodies of most motor neurons are ovoid, with their longitudinal axis parallel to that of the spinal cord, a tendency which is considered to increase in higher species. Other motor neurons, especially at the border towards the white substance, have a somewhat flattened cell body (Aitken and Bridger, 1961). Although the largest neurons (cell body diameter exceeding 40 μm) in this population stand out quite clearly, it has not been possible to provide an accurate morphological definition of all of the cells assumed to be motor neurons. In particular the lower limit of cell body size has been the subject of interest since the physiological recognition of the presence of the gamma motor neurons (Leksell, 1945) innervating the intrafusal muscle fibres of the muscle spindles. Since the diameters of the axons of the gamma motor neurons in the ventral root are between 4–6 μm (Eccles and Sherrington, 1930), as compared with 12–15 μm for the axons of the bigger alpha motor neurons which form about two-thirds of the ventral root fibres, attempts have been made to identify from among the motor neurons a special group of smaller neurons, from which the small gamma axons might originate. Furthermore intracellular recordings from alpha motor neurons have produced a need for more accurate morphological data, which could be used in calculations concerning the electrical properties of these cells. This is particularly important in connection with the proposal (Henneman, Somjen and Carpenter, 1965) that the excitability of motor neurons is inversely related to cell size.

The size-range of the motor neurons

The size-range of the neuron cell bodies in the ventral horn has been investigated light microscopically after a variety of staining procedures. Schadé and v. Harreveld (1961) used consecutive sections, 20 μm thick, to calculate the volumes of 45 large and 96 small cells in the peroneus-tibialis motor pool in the

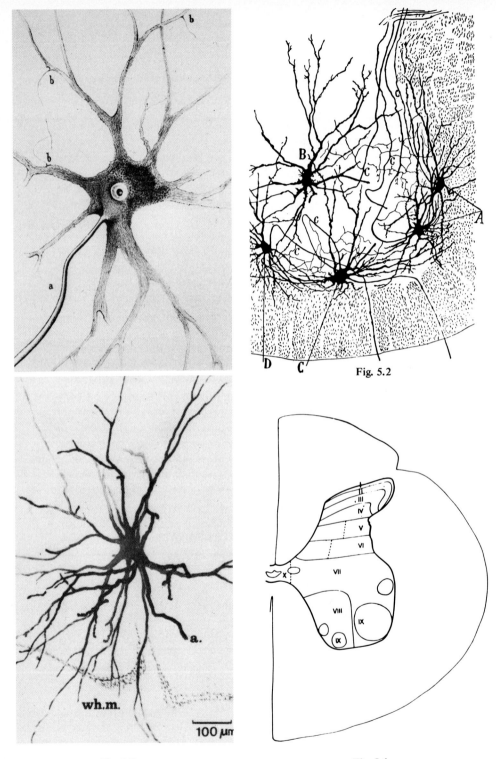

Fig. 5.2

Fig. 5.3

Fig. 5.4

cat. In addition they tested various formulae for calculating the cell body volume from the diameter in single transverse sections in the nucleolar plane, applying the formula $1/6 \, \pi ab\sqrt{(ab)}$, (where a and b are the major and minor cell body diameters), on about 700 nerve cell profiles from the same material, both in the normal state and after sectioning the corresponding motor nerves. Their curve, showing the volume distribution of the neuron cell bodies, with the classes of size used, was continuous and showed two peaks, one at 4000–8000 μm^3, another, much smaller peak at 20 000–28 000 μm^3. The smallest number of neurons was found at 16 000 μm^3. Cells showing retrograde changes after axon section were found in both the smaller and larger groups, but in the highest number around 24 000 μm^3. Micklewright, Kurnick and Hodes (1953), measuring 55 cervical cat spinal motor neurons, also found a peak at 20 000–24 000 μm^3 cell body volume. Mellstrom and Skoglund (1969), (using the same methods as Schadé and v. Harreveld) determined the postnatal growth in single sections through the most cranial neurons in lamina IX of the segments C 7 and L 7 in the cat, and reviewed the older literature. In adult animals they also found a continuous spectrum of cell body size, with a big peak at 6000 μm^3, and another small peak at 30 000 μm^3, with the biggest neurons scattered between 40 000 and 100 000 μm^3.

Naturally investigations such as these involve many difficulties, not least with regard to sampling and shrinkage factors. It is also often very difficult in single sections to distinguish the boundary between the cell body and the base of a stout dendritic stem, arising in the plane of section, and the areas ascribed to the cell bodies may often have been larger than was really the case. In order to avoid such errors and achieve the greatest accuracy, it would seem best to follow the profile of the cell body through several consecutive sections, and make the measurements only on those in which none of the dendrites, or only a single thin one, leaves the cell body in the plane of section. In the author's opinion, such a method nearly always provides sections through the nuclear plane. It cannot be excluded that a failure to discover distinct populations of neurons according to cell body size, is associated with such technical problems. Unfortunately, no figures for the actual diameters are given in the studies already mentioned, and diameters are obviously the only parameters to hand when trying to distinguish

---

Fig. 5.1–5.3   The motor neuron during the last 100 years.

(5.1) (Reproduced from Deiters, 1865.)

(5.2) Kitten motor neurons. (Reproduced from Cajal, 1909.)

(5.3) Reconstruction of a cat spinal motor neuron, injected with radioactive glycine through an intracellular microelectrode. (Reproduced from Lux, Schubert and Kreutzberg, 1970).

Fig. 5 4   Rexed's laminae in the spinal gray matter of lumbosacral segments in the cat. (Reproduced from Rexed, 1952.)

between motor neurons in single sections. Assuming an average major/minor diameter ratio of 1 in these studies, a minimum of neurons would be expected to have a minor diameter of about 30 μm, and the minor diameter of the largest cells should then be in the order of 50 μm or greater. V. Buren and Frank (1965) measured the minor transverse diameter of about 800 neurons in the gastrocnemius-soleus motor pool in the cat and found one peak at about 20 μm and a smaller peak at 40–50 μm. In an electron microscopic investigation, the profiles of large nerve cell bodies, possessing a similar spectrum of apposing boutons, were found to have a minor transverse diameter within a range of 35–65 μm (Conradi, 1969a). With histochemical staining of the ventral horn Campa and Engel (1970) have shown that ventral horn cells having a minor cell body diameter exceeding 30 μm in transverse sections exhibit strong phosphorylase activity, whereas smaller cells are phosphorylase negative and instead show marked succinic dehydrogenase activity.

Gamma motor neurons

Following sectioning of either motor nerves or the ventral roots in adult animals, obvious chromatolysis is restricted to the large ventral horn cells, whereas such changes are difficult to recognize in the smaller cells which are believed to be gamma motor neurons. Nyberg-Hansen (1965) however, using kittens, claimed that small neurons, intermingled with the bigger ones in lamina IX, do undergo retrograde changes. This approach, does not however permit any statements to be made concerning the morphology and dimensions of the gamma motor neurons in the adult state. Gamma motor neurons have recently been investigated in the adult cat following intracellular injection of fluorescent dye (Bryan, Trevino and Willis, 1972). The location of the neurons corresponded to that of the alpha motor neurons to the same muscles, and the diameter of six gamma motor neuron cell bodies were 12.5–20 (minor) and 20–37.5 (major) μm, as compared with 25–50 and 40–50 μm, respectively, for alpha motor neurons in the same study; however it is possible that the staining procedure may have induced volume changes (see p. 288).

Quantitative aspects

It is not believed that cells with any functions other than those of motor neurons belong to the large ventral horn cell population, excepting the big 'spinal border cells' (Cooper and Sherrington, 1940) which are localized in the lateral ventral horn of upper lumbar segments of the cat, and send their axons to the cerebellum. The lower lumbar ventral roots of the cat contain some 5000 myelinated fibres (Holmes and Davenport, 1940; Aitken and Bridger, 1961; Schade, 1964; Gelfan, 1964), implying the presence of a corresponding number of motor neurons (alpha and gamma) on each side. As has been mentioned, almost all of the neurons larger than 16 000 μm^3 in the study of Schadé and v.

Harreveld showed retrograde changes after axon section. This group forms about 25% of the neurons in the peroneus-tibialis motor neuron pool, whereas according to the same authors 10% of the smaller cells also showed retrograde changes. Balthasar (1952), also found that about 25% of the neurons in the peroneus-tibialis pool of the cat were 'motor neurons', whereas Sprague (1951) states that nearly half of the ventral horn cells in the macaque with a diameter exceeding 25 μm are 'proprioceptive'. The total number of neurons in a lumbar spinal cord segment (dog) has been calculated to be 375 000 (Gelfan, 1963), which would mean that the whole spinal cord contains about 14 million neurons (Gelfan, 1963).

In conclusion, then, it is not possible to give a morphological definition of alpha and gamma motor neurons. However the investigations mentioned above, performed mainly in the cat, have provided good reasons for considering the neurons in lamina IX with a minor diameter exceeding 30 μm to be alpha motor neurons, at least in the lower lumbar segments in this animal. In the subsequent sections of this chapter the term 'motor neuron' refers to these cells.

5.2.2 Physiological implications of the size and shape of motor neurons: 'tonic' and 'phasic' motor neurons

'Tonic' and 'phasic' motor neurons

There is evidence that the alpha motor axons to the soleus muscle (cat) are slightly thinner than those to the gastrocnemius muscle (Eccles and Sherrington, 1930). The soleus muscle, containing mainly red muscle fibres with long contraction times, and which show a fused contraction at low frequencies of stimulation, is supplied by motor neurons capable of a maintained tonic discharge in response to muscle stretch. The gastrocnemius muscle, on the other hand, contains high proportion of white muscle fibres which have short contraction-times and are easily fatigued. The motor neurons supplying white muscle fibres operate with short, phasic, bursts of impulses at high frequency (see also Burke, Levine and Zajac, 1971). Recordings made from ventral root filaments have shown that the spike amplitude is smaller in the axons of 'tonic' motor neurons than in those of 'phasic' ones, and further, that the 'tonic' fibres show a slower conduction velocity (Henneman Somjen and Carpenter, 1965). Both of these observations indicate that the axons of the 'tonic' motor neurons are thinner than the axons of 'phasic' motor neurons. Other experiments (Kernell, 1966; Burke, 1967) have shown that the membrane resistance of 'tonic' motor neurons is higher than that of the 'phasic' motor neurons, a finding which has been interpreted to mean that the 'tonic' motor neurons are smaller than the 'phasic' ones, and this interpretation is thought to provide an explanation for the greater excitability of 'tonic' motor neurons upon current injection or synaptic stimulation.

As stated previously, there is no morphological evidence favouring clear delimitation of two sub-groups of alpha motor neurons according to size, and it is therefore impossible at present to recognize 'tonic' and 'phasic' motor neurons from their morphology. Furthermore the evidence that the bigger alpha motor neurons give rise to the thickest axons is scanty. Rexed (1944), among others, points to the fact that proximal muscles in the extremities often receive comparatively thick motor axons, but it is not known whether there is a corresponding difference at the level of the motor neuron cell bodies. In a study of the ventral horn of the Rhesus monkey after mild poliovirus infection (Hodes, Peacock and Bodian, 1949) it was found that destruction of large motor neuron cell bodies (above 40 000 μm^3) predominated when compared to that of smaller (20 000–40 000 μm^3) cell bodies, and at the same time there was a loss of the fastest conducting axons. In a recent study of the growth of motor neuron cell bodies and axons in the rat, Martinez and Friede (1970) concluded that there was a good correlation between the increase in axonal and cell body volume during the development, but, as is easily recognized, this does not necessarily imply a corresponding proportionality between cell body volume and axon diameter in the adult. Since differences have recently been described between 'tonic' and 'phasic' motor neurons with respect to synaptic influences (Burke and ten Bruggencate, 1971), the morphological factors underlying the physiological reasoning described in the preceding paragraph may not relate simply to cell size (see p. 312).

Electrophysiological aspects of the dimensions of motor neurons

From comparisons of figures of the dimensions of various parts of the motor neurons with their electrical parameters, obtained from experiments using the intracellular recording technique, attempts have been made to calculate resistance and capacity per unit membrane area, and the specific resistance of motor neuron cytoplasm. Besides giving information on the electrical properties of excitable membranes, such figures are also of importance in the understanding of the action of the various synapses. Since the nerve impulse is initiated in the first, unmyelinated, part of the axon, the ability of a synapse to influence this part of the motor neuron cell membrane depends, among other things, on the change in membrane potential induced at the synapse, and on the electrical properties of the material situated between this point and the initial axon segment. These properties in turn, depend on several dimensional factors. By assuming certain dimensions for a 'standard' motor neuron cell body (Coombs, Curtis and Eccles, 1959), the electrical properties have been calculated per unit of surface area and volume respectively. However, the diameter of the model used — 70 μm — gives a cell body volume about five times larger than that thought to be contained in the smaller alpha motor neurons (Schadé and v. Harreveld, 1961). As there is also a considerable size-range among the motor neurons, which cannot be left out of account, great care has obviously to be taken when combining morphological data with physiological reasoning!

Neuron model

Attempts to predict the variation in synaptic effects with different locations of the synapses on the motor neuron surface have involved the construction of 'idealized' neuron models (Rall, 1967; Jack and Redman, 1971). The cable model of Rall, based on the anatomical data given by Aitken and Bridger (1961), has the shape of a cylinder, in which one of the sealed ends corresponds to the cell body, including the initial axon segment, the rest of the cylinder being a single hypothetical dendrite representing all of the motor neuron dendrites bundled together (Fig. 5.5). With this model, the actual site of a synapse is represented by a value corresponding to its 'electronic' distance from the site of impulse-origin, and the model presumes, among other things, that at branching points the diameter of the motor neuron dendrites decreases in the ratio 3:2. According to the theory of cable properties, the potential change inside the cell body induced by synapses at large electronic distances on the distal dendrites differs in both amplitude and time-course from that evoked by synapses near the cell body. In addition, the model also emphasizes the functional importance of the synapses located on the more distant dendritic branches, in contrast to the earlier view (see Eccles, 1964), which attributes to the distal synapses insignificant influence on the firing zone of the motor neuron.

In a study in which the motor neurons were labelled with radioactive glycine after physiological recording with an intracellular microelectrode, and were

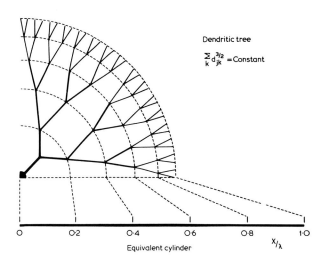

Dendritic tree

$$\sum_k d_{jk}^{3/2} = \text{Constant}$$

Equivalent cylinder

x/λ

Fig. 5.5 The cable model of Rall used in calculations of the action of synapses at varying distances from the initial axon segment. (Reproduced from Rall, 1970.)

A symmetric dendritic tree, and its correspondence to an equivalent cylinder. The dashed lines divide both the tree and the cylinder into five equal increments of electrotonic length. In the equation, subscript j indicates the order of branching and summation over subscript k means to sum over all branches of jth order; when this sum has the same value at all orders of branching, this tree can be transformed into the cylinder.

subsequently studied morphologically (Lux, Schubert and Kreutzberg, 1970), the electrical properties of the motor neuron cytoplasm and cell membrane have been more accurately analysed. In many respects the results obtained confirm the postulates underlying Rall's model. Such staining of neurons with the microelectrode after a study of their physiological properties permit many useful correlations between morphology and function. The most commonly used staining method, involving the deposition of a fluorescent dye (Stretton and Kravitz, 1968), was originally described for light microscopy, a technique which does not allow any statements to be made concerning possible changes inside the neurons, including volume changes, induced by the staining procedure itself. The method has been recently modified for electron microscopy (Kellerth, 1973) using a much smaller amount of dye and a shorter staining time. With this procedure, most stained cells show only minor structural changes, and it is also possible to study the apposed synapses. The changes observed include some swelling of the neurons or, particularly when the neurons seem to have been damaged by the staining procedure, a pronounced shrinkage. The latter very often occurs when a large amount of dye has been used, similar in quantity to that originally described for light microscopy.

In summary, it may be concluded that measurement of the electrical properties of the motor neuron, either in whole or in part, and the application of this information to predictions of synaptic actions still presents many difficulties. Apart from the fact that the precise location on the motor neuron surface of any of the incoming systems is unknown, membrane resistance may well vary with the immediate local relationships of the motor neuron cell membrane.

5.2.3 *The dendritic tree*

The motor neurons send out 5–15 dendrites (Haggar and Barr, 1950; Chu, 1954; Aitken and Bridger, 1961; Sprague and Ha, 1964; Gelfan, Kao and Ruchkin, 1970), which apparently leave the cell body in all directions, although motor neurons near the edge of the white matter possess many dendrites running parallel to this border (v. Buren and Frank, 1965). The diameters of the dendrites adjacent to the cell body vary from 3 to 20 μm, and many dendrites branch one or more times, often dichotomously. The older histologists (see Ramon y Cajal, 1909) had noted that the dendrites may extend 1000 μm or more into adjacent parts of the ventral horn, intermediate grey matter, or the anterior commissure and white substance (see also Aitken and Bridger, 1961). Since the dendrites are probably covered by synapses along their whole course (Gelfan and Rapisarda, 1964; Wyckoff and Young, 1956) the receptive field of an individual motor neuron is very large. It has been calculated that about 80–90% of the motor neuron surface, estimated to be 60 000–80 000 μm^2, is contributed by the dendrites (Aitken and Bridger, 1961; Schadé and v. Harreveld, 1964). Recent studies on Golgi-stained motor neurons have shown that the rostrocaudal ramifications of the dendrites are more extensive than those in the transverse plane (Sterling and Kuypers, 1967; Scheibel and Scheibel, 1970a; Dekker, Lawrence and Kuypers, 1973), and even those dendrites leaving the cell body in the transverse plane often take a rostro-caudal course at their distal extremities. Furthermore it has been recognized that segments of several (5—25) adjacent dendrites from different motor neurons form bundles (Scheibel and Scheibel, 1970a, 1973; Marsh, Matlowsky and Stromberg, 1971; Matthews, Willis and Williams, 1971); that new dendrites enter and leave the bundles along their course; and that each dendrite may accompany the bundle for several hundred micra. Electron microscopy (Matthews, Willis and Williams, 1971), has revealed that adjacent dendrites may be directly apposed within such bundles, and the possibility has been pointed out that their juxtaposition may ensure that the different dendrites in the bundle receive similar synaptic connections.

The dendrites of the motor neurons and other neurons in the grey substance (dog) have recently been subjected to a thorough quantitative study using serially sectioned Golgi stained material (Gelfan, Kao and Ruchkin, 1970; Gelfan, Kao and Ling, 1972). The dendritic tree of big ventral horn cells (diameter exceeding about 35 micra) is claimed to be larger than that of other cells in the grey substance, including the equally big cells in the dorsal horn. Dendrites with a diameter exceeding $10 \mu m$ are sent out only by the largest neurons, i.e. those exceeding $50 \mu m$ in diameter). About 15% of the hypothetical cell body surface is occupied by the origin of the dendrites in the big neurons, and the surface area of the dendritic tree of the large neurons appears to be proportional to the number of parent dendrites leaving the cell body (Gelfan, Kao and Ruchkin, 1970; Gelfan, Kao and Ling, 1972). There seems however to be no clear correlation between cell body size and the number of parent dendrites on the large neurons, and this finding appears to conflict with those of Kernell (1966), who claimed that direct proportionality exists between the diameter of the cell body and the sum of the cross sectional areas of the dendritic stems. Furthermore, Gelfan and his co-workers state that the proportion of unbranched dendrites of the large neurons is surprisingly high, being about 50%, although some sources of error are naturally associated with the serial section method of analysis; in addition the proportion of unbranched dendrites is claimed not to change with the number of parent dendrites. The dendrite to cell body surface ratio is estimated to be between 0.5 and 3, most frequently about 2, or 70% of the total for the largest neurons. Following deafferentation, there is a shortening of the dendrites (Gelfan, Kao and Ling, 1972).

The dendritic tree of the motor neuron thus has proportions commensurate with those of its cell body, and some limited quantitative information concerning its extent is also available. However it is not known whether differences of function between various motor neurons are reflected in differing arrangements of their dendrites. If the data from the quantitative studies by Gelfan and co-workers can be confirmed, it may indicate that measurements of the numbers and diameters of the parent dendrites leaving the motor neuron cell body can be used to predict aspects of the morphology of the whole dendritic tree, a capability which would be of considerable practical value.

5.2.4 *Motor neuron pools*

It has long been known that the location in the ventral horn of the cell bodies of the motor neurons varies according to which muscles the motor neurons innervate (see Bok, 1928). Through careful examination of retrograde changes in the neuron cell bodies after sectioning various motor nerves in the cat, Romanes (1951) showed that motor neurons innervating a group of functionally similar muscles form separate pools or, more correctly, columns (see also Balthasar, 1952; Sterling and Kuypers, 1967). In the lumbosacral cord of the cat, motor neurons innervating proximal muscles are located more ventrally and rostrally than those innervating distal muscles (Fig. 5.6), and motor neurons innervating flexor muscles are situated laterally to the motor neurons innervating their extensor antagonists. The motor neuron columns are aligned rostrocaudally, often extending through more than one segment, and large and small neurons are intermingled. The thickness of the columns seems to vary at regular intervals (Testa, 1964), giving them an appearance of bands of pearls, and sometimes making it difficult to distinguish them in single transverse sections of the cord. There is some evidence that the motor neurons for the different muscles form subgroups within the columns (Eldred *et al.*, 1961), but otherwise nothing is known with regard to whether the location of the motor neurons in the columns, e.g. central or peripheral has any connection with their specific motor functions.

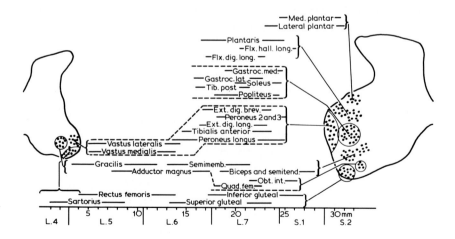

Fig. 5.6 The motor pools in the ventral horn of cat lumbosacral segments (Reproduced from Romanes, 1951.)

5.2.5 *Fine structure of the motor neurons. Structural changes associated with chromatolysis and some other pathological conditions*

Normal state

The cell bodies of the motor neurons are easily recognized embedded in the neuropil when ultrathin sections through the ventral horn are studied in the electron microscope (Fig. 5.7). The neuropil contains densely packed profiles of axons, synapses, dendrites, glial cells and capillaries. (For more detailed descriptions, see Wyckoff and Young, 1956; Bodian, 1964; Conradi, 1969a and McLaughlin, 1972a). The most proximal parts of the dendrites are sometimes continuous with the profiles of the motor neuron cell bodies, but the cellular origin of other profiles of axons or dendrites in the neuropil usually cannot be determined without recourse to an extensive series of consecutive sections. With optimal fixation, for example vascular perfusion with buffered aldehydes (Karlsson and Schulz, 1965), the motor neuron cell bodies and adjacent dendrites have a smooth external contour.

The nucleus of the motor neuron, which has a diameter of about $10-20\ \mu m$ (see Bodian, 1964), is located in the middle of the motor neuron cytoplasm and contains a centrally placed, and prominent, nucleolus. The cytoplasm of the cell body (Fig. 5.8) is filled with aggregates of granular endoplasmic reticulum (Palay and Palade, 1955; Bodian, 1964) which corresponds to the Nissl-bodies of the light microscopists (see Bok, 1928). The ribosomes usually form small rosettes between the membrane sacs of the reticulum (Bodian, 1964) and the endoplasmic reticulum extends for some distance into the proximal parts of the dendrites. Other organelles found in the motor neuron cytoplasm (Fig. 5.8), as in most central neurons, are mitochondria, many neurofilaments, dense bodies and Golgi apparatus, the last being predominantly located in a perinuclear position (Bodian, 1964).

The proximal parts of the motor neuron dendrites contain many neurotubules and neurofilaments, and these are also seen within profiles of small dendrites in the neuropil. Some of these thin dendrites undoubtedly emanate from adjacent motor neurons. It has been claimed that the dendrites of the motor neurons contain a higher proportion of neurofilaments to neurotubules than do the dendrites of neighbouring non motor neurons (Wuerker and Palay, 1969).

Chromatolysis and related conditions

Since much knowledge of the functions and connections of the motor neurons is based upon the morphological changes occurring inside the cell body following axon section, a short note on these changes is included, without entering into other structural aspects of motor neuron cell metabolism. The chromatolytic changes in cat motor neurons after axon section when studied light microscopically, include peripheral dispersion of the Nissl-bodies and Golgi apparatus,

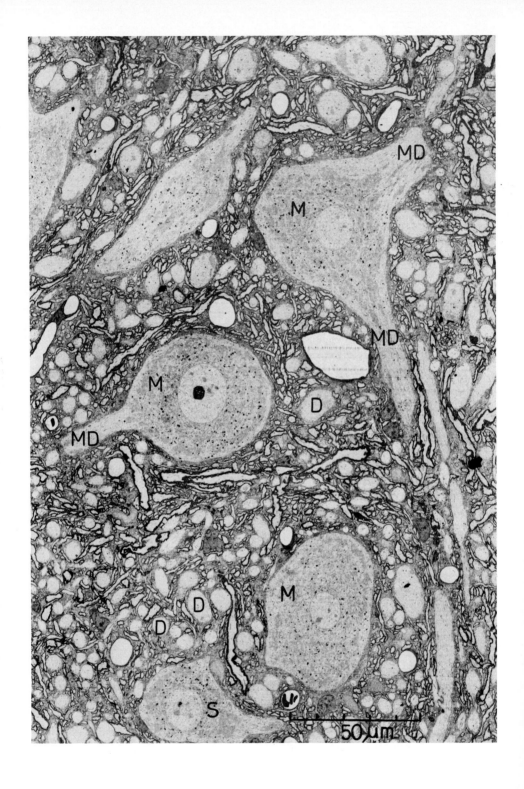

followed by perinuclear reappearance of the Nissl-bodies, displacement of the nucleus to the periphery, and swelling of the whole cell (see Balthasar, 1952; Romanes, 1951; Kirkpatrick, 1968; Barron *et al.*, 1970; for a more detailed account, see Lieberman, 1971). There are marked regional differences in the extent of the reaction, for example between cranial nerve and spinal motor neurons, as well as interspecific variations, the changes inside cat spinal motor neurons being much more obvious than those seen in rabbits, rats and mice (Romanes, 1964).

Ultrastructurally, peripheral dispersion of endoplasmic reticulum and Golgi apparatus have been observed in spinal motor neurons following injury (Bodian, 1964; Barron *et al.*, 1970). Similar changes occur inside facial motor neurons in mice (Torvik and Skjörten, 1971), and the changes here are reported to be reversible after nerve crush, and irreversible, leading to a prolonged process of atrophy, after nerve section. In young mice, the degeneration in facial motor neurons after axon section is much more rapid (Torvik, 1972), and is followed by phagocytosis by means of glial cells. The intense retrograde cellular reaction of bulbar and spinal motor neurons of young animals has been used as the basis for a specific marking technique (Grant, 1970) in which the whole neuron, including dendrites and axon, are impregnated with metal. Around both cranial nerve and spinal motor neurons an intense glial reaction accompanies chromatolysis (see Kirkpatrick, 1968; Blinzinger and Kreutzberg, 1968; Hamberger, Hansson and Sjöstrand, 1970; Torvik and Skjörten, 1971), leading to an extensive displacement and phagocytosis of the synapses on the motor neuron cell bodies.

These changes inside the cell body may be signs of a spectrum of non-specific reactions to injury on part of the motor neuron (Eccles, 1964). Bodian (1964) describes diffuse chromatolysis of the endoplasmic reticulum following infection with a mild strain of poliovirus, but the changes observed differed in some respects from those evoked by axon section. Dissolution of the endoplasmic reticulum also occurs in dorsal vagal neurons (Hansson and Sjöstrand, 1971) in colchicine poisoning, thought to impair axonal and dendritic flow, but in spinal motor neurons this toxin evokes hypertrophy of the neurofilaments (Wisniewski, Shelanski and Terry, 1968). Spinal motor neurons also show disintegration of endoplasmic reticulum after the injection into the motor neuron of fluorescent dye (Kellerth, 1973), while anoxic changes in motor neuron cytoplasm mainly influence mitochondria and the Golgi apparatus (v. Harreveld and Khattab, 1967; Merker, 1969). There are no conclusive reports concerning the ultrastructure of motor neurons in motor neuron disease, but the

---

Fig. 5.7 A survey electron micrograph of the lateral part of the ventral horn in the cat. Three motor neurons (M) are cut through their cell bodies and the proximal parts of dendrites are observed projecting from two of them (MD). At the bottom of the figure, a smaller nerve cell (S) is visible. In the neuropile are profiles of dendrites, (D) glial cells (G), myelinated axons and capillaries. (x 720. Reproduced from Conradi, 1969a.)

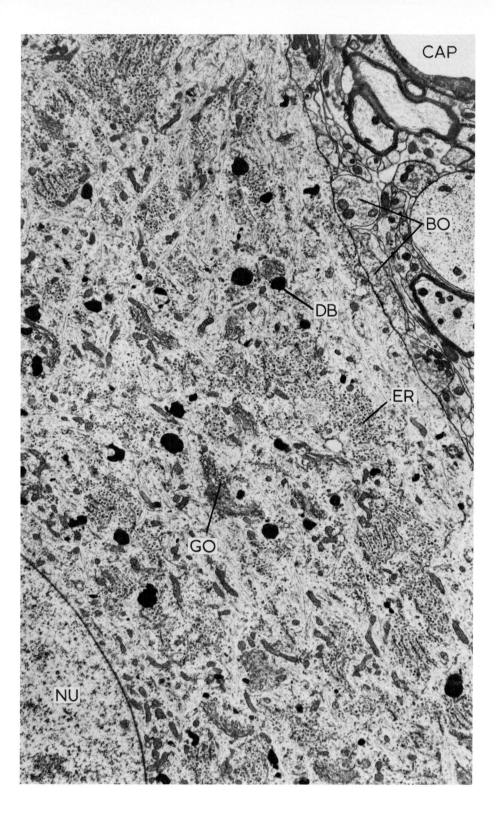

light microscopic changes have recently been reviewed (Norris and Kurland, 1970).

5.2.6 *The central part of the motor axon*

Axon hillock

The axon hillock is the cone-shaped zone of transition between cell body and axon, and is about 10–20 μm long in the motor neurons (Fig. 5.9). Ultrastructurally, this region lacks endoplasmic reticulum, and instead contains mainly neurofilaments and neurotubules (Conradi, 1966, 1969c; Palay *et al.*, 1968). The cell membrane of the motor neuron is covered by synapses and glial cell processes in this region in the same manner as is the rest of the cell body.

Initial axon segment

Since the impulse activity of the motor neuron is initiated in the first unmyelinated part of the motor axon, the initial axon segment, due to a low threshold to excitation of the cell membrane at this site (Fuortes, Frank and Baker, 1957; Coombs, Curtis and Eccles, 1957), the structure of this part of the axon segment is of particular interest.

At the initial segment, which extends for about 25–35 μm, the axon is a uniform thin cylinder, about 3–4 μm in diameter, and often runs in the transverse plane. Ultrastructurally, the cytoplasm contains abundant longitudinal neurotubules and the cell membrane is covered on the inside by a thin layer of amorphous contrast-rich material (Fig. 5.9). Outside the cell membrane, there is a thin rim of extracellular material surrounding the axon (Conradi, 1969c; Kojima and Saito, 1970). The cellular relationships of the motor neuron membrane at the initial axon segment seem to be similar to those seen at the initial segments of the many other types of neurons in the central nervous system (Campos-Ortega, Glees and Neuhoff, 1968; Palay *et al.*, 1968; Peters, Proskauer and Kaiserman-Abramof, 1968), and are also like those found at the central nodes of Ranvier (Andres, 1965; Peters, 1966; Karlsson, 1967; Hildebrand, 1971a). On the whole, the initial motor axon segment is devoid of apposed synaptic boutons (Conradi, 1969c; Kojima and Saito, 1970) as are the central nodes of Ranvier, except for some boutons on the transition to the axon hillock (Conradi, 1969c) or on its most proximal part (Poritsky, 1969; Saito, 1972).

Fig. 5.8   Detail of the cytoplasm of a cat spinal motor neuron. Nucleus (NU); Golgi apparatus (GO); endoplasmic reticulum aggregates (ER), the Nissl-bodies; dense bodies (DB); apposed boutons (BO); capillary (CAP). × 10 000.

The myelinated part of the motor axon

After acquiring its myelin sheath, the diameter of the motor axon increases. Ultrastructurally these thick axons (Conradi, 1969c), like other thick central axons (Hildebrand, 1971a) exhibit some peculiarities when compared to other, thinner, central myelinated fibres (see Bunge, 1968). The myelin sheath possesses incisures of Schmidt—Lantermann and outside the main myelin sheath there are abundant compact bodies of myelin, especially near incisures and nodes. At the nodes of Ranvier of the motor axons there is a thick collar of extracellular material, intermingled with astrocytic projections, around the naked axon (Fig. 5.10). At similar large nodes in the dorsal columns, villi-like astrocytic extensions have been recognized in the nodal gap (Hildebrand, 1971a), producing an arrangement quite similar to that present at the nodes of large peripheral fibres (Landon and Williams, 1963; Berthold, 1968), but no paranodal accumulations of mitochondria are seen at central nodes (see Chapter 1).

Recurrent collaterals of the motor axon

Thin recurrent collaterals leaving the motor axons during their course through the grey matter were described by the light microscopists (see Prestige, 1964). They are considered to form synapses with the Renshaw neurons (Renshaw, 1941), which in turn give inhibitory synapses to the motor neurons (Eccles, Fatt and Koketsu, 1954). As shown by Szentagothai (1967), these collaterals ramify and terminate in the grey substance just inside the point of exit of the ventral root fibres from the spinal cord. The Renshaw cells have been investigated morphologically using the method of intracellular injection of fluorescent dye (see Jankowska and Lindström, 1971), and have been found to be located in the corresponding area of the cord, i.e. the ventral part of Rexed's lamina VII (Fig. 5.4).

5.3 Central connections of the motor neurons

5.3.1 *Ultrastructure of the neuropil of the ventral horn*

The surface of the motor neuron is in contact with glial extensions, dendrites and synaptic boutons (Bodian, 1964; Conradi, 1969a). About one half of the cell membrane of the cell body is covered by astrocytic processes, these are

Fig. 5.9   Axon hillock (AH), initial axon segment (IS), and the first part of the myelinated portion of a cat spinal motor axon. A microglial cell (MG) is apposed to the initial segment, and two oligodendrocytes (OL) are also visible. (x 1900: Reproduced from Conradi, 1969c.)

Fig. 5.10   A central node of Ranvier on the motor axon. Note the collar of extracellular material (asterisk) surrounding the node. (x 9600: Reproduced from Conradi, 1969c.)

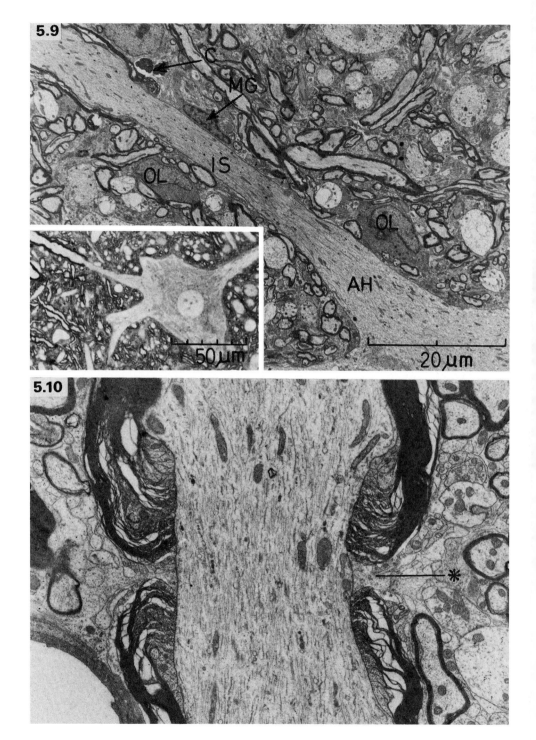

5.9

C

MG

IS

OL

OL

AH

50 μm

20 μm

5.10

*

usually flat and aligned parallel to the cell surface. Thin astrocytic processes are also interwoven between the other constituents of the neuropil and cover the motor neuron dendrites wherever there are no synapses. The cell bodies of the astrocytes are found scattered in the neuropil, whereas the oligodendrocytes, which have an ovoid cell body and dark cytoplasm are often found in a satellite position close to the motor neurons. Microglial cells are also found in the neuropil of the ventral horn. At some places the cell membranes of the motor neurons are directly apposed at adjacent dendritic profiles.

5.3.2 *Ultrastructure of the synapses on the motor neurons*

As judged by electron microscopy, about half of the surface of the motor neuron cell body, and the majority of the dendritic surface are covered by boutons making synaptic complexes (Gray and Guillery, 1966) with the motor neuron. The boutons are mostly half-egg shaped and the cytoplasm contains many synaptic vesicles and mitochondria; some sections also include part of the preterminal axon. The boutons on the motor neurons have been the subject of many light-microscopic studies, mostly involving staining methods which impregnate the mitrochondria (for references, see Illis, 1964), that of Held (1897) providing the first demonstration of boutons in central nervous tissue. It was for long unclear whether the distal dendritic branches of the motor neurons were covered by boutons; such contacts were demonstrated however by Wyckoff and Young (1956) using electron microscopy. The earlier ultrastructural study of motor neurons by Palay and Palade (1955) gave the first description of synapses in the central nervous system, and provided definitive morphological evidence of cytoplasmic discontunuity at the synapse.

The synaptic boutons on the motor neurons have been the subject of many subsequent ultrastructural studies. They have then been divided into several morphological types (Rosenbluth, 1962; Gray, 1963; Bodian, 1964, 1966a, and b; Charlton and Gray, 1966; Uchizono, 1966; Ralston, 1967; Conradi, 1969a,b; Kawana, Akert, and Sandri, 1969; McLaughlin, 1972a; Streit *et al.*, 1972; Kojima, Saito and Kakimi, 1972) on the basis of variations in the size and morphology of both the synaptic vesicles and the synaptic complex, and it has been suggested that this typing may be of a physiological significance, (Bodian, 1966a,b; Uchizono, 1966; Conradi, 1969d) (see below). The descriptions of the various types have varied somewhat, as have their nomenclature. In the following description, the terminology introduced by Bodian will be used (1964, 1966a and b) which is based on studies of aldehyde-fixed material (with some modifications; Conradi 1969a). This typing system has as its basis the recognition of two classes of boutons, widely distributed throughout the central nervous system, having synaptic vesicles of differing shapes. Boutons containing spherical vesicles will be called S-type boutons and those having flattened synaptic vescicles, F-type boutons; the additional types represent variations on this basic pattern.

5.3.3 Morphological types of synapses (Fig. 5.11)

S-type.   Boutons containing spherical synaptic vesicles are about 1–4 µm long and are observed on all regions of the motor neuron surface. The diameter of the vesicles is of the order of 40–50 nm, the synaptic cleft is about 15 nm wide, and there is a comparatively thick layer of dense material beneath the postsynaptic membrane.

T-type.   Some of the boutons with spherical vesicles exhibit dense cytoplasmic bodies beneath the postsynaptic membrane, originally described by Taxi (1961), (T = Taxi). One and the same bouton may establish several synaptic complexes, some with and some without these bodies.

F-type.   Boutons containing flattened vesicles, about 20–30 x 40–60 nm in diameter (Uchizono, 1966; Bodian, 1966a,b), can also be found at all regions of the motor neuron surface. Both the synaptic cleft and the postsynaptic dense material are thinner than at the S-boutons (see Ralston, 1967). The F-boutons are usually slightly bigger than the majority of the S-boutons.

C-type.   Large boutons containing spherical synaptic vesicles and having a flat subsynaptic cistern (C-cistern) situated below the whole region of the postsynaptic motor neuron membrane, (Fig. 5.11) have been described by several authors (Rosenbluth, 1962; Gray, 1963; Bodian, 1964, 1966b; Charlton and Gray, 1966; v. Harreveld and Khattab, 1967; Conradi, 1969a; McLaughlin, 1972a). There is no pre- or postsynaptic density, the synaptic cleft is very narrow, shows histochemical evidence of acetylcholinesterase activity (Lewis and Shute, 1966), and extends below the whole of each of the boutons, which are 3–7 µm long. Several parallel sacs of endoplasmic reticulum are often found within the superficial motor neuron cytoplasm beneath these boutons.

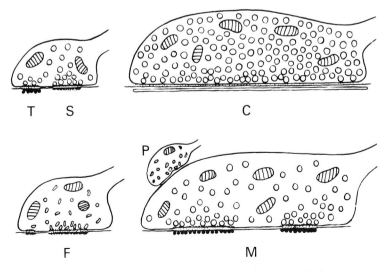

Fig. 5.11   Schematic drawing of the types of synapses on cat spinal motor neurons.

299

M-type. At the proximal parts of the motor neuron dendrites there are a few large boutons, 3–6 μm long, which contain spherical synaptic vesicles and establish large synaptic complexes, usually equipped with the postsynaptic 'Taxi'-bodies. These boutons are formed by terminals of dorsal root afferent fibres (M-monosynaptic), (Conradi, 1969d; McLaughlin, 1972b, see below). On the convex side of these boutons away from the motor neuron, are found small boutons (P-type, presynaptic) containing small synaptic vesicles of varying shape, the majority being flattened.

Several boutons contain dense-cored or granular vesicles, and in these cases the remainder of the vesicles are as a rule spherical; Bodian (1969b) has classified them as a special type, G-type. Some of the boutons, both of the S- and F-types, contain neurofilaments. McLaughlin (1972a) separates these into separate sub-types.

5.3.4 *Discussion of the morphological basis for the typing of boutons*

A system allowing structural classification of boutons on central neurons in general, and of those on the motor neurons in particular, would have many advantages, among which the following seem to be of special importance:

(a) If different synaptic morphologies can be correlated with the origin and functions of various pathways, structural studies will provide a functional dimension to morphological studies on both normal material and on that resulting from experimental procedures and pathological conditions.

(b) Further, if the classification in (a) is achieved, knowledge of the distribution on the neuron surface of the different synaptic inputs will allow more general physiological comparisons, with, for example, the neuron model.

(c) Even if information concerning the origin of the different bouton types is *not* available, knowledge of their distribution on various neurons might still be used as one criterion in a morphological classification of different types of neurons.

(d) If again the origin of the boutons is *not* known, knowledge of their distribution on various neurons in normal material is still of crucial importance to the interpretation of studies of synapses under experimental conditions, or during development.

In the original description of two classes of boutons containing, respectively, flattened and spherical vesicles following aldehyde fixation, Uchizono (1965) claimed that the F-boutons were inhibitory, since their distribution on the Purkinje cells in the cerebellum, i.e. predominantly on the cell bodies, accorded with the pattern predicted for inhibitory synapses from physiological studies; this hypothesis was later applied to synapses on spinal motor neurons (Bodian, 1966a,b; Uchizono, 1966). Since F-boutons have subsequently been found at many places in the central nervous system, the hypothesis has been much discussed (see Gray, 1969; Sotelo, 1971; Akert *et al.*, 1972). Some points concerning the purely morphological aspects of this question will be discussed, and their functional implications will be considered below (Section 5.3.7),

Akert *et al.* (1972) conclude that the S- and F-boutons form two morphologically distinct populations of boutons. This conclusion is based on, amongst other things, observations on tissue impregnated with various metal salts, and after freeze-etching, and they emphasized that the described differences between these two types concern not only the vesicles, but the synaptic complex as a whole. The latter point thus to some degree rebuts criticisms raised against this classification system by Colonnier (1968) and Valvidia (1971), who hold that the flattening of vesicles is merely an artifact of fixation, and that the varying degree of flattening in different boutons, makes it impossible to separate them into only two main types. Akert *et al.* (1972) likewise state that the flattened appearance of the vesicles of the F-boutons after aldehyde fixation probably does not represent the situation present *in vivo*, but they still list six general criteria by which the two bouton types can be differentiated. This distinction is supported by some observations made on motor neurons (Conradi, 1969a,b,d) namely, that the same bouton type is retained in serial sectioning through the boutons; that two boutons seen to emanate from the same preterminal axon always show the same vesicle shape; and, finally, that the S- and F-boutons differ in their mean size and distribution on the motor neuron surface. Bodian (1970, 1972), studying the boutons on the motor neurons after fixation with a variety of solutions, showed that after treatment with cacodylate-buffer, the vesicles of the C-boutons (by him denoted L), P-boutons and even F-boutons show additional flattening, whereas no change was observed in the S-boutons; thus confirming the presence of different, morphologically distinct types of boutons while emphasizing that the definition of individual types may vary with fixation. Dennison (1971) has found two types of F-boutons, one with disc-shaped, the other with cylindrical vesicles, in the goldfish spinal cord using stereomicroscopy, but there are no corresponding reports concerning the mammalian spinal cord.

The available evidence thus strongly indicates that the synapses on the motor neurons can be classified into different morphological types. This typing system, which may have a functional counterpart as discussed in Section 5.3.7, provides a useful basis for studies of the synaptic organization of the motor neurons. There may in addition be further types or sub-types to those described above, which are not distinguishable with present methods.

5.3.5 *The dorsal root synapses*

Dorsal root IA fibres from the muscle spindles establish a monosynaptic excitatory linkage with homonymous motor neurons (Lloyd, 1943). Due to the favourable conditions existing for stimulation and recording, the physiology of the monosynaptic pathway has been extensively studied (see Eccles, 1964). The dorsal root synapses are thought to be subjected to presynaptic inhibition (Frank and Fuortes, 1957), which is considered to be mediated by the activity of small boutons, making synapses on the dorsal root motor neuron synapses. From studies with intracellular microelectrodes, and calculations based on the neuron model (Rall *et al.*, 1967; Mendell and Henneman, 1971), it has been suggested that the dorsal root boutons are located mainly on the motor neuron dendrites, both near to the cell body and more distally. Jack *et al.*, (1971), using a similar technique, have concluded that the majority of the dorsal root boutons are likely to be situated on the proximal parts of the dendrites, while Burke (1968) has presented evidence that the dorsal root boutons are located more distally on the dendrites of 'tonic' than of 'phasic' motor neurons.

There have been several light-microscopic studies of the boutons on the motor neurons of dorsal root origin, which have been based on degeneration experiments (Sprague, 1958; Szentagothai, 1958; Mikeladze, 1966; Illis, 1967; Sterling and Kuypers, 1967; Carpenter, Stein and Shriver, 1968; Scheibel and Scheibel, 1969). The results of these investigations are somewhat inconclusive, ranging from reports of a massive representation over the entire cell surface (Illis, 1967) to the demonstration of a few big boutons on the proximal parts of the dendrites (Szentagothai, 1958). It has been proposed (Sterling and Kuypers, 1967) that the dorsal root axons to the motor neurons run in a longitudinal direction for the last part of their course, and that the boutons contact mainly longitudinal dendrites. In the lower lumbar segments of the cat, the dorsal root fibres reach motor neurons up to two segments below and above the level at which they enter the cord (Sprague and Ha, 1964), and the ramifications of each dorsal root fibre are extensive, resulting in contacts with more than 200 motor neurons per fibre in the cat (Mendell and Hennman, 1971).

The search for the dorsal root boutons on the motor neurons has been performed ultrastructurally following ipsilateral dorsal root section (Bodian, 1966b; Conradi, 1969d; McLaughlin, 1972b). In the monkey, boutons which show clear degenerative changes and are supplied with small boutons on their convex side, have been observed on the proximal parts of the motor neuron dendrites during the first post-operative week (Bodian, 1966b) but no description of the normal morphology of these boutons was included. In the cat, the M-boutons, described above, were found to have disappeared at one week post-operatively (Conradi, 1969d; McLaughlin, 1972b). During this period, most M-boutons were subjected to a rapid process of phagocytosis by adjacent glial cells, or by the motor neurons themselves (Conradi, 1969d). These results have been interpreted to mean that the M-boutons emanate from the dorsal root fibres. In the rat there are M-boutons resembling those in the cat, and such boutons show an accumulation of glycogen-like particles in the early stages of degeneration following dorsal root section (Wuerker, 1971). Whether any of the other boutons on the motor neurons have the same source is difficult to determine, but quantitative evaluation of single sections six weeks after the operation showed no reduction in the numbers of boutons of the other types

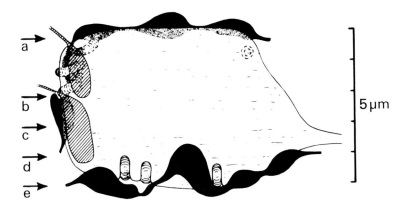

Fig. 5.12 Reconstruction from serial ultrathin sections of an M-bouton on the proximal part of a motor neuron dendrite in a cat. A schematic drawing of the model is seen from the convex side and it is seen that the M-bouton is surrounded by eleven P-boutons (black or striped), some of which are partly covered by the M-bouton when seen from above (stippled). There are seven dendritic spines (concentric circles) along the lateral border of the M-bouton (Reproduced from Conradi 1969d).

(Conradi, 1969d). It must be stressed however that the proportion of M-boutons is so small that if a similar number of boutons of any of the other types had disappeared, their loss would not have been detected in such a study.

Upon examination of serial sections through M-boutons, it is seen that the boutons are usually ovoid, with their long axes parallel to that of the dendrite, one M-bouton occasionally making contact with several dendrites. As a rule several presynaptic boutons, sometimes from the same preterminal axon, are apposed to one M-bouton (Fig. 5.12) and often at its lateral margin, thus making contact with both the motor neuron dendrite and the M-bouton. A synaptic complex is never found at the region of apposition between the P-bouton and the motor neuron surface or any other adjacent neural process, but is always present at the apposition area between the P- and M-boutons (Conradi, 1969d). According to McLaughlin (1972b) however, no synaptic complexes are seen between the P- and M-boutons, which would mean that the P-boutons do not establish synaptic complexes at all!

As mentioned earlier, the synaptic vesicles of the M-boutons are spherical, which would appear to confirm their excitatory character, as discussed below. The shape of the small vesicles of the P-boutons varies, the majority being flattened, although the proposed mechanism for presynaptic inhibition requires an excitatory presynaptic bouton. Hence in this case vesicle shape does not conform to physiological predictions and it may be that axo-axonal synapses have rather special physiological properties.

The M-boutons were found on the proximal parts of the motor neuron dendrites, where they formed 1−2% of the bouton profiles in a quantitative study on single transverse sections (Conradi, 1969a). Since they are bigger than

303

other boutons, their true frequency here may be of the order of 0.5% (see below). The total number of dorsal root boutons per motor neuron has been calculated to be 30 (Gelfan, 1963), or 50–100 (Jack *et al.*, 1971).

5.3.6 *The size and distribution of boutons of different types on the motor neuron surface*

That boutons are not distributed at random on the motor neurons, has been seen already from the description of the dorsal root boutons. There is in fact physiological evidence that the functional differences between various synaptic inputs to the motor neuron can be ascribed to the numbers and localization of the acting boutons, as might be expected from the properties of the neuron model (Granit *et al.*, 1964; Burke, 1968; Burke, Fedina and Lundberg, 1971; Jack *et al.*, 1971). Quantitative morphological studies of the distribution of boutons on the motor neuron surface obviously involve many difficulties, and it is important that methods should be developed which involve a minimum of labour, yet give acceptable information. A complete reconstruction of all the boutons on a motor neuron based on serial ultrathin sections would, for example, require more than a hundred thousand exposures in the electron microscope, the photographic work alone taking several years. Against this background a useful approach seems to be to study strictly delimited areas of single sections in a given plane, and to make small steric reconstructions from serial sections on a part of the material as a control. Two appropriate ways of describing the occurrence of boutons on different parts of a neuron in single ultrathin sections are, first the frequency of boutons of different types, and second, the percentage of the neuron membrane covered by boutons, the latter being expressed either in terms of all of the boutons, or of each of the types separately.

The proportions of different boutons

Cell body and dendrites. On single, transverse sections through the monkey cord, Bodian (1966b) found 46% S-, 40% F- and 4% C-boutons on the motor neuron cell body and dendrites. In a quantitative investigation which the author performed in the cat (Conradi, 1969a), single transverse sections through the peroneus motor pool were used. The material studied comprised sections through 20 motor neuron cell bodies, cut through the nucleolar plane. In addition, the proximal parts of the dendrites arising in the plane of section, and some additional profiles of proximal dendrites, were also studied, as well as 30 profiles of small dendrites in the neuropil; two animals furnished half the material each. The figures for the two animals were quite similar, and some of the observations seem worthy of mention. S-, T-, and F-boutons were found on all regions of the motor neuron surface, and there was an increase in the relative proportion of the F-bouton profiles on the distal dendrites, where they formed about 47% of all profiles to the cell body, where the corresponding value was 57%. The reverse was true for the S- (and T-) boutons, which decreased from about 46% to 34%, respectively. The C-boutons were confined to the cell bodies and the proximal parts of the dendrites. McLaughlin (1972a), studying about 1400 boutons in longitudinal sections through cat lumbar spinal cord, obtained similar values.

The mean size of the F-boutons was somewhat larger than for the S-boutons, and the F-boutons appeared somewhat larger on the cell bodies than on the dendrites, while the S-boutons showed the same mean length everywhere (Conradi, 1969a). Kojima, Saito and Kakimi, (1972), studying the size of the boutons on motor neurons and small neurons in the cervical spinal cord of the cat, found no size-difference that related to location on the motor neuron of the S- and F-boutons, but stated that the boutons are smaller on the small neurons. Since there is a greater chance for large boutons to be included in any single section, figures for proportion of boutons of the different types must therefore be adjusted to take account of the size of the profiles, in order to give a valid estimate of their true proportions. If the percentage of the boutons of any individual type is divided by the mean size of that type, a table of the relative proportions of the various synaptic terminals has the following appearance: (*from* Conradi, 1969a):

Type	Cell body %	prox. dendrite %	distal dendrite %
S-(+T-)	43	45	56
F-	54	52	44
C-	3	2	0.2
M-	—	0.6	0.1

Axon hillock. Using the same material, the author made two studies of the boutons on the axon hillock from complete sets of serial sections (Fig. 5.13). In the first, there were 32 boutons on the whole region; 21 of these, or 66% were F-type, the rest S-type. In the second reconstruction, 46 boutons were located in this region, of which 27, or 59%, were of the F-type, the rest likewise belonging to the S-type. The spectrum of boutons on the axon hillock in this material is thus similar to that of the cell bodies, with a suggestion of a somewhat higher proportion of the F-boutons.

Membrane covering by boutons

Knowledge of the mere proportion of different boutons gives limited information, since nothing is known of the total number of boutons, and it is difficult to make comparisons between normal and experimental material. The relative covering of the membrane by the boutons gives a better understanding in this

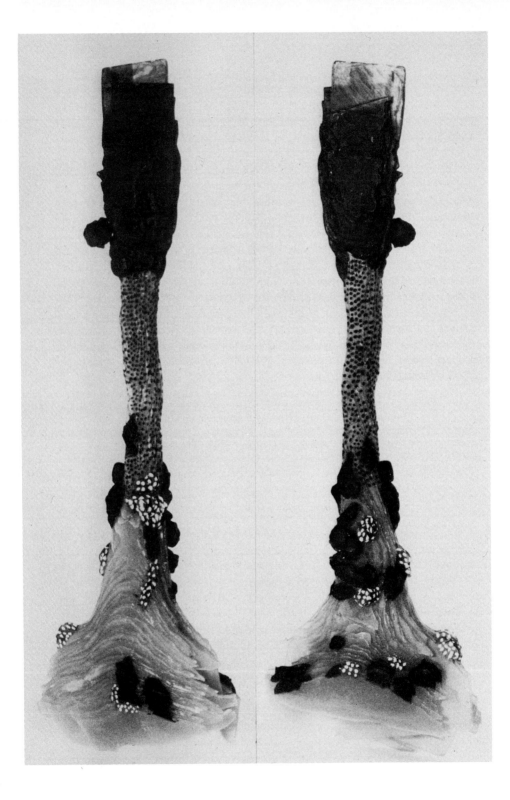

respect, although it requires measurements on the bouton profiles, which is a time-consuming procedure. Green and Pease (1965), while not stating details of the sampling procedure, found a greater covering of the membrane by boutons on motor neuron cell bodies (49%) than on the proximal parts of the dendrites (48%). Kojima, Saito and Kakimi (1972), recently studying the boutons on large and small neurons in the cervical spinal cord of the cat, found 85% and 91% of the cell bodies and proximal parts of the dendrites of the large neurons respectively were covered by boutons. The corresponding figure for the cell bodies of the small cells was 22%, and a similar difference was found for covering of the neuron membrane by the synaptic complexes alone. In the author's own quantitative study on cat (peroneus) motor neurons, mentioned above, the following approximate values for bouton covering on different parts of the motor neuron surface were obtained:

Type	Cell body %	prox. dendrites %	dist. dendrites %
S(+T)-	13	25	24
F-	27	40	24
C-	7	6	0.5
M-	—	2	0.2
Total	47	73	49

Reconstruction from serial sections

In order to investigate the morphology of the boutons further, including their topographic relationships, as well as the reliability of quantitative studies on single sections, the proximal part of a motor neuron dendrite, included in the study on the peroneus motor neurons (Conradi, 1969b), was studied through serial ultrathin sections and a map was constructed of the boutons on the 'unfolded' dendritic surface (Fig. 5.14). It can be seen that all the types of boutons are represented, that there is no distinct pattern of distribution, and that the boutons cover the major part of the dendritic surface. Most boutons are surrounded by thin glial sheaths which cannot be traced in detail at the magnification used. The three-dimensional appearance of astrocytic sheaths around motor neuron cell bodies has been illustrated by Poritsky (1969). There is a considerable size variation between boutons, even among those of the same type, and most boutons establish several synaptic complexes with the dendrite (although this cannot be seen from the figure). The proportion of S (and T)-boutons in the reconstruction is about 42%, as compared to 45% on the

Fig. 5.13 Wax-model from serial ultrathin sections of an axon hillock and initial segment (stippled with black). The model is seen from two aspects: the cell body is at the bottom of the figure. The boutons on the axon hillock are included, black F-type, white stippled S-type. (Reproduced from Conradi, 1969b.)

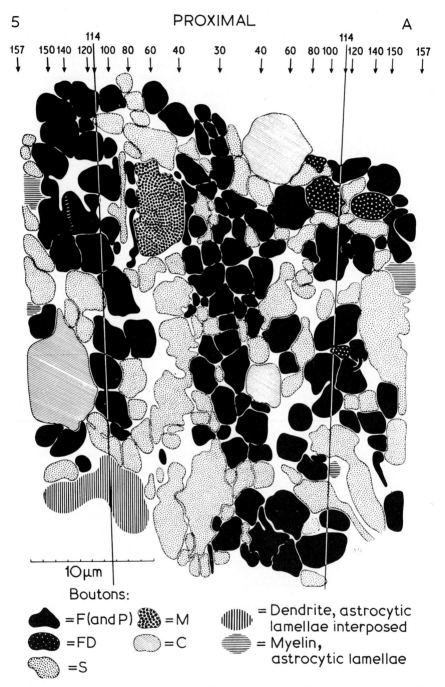

Fig. 5.14 Membrane relationships of the proximal part of a motor neuron dendrite derived from a complete series of consecutive ultrathin sections. The dendrite mantle surface is shown 'unfolded'. (Reproduced from Conradi, 1969b.)

proximal parts of the dendrites in the material from single sections. Corresponding values for the F-boutons are 57% and 52%, respectively, and the values for bouton covering are quite similar in the two sets of material. The packing density of the boutons on the reconstruction is of the order of 20 boutons per $100 \, \mu m^2$ of dendritic surface, a figure which agrees well with earlier light-microscope observations (see Gelfan and Rapisarda, 1964).

Conclusion

The synapses of different morphological types are thus not uniformly distributed over the motor neuron surface. Synapses seem to be more abundant on the dendrites than on the cell body, and synapses containing flattened synaptic vesicles after aldehyde-fixation, F-type, occur more frequently on the cell body and axon hillock than on the dendrites, whereas the reverse is true for synapses containing spherical synaptic vesicles, the S-type. Large synapses having a sub-synaptic cistern, C-type, are confined to the cell body and proximal parts of the dendrites. Due to the time-consuming procedures required to make quantitative studies of synapses, only very small amounts of material have been studied, usually from single ultrathin sections, and caution must be exercised in the interpretation of such data. Indeed, very little is known either of the synaptology of the single cell or of possible differences between cells, and therefore we have in this laboratory begun to make counts of synapses on sections taken at regular intervals through single motor neurons. With this method, individual dendrites can also be traced and comparisons can be made between different dendrites: the spectrum of boutons on the motor neuron cell body appears to be about the same, regardless of the level along the rostrocaudal axis.

5.3.7 *Discussion of the origin and function of the synapses on the motor neurons*

Origin of the boutons

Much work remains before the synaptic boutons, as seen in the microscope, can be classified with confidence according to their origin and functions, if, indeed, that ideal can ever be attained. The three main sources of the synapses are the dorsal root; the higher centres and the interneurons in the cord. Of these three the vast majority of the boutons are derived from spinal interneurons, the short course of whose fibres rendering them difficult of access for neuroanatomical studies, at least using traditional degeneration experiments.

Most tracts descending in the spinal cord terminate in laminae IV–VII, probably in the main on interneurons (Nyberg-Hansen 1966, 1969; see Kuypers, 1973). Monosynaptic excitation of lumbar alpha motor neurons in the cat has been described from the vestibulospinal and reticulospinal tracts (Lund and Pompeiano, 1968; Grillner and Lund, 1968; Grillner, Hongo and Lund, 1966, 1970), and both flexor and extensor motor neurons receive such contacts. The vestibulospinal synapses are thought to be located on or near the cell bodies (Grillner, Hongo and Lund, 1970), whereas the reticulospinal synapses are believed to be located distally on the dendrites. Descending tracts also form inhibitory monosynaptic contacts with the motor neurons (see Wilson and Yoshida, 1969). In regard to links with the pyramidal tract and the red nucleus, monosynaptic connections with the spinal motor neurons seem to be formed to a higher degree in primates than in subprimates (see Granit, 1970 p. 203; Shapovalov, 1972). The pyramidal tract of the cat terminates in laminae V—VII (Scheibel and Scheibel, 1966) and it has not been possible to determine anatomically whether it makes direct contacts with the dendrites of the motor neurons passing through these regions.

Ultrastructural studies of the boutons on cat lumbosacral motor neurons have been performed after hemisection of the spinal cord (McLaughlin 1972c; Rogers, 1972). After a thoracic hemisection (Rogers, 1972), there was a sparse ipsilateral degeneration of boutons, mainly of the S-type, although some obviously degenerating F-boutons were also seen. The degeneration observed occurred on cell bodies as well as on proximal, and presumably also on distal, parts of the dendrites. Following cord transection at the second lumbar segment (McLaughlin, 1972c), there was massive degeneration of boutons of both the S- and F-types on the motor neurons in the segments just below the level of the transection, while at lower lumbar segments, there was a sparse degeneration, similar to that described above. In none of the cases were the C- or M-boutons affected. The massive degeneration was thought to be due to interruption of the axons of interneurons with short axons (see Sterling and Kuypers, 1968), but in both accounts it is pointed out that the remote degeneration was probably due to interruption of both the tracts of supraspinal origin and the long propriospinal tracts, the light-microscopic appearance of which have been studied by Barilari and Kuypers (1969). Matsushita and Ikeda (1973), studying the synapses on cervical motor neurons in the cat after thoracic or lower cervical lesions, found degeneration of S-, F-, and some C-boutons: these are thought to be derived from ascending propriospinal fibres.

In conclusion, it seems clear from these studies that both the S- and F-boutons found on the motor neurons are of heterogenous origin. Mapping out the distribution on the motor neuron surface of its various synaptic inputs will require quantitative studies of synaptic degeneration after a wide range of lesions, or the use of refined tracer techniques.

The functions of the different types of synapses

As mentioned earlier, there are some arguments in favour of the concept that F-boutons are inhibitory, and it is certainly true that this hypothesis has not yet been disproved. On the contrary, the recent demonstration of the labelling of F-boutons in spinal cord slices with radioactive glycine (Matus and Dennison, 1971), thought to be an inhibitory transmitter in the spinal cord, favours such an idea. This correlation of F-boutons with an inhibitory transmitter would therefore imply a predominance of inhibitory synapses on the motor neuron cell bodies. Asphyxia of the spinal cord is followed by rigidity of the hind limbs and this is thought to be the result of mass destruction of largely inhibitory interneurons. Light-microscopically, there is a marked loss of boutons on the motor neurons, which is most obvious on the cell bodies (Gelfan and Rapisarda, 1964), and this accords with the presumed predominance of inhibitory synapses in this location.

If there is a tendency for inhibitory synapses to predominate on the cell body, decreasing distally along the dendrites, then the localizaton of the C-boutons is compatible with their also having an inhibitory function. The assumption that inhibitory boutons contain flattened vesicles after aldehyde fixation does not necessarily imply that all the boutons containing spherical vesicles are excitatory, and boutons, similar to the C-boutons, are formed by the presumed inhibitory endings of the olivocochlear bundle (Smith and Rasmussen, 1965; Wersäll, 1968).

Physiological aspects of the localization of synapses on the motor neurons

The physiological evidence for the localization of inhibitory synapses on the motor neuron surface is conflicting. Eccles (1964) has argued that these synapses are restricted to the cell bodies, and computations based on the neuron model (Rall *et al.*, 1967), likewise lead to the assumption that the inhibitory synapses should be located on or near to the cell bodies, whereas the excitatory synapses should be distributed over the entire cell surface. Somewhat different predictions concerning the location of synapses have been derived from physiological experiments concerned with recording changes in the impulse frequency of the motor neurons rather than their intracellular potential changes. It has also been stated that inhibitory synapses may be located on the distal dendrites, possibly exerting different effects on the impulse-frequency characteristics of the motor neuron than when located on, or near, the cell body (Granit, Kernell and Lamarre, 1966; Kernell, 1971).

The location of the inhibitory synapses on the motor neurons may, however, vary with different inhibitory synaptic inputs to the motor neuron. It has been argued that the inhibitory Renshaw synapses are located mainly on the proximal parts of the motor neuron dendrites, while the inhibitory synapses mediating the reciprocal inhibition to antagonists in the stretch reflex, usually called IA inhibition, are located on the motor neuron cell bodies (Burke, Fedina and Lundberg, 1971). Through the use of intracellular dye injection, the IA interneurons have been recognized morphologically and have been found to be situated in lamina VII, just dorsomedial the motor neurons (Jankowska and Lindström, 1972). The description of site and morphological characteristics of these interneurons and the Renshaw cells may facilitate future morphological investigations of their connections.

Excitatory and inhibitory synapses are probably not distributed uniformly on all motor neurons. 'Tonic' motor neurons are believed to be subjected to a stronger influence from both Renshaw (Granit *et al.*, 1957) and IA (Burke, Jankowska and ten Bruggencate, 1970) inhibition, as well as from the dorsal roots (Burke, 1968), than are 'phasic' motor neurons. Inhibition from cutaneous afferents and the red nucleus also show a tendency to exceed excitation from these sources on 'tonic' motor neurons, whereas the reverse is true for the 'phasic' motor neurons (Burke, Jankowska and ten Bruggencate, 1970). Thus when studying the anatomical counterparts of excitatory and inhibitory influences, it is an advantage to be able to recognize motor neurons with different physiological properties. In a study at present in progress, an attempt is being made to characterize morphologically individual cat motor neurons with different functions, using ultrastructural studies of serial sections of neurons identified by intracellular deposition of the fluorescent dye 'Procion yellow', following physiological recording with an intracellular microelectrode (Berthold, Kellerth and Conradi in progress). Studies of the central parts of two 'tonic' soleus motor neurons and two 'phasic' gastrocnemius motor neurons have revealed a drastic difference in the occurrence of the C-boutons between the two kinds of neurons. These boutons occur only sporadically on the 'tonic' neurons, whereas they form clusters around the dendritic roots and on the axon hillock of the 'phasic' neurons.

5.4 Some aspects of the morphology of the motor neurons during development

As has been mentioned earlier, the motor neurons offer a favourable field for developmental studies since the knowledge of the physiology of these cells in the adult stage is comparatively extensive. Correlations betwen disciplines on developmental material are however limited due to the fact that the changing situation during development has received much less study than have the corresponding phenomena in the adult state. There are also species differences in regard to both the speed and the sequence of the various developmental stages, leading to terminological difficulties. More information will be gained from a number of studies on one species, for example the cat, knowledge of the adult stage of which is outstanding, rather than from a corresponding effort directed towards many species (Skoglund, 1969).

Those features of motor neuron morphology which, from a functional point of view, seem most pertinent in the adult, namely the morphological definition of the cells, their dimensions, and the architecture and distribution of boutons on the cell surface, will also be of interest in developmental studies. Their signficance may differ however due to the dynamic nature of the relationships existing between the constituents of developing tissues. A brief description will be given, with emphasis on these points and attention will be concentrated on the cat lumbosacral motor neurons and the changes therein during the first postnatal weeks, during the course of which the animal acquires the ability to use its hind limbs to stand and walk.

5.4.1 *Embryology*

The motor neurons are the first cells to be detached from the neuroepithelium in the embryonic spinal cord. Studies such as those of Nornes and Das (1972), employing thymidine labelling in the rat, have shown that the motor neurons are formed in a rostrocaudal order, with the detachment beginning ventrally in each segment. The first formed neurons are subsequently pushed laterally by the continuing central cellular proliferation. At first the motor neurons are densely packed, but with the subsequent formation of the axon and small dendrites their separation gradually increases throughout that long period during which the constituents of the neuropil are formed and grow. The fine structure of such embryonic motor neurons has been studied in the monkey by Bodian (1966d), who paid particular attention to correlations between the formation of synapses and the occurrence of first limb movements. The embryonic motor neurons have a comparatively large nucleus and the cytoplasm contains abundant endoplasmic reticulum. In the early stages, when no movements can be elicited, there are no boutons on the motor neurons, but in the neuropil many 'growth cones' are visible, i.e. swollen bulbs containing large vesicles at the ends of axons and dendrites. Somewhat later, with the onset of local spontaneous and reflex movements, some boutons containing a few synaptic vesicles can be found on the proximal parts of the primitive motor neuron dendrites; these vesicles are spherical following aldehyde fixation, a finding which has been interpreted to indicate an excitory character for these synapses; some of these boutons are apparently formed by growth cones. It is known from studies on tissue cultures (Bunge, Bunge and Peterson, 1967) that the electrical activity of the tissue changes markedly when the first synaptic complexes are formed. By the time at which long intersegmental reflexes and co-ordinated movements can be detected (Bodian, Melby and Taylor, 1968) the majority of the motor neurons had been pushed apart, although some cell bodies were still apposed. Fewer growth cones were visible and the boutons were somewhat larger and could be found on both the cell bodies and dendrites, although well separated. About 1/3 of the boutons at this stage belonged to the F-type, and the authors have pointed out the coincidence between the time of appearance of these boutons and the animal's ability to perform alternate movements. Vaughn and Grieshaber (1973), studying rat motor neurons, likewise observed that the earliest synapses are found on the proximal parts of the dendrites, with a predominance of S-boutons during the pre-reflex period. They followed the subsequent formation of synapses quantitatively, and found that the development of synapses on the motor neurons is always in advance of that seen on more dorsally placed interneurons.

5.4.2 *Postnatal development of spinal motor neurons in the cat*

The structure and connections of cat spinal motor neurons in the period when the major skeletomotor abilities are acquired will be described in some detail in this and the following sections. Unless it is specifically indicated otherwise the results refer to an ultrastructural study of cat motor neurons (Conradi and Skoglund, 1969a, b), which formed part of a larger series of functional studies on this animal, directed by the late S. Skoglund (see Skoglund, 1966).

Physiological background

The gradually acquired ability to stand and walk during the first three postnatal weeks parallels the development of the tonic stretch reflex (Skoglund, 1960a), which proceeds according to the cranio-caudal rule (Kingsbury, 1932), and in a proximo-distal direction in the extremities. This tonic stretch reflex is absent in the newborn kitten. Apart from the lack of tonic discharge from the muscle spindles in the newborn kitten (Skoglund, 1960a), the afferent fibres are not able to transmit impulses at high frequency (cf. Wilson, 1962), and as has been shown ultrastructurally, the future large myelinated peripheral fibres in the roots have to pass through a period of loss of internodes and remodelling of the nodes of Ranvier (Berthold, 1968), before attaining adult electrical properties.

Despite being unable to transmit the tonic stretch reflex, extensor motor neurons in the hindlimbs can be activated from other sources in the newborn kitten, for example in the crossed extensor reflex (Skoglund, 1960a). The monosynaptic connection from the dorsal root is also present in the newborn kitten (Skoglund, 1960b), but cannot sustain impulses with the same frequency as in the adult (Mellström, 1971a). Indeed the motor neurons are more readily excitable through the dorsal root than are adult motor neurons (Kellerth, Mellström and Skoglund, 1971), and this excitability decreases with age. Progress in this respect proceeds faster in flexor motor neurons than in extensor motor neurons (Mellström, 1971a), and measurements of calibre spectra of motor nerves also show an earlier growth of those supplying flexor muscles (Mellström, 1971b). There is in general a dominance of flexor motor neurons in the newborn kitten, with a strong and long-lasting late inhibition of the extensors from the flexors (Skoglund, 1960c), and easily elicited flexor reflexes (Ekholm, 1967). Renshaw inhibition is also detectable in the newborn stage (Naka, 1964b; Mellström, 1971b).

Ultrastructure of cat motor neurons from birth onwards

At birth, the nerve cells in the ventral horn are densely packed, and in some cases there is direct apposition between adjacent motor neuron cell bodies. Two

314

classes of cells can be distinguished by size and the cell bodies of the bigger ones, assumed to be alpha motor neurons, have a diameter of 25–40 μm. At one month postnatally, the motor neurons have still not achieved their adult separation. The nucleus of the motor neurons of young animals is prominent, the cytosplasm often containing glycogen-like particles, while the mitochondria are small during the first postnatal weeks. During the entire first postnatal month, the dendrites seen to project from the motor neurons are comparatively thin. The axon hillock has the same diameter as the initial axon segment in the early stages and both are again comparatively thin, the latter having about half the diameter, but the same length, in the newborn as in the adult. Physiologically, the motor neurons of young kittens resist invasion with antidromic impulses (Naka, 1964), which may be a consequence of the small diameter of the initial axon segment when compared to the size of the cell body. Even at birth, the central part of the motor axon is myelinated (cf. Windle, 1930), in contrast to nearly all the other fibres in the ventral horn. Only a thin rim of extracellular material is present around the nodes of Ranvier at birth, the adult appearance being reached at about one month of age (see also Hildebrand, 1971b).

Neuropil. The most characteristic feature of the neuropil at birth is the absence of myelin and the majority of the fibres are not myelinated until the end of the first postnatal month, or even later. The densely packed neuropil contains the same cellular elements as in the adult. The glial cells are still immature during the first period after birth (see Vaughn, 1969), and some glial mitoses can be observed in the earlier developmental stages.

Synapses. At birth, boutons contact the motor neuron cell membrane at all points. They appear to be evenly distributed and are as a rule tightly packed and much smaller than in the adult. During the first postnatal period, boutons are apposed to the initial motor axon segment, in contrast to the situation seen in the adult (see below). In addition to the synaptic vesicles, the boutons contain a few small mitochondria and, often, glycogen-like particles (see Vaughn and Grieshaber, 1972). Small synaptic complexes are usually found, and unlike the situation in the adult, many of the boutons on motor neuron cell bodies and proximal parts of the dendrites establish synaptic contact with yet another neural profile, usually a small dendrite. By three weeks the boutons have grown considerably and those establishing double contacts are observed less frequently. Neither in the newborn nor at later stages are any growth cones visible in the neuropil or signs of the formation of new synaptic complexes (for criteria for distinguishing the latter, see Bodian, 1966d; Wechsler, 1966). Even in the newborn the boutons can be classified according to the same criteria as those used in the adult, and definite S-, T-, F- and C-type boutons are present at birth. M-boutons are not observed until the third postnatal week.

5.4.3 *Quantitative aspects of the growth of cat spinal motor neurons and the distribution of synapses*

Motor neuron size

Since the size of a neuron is thought to influence its excitability (Henneman, Somjen and Carpenter, 1965), the small volume of the motor neurons at birth might provide one reason for their high excitability at that time. This possibility has stimulated quantitative studies of volume changes of the motor neuron cell bodies in the cat during their development (Mellström and Skoglund, 1969). At birth the size range of the neuron cell bodies in lamina IV of L7 in the kitten is very limited, and the volumes of most cell bodies do not exceed $3000 \, \mu m^3$. Considerable growth occurs during the first two postnatal months, the biggest neurons growing much more rapidly than the smaller ones, and from birth on, the mean cell body volume increases six times or more. Growth is very slight during the first two postnatal weeks, and is at its most rapid between the third and sixth weeks after birth, during which period there is a rapid decrease in motor neuron excitability.

There are no quantitative studies on the growth of the motor neuron dendrites after birth, although Sakla (1959), in a study on the mouse, has reported a considerable postnatal growth. From Golgi studies in the kitten, Scheibel and Scheibel (1970b, 1971), have stated that the dendrite bundles (see above) are already formed at birth in the cervical spinal cord of the cat, whereas they develop during the second postnatal week in the lumbosacral region.

Synaptology

The dorsal root boutons. In the newborn kitten there are no clearcut M-boutons, but on the proximal parts of the dendrites some comparatively big boutons can be observed, $1-3 \, \mu m$ in diameter and containing spherical synaptic vesicles. On the convex side of these boutons, another bouton is apposed, having small synaptic vesicles of irregular shape. After dorsal root section in newborn animals, the big boutons appear to undergo the dense type of degeneration (for details see Walberg, 1964; McMahan, 1967), which is not seen in the adult cat. The location of these boutons appeared to be similar to that of the M-boutons in the adult. From three weeks onwards, identifiable M-boutons appear, reacting to dorsal root section as they would in the adult. No signs could be found of a marked change in the number and distribution of the dorsal root boutons on the motor neurons during the development.

Size and distribution of boutons of different types

In an attempt to discover whether there are any changes in the size and distribution of the boutons on the motor neurons which might parallel the changes in reflex behaviour with age, a quantitative study was carried out on single transverse sections through peroneus motor neurons at the seventh lumbar segment in two newborn kittens (Conradi and Skoglund, 1969a), in a similar fashion to that performed in the adult (see above).

Cell body and dendrites. It was found that even at birth, there is a higher proportion of F-boutons on the cell bodies than on the dendrites, just as in the adult, and the reverse is likewise true for the S-boutons. The C-boutons are restricted to cell bodies and proximal parts of the dendrites, again as in the adult. The mean lengths of apposition of the S- and F-bouton profiles differ little in the newborn, being 0.7 and 0.9 μm respectively, as compared to 1.7 to 2.1 μm in the adult, implying that while the mean length increases about twice, the increase is somewhat greater in the F-boutons. The growth of the C- and M-boutons after birth is somewhat greater. If the proportion of the different bouton types is corrected for mean length of the profiles, there are only slight changes in the proportion of different types of boutons during development at the regions studied. Generally, the increase in mean length of the bouton profiles exceeds that of the motor neuron cell body outline. The mean minor diameter of the motor neuron cell bodies at birth was found in the present material to be 29 μm (20 profiles), as compared to 49 μm in the adult. If it can be assumed that the postnatal growth of a structure reflects its maturity at birth, it would appear that the S-boutons are somewhat more developed than the F-boutons at birth.

The membrane covered by boutons is the greatest on the proximal parts of the dendrites in the newborn. When the values for the cover provided by the different bouton types are studied and compared with the adult, some unexpected tendencies are revealed (From Conradi and Skoglund, 1969a approximate values):

	Cell body		Prox. dendrite		Dist. dendrite	
Bouton type	newb. %	adult %	newb. %	adult %	newb. %	adult %
S(+T)-	20	13	27	25	23	24
F-	28	27	30	40	20	24
C-	3	7	2	6	0.2	0.5
M-	0.3		1.3	1.9	0.1	0.2
Total	51	47	60	73	43	49

It will be seen that the covering of the F-boutons increases on the proximal parts of the dendrites, whereas there is a small decrease on the cell bodies; and the covering of the S-boutons decreases noticeably on the cell bodies. There is also a higher mean total of bouton profiles apposed at the motor neuron cell bodies in single sections through the nuclear plane in the newborn (53) than in the adult (34).

In analyses of serial sections through the proximal part of a motor neuron dendrite in the newborn, the boutons seemed to be distributed at random, as in the adult, but about one-fifth of the boutons established double synaptic contacts, whereas very few do so in the adult. Within an area of 100 μm^2, there were about 80 boutons in the newborn, compared to about 20 in the adult.

Axon hillock, initial axon segment

As has been previously mentioned boutons are found on the initial axon segment in the newborn, and these have disappeared by three weeks. In order to study the proportion of boutons on these regions, reconstructions were made from serial sections on material from two newborn kittens. On the axon hillock, the total number of boutons was comparable to that in the adult, and the proportions of the synaptic types were also similar about two-thirds of the boutons being of the F-type. On the initial axon segment, there were 19 and 15 boutons, respectively, in two cases, about half being F-type and the rest S-type.

5.4.4 Discussion of postnatal changes in motor neuron synaptology of the cat. Removal of boutons

There are considerable difficulties connected with quantitative estimations of boutons during development. For practical reasons, the material has to be small, and this factor, together with contingent sampling difficulties, renders precise quantitation impossible. However some of the tendencies observed in our study appeared to be quite consistent, and will be discussed.

Growth of the motor neurons may in itself have physiological implications, and the fact that the dendrites are very thin at early stages could point to a comparatively greater influence of the boutons on the cell body at that time. It is possible that the relative predominance of S-boutons on the cell bodies and the proximal parts of the dendrites of motor neurons assumed to belong to the peroneus nucleus, could provide the basis for the high excitability and functional predominance of flexor motor neurons in the early postnatal state (see Skoglund, 1966); however nothing is known at present about the spectrum of boutons on extensor motor neurons, either in the adult or during development.

The significance of the presence of boutons on the initial axon segment in younger animals is not clear but these boutons must be very effective in governing the impulse-activity of the motor neurons. There are no clear physiological findings which might provide confirmatory evidence for the presence of these boutons, although Purpura, Shofer and Scarff (1965), studying postsynaptic potentials in immature neocortex of the cat, point to the possibility of the presence of such synapses, but no morphological evidence was included. There are thus several boutons localized on the initial axon segment of the motor nerons of the newborn kitten, in contrast to the situation at three weeks or in the adult. From studies of a large number of completely serially sectioned initial motoraxon segments taken during the first three postnatal weeks

(Ronnevi, to be published), it seems clear, that the boutons become removed during the second week after birth. As to the mode of operation of the process of removal, the boutons seem to undergo a spontaneously occurring phago-cytosis by means of extensions of immature astrocytes (see Ronnevi and Conradi, 1974). Thus, boutons can be observed during this period to be partly detached from the motor neuron surface through the intervention of thin astrocytic processes, and some boutons can be shown by serial sectioning to be completely engulfed by astrocytes. Astrocytic extensions containing boutons undergoing dissolution can also be seen during this period. Interestingly, exactly the same phenomena can be observed on the motor neuron cell bodies and dendrites during the same period of time, why there seems to be a generalized phagocytosis of boutons on the motor neuron surface during the second postnatal week, which is just before the period of rapid growth of the motor neurons.

In an attempt to quantify the total loss of boutons from the motor neuron cell body from birth on, the previously mentioned data on mean size and covering of the boutons and the mean size of the motor neuron cell bodies in the newborn and adult stages can be used. It has been calculated that altogether about half of the S- and F-boutons get lost after birth, whereas the postnatal loss of the C-boutons is probably somewhat smaller (Conradi and Ronnevi, 1975). Whether the whole of this calculated loss of boutons on the motor neuron cell bodies occurs during the second postnatal week, as it does on the initial motoraxon segment, could, however, not be stated with certainty.

Although the exact functional counterpart of this massive elimination of boutons on the motor neurons after birth is not known, the process must influence the impulse-activity of the motor neurons, particularly when removing boutons from the initial axon segment.

The presence of degenerative processes operating in the central nervous system during the development has been recognized since Long (see Levi-Montalcini, 1964; Källén, 1965; Bodian, 1966c; Wechsler, 1966). The observa-tions refer to the embryonic period, when there occurs massive death of neurons in varying regions, including the spinal cord. Recently, Das and Hines (1972) have also described degeneration of a reticulospinal fibre system in embryonic rats. Since all these observations have been made at earlier developmental stages than the one dealt with above, the postnatal removal of boutons on cat spinal motor neurons might not be a reflection of massive neuronal death – such a neuronal death has not been described at least in the spinal cord, during the weeks after birth in the cat. It would indeed be of interest to know whether there is a considerable loss of boutons after birth also in other regions of the CNS. The process of bouton elimination could be a mechanism for the uncoupling of connections, being present only at earlier developmental stages.

5.5 Conclusion

It will be evident from the preceding discussion that accurate morphological data are of great importance to the study of a variety of aspects of the functions of central nervous tissue. A quantitative approach to such morphology is often needed, and a wider application of quantitative methods to studies of neuronal circuitry is urgently required. The spinal motor neuron is a suitable subject for such studies, particularly that of the cat in which there are many possibilities for correlations between morphology and physiological observations. While it is today technically possible to map the distribution of synapses on relatively large areas of the surface membrane of individual neurons, using single or serial ultrathin sections in the electron microscope, little work of this kind has been published to date. Perhaps surprisingly the major obstacle to progress in this field seems, at present, to be the large amount of time and labour required for such studies. However, the introduction of semi-automatic analytical systems presents a prospect of the extension of quantitative neuro-anatomical studies into many new and fascinating dimensions.

References

Aitken J. and Bridger, J. (1961) Neuron size and neuron population density in the lumbosacral region of cat spinal cord. *Journal of Anatomy*, 95, 38–53.

Akert, K., Pfenninger, K., Sandri, C. and Moor, H. (1972) Freeze-etching and cytochemistry of vesicles and membrane complexes in synapses of the central nervous system. In *Structure and function of synapses*, (eds.) Pappas, G. D. and Purpura, D. P., pp. 67–86, Raven Press, New York.

Andres, K. H. (1965) Über die Feinstruktur besonderer Einrichtungen in markhaltigen Nervenfasern des Kleinhirns der Ratte. *Zeitschrift für Zellforschung und Mikroskopische Anatomie*, 65, 701–702.

Balthasar, K. (1952) Morphologie der spinalen Tibialis- under Peroneus-Kerne bei der Katze. *Archiv für Psychiatrie und Neurologie*, 188, 345–378.

Barilari, M. G. and Kuypers, H. G. J. M. (1969) Propriospinal fibers interconnecting the spinal enlargements in the cat. *Brain Research*, 14, 321–330.

Barr, M. L. (1939) Some observations on the morphology of the synapse in the cat's spinal cord. *Journal of Anatomy*, 74, 1–11.

Barrett, J. N., Grill, W. E. (1971) Specific membrane resistivity of dye-injected cat motoneurons. *Brain Research*, 28, 556–561.

Barrett, J. N., Graubard, K. (1970) Fluorescent staining of cat motoneurons in vivo with beveled micropipettes. *Brain Research*, 18, 565–568.

Barron, K. D., Daniels, A. C., Chiang, T. Y. and Doolin, P. F. (1970) Fine structure of chromatolytic motoneurons. *Experimental and Molecular Pathology*, 12, 46–57.

Berthold, C.-H. (1963) Ultrastructure of the node-paranode region of mature feline ventral lumbar spinal-root fibres. *Acta Societatis Medicorum Upsaliensis*, Suppl. 9, 37–70.

Berthold, C. -H. (1968) Ultrastructure of postnatally developing peripheral nodes of Ranvier. *Acta Societatis Medicorum Upsaliensis*, 73, 145–168.

Berthold, C. -H., Conradi, S. and Kellerth, J. -O. To be published.

Blinzinger, K. and Kreutzberg, G. (1968) Displacement of synaptic terminals from regenerating motoneurons by microglial cells. *Zeitschrift für Zellforschung und Mikroskopische Anatomie*, 85, 145–157.

Bodian, D. (1964) An electron microscopic study of the monkey spinal cord. *Bulletin of Johns Hopkins Hospital*, 114, 13–119.

Bodian, D. (1966a) Electron microscopy: Two major synaptic types on spinal motoneurons. *Science*, 151, 1093–1094.

Bodian, D. (1966b) Synaptic types on spinal motoneurons. An electron microscopic study. *Bulletin of Johns Hopkins Hospital*, 119, 16–45.

Bodian, D. (1966c) Spontaneous degeneration in the spinal cord of monkey fetuses. *Bulletin of Johns Hopkins Hospital*, 119, 212–234.

Bodian, D. (1966d) Development of fine structure of spinal cord of monkey fetuses. I: The motoneuron neuropile at the time of onset of reflex activity. *Bulletin of Johns Hopkins Hospital,* 119, 129–149.

Bodian, D. (1970) An electron microscopic characterization of classes of synaptic vesicles by means of controlled aldehyde fixation. *Journal of Cell Biology,* **44** 115–124.

Bodian, D. (1972) Synaptic diversity and characterization by electron microscopy. In *Structure and function of synapses,* (eds.) Pappas, G. D. and Purpura, D. P., p. 45–65, Raven Press, New York.

Bodian, D., Melby, E. C. jr. and Taylor, N. (1968) Development of fine structure of spinal cord in monkey fetuses II: Pre-reflex period to period of long intersegmental reflexes. *Journal of Comparative Neurology,* 133, 113–166.

Bok, S. T. (1928) Das Rückenmark. In *Möllendorffs Handbuch der mikroskopischen Anatomie des Menschens.* Bd. IV/1, s. 478–578.

Bryan, R. N., Trevino, D. L. and Willis, W. D. (1972) Evidence for a common location of alpha and gamma motoneurons. *Brain Research,* 38, 193–196.

van Buren, J. M. and Frank, K. (1965) Correlation between the morphology and potential field of a spinal motor nucleus in the cat. *Electroencephalography and Clinical Neurophysiology,* 19, 112–126.

Bunge, M. B., Bunge, R. P. and Peterson, E. R. (1967) The onset of synapse formation in spinal cord cultures as studied by electron microscopy. *Brain Research,* 6, 728–749.

Bunge, R. P. (1968) Glial cells and the central myelin sheath. *Physiological Reviews,* 43, 197–251.

Burke, R. E. (1967) Motor unit types of cat triceps surae muscle. *Journal of Physiology,* 193, 141–160.

Burke R. E. (1968) Group IA synaptic input to fast and slow twitch motor units of cat triceps surae. *Journal of Physiology,* 196, 605–630.

Burke, R. E. (1973) On the central nervous control of fast and slow twitch motor units. In *New Developments in Electromyography and Clinical Neurophysiology,* (ed.) Desmedt, J. E., Vol. 3, pp. 69–94. Karger: Basel.

Burke, R. E and ten Bruggencate, G. (1971) Electronic characteristics of alpha motoneurons of varying size. *Journal of Physiology,* 212, 1–20.

Burke, R. E., Fedina, L. and Lundberg, A. (1971) Spatial synaptic distribution of recurrent and group IA inhibitory systems in cat spinal motoneurons. *Journal of Physiology,* 214, 305–326.

Burke, R. E., Jankowska, E. and ten Bruggencate, G. (1970) A comparison of peripheral and rubrospinal synaptic input to slow and fast twitch motor units of triceps surae. *Journal of Physiology,* 207, 709–732.

Burke, R. E., Levine, D. N. and Zajac, F. E. III (1971) Mammalian motor units: Physiological histochemical correlation in three types in cat gastrocnemius. *Science,* 174, 709–732.

Campa, J. F. and Engel, W. K. (1970) Histochemistry of motor neurons and interneurons in the cat lumbar spinal cord. *Neurology,* 20, 559–568.

Campos-Ortega, J. A., Glees, P. and Neuhoff, V. (1968) Ultrastructural analysis of individual layers in the lateral geniculate body of the monkey. *Zeitschrift für Zellforschung und Mikroskopische Anatomie,* 87, 82–100.

Carpenter, M. B., Stein, B. M. and Shriver, J. -E. (1968) Central projections of spinal dorsal roots in the monkey. II: Lower thoracic, lumbosacral and coccygeal dorsal roots. *American Journal of Anatomy,* 123, 75–118.

Charlton, B. T. and Gray, E. G. (1966) Comparative electron microscopy of synapses in the vertebrate spinal cord. *Journal of Cell Science,* 1, 67–80.

Chu, L. W. (1954) A cytological study of anterior horn cells isolated from human spinal cord. *Journal of Comparative Neurology,* 100, 381–413.

Colonnier, M. (1968) Synaptic patterns on different cell types in the different laminae of the cat visual cortex. An electron microscopic study. *Brain Research,* 9, 268–287.

Conradi, S. (1966) Ultrastructural specialization of the initial axon segment of cat lumbar motoneurons. Preliminary observations. *Acta Societatis Medicorum Upsaliensis,* 71, 281–284.

Conradi, S. (1969a) Ultrastructure and distribution of neuronal and glial elements on the motoneuron surface in the lumbosacral spinal cord of the adult cat. *Acta Physiologica Scandinavica,* Suppl. 332, 5–48.

Conradi, S. (1969b) Ultrastructure and distribution of neuronal and glial elements on the surface of the proximal part of a motoneuron dendrite as analyzed by serial sections. *Acta Physiologica Scandinavica,* Suppl. 332, 49–64.

Conradi, S. (1969c) Observations on the ultrastructure of the axon hillock and initial axon segment of lumbosacral motoneurons in the cat. *Acta Physiologica Scandinavica.* Suppl. 332, 65–84.

Conradi, S. (1969d) Ultrastructure of dorsal root boutons on lumbosacral motoneurons of the adult cat, as revealed by dorsal root section. *Acta Physiologica Scandinavica,* Suppl. 332, 85–115.

Conradi, S. and Skoglund, S. (1969a) Observations on the ultrastructure and distribution of neuronal and glial elements on the motoneuron surface in the lumbosacral spinal cord of the cat during postnatal development. *Acta Physiologica Scandinavica,* Suppl. 333, 5–52.

Conradi, S. and Skoglund, S. (1969b) Observations on the ultrastructure of the initial motoraxon segment and dorsal root boutons on the motoneurons in the lumbosacral spinal cord of the cat during postnatal development. *Acta Physiologica Scandinavica,* Suppl. 333, 53–76.

Conradi, S. and Ronnevi, L.-O. (1975) Spontaneous elimination of synapses on cat spinal motoneurons after birth: Do half of the synapses on the cell bodies disappear? *Brain Research,* 92, 505–510.

Coombs, J. S., Curtis, D. R. and Eccles, J. C. (1957) The generation of impulses in motoneurons. *Journal of Physiology* 39, 232–249.

Coombs, J. S., Curtis, D. R. and Eccles, J. C. (1959) The electrical constants of the motoneurone membrane. *Journal of Physiology,* 145, 505–528.

Cooper, S. and Sherrington, C. S. (1940) Gower's tract and the spinal border cells. *Brain,* 63, 123–134.

Das, G. D. and Hines, R. J. (1972) Nature and significance of spontaneous degeneration of axons in the pyramidal tract. *Zeitschrift für Anatomie und Entwicklungsgeschichte,* 136, 98–114.

Deiters, O. (1865) *Untersuchungen über Gehirn und Rückenmark des Menschen und der Säugethiere.* Vieweg u. Sohn, Braunschweig.

Dekker, J. J., Lawrence, D. G. and Kuypers, H. G. J. M. (1973) The location of longitudinally running dendrites in the ventral horn of the cat spinal cord. *Brain Research,* 51, 319–325.

Dennison, E. M. (1971) Electron microscopy as a means of classifying synaptic vesicles. *Journal of Cell Sciences,* 8, 525–539.

Eccles, J. C. (1957) *The Physiology of Nerve Cells.* Johns Hopkins Press, Baltimore.

Eccles, J. C. (1964) *The Physiology of synapses.* Springer Verlag, Heidelberg.

Eccles, J. C., Fatt, P. and Koketsu, K. (1954) Cholinergic and inhibitory synapses in a pathway from motor-axon collaterals to motoneurones. *Journal of Physiology,* 126, 524–562.

Eccles, J. C. and Sherrington, C. (1930) Numbers and contraction values of individual motor-units examined in some muscles of the limb. *Proceedings of the Royal Society London (Series B),* 106, 326–357.

Ekholm, J. (1967) Postnatal changes in cutaneous reflexes and in the discharge pattern of cutaneous and articular sense organs. *Acta Physiologica Scandinavica,* Suppl. 297, 1–130.

Eldred, E., Swett, J. E., Buchwald, J. S. and Bridgman, C. F. (1961) Relationships of spinal efferent outflow to position of motor units in medial gastrocnemius. *Federation Proceedings,* 20/1, Part II, s. 346.

Frank, K. and Fuortes, M. G. F. (1957) Presynaptic and postsynaptic inhibition of monosynaptic reflexes. *Federation Proceedings,* 16, 39–40.

Fuortes, M. G. F., Frank, K. and Baker, M. C. (1957) Steps in the production of motoneuron spikes. *Journal of General Physiology,* 40, 735–752.

Gelfan, S. (1963) Neurone and synapse populations in the spinal cord: indication of role in total integration. *Nature,* 198, 162–163.

Gelfan S. (1964) Neuronal interdependance. *Progress in Brain Research,* 11, 238–258.

Gelfan, S., Kao, G. and Ling, H. (1972) The dendrite tree of spinal neurons in dogs with experimental hind-limb rigidity. *Journal of Comparative Neurology,* 146, 143–174.

Gelfan, S., Kao, G. and Ruchkin, D. S. (1970) The dendritic tree of spinal neurons. *Journal of Comparative Neurology,* 139, 385–412.

Gelfan, S. and Rapisarda, A. F. (1964) Synaptic density on spinal neurons of normal dogs and dogs with experimental hindlimb rigidity. *Journal of Comparative Neurology,* 123, 73–96.

Granit, R. (1970) *The Basis of Motor Control,* Academic Press: London and New York.

Granit, R., Kellerth, J. -O. and Williams, T. D. (1964) 'Adjacent' and 'remote' postsynaptic inhibition in motoneurones stimulated by muscle stretch. *Journal of Physiology,* 174, 453–472.

Granit, R., Kernell, D. and Williams, T. D. (1966) Algebraic summation in synaptic activation of motoneurons firing within the 'primary range' to injected currents. *Journal of Physiology,* 187, 379–399.

Granit, R., Pascoe, J. E. and Steg, G. (1957) The behaviour of tonic alpha and gamma motor neurons during stimulation of recurrent collaterals. *Journal of Physiology,* 138, 381–400.

Grant, G. (1970) Neuronal changes central to the site of axon transection. A method for the identification of retrograde changes in perikarya, dendrites and axons by silver impregnation. In *Contemporary Research Methods in Neuroanatomy,* (eds.) Nauta, W. J. H. and Ebbesson, S. O. E., pp. 173–185, Springer-Verlag, Berlin.

Gray, E. G. (1963) Electron microscopy of presynaptic organelles of the spinal cord. *Journal of Anatomy,* 97, 101–106.

Gray, E. G. (1969) Electron microscopy of excitatory and inhibitory synapses: a brief review. In *Progress in Brain Research,* Vol. 31, (eds.) Akert, K. and Waser, P. G., pp. 141–156, Elsevier: Amsterdam.

Gray, E. G. and Guillery, R. W. (1966) Synaptic morphology in the normal and degenerating nervous system. In *International Review of Cytology,* (eds.) Bourne, G. H. and Danielli, J. F., Vol. 19, pp. 111–181. Academic Press: New York.

Green, J. D. and Pease, D. C. (1965) cited by Terzuolo, C. A. and Llinas, R. in *Distribution of synaptic impulse in the spinal motor neuron and its functional significance.* In *Muscular afferents and motor control,* Nobel Symposium I, (ed.) Granit, R., p. 373–384, Almqvist & Wiksell: Stockholm.

Grillner, S., Hongo, T. and Lund, S. (1966) Descending pathways with monosynaptic action on motoneurones. *Acta Physiologica Scandinavica,* Suppl. 277, 1–60.

Grillner, S., Hongo, T. and Lund, S. (1970) The vestibulospinal tract. Effects on alpha-motoneurones in the lumbosacral spinal cord in the cat. *Experimental Brain Research,* 10, 94–120.

Grillner, S. and Lund, S. (1968) The origin of a descending pathway with monosynaptic action of flexor motoneurones. *Acta Physiologica Scandinavica,* 74, 274–284.

Haggar, R. A. and Barr, M. L. (1950) Quantitative data on the size of synaptic endbulbs in the cat's spinal cord. *Journal of Comparative Neurology,* 93, 17–32.

Hamberger, A., Hansson, H. -A. and Sjöstrand, J. (1970) Surface structure of isolated neurons. Detachment of nerve terminals during axon regeneration *Journal of Cell Biology,* 47, 319–331.

Hansson, H. -A. and Sjöstrand, J. (1971) Ultrastructural effects of colchicine on the hypoglossal and dorsal vagal neurons of the rabbit. *Brain Research,* 35, 379–396.

van Harreveld, A. and Khattab, F. J. (1967) Electron microscopy of asphyxiated spinal cords of cats. *Journal of Neuropathology and experimental Neurology,* 26, 521–536.

Held, H. (1897) Beitrage zum Structur der Nervenzellen under ihrer Fortsätze. *Archiv für Anatomie und Entwicklungsgeschichte,* Suppl. 21, p. 273–312.

Henneman, E., Somjen, G. and Carpenter, D. O. (1965) Functional significance of cell size in spinal motoneurons. *Journal of Neurophysiology,* 28, 560–580.

Hildebrand, C. (1971a) Ultrastructural and light-microscopic studies of the nodal region in large myelinated fibres of the adult feline spinal cord white matter. *Acta Physiologica Scandinavica,* Suppl. 364, 43–81.

Hildebrand, C. (1971b) Ultrastructural and light-microscopic studies of the developing feline spinal cord white matter. I. The nodes of Ranvier. *Acta Physiologica Scandinavica,* Suppl. 364, 81–109.

Hildebrand, C. (1971c) Ultrastructural and light-microscopic studies of the developing feline spinal cord white matter. II. Cell death and myelin sheath disintegration in the early postnatal period. *Acta Physiologica Scandinavica,* Suppl. 364, 109–145.

Hodes, R., Peacock, S. M. and Bodian, D. (1949) Selective destruction of large motoneurons by poliomyelitis virus. II. Size of motoneurons in the spinal cord of Rhesus monkeys. *Journal of Neuropathology*, 8, 400–410.

Holmes, F. W. and Davenport, H. (1940) Cells and fibres in spinal nerves. IV. The number of neurites in dorsal and ventral roots of the cat. *Journal of Comparative Neurology*, 73, 1–5.

Illis, L. (1964) Spinal cord synapses in the cat. The normal appearance by the light microscope. *Brain*, 87, 543–554.

Illis, L. (1967) The relative densities of monosynaptic pathways to the cell bodies and dendrites of the cat ventral horn. *Journal of the Neurological Sciences*, 4, 259–270.

Jack, J. J. B., Miller, S., Porter, R. and Redman, S. J. (1971) The time course of minimal excitatory post-synatic potentials evoked in spinal motoneurones by group IA afferents. *Journal of Physiology*, 215, 353–380.

Jack, J. J. B. and Redman, S. J. (1971) The propagation of transient potentials in some linear cable structures. *Journal of Physiology*, 215, 283–320.

Jacobson, M. (1970) *Developmental Neurobiology*, p. 271–286. Holt, Rinehart and Winston, Inc: New York.

Jankowska, E. and Lindström, S. (1971) Morphological identification of Renshaw cells. *Acta Physiologica Scandinavica*, 81, 428–430.

Jankowska, E. and Lindström, S. (1972) Morphology of interneurones mediating IA reciprocal inhibition of motoneurons in the spinal cord of the cat. *Journal of Physiology*, 226, 805–823.

Källén, B. (1965) Degeneration and regeneration in the vertebrate central nervous system during embryogenesis, In *Progress in Brain Research: Degeneration patterns in the nervous system*, (eds.) Singer, M. and Schadé, J. P., Vol. 15, p. 77–97, Elsevier: Amsterdam.

Karlsson, U. L. (1967) Three dimensional studies of neurons in the lateral geniculate nucleus of the rat. III. Specialized neuronal contacts in the neuropil. *Journal of Ultrastructure Research*, 17, 137–157.

Karlsson, U. and Schultz, R. L. (1965) Fixation of the central nervous system for electron microscopy by aldehyde perfusion: I. Preservation with aldehyde perfusates versus direct perfusion with osmium tetroxide with special reference to membranes and the extracellular space. *Journal of Ultrastructure Research*, 12, 160–186.

Kawana, E., Akert, K. and Sandri, C. (1969) Zinciodide-osmium tetroxide impregnation of nerve terminals in the spinal cord. *Brain Research*, 16, 325–331.

Kellerth, J. -O. (1973) Intracellular staining of cat spinal motoneurons with Procion Yellow for ultrastructural studies. *Brain Research*, 50, 415–418.

Kellerth, J. -O., Mellström, A. and Skoglund, S. (1971) Postnatal excitability changes of kitten motoneurones. *Acta Physiologica Scandinavica*, 83, 31–41.

Kernell, D. (1970) Input resistance, electrical excitability and size of ventral horn cells in cat spinal cord. *Science*, 152, 1637–1640.

Kernell, D. (1971) Effects of synapses of dendrites and soma on the repetitive impulse firing of a compartmental neuron model. *Brain Research*, 35, 551–555.

Kingsbury, B. F. (1932) The 'law' of cepahlocaudal differential growth in its application to the nervous system. *Journal of Comparative Neurology*, 56, 431–464.

Kirkpatrick, J. B. (1968) Chromatolysis in the hypoglossal nucleus of the rat. An electron microscopic analysis. *Journal of Comparative Neurology*, 132, 189–212.

Kojima, T. and Saito, K. (1970) A Photographic presentation on the initial axon segment of an anterior horn neuron in the cat. *Journal of Electron Microscopy*, 19, 384–385.

Kojima, T., Saito, K. and Kakimi, S. (1972) Electron microscopic quantitative observations on the neuron and the terminal boutons contacted with it in the ventrolateral part of the anterior horn (C6-C7) of the adult cat. *Okajimas Folia Anatomica Japonica*, 49, 175–226.

Kuypers, H. G. J. M. (1973) The anatomical organization of the descending pathways and their contributions to motor control especially in primates. In *New Developments in Electromyography and Clinical Neurophysiology*, (ed.) Desmedt, J. E., Vol. 3, pp. 38–68, Karger: Basel.

Landon, D. N. and Williams, P. L. (1963) Ultrastructure of the node of Ranvier. *Nature*, 199, 575–577.

Leksell, L. (1945) The action potential and excitatory effects of the small ventral root fibres to skeletal muscle. *Acta Physiologica Scandinavica,* suppl. **31**.

Levi-Montalcini, R. (1964) Events in the developing nervous sysem. *Progress in Brain Research: Growth and Maturation of the Brain* (ed.) Purpura, D. P. and Schadé, J. P., Vol. 4, p. 1–29. Elsevier, Amsterdam.

Lewis, P. R. and Shute, C. C. D. (1966) The distribution of cholinesterase in cholinergic neurons demonstrated with the electron microscope. *Journal of Cell Science,* **1**, 381–390.

Lhermitte, J. and Kraus, W. M. (1925) On the form of the anterior horn cells. *Anatomical Record,* **31**, 123–129.

Lieberman, A. R. (1971) The axon reaction: A review of the principle features of perikaryal responses to axon injury. In *International Review of Neurobiology,* (eds.) Pfeiffer, C. C. and Smythies, J. R., Vol. 14, p. 49–124. Academic Press: London and New York.

Lloyd, D. P. C. (1943) Conduction and synaptic transmission of reflex response to stretch in spinal cats. *Journal of Neurophysiology,* **6**, 317–326.

Lund, S. and Pompeiano, O. (1968) Monosynaptic excitation of alpha motor neurones from supraspinal structures in the cat. *Acta Physiologica Scandinavica,* **73**, 1–21.

Lux, H. D., Schubert, P. and Kreutzberg, G. W. (1970) Direct matching of morphological and electrophysiological data in cat spinal motor neurones. In *Excitatory Synaptic Mechanisms,* (eds.) Anderson, P. and Jansen, J. K.. S., pp. 189–198, Universitetsforlaget: Oslo.

McLaughlin, B. J. (1972a) The fine structure of neurons and synapses in the motor nuclei of the cat spinal cord. *Journal of Comparative Neurology,* **144**, 429–460.

McLaughlin, B. J. (1972b) Dorsal root projections to the motor nuclei in the cat spinal cord. *Journal of Comparative Neurology,* **144**, 461–474.

McLaughlin, B. J. (1972c) Propriospinal and supraspinal projections to the motor nuclei in the cat spinal cord. *Journal of Comparative Neurology,* **144**, 475–500.

McMahan, V. J. (1967) Fine structure of synapses in the dorsal nucleus of the lateral geniculate body of normal and blinded rats. *Zeitschrift fur Zellforschung und Mikroskopische Anatomie,* **76**, 116–146.

Marsh, R. C., Matlowsky, L. and Stromberg, M. W. (1971) Dendritic bundles exist. *Brain Research,* **33**, 273–277.

Martinez. A. J. and Friede, K. (1970) Changes in nerve cell bodies during the myelination of their axons. *Journal of Comparative Neurology,* **138**, 329–338.

Matsushita, M. and Ikeda, M. (1973) Propriospinal fiber connections of the cervical motor nuclei in the cat: A light and electron microscope study. *Journal of Comparative Neurology,* **150**, 1–32.

Matthews, M. A., Willis, W. D. and Williams, V. (1971) Dendrite bundles in lamina IX of cat spinal cord: A possible source for electrical interaction between motoneurons. *Anatomical Record,* **171**, 313–328.

Matus, A. J. and Dennison, M. E. (1971) Autoradiographic localization of tritiated glycine at 'flat-vesicle' synapses in spinal cord. *Brain Research,* **32**, 195–197.

Mellström, A. (1971a) Postnatal excitability changes of the ankle monosypaptic reflexes in the cat. *Acta Physiologica Scandinavica,* **82**, 477–489.

Mellström, A. (1971b) Postnatal difference in calibre spectra between ankle extensor and flexor muscle nerves in the cat. *Acta Neurologica Scandinavica,* **47**, 331–334.

Mellström, A. (1971c) Recurrent and antidromic effects on the monosynaptic reflex during postnatal development in the cat. *Acta Physiological Scandinavica,* **82**, 490–499.

Mellström, A. and Skoglund, S. (1969) Quantitative morphological changes in some spinal cord segments during postnatal development. A study in the cat. *Acta Physiologica Scandinavica,* Suppl. **331**, 1–84.

Mendell, L. M. and Henneman, E. (1971) Terminals of single IA fibres: Location, density and distribution within a pool of 300 homonymous motor neurons. *Journal of Neurophysiology,* **34**, 171–187.

Merker, G. (1969) Ultrastrukturveränderungen motorischer Vorderhornzellen des Kaninchens unter abgestufter Ischämie. *Zeitschrift für Zellforschung und mikroskopische Anatomie,* **95**, 568–593.

Micklewright, H. L., Kurnick, N. B. and Hodes, R. (1953) The determination of cell volume. *Experimental Cell Research*, 4, 151–158.

Mikeladze, A. C. (1966) Endings of afferent nerve fibres in lumbosacral region of spinal cord. *Federation Proceedings*, 25, 1211–1216.

Motor neuron diseases (1969) (eds.) Norris, F. H. and Kurland, L., Grune and Stratton: New York.

Mugnaini, E. and Walberg, F. (1964) Ultrastructure of neuroglia. *Ergebnisse der Anatomie und Entwicklungsgeschichte*, 37, 194–236.

Naka, K. – I.(1964a) Electrophysiology of the fetal spinal cord. I. Action potentials of the motoneuron. *Journal of General Physiology*, 47, 1003–1022.

Naka, K. – I. (1964b) Electrophysiology of the fetal spinal cord. II. Interaction among peripheral inputs and recurrent inhibition. *Journal of General Physiology*, 47, 1023–1038.

Nornes, H. O. and Das, G. D. (1972) Temporal pattern of neurogenesis in spinal cord: Cytoarchitecture and directed growth of axons. *Proceedings of the National Academy of Sciences*, 69, 1962–1966.

Nyberg-Hansen, R. (1965) Anatomical demonstration of gamma motoneurons in the cat's spinal cord. *Experimental Neurology*, 13, 71–81.

Nyberg-Hansen, R. (1966) Functional organization of descending supraspinal fibre systems to the spinal cord. Anatomical observations and physiological correlations. *Ergebnisse der Anatomie under Entwicklungsgeschichte*, 39, 1–48.

Nyberg-Hansen, R. (1969) Do cat spinal motoneurons receive direct supraspinal connections? *Archives Italiennes de Biologie*, 107, 67–78.

Palay, S. L. and Palade, G. E. (1955) The fine structure of neurons. *Journal of Biophysical and Biochemical Cytology*, 1, 69–88.

Palay, S. L., Sotelo, C., Peters, A., and Orkand, P. M. (1968) The axon hillock and initial axon segment. *Journal of Cell Biology*, 12, 193–210.

Peters, A. (1966) The node of Ranvier in the central nervous system. *Quarterly Journal of Experimental Physiology*, 51, 229–236.

Peters, A., Proskauer, C. C. and Kaiserman-Abramof, J. R. (1968) The small pyramidal neuron of the rat cerebral cortex. The axon hillock and initial segment. *Journal of Cell Biology*, 39, 604–619.

Poritsky, R. (1969) Two- and three-dimensional ultrastructure of boutons and glial cells on the motoneuronal surface in the cat spinal cord. *Journal of Comparative Neurology*, 135, 423–452.

Prestige, M. C. (1966) Initial collaterals of motor axons within the spinal cord of the cat. *Journal of Comparative Neurology*, 126, 123–135.

Purpura, D. P., Shofer, R. J. and Scarff, T. (1965) Properties of synaptic activities and spike potentials of neurons in immature neocortex. *Journal of Neurophysiology*, 28, 925–942.

Rall, W. (1967) Distinguishing theoretical synaptic potentials computed for different soma-dendritic distributions of synaptic input. *Journal of Neurophysiology*, 30, 1138–1168.

Rall, W. (1970) Cable properties of dendrites and effects of synaptic location. In *Excitatory Synaptic Mechanism*, (eds.) Andersen, P. and Jansen, J. K. S., p. 175–187, Universitetsforlaget, Oslo.

Rall, W., Burke, R. E., Smith, T. G., Nelson, P. G. and Frank, K. (1967) Dendritic location of synapses and possible mechanisms for the monosynaptic EPSP in motoneurons. *Journal of Neurophysiology*, 30, 1169–1193.

Ralston, H. J. III (1967) Synaptic morphology in the ventral horn of cat spinal cord. *Anatomical Record*, 157, 305–306.

Ramon y Cajal, S. (1909) Histologie du système nerveux de l'homme et des vertebrés. Maloine, Paris.

Renshaw, B. (1941) Influence of the discharge of motor neurons upon excitation of neighbouring motor neurons. *Journal of Neurophysiology*, 4, 167–183.

Rexed, B. (1944) Contributions to the knowledge of the postnatal development of the peripheral nervous system in man. *Acta Psychiatrica et Neurologica*, suppl. 33.

Rexed, B. (1952) The cytoarchitectonic organization of the spinal cord in the cat. *Journal of Comparative Neurology*, 96, 415–495.

Rogers, D. C. (1972) Ultrastructural identification of degenerating boutons of mono-synaptic pathways to the lumbosacral segments in the cat after spinal hemisection. *Experimental Brain Research*, 14, 293–311.

Romanes, G. J. (1951) The motor cell columns of the lumbosacral spinal cord of the cat. *Journal of Comparative Neurology*, 94, 313–363.

Romanes, G. J. (1964) The motor pools of the spinal cord. In *Organization of the Spinal Cord*, (eds.) Eccles, J. C. and Schadé J. P., *Progress in Brain Research*, 11, 93–116. Elsevier, Amsterdam.

Ronnevi, L.- O. Unpublished studies in progress.

Ronnevi, L.- O. and Conradi, S. (1974) Ultrastructural evidence for spontaneous elimination of synaptic terminals on spinal motor neurons in the kitten. *Brain Research*, 80, 335–339.

Rosenbluth, J. (1962) Subsurface cisterns and their relationship to the neuronal plasma membrane. *Journal of Cell Biology*, 13, 405–421.

Saito, K. (1972) Electron microscopic observations on terminal boutons and synaptic structures in the anterior horn of the spinal cord in the adult cat. *Okajimas Folia Anatomica Japonica*, 48, 361–412.

Sakla, F. B (1959) Postnatal growth of the cervical spinal cord of the albino mouse and the dendritic organization of its ventral horn cells. *Journal of Comparative Neurology*, 113, 491–508.

Sakla, F. B. (1965) Postnatal growth of neuroglia cells and blood vessels of the cervical spinal cord of the albino mouse. *Journal of Comparative Neurology*, 124, 189–202.

Schadé, J. P. (1964) On the volume and surface area of spinal neurons. In *Organization of the Spinal Cord*, (eds.) Eccles, J. C. and Schadé J. P., *Progress in Brain Research*, 11, 261–277. Elsevier: Amsterdam.

Schadé, J. P. and V. Harreveld, A. (1961) Volume distribution of moto- and interneurons in the peroneus-tibialis neuron pool in the cat. *Journal of Comparative Neurology*, 117, 387–398.

Scheibel, M. E. and Scheibel, A. B. (1966) Terminal axonal patterns in cat spinal cord. I. The lateral cortico-spinal tract. *Brain Research*, 2, 333–350.

Scheibel, M. E. and Scheibel, A. B. (1969) Terminal axonal patterns in cat spinal cord. III. Primary afferent collaterals. *Brain Research*, 13, 417–443.

Scheibel, M. E. and Scheibel, A. B. (1970a) Organization of spinal motor neuron dendrites in bundles. *Experimental Neurology*, 28, 106–112.

Scheibel, M. E. and Scheibel, A. B. (1970b) Developmental relationship betwen motoneuron dendrite bundles and patterned activity in the hindlimb of cats. *Experimental Neurology*, 29, 328–356.

Scheibel, M. E. and Scheibel, A. B. (1971) Developmental relationship between spinal motor neuron dendrite bundles and patterned activity in the forelimb of cats. *Experimental Neurology*, 30, 367–373.

Scheibel, M. E. and Scheibel, A. B. (1973) Dendrite bundles in the ventral commissure of cat spinal cord. *Experimental Neurology*, 39, 482–488.

Shapovalov, A. J. (1972) Extrapyramidal monosynaptic and disynaptic control of mammalian motor neurons. *Brain Research*, 40, 105–115.

Skoglund, S. (1960a) On the postnatal development of postural reflexes as revealed by electromyography and myography in decerebrate kittens. *Acta Physiologica Scandinavica*, 49, 299–317.

Skoglund, S. (1960b) The spinal transmission of proprioceptive reflexes and the postnatal development of conduction velocity in different hindlimb nerves in the kitten. *Acta Physiologica Scandinavica*, 49, 318–329.

Skoglund, S. (1960c) Central connexions and functions of muscle nerves in the kitten. *Acta Physiologica Scandinavica*, 50, 222–237.

Skoglund, S. (1966) Muscle afferents and motor control in the kitten. In *Muscular afferents and Motor Control*, Nobel Symposium I, (ed.) Granit, R., p. 45–59, Almqvist and Wiksell: Stockholm.

Skoglund, S. (1969) Growth and differentiation with special emphasis on the central nervous system. *Annual Review of Physiology*, 31, 19–42.

Smith, C. A. and Rasmussen, G. L. (1965) Degeneration in the efferent nerve endings in the cochlea after axonal section. *Journal of Cell Biology*, 26, 63–77.

Sotelo, C. (1971) General features of the synaptic organization in the central nervous system. In *Chemistry and Brain Development*, (eds.) Paoleth, R. and Davison, A. N., Plenum Press, New York.

Sprague, J. M. (1951) Motor and propriospinal cells in the thoracic and lumbar ventral horn of the Rhesus monkey. *Journal of Comparative Neurology*, **95**, 103–124.

Sprague, J. M. (1958) The distribution of dorsal root fibres on motor cells in lumbosacral spinal cord of the cat and the site of excitatory and inhibitory terminals in monosynaptic pathways. *Proceedings of the Royal Society London (Series B)*, **149**, 534–556.

Sprague, J. M. and Hongchien, Ha (1964) The terminal fields of dorsal root fibres in the lumbosacral spinal cord of the cat and the dendritic organization of the motor nuclei. *Progress in Brain Research*, **11**, 120–152.

Sterling, P. and Kuypers, H. G. J. M. (1967) Anatomical organization of the brachial spinal cord of the cat. I. The distribution of dorsal root fibres. *Brain Research*, **41**, 1–15. II. The motoneuron plexus. *Brain Research*, **4**, 16–32.

Sterling, P. and Kuypers, H. G. J. M. (1968) Anatomical organization of the brachial spinal cord of the cat. III. The propriospinal connections. *Brain Research*, **7**, 419–443.

Stensaas, L. J. and Stensaas, S. S. (1968) Astrocytic neuroglial cells, oligodendrocytes and microgliacytes in the spinal cord of the toad. II. Electron microscopy. *Zeitschrift für Zellforschung*, **86**, 184–213.

Streit, P., Akert, K., Sandri, C., Livingston, R. B. and Moor, H. (1972) Dynamic ultrastructure of presynaptic membranes at nerve terminals in the spinal cord of rats. Anesthetized and unanesthetized preparations compared. *Brain Research*, **48**, 11–26.

Stretton, A. O. W. and Kravitz, E. A. (1968) Neuronal geometry: Determination with a technique of intracellular dye injection. *Science*, **162**, 132–134.

Szentágothai, J. (1958) The anatomical basis of synaptic transmission of excitation and inhibition in motoneurons. *Acta Morphologica Academiae Scientificae Hungarica*, **8**, 287–309.

Szentágothai, J. (1967) Synaptic architecture of the spinal motoneuron pool. In *Recent advances in clinical neurophysiology*, (ed.) Widén, L., p. 4–19. Elsevier, Amsterdam.

Taxi, J. (1961) Etude de lúltrastructure des zones synaptiques dans les ganglions sympathiques de la grenouille. *Comptes Rendues de l' Academie des Sciences*, **252**, 174–176.

Testa, C. (1964) Functional implications of the morphology of spinal ventral horn neurons of the cat. *Journal of Comparative Neurology*, **123**, 425–444.

Torvik, A. (1972) Phagocytosis of nerve cells during retrograde degeneration. *Journal of Neuropathology and Experimental Neurology*, **31**, 132–146.

Torvik, A. and Skjörten, F. (1971) Electron microscopic observations on nerve cell regeneration and degeneration after axon lesions. I. Changes in the nerve cell cytoplasm. *Acta Neuropathologica*, **17**, 243–264. II. Changes in the glial cells. *Acta Neuropathologica*, **17**, 265–282.

Uchizono, K. (1965) Characteristics of excitatory and inhibitory synapses in the central nervous system of the cat. *Nature*, **207**, 642–643.

Uchizono, K. (1966) Excitatory and inhibitory synapses in the cat spinal cord. *Japanese Journal of Physiology*, **16**, 570–575.

Valvidia, O. (1971) Methods of fixation and the morphology of synaptic vesicles. *Journal of Comparative Neurology*, **142**, 257–274.

Vaughn, J. E. (1969) An electron microscopic analysis of gliogenesis in rat optic nerves. *Zeitschrift für Zellfoschung und Mikroskopische Anatomie*, **94**, 293–324.

Vaughn, J. E. and Grieshaber, J. A. (1972) An electron microscopic investigation of glycogen and mitochondria in developing and adult rat spinal motor neuropil. *Journal of Neurocytology*, **1**, 397–412.

Vaughn, J. E, and Grieshaber, J. A. (1973) A morphological investigation of an early reflex pathway in developing rat spinal cord. *Journal of Comparative Neurology*, **148**, 177–210.

Walberg, F. (1964) The early changes in degenerating boutons and the problem of argyrophilia. *Journal of Comparative Neurology*, **122**, 113–127.

Wechsler, W. (1966) Elektronenmikroskopischer Beitrag zur Nervenzell-differenzierung und

Histogenese der grauen Substanz des Rückenmarks von Hühnerembryonen. *Zeitschrift für Zellforschung und Mikroskipische Anatomie,* **74**, 401–422.

Weil, A. (1927) The form of the anterior horn cells of vertebrates. *Archives of Neurology and Psychiatry,* **17**, 783–793.

Wersäll, J. (1968) Efferent innervation of the inner ear. In *Structure and function of inhibitory neuronal mechanisms,* (eds.) v. Euler, C., Skoglund, S. and Söderberg, U., p. 123–139. Pergamon Press, Oxford.

Wilson, V. J. (1962) Reflex transmission in the kitten. *Journal of Neurophysiology,* **25**, 263–275.

Wilson, V. J. and Yoshida, M. (1969) Comparison of the effects of stimulation of Deiter's nucleus and the ventral longitudinal fasciculus on neck, forelimb and hindlimb motor neurons *Journal of Neurophysiology,* **32**, 743–758.

Windle, W. F. (1930) Normal behavioural reactions of kittens correlated with the postnatal development of nerve fiber density in the spinal gray matter. *Journal of Comparative Neurology,* **50**, 479–503.

Wisniewski, H., Shelanski, M. L. and Terry, R. D. (1968) Effects of mitotic spindle inhibitors on neurotubules and neurofilaments in anterior horn cells. *Journal of Cell Biology,* **38**, 224–229.

Wuerker, R. B. (1971) Monosynaptic terminals on ventral horn cells of the rat. *International Journal of Neurosciences,* **1**, 339–346.

Wuerker, R. B. and Palay, S. L. (1969) Neurofilaments and microtubules in anterior horn cells of the rat. *Tissue and Cell,* **1**, 387–402.

Wyckoff, R. W. G. and Young, J. Z. (1956) The motor neuron surface. *Proceedings of the Royal Society London (Series B),* **144**, 440–450.

SPINAL AND CRANIAL NERVE ROOTS

H.J. Gamble

6.1 Introduction

In most of their extent spinal nerve roots are of similar but not identical construction to the spinal nerves proper which they form. There are differences in their connective tissue content and in their cellular sheaths and a very substantial change in their structure occurs close to their attachment to the spinal cord where an organization typical of the peripheral nervous system abruptly changes to that typical of the central nervous system. This transitional zone has received little attention, whether from light or electron microscopists, even less than have the more distal parts of the roots.

Spinal nerve roots, meanwhile, are coming to be recognized as valuable models for physiological and other experimentation (e.g. Whitehorn and Burgess, 1973) and are, of course, the focus of experimentation designed to elucidate the significance of the dorsal root potential, first described by Barron and Mathews (1938) and subsequently studied by many others (e.g. Mendell and Wall, 1964; Melzak and Wall, 1965; Zimmermann, 1968; Grinnell, 1970). The initial exposure of the *cauda equina* is more difficult than that of a nerve trunk but once exposed in the subarachnoid space, the roots are accessible to recording or stimulating electrodes or to drugs and other substances without the need of careful, but still damaging, dissection of fascia and dense connective tissue epineurium. In these circumstances it may be useful to review what is known of the structure of nerve roots in the hope that it may be related to what is becoming known of their behaviour.

Cranial nerves have often less clearly defined roots and where the term is usually applied to them it corresponds more nearly with the rootlets of spinal roots. For convenience, cranial nerve roots will be taken to consist of those parts of the cranial nerves which extend from their attachments to the brain stem, or olfactory bulb, to the point at which they perforate the inner or meningeal layer of the cranial dura mater: within this definition they resemble spinal nerve roots in these particulars: they are bathed in cerebro-spinal fluid throughout their length; they undergo a transformation in their structure at some point along their length; and they have received little attention from anatomists in recent years.

In the account which follows it will be apparent that much information originally acquired from the study of peripheral nerve trunks is applicable also to

330

spinal nerve roots and that a very extensive literature is available for reference. There are a very few recent accounts of the structure of cranial nerve roots (as defined above) but it appears that the olfactory nerve roots represent an essentially embryonic condition persisting into maturity, that the vestibulo-acoustic nerve roots are, in truth, tracts of fibres of the central nervous system for the greater part of their lengths and that even the trigeminal nerve root, in some respects the most 'ordinary' of those studied, differs from spinal nerve roots in the important matter of the manner of its ensheathing. It is convenient, consequently, to deal first with the better documented spinal nerve roots and then to deal in detail with the three cranial nerve roots mentioned above. Of the other cranial nerve roots there will be very little to say.

6.2 Spinal nerve roots

6.2.1 *Development of nerve roots*

It is well established from the study of normal embryos and confirmed experimentally, that cells of the neural crest give origin to the nerve cells of dorsal root ganglia and cranial nerve ganglia as well as to the Schwann cells associated with them. Axons of the ventral spinal roots, and efferent cranial nerves, are outgrowths from neuroblasts of the basal lamina of the neural tube and it seems almost certain that some of their associated Schwann cells derive from glioblasts migrating from the neural tube towards the periphery; other Schwann cells of efferent fibres may originate in the neural crest.

While so much appears certain, doubts remain over the sequence in which these events occur. To some observers, spinal nerve roots are first recognizable as slender strands of tissue linking the alar part of the neural tube to local aggregations of the neural crest, and linking the basal part of the tube to somites. To some investigators ventral roots are substantially the earlier to appear (e.g. Hamilton, Boyd and Mossman, 1972) to others, dorsal roots are the earlier (e.g. Balfour, 1885; Marshall, 1893). At these early stages of development the roots are of uncertain composition, being 'protoplasmic' and lacking nuclei in some accounts (e.g. Hamilton *et al.*) or composed of spindle-shaped cells in others (e.g. Balfour). It is interesting that Schwann (1847) referred to Remak, and quoted him as stating that 'the substance of the cerebro-spinal nerves of the rabbit, in the third week of embryonal existence, consists of corpuscles, some of which are irregularly spherical, others slightly elongated, having a very delicate filament adhering: they are mostly transparent and arranged in rows without, however, presenting any distinctly perceptible fibrous structure'. His own observations regarding these 'corpuscles' was to the effect that they were 'the primitive structure of nerve, for the younger the fetus, the greater is their relative quantity, and in a pig's fetus of three inches in length, I found them the sole constituent'. However, where protoplasmic strands were described as the earliest form of nerve root, a later 'fibrillation' was said to occur, followed by the appearance of nuclei.

Harrison's (1907) tissue culture experiments demonstrated that embryonic nerve cells, in culture, are capable of growing axonal processes of relatively considerable length and led to the assumption, still widely accepted, that the primitive nerve roots were formed by axonal processes growing from neuroblasts of the dorsal root ganglia, or from the basal lamina of the neural tube. A similar, but peripherally directed, axonal outgrowth from the peripherally directed, axonal outgrowth from the dorsal root ganglion neuroblast completed the early bipolar form of these cells. The further assumption was then made that subsequent migrations of neural crest cells, and of glioblasts from the neural tube, along the pre-existing nerve fibres, allowed the primitive Schwann cells to assume their satellite relationships and undergo proliferation and morphological change until the adult condition had been achieved.

Recent electron microscopic studies raise some doubts about this sequence of events. In the earlier stages of its development the human sciatic nerve contains some fascicles formed by cords of Schwann cells in direct contact with each other but only rarely in contact with any of the few axons usually also present in the fascicle (Cravioto, 1965). At the same stage of development other fascicles of the nerve might consist of isolated Schwann cells enveloping large bundles of axons, but the possibility appears to exist that Schwann cells may be present in the peripheral nerve before axonal processes have extended so far.

More recently (1970) Tennyson has shown that the growth cones of developing dorsal roots in the rabbit do not perforate the neural tube until the early part of the eleventh day of development. Even at this stage they are invested, if incompletely, by satellite Schwann cell processes and it seems likely that a 'dorsal root' had been present for some two days before any perforation occurred (see Marshall, 1893, Chapter V). The nature of this root is not known but it seems improbable that growth cones would remain, inactive, for rather more than two days at the surface of the neural tube: the possibility clearly exists that the earliest root may consist of Schwann cells.

Finally it may be remarked that in the repair of injured peripheral nerve, where regeneration involves the bridging of a gap between proximal and distal stumps, the outgrowth of axonal sprouts is always, and apparently necessarily, preceded by a migration of proliferated Schwann cells to bridge the gap (Thomas, 1966). Once these pioneering cells achieved a union a suitable sequence of cell surfaces is apparently available for axonal growth. It may be that in this, as in other respects, axonal regeneration and maturation mimic the events which lead to the development and maturation of developing nerves.

6.2.2 *Maturation of nerve root fibres*

The development of progressively more complex interrelationships between Schwann cells and axons have been studied more extensively by electron microscopy in spinal nerves than in spinal nerve roots. Such findings as have been reported in roots, however, correspond closely with those made in nerves at similar, relatively late, stages of development and maturation so that it seems likely that essentially the same processes occur in both situations.

The earliest stage of the developing interrelationship appears to have been observed by Cravioto (1965) in a study of the fetal human sciatic nerve. Here, at 12 weeks of intra-uterine life, some fascicles consisted largely of cords of closely-packed Schwann cells not all of which contacted the few axons present in the fascicles (Fig. 6.1a). Other fascicles consisted of Schwann cells from which sheets of cytoplasm extended to embrace bundles of closely-packed and numerous axons (Fig. 6.1b). Only this latter arrangement was seen by Gamble (1966) in human fetal ulnar nerves of similar and slightly lesser ages. The first arrangement was assumed to represent an earlier stage of development reflecting precocious development in the upper as compared with the lower limb. At these stages all axons were of very small calibre (ranging from 0.1–1.0 μm) most being far too small to be resolved by techniques of light microscopy. As many as 450 tiny axons have been seen in one bundle, communally invested by cytoplasmic sheets, or processes, of a single Schwann cell.

Perhaps stimulated by this massive ingrowth of axons into the nerve, Schwann cells undergo a series of mitotic divisions, each daughter cell of the division becoming associated with some of the previous complement of associated axons and, by elaborating additional sheets of cytoplasm, breaking up the axons into progressively smaller bundles (Figs. 6.1b–g). Even as early as about 11 weeks menstrual age, the human fetal ulnar nerve may show single axons, isolated from their fellows by small sheets of Schwann cell cytoplasm. The incidence and the size of such isolated axons increases during the following weeks but at 10–12 weeks incipient myelination of isolated axons may occasionally be seen. It occurs only where an isolated axon is related uniquely to a Schwann cell and is recognizable by the elongation and some spiralling of the mesaxon (Fig. 6.1e). This process was first recognized by Geren in 1954 in the chick embryo and has since been observed in many other species.

An essentially similar course of events was described by Cravioto (1965) in the human fetal sciatic nerve although it occurred some weeks later. In both ulnar and sciatic nerves from human fetuses myelination extended over a prolonged period. The myelination achieved at about 14 weeks in the human fetal ulnar nerve (Gamble and Breathnach, 1965) corresponds closely with that achieved in rat fetuses at about 20 days (Peters and Muir, 1959); the further attainment of a diameter of about 2.5 μm requires a period of about 10 weeks in human fetuses (Gamble, 1966) while, by contrast, four days suffice for a similar attainment in the rat (Peters and Muir, 1959).

It is to be expected that the activities of Schwann cells in these circumstances should be reflected in an 'active' appearance of their cytoplasm. This is manifested by abundant endoplasmic reticulum (often with dilated cisternae), numerous free ribosomes, numerous mitochondria and a large and prominent Golgi apparatus, and is particularly marked in those cells which had invested a single axon, whether or not myelination had begun (Allt, 1969). None of these

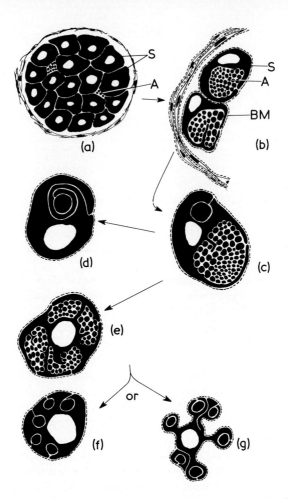

Fig. 6.1 Consists of diagrams representing cross-sections from bundles of developing nerve fibres of the peripheral nervous system (*After* Cravioto, 1965; Gamble, 1966 and Gamble and Breathnach, 1965.) **(a)** Shows the earliest stage observed, where Schwann cells (S) are numerous. Only a few of them contact the few axons (A) which are present, and do so without in any way ensheathing them. Perineurial cells resemble fibroblasts. No basement membranes (basal laminae) are present. **(b)** Shows a slightly later stage where axons are relatively much more numerous, large bundles of them being invested communally by processes of Schwann cell cytoplasm. Basement membranes (BM) cover surfaces of Schwann cells and of perineurial cells. **(c)** Shows a slightly later stage where one axon is enlarged and is separately ensheathed by a Schwann cell which, by other cytoplasmic processes, communally ensheaths many smaller axons. **(d)** Shows a later stage where, after mitotic division of the Schwann cell in (c), one daughter cell ensheaths the large axon and, by the extension of a spiralling cytoplasmic process about the axon, has begun to form a myelin sheath upon it. **(e)** Shows the other daughter cell derived from the mitotic division of the Schwann cell shown in (c). It now envelops its complement of axons in four separate bundles, by the elaboration of additional cytoplasmic processes. **(f)** Shows the effect of further mitotic divisions of the Schwann cell shown in (e). There are many fewer axons associated with the cell and each is separately invaginated from the cell surface. This arrangement is common in small laboratory animals. **(g)** Shows the effect of further mitotic divisions of the Schwann cell shown in (e) together with a remodelling in the form of the Schwann cell. This arrangement of Schwann cell and unmyelinated axons is found in the adult human peripheral nervous system.

organelles is conspicuous in the normal adult Schwann cell whether associated with a myelinated fibre or with unmyelinated fibres.

Matheson and Cavanagh (1967) and Matheson (1968) have shown, by means of biochemical studies of glycine incorporation into the sciatic nerve of the rat, that the rate of amino-acid incorporation, relative to DNA content, is extremely high at or soon after birth, and shows a steady decline during maturation. This suggests a high rate of protein synthesis in the immature Schwann cell which, indeed, is an obvious corollary of its observed role in the elaboration of the partly protein myelin sheath. Some figures are given by Gamble (1973) relative to the increase in the surface area of the Schwann cell plasma membrane during the growth of a Schwann cell from about 200 μm in length with 6 myelin lamellae to 1000 μm in length with 60 myelin lamellae, and an increase in diameter from 1.2 to 10 μm: the increase in surface area would be of the order of 330 times. Even the Schwann cell of unmyelinated fibres, despite its less dramatic role, must enlarge itself many times over to provide separate axonal investments in place of the communal axonal investment of earlier stages.

At the outset of myelination in the peripheral nervous system, the myelinating Schwann cell is some 200—400 μm in length. The subsequent spinning of the myelin sheath about the axon is accompanied by elongation of the Schwann cell; in some situations this elongation conforms closely with the growth and elongation of the region through which the nerve fibre runs (Vizoso and Young, 1948) There is also evidence, however, that some Schwann cells, and the associated segments of myelin of which they are parts, being surplus to the final complement of Schwann cells associated with the axon, may degenerate and disappear without ever reaching the normal basic length of 200—400 μm. This explanation is advanced by Berthold and Skoglund (1968a and b) in relation to 'myelin monsters', 10—50 μm long, observed in maturing myelinated nerve fibres in lumbar spinal nerve roots and some peripheral nerves in kittens. If such changes in lumbar nerve roots occur for the reason suggested, then they might be expected to be more numerous in cervical or even thoracic roots where there is less disparity between segmental level of cord and the vertebral level of the skeleton i.e. where the roots have undergone far less elongation. Cervical roots have not been investigated in the kitten, and while Fraher (1972) did not describe 'myelin monsters' in cervical roots of neonatal and infant rats, he did describe a number of 'significant artefacts or unusual myelin forms'.

Elongation of the myelinating Schwann cell is accompanied by the elaboration of a complex paranodal apparatus at its axial extremities (Fig. 6.2) This process of elaboration as observed in the kitten, includes a build-up of mitochondria in the paranodal Schwann cell cytoplasm more or less concurrent with a build-up of enzyme activity sometimes associated with efficient nerve impulse conduction (Berthold and Skoglund, 1967). The myelin sheath at first appears to throw out irregular swellings and pockets (containing smaller outpocketings of the axon and inner Schwann cell cytoplasm) which later become detached and disappear, while the remaining myelin reforms itself into

335

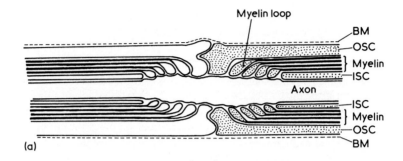

(a)

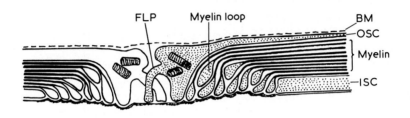

(b)

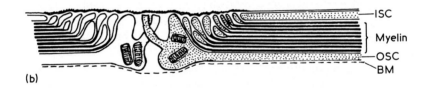

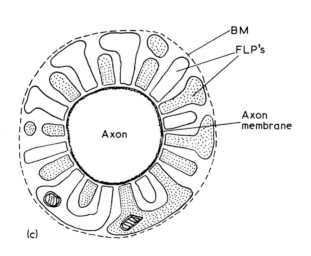

(c)

the typically crested or crenated form of the paranodal region (Berthold and Skoglund, 1968a and b, and Chapter 1). It is difficult to visualize means by which parts of the spiralled myelin, having been broken, might realign and then reform the concentric lamellae and it is to be hoped that further study of this region may provide a fuller explanation.

Another process involved in the maturation of the paranodal apparatus is the development of finger-like processes from the outermost turn of the Schwann cell to lie in a gap substance surrounding the nodal axon and contained within the basal membrane sheath (Fig. 6.2b). Finger-like processes are arranged in an apparently random fashion in peripheral nerve of the frog (Robertson, 1959) but in mammals they display a precise ordering where processes from the two Schwann cells limiting the node alternate to interdigitate and turn in upon the nodal axon (Fig. 6.2c), from which they then appear to radiate (Chapter 1; Landon and Williams, 1963). The steps leading to this ordered pattern were studied by Berthold (1968a) in ventral spinal nerve roots and sural nerves of newborn and older kittens confirming results obtained in an earlier study of nerve roots from a full-term stillborn child (Hildebrand and Skoglund, 1967).

At all stages studied in the kitten, the nodal axon contains an electron-dense undercoating of the plasma membrane. In small fibres (about 1 μm diameter, 5—6 myelin lamellae) in the newborn kitten successive Schwann cells merely overlap at the node, but in larger fibres (up to 5—6 μm in diamter) there is a spacious nodal gap limited by the basal membrane and containing a few irregularly evaginated processes of the outermost layer of the two related Schwann cells. At these stages the nodal axon shows no constriction.

In kittens of 7 days of age a near adult arrangement of finger-like processes is found at the node, where their radial orientation is conspicuous. Thereafter there is an increase in the size of the fibre (see, for example, Nyström and Skoglund, 1965) and in the number of finger-like processes while from about the fourteenth day a nodal constriction appears in the axon and increases. An essentially similar sequence of events has been described by Allt (1969) in the developing nerves of the rat. The gap substance in which the finger-like processes

---

Fig. 6.2 Consists of diagrams representing myelinating axons of the peripheral nervous system where two Schwann cells meet at a node of Ranvier. (a) In a longitudinal section, Schwann cell cytoplasm occurs as an inner layer (ISC) lying beside the axon (o), as 'myelin loops' at the extremities of the myelin lamellae, and as an outer layer (OSC) enveloping the myelin sheath. The axon membrane tends to conform with contours of overlying Schwann cell processes and the basement membrane (BM) extends from one Schwann cell to the next. (b) With myelination further advanced, a longitudinal section shows more myelin lamellae which in some cases are insufficiently elongated to overlap the layer next within, so that the cytoplasmic loop may fall short of contact with the paranodal axon. A gap now separates the two Schwann cells, the outer layers of which are provided with mitochondria and with finger-like processes whose extremities contact the nodal axon. (c) A transverse section through the node of Ranvier shown in (b) illustrates finger-like processes from the two Schwann cells, interdigitating and converging upon the nodal axon. They are contained within a space bounded externally by basement membrane.

of the node lie has been shown to bind cations (Landon and Langley, 1971) and is considered to be mainly protein-linked carboxylated mucopolysaccharide.

While the rather dramatic activities of one population of Schwann cells, associated with an increase in the calibre of axons, leads to the formation and maturation of myelinated nerve fibres, the majority of the axons in the nerve roots remain unmyelinated and of small diameter. Even by the techniques of light microscopy it had been shown long ago that unmyelinated fibres outnumbered the myelinated by about four to one in peripheral nerves (Duncan, 1932; Ranson and Davenport, 1931) and this has since been confirmed by electron microscopy.

In the early stages of human development (e.g. at about 10 weeks) a single Schwann cell may invest many hundreds of tiny axons (Gamble, 1966), providing individual invaginations for a few by minor processes of its cytoplasm, but enveloping the great majority into one or two large bundles. At later stages the number of axons related to a Schwann cell is progressively reduced until some 12 weeks later a condition closely resembling that of mature human unmyelinated nerve fibres is seen. Since it may be assumed that some ingrowth of new axons has occurred during this time the reduction in the axon/Schwann cell ratio must result from Schwann cell mitosis or immigration of Schwann cells, or both of these processes.

The presence of extensive sheets of Schwann cell cytoplasm around bundles of axons or projecting into a bundle might seem likely to hinder migration of the cell but in fact the true extent of such sheets is not known, and their permanence or otherwise are equally unknown. It seems clear that the Schwann cells of unmyelinating axons must be extremely active cells, not only in mitosis but in elaborating cytoplasmic processes in increasing numbers required to permit the individual rather than communal ensheathing of axons characteristic of their maturity. In most small mammalian and in some adult human nerves the simple invagination of each of some ten to fifteen axons is the rule, the Schwann cell assuming a fluted form (see Fig. 6.1f). In human nerve roots and some peripheral nerves (more particularly cutaneous nerves) the Schwann cell assumes a far more complex form. Cytoplasmic processes extend laterally from the nuclear region and then bifurcate to be elongated proximally and distally along the axis of the nerve. Each elongated process so formed is invaginated by one axon and the apparently independent units (each an axon plus invaginating Schwann cell cytoplasm) so formed is invested by basement membrane (see Fig. 6.1g). Often two or three such units may share investment by basement membrane but only serial sections show that ultimately they belong to one Schwann cell (Gamble and Eames, 1964; Eames and Gamble, 1970). It is clear that in the achievement of their mature form Schwann cells of this kind must be extremely active in the production of extensive cytoplasm as in the production of plasma membrane. The further elaboration of sheaths about bundles of collagen (Gamble, 1964; Gamble and Eames, 1964) in nerves, and in nerve roots to a lesser extent, is further proof of their activity (Gamble and Eames, 1966). It is reflected in the occurrence in their cytoplasm of relatively conspicuous granular endoplasmic reticulum, often closely associated with mitochondria, organelles not frequently seen in Schwann cells of adult unmyelinated nerve fibres.

In their development, then, the axon-Schwann cell relationships of spinal nerve roots are identical with those found more peripherally in the more frequently studied spinal nerves. The connective tissues of nerve roots also resemble those of spinal nerves but are markedly more scanty and it is not possible to demonstrate either the inner reticulin sheath of Plenk-Laidlaw or the outer, collagenous sheath of Key and Retzius (Gamble, 1964) which are often conspicuous in peripheral nerves (Thomas, 1963). This lack of collagen accounts for the extreme fragility of root fibres when attempts are made to tease them apart, and reflects the sheltered nature of their situation. In fact, the total absence of collagen from their points of attachment to the spinal cord (see below) would render useless any substantial quantity of collagen along their length. Under tension nerve roots are likely to detach from the cord, their weakest point.

6.2.3 *The nerve root endoneurial tissues*

When studied by the techniques of light microscopy, the endoneurium of nerve roots has appeared to be the same as that of peripheral nerve (Tarlov, 1937a), although Laidlaw (1930) thought that both 'the longitudinal fibres and the web' (corresponding to the sheaths of Key and Retzius and of Plenk-Laidlaw, respectively) were 'heavier and more prominent' in nerve roots than in peripheral nerve. While there is a possibility that species differences explain this finding, it has been shown by Gamble (1964) that the extreme fragility of rat dorsal nerve root fibres is to be attributed to the paucity of endoneurial collagen: what little collagen is present is not organized as sheaths about the nerve fibres. Human dorsal nerve roots are similarly deficient in endoneurial collagen (Gamble and Eames, 1966) except after injury; crush injury is followed by collagen proliferation as in peripheral nerve trunks.

Endoneurial fibroblasts are present in nerve roots (as in peripheral nerves) but no estimates are available as to their numbers. Mast cells occur in the endoneurium of rat peripheral nerve (Gamble and Goldby, 1961; Gamble, 1964) but are apparently wholly absent from their roots. The incidence of mast cells in the endoneurium of other species is not known in detail, save that they occur in man, the baboon and cat amongst mammals, and in the bony fish *Orthagoriscus mola* (Romieu, 1924); their precise function in this situation is at present obscure.

The blood vessels of nerve roots appear not to have been studied in any systematic way except in relation to their origins and the grosser aspects of their distribution (Gillilan, 1958). It is only as components of an endoneurium essentially similar to that of peripheral nerve that capillaries are mentioned by

Nathaniel and Pease (1963), Gamble (1964) and Steer (1971). Berthold (1968b and c) reported that endoneurial vessels are scarce and small in nerve roots of mature cats but abundant and large in the roots of newborn kittens. He gave no further account of them and it is impossible to judge from his figures (which are light micrographs) whether arterioles, venules or capillaries are present. In any event, some of the vessels appear to reside in the perineurial or root sheath tissues. Most of the nerve root vessels figured by Haller, Haller and Low (1972) lie just outside or in the substance of the root sheath, or on the surface of the spinal cord and do not appear to be endoneurial in their distribution. All appear to be very thin-walled but no certain identification of their nature can be made. The vessel lying just within the root sheath in Fig. 14 of McCabe and Low's (1969) publication appears to have a lumen of some $15 \times 10 \mu m$ and to have a pericyte covering a large part of its periphery but again identification is uncertain and it might be argued that this, in any event, is a vessel penetrating into, but not yet of, the endoneurium.

Such little evidence as is available, then, suggests that the vessels penetrating into nerve root endoneurium are capillaries, as they are reported to be in peripheral nerves (Thomas, 1963). Although they are often associated with pericytes the significance of this is not known. The properties of nerve root blood vessels in relation to their permeability, and as barriers between blood and the root nerve fibres, do not appear to have been investigated. Olsson (1966) and Aker (1972) observed marked permeability in perineurial and epineurial vessels, as compared with impermeability in endoneurial vessels, in normal nerves of the rat and rabbit; Olsson also suggested that the permeability which appeared in the endoneurial vessels after injury to the nerve might be in some way related to the release of biogenic amines from mast cells located in the endoneurium. Mast cells however, are absent from rat nerve roots (Gamble and Goldby, 1961; Gamble, 1964) although nerve roots react to injury in ways very similar to peripheral nerves.

6.2.4 *The nerve root sheaths (Perineurium and Pia mater)*

In peripheral nerves a multilamellar perineurial sheath is a conspicuous feature of every fascicle, and branches of the sheath are prolonged over branches of the nerve. It consists of flattened cells, joined tightly edge-to-edge, covered on both inner and outer aspects by basal membranes and incorporating longitudinally orientated collagen fibrils between the cellular layers. In some branches, as in those to the more complex encapsulated sensory nerve endings (Pease and Pallie, 1959) the sheath, though reduced in thickness, is apparently in continuity with the capsule. In other branches it apparently ends by opening into the surrounding connective tissue spaces, the contained nerve fibres emerging through its open end. The presence of this multilamellar covering in essentially similar form on both spinal nerve roots and peripheral nerves, was first noted by Key and Retzius (1876), and the alternation of cellular and fibrous layers described by Ranvier in 1878. Continuity of the sheath from root to spinal nerve was described by Shanthaveerappa and Bourne (1962) in a light microscopic study of serial sections, a finding recently supported by the electron microscope study of Haller and Low (1971), but with the reservation that there are ways in which the sheath of the root differs from that of the nerve (cf. Chapter 3).

The epineurium, the dense connective tissue outer covering of peripheral nerve trunks, is apparently continuous with the dura mater at the union of spinal nerve with spinal roots, and the scattered collagen fibrils and fibroblast-like cells associated with nerve roots, outside the cellular sheath, are of leptomeningeal tissue, to be called pial or arachnoidal as seems most fitting.

It is only in recent years that much attention has been given to the perineurial and epineurial sheaths of peripheral nerve, since demonstrations that they, or some of their components, may form effective barriers to the entry of some drugs capable of blocking nerve impulse conduction (Crescitelli, 1951) or to the diffusion of certain ions active physiologically in nerve impulse conduction (Huxley and Stampfli, 1951). It has usually been assumed that it is the cellular component of the perineurium that is the site of the barrier (e.g. Huxley and Stampfli, 1951; Krnjevic, 1954) but there is some evidence that the epineurium cannot be wholly excluded from consideration in this respect (Evans, 1968).

The sheaths of spinal nerve roots of the rat have been studied electron microscopically by Benke and Röhlich (1963) and by Gamble (1964) who found essential similarity there and in the perineurium of peripheral nerve. Haller and Low (1971) found some of these features in the nerve roots of various small mammals but basal membrane, although haphazardly variable, was often present only on the inner aspect of the innermost cellular layer. The outer cells were often somewhat irregularly arranged, and were, perhaps, rather leptomeningeal cells than perineurial. In the frog spinal nerve root, Pick, Gerdin and Delemos (1963) classified the several layers of ensheathing cells as fibrocytes; but since basement membranes were not always present on the Schwann cells of the root fibres (normally a prime characteristic of the Schwann cell) one must suspect that preservation of the tissue was in some way defective.

A study of the proximal end of rat spinal nerve rootlets (Steer, 1969; 1971) suggests that the flattened cellular layers of the root sheath terminate successively as they approach the cord, outer layers first, until almost at the point of attachment of rootlet to cord the the innermost layer also ends, allowing the root fibres to run through its open end to enter the spinal cord (Fig. 6.3). At the same time loosely arranged collagen fibrils and an interwoven layer of fibroblast-like cells on the outer aspect of the organized sheath become continuous with similar fibrils and cells on the surface of the cord, i.e. with epipial tissue or pia mater depending upon the terminology employed. This last prolongation of tissue from rootlet to cord was described also by Haller *et al.* (1972), but as forming no more than an extensively fenestrated membrane so that there is free communication between the endoneurial spaces within the root sheath and the sub-arachnoid space in which the root lies. It would follow from what has been said of the continuity of root sheaths and perineurial sheaths of spinal nerves and their peripheral branches that cerebro-spinal fluid is, ultimately, in continuity with tissue spaces associated at least with unencapsulated nerve endings. There is no evidence that continuity of space is normally accompanied by flow of fluid in either direction, although some evidence has recently been presented (Steer and Horney, 1968) that particulate matter

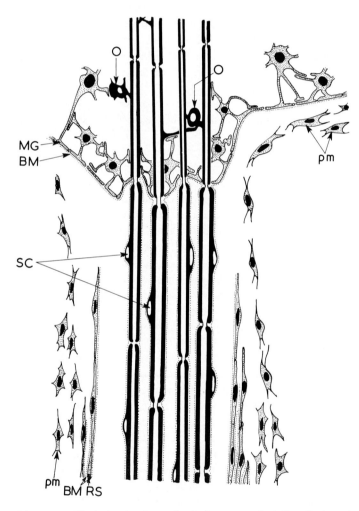

Fig. 6.3   Diagram to illustrate structure of spinal nerve root at the attachment to the spinal cord. Four axons are myelinated by oligodendrocytes (o) within the central nervous system, i.e. up to the point where they pass through gaps between astrocytes of the marginal glia (MG). The basement membrane covering the marginal glia is prolonged onto the Schwann cells (SC) which invest the axons with myelin after their entry into the peripheral nervous system. Fibroblast-like cells of the pia mater (pm) form a discontinuous covering of spinal cord and nerve root alike. More distally on the root an organized root sheath (RS), of flattened cells, associated with basement membrane, lies within the pial investment.

injected into the sub-arachnoid space can extend peripherally into the endoneurial spaces of spinal nerves.

Assuming that this interpretation of the sheathing arrangements of spinal roots and nerves is correct, and of general application, then it may be that analgesics applied to dorsal nerve root fibres through the medium of the cerebro-spinal fluid may reach the endoneurial spaces of the root directly through the open proximal end of the root sheath and without need to traverse a cellular or any other sheath. So direct an access to the nerve fibres might explain why some analgesics act so much more rapidly, and in so much smaller doses, when injected into the sub-arachnoid space than when injected into the epidural space or alongside peripheral nerve trunks. (In this context it is interesting to see how vulnerable are the C fibres of dorsal roots to alterations in the ionic content of the fluid in which they are normally bathed (Jewett and King, 1971; King, Jewett and Sundberg, 1972).) However, there are substantial differences between the susceptibility of spinal root fibres and that of spinal nerve fibres to the effects of certain toxins even when these are applied in circumstances which, most probably, prevent any possibility of their entry into the root save by traversing the cells of its investing sheath (Evans, 1968). It should be borne in mind also that central and peripheral processes of a dorsal root ganglion cell do not always behave identically in relation to apparently identical insults applied to each. For example, Nathan and Sears (1961) have shown that while chemical blocking of peripheral nerve first affects C fibres (before myelinated fibres fail) in posterior roots small myelinated fibres fail before unmyelinated. It is true, however, that epineurium was present upon the surface of the peripheral nerve tested, and absent from the root and that the similarity of the cellular sheaths may be more apparent than real. It is also claimed that unmyelinated fibres of dorsal roots are of smaller calibre than their counterparts in the peripheral nerve and yet must be processes of the same dorsal root ganglion cell (Gasser, 1955, but denied by Rexed and Sourander, 1949). Whether any disparity in size is found in myelinated fibres is not known.

The origins of the flattened cells of the perineurium and their proximal extensions onto spinal nerve roots are uncertain Shanthaveerappa and Bourne (e.g. 1963) are strongly of the opinion that the cells are of ectodermal origin, basing their belief, apparently, largely on experiments on the neural crest by Harvey and Burr (1926) and by Harvey, Burr and van Campenhout (1933). These experimental findings have yet to be confirmed and the possibility of another origin, in mesodermal tissues, was discussed by Gamble and Breathnach (1965) who observed that the perineurial cells of human fetal nerves resemble active fibroblasts and in early stages wholly lack the basement membranes which later become one of their major characteristics. Allt's (1969) Fig. 1 shows perineurial cells, in five-day-old rat sciatic nerve, where basement membrane is perhaps present over small parts of the cells' surfaces but is certainly absent from the greater part. In 1966, Gamble further remarked that the restoration of a perinurial investment of the repaired segment of a transected peripheral nerve involves changes which closely resemble those observed in fetal nerves, being

accomplished by the differentiation and ordering of cells originally indistinguishable from active fibroblasts. Shanthaveerappa and Bourne (1966) argue, in
relation to the capsular cells of the Pacinian corpuscle that 'it is important to
point out that if these lamellar cells were fibroblasts, the corpuscle would
contain much fibrous tissue. On the contrary, little collagen is found between
lamellar cells'. Their argument is two-edged. They claim identity between
lamellar cells of Pacinian corpuscle and of perineurium and the perineurium does
contain collagen, often in substantial quantity, between its concentric cellular
layers. (See Chapter 3 for a detailed discussion of the structure and homologies
of peripheral nerve connective tissues.)

6.2.5 *Junction of nerve roots with spinal cord*

It is commonly accepted that oligodendrocytes form the myelin sheaths of the
central nervous system, one oligodendrocyte providing an inter-nodal segment of
myelin on each of several (in fact, an unknown number) of adjacent axons (see,
for example, Bunge, 1968). There is also some evidence that astrocytes may be
involved in situations where oligodendrocytes are rare (e.g. Blunt, Paiseley and
Wendell-Smith, 1972). Ensheathment or other means of supporting unmyelinated axons of the central nervous system is very far from being fully
understood at present, but it is unlikely that anything comparable with the unit
of peripheral nervous system unmyelinated fibres i.e. a satellite (Schwann cell)
providing separate sheaths for each of several axons, occurs in the central
nervous system. However this may be, it is certain that extracellular spaces in the
central nervous system occur only between cells and their processes of a
common origin in neurectoderm and that basement membranes (basal laminae)
and extracellular collagen fibrils occur only where such cells and processes
confront penetrating blood vessels. It follows that where nerve root axons enter
or leave the central nervous system, there is an abrupt change in the manner of
their investment by satellite cells, from that by neuroglia alone to that by
Schwann cells associated with connective tissue.

The zone of transition between the central glial and the peripheral non-glial
segment of nerve roots was first described by Thomsen in 1887; subsequent light
microscopic studies were reviewed and augmented by Tarlov (1937a and b). The
transition occurs at the 'glial dome' usually marked by a local accumulation of
glial cells at the extremity of the glial segment a short distance beyond the
surface of the spinal cord. The length of the glial segment is always short but
may be as much as two to three millimetres in the roots of the *cauda equina* of
large animals. Besides the changes in satellite cells and connective tissue
infiltration already mentioned, abrupt increases in axonal diameter and myelin
thickness mark the transition from central to peripheral myelinated nerve fibres.

Electron microscopy, although rarely applied to the study of the transitional
zone, has confirmed some of the findings of light microscopy and has added

much detailed information (Steer, 1969 and 1971; Haller *et al.*, 1972). It has been shown that sub-pial astrocytes (marginal glia) and their cytoplasmic processes which everywhere form a mosaic on the outer surface of the spinal cord, constitute the majority of the cells of the glial dome. Here they are arranged with many gaps in the surface mosaic through which nerve root axons perforate to leave, or enter the spinal cord. It is clear that the 'dome' of light microscopy in fact forms a very jagged frontier; glial salients projecting into non-glial territory are themselves indented by minor salients and, besides this, small outlying islands of glial tissue often occur more distally in the root. The basement membrane which covers the outer aspect of the sub-pial astrocytes or their processes (Fig. 6.3) is reflected onto the surface of the perforating nerve root fibres (more precisely, onto the surface of their associated Schwann cells) rather in the manner that the material of a glove covering the hand is prolonged as cylinders upon each of the fingers. Fibrous astrocytes seem to predominate at the transitional zone (a finding at variance with Tarlov (1937a) who believed that oligodendrocytes did so) perhaps in part making good the deficiency in tensile strength which presumably results from the abrupt deficiency in collagen fibrils.

Oligodendrocytes apparently maintain their characteristic relationships with the central myelinated axons up to the point where these perforate the astrocytic layer. Since these oligodendrocytes are relatively few in number, and unusually large, it must be assumed that each has a myelin-forming role in relation to an unusually large number of axons. Beyond this oligodendrocyte-formed segment of myelin there is a node of Ranvier whose other boundary derives from a Schwann cell. While it appears certain that this node is contained within a tube of basement membrane continuous with that covering sub-pial astrocytes proximally and with that covering the Schwann cell distally, nothing is known in detail of its structure, nor of the paranodal regions of the bounding cells. Electron microscopy tends to confirm that axons are of larger diameter and provided with thicker myelin sheaths after entering into the peripheral segment. Figures illustrating this region (Haller *et al.*, 1972) certainly show such differences and the measurements of axonal diameter (myelinated and un-myelinated) given by Steer (1969) give some further support. It is not known whether mere enlargement at the node is accompanied by undercoating of the nodal axolemma, whether the paranodal axon is indented by paranodal Schwann cell processes or fluted by a similar fluting of the paranodal Schwann cell. Equally it is not known whether finger-like processes occur at this node, and if they do occur, whether they arise only from the Schwann cell. It is clear that this node of Ranvier is worthy of special attention from electron microscopists.

The transition from central to peripheral unmyelinated fibre is attended by at least equal ignorance. The same assumption concerning basement membrane continuity (frrom that covering the sub-pial astrocytes to that investing Schwann cell) that is made for myelinated fibres is probably justified for the un-myelinated fibres also; beyond this, nothing is known.

345

6.3 Particular properties of cranial nerve roots

It appears to be beyond dispute that the bulk of the components of the cranial nerves develop in essentially the same way as spinal nerves, neural crest being the source of most of the afferent and neural tube the source of all the efferent fibres. In the absence of any certain information one may suppose that the associated satellite (Schwann) cells are derived from the same sources.

There are, however, special ectodermal structures associated with the developing brain, the olfactory and otic placodes, which do or may, respectively play a part as sources of cranial nerve root fibres. As it happens, the nerve roots concerned, olfactory and auditory, have been the subjects of electron microscopic study as has the more 'ordinary' trigeminal nerve root. Other cranial nerve roots have been studied by Němeček, Pařizek, Špaček and Němečková (1969) and appear to resemble spinal roots although it is not possible to tell which roots were studied.

The olfactory nerve roots are unique in being the processes of neurons which have developed and remained (in olfactory epithelium) at the outer surface of the body; neurectoderm indeed. They maintain their primitive character at the ultrastructural level also, occurring as large bundles of very small axons (about 0.2 μm in diameter) invested communally by Schwann cells (Gasser, 1958). One Schwann cell may invest some hundreds of axons in adult olfactory nerve roots, thus resembling the condition found in the human ulnar nerve of embryos of some 10 weeks of intra-uterine life (Gamble, 1966), but not for long thereafter. The significance of this primitive arrangement is obscure. No information is available regarding the presence or absence of sheaths upon olfactory nerve roots and nothing is known of the entry of the axons into the olfactory bulb.

The auditory nerve, by contrast, in most of its length consists essentially of a fibre tract of the central nervous system i.e. its central glial segment is unusually long. In the rat the glial component extends well into the modiolus (Němeček, *et al.*, 1969; Ross and Burkel, 1971) but detailed information is lacking in respect of other species.

The central segment consists of the axons, oligodendrocytes and astrocytes which might be expected to be present in a fibre tract of the central nervous system, bounded by sub-pial astrocytes and covered externally by a basement membrane (Fig. 6.4). In addition it contains large and medium-size multipolar neurons of slightly unusual fine structure in that dendrites are distinguishable from the axon rather by their size and pattern of branching than by their content of organelles. Their function is not known but it seems possible that they represent outlying cells of the cochlear nuclei.

The central segment of the nerve root terminates in a 'glial dome' essentially similar to that described in spinal nerve roots. Ross and Burkel show an electron micrograph from a longitudinal section through a mode of Ranvier at the interface between central and peripheral segments (their Fig. 9) where finger-like processes may be present (certainty is not possible). The axon appears to

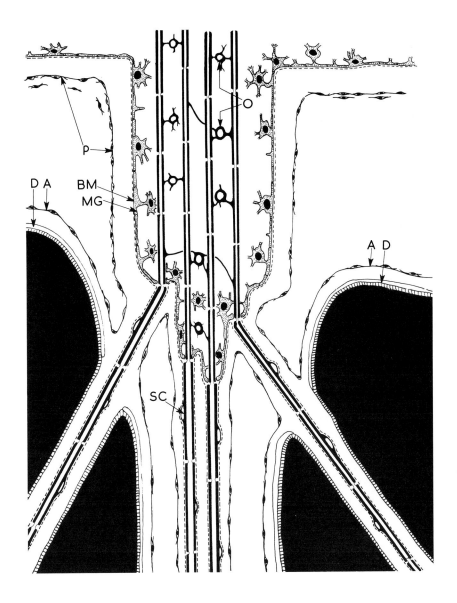

Fig. 6.4 Diagram to illustrate structure of auditory division of eighth cranial nerve. In most of its extent, the nerve has the structure of a fibre tract of the central nervous system, i.e. myelin sheaths are formed by oligodendrocytes, while astrocytes form the marginal glia (mg). The transition to Schwann cell investment of axons occurs at the base of the modiolus with (as in spinal roots) beasement membrane of marginal glia continuous with that of Schwann cells. The nerve is further invested by pial cells (P) which are continuous peripherally with he arachnoid mater (A) but there is no 'root sheath' present comparable with that found on spinal nerve roots. After nerve fibres enter into bony canals only the periosteum separates them from bone; the inner layer of the dura mater (D) ends at the margins of the bony foraminae.

increase in diameter just distal to the node, and the myelin is said to become thicker distally. From this one figure, it is not possible to determine whether or not axonal crenation, and mitochondrial accumulations occur in the Schwann cell cytoplasm paranodally.

The peripheral, non-glial segment of the nerve root is short but its structure resembles that of the peripheral parts of spinal nerve roots except for the absence of any sheath comparable with the perineurium. Scattered pial cells and collagen surround the branches as they pass toward the modiolar foramina but at the inner ends of the foramina pia is reflected onto arachnoid mater lining the dural wall of the modiolus. The meningeal layer of the dura mater also ends abruptly at the inner end of the modiolar foramen, and so, by the definition of cranial nerve roots used here, does the auditory nerve root also. The auditory nerve proper i.e. beyond the rather artificial termination of its root, is outside the proper scope of this chapter, but it is worth mentioning that it (in the form of many small branches perforating into the modiolar foramina) lacks both of the layers of connective tissue which usually invest nerves: the meningeal layer of the dura mater is not prolonged into an epineurium and nor is there a perineurium. The Schwann cell invested axons of the nerve and the similarly invested bipolar cells of the spiral ganglion (cf. Chapter 4) are surrounded only by the periosteal layer of the dura mater in the modiolar foramina, the spiral tract and the osseous spiral laminae, although a few wisps of pia mater-like tissue are described as surrounding groups of nerve fibres and ganglion cells in the spiral tracts. In most respects it seems that the relations of pia mater to the auditory nerve root closely resemble those of the pia mater to spinal nerve roots. There may be an exception of some importance, however. Ross and Burkel describe the pial investment of the auditory nerve as being by a 'thin continuous sheet of flattened cells', in this resembling Steer's (1971) description of an arachnoid membrane extending onto the outer aspect of the spinal nerve root sheath and consisting of 'very thin closely packed cells which branch to form a neatly interwoven layer'. Haller *et al.* (1972) however, were of the opinion that the spinal cord's covering of pia mater extended onto spinal nerve roots as a fenestrated membrane permitting free communication between cerebro-spinal fluid and the endoneurial fluids of the nerve root. It is difficult to judge between the validity of the interpretations of Steer on the one hand and Haller *et al.* on the other. In any event, nothing is known of the physiological properties of pial cells, nor of their effectiveness as a container of cerebro-spinal fluid when forming a continuous sheet of cells. Some investigation of these properties might prove to be of interest.

There remains for consideration an account of the trigeminal nerve root by Maxwell, Kruger and Pineda (1969). In general, it may be said that the structure of the trigeminal nerve root closely resembles that of a spinal nerve root in the central segment and in the transitional zone, and differs in the peripheral segment only by lacking a lamellated perineurium. The loose connective tissue described as investing this part of the root probably corresponds with the pial investment of spinal and auditory nerve roots, although its continuity with pontine pia mater proximally and with arachnoid mater peripherally have not been demonstrated. How effective a barrier it might be between cerebro-spinal fluid and endoneurial connective tissue spaces is uncertain.

6.4 Degeneration and regeneration in nerve roots

Transection or severe crushing of spinal nerve roots result in degenerative changes in axons and Schwann cells (myelin sheaths) distal to the lesion which are precisely similar to those constituting Wallerian degeneration in peripheral nerves. These changes are usually accompanied by a marked proliferation of the endoneurial connective tissues (Gamble 1964). In the case of dorsal nerve roots, of course, the term 'distal to the lesion' is applied to that part of the root more distant from the cell of origin in the dorsal root ganglion so that the degenerative changes extend into the spinal cord to involve glial cells in the degenerative phenomena.

The degenerative changes occurring in a ventral root as the result of crushing may be followed by successful regeneration of axons growing through the lesion and into the bands of Büngner where proliferated Schwann cells provide an ordered sequence of surfaces suitable for axonal growth, contained within a basement membrane sheath leading to nerve terminals appropriate to the nature of the regenerated axon. In such cases regeneration can be extensive and valuable and can occur, for example, when pressure upon a ventral root (by a prolapsing intervertebral disc, or by a neuroma upon an adjacent root of the *cauda equina* (Gamble and Eames, 1966)) is relieved by operation. Transection of ventral roots is likely to be accompanied by passive separation of the cut ends, which are in any event fragile and not easily sutured or otherwise rejoined. The chancey nature of functional repair which may occur in cut and sutured peripheral nerves is exaggerated by these features of nerve roots.

Similar factors limit the likelihood of functional repair of transected dorsal nerve roots but with the additional difficulty, applicable equally to crushed fibres, that regenerating axons are apparently unable to enter the central nervous system in any numbers. The few that may do so are unable to effect useful connections with other neurons, being impeded by the glial proliferation which follows the degeneration of the original axons (in the absence of basement membranes about the satellite cells of axons in the central nervous system, there is no basis for the segregation of proliferated glial cells into columns resembling the bands of Büngner. Such cells apparently form a largely impenetrable glial 'scar'). Other regenerating axons apparently enter, but cannot leave, peri-vascular spaces of the central nervous system (Moyer, Kimmel and Wimborne, 1953), and still others extend into leptomeningeal spaces: in either event useful connections with other neurons are not made.

In traction lesions of the brachial plexus, nerve roots may be avulsed from the cord at the transitional zone between their non-glial components, a point which coincides with transition from collagen-associated Schwann cells to glial cells unassociated with collagen. Although the majority of the glial cells at the transition are fibrous astrocytes, their tensile strength appears to be much less than that of collagen reinforced endoneurium. Degenerative and regenerative changes following such lesions conform to the pattern set out above, so that functional recovery is unknown in the sensory fibres and extremely rare, if it occurs at all, in the motor fibres. At the same time dorsal root ganglion cells show no more than transient changes and maintain apparently normal fibres extending through spinal nerves to the periphery.

It is difficult to find other examples of pathological change in nerve roots which are to be attributed to particular features of their structure, although their close investment by pia mater is liable to involve them in pathological processes originating in the leptomeninges. It is possible that the degeneration in dorsal nerve root fibres and in the dorsal columns of the cord, which occurs in Tabes dorsalis, originates in a disorder of the pial investment of the roots. Such an explanation fails to account for the apparent sparing of some fibres entering through the affected roots: dorsal root ganglia of affected roots are often found to be small but whether as a primary or as a secondary event is not known.

Other injuries to spinal roots are attributable to their location in cerebro-spinal fluid within the sub-arachnoid space and to the use that has been made of this fluid as a medium by which spinal anaesthetics may be brought into contact with dorsal nerve root fibres. On occasion injurious detergents and antiseptics have followed the same route from syringes to sensory (and motor) fibres (see Mayer, 1958). It is possible that only epineurium and perineurium have saved peripheral nerves from similar hazards when being infiltrated with locally injected anaesthetics.

A very large number of pathological conditions are cited by Greenfield (1958a and b) and by Mayer (1958) where degerative changes in axons, or Schwann cells, or both are found in nerve roots and are variously attributed to dietary deficiencies, to metallic poisons, to toxins and to infections of different kinds. These never, apparently, affect nerve roots in isolation and indeed nerve roots appear often to be unscathed (more precisely, unmentioned) in conditions where perpheral nerves may be seriously affected.

It seems that degenerative changes in cranial nerve roots are, like those in spinal nerve roots, only rarely directly referable to their characteristic structure, although like the latter their course through the sub-arachnoid space and their investment by pia mater may involve them in pathological processes affecting the leptomeninges. However, it is said that the eighth cranial nerve is more liable than other cranial nerves to be torn by direct blows to the head (even by loud noises) and its weakness has been attributed to this aspect of its structure (e.g. Gray, 1967) namely the presence of a long glial segment. As has been pointed out, however, all nerve roots have glial segments, however short, and there is no particular feature of the glial segment of the eighth nerve to which its apparent weakness is to be attributed. It may be that the non-glial segment, ordinarily capable of some elongation without tearing, is simply too short.

Finally one may note the constant close relationship between the root of the third cranial nerve and the posterior cerebral and superior cerebellar arteries; and the chance that the nerve root may be involved in periarteritis affecting these vessels.

References

Aker, F. D. (1972) A study of hematic barriers in peripheral nerves of albino rabbits. *The Anatomical Record,* **174,** 21–38.

Allt, G. (1969) Ultrastructural features of the immature peripheral nerve. *Journal of Anatomy,* **105,** 283–293.

Balfour, D. H. (1885) *Comparative Embryology.* Ch. XV, pp. 400–469. Macmillan and Company: London.

Barron, D. H. and Mathews, B. H. C. (1938) The interpretation of potential changes in the spinal cord. *Journal of Physiology,* **92,** 276–321.

Benke, B. and Röhlich, P. (1963) Elektronmikroskopische Untersuchungen an den Hüllen der Ruckenmarks-wurzeln. I Hintere Wurzel. *Journal für Hirnforschung,* **7,** 87–93.

Berthold, C. H. (1968a) Ultrastructure of postnatally developing feline peripheral nodes of Ranvier. *Acta Societatis Medicorum Upsaliensis,* **73,** 145–168. (1968b) A study of fixation of large mature feline myelinated ventral lumbar spinal-root nerve fibres. *Ibid.,* **73,** suppl. 9, 1–36. (1968c) Ultrastructure of the node-paranode region of mature feline ventral lumbar spinal-root fibres. *Ibid.,* **73,** Suppl. 9, 37–70.

Berthold, C. H. and Skoglund, S. (1967) Histochemical and ultrastructural demonstration of mitochondria in the paranodal region of developing feline spinal roots and nerves. *Ibid.,* **72,** 37–70. (1968a) Postnatal development of feline paranodal myelin sheath segments. I. Light microscopy. *Ibid.,* **73,** 113–126. (1968b) Postnatal development of feline paranodal myelin sheath segments. II. Electron microscopy. *Ibid.,* **73,** 127–144.

Blunt, M. J., Paisley, P. B. and Wendell-Smith, C. P. (1972) Oxidative enzyme histochemistry of immature neuroglia during myelination. *Journal of Anatomy,* **110,** 421–433.

Bunge, R. P. (1968) Glial cells and the central myelin sheath. *Physiological Reviews,* **48,** 197–251.

Cravioto, H. (1965) The role of Schwann cells in the development of human peripheral nerves. An electron microscope study. *Journal of Ultrastructure Research,* **12,** 634–651.

Crescitelli, F. (1951) Nerve sheath as a barrier to the action of certain substances. *American Journal of Physiology,* **166,** 229–250.

Duncan, D. (1932) A determination of the number of unmyelinated fibres in the ventral roots of the rat, cat and rabbit. *Journal of Comparative Neurology,* **55,** 459–471.

Eames, Rosemary A. and Gamble, H. J. (1970) Schwann cell relationships in normal human cutaneous nerves. *Journal of Anatomy,* **106,** 417–435.

Evans, M. H. (1968) Topical application of saxitoxin and tetrodotoxin to peripheral nerves and spinal roots in cat. *Toxicon,* **5,** 289–294.

Fraher, J. P. (1972) A quantitative study of anterior root fibres during early myelination. *Journal of Anatomy,* **112,** 99–124.

Gamble, H. J. (1964) Comparative electron microscope observation on the connective tissue of a peripheral nerve and a spinal root in the rat. *Journal of Anatomy,* **98,** 17–25. (1966) Further electron microscope studies of human foetal peripheral nerves. *Journal of Anatomy,* **100,** 487–502. (1974) In *The Cell in Medical Science,* (eds.) Beck, F. and Lloyd, J. B., Vol. 1, Chapter 13, Academic Press Inc.: London.

Gamble, H. J. and Breathnach, A. S. (1965) An electron microscope study of human foetal peripheral nerves. *Journal of Anatomy,* **99,** 573–584.

Gamble, H. J. and Eames, Rosemary, A. (1964) An electron microscope study of the connective tissues of human peripheral nerve. *Ibid.,* **98,** 655–663.

Gamble, H. J. and Eames, Rosemary, A. (1966) Electron microscopy of human spinal nerve roots. *Archives of Neurology,* 14, 50–53.

Gamble, H. J. and Goldby, S. (1961) Mast cells in peripheral nerve trunks. *Nature (London),* 189, 766–767.

Gasser, H. S. (1955) Properties of dorsal root unmedullated fibres on the two sides of the ganglion. *Journal of General Physiology,* 38, 709–728. (1958) Comparison of the structure, as revealed by the electron microscope, and the physiology of the unmedullated fibers in the skin nerves and in the olfactory nerves. *Experimental Cell Research Supplement,* 5, 3–17.

Geren, B. B. (1954) The formation from the Schwann cell surface of myelin in peripheral nerves of chick embryos. *Experimental Cell Research,* , 7, 558–562.

Gillilan, Lois A. (1958) The arterial blood supply of the human spinal cord. *Journal of Comparative Neurology,* 110, 75–103.

Gray's *Anatomy* (1967) (ed.) Davies, D. V., 34 th edition, Longmans, Green & Co.: London.

Greenfield, J. G. (1958) Infectious diseases of the nervous system, In *Neuropathology,* (eds.) J. G. Greenfield, W. Blackwood, W. H. McMenemey, A. Mayer and R. M. Norman. Chapter 3, 132–229. Edward Arnold: London. (1958) Diseases of the lower motor and sensory neurons (peripheral neuritis and neuropathy) in *Ibid.,* Chapter 12, 583–615.

Grinnell, A. D. (1970) Electrical interaction between antidromically stimulated frog motoneurons and dorsal root afferents: enhancement by gallamine and TEA. *Journal of Physiology,* 210, 17–43.

Haller, F. R., Haller, Ann C. and Low, F. N. (1972) The fine structure of cellular layers and connective tissue space at spinal nerve root attachments in the rat. *American Journal of Anatomy,* 133, 109–124.

Haller, F. R. and Low, F. N. (1971) The fine structure of the nerve root sheath in the sub-arachnoid space in the rat and other laboratory animals. *American Journal of Anatomy,* 131, 1–20.

Hamilton, W. J., Boyd, J. D. and Mossman, H. W. (1972) *Human Embryology (Prenatal development of form and function)* 4th edn., Ch. XIII, 437–525. W. Heffer and Sons: Cambridge.

Harrison, R. G. (1907) Obervations of the living developing nerve fibre. *Anatomical Record,* 1, 116–118.

Harvey, S. C. and Burr, S. H. (1926) The development of meninges. *Archives of Neurology and Psychiatry, Chicago,* 15, 545–567.

Harvey, S. C., Burr, S. H. and Van Campenhout, E. (1933) Development of meninges. *Archives of Neurology and Psychiatry, Chicago,* 29, 683–690.

Hildebrand, A. F. and Skoglund, S. (1967) Ultrastructural features of the nodal region in lumbar spinal roots of newborn man. *Acta Societas Medicorum Upsaliensis,* 72, 71–75.

Huxley, A. F. and Stampfli, R. (1951) Effects of potassium and sodium on resting and action potentials of single myelinated nerve fibres. *Jounal of Physiology,* 112, 496–508.

Jewett, D. L. and King, J. S. (1971) Conduction block of monkey dorsal rootlets by water and hypertonic saline solutions. *Experimental Neurology,* 33, 225–237.

Key, A. and Retzius, G. (1876) *Studien in der Anatomie des Nervensystems und des Bindegewebes.* Samson and Wallin: Stockholm.

King, J. S., Jewett, D. L. and Sundberg, H. R. (1972) Differential blockade of cat dorsal root C fibers by various chloride solutions. *Journal of Neurosurgery,* 36, 569–583.

Krnjevic, K. (1954) The connective tissue of frog sciatic nerve. *Quarterly Journal of Experimental Physiology,* 39, 55–72.

Laidlaw, G. (1930) Silver staining of the endoneurial fibres of the cerebro-spinal nerves. *American Journal of Pathology,* 6, 435–444.

Landon, D. N. and Langley, O. K. (1971) The local chemical environment of nodes of Ranvier: a study of cation binding. *Journal of Anatomy,* 108, 419–432.

Landon, D. N. and Williams, P. L. (1963) Ultrastructure of the node of Ranvier. *Nature, London,* 199, 575–577.

McCabe, J. S. and Low, F. N. (1969) The sub-arachnoid angle: an area of transition in peripheral nerve. *The Anatomical Record,* 164, 15–33.

Marshall, A. M. (1893) *Vertebrate Embryology,* Chapter V, pp. 341–447, Chapter VI, pp. 448–619. Smith, Elder & Co.: London.

Matheson, D. F. (1968) Influence of age in the incorporation of ^{14}C-Glycine into isolated rat nerve segments *in vitro*. *Journal of Neurochemistry* **15**, 187–194.

Matheson, D. F. and Cavanagh, J. B. (1967) Protein synthesis in peripheral nerve and susceptibility to diphtheritic neuropathy. *Nature, London,* **214**, 721–722.

Maxwell, D. S., Kruger, L. and Pineda, A. (1969) The trigeminal nerve root with special reference to the central-peripheral transition zone: an electron microscope study in the Macaque. *Anatomical Record,* **164**, 113–126.

Mayer, A. (1958) Anoxias, Intoxications and Metabolic Disorders, in *Neuropathology,* (eds.) J. G. Greenfield, W. Blackwood, W. H. McMenemey, A. Mayer and R. M. Norman. Chapter 4, pp. 230–299. Edward Arnold: London.

Melzack, R. and Wall, P. D. (1965) Pain mechanisms: a new theory. *Science,* **150**, 970–979.

Mendell, L. M. and Wall, P. D. (1964) Presynaptic hyperpolarisation: a role for fine afferent fibers. *Journal of Physiology,* **172**, 274–294.

Moyer, E. K., Kimmel, D. L. and Wimborne, L. W. (1953) Regeneration in sensory spinal roots in young and senile rats. *Journal of comparative Neurology,* **98**, 283–307.

Nathan, P. W. and Sears, T. A (1961) Some factors concerned in differential block by local anaesthetics. *Journal of Physiology,* **157**, 565–580.

Nathaniel, E. J. H. and Pease, D. C. (1963) Degenerative changes in rat dorsal roots during Wallerian degeneration. *Journal of Ultrastructure Research,* **9**, 511–532.

Němeček, S., Pařizek, J., Špaček, J. and Němrčková, J. (1969) Histological, Histochemical and Ultrastructural appearance of the transitional zone of the cranial and spinal nerve roots. *Folia Morphologica,* **17**, 171–181.

Nyström, B. and Skoglund, S. (1965) Calibre spectra of spinal nerves and roots in newborn man. *Acta Morphologica Neerlando – Scandinavica,* **6**, 115–127.

Olsson, Y. (1966) Studies on vascular permeability in peripheral nerves. I. Distribution of circulating fluorescent serum albumin in normal, crushed and sectioned rat sciatic nerve. **7**, 1–15.

Pease, D. C. and Pallie, W. (1959) Electron microscopy of digital tactile corpuscles and small cutaneous nerves. *Journal of Ultrastructure Research,* **2**, 352–365.

Peters, A. and Muir, A. R. (1959) The relationship between axons and Schwann cells during development of peripheral nerves in rat. *Quarterly Journal of Experimental Physiology,* **44**, 117–130.

Pick, J., Gerdin, C. and Delemos, C. (1963) On the ultrastructure of spinal nerve roots in the frog (*Rana pipiens*). *Anatomical Record,* **146**, 61–84.

Ranson, S. W. and Davenport, H. K. (1931) Sensory unmyelinated fibers in the spinal nerves. *American Journal of Anatomy,* **48**, 331–353.

Ranvier, M. L. (1878) *Leçons sur l'histologie du système nerveux.* E. Savy: Paris.

Rexed, B. and Sourander, P. (1949) The calibre of central and peripheral neurites of spinal ganglion cells and variations at different levels of dorsal spinal roots. *Journal of Comparative Neurology,* **91**, 297–306.

Robertson, J. D. (1959) Preliminary observations on the ultrastructure of Nodes of Ranvier. *Zeitschrifft für Zellforschung und mikroskopische Anatomie,* **50**, 553–560.

Romieu, M. (1924) Contribution a l'étude des mastocytes des poissons osseux. *Compte Rendu de la Société de Biologie,* Paris, **91**, 655–657.

Ross, Muriel D. and Burkel, W. (1971) Electron microscopic observations of the nucleus, glial dome and meninges of rat acoustic nerve. *American Journal of Anatomy,* **130**, 73–92.

Schwann, T. (1847) *Microscopic researches into the accordance in the structure and growth of animals and plants.* Translated Smith, H. Sydenham Society: London.

Shanthaveerappa, T. R. and Bourne, G. H. (1962) A perineurial epithelium. *Journal of Cell Biology.* **14**, 343–346.

Shanthaveerappa, T. R. and Bourne, G. H. (1963) New observations on the structure of the Pacinian corpuscle and its relation to the perineurial epithelium of peripheral nerves. *American Journal of Anatomy,* **112**, 97–109. (1966) Histochemical studies on the Pacinian corpuscle. *American Journal of Anatomy,* **118**, 461–470.

Steer, J. C. and Horney, F. D. (1968) Evidence for passage of cerebro-spiral fluid along spinal nerves. *Journal of the Canadian Medical Association,* **98**, 71–78.

Steer, Janet M. (1969) *An investigation into the fine structure of spinal dorsal nerve roots at the junction of peripheral and central nervous systems.* A Thesis accepted for the Degree of Master of Science, University of London.

Steer, Janet M. (1971) Some observations on the fine structure of rat dorsal spinal nerve roots. *Journal of Anatomy,* **109**, 467–485.

Tarlov, I. M. (1937a) Structure of the nerve root. I. Nature of the junction between the central and peripheral nervous system. *Archives of Neurology and Psychiatry,* **37**, 555–583. (1937b) Structure of the nerve root. II. Differentiation of sensory from motor roots: observations on identification of function in roots of mixed cranial nerves. *Ibid.,* **37**, 1338–1355.

Tennyson, Virginia M. (1970) The fine structure of the axon and growth cone of the dorsal root neuroblast of the rabbit embryo. *Journal of Cell Biology,* **44**, 62–79.

Thomas, P. K. (1963) The connective tissue of peripheral nerve: an electron microscope study. *Journal of Anatomy,* **97**, 35–44.

Thomas, P. K (1966) The cellular response to nerve injury I. The cellular outgrowth from the distal stump of transected nerve. *Journal of Anatomy,* **100** , 287–303.

Thomsen, R. (1887) Ueber eigenthümliche aus veränderten Ganglien Zellen hervorgegangene Gebilde in dem Stämmen der Hirnnerven des Menschen. *Virchow's Archives für Pathologisches Anatomie,* **109**, 459–503.

Vizoso, A. D. and Young, J. Z. (1948) The internodal length and fibre diameter in developing and regenerating nerves. *Journal of Anatomy,* **82**, 110–124.

Whitehorn, D. and Burgess, P. R. (1973) Changes in polarization of central branches of myelinated mechanoreceptor and nociceptor fibres during noxious and innocuous stimulation of the skin. *Journal of Neurophysiology,* **36**, 226–237.

Zimmermann, M. (1968) Dorsal root potentials after C-fiber stimulation. *Science,* **160**, 896–898.

GANGLIA OF THE AUTONOMIC NERVOUS SYSTEM

G. Gabella

In this chapter a survey is presented of the structure of the better known ganglia of the autonomic (vegetative) nervous system. This part of the peripheral nervous system provides the innervation to the viscera, the cardio-vascular system, and the smooth muscles of the eye and the skin. Attention is focused on the mammalian ganglia, where the available morphological and physiological data are more numerous, but the sympathetic ganglia of amphibia and the ciliary ganglion of birds are also briefly discussed. This presentation does not therefore cover the whole area of the vegetative nervous system systematically, nor does it attempt to interpret the general lines of its organization and evolution. However, even within the field chosen for review, the information available appears strikingly small in relation to the structural complexity of the system and its great variability between different classes, species and individuals.

7.1 Sympathetic ganglia

The sympathetic ganglia can be divided into two anatomical categories, paravertebral and prevertebral. The paravertebral ganglia and their connecting trunks constitute the sympathetic chains and are situated bilaterally along the ventro-lateral aspect of the spinal column, from the sacral to the upper cervical level, while the prevertebral ganglia lie close to the median sagittal plan of the body anteriorly to the abdominal aorta.

In the sympathetic chain of mammals the thoracic and the lumbar regions have approximately one ganglion for each metameric segment of the body, whereas at the cervical level there is an upper ganglion (the superior cervical ganglion), a lower (the stellate ganglion, which usually incorporates the first thoracic ganglion), and a small intermediate ganglion. In the lumbo-sacral region the right and left chains are connected by branches across the midline, and in front of the coccyx the two chains converge to form a small *ganglion impar* in the midline. Variations in the number, size and distribution of the sympathetic ganglia between different species and individuals are common, and in man variations in the pattern of ganglia are particularly obvious in the neck (Becker and Grunt, 1957).

Connections between sympathetic ganglia and spinal cord are provided by nerves called *white rami communicantes*. They are composed of preganglionic

but counts have been performed on individual ganglia, and in particular upon the superior cervical ganglion. This ganglion is well defined and easily isolated, with afferent and efferent nerves, and has therefore been the ganglion most used for structural and functional studies of sympathetic neurons. However, this ganglion is no more a *typical* ganglion than is any other, and the data derived from it are not always applicable to other sympathetic ganglia, or vice versa.

In man between 760 000 and 1 000 000 neurons were estimated to be present in six superior cervical ganglia examined by Ebbeson (1968a). In other primates the numbers of neurons found are smaller and this correlates with body size; progressively smaller numbers of neurons were found in primates of decreasing body size (for example 838 000 in a chimpanzee of 50 kg, 325 000 in a baboon of 15 kg, 205 000 in a stumptail monkey of 5 kg, and 64 000 in a squirrel monkey of 0.6 kg). Parallel to the increase in the total number of ganglion cells, with increase in body size, there is a decrease in the mean cell density, i.e. an increase in the so called cell territory. In the superior cervical ganglion Ebbeson (1968b) found 32 000 ganglion cells/mm^2 in a squirrel monkey (mean cell territory about 3×10^{-5} mm^3) and 4500 and 7000 ganglion cells/mm^3 in two human subjects (mean cell territory about 22 and 14×10^{-5} mm^3 respectively). The occurrence of larger neurons with greater arborization of dendrites in large animal species, notably in man, and particularly in the superior cervical ganglion, has been known for a long time (Cajal, 1911; Terni, 1922; De Castro, 1932). The spaces between ganglion cells are mainly occupied by investing satellite cells, dendrites and axons and collagen fibrils. In addition the ganglia contain granular cells (see below), mast cells (about 24 000 in the superior cervical ganglion of the cat, Hollinshead and Gertner, 1969), fibroblasts and blood vessels. Other published counts of neuron numbers have given the following results: superior cervical ganglion of mouse 15 000 neurons (average of 12 ganglia) (Levi-Montalcini and Booker, 1960; Klingman and Klingman, 1967); stellate ganglion of the mouse 19 000 (seven cases) (Klingman and Klingman, 1967); superior cervical ganglion of the cat: 123 000 (one case) (Billingsley and Ransom, 1918), 66–96 000 (two cases) (Wolf, 1941); coeliac and superior mesenteric ganglia of the mouse each about 25 000 (Klingman and Klingman, 1967).

In the superior cervical ganglion of the rat the number of neurons was found to range between 52 000 and 54 000 in male rats (three cases) and between 41 000 and 45 000 in female rats (three cases) (Gabella and Millar, 1974). Number variations between individuals were smaller than observed in other species. The numerical difference between male and female rats is statistically significant and does not correlate with the body weight of the adult animals.

All ganglion cells are invested by satellite cells (glial cells) which completely enwrap them, so that no part of the perikaryal surface is in direct contact with connective tissue. There are several satellite cells for every neuron, and their small, dense nuclei are flattened and close to the surface of the ganglion cells. In electron micrographs, satellite cells are conspicuous in the region of the nuclei, but in other regions they are often reduced to slender lamellae, consisting of a layer of cytoplasm only a fraction of a micron thick and two plasma membranes. The lamellae from neighbouring satellite cells can overlap, but in general only a single thin lamella intervenes between the perikaryal surface and the surrounding connective tissue. The gap between the apposed membranes of satellite and nerve cells is 15—20 nm (Elfvin, 1963a; Cravioto and Merker, 1963). The outer surface of the satellite cells, or of the outmost lamella when several of them overlap, is covered by a basal lamina. Ganglion cells are usually mono-nucleated, but cells with two or more nuclei are also found, notably in the rabbit (Huber, 1899); binucleated cells are said to be more numerous in young subjects. The nucleus is round, poor in chromatin and not always situated in the centre of the cell. Neurons in the mammalian sympathetic ganglia are multipolar (De Castro, 1932). The dendrites, as visualized by silver impregnation, are numerous, relatively thick, long and branched, but they display a great morphological variability. They can be smooth-surfaced or varicose, and sometimes several of them appear to converge upon a single neighbouring neuron. In some species dendrites from two or more (sometimes up to a hundred) ganglion cells form a dendritic glomerulus, to which preganglionic fibres also contribute terminals (De Castro, 1932). Such glomeruli are common in man (Cajal, 1911, Ranson and Billingsley, 1918; Gairns and Garven 1953), less frequent in cattle and horses (De Lorenzi, 1931), and are rare or absent in small mammals (De Castro, 1932; McLachlan, 1973); their number and complexity increases with age but a few can be found even in embryonic ganglia (De Castro, 1932). McLachlan (1974) has found, by intracellular injection of a flourescent dye after electrical recording, 13 dendrites per ganglion cell on average in the superior cervical ganglion of the guinea-pig: the ration of dendritic to perikaryal surface area was calculated to be about 2.16:1. Other ganglion cell processes, the accessory or secondary dendrites or intracapsular processes, are short and thin and are contained entirely within the satellite cell sheath of perikarya.

An attempt to distinguish different classes of neurons was made by Dogiel (1896); this was initially based upon observations on cardiac and intestinal ganglia of the cat, but was subsequently considered to have a more general validity. Three classes of neurons were recognized: type I, with many short processes, were motor neurons; type 2, with only long processes, were sensory neurons (their long branched dendrites ending as sensory receptors, the axon arborizing within the ganglion); and type 3, with dendrites of medium length that branch around other ganglion cells.

This classification, and in particular its generalization to the entire vegetative nervous system, and to species other than cat, has not been fully substantiated, although ganglion cells can be found which correspond to three types described by Dogiel and many of his successors. Cajal (1911) proposed an alternative classification: (a) cells with short intracapsular processes only; (b) cells with long processes only; and (c) cells with both short and long processes. However, Amprino (1938) has subsequently shown that the structural characteristics of

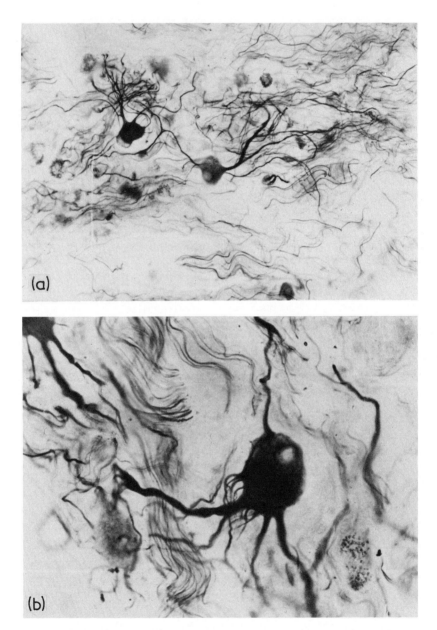

Fig. 7.2a and **b**   Human superior cervical ganglia, silver impregnated (Bielschowsky-Gros method). Complex arborization of the cell processes. (Reproduced by courtesy of Professor R. Amprino.)

the processes of human ganglion neurons dramatically change during the life span of the individual, especially in the superior cervical ganglion. In the newborn and the young for example all of the ganglion neurons have long processes only, the short intracapsular processes developing later in life. Other age-related changes include the accumulation of pigment, which can be very extensive in the superior cervical ganglion of man (De Lorenzi, 1931; Amprino, 1938), and the horse (De Lorenzi, 1931), but is virtually non-existent in cattle (De Lorenzi, 1931). Many authors report that age-related changes are far more striking in man than in other mammals, and more so in the superior cervical ganglion than in other sympathetic ganglia. It is unfortunate that these early attempts to analyse age-related changes in ganglion morphology with silver impregnation methods (Terni, 1922; De Castro, 1932; Amprino, 1938) have not been followed up using electrophysiological and electronmicroscopical techniques.

De Castro and Herreros (1945) classified the neurons of the superior cervical ganglion of the cat and man on the basis of cell body size, and their suggestion that large neurons (33–60 μm in diameter) provide the intrinsic innervation of the eye, whereas medium-sized neurons (25–32 μm) provide vaso- and pilomotor fibres, is indirectly supported by electrophysiological evidence (Bishop and Heinbecker, 1932; Eccles, 1935). No function was suggested for the small neurons; these measure 15–24 μm in diameter, are oval or pear-shaped, contain argentophilic granules, and have only a few dendrites which, although of the long type, are shorter than those of the other ganglion neurons. Some of these dendrites ended in the glomeruli, but no mention was made of their axons. These small ganglion neurons persist throughout life, and they were interpreted by De Castro and Herreiros (1945) to be nerve elements retarded in their development; some of them, however, probably correspond to the small intensely fluorescent cells which have been described more recently (see below). The number of small neurons observed by De Castro and Herreiros (22 per cent of all the ganglion cells in the superior cervical ganglion; 10–17 per cent in the thoracic and lumbar ganglia) is, however, higher than that reported for the small fluorescent cells, and it is thus possible that some of them do indeed represent immature elements which persist throughout life. Botar (1966), using the Bielschowky–Gros silver impregnation method, found that in the coeliac ganglia of adult dogs 10 per cent of the ganglion cells were immature neurons (e.g. sympathicoblasts), while the remainder of the neurons had numerous large processes (10–30 per cell), amongst which the axon could not be identified on the basis of its structure.

In the cat prevertebral ganglia the ganglion cells are larger than in paravertebral ganglia and more frequently possess accumulations of lipofuscin granules (Fredricsson and Sjöqvist, 1962).

In the electron microscope the sympathetic ganglion cells show many of the usual features of nerve cells. The nucleus is poor in chromatin, Nissl bodies are clumped in the deeper part of the cell, and there are numerous mitochondria,

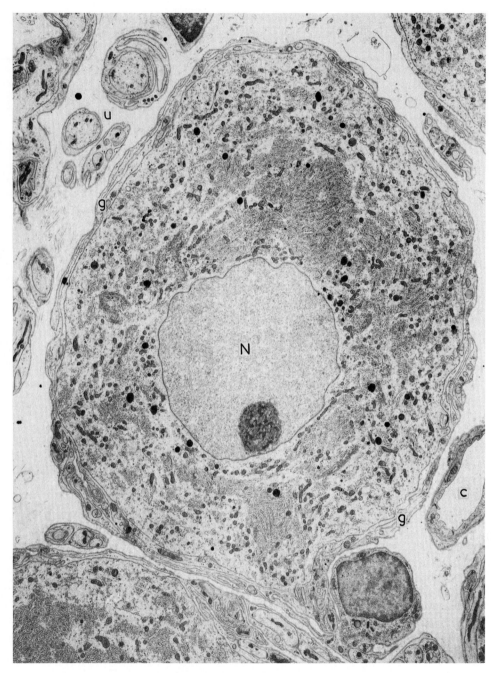

Fig. 7.3 A neuron of the superior cervical ganglion of the rat, fixed by immersion in osmium tetroxide. N – nucleus with nucleolus; u – unmyelinated axons; g – lamellae of satellite cells' cytoplasm; c – capillary. (Reproduced by courtesy of Dr Margaret Matthews.)

Golgi profiles and dense bodies (Elfvin, 1963a 1963b; Matthews and Raisman, 1972). In the most superficial part of the cells clusters of small granulated vesicles (i.e. of the adrenergic type) are observed (Hökfelt, 1969), and these sometimes occupy a mushroom-shaped process evaginated from the cell surface (van Orden *el al.*, 1970). The granules of these vesicles are difficult to preserve and are not seen in most preparations of sympathetic ganglia fixed with gluteraldehyde or osmium, and only after permanganate fixation (as recommended by Richardson, 1966) are they consistently observed. Other granulated vesicles, usually larger, are scattered in the cytoplasm, particularly near the Golgi vesicles (Taxi, 1965; Grillo, 1966).

Long cylindrical processes originate fron the ganglion cells. No specific structural features have been found that will permit the different types of process to be distinguished at their origins. Even at some distance from the cell body it is frequently not possible to tell an axon from a dendrite (though no author has questioned the validity of this classification of cell processes). Axons contain mainly microtubules and neurofilaments, while dendrites show inclusions of a kind usually found in the cytoplasm of the cell soma, such as ribosomes; some dendrites also have spines. Clusters of small vesicles (30–50 nm in diameter), granulated or more frequently non-granulated (in gluteraldehyde fixed tissues), are observed in dendrites similar in appearance to those near the surface of the cell body. They probably represent the catecholamine stores which give the dendrites their beaded and fluorescent appearance in fluorescent microscopy. The significance of these accumulations of vesicles is not clear, nor indeed is it clear why there should be large amounts of neurotransmitter in the dendrites. Cell processes are enwrapped by glial cells and their thin processes, the surface of a dendrite only rarely lying directly beneath the basal lamina, but at such areas clusters of vesicles are common (Taxi *et al.*, 1969).

Elfvin (1963b), studying serial sections in electron microscopy, observed numerous areas of intimate contact between dendrites in the superior cervical ganglion of the cat. Some were juxtapositions of two dendrites with a gap of about 7 nm; in other contacts there were accumulations of dense material on the cytoplasmic side of both membranes.

Preganglionic fibres provide the ganglion neurons with a large number of synapses. The fibres run parallel or wind around the dendrites, each forming several axodendritic synapses *en passage* (Elfvin, 1963b). All authors agree that in mammalian sympathetic ganglia synapses on the soma are far less numerous than on dendrites (Elfvin, 1963b; Forssmann, 1964; Taxi, 1965; Pick, 1970). In the superior cervical ganglion of the rat only 14 per cent of the synapses are axo-somatic; 71 per cent are on dendrites less than $0.5 \mu m$ in diameter (Tamarind and Quilliam, 1971). Preganglionic nerve endings are about $0.1–0.3 \mu m$ in diameter. They contain round, agranular synaptic vesicles, 30–50 nm in diameter, some of which lie clustered on the preganglionic membrane and its dense material. A few large granulated vesicles, mitochondria, and smooth endoplasmic reticulum are also present. Tamarind and Quilliam

(1971) observed in the superior cervical ganglia of the rat and the cat, a small proportion (6 per cent and 2 per cent respectively) of endings containing small granulated vesicles of the adrenergic type; in the rabbit this type of ending amounts to about 25 per cent of the total. These endings were interpreted to be recurrent axon collaterals of postganglionic fibres. These interesting observations need to be confirmed, paying particular attention to the fact that dendrites also contain small granulated vesicles, store noradrenaline and have membrane contact specializations. Only few synaptic junctions are observed in the superior cervical ganglion following preganglionic denervation. For the prevertabral ganglia, however, there is physiological and histological evidence that the ganglion cells receive, in addition to a synaptic input from the preganglionic neurons, also synapses from other prevertebral ganglion cells and synapses from neurons located within the wall of the viscera (Kuntz, 1938, 1940). These observations have been recently confirmed by intracellular recordings from the inferior mesenteric ganglion of the guinea-pig (Crowcroft and Szurszewski, 1971).

A limited number of synapses in sympathetic ganglia of various mammalian species exhibit a subsynaptic formation in the shape of a row of electron dense dots (Taxi, 1965; Taxi and Babmindra, 1972). This is similar to the subsynaptic apparatus found in sympathetic ganglia of the frog (Taxi, 1961) and in various regions of the central nervous system (Gray, 1963; Milhaud and Pappas, 1966).

Most of the neurons of the sympathetic ganglia display the formaldehyde-induced fluorescence specific for catecholamines (Falck and Hillarp method, described in Falck and Owman, 1965), and are therefore considered to be adrenergic neurons releasing a catecholamine at their terminals. In mammalian sympathetic neurons this catecholamine is noradrenaline. The fluorescence is intense in some 5–10 per cent of the ganglion cells, while the majority of the remainder show a moderate reaction.

Fluorescence is also observed in the dendrites, sometimes smooth and sometimes varicose, which impinge on neighbouring fluorescent or non-fluorescent neurons (Jacobowitz and Woodward, 1968). The intensity of fluorescence in cell bodies is consistently less than that of the corresponding terminals in the peripheral organs. It has in fact, been estimated that the nerve terminals originating from one neuron of the superior cervical ganglion of the cat contain about 300 times more noradrenaline than their corresponding perikaryon (Dalhström and Häggendal, 1966).

A minority of non-fluorescent neurons are also present in the sympathetic ganglia of many species (Norberg, 1967), but their proportions have not yet been determined under adequate technical conditions. It has been reported that non-fluorescent cells possess intense acetylcholinesterase activity (Yamauchi and Lever, 1971): they may therefore be the cholinergic sympathetic postganglionic neurons that innervate blood vessels (vaso-dilator fibres) and sweat glands.

In addition, varicose fluorescent fibres have been described among the fluorescent and non-fluorescent cell bodies in some sympathetic ganglia. In the superior cervical ganglion of the cat such fibres appear to abut on dendrites at a short distance from the perikarya or to form pericellular nets around some ganglion cells (Csillik, Kalman and Knyihar, 1967; Jacobowitz and Woodward, 1968), but it is not clear whether they are fluorescent dendrites or axon collaterals of postganglionic fibres. Such pericellular nets of fluorescent fibres are more prominent in the prevertebral ganglia than in the sympathetic chain ganglia (Norberg, 1967). They are particularly well developed in the rabbit, but less so in the cat and rat (Hamberger and Norberg, 1965; Norberg and Ungerstedt, 1965).

The histochemical reaction for acetylcholinesterase is negative or of only moderate intensity in the majority of the sympathetic ganglion cells. A minority of neurons display an intense reaction — rat superior cervical ganglion: 10 per cent of the ganglion cells (Giacobini, 1956); cat superior cervical ganglion: 0.5 per cent (Holmstedt and Sjoqvist, 1957); cat stellate ganglion: 7 per cent (Holmstedt amd Sjöqvist, 1957); rat, sheep and pig superior cervical ganglion: 4 per cent, 5 per cent and 6 per cent respectively (Yamauchi and Lever, 1971). It is likely that ganglion cells with an intense acetycholinesterase activity are cholinergic neurons, and correspond to the sympathetic cholinergic post-ganglionic neurons that provide the sudimotor and vasodilator fibres to the limbs. In the prevertebral ganglia of the cat less than 1 per cent of the ganglion cells show an intense acetylcholinesterase activity (Holmstedt and Sjöqvist, 1957; Taxi, 1965), the remainder of the population giving a negative reaction.

7.1.1 *Chromaffin cells*

Sympathetic ganglia also contain chromaffin cells, i.e., those which stain with bichromate salts, similarly to the adrenal medullary cells, although less intensely. Such cells have been described in a number of ganglia (see review in Coupland, 1965), including the superior cervical ganglion of the cat (Bülbring, 1944). Stöhr (1939), using a silver impregnation method reported that in the prevertebral ganglia chromaffin cells are innervated by preganglionic fibres.

More recently cells of similar description have been identified in sympathetic ganglia by means of the fluorescence histochemical method for catecholamines, and labelled with the descriptive term of *small intensely fluorescent (S.I.F.) cells*. In the electron microscope these cells are characterized by the presence of numerous large granulated vesicles, and have therefore been labelled *granular cells*. 'Chromaffin cells', 'small intensely fluorescent cells' and 'granular cells' are probably all the same type of cell, as seen with different histological methods. The term 'chromaffin cells' is preferred here, since it is felt that no ambiguity is involved in its use, although the chromaffin reaction is the least reliable and the least used of the three methods mentioned. Indeed, some ganglia give no clear chromaffin reaction (although they can be shown to contain small intensely fluorescent cells), which is explained by the low sensitivity of this method. For the reasons discussed below, the terms 'interneurons' and 'small neurons', also used by some authors, are considered less satisfactory. Chromaffin cells of sympathetic ganglia are clustered in small groups, particularly around blood vessels. Between 400 and 1000 chromaffin cells (small intensely fluorescent cells) per ganglion have been found by Eränkö and Eränkö (1971) in superior cervical ganglia of rats, with little numerical change from birth to maturity.

The chromaffin cells are characterized by an intense yellow-green form-aldehyde-induced fluorescence (method of Falck and Hillarp), which indicates the presence of biogenic amines in high concentration. The cell bodies which are more intensely fluorescent than the surrounding adrenergic ganglion cells, measure $10-15\,\mu m$ in diameter, and from them emerge few short varicose processes — up to $40\,\mu m$ long in the superior cervical ganglion of the rat — (Norberg, Ritzén and Ungerstedt, 1966).

There is still some uncertainty as to the type of amine stored by chromaffin cells in various ganglia and species. It has been shown biochemically that chromaffin cells of the dog inferior mesenteric ganglion (Muscholl and Vogt, 1964), and those of the pelvic ganglia of dog, cat and rabbit (Owman and Sjöstrand, 1965) contain adrenaline. Björklund *et al.* (1970) found dopamine in the small intensely fluorescent cells of the sympathetic ganglia of the pig, cat and rat, whereas Eränkö and Eränkö (1971) showed by microspectrofluorimetry that those of the rat superior cervical ganglion contain noradrenaline. Libet and Owman (1974) reported that in the superior cervical ganglion of the rabbit small intensely fluorescent cells contain dopamine; moreover, when experimentally depleted, these cells are able to take up exogenous dopamine and restore their fluorescence. S.I.F. cells, in the superior cervical ganglion of the rat, lack any histochemically demonstrable dopamine-beta-hydroxylase, the enzyme which catalyzes the symthesis of noradrenaline from dopamine (Fuxe, Goldstein, Hökfelt and Joh, 1971).

Comparing fluorimetric assays with fluorescence observations and electron microscopy, van Orden *et al.* (1970) estimated that of the total amount of amines in the rat superior cervical ganglion 70 per cent was associated with adrenergic ganglion neurons and 30 per cent with intensely fluorescent cells.

The chromaffin cells of the sympathetic ganglia are readily identifiable in the electron microscope, because of their small diameter $(6-12\,\mu m)$ and the presence of numerous large granulated vesicles (Grillo 1966; Siegrist, *et al.*, 1968; Hökfelt, 1968; Matthews and Raisman, 1969; Taxi, Gautron and L'Hermite, 1969; Williams and Palay, 1969; Matthews and Nash 1970; van Orden *et al.*, 1970; Tamarind and Quilliam, 1971; Yokota, 1973; all working on the superior cervical ganglion of the rat). They are round or polyhedral in shape and have a central nucleus usually without a nucleolus and rich in chromatin (Matthews and Raisman, 1969). They are sheathed by satellite cells similar in structure to those around the ordinary ganglion cells, but when clustered together granule-containing cells are often directly apposed and interdigitate with a gap of 15–20 nm without the intervention of satellite cells (Siegrist *et al*,

1968; Matthews and Raisman, 1969; Williams and Palay, 1969; Yokota, 1973).

Nerve endings filled with agranular synaptic vesicles, 30–40 μm in diameter, synapse on the cell body, and to a lesser extent on the processes (Yokota, 1973), of the granule-containing cells (Grillo, 1966; Siegrist *et al.*, 1968; Matthews and Raisman, 1969; Williams and Palay, 1970; Yokota, 1973). These nerve endings originate from the spinal cord, as do other preganglionic fibres (Taxi *et al.*, 1969; Matthews, 1971; Quilliam and Tamarind, 1972), and are probably cholinergic.

In addition to afferent synapses some granule-containing cells of the rat superior cervical ganglion possess specialized contacts having thickening of the cell membrane and a limited clustering of granulated vesicles (efferent synapses?) (Siegrist *et al.*, 1968; Matthews and Raisman, 1969; Williams and Palay, 1969; Yokota, 1973). The majority of these contacts seem to arise from the cell body (Matthews and Raisman, 1969), but only in a few cases has the post-junctional element been identified as a sympathetic adrenergic ganglion cell by the presence of small granulated vesicles (Taxi *et al.*, 1969; Yokota, 1973). Taxi *et al.* (1969) have been cautious in their identification of efferent contacts arising fron the small granular cells, however, and have argued that there is as yet insufficient evidence to justify the labelling of such junctions as synapses, and preferred the term 'zone synaptoide'. Moreover, several authors have reported that after section of the superior cervical sympathetic trunk all synapses disappear from the superior cervical ganglion (Ceccarelli *et al.*, 1971, in the cat; Hamori *et al.*, 1968, in the cat; Taxi *et al.*, 1969, in the rat; Babmindra and Diatchkova, 1970, in the dog; Lakos, 1970, in the cat). Only in the rat have Grillo (1966) and Lakos (1970) reported that some rare synapses were present several days after preganglionic denervation. Recently Raisman *et al.* (1974), in a quantitative study of the synapses in normal and preganglionically denervated superior cervical ganglia of rats, observed only a few synapses after denervation, and none of these showed the expected morphological characteristics of the processes of the small cells.

Thus the evidence available is as yet insufficient to warrant the conclusion that chromaffin cells in the sympathetic ganglia are interneurons. Further studies are obviously needed, particularly of other ganglia than the superior cervical ganglion of the rat. While by definition interneurons are neurons with afferent and efferent synapses, the absence of efferent synapses from granule-containing cells would not rule out their function as 'modulators' of ganglionic trans-mission. It has been suggested that granule-containing cells act as endocrine cells, releasing catecholamines that would reach the ganglion neurons either by diffusion or through the capillaries (Grillo, 1966; Siegrist *et al.*, 1968; Matthews and Raisman, 1969), and the possibility of such a rôle is supported by recent experimental studies (Libet and Owman, 1974). Eränkö and Eränkö (1971) and Tamarind and Quilliam (1971) have suggested that the granule-containing cells may also act as chemoreceptors.

The great interest directed towards the small cells in sympathetic ganglia during the past ten years is in part related to the observation by Marrazzi (1939) and Bülbring (1944) that catecholamines affect ganglionic transmission, (see reviews in Volle, 1966; Kosterlitz and Lees, 1972), and a variety of findings suggest that catecholamines have a physiological inhibitory rôle in sympathetic ganglia (De Groat and Saum, 1971). The relative importance of the various sources of catecholamines in the sympathetic ganglia: the chromaffin cells, recurrent adrenergic axons, the circulating blood, the perikarya and, in particular, the dendrites remains to be determined Recent histological studies (e.g., Williams *et al.*, 1975), in various ganglia and species, have shown that there are different types of chromaffin cell. Some cells show reciprocal synapses with the ganglion neurons (Yamauchi *et al.*, 1975).

7.1.2 *Preganglionic fibres*

The preganglionic fibres to the sympathetic ganglia originate in the spinal cord and reach the paravertebral ganglia through the ventral roots and the white rami communicantes. They end in the paravertebral ganglia of the corresponding level, or ascend or descend along the sympathetic chain to more cranial or more caudal ganglia, or pass to the prevertebral ganglia by means of the splanchnic nerves. Preganglionic fibres branch and can thus provide terminal branches to different ganglia. The details of this arrangement are not known but there is physiological evidence of preganglionic fibres supplying branches that synapse on ganglion cells of the V lumbar sympathetic ganglion of the cat and pass to more distally located ganglia (Obrador and Odoriz, 1936).

Preganglionic fibres represent a heterogeneous population of fibres in terms of size, presence of myelin sheath, and conduction velocity. Foley and Dubois (1940) calculated that the percentage of unmyelinated preganglionic fibres ranges from 5 to 60 per cent, with an average of 23 per cent, in the white rami communicantes contributing fibres to the superior cervical trunk of the cat. Myelinated fibres are very few in the sympathetic chain and in the rami communicantes of the rat (DeLemos and Pick, 1966).

Foley and Dubois (1940) also counted the preganglionic fibres in the cervical sympathetic trunk in cats, dogs and rats (Table 7.1) and found a difference in the numbers of fibres up to one hundred per cent between different cats (sex, age, and body weight not given), greater (up to 300 per cent) and smaller (up to 50 per cent) differences being found in dogs and rats respectively. Unmyelinated fibres provide 96–99 per cent of the total in the cervical sympathetic trunk of the rat (Foley and Dubois, 1940; Forssmann, 1964; Bray and Aguayo, 1974), whereas in the cat (Williams, Jew and Palay, 1973), and in the dog they constitute about 50 per cent of the total (Table 7.1) (Foley and Dubois, 1940). De Castro (1951) classified the preganglionic fibres in the superior cervical trunk of the cat into three groups on the basis of their diameters, while Eccles (1935) found that four groups of fibres were identifiable by their excitability and conduction velocity. Folkow, Johansson and Oberg (1958) differentiated three groups of preganglionic sympathetic fibres; they were, in order of increase in their threshold (i.e. of decrease of their diameter): 1.fibres to the artero-venous

Table 7.1   Numbers of axons in cervical sympathetic trunks of the cat, dog and rat; pyridine silver and osmic acid stains. (From Foley and DuBois, 1940)

	Right		Left	
	Axons	% unmyelinated	Axons	% unmyelinated
		CAT		
1	6 136	44	6 279	42
2	6 137	40	7 378	47
3	9 635	50	8 592	42
4	7 387	68	7 690	61
		DOG		
1	11 869	66	10 939	64
2	9 652	56	10 617	60
3	12 562	55	12 839	51
4	5 374	42	5 605	45
		RAT		
1	3 287	99	2 543	98
2	2 618	98	3 875	98
3	2 898	98	2 747	98
4	2 746	98	2 909	98

anastomoses of the skin, to the nictitating membrane and to the pupil; 2. vasoconstrictor fibres of the skin, skeletal muscles and tongue; 3. sympathetic vasodilator fibres of skeletal muscles. Three types of myelinated fibres were identified by Williams, Jew and Palay (1973) in the cat cervical sympathetic trunk, on the basis of their diameter and myelin thickness, intermingled with the unmyelinated fibres constituting about 50 per cent of the axons, and while most preganglionic, unmyelinated axons have a thin individual sheath of Schwann cell cytoplasm, up to 20 postganglionic axons are wrapped up by each Schwann cell (Williams, Jew and Palay, 1973). A wide range of sizes and conduction velocities has also been found in the rat cervical sympathetic trunk (Dunant, 1967).

Preganglionic fibres are many times less numerous than ganglion neurons. The ratio was found to vary betweeen 1:11 and 1:17 in the superior cervical ganglion of the cat (Wolff, 1941), which corresponds to the ratio 1:32 calculated for the myelinated fibres only by Billingsley and Ranson (1918), these being about 50 per cent of the total. The ratio between preganglionic fibres and ganglion neurons for the superior cervical ganglion ranges in various species of primates from 1:28 to 1:196, with wide variations even between individuals of the same species (e.g. in man from 1:63 to 1:196) (Ebbeson, 1968a). In this group of species the numbers of preganglionic fibres seem to vary less than the numbers of ganglion cells, and Ebbeson (1968a) has postulated that the numbers of preganglionic fibres serving specific functions are of the same order of magnitude in species of different body size, but they are related to a different number of ganglion cells. This interesting conclusion should be confirmed by more accurate counts of the preganglionic fibres (i.e. by electron microscopy), of which between 6 and 80 per cent were unmyelinated in Ebbeson's material.

All counts indicate that the numbers of preganglionic fibres exceed the numbers of ganglion cells. While the reported ratios can only be taken to be approximations, they indicate a divergence of impulses along the efferent pathway which is substantially greater than that found in parasympathetic ganglia (see below). It is however not known how much the preganglionic fibres branch before reaching the ganglia, i.e. how many of the preganglionic fibres entering one ganglion have issued from one spinal preganglionic neuron. Similarly little is known of the changes in axonal diameter and myelin thickness along the length of individual preganglionic fibres. Finally, such counts give an *average* ratio between pre- and postganglionic fibres *as if* all ganglion cells recieved an identical preganglionic input.

7.1.3 *Post-ganglionic fibres*

These leave the paravertebral ganglia, and form the *grey rami communicantes*, through which they reach the spinal nerves, and thus pass to the periphery. The post-ganglionic fibres from the prevertebral ganglia and the superior cervical ganglion reach the peripheral organs in small nerves that are satellites to arteries. Postganglionic fibres are usually unmyelinated axons, but in the cat a considerable number of postganglionic fibres in the grey rami and in the carotid nerves are myelinated (Langley, 1896). The motor nerve fibres supplying the medial muscle of the nictitating membrane of the cat are myelinated adrenergic axons issuing from the superior cervical ganglion (Kosterlitz, Thompson and Wallis, 1964), and in birds the very great majority of postganglionic sympathetic fibres are myelinated (Langley, 1904).

After repeatedly branching the postganglionic adrenergic fibres reach the peripheral organs, where they acquire a characteristic structure. In what is called their terminal portion they have a beaded appearance, due to the alternation of thin and thick components; the thick portions, or varicosities, measure 1 μm or more in diameter, and are filled with small granulated vesicles and mitochondria, whereas the thin inter-varicose parts can be as thin as 0.1 μm in diameter and mainly contain microtubules. There are on average 25–30 varicosities per 100 μm of terminal length (Dahlström and Häggendal, 1966). From histo-chemical and biochemical studies of the superior cervical ganglion and the adrenergic fibres in the head of the rat, Dahlström and Häggendal (1966) have calculated that each neuron has about 26 000 varicosities spread over a total of about 100 mm of axon terminal length. The total number of varicosities in the rat iris alone has been calculated to be over 1 x 10^6, and in a 10 mm length of vas deferens over 5 x 10^7 (Dahlström, Häggendal and Hökfelt, 1966).

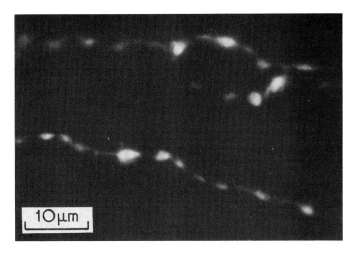

Fig. 7.4 Two intramuscular fluorescent fibres displaying their characteristic beaded structure. (Reproduced from Gabella and Costa. 1967.)

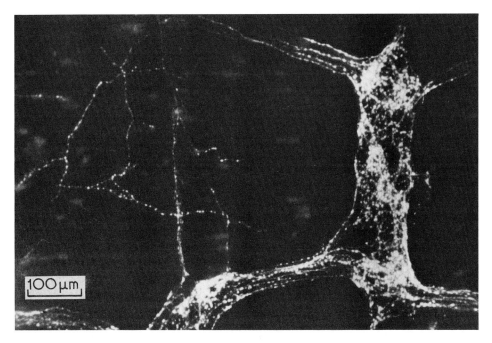

Fig. 7.5 Stretch preparation of the ileum of guinea-pig, processed with the Falck-Hillarp histochemical method for catecholamines. It shows a thick feltwork of fluorescent fibres in a ganglion of the myenteric plexus (to the right) and several individual varicose fluorescent fibres. (Reproduced from Gabella and Costa, 1967.)

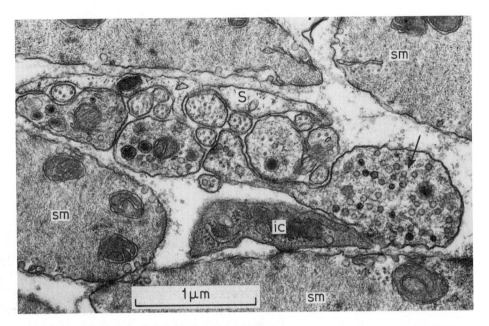

Fig. 7.6   Adrenergic nerve ending at some distance from a smooth muscle cell of the circular layer of the ileum of guinea-pig (glutaraldehyde-osmium fixation). Small granulated vesicles are visible in the adrenergic ending (arrow). sm – smooth muscle cells; ic – interstitial cells; S – Schwann cell process. (Reproduced from Gabella, 1972.)

Adrenergic fibres end either in close relation to muscular and glandular effectors (e.g. the salivary glands, and the muscles of the iris, of the blood vessels, of the sphincteric part of the alimentary canal, of the genital organs), or by synapsing on ganglion neurons of the submucous and myenteric plexuses (see intramural ganglia of the alimentary tract).

7.2 Sympathetic ganglia in Amphibia

The ganglion cells are unipolar with a single large process forming the postganglionic fibre. The preganglionic fibres branch within the ganglia, and each branch spirals around the initial tract of the axon and the neighbouring part of one ganglion cell soma (Johnson, 1918). In the electron microscope synapses are found on the cell body, and to a lesser extent over the remainder of the cell surface (Taxi, 1965). The cell body appears smooth in silver preparations, but in

Fig. 7.7   Adrenergic nerve ending synapsing on an intramural neuron of the myenteric plexus in the guinea-pig. Mitochondria, large granulated vesicles, agranular vesicles and small dense core vesicles are visible; some of the vesicles display a very dense membrane.

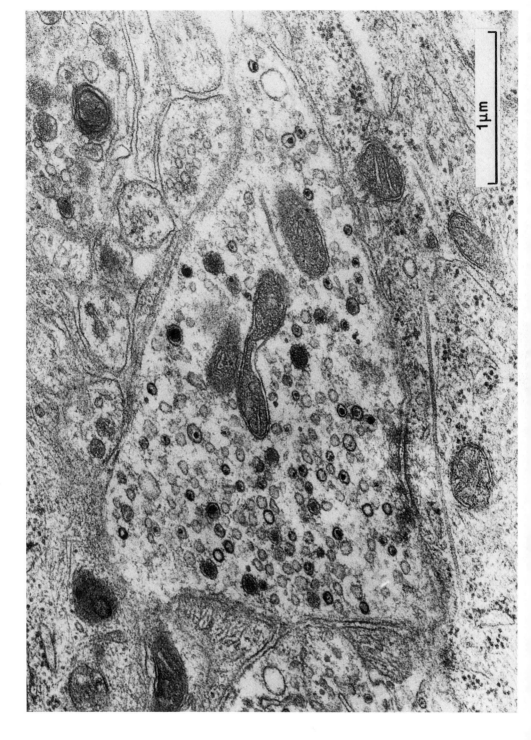

1 µm

electron micrographs shows short processes (Pick, 1961), on both the soma and the initial tract of the axon (Taxi, 1965), which remain beneath the satellite cells ensheathing the ganglion cells. The nuclei of the ganglion cells are eccentrically located, and a large crescent-shaped accumulation of glycogen granules occupies the superficial region at one pole of the cytoplasm (Pick, 1963; Yamamoto, 1963).

Two classes of neurons are described in the sympathetic ganglia of the frog: large neurons in the cortex of the ganglion, with poorly developed Nissl bodies, and small neurons, more deeply situated with abundant Nissl bodies (Fujimoto, 1967); in light microscopy the two types are recognizable as light and dark neurons. Nishi, Soeda and Koketsu (1965) have identified two types of neuron by electrophysiological means, which have been called 'B' and 'C' neurons, since they give origin to postganglionic fibres with conduction velocities typical of B and C fibres respectively. 'C' neurons are smaller (about 18 μm in diameter) than 'B' neurons (about 35 μm in diameter), and receive synaptic input from two or three spinal roots; the conduction velocity of their preganglionic fibres is about 0.20–0.30 m s^{-1}.

On the other hand most of the 'B' neurons receive synaptic inputs from one spinal level only (mono-segmental innervation), the preganglionic fibres conducting at about 5 m s^{-1}. Honma (1970b) has confirmed the bimodal distribution of ganglion cells sizes in the 10th lumbar sympathetic ganglion of the toad, and has obtained evidence suggesting that 'B' neurons innervate the toxic glands of the skin and that the 'C' neurons innervate the vascular system of the lower limbs. These findings are in agreement with previous electrophysiological evidence (Hutter and Loewenstein, 1955).

Numerous postganglionic fibres are myelinated to such an extent that certain 'grey' (postganglionic) rami communicantes to the somatic nerves consist chiefly of myelinated fibres (Bishop and O'Leary, 1938). In total the post-ganglionic fibres are said to outnumber the preganglionic fibres by about 7 to 1 (Huber, 1899).

All the amphibian sympathetic ganglion cells show specific fluorescence for catecholamines (Norberg and McIsaac, 1967; Honma, 1970a; Woods, 1970a). The intensity of this reaction varies between cells but it is not related to cell size, and no non-fluorescent ganglion cells have been observed. Since the work of von Euler (1946) it has been generally accepted that the catecholamines involved is adrenaline, as demonstrated by Loewi (1921). This finding has been confirmed in several species of frog and toad (Azuma, Binia and Vissher, 1965; Angelakos, Glassman, Millar and King, 1965), but newts, on the other hand, possess only noradrenaline (Angelakos *et al.*, 1965). Although the postganglionic fibres store adrenaline and release it upon stimulation (Azuma *et al.*, 1965), the sympathetic ganglia of the frog contain larger amounts of noradrenaline than of adrenaline (in the ratio of approximately 5:1, Azuma *et al.*, 1965), the content of noradrenaline probably being accounted for by the granulated cells (see p. 367). Seasonal changes in catecholamine content occurs in the nerves of Amphibia,

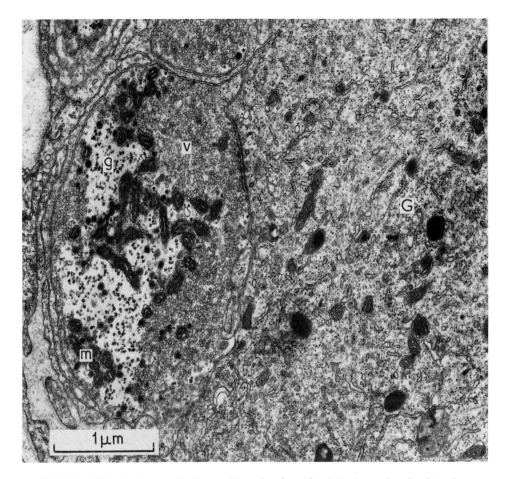

Fig. 7.8 Abdominal sympathetic ganglion of a frog (fixed by immersion in glutaraldehyde). A preganglionic fibre synapses on a ganglion cell soma. Besides many small agranular vesicles (v) and mitochondria (m) the nerve ending contains a few large granulated vesicles and abundant glycogen (g). G – ganglion cell body.

with values significantly higher in summer than in winter, but there is no concomitant change in the velocity of the distally directed transport of catecholamines along the axons (Rodriguez-Echandia, Donoso and Pedroza, 1972).

The fine structure of nerve endings in amphibian sympathetic ganglia has been reported by several authors since the first description by De Robertis and Bennett (1954, 1955). Numerous synapses are found on the axon hillock and the proximal part of the axon (Uchizono, 1964; Taxi, 1965; Hunt and Nelson, 1965; Nishi, Soeda and Koketsu, 1967). Other terminals, much larger than those found on the axon, synapse on the perikaryon (Fig. 7.8). Nishi, Soeda and Koketsu (1967) calculate that in the toad lumbar sympathetic ganglion neurons approximately 10 per cent of the cell surface is covered by nerve terminals, approximately 55 nerve terminals being found on a 'B' neuron and 15 on a 'C' neuron. The nerve terminals contain electron-lucent vesicles with a diameter of approximately 50 nm (Uchizono, 1964), together with a few large granulated vesicles. Many of the terminals contain large numbers of glycogen granules, and these can be so abundant that some terminals appear to be completely filled with them (Pick, 1963; Fujimoto, 1967). In the sympathetic neurons of the frog (*Rana esculenta*) and axolotl there is frequently a sub-synaptic apparatus (Taxi, 1965), formed by a band of electron-dense material approximately 25 nm thick lying a few tens of nanometers beneath the post-synaptic membrane.

A high activity of acetylcholinesterase is detectable histochemically in the preganglionic fibres of the frog (Giacobini, 1956). This cholinesterase activity is intense in about 10 per cent of the neurons, and moderate or absent in the others, a pattern not dissimilar to that seen in the cat and the rat. The intracellular distribution of acetylcholinesterase has been studied by Brzin, Tennyson and Duffy (1966), who found the reaction end product to be concentrated mainly in the sacs of the rough endoplasmic reticulum.

In addition to the ganglion cells the sympathetic ganglia always contain some granulated cells grouped into clumps or short cords, and frequently in close proximity to blood vessels (Fujimoto, 1967), their cytoplasm being filled with granulated vesicles 20—60 nm in diameter. These vesicles are round and dense in osmium fixed ganglia and oval or rod-shaped and less dense in glutaraldehyde fixed ganglia; furthermore a distinct clear halo surrounds the granule after osmium but this is barely visible following glutaraldehyde (Fujimoto, 1967). Such granular cells are closely associated with nerve fibres, and although neither afferent nor efferent synapses have been seen to end upon them, Fujimoto (1967) suggests that their secretion is under direct nervous control. The granular cells correspond to the cells with intense yellow, formaldehyde-induced fluorescence, and therefore contain a high concentration of catecholamines (Norberg and McIsaac, 1967; Honma, 1970; Jacobowitz, 1970). The histo-chemical properties of these cells indicate that they contain nor-adrenaline rather than adrenaline (Woods, 1970).

7.3 The ciliary ganglion in mammals

The ciliary ganglion is a small ganglion, up to 2 mm in its antero-posterior diameter in man, situated behind the eyeball, lateral to the optic nerve. It receives nerves (its *roots*) from the oculomotor nerve (generally through the branch to the inferior oblique muscle), and sends nerves (the short ciliary nerves) to the eyeball. In some species it also contains sensory fibres from the trigeminal nerve and sympathetic postganglionic fibres from the superior cervical ganglion; both these orders of fibres pass through the ciliary ganglion without interruption. In the small rodents the ganglion is composed of microscopic clusters of neurons in proximity to the optic nerve.

The ganglion neurons are spheroidal and measure about $25-36 \mu m$ in diameter in man, $11-15 \mu m$ in the mouse, $34-50 \mu m$ in the dog (Slavich, 1932), and $30-40 \mu m$ in the guinea-pig (Watanabe, 1972). In the cat the number of ganglion cells in four individuals ranged between 4250 and 5100 (Wolf, 1941). The ciliary ganglion neurons are closely packed and individually ensheathed by satellite cells, and in all species investigated are larger than the neurons of the corresponding sympathetic ganglia (for example those of the superior cervical ganglion); furthermore, they never show accumulation of pigment, even in old subjects (Slavich, 1932).

Slavich (1932) has studied the cell processes in the ciliary ganglia of several species by silver impregnation methods. A few ganglion cells, particularly in human ganglia, have long dendrites, whereas the majority of cells have only short processes which are confined within the pericellular sheath.

These short processes, also called intracapsular processes, become thicker and coarser in old subjects, and may, notably in man and dog, form pericellular nests together with the preganglionic fibres. The axons from the ganglion cells are clearly identifiable in silver preparations: they cross the sheath and proceed undivided among other neurons. The initial tract of the axon sometimes shows short fine collaterals.

In the electron microscope the ganglion cells of the ciliary ganglion of the guinea-pig show many protrusions $0.1-2.0 \mu m$ long and $0.2-0.5 \mu m$ wide, which are covered by satellite cells, as are the perikarya. The endings of the preganglionic fibres contain agranular vesicles of 50 nm in diameter and synapse with cell bodies and processes (Watanabe, 1972). In man, using silver impregnation and Golgi methods, preganglionic fibres are seen to form complicated terminal nets around the great majority of neurons. Classifications of neurons into different categories on morphological bases were attempted by Pines (1927) and Pines and Friedman (1929). Whitteridge (1937) and Nishi and Christ (1971) obtained electrophysiological evidence that there are two types of neuron in the ciliary ganglion of the cat, B- and C-neurons. There are therefore two transmission pathways through the ganglion: one characterized by a higher excitability of the preganglionic fibres, a shorter synaptic delay and a higher postganglionic conduction than the other. In the monkey only the fast transmission pathway is found (Whitteridge, 1937).

The histochemical reaction for acetylcholinesterase is positive in all of the neurons of the ciliary ganglion of the cat and in their pericellular nets (preganglionic terminals and short processes) (Koelle, 1951; Koelle and Koelle, 1959; Taxi, 1965).

The intensity of the reaction is the same in all of the ganglion cells and much higher than that seen in any sympathetic ganglion cell (Sjöqvist, 1962). Choline acetylase activity per unit weight is more than twice that found in the stellate and lumbar sympathetic ganglia (Buckley, Consolo, Giacobini and Sjöqvist, 1967).

Perry and Talesnik (1953), working on the cat, have provided pharmacological evidence that the synapses between preganglionic fibres and ganglion neurons are cholinergic (nicotinic). Most of the cells are innervated by two or more preganglionic fibres, but B-neurons are exclusively innervated by B fibres, and C-neurons by C fibres (Nishi and Christ, 1971).

No adrenergic perikarya are present in ciliary ganglia of rats, cats, guinea-pigs and monkeys (Ehinger and Falck, 1970; Watanabe, 1972). A few varicose fibres with specific fluorescence for catecholamines are found in mammalian ciliary ganglia (Hamberger, Norberg and Ungerstedt, 1965), and they probably represent perivascular adrenergic fibres (Ehinger and Falck, 1970; Watanabe, 1972). However fluorescent neurons were present in the ciliary ganglion, in rats

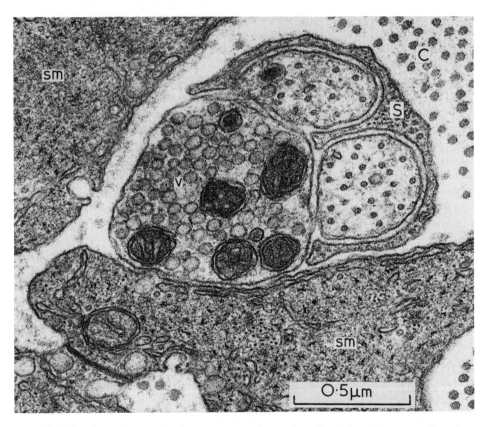

Fig. 7.9   A small nerve bundle among smooth muscle cells of the sphincter pupillae of guinea-pig (fixed in glutaraldehyde and osmium). One axon is filled with mitochondria and agranular vesicles (v); its distance from the nearest muscle cell is about 20 nm. The other two axons contain mainly microtubules and are enwrapped by a Schwann cell cytoplasm process (S). C – collagen fibrils; sm – smooth muscle cells.

which died under severe stress or were injected high doses of Nialamide or L-DOPA, (Ehinger and Falck, 1970).

Preganglionic fibres are myelinated and originate in the mesencephalon in the nucleus of Edinger–Westphal. This contains multipolar neurons, $15-25\ \mu m$ in diameter in the monkey, with few Nissl bodies (Warwick, 1954). In the rat these neurons show an intense acetylcholinesterase activity (Koelle, 1954). Warwick (1954) observed chromatolysis in the neurons of Edinger–Westphal nucleus and its cephalic prolongation in monkeys 8–16 days after removal of the ciliary ganglion. In the cat the ratio between preganglionic fibres and ganglion neurons ranges between 1:1.7 and 1:2.6 (Wolf, 1941).

Some of the postganglionic fibres, possibly the majority, are myelinated for some of their length, although it is not known where they loose their myelin sheaths. Postganglionic fibres innervate the ciliary muscle and the sphincter pupillae of the iris. In the iris the terminal arborization of ciliary fibres is very extensive, with the fibres becoming varicose and having numerous 'endings' along their terminal lengths. Such endings contain agranular vesicles about 50 nm in diameter, and come into close relation with the muscle cells. A gap of only 20 nm is present in most of the junctions, and pre- and post-junctional membrane specializations are frequently observed (Gabella, 1974).

7.4 The ciliary ganglion in birds

The ganglion contains about 6000 neurons in the turkey (Terzuolo, 1951) and pigeon (Marwitt, Pilar and Weakley, 1971), subdivided into two populations of neurons, large and small (Carpenter, 1911; Terzuolo, 1951; Hess, 1965). In the turkey the small neurons are less numerous, more tightly packed, and occupy the upper and more distal part of the ganglion (Terzuolo, 1951), while in the pigeon they represent 50 per cent of the total ganglion cells (Marwitt et al., 1971). The large neurons provide the motor innervation to the ciliary muscle and the iris (and are therefore also called 'ciliary neurons'), whereas the small neurons form the choroid nerves ('choroid neurons') (Marwitt et al., 1971). All ganglion cells are round, have one axon and only very short, intracapsular dendrites (unipolar neurons); the nucleus is often eccentric (De Lorenzo, 1960; Takahashi and Hama, 1965b). The short dendrites and the arborization of the preganglionic fibres around the large neurons show a remarkable increase in complexity throughout life (fowls up to 12 years old were studied) (Terzuolo 1951).

The ganglion cells are ensheathed by glial satellite cells. In the large neurons the sheath consists of 3–20 lamellae of loose, semi-compact or compact myelin (Hess, 1965); this myelin sheath is provided by satellite glial cells, many of which are present around each ganglion cell.

The endings of preganglionic fibres are situated inside the myelin sheath, synapsing on the perikaryon. The characteristic synapse of the avian ciliary ganglion, first described by Carpenter (1911), is formed by calyciform (or cup-shaped) nerve terminals (De Lorenzo, 1960). They are found only on the large neurons (Hess, 1965) and cover as much as 65 per cent of the ganglion cell surface in 1 month-old chickens (De Lorenzo, 1966). In the chick during the first months, post-hatching, all large neurons are surrounded by a calyx, each calyx originating from one axon. At around six months few calyces remain, but on the majority of cells numerous small bouton-like synapses are seen in their stead. The calyx, and the numerous boutons which are formed as a result of its cleavage, provide the only synaptic input to the perikaryon. The short intracapsular dendrites originate as interdigitations between the nerve endings and the perikarya during post-hatching life (Koenig, 1967). Rarely, the perikaryon protrudes into the calyciform nerve terminal with a process about 1 μm long and 1.5 μm in diameter, having an expanded end and post-synaptic differentiations on the lateral aspects of such a somatic spine (Takahashi and Hama, 1967a; Koenig, 1967). Other nerve terminals, independent of the calyx and possibly originating from another preganglionic fibre, are found in great numbers on the axon hillock (Hess, 1965). De Lorenzo (1966) does not make this distinction and considers the nerve terminals on the axon hillock to be part of the calyx, although the calyx was originally described to occur around the opposite pole of the ganglion cell (Carpenter, 1911). On the small neurons only the second (non-calyciform) type of synapse is found (Hess, 1965). In this type of endings, the preganglionic axon divides before reaching the ganglion cell and produces many small terminal knobs (De Lorenzo, 1960). The occurrence of pre-synaptic endings on the calyx and on the axon hillock has been suggested by De Lorenzo (1966), but there is as yet no other convincing evidence for this.

The opposed membrane of ganglion cell and calyciform ending possess a great number of synaptic complexes, with thickening of the adjacent membranes and clustering of agranular vesicles (De Lorenzo, 1960). There are also frequent desmosome-like contacts, with symmetrical thickenings of the membranes, no vesicles and an intercellular cleft of approximately 30 nm (Takahashi and Hama, 1965a). A rare occurrence is the presence of round areas of close apposition of the adjacent cell membranes; at such points there is no clustering of vesicles and the gap between the cells is less than 8 nm (in osmium fixed preparations) (Takahashi and Hama, 1965a; Koenig, 1967). These junctions are not found in embryonic or newly-hatched chicks, but first appear in chicks of several days of age. They probably correspond to the junctions described by De Lorenzo (1966) as 'tight junctions' at which there is partial fusion of the adjacent membranes.

All of the nerve endings on the ganglion cells contain agranular vesicles 30—60 nm in diameter, together with a few large granulated vesicles. Preganglionic nerve terminals store and release acetylcholine, more than half of the total content of acetylcholine, measured gas-chromatically, being in the presynaptic nerve terminals, and less than a quarter in the ganglion cells (Pilar, Jenden and Campbell, 1973). Preganglionic denervation causes a great fall in the acetylcholine of nerve terminals as might be expected, but the acetylcholine in the ganglion cells and postganglionic nerves also falls to as little as one tenth of their control values. The acetylcholine levels of the ganglion cells tend to return to their control values upon reinnervation (after 15 days), providing an example of a trans-synaptic orthograde influence. The great effect of section of the oculomotor nerve on the ciliary ganglion cells is also related to the fact that these fibres provide their only synaptic input, the section of the oculomotor nerve causing all preganglionic terminals to disappear (Terzuolo, 1951; Pilar *et al.*, 1973). On the other hand no degenerating fibres are found in the ciliary nerves after oculomotor section, i.e. all fibres from the oculomotor which reach the ganglion end in it (Terzuolo, 1951). In some ganglion cells post-synaptic membrane thickening appear still to be present even when pre-synaptic terminals have disappeared some 3–5 days after denervation (Pilar *et al.*, 1973), and post-synaptic structures were clearly seen by Koenig (1967) as late as 12 days after preganglionic denervation in the chick. Such structures may correspond to the spots of intense acetylcholinesterase activity seen on the surface of ciliary ganglion neurons after axotomy (Taxi, 1965).

Acetylcholinesterase activity of medium intensity is histochemically detectable in all ganglion cells (Szentagothai, Donhaffer and Rajkovits, 1954; Taxi, 1965; Koenig, 1965). In 20–30 per cent of the ganglion cells one pole of the cell is capped by an area with intense acetylcholinesterase activity, corresponding to the calyciform terminal. These caps disappear after preganglionic nerve section, whereas a significant increase in their number follows postganglionic section (Taxi, 1965; Koenig, 1967).

Ehinger (1967) found fine varicose non-vascular adrenergic terminals throughout the ganglion in the chick, pigeon and duck. They were particularly numerous in the region of the small (choroid) neurons and occasionally such adrenergic fibres formed a pericellular net around a ganglion cell, but adrenergic perikarya were absent. Cantino and Mugnaini (1974) confirmed these observations, and found by electron microscopy that adrenergic fibres, whose varicosities are filled with dense-core vesicles, are never in direct contact with the ganglion neurons beneath the glial satellite cells.

Preganglionic impulses to the large and myelinated ciliary neurons are transmitted by a dual mechanism, both electrical and chemical. The small choroid neurons receive only chemically transmitted impulses. Chemical transmission is cholinergic in both cases, although the mechanisms are not pharmacologically identical, the choroid cells being more suceptible to block by hexamethonium than are the ciliary neurons. The two systems of cells appear connected to two separate sets of preganglionic fibres (Merwitt *et al.*, 1971). Moreover the axons (postganglionic fibres) of the large neurons are myelinated, whereas those of the small neurons are unmyelinated.

The electrical synaptic transmission in chick and pigeon ciliary ganglia has been studied by Pilar and collaborators (Martin and Pilar, 1963; Marwitt *et al.*, 1971). It was first suggested that the close apposition of pre- and postganglionic membranes explained the occurrence of electrical transmission (De Lorenzo, 1966), since in several tissues, both nervous and non-nervous, apposition of

381

junctional membranes has been thought to provide a low resistance pathway for electrical coupling. Hess, Pilar and Weakley (1969) have shown, however, that the time of appearance of electrical coupling (before hatching in the chick; during the second post-hatching week in the pigeon) correlates better with the presence of myelin lamellae than with the occurrence of close apposition junctions. Although it is not known to what extent the rather loose myelin around ganglion cells has electrical properties (resistance value) comparable to those of myelin in peripheral nerves, the authors suggest that 'the so-called saltatory conduction of nerve impulses that oocurs in myelinated nerve fibres might also occur through the ciliary ganglion. That is, the synaptic apparatus with its myelin envelope may behave as an "internode".'

7.5 Intramural ganglia

Ganglia situated inside the organ they innervate are characteristically associated with the alimentary tract and constitute the 'enteric nervous system' (Langley, 1921), which is connected with both the parasympathetic and the sympathetic outflows (extrinsic nerves). The ganglia start in the oesophagus and extend as continuous plexuses down to the anal canal. They are co-extensive with the smooth musculature, including that of the biliary extra-hepatic pathways. The ganglia are flattened and connected by strands of varying thickness to form a meshwork whose pattern is characteristic of the various portions of the tract and varies from species to species. Two main plexuses are described, one situated between the two muscle layers of the muscularis externa (myenteric or Auerbach's plexus), the other situated in the submucosa (submucous or Meissner's plexus). The two plexuses are interconnected and send branches to the muscle layers, to the blood vessels and to the mucosa. The ganglia, which contain from a few up to tens of neurons, are ensheathed by a thin collagen capsule, but this usually does not penetrate into the ganglia or around individual ganglion cells (Taxi, 1965).

The number of neurons in the intestinal intramural ganglia is considerable, but varies from species to species, with different densities of neurons per unit of surface in the various segments of the alimentary canal (see Gabella, 1971). In the myenteric plexus of the guinea-pig ileum about 7500 neurons have been counted in the ganglia corresponding to 1 cm^2 of serosal surface (Irwin, 1931; Matsuo, 1934). Higher values were found in the colon (15–19 000), rectum (18 000) and pyloric part of the stomach (20 000). In the caecum, neurons are nearly three times more numerous beneath the taeniae coli than between them. In the rat it has been calculated that nearly two million neurons are present within the wall of the alimentary canal (Gabella, 1971). The packing density of intramural neurons is higher in species of small body size, whereas the average perikaryon size is larger in larger species.

Dogiel's (1896) classification of autonomic neurons reported on p. 359 was originally devised for the intestinal plexuses. Although the problem has been

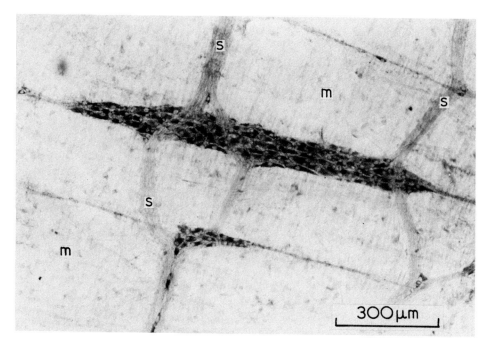

Fig. 7.10 Ganglia of the myenteric plexus in the duodenum of guinea-pig, stained with the histochemical reaction for NADH-diaphorase. s – strands of unmyelinated fibres connecting the ganglia; m – the longitudinal musculature, virtually unstained.

extensively debated since then, no clear cut classification of intramural neurons is at present available. There is no doubt that the cells of the intramural ganglia constitute a heterogeneous population, as can be clearly seen from their morphology (e.g. from their sizes and the size and pattern of their cell processes (see Schofield, 1968)), and more recently from electrophysiological studies (Nishi and North, 1973; Hirst, Holman and Spence, 1974). However, it is not as yet possible, to identify which neurons are motor, which are sensory, and which are interneurons.

With few exceptions (described on p. 384) the intramural neurons are not adrenergic, but they receive an abundant supply of adrenergic fibres (containing noradrenaline) mainly from the prevertebral ganglia. The sites of termination of adrenergic fibres in the alimentary canal, which had been interpreted in contrasting ways when studied by means of silver impregnation methods, have been clarified by the fluorescence microscopy method for catecholamines. Numerous adrenergic fibres are seen by fluorescence microscopy in the myenteric and submucous plexuses (Norberg, 1964; Jacobowitz, 1964). Individual varicose fluorescent fibres can be followed in the connecting meshes, but in the ganglia they form thick networks, sometimes in the form of pericellular nests, and cannot be followed as individual fibres. A similar distribution of adrenergic fibres has been seen throughout the entire length of the alimentary canal (Gabella and Costa, 1967; Read and Burnstock, 1969). Other adrenergic fibres, as identified in fluorescence microscopy, lie directly among the muscle cells and in the tunica propria, close to the glands; and abundant fluorescent fibres accompany the blood vessels, particularly in the submucosa (Furness, 1971). After extrinsic denervation all fluorescent fibres in the intestinal wall disappear (Furness, 1969) and the noradrenaline content falls to close to zero (Juorio and Gabella, 1974). The only exception to this arrangement is the myenteric plexus in the proximal colon of the guinea-pig, where a minority of adrenergic neurons is consistently observed in fluorescence microscopy (Costa, Furness and Gabella, 1971; Furness and Costa, 1971); these ganglia adrenergic fibres are therefore partly intrinsic and partly extrinsic in origin.

In the electron microscope the adrenergic nerve endings, which are identified by the presence of small dense-core vesicles, are seen synapsing on the perikarya and processes of ganglion neurons. The intramuscular adrenergic nerve endings lie within a distance of 50 nm or more from a muscle cell and do not show pre-junctional specializations.

Adrenergic synapses on intramural ganglion cells are considered to be inhibitory, since catecholamines inhibit acetylcholine output from the myenteric plexus of the guinea-pig (Paton and Vizi, 1969) and noradrenaline reduces the amplitude of evoked potentials (Holman, Hirst and Spence, 1972; Nishi and North, 1973). The synapses are found on the perikarya and on the dendrites: axo-axonic synapses are hard to identify since we do not have criteria for recognizing the initial tract of the axons. Adrenergic synapses seem to be present on the majority of ganglion neurons in agreement with the observed pattern of fluorescent fibres. It is not known, however, whether all of the varicosities, which give the adrenergic fibre a fairly regular beaded appearance, are in synaptic contact with a ganglion neuron.

Another type of nerve ending synapsing on myenteric neurons contains a heterogeneous population of agranular and granulated vesicles (Baumgarten, Holstein and Owman, 1970, in the large intestine of the rhesus monkey, guinea-pig and man; Gabella, 1972, in the small intestine of the guinea-pig) (Fig. 7.11): most of the vesicles are about 100 nm in diameter and are filled with a material of medium electron density, but it is characteristic that only agranular vesicles about 50 nm in diameter are found adjacent to the presynaptic membrane (Gabella, 1972). The nature of the neurotransmitter released by these endings (which originate from neurons within the intestinal wall) is unknown, as are the relationships between the various types of vesicles these endings contain. Besides cholinergic and adrenergic neurons, at least one other type of fibre has been identified which is both inhibitory and intramural (Burnstock, Campbell, Bennett and Holman, 1964). Evidence has been obtained by Burnstock and collaborators that its transmitter may be ATP (Burnstock, Campbell, Satchell and Smythe, 1972; see Burnstock, 1972), but these intramural inhibitory fibres have not yet been identified histologically.

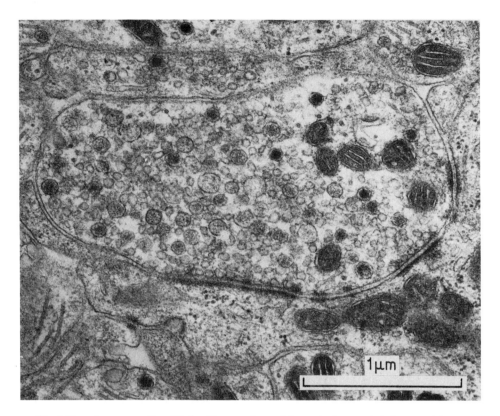

Fig. 7.11   A nerve ending filled with granular vesicles and characteristic large vesicles containing a finely granular material of medium electron density with no electron clear halo around it. This type of nerve ending is morphologically different from the cholinergic and adrenergic endings, and it is found synapsing on the intramural neurons of the intestine.

A third type of nerve ending synapsing on intramural neurons contains only granular vesicles (apart from occasional large granulated vesicles). Nerve varicosities with agranular vesicles are found not only synapsing on intramural neurons but also at the surface of ganglia, directly underneath the basal lamina. Such nerve endings containing agranular vesicles constitute the majority of endings in the myenteric plexus. They originate mainly from other intrinsic ganglion neurons and are considered to be cholinergic. In fact the content of acetylcholine in the myenteric plexus is higher than that of any other mammalian nervous tissue (Welsh and Hyde, 1944), and large amounts of acetylcholine are released from the plexus upon stimulation (Feldberg and Lin, 1950; Paton and Zar, 1968). Neurons are found in the myenteric plexus of the guinea-pig ileum which receive synapses from all the three types of ending described above.

Other nerve endings are characterized by flat agranular vesicles. Some of these synapse on intramural neurons, others lie at the surface of the ganglia. It is still

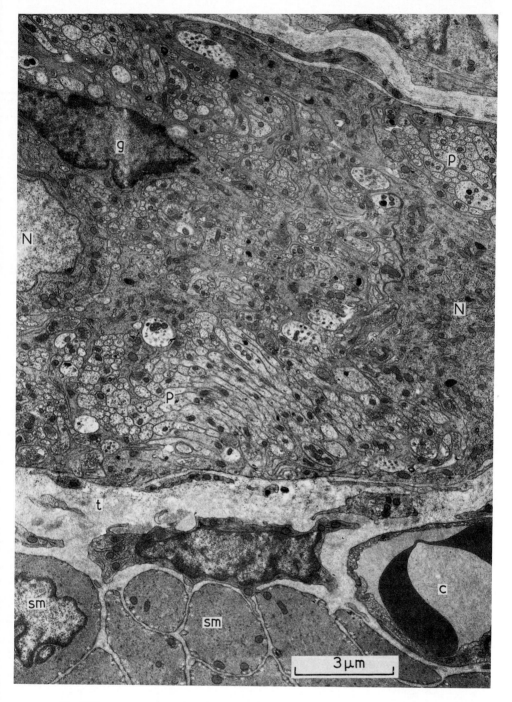

Fig. 7.12 Low power electron micrograph of a ganglion of the myenteric plexus. N – neuron; g – glial cell; p – nerve and glial processes tightly packed; c – capillary; sm – smooth muscle cells of the circular layer; t – connective tissue surrounding the ganglion. (Reproduced from Gabella, 1972.)

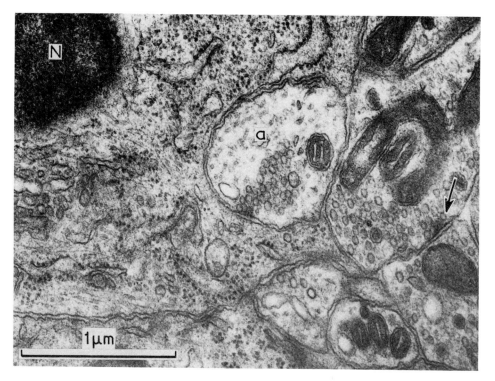

Fig. 7.13 Glial cell from a ganglion of the Myenteric plexus of guinea-pig. A nerve ending (a) has a specialized contact with the glial cell, with clustering of vesicles. Other axons are visible to the right. The arrow points to a specialized contact (a synapse?) between two axons. N – nucleus.

not clear whether or not these flat vesicles arise from round vesicles during the histological preparation procedure, but it seems likely that they characterize a different type of ending.

Numerous varicosities in the myenteric plexus, usually containing agranular vesicles, show contact specializations with glial cells: clustering of vesicles, thickening of an area of the axolemma, and a wider and more regular intercellular gap (Fig. 7.13). The significance of these neuro-glial junctions is unknown. Symmetrical contacts (attachment plaques) are also found between glial and nerve elements, without clustering of vesicles.

Glial cells are numerous in the intestinal plexuses. In the guinea-pig and rat they outnumber the ganglion cells by three to one. They cover part of the surface of the ganglion cells and penetrate between the various axonal and dendritic processes, moulding their shape to the spaces left among them. The ganglia are, therefore, compact structures where the only 'extracellular' space of a gap of 20–30 nm between adjacent structures. A characteristic feature of intramural neurons is that part of their cell membrane lies directly underneath the basal lamina and faces the connective tissue and interstitial space surrounding the ganglia. A layer, or patches, of microfilamentous material can be observed on the inner aspect of the plasma membranes of both glial and nerve cells, where they are in contact with the basal lamina.

In the intramural ganglia a direct study of pre- and postganglionic fibres is more difficult than in sympathetic ganglia. Postganglionic fibres from prevertebral sympathetic ganglia are preganglionic to the intramural ganglia (and are part of a pathway made of at least three neurons); vagal parasympathetic fibres are also preganglionic to the intramural ganglia of the stomach and probably to part of the intestine as well, but the actual endings of vagal fibres have not yet been identified by electron microscopy, and as silver impregnation methods have given conclusive results, the evidence that vagal fibres end on the intramural neurons is based mainly on physiological studies. Postganglionic fibres from intramural ganglion cells pass to the smooth musculature and to glands. Other ganglion neurons are interneurons and their fibres lie entirely within the plexuses.

References

Amprino, R. (1938) Modifications de la structure des neurones sympathiques pendant l'accroissement et la sénéscence. Recherches sur le ganglion cervical supérieur *Comptes Rendus de l'Association des Anatomistes.* 33, 3–18.

Angelakos, E. T. Glassman, P. M., Millard, R. W. and King, M. (1965) Regional distribution and subcellular localization of catecholamines in the frog heart. *Comparative Biochemistry and Physiology,* 15, 313–324.

Azuma, T., Binia, A and Visscher, M. B. (1965) Adrenergic mechanisms in the bullfrog and turtle. *American Journal of Physiology,* 209, 1287–1294.

Babmindra, V. P. and Biatchkova (1968) (quoted by Taxi and Babmindra, 1972).

Baumgarten, H. G., Holstein, A. F. and Owman, Ch. (1970) Auerbach's plexus of mammals and man: electron microscopic identification of three different types of neuronal processes in myenteric ganglia of the large intestine from rhesus monkeys, guinea-pigs and man. *Zeitschrift für Zellforschung,* 106, 376–397.

Becker, R. F. and Grunt, J. A. (1957) The cervical sympathetic ganglia. *Anatomical Record,* 127, 1–14.

Billingsley, P. R. and Ranson, S. W. (1918) On the number of nerve cells in the ganglion cervicale superius and of nerve fibers in the cephalic end of the truncus sympathicus in the cat and on the numerical relations of preganglionic and postganglionic neurones. *Journal of Comparative Neurology,* 29, 359–366.

Bishop, G. H. and Heinbecker, P. (1932) A functional analysis of the cervical sympathetic nerve supply to the eye. *American Journal of Physiology,* 100, 519–532.

Bishop, G. H. and O'Leary, J. (1938) Pathways through the sympathetic nervous system in the bull frog. *Journal of Neurophysiology,* 1, 442–454.

Björklund, A., Cegrell, L., Falck, B., Ritzen, M. and Rosengren, E. (1970) Dopamine-containing cells in sympathetic ganglia. *Acta physiologica scandinavica,* 78, 334–338.

Botar, J. (1966) The autonomic nervous system. Akadémiai Kiado, Budapest.

Bray, G. M. and Aguayo, A. J. (1974) Regeneration of peripheral unmyelinated nerves. Fate of the axonal sprouts which develop after injury. *Journal of Anatomy,* 117, 517–529.

Brzin, M., Tennyson, V. M. and Duffy, P. E. (1966) Acetylcholinesterase in frog sympathetic and dorsal root ganglia. A study by electron microscope cytochemistry and microgasometric analysis with the magnetic diver. *Journal of Cell Biology,* 31, 215–242.

Buckley, G., Consolo, S., Giacobini, E. and Sjöqvist, F. (1967) Cholinacetylase in innervated and denervated sympathetic ganglia and ganglion cell of the cat. *Acta physiologica scandinavica,* 71, 348–356.

Bülbring, E. (1944) The action of adrenaline on transmission in the superior cervical ganglion. *Journal of Physiology*, 103, 55–67.

Burnstock, G. (1972) Purinergic nerves. *Pharmacological Reviews*, 24, 509–581.

Burnstock, G., Campbell, G., Bennet, H. and Holman, M. E. (1964) Innervation of the guinea-pig taenia coli: are there intrinsic inhibitory nerves which are distinct from sympathetic nerves? *International Journal of Neuropharmacology*, 3, 163–166.

Burnstock, G., Campbell, G., Satchell, D. and Smythe, A. (1970) Evidence that adenosine triphosphate or a related nucleotide is the transmitter released by non-adrenergic inhibitory nerves in the gut. *British Journal of Pharmacology*, 40, 668–688.

Cajal, S. R. (1911) Histologie du système nerveux de l'homme et des vertébres, Vol. II. Maloine, Paris.

Cantino, D. and Mugnaini, E. (1974) Adrenergic innervation of the parasympathetic ciliary ganglion in the chick. *Science*, 185, 279–281.

Carpenter, F. W. (1911) The ciliary ganglion of birds. *Folia neuro-biologica*, 5, 738–754.

Ceccarelli, B., Clementi, F. and Mantegazza, P. (1971) Synaptic transmission in the superior cervical ganglion of the cat after re-innervation by vagus fibres. *Journal of Physiology*, 216, 87–98.

Costa, M., Furness, J. B. and Gabella, G. (1971) Catecholamine containing nerve cells in the mammalian myentric plexus. *Histochemie*, 25, 103–106.

Coupland, R. E. (1965) The natural history of the chromaffin cell. Longmans; London.

Cravioto, H. and Merker, H. (1963) Elektronenmikroskopische Untersuchungen an Satellitenzellen der sympatischen Ganglien des Menschen. *Archiv für Psychiatrie und Nervenkrankheiten*, 204, 1–10.

Crowcroft, P. J. and Szurszewski, J. H. (1971) A study of the inferior mesenteric and pelvic ganglia of guinea-pigs with intracellular electrodes. *Journal of Physiology*, 219, 421–441.

Csillik, B., Kalmàn, G. and Knyihar, E. (1967) Adrenergic nerve endings in the feline cervicale superius ganglion. *Experientia*, 23, 477–478.

Dahlström, A. and Häggendal, J. (1966) Some quantitative studies on the noradrenaline content in the cell bodies and terminals of a sympathetic adrenergic neuron system. *Acta physiologica scandinavica*, 67, 271–277.

Dahlström, A., Häggendal, J. and Hökfelt, T. (1966) The noradrenaline content of the varicosities of sympathetic adrenergic nerve terminals in the rat. *Acta physiologica scandinavica*, 67, 289–294.

De Castro, F. (1932) Sympathetic ganglia, normal and pathological. In: *Cytology and cellular pathology of the nervous system*. (ed.) Penfield W., Vol. I, 319–379. Hoeber: New York.

De Castro, F. (1951) Aspects anatomiques de la transmission synaptique ganglionnaire chez les mammiferes. *Archives internationales de Physiologie et de Biochimie*, 59, 479–511.

De Castro, F. and Herreros, M. L. (1945) Actividad funcional del ganglio cervical superior, en relacion al numero y modalidad de sus fibras preganglionicas. Modelo de la sinapsis. *Trabajos del Instituto Cajal de Investigationes Biologicas*, 37, 287–342.

De Groat, W. C. and Saum, W. R. (1971) Adrenergic inhibition in mammalian parasympathetic ganglia. *Nature*, 231, 188–189.

De Lemos, C. and Pick, J. (1966) The fine structure of thoracic sympathetic neurons in the adult rat. *Zeitschrift für Zellforschung*, 71, 189–206.

Delorenzi, E. (1931) Modificazioni dei neuroni simpatici dei Mammiferi domestici in relazione all'accrescimento somatico e alla senescenza. *Archivo italiano di Anatomia*, 28, 529–552.

De Lorenzo, A. J. (1960) The fine structure of synapses in ciliary ganglion of the chick. *Journal of biophysical and biochemical Cytology*, 7, 31–36.

De Lorenzo, A. J. (1966) Electron Microscopy: tight junctions in synapses of the chick ciliary ganglion. *Science*, 152, 76–78.

De Robertis, E. D. P. and Bennett, H. S. (1954) Submicroscopic vesicular component in the synapse. *Federation Proceedings*, 13, 35.

De Robertis, E. D. P. and Bennett, H. S. (1955) Some features of the submicroscopic morphology of synapses in frog and earthworm. *Journal of biophysical and biochemical Cytology*, 1, 47–58.

Dogiel, A. S. (1896) Zwei Arten sympathischer Nervenzellen. *Anatomische Anzeiger,* 11, 679–687.

Dunant, Y. (1967) Organisation topographique et fonctionelle du ganglion cervical supérieur chez le rat. *Journal de Physiologie,* 59, 3–24.

Ebbeson, S. O. E. (1968a) Quantitative studies of superior cervical sympathetic ganglia in a variety of primates including man. I. The ratio of preganglionic fibres to ganglionic neurons. *Journal of Morphology,,* 124, 117–132.

Ebbeson, S. O. E. (1968b) Quantitative studies of superior cervical sympathetic ganglia in a variety of primate including man. II. Neuronal packing density. *Journal of Morphology,* 124, 181–186.

Eccles, J. C. (1935) The action potential of the superior cervical ganglion. *Journal of Physiology,* 85, 179–206.

Ehinger, B. (1967) Adrenergic nerves in the avian and ciliary ganglion. *Zeitschrift für Zellforschung,* 82, 577–588.

Ehinger, B. and Falck, B. (1970) Uptake of some catacholamines and their precursors into neurons of the rat ciliary ganglion. *Acta physiologica scandinavica,* 78, 132–141.

Elfvin, L. G. (1963a) The ultrastructure of the superior cervical sympathetic ganglion of the cat. I. The structure of the ganglion cell processes as studied by serial sections. *Journal of Ultrastructure Research,* 8, 403–440.

Elfvin, L. G. (1963b) The ultrastructure of the superior cervical sympathetic ganglion of the cat. II. The structure of the preganglionic end fibers and the synapses as studied by serial sections. *Journal of Ultrastructure Research,* 8, 441–476.

Eränkö, O. and Eränkö, L. (1971) Small, intensely fluorescent granule-containing cells in the sympathetic ganglion of the rat. *Progress in Brain Research,* 34, 39–51.

Euler, U. S. V. (1946) A specific sympathomimetic ergone in adrenergic nerve fibres (sympathin) and its relation to adrenaline and noradrenaline *Acta physiologica scandinavica,* 12, 73–97.

Falck, B. and Owman, B. (1965) A detailed methodological description of the fluorescence method for cellular localization of biogenic amines. *Acta Universitatis Lundiensi,* Section II, N.7.

Feldberg, W. and Lin, R. C. Y. (1950) Synthesis of acetylcholine in the wall of the digestive tract. *Journal of Physiology,* 163, 475–487.

Foley, J. O. and DuBois, F. S. (1940) A quantitative and experimental study of the cervical sympathetic trunk. *Journal of comparative Neurology,* 72, 587–603.

Folkow, B., Johansson, B. and Öberg, B. (1958) The stimulation threshold of different sympathetic fibre groups as correlated to their functional differentiation. *Acta physiologica scandinavica,* 44, 146–156.

Forssman, W. G. (1964) Studien über den Feinbau des Ganglion cervicale superius der Ratte. I. Normale Struktur. *Acta anatomica,* 59, 420–433.

Fredricsson, B. and Sjöqvist, F. (1962) A cytomorphological study of cholinesterase in sympathetic ganglia of the cat. *Acta morphologica neerlando-scandinavica,* 5, 140–166.

Fujimoto, S. (1967) Some observations on the fine structure of the sympathetic ganglion of the toad, *Bufo vulgaris japonicum. Archivium histologicum japonicum,* 28, 313–335.

Furness, J. B. (1969) The presence of inhibitory nerves in the colon after sympathetic denervation. *European Journal of Pharmacology,* 6, 349–352.

Furness, J. B. (1971) The adrenergic innervation of the vessels supplying and draining the gastrointestinal tract. *Zeitschrift für Zellforschung,* 113, 67–82.

Furness, J. B. and Costa, M. (1971) Morphology and distribution of intrinsic adrenergic neurones in the proximal colon of the guinea-pig. *Zeitschrift für Zellforschung,* 120, 346–363.

Fuxe, K., Goldstein, T., Hökfelt, T. and Joh, T. H. (1971) Cellular localization of dopamine-hydroxylase and phenylethanolamine-N-methyl transferase as revealed by immunohistochemistry. *Progress in Brain Research,* 34, 127–138.

Gabella, G. (1971) Neuron size and number in the myenteric plexus of the newborn and adult rat. *Journal of Anatomy,* 109, 81–95.

Gabella, G. (1972) Fine structure of the myenteric plexus in the guinea-pig ileum. *Journal of Anatomy,* 111, 69–97.

Gabella, G. (1974) The sphincter pupillae of the guinea-pig: structure of muscle cells, intercellular relations and density of innervation. *Proceedings of the Royal Society of London Series B,* 186, 369–386.

Gabella, G. and Costa, M. (1967) Le fibre adrenergiche nel canale alimentare. *Giornale dell'Accademia di Medicina di Torino,* 130, 199–221.

Gabella, G. and Millar, J. (1975) (in preparation).

Gairns, F. W. and Garven H. S. D. (1953) Ganglion cells and their relationships with on another in the human lumbar sympathetic ganglia. *Journal of Physiology* 122, 16–17.

Giacobini, E. (1956) Demonstration of AChE activity in isolated nerve cells. *Acta physiologica scandinavica,* 36, 276–290.

Gray, E. G. (1963) Electron microscopy of presynaptic organelles of the spinal cord. *Journal of Anatomy,* 97, 101–106.

Grillo, M. A. (1966) Electron microscopy of sympathetic tissues. *Pharmacological Reviews,* 18, 387–399.

Hamberger, B., Norberg, K. A. and Ungerstedt, U. (1965) Adrenergic synaptic terminals in autonomic ganglia. *Acta physiologica scandinavica,* 64, 285–286.

Hamori, J., Lang, E. and Simon, L. (1968) Experimental degeneration of the preganglionic fibers in the superior cervical ganglion of the cat. *Zeitschrift für Zellforschung,* 90, 37–52.

Harris, A. J. (1943) An experimental analysis of the inferior mesenteric plexus. *Journal of comparative Neurology,* 79, 1–17.

Hess, A. (1965) Developmental changes in the structure of the synapse on the myelinated cell bodies of the chicken ciliary ganglion. *Journal of Cell Biology,* 25, 1–19.

Hess, A., Pilar, G. and Weakley, J. N. (1969) Correlation between transmission and structure in avian ciliary ganglion synapses. *Journal of Physiology,* 202, 339–354.

Hirst, G. D. S., Holman, M. E. and Spence, I. (1974) Two types of neurones in the myenteric plexus of the duodenum in the guinea-pig. *Journal of Physiology,* 236, 303–326.

Hökfelt, T. (1968) *In vitro* studies on central and peripheral monoamine neurons at the ultrastructural level. *Zeitschrift für Zellforschung,* 91, 1–74.

Hökfelt, T. (1969) Distribution of noradrenaline storing particles in peripheral adrenergic neurons as revealed by electron microscopy. *Acta physiologica scandinavica,* 76, 427–440.

Hollinshead, M. B. and Gertner, S. B. (1969) Mast cell changes in denervated sympathetic ganglia. *Experimental Neurology,* 24, 487–496.

Holman, M. E., Hirst, G. D. S. and Spence, I. (1972) Preliminary studies of the neurones of Auerbach's plexus using intracellular microelectrodes. *Australian Journal of experimental Biology and medical Science,* 50, 795–801.

Holmstedt, B. and Sjöqvist, F. (1957) Distribution of acetycholinesterase in various sympathetic ganglia. *Acta physiologica scandinavica,* Suppl. 145, 72–73.

Honma, S. (1970a) Histochemical demonstration of catecholamines in the toad sympathetic ganglia. *Japanese Journal of Physiology,* 20, 186–197.

Honma, S. (1970b) Functional differentiation in sB and sC neurons in toad sympathetic ganglia. *Japanese Journal of Physiology,* 20, 281–295.

Huber, G. C. (1899) A contribution on the minute anatomy of the sympathetic ganglion of the different classes of vertebrates. *Journal of Morphology,* 16, 27–86.

Hunt, C. C. and Nelson, P. G. (1965) Structural and functional changes in the frog sympathetic ganglion following cutting of the presynaptic nerve fibres. *Journal of Physiology,* 177, 1–20.

Hutter, O. F. and Loewenstein, W. R. (1955) Nature of neuromuscular facilitation by sympathetic stimulation in the frog. *Journal of Physiology,* 130, 559–571.

Irwin, D. A. (1931) The anatomy of Auerbach's plexus. *American Journal of Anatomy,* 49, 141–166.

Jacobowitz, D. (1965) Histochemical studies of the autonomic innervation of the gut. *Journal of Pharmacology and experimental Therapeutics,* 149, 358–364.

Jacobowitz, D. (1970) Catecholamine fluorescence studies of adrenergic neurons and chromaffin cells in sympathetic ganglia. *Federation Proceedings,* 29, 1929–1944.

Jacobowitz, D. and Woodward, J. K. (1968) Adrenergic neurons in the cat superior cervical ganglion and cervical sympathetic nerve trunk. A histochemical study. *Journal of Pharmacology and experimental Therapeutics,* 162, 213–226.

Johnson, S. E. (1918) On the question of commissural neurones in the sympathetic ganglia. *Journal of comparative Neurology,* 29, 385–404.

Juorio, A. V. and Gabella, G. (1974) Noradrenaline in the guinea-pig alimentary canal: regional distribution and sensitivity to denervation and reserpine. *Journal of Neurochemistry,* 22, 851–858.

Klingman, G. I. and Klingman, J. D. (1967) Catecholamines in peripheral tissues of mice and cell counts of sympathetic ganglia after the prenatal and postnatal administration of the nerve growth factor antiserum. *International Journal of Neuropharmacology,* 6, 501–508.

Koelle, G. B. (1951) The elimination of enzymatic diffusion artifacts in the histochemical localization of cholinesterases and a survey of their cellular distribution. *Journal of Pharmacology and experimental Therapeutics,* 103, 153–171.

Koelle, G. B. (1954) The histochemical localization of cholinesterase in the central nervous system of the rat. *Journal of comparative Neurology,* 100, 211–228.

Koelle, W. A. and Koelle, G. B. (1959) The localization of external or functional acetylcholinesterase at the synapses of autonomic ganglia. *Journal of Pharmacology and experimental Therapeutics,* 126, 1–8.

Koenig, H. L. (1965) Relations entre la distribution de l'activité acétylcholinestérasique et celle de l'ergastoplasme dans les neurones du ganglion ciliaire du poulet. *Archives d'Anatomie microscopique et de Morphologie expérimentale,* 54, 937–964.

Koenig, H. L. (1967) Quelques particularités ultrastructurales des zones synaptiques dans le ganglion ciliaire du poulet. *Comptes Rendus de l'Association des Anatomistes* 52, 711–719.

Kosterlitz, H. W. and Lees, G. W. (1972) Interrelationship between adrenergic and cholinergic mechanisms. Handbook of Experimental Pharmacology, Vol. XXXIII (eds.) Blashko, H. Muscholl, E.,) pp. 762–812.

Kosterlitz, H. W., Thompson, J. W. and Wallis, D. I. (1964) The compound action potential in the nerve supplying the medial smooth muscle of the nictitating membrane of the cat. *Journal of Physiology,* 171, 426–433.

Kuntz, A. (1938) The structural organization of the celiac ganglia. *Journal of comparative Neurology,* 69, 1–12.

Kuntz, A. (1940) The structural organization of the inferior mesenteric ganglia. *Journal of comparative Neurology,* 72, 371–382.

Lakos, I. (1970) Ultrastructure of chronically denervated superior cervical ganglion in the cat and rat. *Acta biologica Academiae Scientiarum hungaricae,* 21, 425–427.

Langley, J. N. (1896) Observations on the medullated fibres of the sympathetic system and chiefly on those of the gray rami communicants. *Journal of Physiology,* 20, 55–76.

Langley, J. N. (1904) On the sympathetic system of birds, and on the muscles which move the feathers. *Journal of Physiology,* 30, 221–252.

Langley, J. N. (1921) The autonomic nervous system. Cambridge: Heffer.

Levi-Montalcini, R. and Booker, B. (1960) Excessive growth of the sympathetic ganglia evoked by a protein isolated from mouse salivary glands. *Proceedings of the National Academy of Sciences of the USA,* 46, 373–384.

Libet, B. and Owman, C. (1974) Concomitant changes in formaldehyde-induced fluorescence of dopamine interneurones and in slow inhibitory post-synaptic potentials of the rabbit superior cervical ganglion, induced by stimulation of the preganglionic nerve or by a muscarinic agent. *Journal of Physiology,* 237, 635–662.

Loewi, O. (1921) Ueber humorale Uebertragbarkeit der Herznervenwirkung. *Archiv für die gesamte Physiologie,* 189, 239–242.

Marrazzi, A. S. (1939) Adrenergic inhibition at sympathetic synapses. *American Journal of Physiology,* 127, 738–744.

Martin, A. R. and Pilar, G. (1963) Dual mode of synaptic transmission in the avian ciliary ganglion. *Journal of Physiology,* 168, 443–463.

Marwitt, R., Pilar, G. and Weakley, J. N. (1971) Characterization of two ganglion cell populations in avian ciliary ganglia. *Brain Research,* 25, 317–334.

Matuso, H. (1934) A contribution on the anatomy of Auerbach's plexus. *Japanese Journal of Medical Sciences, Anatomy,* 4, 417–428.

Matthews, M. R. (1971) Evidence from degeneration experiments for the preganglionic origin of afferent fibres to the small granule-containing cells of the rat superior cervical ganglion. *Journal of Physiology,* **218**, 95–96.

Matthews, M. R. and Nash, J. R. G. (1970) An efferent synapse from small granule-containing cells to a principle neuron in the superior cervical ganglion. *Journal of Physiology,* **210**, 11–13.

Matthews, M. R. and Raisman, G. (1969) The ultrastructure and somatic efferent synapses of small granule-containing cells in the superior cervical ganglion. *Journal of Anatomy,* **105**, 255–282.

Matthews, M. R. and Raisman, G. (1972) A light and electron microscopic study of the cellular response to axonal injury in the superior cervical ganglion of the rat. *Proceedings of the Royal Society of London (Series B),* **181**, 43–79.

McLachlan, E. M. (1974) The formation of synapses in mammalian sympathetic ganglia reinnervated with preganglionic or somatic nerves. *Journal of Physiology,* **237**, 217–242.

Milhaud, M. and Pappas, G. (1966) The fine structure of neurons and synapses of the habenula of the cat with special reference to subjunctional bodies. *Brain Research,* **3**, 158–173.

Muscholl, E. and Vogt, M. (1964) Perfusion of extramedullary chromaffine tissue. *Journal of Physiology,* **169**, 93–94.

Nishi, S. and Christ, D. (1971) Electrophysiological properties and activities of mammalian parasympathetic ganglion cells. *Federation Proceedings,* **30**, 489.

Nishi, S. and North, R. A. (1973) Presynaptic action of noradrenaline in the myenteric plexus. *Journal of Physiology,* **231**, 29–30.

Nishi, S., Soeda, H. and Koketsu, K. (1965) Studies on sympathetic B and C neurones and patterns of preganglionic innervation. *Journal of cellular and comparative Physiology,* **66**, 19–32.

Nishi, S., Soeda, H. and Koketsu, K. (1967) Release of acetylcholine from sympathetic nerve terminals. *Journal of Neurophysiology,* **30**, 114–134.

Norberg, K. A. (1964) Adrenergic innervation of the intestinal wall by fluorescence microscopy. *International Journal of Neuropharmacology,* **3**, 379–382.

Norberg, K. A. (1967) Transmitter histochemistry of the sympathetic adrenergic nervous system. *Brain Research,* **5**, 125–170.

Norberg, K. A. and McIsaac, R. J. (1967) Cellular localization of adrenergic amines in frog sympathetic ganglia. *Experientia,* **23**, 1052.

Norberg, K. A., Ritzen, M. and Ungerstedt, U. (1966) Histochemical studies on a special catecholamine-containing cell type in sympathetic ganglia. *Acta physiologica scandinavica,* **67**, 260–270.

Obrador, S. and Odoriz, J. B. (1936) Transmission through a lumbar sympathetic ganglion. *Journal of Physiology,* **86**, 269–276.

Owman, C. and Sjöstrand, N. O. (1965) Short adrenergic neurons and catecholamine-containing cells in vas deferens and accessory male genital glands of different mammals. *Zeitschrift für Zellforschung,* **66**, 300–320.

Paton, V. D. M. and Vizi, E. S. (1969) The inhibitory action of noradrenaline and adrenaline on acetylcholine output by guinea-pig ileum longitudinal muscle strip. *British Journal of Pharmacology,* **35**, 10–28.

Paton, W. D. M. and Zar, M. A. (1968) The origin of acetylcholine released from guinea-pig intestine and longitudinal muscle strips. *Journal of Physiology,* **194**, 13–33.

Pera, L. (1971) Sui rapporti tra nervo vago e gangli prevertebrali nel gatto. *Archivio italiano di Anatomia e Embriologia,* **76**, 7–17.

Perry, W. L. M. and Talesnik, J. (1953) The role of acetylcholine in synaptic transmission at parasympathetic ganglia. *Journal of Physiology,* **119**, 455–469.

Pick, J. (1963) On the submicroscopic organization of the sympathetic ganglion in the frog (Rana pipiens). *Journal of comparative Neurology,* **120**, 409–462.

Pick, J. (1970) *The autonomic nervous system.* Lippincott: Philadelphia and Toronto.

Pilar, G., Jenden, D. J. and Campbell, B. (1973) Distribution of acetylcholine in the normal and denervated pigeon ciliary ganglion. *Brain Research,* **49**, 245–256.

Pines, J. L. (1927) Die Morphologie des Ganglion ciliare beim Menschen *Zeitschrift für mikroskopisch-anatomische Forschung,* **10**, 313–380.

Pines, L. and Friedman, E. (1929) Zur vergleichenden Histologie des Ganglion ciliare bei Säugetieren. *Zeitschrift für mikroskopisch-anatomische Forschung*, 16, 259–294.

Quilliam, J. P. and Tamarind, D. L. (1972) Electron microscopy of degenerative changes in decentralized rat superior cervical ganglia. *Micron*, 3, 454–472.

Raisman, G., Field, P. M., Ostberg, A. J. C., Iversen, L. L. and Zigmond, R. E. (1974) A quantitative ultrastructural and biochemical analysis of the process of reinnervation of the superior cervical ganglion in the adult rat. *Brain Research*, 71, 1–16.

Ranson, S. W. and Billingsley, P. R. (1918) The superior cervical ganglion and the cervical portion of the sympathetic trunk. *Journal of comparative Neurology*, 29, 313–358.

Read, J. B. and Burnstock, G. (1969) Adrenergic innervation of the gut musculature in Vertebrates. *Histochemie*, 17, 263–272.

Richardson, K. C. (1966) Electron microscopic identification of autonomic nerve endings. *Nature*, 210, 756.

Rodriguez Echandia, E. L., Donoso, A. O. and Pedroza, E. (1972) A further contribution to the study of catecholamine flow in amphibian nerves. *Acta physiologica latino-americana*, 22, 161–165.

Schofield, G. C. (1968) Anatomy of muscular and neural tissues in the alimentary canal. In *Handbook of Physiology*, (ed.) Code, C. F., Section 6, Vol. IV, pp. 1579–1627. American Physiological Society, Washington.

Siegrist, G., Dolivo, M., Dunant, Y., Forogloukerameus, C., De Ribaupierre, Fr. and Rouiller, Ch. (1968) Ultrastructure and function of the chromaffin cells in the superior cervical ganglion of the rat. *Journal of Ultrastructure Research*, 25, 381–407.

Slavich, E. (1932) Confronti fra la morfologia di gangli del parasimpatico encefalico e del simpatico cervicale con speciale riguardo alla struttura del ganglio ciliare. *Zeitschrift für Zellforschung*, 15, 688–730.

Stöhr, P. (1939) Uber "Nebenzellen" und deren Innervation in Ganglien des vegetativen Nervensystem, zugleich ein Beitrag zur Synapsenfrage. *Zeitschrift für Zellforsch*, 29, 569–612.

Szentagothai, J., Donhoffer, A. and Rajkovits, K. (1954) Die Lokalisation der Cholinesterase in der interneuronalen Synapse. *Acta histochemica*, 1, 272–281.

Takahashi, K. and Hama, K. (1965a) Some observations on the fine structure of the synaptic area in the ciliary ganglion of the chick. *Zeitschrift für Zellforschung*, 67, 174–184.

Takahashi, K. and Hama, K. (1965b) Some observations of the fine structure of nerve cell bodies and their satellite cells in the ciliary ganglion of the chick. *Zeitschrift für Zellforschung*, 67, 835–843.

Tamarind, D. L. and Quilliam, J. P. (1971) Synaptic organisation and other ultrastructural features of the superior cervical ganglion of the rat, kitten and rabbit. *Micron*, 2, 204–234.

Taxi, J. (1961) Etude de l'ultrastructure des zones synaptiques dans les ganglions sympatiques de la Grenouille, *Comptes Rendus Academie des Sciences de Paris*, 252, 174–176.

Taxi, J. (1965) Contribution a l'étude des connexions des neurones moteurs due système nerveux autome. *Annales des Sciences naturelles, Zoologie*, 7, 413–674.

Taxi, J. and Babmindra, V. P. (1972) Light and electron microscopic studies of normal and heterogeneously regenerated ganglionic synapses in dog. *Journal of Neural Transmission*, 33, 257–274.

Taxi, J., Gautron, J. and L'Hermite, P. (1969) Données ultrastructurales sur une éventuelle modulation adrénergique de l'activité du ganglion cervical supérieur du rat. *Comptes Rendus Academie des Sciences de Paris*, 269, 1281–1284.

Terni, T. (1922) Ricerche sulla struttura e sull'evoluzione del simpatico dell'uomo. *Monitore zoologico italiano*, 33, 63–72.

Terzuolo C. (1951) Ricerche sul ganglio ciliare degli uccelli. Connessioni, mutmenti in relazione all'età a dopo recisione delle fibre prepangliari. *Zeitschrift für Zellforschung*, 36, 255–267.

Uchizono, K. (1964) On different types of synaptic vesicles in the sympathetic ganglia of amphibia. *Japanese Journal of Physiology*, 14, 210–219.

Van Orden, L. S. III, Burke, J. P., Geyer, M. and Lodden, F. V. (1970) Localization of depletion-sensitive and depletion-resistant norepinephrine storage sites in autonomic ganglia. *Journal of Pharmacology and experimental Therapeutics,* 174, 56–71.

Van Orden, L. S. III, Schaefer, J. M., Burke, J. P. and Lodden, F. V. (1970) Differentiation of norepinephrine storage compartments in peripheral adrenergic nerves. *Journal of Pharmacology and experimental Therapeutics,* 174, 357–368.

Volle, R. L. (1966) Modification by drugs of synaptic mechanisms in autonomic ganglia. *Pharmacological Reviews,* 18, 199–200.

Warwick, R. (1954) The ocular parasympathetic nerve supply and its mesencephalic sources. *Journal of Anatomy,* 88, 71–93.

Watanabe, H. (1972) The fine structure of the ciliary ganglion of the guinea-pig. *Archivium histologicum japonicum,* 34, 261–276.

Welsh, J. H. and Hyde, J. E. (1944) Acetylcholine content in the myenteric plexus and resistance to anoxia. *Proceedings of the Society for experimental Biology and Medicine,* 55, 256–257.

Whitteridge, D. (1937) The transmission of impulses through the ciliary ganglion. *Journal of Physiology,* 89, 99–111.

Williams, T. H., Black, A. C. jr., Chiba, T. and Bhalla, R. C. (1975) Morphology and biochemistry of small, intensely fluorescent cells of sympathetic ganglia. *Nature,* 256, 315–317.

Williams, T. H., Jew, J. and Palay, S. L. (1973) Morphological plasticity in the sympathetic chain. *Experimental Neurology,* 39, 181–203.

Williams, T. H. and Palay, S. L. (1969) Ultrastructure of the small neurons in the superior cervical ganglion. *Brain Research,* 15, 17–34.

Wolf, G. A. (1941) The ratio of preganglionic neurons in the visceral nervous system. *Journal of comparative Neurology,* 75, 235–243.

Woods, R. I. (1970a) The innervation of the frog's heart. I. An examination of the autonomic postganglionic nerve fibres and a comparison of autonomic and sensory ganglion cells. *Proceedings of the Royal Society of London (Series B),* 176, 43–54.

Yamamoto, T. (1963) Some observations on the structure of the sympathetic ganglion of the bullfrog. *Journal of Cell Biology,* 16, 159–170.

Yamauchi, A. and Lever, J. D. (1971) Correlations between formol fluorescence and acetylcholinesterase (AChE) staining in the superior cervical ganglion of normal rat, pig and sheep. *Journal of Anatomy,* 110, 435–443.

Yamauchi, A., Fujimaki, Y. and Yokota, R. (1975) Reciprocal synapses between cholinergic postganglionic axon and adrenergic interneuron in the cardiac ganglion of the turtle. *Journal of Ultrastructure Research,* 50, 47–57.

Yokota, R. (1973) The granule-containing cell somata in the superior cervical ganglion of the rat, as studied by a serial sampling method for electron microscopy. *Zeitschrift für Zellforschung,* 141, 331–345.

8 SENSORY TERMINALS OF PERIPHERAL NERVES

L.H. Bannister

8.1 Introduction

8.1.1 *Historical aspects of sensory studies*

Philosophers have been grappling with the problems posed by our conscious awareness of an outside world since ancient times, and even in the twentieth century seem to have advanced very little towards unravelling the threads of this aspect of our experience. In terms of understanding the mechanism of sensation, a more modest goal, scientists in the last one and a half centuries have succeeded in explaining many of the features of sensory systems, and with the advent of new techniques in electrophysiology, histology and experimental psychology, the sensory pathways have been explored in increasing detail. This chapter is an attempt to survey some areas of research into the structure and functions of receptor endings. For reasons of space the approach will inevitably be superficial, and some major sensory systems – the visual and acoustico-vestibular pathways, for example – have been omitted altogether. For more detailed accounts the reader is referred to the reference list and to such comprehensive surveys as the multi-volume 'Handbook of Sensory Physiology' (Springer: Berlin, 1971 onwards).

A detailed history of sensory studies is also beyond the scope of this chapter, but some reference to the development of the subject is required since the arguments of the past to some extent determine the outlook of modern investigators (see also Brazier, 1957, Sinclair, 1967). Apart from early attempts to categorise our sensory experience in terms of 'the senses' – sight, hearing, touch, taste and smell, which stem from Aristotle (temperature sense was apparently no great problem in the sunny Aegean), the modern era of experimental studies on the mechanism of sensation can be traced back only about two hundred years. Restricting ourselves to the field of general sensation, Bell, Müller and Helmholtz writing in the eighteenth and early nineteenth centuries, are key figures in the development of perceptual studies. The recognition that particular types of subjective sensation are related to the type of nerve ending being stimulated rather than to the nature of the stimulus (Müller's theory of specific nervous energy), was a major step. In his proposal of the existence of distinct 'modalities of sensation', Helmholtz recognized that while a single type of receptor may respond to a limited range of stimuli having a similar energy form – different smells, for example, stimulating many olfactory receptors, further discrimination may be possible due to specialization within a population of similar receptors.

The development of neurohistological techniques during the second half of the nineteenth century, in particular the silver and gold impregnation methods of Golgi and Cajal, allowed the detailed study of nerve endings and demonstrated their wide variety of form. It was natural to speculate about the possible specific functions of such nerve endings, and, like von Frey (1894, 1906), to attempt to relate different types of structure to known sensory specificities. However, the idea that different encapsulated cutaneous end organs mediated specific stimulus qualities – touch, cold, warmth, and pain – lacked any conclusive supporting evidence, and it subsequently became clear that the sensory endings possessed such a diversity of structure that no such simple correlation was possible. The electrophysiological recording of sensory nerve impulses from the 1920's onwards opened a new era of sensory studies, and the pioneering work of Adrian, Zotterman, B. H. C. Matthews and others revealed the chief functional characteristics of the various receptor systems. It soon became obvious that while the different receptors showed basically similar patterns of response, they varied greatly in the types of stimulus to which they were most sensitive and in their rates of adaptation, maximum response frequency, stimulus thresholds and the like.

The relevance of subsequent studies of the detailed structure of cutaneous endings to the problem of sensory discrimination was called into question by Weddell and his associates (see Weddell and Miller, 1962; Sinclair, 1967), who had recognized that in certain situations – the ear skin of rabbits, for example, a wide range of sensitivities exist in the absence of any apparent differentiation of the cutaneous nerve endings comprising the 'free ending' dermal plexus. Weddel et al. suggested a possible explanation for this seeming inconsistency in their 'pattern' theory of cutaneous sensation in which they proposed that in general each afferent fibre was relatively non-specific, and that while there was some degree of differential response to mechanical, thermal and traumatic stimuli, the central perception of any particular stimulus was signalled by the complex pattern of responses carried by the total population of cutaneous nerve fibres involved. Recordings from single afferent fibres have since shown that the thresholds of most fibres are orders of magnitude lower to some stimuli than to others, each fibre appearing to be 'tuned' to a particular physiological mode of excitation. Furthermore, recent electron microscopical and other morphological studies appear to show differences between what appear to be identical nerve endings according to classical histological criteria. Exceptions to this high degree of specificity are to be found in some high-threshold cutaneous receptors, which appear to be equally sensitive to both noxious mechanical and thermal stimuli, and certain alimentary and respiratory tract receptors which are unable to discriminate between noxious chemicals, change in pH, or mechanical irritation.

Although Weddell's 'pattern' theory does not in itself provide an adequate explanation for sensory receptor mechanisms, the criticisms he levelled at previous theories have injected a healthy note of caution into subsequent attempts to correlate details of structure with function, and it must be remembered that many sensory endings in relatively unexplored sites, such as the alimentary and respiratory tracts, are known solely from either physiological, of from morphological studies, and that correlation between the two is lacking. In conclusion it must be mentioned that much information about the behaviour of the sensory endings has also been gleaned from comparative studies on lower vertebrates and invertebrates, but a review of these findings is beyond the scope of this account.

8.1.2 *General features of receptor systems*

Receptor classification

Receptors are customarily classified in a number of different ways. First, they may be divided up on the basis of their adequate stimulus, that is the type of energy to which they normally respond in life; there are therefore mechano-receptors, thermoreceptors, chemoreceptors, photoreceptors, and, in some types of electrogenic fish, electroreceptors. Second, it is common to classify them according to their anatomical position, exteroceptors responding primarily to external stimuli, entoreceptors to visceral and vascular stimuli, and proprioceptors to changes in the locomotor system (muscles tendons and joints). Third, receptors with high thresholds, responding only to noxious or potentially damaging stimuli are often referred to as nociceptors. Within these general categories, receptor types may be further sub-divided according to their functional or morphological organization and these subdivisions will be outlined in Section 8.3.

Stages in the sensory process

When a stimulus large enough to activate a sensory channel arrives at a receptor terminal, it sets in train a sequence of electrical events which eventually results in a change in the continuum activity of the central nervous system. In most sensory systems such events are separable into a number of distinct stages, as follows (see Fig. 8.1).

(1) Since in most cases the sensory ending is not in direct contact with the external environment, the stimulus must pass through intervening tissues or substances before it can affect the receptor surface; this is the stage of *stimulus accession*.

(2) The energy of the stimulus, of whatever type, must then be converted into electrical energy, in the form of an initial graded change in the electrochemical polarity of the receptor membrane; this process is termed *stimulus transduction*.

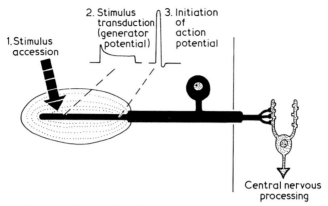

Fig. 8.1 A diagram indicating the chief events that occur when a stimulus activates a sensory nerve ending. For details, see text.

(3) The graded potential initiates a series of *action potentials* in the nerve fibre close to the receptor ending, and these are conducted to the central nervous system.

(4) Higher order neurons within the spinal cord and brain are excited and many interactions occur which result in sensory analysis, the integration of different sensory inputs, and a host of other neural activities; we can call this the stage of *neural processing*. Each of these stages will be considered in greater detail.

Stimulus accession

The cells and extracellular materials surrounding receptors may profoundly modify the nature of stimuli which pass through them, serving to amplify or organize them as in the eye and auditory apparatus, or to act in more subtle ways. In the Pacinian corpuscle for example, mechanical stimuli reach the nerve ending through concentric layers of flattened cells interleaved with collagen fibres and fluid; this arrangement absorbs the energy of all except very rapidly changing deformations, by the displacement of fluid between cells, and thus acts as a 'high pass' filter (Hubbard, 1958; Loewenstein and Mendelson, 1965; Loewenstein, 1971). Likewise, odours and gustatory stimuli must pass into and diffuse through mucus layers before affecting sensory endings, and their maximum concentrations and duration of action will be affected by their solubilities and diffusion speeds in such liquids. Many other examples of related phenomena are also seen in the behaviour of other sensory endings (see Section 3.3).

Stimulus transduction

All types of sensory ending exhibit a resting potential (see Chapter 12), the interior of the cell being negative with respect to the outside. When stimulated,

399

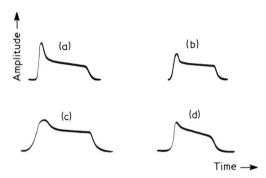

Fig. 8.2 Generator potentials of various sensory endings showing the general similarity in their form: (a) – frog muscle spindle; (b) – crayfish stretch receptor; (c) – frog olfactory epithelium (EOG); (d) – pacinian corpuscle (mammalian) (a)–(c) (After Ottoson 1974); (d) (After Loewenstein, 1971).

the usual response is a partial or total depolarisation, the extent of which is related to the strength and duration of the stimulus. Such a graded response, called the *generator* or *receptor potential* was first recorded extracellularly by Katz (1950) in muscle spindles, and has since been demonstrated for every major receptor system (see Granit, 1955, Grundfest, 1971). The shape of the response waveform of all receptor potentials appears to be similar, consisting typically of an initial rapid depolarization which adapts quickly to a plateau of reduced polarization (Fig. 8.2). The relative sizes of these two parts of the wave, termed respectively the dynamic and static components are of great significance since they determine the degree to which a receptor reacts differentially to rapidly changing or steadily maintained stimulus strengths (see p. 403).

As in all bioelectric activity, the receptor potential reflects sudden changes in the conductance of the membrane to small inorganic ions. Diamond, Gray and Inman (1958), and others, have shown that in Pacinian corpuscles the generator potential is largely sodium-dependent, and this has in general been confirmed to be the case in other types of receptor (see Lipetz, 1971). Recent evidence has suggested that the dynamic component of the generator potential is caused by an influx of K^+ and the static component by an influx of Na^+ (Husmark and Ottoson, 1971; Ottoson, 1973, 1974).

Responses other than depolarization are shown by some receptors. In retinal rods the inner segment is partially depolarized in the resting state and becomes hyperpolarized when illuminated, so causing the depolarization of other parts of the cell. Lateral line mechanoreceptors in fishes are depolarized when their apical projections are bent in one direction, and hyperpolarized when bent the opposite way (Flock, 1965). A similar phenomenon probably occurs in the Ruffini endings in joint capsules and other connective tissue sites, since their resting impulse activity may be either increased or decreased according to the direction in which stresses are applied (Skoglund, 1973). In some types of receptor, hyperpolarization is seen at the end of stimulation, caused perhaps by

400

an over-shoot in the activity of the regenerative sodium pump (Ottoson, 1974), as in the lateral eye of the King Crab *Limulus*, a classical sensory experimental preparation (Hartline and Ratcliff, 1957).

The molecular events in the receptor that initiate such conductance changes, are not yet known for any receptor, although there has been no shortage of speculation. In visual cells, the chemistry of the visual pigments, their association within membranes with globular proteins, and their structural organization have all been studied (e.g. Shields, Dinovo, Henrickson, Kimbel and Millar, 1967), but the final link with electrical activity is still lacking. A number of workers have isolated proteins that are capable of binding sweet and bitter tasting substances from gustatory endings, but these have yet to be proved specific to gustation (Price, 1974), and analogies have been drawn between chemoreception and the activity of acetylcholine at the receptor surfaces of muscle cells and the electroplaxes of electrogenic fishes from which specific receptor proteins have also been isolated; chemoreception in bacteria also appears to be dependent upon proteins at the cell surface (Adler,1969; Anraku, 1968). It is tempting to speculate that all receptor activity may be related to the presence of specific proteins in the receptor membrane, and that these undergo configurational changes when subjected to mechanical stress, temperature change, the presence of particular chemicals and so forth, depending upon the type of sensory ending involved, and so opening up ion channels in the membrane. Small differences in the tertiary structure of such molecules and variations in their numbers could be responsible for the wide range of adaptation rates, threshold levels and other similar characteristics which are known to vary greatly between the different types of receptor terminal.

More direct models have also been proposed for some receptors, in which molecular disruption at the receptor membrane leading to ion influx is thought to be caused by mechanical stretching of the receptor surface (see Catton, 1970), or by the action of lipid-soluble chemicals (Davies, 1971). While it is difficult to envisage how such processes could be responsible for all of the complex properties of the generator potential, it must be admitted that there is equally little firm evidence to support any of the other theories of transduction.

Graded potentials may be conducted along short lengths of receptor ending before impulses are triggered, as in olfactory dendrites and Pacinian axons. In gustatory cells, the generator potential probably invades the whole receptor, and the impulse is initiated only in the axons innervating its base (Kimura and Beidler, 1961).

Action potential initiation

Apart from the example mentioned above, impulses are triggered by the generator potential reaching a specialized 'pacemaker' region of the sensory fibre situated adjacent to the terminal. The frequency at which impulses are initiated depends upon the amplitude of the generator potential, which is in turn related to both the stimulus size and its duration. The impulse activity is therefore a frequency coded response to a graded stimulus, and from this point in the sensory pathway onwards, all stimulus information is dealt with in terms of impulse frequency.

Important features of this step are, firstly, that there is a linear relationship between generator potential amplitude and impulse frequency, and secondly, that adaptation can occur so that a sustained generator potential may only initiate a few impulses, as in experimentally decapsulated Pacinian endings (Loewenstein, 1971). Thirdly, the maximum frequency of impulses depends upon the size of the fibre, the refractory period between successive impulses being several times shorter in a large group Ia fibre than in a C fibre (Sassen and Zimmermann, 1971); since the maximum firing rate determines the range of information which a fibre can carry, large diameter fibres therefore have a greater dynamic range than small ones. Lastly, where the terminal is branched, impulses from one limb can invade others to 're-set' their resting potentials, thus ensuring synchronization of their responses (Iggo and Muir, 1969). The regularity of firing in afferent fibres varies in a characteristic manner. Type II S.A. mechanoreceptors (see p. 422) are highly regular in their activity, whereas Type I S.A. units are irregular in their responses, perhaps because of convergent activity from several terminal collaterals. Since sensory analysis must depend in part upon an assessment of impulse frequency, regular firing is probably more rapidly sampled than are irregular trains of impulses (Burgess and Perl, 1973).

Neural processing

The sensory fibres of different types of receptors pass to the spinal cord or brain where their anatomical pathways and connections with higher order neurons differ according to the sensory modalities they subserve and their topographical position within the body. Although the structure and functions of the central connections are understood in outline only in a few cases, certain resemblances have emerged which may indicate a common pattern of organization. In the visual system, for example, certain hierarchies of neural organization have been demonstrated (Hubel and Wiesel, 1961, 1968). The retinal receptors initially converge onto a smaller number of neurons which, by inhibiting surrounding elements in a directional manner, collectively form a means of detecting contrasts and movements. Similar arrangements of convergence and differential inhibition occur at a series of levels of higher order neuronal organization, enabling both moving and static visual patterns to be detected.

The essence of the process of 'lateral inhibition' is that an excitatory unit, when activated, depolarizes neighbouring inhibitory cells which in turn tend to inhibit other surrounding excitatory units. In this way, only the most active of the excitatory units remain uninhibited and contrasts of activity are therefore enhanced. This effect is particularly important where there is topographical representation of a sensory surface within a group of neurons, since the precise location of the site of maximum stimulation is greatly improved by the suppression of the more weakly stimulated surrounding pathways. Lateral inhibition is a feature of a number of other sensory systems, and may indeed be a characteristic element of all sensory pathways. In the olfactory bulb, granule cells – small inhibitory interneurons – surround the second order excitatory (mitral) cells, and small interneurons with a similar structure are also numerous in the ventrobasal thalamic nuclei which serve the main somatosensory system.

The representation of the peripheral position of receptor endings as a kind of two- or three-dimensional map within the central nervous system is also a general feature of sensory pathways. In the spinal somatosensory system, for example, such somatotopic representation occurs at several levels, including the laminar grouping of neurons in the dorsal grey columns, the dorsal column nuclei of the brain stem, the ventrobasal thalamic nuclei and the final projection areas of the somatosensory cortex.

Finally, centrifugal control of sensory pathways is of great importance in regulating sensory activity. Particular pathways can be facilitated or inhibited by centrifugal action at several levels in the nervous system. In the somatosensory pathways this may occur either presynaptically at the central termination of the primary sensory neuron, or post-synaptically on second or higher order cells. Where several different types of sensory fibre converge upon a single channel, as in laminae of the spinal cord dorsal grey, sequential inhibition of different primary fibres occurs, providing a mechanism for search and selection among the different types of sensory information. Centrifugal inhibition may also be present in more peripheral situations, as in mechanoreceptive hair cells of the cochlea (Fex, 1962, 1967), and it has been demonstrated physiologically in carotid chemoreceptor function. Whether or not other sensory endings receive centrifugal terminals remains to be shown.

Receptor adaptation

It has already been mentioned that receptors adapt to a maintain stimulus at varying speeds, and that the rate of adaptation determines whether a receptor is primarily responding to a change in stimulus strength or to its steady level – that is, whether it is a dynamic or a static receptor. Most receptors show varying mixtures of these two features, ranging from the Pacinian ending which adapts so rapidly that the static component is missing in its final response, the receptor providing information solely about the rate of acceleration of the mechanical deformation (see Loewenstein, 1971), to the Golgi tendon organ which is virtually non-adapting (B. H. C. Matthews, 1933). Between these two extremes lies a spectrum of responses (Fig. 8.3), allowing central analysis of the different aspects of a single stimulus. The dynamic and static modes of behaviour are most clearly distinguishable experimentally when receptors are

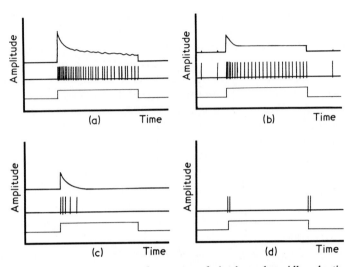

Fig. 8.3 Response characteristics of a range of slowly and rapidly adapting sensory endings. (a) is typical of a Type I slowly adapting cutaneous endings, with dynamic and static components both strongly demonstrated and an irregular discharge pattern; (b) represents the discharge of a Type II S.A. cutaneous mechanoreceptor, with smaller dynamic and more marked static features; (c) is a rapidly adapting mechanoreceptor unit of the 'down hair' type, and (d) is typical of the very rapidly adapting discharge of a Pacinian ending, with spike discharges at both the onset and termination of the stimulus.

In each case the lower line represents the stimulus, the middle line the action potentials of the afferent unit and the upper line the rate of firing. (a) After Iggo and Muir, 1969; (b) after Chambers *et al.*, 1972; (c) and (d) after various sources.

presented with an oscillating stimulus, since dynamic receptors respond primarily to rates of change rather than to amplitude, whilst in the static variety, the response is directly related to the magnitude of the stimulus.

In mechanoreceptors, the static response permits the additional possibility of detecting the position of associated tissues, so that the receptor may be directionally sensitive. Such receptors are seen in the Ruffini terminals of joints (Skoglund, 1973) and in the type II slowly adapting receptors of vibrissal hairs (Gottschaldt, Iggo and Young, 1973). Dynamic receptors, conversely, often respond equally to a change in position in any direction (see Burgess and Perl, 1973).

The underlying causes of receptor adaptation are complex and not yet fully understood. Some degree of adptation is found in the excitable properties of all biological membranes, and is predicted by the Hodgkin-Huxley model of nerve conduction and general membrane excitability (Catton, 1970). Another source of adaptation is provided by the presence of non-neural cells surrounding the nerve terminal, as already described in the Pacinian ending, and it is interesting that several rapidly adapting endings are associated with complex lamellar capsules. In other situations the reverse may apply, as in Golgi tendon organs where the terminal branches of the axon ramify amongst non-deformable

404

collagen fibres which may prevent relaxation of tension at the receptor surface. The mechanical properties of the intrafusal muscles of neuromuscular spindles may also affect the adaptation rates of their receptor endings (see Section 3.3). However, high rates of adaptation are still seen in Pacinian endings from which most of the capsule has been stripped, and also in unencapsulated chemoreceptor endings, implying that some fundamental property of the receptor membrane is involved: the adaptation detected at the transducer-pacemaker interface in receptor endings also supports this view. An adequate explanation of these phenomena remains to be found.

Stimulus-response relationships: transfer functions

In all sensory systems the stimulus strength is signalled by the generator potential amplitude and subsequently by the impulse frequency in the afferent fibre. As might be expected, a predictable relationship exists between these parameters, although there has been some argument as to its precise form.

It has long been known that a perceived change in stimulus strength is a function of the proportional change in actual stimulus strength, that is, of $\Delta S/S$ (where S is the previous suprathreshold stimulus strength, and ΔS the change in intensity), or to the logarithm of the stimulus intensity, $\log_{10} S$ – the Weber-Fechner rule (Fechner, 1860). More recently it has been suggested that the relationship is more accurately described as a power function, that is $R = aS^n$ (a and n being constants, n numerically 1 or less, and R the magnitude of the perceived response). Such a phenomenon is presumably a reflection of neural behaviour, relating either to peripheral sensory transduction or central nervous transmission; of the two, the former seems to be more likely, since electrophysiological measurements have demonstrated power function or similar relationships between stimulus and generator potential amplitudes in many different sensory endings (see Mackay, 1963, Lipetz, 1971). Furthermore, precise measurements indicate that in many cases a hyperbolic function provides a more exact description, as for example in gustatory endings (Kimura and Beidler, 1961) and olfactory terminals (Poynder, 1974), that is, $R = aS/(1 + bS)$ (a and b being constants; see Fig 8.4).

Measurements of impulse frequencies, inter-impulse intervals, or the total numbers of impulses resulting from a single stimulus have demonstrated the existence of a variety of relationships between stimulus strength and impulse output, ranging from linear responses ($R = bS$, b being a constant) to the familar power responses, depending upon the range of stimulus strengths investigated (see Werner and Mountcastle, 1965). It is probable that impulse frequency is linearly related to generator potential amplitude, and that the linear and power functions described represent only portions of a fundamentally hyperbolic phenomenon, the available range of stimulus strengths being insufficient to demonstrate the true nature of the relationship.

Hyperbolic functions of this kind, in chemoreceptors, have been taken to

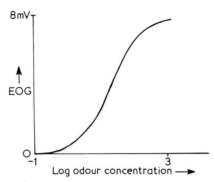

Fig. 8.4   A typical curve relating the stimulus strength and the output of the transducer, in this case the amplitude of the Electro-olfactogram (EOG) of a frog. Note the hyperbolic shape of the curve relating the logarithm of the concentration of odorant with the voltage of the EOG (After Poynder, 1974.)

reflect the kinetics of competition between stimulant molecules for a limited number of receptor sites (Kimura and Beidler, 1961), but in view of their widespread occurrence, they are also likely to represent some fundamental property of receptor membranes in general. Lipetz (1971) has described an electrical analogue possessing similar 'self-shunting' behaviour dependent on current flow through an excitable membrane. Whether such a simple model is applicable to the entire range of transduction phenomena remains to be determined (see Poynder, 1974).

Receptor cytology

Receptors, as well as being sensory structures, carry out the normal functions common to all cells, and many of their structural features have little to do with reception, and merely reflect the local 'domestic' demands of cell metabolism. Characteristic features of the cytoplasm of sensory cells are microtubules and microfilaments, although these cellular components are found in all neurons, and probably in most other cells, where they are believed to be related to cytoplasmic movements, structural support and similar associated functions (see Chapter 1). Their presence in sensory cells has led to some speculation that they may be directly involved in the transduction process (Atema, 1973), but the evidence supporting this view is slender, and it seems far more likely that these components have the same functions in these cells as in those incapable of sensory reception. Other common structural features are the presence of a well developed golgi complex, numerous lysosomes, transport vesicles and smooth endoplasmic reticulum, components which may be associated with a rapid turnover of sensory membranes. Such features have not attracted much attention in the past, but may be important to an understanding of receptor cell biology.

The organelles close to the receptor surface itself are more likely to be implicated in specialized sensory activities. Mitochondria are always numerous, as might be expected from the energy demands of re-setting the polarity of the membrane after stimulation. Small vesicles with lucent or dense cored contents are also common, although the significance of these is not obvious; some authors have suggested they might contain transmitters released during stimulation to excite the cell surface (e.g. Spencer and Schaumberg, 1973). In the olfactory receptor, particulate material is taken into such vesicles from the cell surface (Kristenssen and Olsson, 1972), and they seem to be part of an endocytotic system, perhaps a mechanism for membrane renewal. In many receptor endings, particularly those of mechanoreceptors, fine microfilaments form the matrix of the cytoplasm; in other, non-sensory situations such as in embryonic cells, similar structures appear to be associated with the maintenance of cell shape, and it is probable that they carry out similar functions in sensory receptors.

Relationships between receptors and other cells

The finding, at many sites, of a variety of specialized nonsensory cells around sensory endings appears to point to a form of cooperative interaction between these two types of cell. In some cases, as in the neuromuscular spindle, where muscle cells lie close to the receptor endings, and in the Pacinian corpuscle (see above), the adjacent cells directly influence the form of the receptor response. Metabolic and organizational relationships are also involved in these and in other receptor systems, since degeneration of one of the components usually causes atrophy in the other. The epidermal Merkel cell, for example, when denervated, becomes abnormal in form and remains so until neural regeneration occurs (Brown and Iggo, 1962). The intrafusal muscle fibres of neuromuscular spindles also change in structure when their related dorsal root ganglia are removed (Tower, 1932; Boyd, 1962). Such interactions are also seen in the original embryonic development of sensory endings. The first intrafusal muscle fibres begin to differentiate when the sensory fibres reach them and once this contact has been made, the two elements become trophically dependent upon one another. This particular example is of especial interest since the intrafusal muscles are also trophically dependent upon their fusimotor innervation (Boyd, 1962). Neither the mechanisms of such peripheral interactions nor the relationship between the neuron somata and adjacent non-nervous cells are fully understood, although in the latter case it is known that the two types of cells are to some extent metabolically interdependent. The question as to whether or not a similar relationship exists in the peripheral receptors deserves further investigations.

Developmental and trophic aspects of sensory cells

During embryonic development, each sensory receptor must establish appropriate connections both with peripheral tissues and with the central nervous system, and these must be maintained throughout postnatal life. Often, specialized non-nervous end-organs are also under the trophic influence of sensory nerves associated with them.

The primary somatosensory cells are the neurons, developing from neural crest neuroblasts of the spinal and cranial nerve ganglia, the neurites of which grow out during embryogenesis to their peripheral positions. Their final destination appears in many cases to be determined by the structures which they innervate; taste bud primordia for example begin to differentiate before they are actually innervated (see Jacobson, 1970). Full differentiation and maintenance of end-organ structure is, however, usually dependent upon the nerve supply, so that, for example, muscle spindles de-afferented before birth rapidly atrophy (Zelená, 1957, 1964). In postnatal life, Merkel cells, Pacinian corpuscles, Grandry and Herbst corpuscles, and taste buds all degenerate when their afferent nerves are cut, regaining their normal appearance and functions only when reinnervated (see Dijkstra, 1933; Brown and Iggo, 1962; Quilliam, 1962, Burgess, English, Horsch and Stensaas, 1974). Muscle spindles also atrophy to some extent when de-afferented although the effect is much reduced if operation is delayed until two weeks after birth (Zelená, 1957), and the intrafusal muscle fibres are again of especial interest since they are also innervated by motor nerves which undoubtedly exert trophic influences upon their polar regions (Tower, 1932; Boyd, 1962). Whether a peripheral end organ needs to be innervated by its own specific type of afferent nerve fibre for full differentiation is still a matter for debate. Vibrissal follicles transplanted to the hairless feet in mice are re-innervated by cutaneous nerves which would normally not end on hair follicles (Kadanoff, 1925), but taste buds in mammals regenerate only in the presence of true gustatory nerves (Olmsted, 1920; Zalewski, 1969; Guth, 1971); however, receptor responses are found when the facial nerve is caused to re-innervate the taste buds of the posterior tongue, although this is normally supplied by IXth nerve fibres; the responses appear to retain the characteristics of posterior tongue receptors and are therefore not affected by the foreign innervation (Oakley, 1967). In lower vertebrates trophic relationships are less specific, but seem to follow the same general pattern.

In the somatosensory system the receptors, being primary neurons, do not multiply in postnatal life, and regeneration is restricted to regrowth of the peripheral axon. In taste buds it is remarkable that the actual receptor elements themselves are constantly being lost and replaced throughout life, by the mitotic activity of basally-situated 'blastema' cells within the epithelium (Walker, 1960: Beidler and Smallman, 1965). The same kind of receptor cell turnover has also been demonstrated in the olfactory epithelium of mammals (see Moulton, Çelebi and Fink, 1970; Graziadei, 1973) where the receptor is a primary sensory neuron. When the axons are damaged the olfactory receptors degenerate completely and are replaced by multiplication of basal cells (see Graziadei, 1973) which subsequently re-establish their central connections. The mechanisms responsible for continued cell differentiation and the formation of new central connections pose interesting problems; in biological terms such cell turnover may be of great advantage where the receptors are exposed to the hazards of the external environment, as they are in epithelia, and the total replacement of damaged cells is required rather than limited regrowth.

8.2 Structure and functions of individual sensory endings

8.2.1 *Mechanoreceptors*

Receptors responding primarily to mechanical forces are distributed widely throughout all tissues except those within the brain and spinal cord. They are particularly numerous in the skin, fasciae, and joint capsules, and are also of considerable importance in muscles, tendons, ligaments, meninges and the linings of large blood vessels, and of the alimentary, respiratory and urino-genital tracts.

Mechanoreceptors can be classified in several ways. Structurally, it is usual to distinguish between encapsulated and 'free' terminals, although such a division may obscure important morphological differences. Functionally, speeds of adaptation, physiological relationships with non-neural elements, and other features are used to classify receptors. In the present account, morphological features will be emphasized, and the mechanoreceptors will be grouped as follows:

Mechanoreceptors with complex lamellar capsules:
    Pacinian, paciniform and other encapsulated endings with concentric lamellae; Meissner's corpuscles.
Lanceolate endings of hair follicles.
Mechanoreceptors associated with one or a few specialized cells;
    Merkel's disc endings; Grandry's corpuscles.
Mechanoreceptors within capsules enclosing other tissues
Ruffini terminals of skin and joints;
    Golgi tendon organs
    Neuromuscular spindles
Mechanoreceptor endings with no specialized encapsulating structures.

In addition to these types of receptor, neural responses from structurally unknown receptors have been recorded from a number of situations, and these will be considered separately.

Mechanoreceptors with with complex lamellar capsules

This category is comprised of terminals that are ensheathed by many layers of flattened non-nervous cells (Fig. 8.5). These may be arranged concentrically as in Pacinian endings, or piled up on each other as in Meissner terminals. There are also forms intermediate between these two types, but functionally, all of those that have been investigated have shown rapidly adapting receptor characteristics,

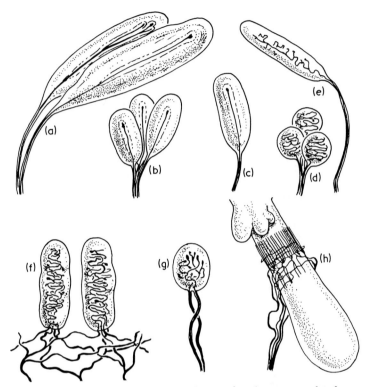

Fig. 8.5 A diagram showing the range of forms of various encapsulated or complex cutaneous sensory endings, including (a) Pacinian, (b) paciniform, (c) Herbst, (d) bulbous (e) Krause, (f) Meissner, (g) Golgi-Mazzoni, (h) palisade (hair) types.

a feature which may be attributed, at least in part, to their lamellar construction.

Pacinian corpuscles (corpuscles of Vater-Pacini), are amongst the largest receptor structures of the general sensory system, and because of their accessibility to recording electrodes have provided valuable data concerning the functions of receptors in general. They are present in subcutaneous tissue of all types of skin, in mesenteries, and in various other connective tissue sites, (Cauna and Mannan, 1958). They are ovoid, cylindrical, or spheroidal structures measuring up to 20 x 0.5 mm, often occurring in small groups (Figs. 8.5, 8.6).

Fig. 8.6(a−c) Micrographs illustrating the structure of the Pacinian corpuscle.
(a) transverse section showing the corpuscle from a Rhesus monkey, surrounded by a densely staining sheath, and containing outer and inner core regions. Resin section stained with toluidine blue.
(b) longitudinal section showing the axon of a corpuscle in a late human fetus, surrounded by inner and outer core elements. (Bielschowsky silver impregnation x 350: Kindly provided by Mr. R. Bilhous.)
(c) An electron micrograph of the axon, and surrounding inner core cells (Rhesus monkey). Note the peripheral, mitochondria rich zone of the axon and the microtubules and microfilaments in its interior. (x 5000.)

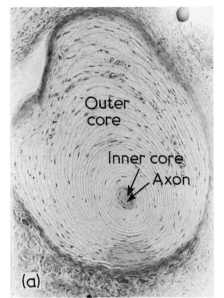

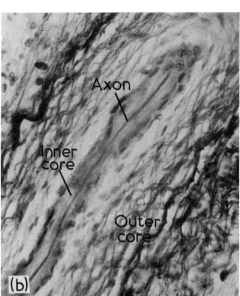

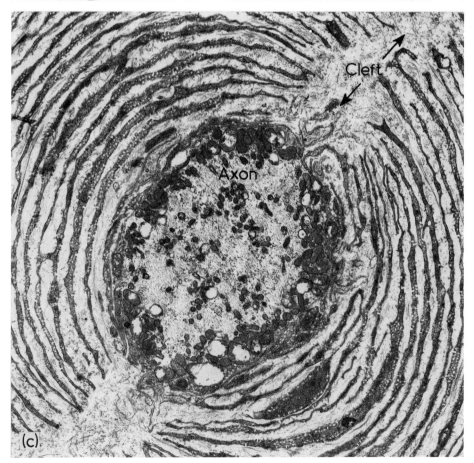

Each is served by a single large unbranched myelinated axon of the group Aα in Gassers classification, which courses for some distance within the capsule before losing its myelinated sheath, often branching at this point into two or more parallel terminals, the ends of which are slightly expanded. The terminal region is surrounded by an inner core of closely packed flattened cells, and this in turn is enclosed in a more loosely constructed outer core of similar elements. The whole capsule is bounded by a connective tissue sheath rich in elastin. One or more vascular loops are enclosed by the capsule (Cauna and Mannan, 1958) and small, non-myelinated nerve fibres may also pass into it.

Several fine structural studies of the Pacinian ending have been published (Pease and Quilliam, 1957; Nishi, Oura and Pallie, 1969; Chouchkov, 1971: Munger, 1971; Spencer and Schaumberg, 1973, and others). It has been shown that within the confines of the corpuscle, the axon is divisible into three regions: a myelinated *preterminal* segment, an unmyelinated, flattened *terminal* segment, and an expanded 'ultraterminal' segment. The preterminal region is often relatively long, extending for several internodes, and is surrounded by the 'outer core' which is continuous outside the capsule with the perineural sheath of the axon. The terminal portion is, in addition, ensheathed by the inner core lamellae in a distinctive manner (Fig. 8.6a–c), the cells forming this structure being arranged in two rows, with intervening radial clefts into which pass finger-like extensions of the axon surface. In the 'ultraterminal' region this bilaterally symmetrical arrangement is replaced by an irregular pattern of core cells. The cells of the inner core are closely spaced and each is surrounded by a basal lamina and fine collagen fibres; their cytoplasm, of variable electron density, contains granular endoplasmic reticulum, and their surfaces are marked by numerous pinocytotic vesicles. The innermost of these cells provide finger-like extensions which abut against the axon surface. The outer core cells, in contrast, are larger and more widely spaced, with prominent intervening layers of collagen fibres and intercellular mucosubstance. The cells contain few organelles, and their flattened nuclei are situated randomly within the outer core (Fig. 8.6).

The terminal portion of the central axon is bilaterally flattened; numerous mitochondria, and clear and dense-cored vesicles are situated immediately beneath the axolemma, and the central axoplasm contains microfilaments and microtubules. The 'ultraterminal' region is similar in structure, except that it is much expanded and irregular in cross section with multiple axonal branches; mitochondria and vesicles are also more numerous and fill the axoplasm.

Fine unmyelinated fibres have also been described as terminating within the inner core, either amongst the lemmal cells, or elsewhere; it has been suggested that such fibres may exert centrifugal control of receptor activity, but it is also possible that they are vasomotor (Santini, 1969; Santini, Ibata and Pappas, 1971), or that they are branches of the main afferent axon (Spencer and Schaumberg, 1973).

Pacinian corpuscles appear relatively early in embryonic development, and alter their shape throughout postnatal life, in old age becoming greatly elongated and often tortuous in form (Cauna and Mannan, 1958).

Paciniform endings.   This term is used to denote encapsulated terminals similar in appearance to Pacinian endings but of much smaller dimensions. Such receptors occur singly or in groups in many connective tissue sites, including the dermis, fascial planes, joint capsules, meninges and periosteum. They have also been found at the bases of vibrissae in some mammals (Andres, 1966). Their fine structure appears also to be similar to that of Pacinian endings, although the capsules contain fewer lamellar units (Andres, 1969; Polaček and Hilata, 1970). The term 'Paciniform ending' has also been used of other lamellar endings in which the axons appear to be multiple or highly branched and coiled (see Fig. 8.5).

Herbst corpuscles are again similar to Pacinian endings; they occur in birds, their classical location being the dermis of the bill in ducks; their ultrastructure appears to be similar, differing only in some details of arrangements of the inner core cells (Nafstad and Andersen, 1970; Munger, 1971).

Other forms of concentrically organized capsular endings.   A wide variety of relatively small lamellar endings has been described by light microscopists, and the fine structure of some of these has also been described. The terminology applied to them is somewhat confused, and it is not at present possible to provide a clear-cut description of either their classification or distribution. Such simple encapsulated endings appear to be common at mucocutaneous junctions, where they take the form of spherical, ellipsoidal or cylindrical structures containing flattened capsular cells arranged loosely around highly coiled, branching nerve terminals. The largest of these are the end bulbs of Krause, present around the mouth (Krause, 1881; Cauna, 1965). The bulbous corpuscles of Dogiel (1903) and other investigators are smaller and less regular in their organization, and the 'genital corpuscles', occurring in the mammalian penis and clitoris (Patrizi and Munger, 1965; Polaček and Malinowsky, 1971) may also be included in this category. The 'innominate corpuscles' of sheep (Quilliam, 1966), and the narrow lamellar endings of murine dermis (Cunningham and Fitzgerald, 1972) also probably belong to this group. Small lamellated endings enclosing two or more afferent fibres have been described in glabrous skin and in connective tissue sites, and are known as the corpuscles of Golgi-Mazzoni: typically their nerve terminals branch profusely and coil within the corpuscle, ending in bulbous expansions (Lambertini, 1961; Chouchkov, 1973).

Apart from the Pacinian, paciniform and Herbst endings, the physiology of these various structures is unknown, and in the absence of contrary data it can only be guessed that they are mechanoreceptors from their resemblance to Pacinian terminals.

Physiological responses of Pacinian and related endings.   When Pacinian corpuscles are mechanically stimulated with a single deformation, a short train of one to three impulses is recordable in the afferent fibre at its onset, and again

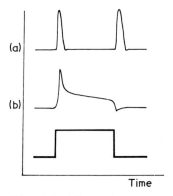

Fig. 8.7   Generator potentials of Pacinian endings: (a) with capsule intact, showing transient 'on' and 'off' peaks; (b) with capsule experimentally removed, indicating the part played by the capsule in accentuating adaptation and in causing the 'off' response. The lower trace represents the stimulus. (After Loewenstein, 1971.)

when the deformation is removed (Figs. 8.3, 8.7). With rapid repetitive stimulation at a frequency of 150–300 Hz the receptor responds with one impulse for each cycle (Fig. 8.8), independently of the amplitude above a constant threshold (Hunt, 1961; Sato, 1961; Lindblom and Lund, 1966; Lynn, 1969). This type of ending is therefore a rapidly adapting receptor, with a rate of adaptation so high that it only responds to very rapid transient accelerations or jerks (Burgess and Perl, 1973) rather than simply to velocity. The suggested reasons for these characteristics have already been discussed (Section 8.2). It is also interesting that whereas intact receptors have no directional sensitivity, decapsulated endings are most sensitive to stimuli applied to the flattened sides of the axon terminal, that is, in a manner most likely to stretch the axolemma (Loewenstein, 1971) and hyperpolarization results from deformation applied to the edges (Nishi and Sato, 1968). The site of stimulus transduction is known to be the unmyelinated portion of the axon, and it is thought that this region is also responsible for impulse initiation (Ozeki and Sato, 1964), although earlier results suggested that this occurred at the first node of Ranvier (Diamond, Gray and Sato, 1956).

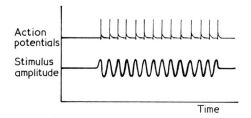

Fig. 8.8   Response of a Pacinian ending to a vibrational stimulus at 300 Hz.

Paciniform endings in joint capsules show similar responses (Skoglund, 1973), and rapidly adapting impulse activity has also been attributed to lamellar endings of vibrissal follicles (Gottschaldt, Iggo and Young, 1973) although the adaptation rates of these are somewhat slower. Herbst corpuscles in birds show a similar range of sensitivities (Skoglund, 1960).

In all of these types of ending, it is likely that the chief biological role is to detect rapidly fluctuating mechanical forces acting on the connective tissues within which they are embedded, and in particular to signal vibrational or 'fluttering' stimuli (see Talbot, Darian-Smith, Kornhuber and Mountcastle, 1968).

Meissner corpuscles. These are prominent corpuscular endings situated in the dermal papillae of glabrous skin (Figs. 8.5, 8.10) and were first described by Meissner in 1853. Von Frey (1906) considered them to be touch endings because of their frequency in such regions as the finger tips and other sites with a high tactile sensitivity.

The corpuscles are found in the plantar, palmar and volar surfaces of glabrous skin, and have also been identified in the hairless skin covering the snouts of some mammals (Cauna, 1966). On the extremities of limbs they are placed in rows in the dermal papillae underlying the friction ridges, achieving a high density in human finger tips. Their precise size and shape varies with age and with the amount of wear and tear to which the skin is subjected (Cauna, 1965). In mature primates including man, they are oval in longitudinal section, being about 200 μm long by 80 μm wide, and are orientated at right angles to the skin surface. In later years they increase in length and become vermiform in appearance. The base of each corpuscle is penetrated by up to nine myelinated fibres, each being the branch of axons which serve other Meissner's corpuscles in the neighbourhood. Once inside the capsule, the myelin sheaths are lost and the terminals spiral and branch amongst the flattened processes of the capsule cells, the nuclei of which lie around the periphery of the whole structure. These cells are apparently discoidal and their intervening intercellular spaces are occupied by ground substance and thin sheets of fibrillar material similar to collagen in its periodic structure. A thin layer of collagenous matrix also surrounds the capsule which is anchored to the surrounding epidermis by connective tissue rich in elastin fibres (Cauna and Ross, 1960; Cauna, 1966).

The unmyelinated terminals contain clusters of mitochondria and clear vesicles of about 50 nm diameter, and partially invaginate the capsule cells, the surfaces of which show many pinocytotic vesicles: the capsule cells themselves contain few organelles, but the enzyme butyrylcholinesterase has been demonstrated in them in abundance using light microscope histochemical methods, and this may imply some specific metabolic activity (Montagna, 1960).

The physiology of Meissner's endings is not known with any certainty, since correlative functional and structural studies remain to be carried out. Their afferent axons appear from histological examination to belong to Group Aα category, and their responses to stimulus should therefore be sought amongst

415

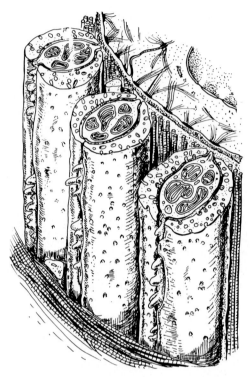

Fig. 8.9   Diagram of the organization of lanceolate terminals of down or guard hairs. Each sensory terminals is partially enshrouded by two sleeves of Schwann cell origin, and associated with the surface of the hair follicle and with numerous collagen fibres. (After electron micrographs of Cauna, 1969.)

fibres with an appropriate conduction velocity. Recordings of the afferent fibres from the glabrous skin of foot pads of cats have shown rapidly adapting responses which are elicited from small cutaneous fields, and cannot be attributed to any other known receptor ending: Meissner's endings have been suggested as their origin (Jänig, Schmidt and Zimmermann, 1968; Jänig, 1971; Lynn, 1969). However, similar responses have been seen in afferents from hairy skin (the Type 1 Field) receptors of Burgess, Petit and Warren, 1968) from which Meissner's corpuscles are apparently absent.

Lanceolate endings in hair follicles

It has long been known that hair follicles are richly innervated (Gegenbauer, 1851; Retzius, 1892), and recent work on their structure and physiology has shown that several distinct varieties of innervation may be associated with hairs of different types (see Section 8.4.1). Some of these sensory endings are similar to those found elsewhere in the skin, but one type, the lanceolate ending, appears to be peculiar to the innervation of hairs (Andres, 1966).

Lanceolate terminals are fine, radially flattened endings of myelinated fibres which pass into the dermal tunic of the hair follicle in multiples and branch into a number of parallel unmyelinated terminals which run up or down the perimeter of the follicle (palisade endings: Weddell and Pallie, 1955; Cauna, 1969) or encircle it spirally (Figs. 8.8, 8.9). These terminals – or more probably their Schwann sheaths – are strongly positive to tests for butyrylcholinesterase activity (Cauna, 1969). The terminal portions of these fibres lie close to the epidermal basal lamina, sandwiched between two sleeves of Schwann cell cytoplasm, fingers of receptor axoplasm protruding through occasional gaps. Fine collagen fibres surround the endings and probably serve to couple them mechanically to the follicle. Within the sensory endings lie numerous mitochondria, vesicles, microfilaments and other components typical of receptor terminals.

Andres (1966) has also described lanceolate endings in vibrissal follicles which differed from those of the palisade terminals of smaller hairs in their arrangement, and in the presence of longer axolemmal fingers; these endings have been associated by Gottschaldt et al. (1973) with a different type of receptor response. The lanceolate endings of the palisade array are present in those hair follicles in which stimulation of the relevant hair shaft by bending elicits a rapidly adapting response from Aa and Ad cutaneous afferents (Adrian, 1931; Iggo, 1966: also see Section 8.4.1). In vibrissal hairs, both a rapidly adapting and a slowly adapting response are recordable, and it is thought that the secondary type of lanceolate ending mentioned above may be responsible for the slow response.

Mechanoreceptors associated with one or a few specialized cells

Merkel disc endings are an important feature of both glabrous and hairy skin. They are expanded plate-like nerve terminals that lie in close proximity to specialized epidermal (Merkel) cells, an association which was first recognized in birds (Merkel, 1875). They are particularly numerous among the rete pegs of the fingers and toes, and other volar and plantar surfaces, as well as in the glabrous skin of the snout in certain mammals, for example the opossum (Munger, 1965) and the mole, where they form part of Eimer's organ (see Quilliam, 1966). In hairy skin they are grouped in small circular patches or, in some species, in elevated 'touch domes' (Iggo, 1963) which may often be found at the bases of large hairs ('tylotrichs': Straile, 1960); Pinkus (1902) named them 'Haarschieben' for this reason. Up to 120 single terminals have been counted in one touch done (Iggo and Muir, 1969), all of them the end branches of an axon which may in turn be a branch of an afferent fibre serving a number of different receptor groups. Similar clusters of Merkel disc endings have also been described in vibrissal follicles (see Section 8.4.1).

Merkel discs are unmyelinated disc-like expansions of Group Aα axons which having lost their myelin and Schwann sheaths, and invaginate the bases of

417

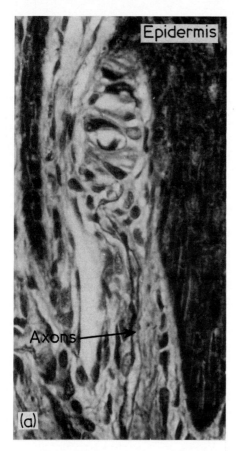

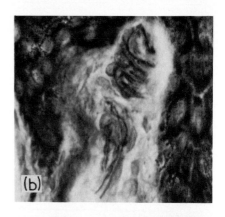

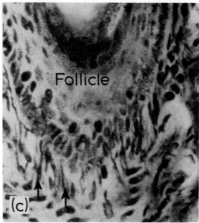

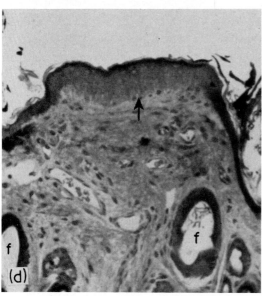

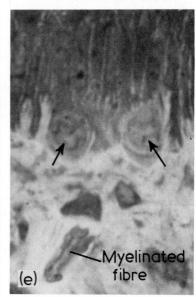

specialized Merkel cells situated at or near the basal layer of the epidermis (Figs. 8.10d—e, 8.11). Each terminal contains mitochondria, clear vesicles, microfilaments and occasional lysosome-like bodies (Iggo and Muir, 1969; Smith, 1969, 1970). The Merkel cell is rounded or elliptical in profile, and contains palely staining cytoplasm and an elongated, irregular nucleus (Figs. 8.10, 8.11). The surface bears stout finger-like extensions which interdigitate with the surrounding keratinocytes and contain numerous microfilaments; desmosomal attachments exist between the neighbouring cell surfaces, and also between the Merkel cell and its nerve terminal. The cytoplasm contains granular endoplasmic reticulum, mitochondria and other organelles, glycogen, and numerous irregular dense-cored vesicles, many of them clustered near the nerve ending. A variety of cytochemical tests have failed to demonstrate the expected presence of catecholamines in Merkel cells (Smith and Creech, 1967), but this negative result does not rule out the presence of some other kind of transmitter.

The curious association between the nerve ending and the Merkel cell appears to imply the existence of some form of trophic relationship, but its functional significance is otherwise obscure. Merkel cells are not of epidermal origin and have been shown to invade the epithelium from the underlying connective tissue during embryonic development (Breathnach and Robins, 1970, Hashimoto, 1972), and they may share with Schwann cell an origin from the neural crest.

Much intensive work by Iggo's research group, and others, has shown the Merkel endings to be slowly adapting mechanoreceptors (Type I S.A. Cutaneous mechanoreceptors) in which both the dynamic and static features are well developed (see Iggo and Muir, 1969; see also Fig. 8.3). The afferent unit is usually more or less silent before stimulation and responds to vertical or shearing deformation of the skin with a dynamic burst tailing away to an irregular static discharge. Both the velocity and the amplitude of displacement are therefore important components of the stimulus. Stimulation of one group of endings causes the threshold of others innervated by the same unit to rise, probably as a consequence of retrograde depolarization: simultaneous stimulation, in contrast, summates in the afferent unit. Directional sensitivity may be related in some instances to the presence of neighbouring hairs which may lie

---

Fig. 8.10(a—e)

(a) A vertical section through a Meissner's corpuscle in a dermal papilla, showing two axons emerging from the encapsulated complex. Rhesus monkey finger, Glees and Marsland technique (x 700).

(b) Section similar to (a) showing another Meissner's ending supplied by four axons. The spiral terminals can be seen clearly.

(c) A hair follicle in a monkey's finger, cut in oblique section to show parallel palisade endings (arrows). Glees and Marsland method (x 450).

(d) A haarschiebe from a rabbit's hind limb showing the typical patch of thickened epidermis overlying a region of highly vascular dermis. Note the hair follicles (f) cut obliquely. The arrow marks the position of the Merkel cells shown in the next micrograph. (Resin section, stained with toluidine blue. x 250.)

(e) Two Merkel cells situated at the base of the epidermis of a haarschiebe. The afferent fibre, approaching from beneath, is visible. (Resin section, stained with toluidine blue, x 1000.)

419

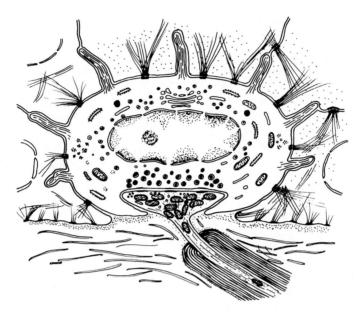

Fig. 8.11   Diagram of the organization of Merkel ending, showing a Merkel cell with dense cored vesicles and an associated sensory terminal (After Iggo and Muir, 1969, and others).

across the touch dome and so deform it when deflected appropriately; Merkel cells around vibrissal follicles are also directionally sensitive (see Section 3.3.1).

Grandry corpuscles are conspicuous end-organs of myelinated nerve fibres, found in the dermis of the beak in birds. Each corpuscle consists of a group of two or more large cylindrical cells in association with the ends of branched axon terminals (see Quilliam, 1966; Gottschaldt and Lausmann, 1974). In their detailed structure, Grandry corpuscles bear a strong resemblance to Merkel endings, the flattened nerve terminals being apposed to the surfaces of the large corpuscular cells which contain numerous dense-cored vesicles (Halata, 1971; Munger, 1971).

It might be expected from their similarity to Merkel endings that Grandry terminals would be slowly adapting mechanoreceptors with Type I character- istics. Gottschaldt and Lausmann (1974) have shown electrophysiologically, however, that in geese they are rapidly adapting terminals responding optimally to tangential deformations of moderate to low velocity, so that the structural resemblance to Merkel endings must be related to some property other than rate of adaptation.

Mechanoreceptors within capsules enclosing other tissues

Receptors included in this class show more than a superficial resemblance to each other in their general response characteristics and their structural

420

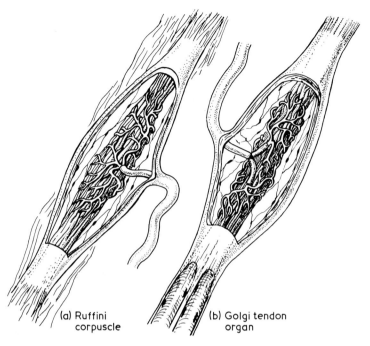

Fig. 8.12 Diagram showing the organization of (a) a Ruffini end organ and (b) a Golgi tendon organ. Note the similar arrangement of terminals around the connective tissue cores, and the outer capsule, diagramatically cut away to show the interior. ((a) After Chambers *et al.*, 1972; (b) after Schoultz and Swett, 1972).

arrangement. All of them are stimulated by the stresses transmitted from adjacent tissues, and all show strongly non-adaptive responses, although more dynamic response features are also often present. *Ruffini terminals* are encapsulated end organs of Group Aα or IIa myelinated afferents, situated in the connective tissue of skin, joint capsules and other structures. They show a characteristic structure (Ruffini, 1894), the terminal branches of the nerve fibres ramifying extensively in and around small bundles of collagen fibres (Fig. 8.12a). Recently, the ultrastructure and physiology of these terminals have been described in detail in the hairy skin of cats by Chambers, Andres, von Duering and Iggo (1972). Each corpuscle is an elongate spindle, 0.5–2.0 mm long by about 0.1 mm wide. The capsule is several layers thick, and is composed of flattened perineural elements continuous with the sheath of the afferent nerve. The axis is formed by an inner core of longitudinal collagen fibres which are continuous at either end of the capsule with collagen fibre bundles in the surrounding tissues, and the space around this axis is filled with delicate fibroblastic elements and ground substance. The nerve fibre (Group Aα) penetrates the capsule at its equator or at one pole and continues to the central core where it breaks up into numerous fine unmyelinated branches which

421

surround, and penetrate between, the delicate collagen bundles of this region (Fig. 8.12a). Schwann cells cover these terminal branches except at their ends where they may come into direct contact with the adjacent collagen fibres. Within these terminals are found microtubules, microfilaments, mitochondria and clear vesicles. They finally end in narrow processes about 0.1 μm wide, packed with microfilaments.

Their responses are typically slowly adapting and highly regular in frequency, with a minimal dynamic component. In the absence of overt stimuli they show a steady low level of resting activity which may be related to the state of tension of the surrounding tissues; they are thus ideally suited to be position or stress detectors, and they are important elements in cutaneous and joint sensation for these reasons. In the skin they have been classed as Type II S.A. cutaneous mechanoreceptors by Chambers *et al.* (1972), and there seems little doubt that they are identical to the joint receptors in structure and responses.

Golgi tendon organs (Fig. 8.12b) are present in the terminal portions of tendons close to their myo-tendinal junctions, and in ligaments of joint capsules; they are innervated by large myelinated muscle afferent nerves (Class Ib) which ramify finely within encapsulated tendon fasciculi, insinuating their terminal branches between and around their component collagen bundles (Golgi, 1880a,b; Wohlfart and Henriksson, 1960). The capsule is composed of several layers of flattened cells similar to, and continuous with, the perineurium of the afferent fibre, and contains, besides the tendon fibres, fluid filled spaces amongst which lie fibroblasts and delicate connective tissue elements. They are similar to Ruffini endings in their fine structure, the myelinated fibre giving off numerous unmyelinated end branches which lie close to or in contact with the collagen fibres, often with no intervening Schwann sheath. Their organelle content is also very similar (Merilees, 1962; Schoultze and Swett, 1972, 1974). Capillaries are usually present within the capsule.

It has been suggested (Bridgeman, 1968) that when tension is applied to the rather loosely arranged fasciculi of collagen in the tendon organ, they tighten upon the nerve endings which penetrate between them deforming their receptor surfaces and so stimulating them. Ultrastructural evidence supports this view (Schoultze and Swett, 1972). Since collagen does not stretch appreciably, it appears that tendon receptors respond to tension rather than to stretch. Their sensory responses are typical of slowly adapting mechanoreceptors, as B. H. C. Matthews first demonstrated in 1933. A predominant reflex effect induced by the stimulation of tendon receptors is the inhibition of motor activity in the attendant muscle, and since the early experimentors could only fire the tendon receptors with externally applied loads of 200 g or more, it was thought that their main function was to prevent the development of excessive contraction in associated muscles. It was later shown that when such endings are stimulated by active muscle contraction their sensitivity is much increased and that they will even respond to the contraction of single muscle fibres (Alnaes, 1967; Jansen and Rudjford, 1967; Houk and Henneman, 1967; see also P. B. C. Matthews,

1973). Such experiments as these have shown the Golgi tendon organs to be highly sensitive tension receptors, responding to a steady stimulus with a very regular, very slowly adapting discharge in which the dynamic component although visible, is inconspicuous. Tendon organs are obviously important components of the proprioceptor system, working cooperatively with other endings in muscles and joints to signal the forces acting in these structures during motor activity.

Neuromuscular spindles. The presence within muscles of specialized small muscle fibres, grouped within connective tissue capsules and innervated by complicated axon terminals, has been known for many years (Weismann, 1861; Ruffini, 1898). It was conclusively demonstrated by Sherrington (1894, 1898) that these structures were stretch receptors and were involved in the reflex control of muscle tension and length. They are present in varying numbers in the muscles of all mammals, with the exception of a few specialized eye muscles of some species, and although some variation in structure occurs, they have a broadly similar construction in all mammals (see the excellent and comprehensive review by Matthews, 1973).

The muscle fibres of the neuromuscular spindle (intrafusal muscles) are from 2 to 12 in number, and possess the normal contractile apparatus of striated muscle fibres except in their equatorial region where the myofibrils are confined to a thin sub-sarcolemmal layer and the middle of the fibre is occupied by muscle cell nuclei (Fig. 8.13). In most species, two types of fibre are distinguishable by the arrangement of these nuclei: *nuclear bag fibres* in which the equatorial nuclei form several rows, and *nuclear chain fibres*, with a single

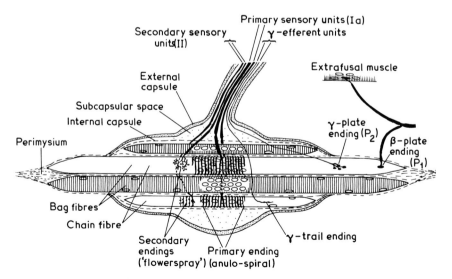

Fig. 8.13 A simple diagram showing some of the features of a mammalian muscle spindle and its innervation. For details, see text.

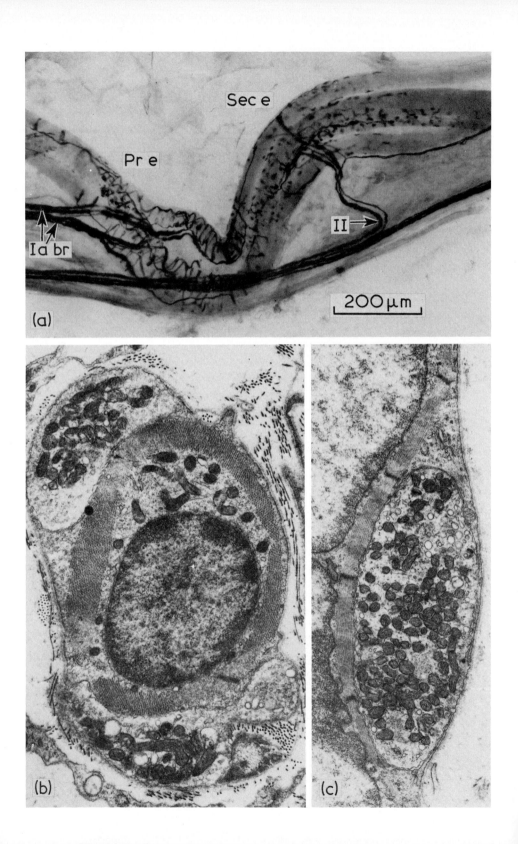

(a)

Sec e

Pr e

Ia br

II→

200 μm

(b)

(c)

file of equatorial nuclei (Boyd, 1962). In both fibres, myonuclei elsewhere are found in the more usual subsarcolemmal position. Other differences also exist between bag and chain fibres, the former being wider, and several times longer than the latter. The sarcomere ultrastructure is also different; in bag fibres the myofibrils are more uniform in diameter than in the chain fibres, the sarcomeres are longer, M lines are absent, mitochondria are fewer than in chain fibres, and more myoglobin is present (Landon, 1966; Adal, 1969; Corvaja, Marinozzi and Pompeiano, 1969). The significance of these differences is not entirely clear, but various lines of evidence indicate that bag and chain fibres contract at different rates when stimulated by their fusimotor axons (see below), and no doubt such different rates of activity are related to the observed structural dissimilarities.

The sensory innervation of the spindle (Figs. 8.13 and 8.14) is twofold and complex. Unmyelinated endings of a large myelinated (group Ia) fibre bifurcate to form two spirals around the equatorial zone of each intrafusal muscle fibre: these form the *primary* or *annulo-spiral* endings (the spirals often fusing to form loops). Secondly, unmyelinated terminals of somewhat smaller fibres (group IIa) branch to supply a zone on either side of the equatorial region; this is the *secondary* ending, which is more common on chain fibres, where it is often spiralized, than on bag fibres where the endings when present are finely branched (the flower-spray endings of Ruffini, 1898). Sometimes several such endings are seen on a single fibre. Ultrastructurally these terminals resemble each other; both invaginate the sarcolemma to some extent, lie within its basal lamina boundary, and are elliptical in section. In some species specialized attachment zones are found between the muscle and nerve cell membranes. Within the cytoplasm of the nerve endings, mitochondria and small, rounded vesicles are prominent features, and the terminal expansions are filled with a finely filamentous material. Microtubules are also usually present.

The muscle spindles are also innervated by motor fibres. Fine, thinly myelinated axons terminate on the polar regions of the intrafusal muscles. It has been claimed on structural grounds that the 'bag' and 'chain' fibres receive fibres of different diameter (gamma 1 and gamma 2) and that these terminate in a

---

Fig. 8.14(a–c) Sensory endings of neuromuscular spindles.
(a) Teased preparation of a neuromuscular spindle from the peroneus longus muscle of a cat, stained with silver to show anulo-spiral primary ending (left: Pr e.) of a branch of a type Ia afferent fibre (Ia br.), and secondary endings (right: Sec e) of a type II afferent (2). Note that the secondary endings are of the flower-spray type and are unusual in being distributed to both bag and chain fibres (see p. 425). (x 125: Reproduced from D. Barker, 1974, in *'Muscle Receptors': Handbook of Sensory Physiology*, Vol. 3, Pt. 2 (ed, C. C. Hunt), p. 41, by kind permission of Springer-Verlag, Berlin.)
(b) Electron micrograph of a transverse section through the para-equatorial region of a nuclear chain fibre (rat) showing profiles of a secondary ending on each side of myofilaments surrounding a central myonucleus. Note the large number of mitochondria in the expanded segments of the terminal. (x 12 000.)
(c) Part of the equatorial region of a nuclear bag fibre (rat) in longitudinal section, showing part of a primary ending deeply invaginated within the sarcolemma, and to the left, a few sarcomeres abutting the myonuclei. (x 12 000: b and c provided by Dr. D. N. Landon.)

different manner, gamma 1 fibres ending in 'en grappe' terminals on nuclear bag fibres and gamma 2 axons in more extensive 'trail' endings on nuclear chain fibres. This distinction has been disputed by others (see Matthews, 1973), but in spite of the observed structural ambiguities, the available physiological evidence favours separate motor control of the 'chain' and 'bag' fibres. A third type of motor ending is provided by collaterals of small extrafusal motor fibres (group IIb) which enter the polar regions of the spindle to terminate as small motor end plates on the extracapsular extremities of the bag fibres.

The capsule surrounding the neuromuscular complex is a multi-layered structure, the outer regions being derived from the perineurium of the main nerve of supply, the inner regions resembling endoneurium in construction. In the equatorial region a large fluid filled space separates the outer and inner parts of the capsule (the 'lymph space' of Sherrington) and gives the capsule its spindle-like shape. This space is filled with mucosubstance which possibly serves to protect the sensory endings from responding to mechanical forces other than those acting along the length of the intrafusal fibre. Some elastin fibres are present around the intrafusal fibres and capillaries and autonomic nerve fibres have also been described within the capsule. The outer sheath extends only to the limits of the nuclear chain fibres and beyond this point the bag fibres enter the general tissue space of the muscle sheath.

Responses of neuromuscular spindle endings. During the early years of muscle spindle investigations, it was undecided whether these structures were of pathologicial, embryological or neurological importance. The final proof came with the demonstration by Sherrington (1909) of their role in postural reflexes and since that time much has been done to clarify the mechanisms by which the sensory endings detect and signal changes in the length and tension of skeletal muscles. To the pioneering work of B. H. C. Matthews (e.g. 1933) and later P. B. C. Matthews, we owe much of our understanding of their function. In recent years this subject has attracted many physiologists and the recent contributions have been numerous (see the reviews by Barker, Stacey and Adal, 1970; Granit, 1970; P. B. C. Matthews, 1971, 1973).

Experiments have shown that although both the primary and secondary endings are tension receptors, they provide the central nervous system with different types of sensory information (Fig. 8.15). The dynamic component of the signal predominates in the primary endings, although a static component is also present, so that the response to change of length contains information relating to both the velocity of the stretch and its amplitude. As the velocity component adapts very rapidly, acceleration rather than linear speed of stretch appears to be the most important parameter of the stimulus. The secondary ending gives only a small dynamic response, the static component being dominant, so that it functions primarily as a detector of stretch amplitude, giving a regular, virtually non-adapting, discharge pattern very similar to that originating from a Golgi tendon organ or a Ruffini (Type II S.A.) ending. The reasons for the observed differences in the response of the primary and secondary

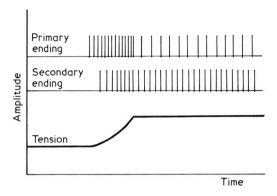

Fig. 8.15 Typical response patterns of (a) the primary and (b) the secondary terminals of a mammalian muscle spindle to a single ramped stretch (bottom trace). Note that the primary ending adapts more rapidly than the secondary. (After Matthews, 1973.)

endings to identical stimuli have been sought in the structural organisation of the intrafusal muscles (see P. B. C. Matthews, 1973). When these fibres are stretched it seems likely that the more viscous regions of the muscle, that is, those portions in which myofibrils occupy the majority of the cross sectional area will stretch more slowly than the more elastic equatorial region containing the central nuclei. A stretch will initially result in lengthening the equatorial region and hence stimulate the primary endings. After a short time the sarcomeres will stretch, and relax the tension on the primary endings. It is to be expected that the bag fibres would be predominantly dynamic elements because of their larger and presumably less viscous equatorial region, and because their secondary endings are less frequent anyway, whereas the chain fibres would be related to static responses for the opposite reasons. Differences in the myofibril structure between these two types of intrafusal fibre may be related to differences in contractile activity which may in turn accentuate their dynamic and static characteristics. Ottoson and Shepherd (1968) failed to find any tendency for the equatorial regions to stretch earlier or faster than the polar regions in isolated frog spindle fibres, but in mammals this question has yet to be adequately explored.

The efferent nerves also play a vital role in spindle function. When the spindle afferents discharge under tension they induce motor activity in the extrafusal efferents by way of a monosynaptic reflex arc. This in turn causes the extrafusal muscle fibres in parallel with the spindle to contract to an extent sufficient to reduce the tension on the intrafusal fibres, and thus reduce afferent activity. This process hence results in the maintenance of a constant muscle tone, oscillating somewhat around a mean value. Extrafusal muscle contraction is followed by intrafusal contraction by which the spindle length is adjusted to the new muscle length, thus resetting the base-line activity of the sensory endings. It has been suggested that this control mechanism may also be used to drive

427

extrafusal contraction, since active shortening of the contractile ends of the intrafusal fibres would excite the sensory endings in the same manner as if the spindle as a whole had been passively stretched, and thus initiate reflex motor activity in the extrafusal efferents (Merton, 1953). Much evidence has been adduced in support of this concept of a 'servo' type of control of muscle contraction (see Granit, 1970), but more recent evidence obtained from human volunteers suggests that the 'servo-loop' may be used chiefly as an aid to monitoring the progress of extrafusal muscle contraction rather than driving it; that is, volitional movements may involve 'servo-assisted' control rather than a simple, direct 'servo' system (see Matthews, 1973). The independent motor innervation of 'bag' and 'chain' intrafusal muscle fibres may also be of significance in potentiating the dynamic and static discharges of their respective sensory endings. The 'chain' fibres appear to be capable of rapid twitch contractions, whereas the 'bag' fibres undergo more sustained localized propagated contractions (Smith, 1966), and such differences may serve to increase the respective sensitivity of the 'static' and 'dynamic' sensory endings on the two types of fibres.

The mechanoreceptor activities of the different types of spindle afferents are related to various forms of locomotor response. Firstly at the segmental level, they are associated with reflex contractions of relevant muscles, the primary endings driving contraction in their surrounding extrafusal muscle fibres by way of the monosynaptic reflex, while simultaneously inhibiting contraction in the antagonistic muscles, through polysynaptic pathways. The secondary endings have classically been considered to have an inhibitory effect on antagonistic muscles, but recently obtained evidence indicates that they may in fact be excitatory to their own extrafusal muscles. The various structures affected by the actions of a single afferent ending have been termed a 'myotatic unit', but it is now known that this is not as clearly delimited an entity as was once imagined, and it is also clear that the precise roles of these two types of endings with respect to reflex motor activity are not yet fully understood.

In addition to these fairly local spinal actions, spindle afferents send information to the brain by a variety of routes. The large Ia axons of the primary afferents pass via the dorsal funiculi to synapse in the dorsal column nuclei, whence successive relay neurons pass to the ventrobasal thalamus, and radiate from thence to the somato-sensory cortex including area 3a; secondary endings send impulses via a similar route to related areas of cortex. In spite of this cortical representation, spindles apparently do not provide conscious sensation of muscle or limb movement (kinaesthesia), this being the province of joint receptors and Group III afferents from muscle sheaths.

As might be expected, afferent impulses are conducted by both direct and polysynaptic pathways to the cerebellum via the spinocerebellar, cuneocerebellar, spino-olivary and other tracts, and to the reticular formation and other parts of the cord and brain stem. These centres in turn control the activity of neurons innervating both the extrafusal and intrafusal (gamma efferent) motor endings in a complex manner, providing the possibility of precise control of both spindle sensitivity and extrafusal muscle contraction.

The development of muscle spindles has been described in some detail by several authors (e.g. Tello, 1917; Zelená, 1957), and at the fine structural level by Landon (1972) and by Milburn (1973). In the rat the intrafusal muscle fibres form in the same manner as the extrafusal fibres by the progressive fusion of myoblasts to form a myotube, the nuclear bag fibres being formed first; sensory nerve endings begin to associate with the equatorial region at this stage, and their branches enwrap nuclear chain muscle fibres as these begin to differentiate in close cellular approximation to the nuclear bags. The capsule is formed as an extension of the perineurium. After birth, efferent nerves make contact with the ends of the muscle fibres, the final cytological differentiation and growth of which are to some extent controlled by this motor innervation.

Mechanoreceptors with no specialized encapsulating structures ('free' endings)

Fine terminal branches of small myelinated or unmyelinated fibres are present in many tissues of the body. Mechanoreceptor responses, conducted at low speeds (less than 15 m/sec) are recordable from nerves to such regions, and since encapsulated receptors always possess large diameter, fast conducting axons it seems reasonable to associate the slower activity with the free endings.

Cutaneous endings. Terminal plexuses of afferent fibres with unencapsulated end branches are present near the base of the epidermis (the subpapillary or superficial corial plexus), and around hair follicles and nail beds (see Sinclair, 1967). Free sensory endings also occur in other situations such as the cornea, where no other class of terminals is present (Whitear, 1960). At present it is not possible to determine which of the various types of fibre that can be distinguished on the basis of their fine structure (see 8.4.1) are mechanoreceptors, but we know from electrophysiological records that such fibres must exist. One of the most important categories of such afferents are the slowly responding low threshold C fibres which make up as much as 50% of all unmyelinated fibres in proximal afferent nerves (Bessou, Bergess, Perl and Taylor, 1971). Such fibres give an initial dynamic response, adapting to a low level static discharge which may persist for some time after the stimulus has been removed. These fibres are only stimulated by low velocity deflections of the skin and the stimulus must be maintained for some hundreds of milliseconds before a response can be elicited; such endings fatigue rapidly, and after prolonged stimulation may take a minute or more to recover their initial sensitivity. Another interesting feature of these endings is their positive response to cooling, implying that they could constitute an important array of polymodal receptors. However, their sensitivity to temperature is too low to account for observed levels of thermal discrimination and this aspect of their response may not be of functional importance. Similar slow conducting mechanoreceptive afferents have been explored in skeletal muscle (see P. B. C. Matthews, 1973), and in the viscera and blood vessels.

Alimentary receptors are important in the reflex regulation of digestive processes, but are known almost entirely from physiological studies (see the extensive reviews of this subject by Leek, 1972; Paintal, 1972, 1973). Although a large proportion of the fibres in the vagus nerve are afferent in nature, their fine terminals are relatively sparsely distributed in the alimentary walls, and are impossible to distinguish from efferent terminals by normal light microscopy.

Both rapidly and slowly adapting alimentary receptors have been found by physiological means. Rapidly adapting endings are present in the muscularis mucosa where they probably act as flow detectors, and similar terminals in the serosa respond to both active and passive gut movements. The activities of Pacinian corpuscles, situated in the mesentery, may also possibly be related to gut movement.

Slowly adapting tension receptors, placed in series with smooth muscle fasciculi of the muscularis externa of the alimentary tract are active during distension and contraction. These receptors appear to initiate both local gut reflexes via the parietal plexuses, and vagal efferent reflexes. Slowly adapting receptor terminals that respond to both mechanical and low pH stimulation of the gastric and duodenal mucosae are thought to be present in the epithelial lining of these regions. Such vagal afferent fibres from the alimentary tract are mostly small (A) myelinated and unmyelinated fibres.

Urinary mechanoreceptors. Rapidly adapting units excited by the flow of urine and changes in mural tension have been described in the bladder and urethra (Todd, 1964; Iggo, 1955: see Paintal, 1972) as have slowly adapting, 'in series', tension receptors within the muscular coat of the bladder. These endings, having similar response characteristics to their equivalents in the alimentary tract, are involved in the reflex control of micturition.

Receptors of the respiratory tract. As with the alimentary tract, the receptors of this system have been studied chiefly from a physiological view-point (Fillenz and Widdicombe, 1972; Paintal, 1973). Reflex control of ventilation, protection of the respiratory tract against obstruction, congestion and abrasion are among the important functions of such receptor endings.

Three types of receptor have been distinguished physiologically. *'Irritant' terminals*, situated in or close to the epithelial lining of both upper and lower respiratory tracts, are rapidly adapting units responding to both mechanical and chemical stimulation of the epithelial surface, and to distension or collapse of the respiratory passages. In the upper part of the tract, stimulation initiates an inspiratory reflex, whereas in the trachea and larynx, a cough reflex is elicited. Deeper in the tract, stimulation causes an increase in amplitude and frequency of ventilation movements. These endings may correspond to unmyelinated terminals of myelinated fibres, which have been found in close association with the bronchial epithelial cells; it is possible that the receptor endings proper may include specialized epithelial elements (Fillenz and Woods, 1970).

Stretch receptors, playing a major role in the Hering-Breuer reflex, are situated in the smooth muscle surrounding the pulmonary passages. They are slowly adapting endings which are stimulated when the walls are distended by increased pulmonary pressure, but their structural homologues have not been identified with any confidence.

Juxtapulmonary capillary ('J') receptors (Paintal, 1973) are found in the alveolar walls. They respond to a wide variety of mechanical stimuli, particularly pulmonary congestion. Fine unmyelinated terminals have been described close to capillaries, electron microscopically (Fillenz and Widdicombe, 1972), and these may correspond to 'J' receptor terminals. Their conduction velocities indicate the afferent fibres to be of the C and A types.

Vascular baroreceptors. Stretch receptors signalling changes in blood pressure are present in the walls of the atria and ventricles of the heart and in the great arteries near their origins (see the reviews by Paintal, 1972, 1973). Around the bases of the common carotid arteries special zones of nerve endings are associated with the carotid sinuses, lying chiefly within the adventitia (de Castro, 1928). In the carotid sinus, these endings consist of unmyelinated terminals of myelinated (Aδ) and unmyelinated fibres (Fidone and Sato, 1969), but in aortic and brachiocephalic arterial walls their afferent fibres are all myelinated. These endings are surrounded by Schwann cell processes and ramify amongst the collagen fibres of the adventitia (Rees, 1967), and contain densely clustered mitochondria and small clear vesicles. Their parent afferent fibres enter the vagus and glossopharyngeal nerves.

All of these mechanoreceptors are of the slowly adapting type, responding experimentally to an artificial square pressure pulse with an initial dynamic burst of activity which is rapidly succeeded by a steady, slowly adapting series of impulses. In the natural state, the behaviour of most of these pressure receptors closely parallels that of the pressure pulse, showing a transient rise in activity for a brief period shortly after the beginning of the systolic wave. In the heart, physiological experiments have demonstrated the existence of atrial receptors on the posterior (dorsal) atrial wall and of ventricular receptors along the interventricular septum. Within the atrial group of receptors, two subclasses (A and B) have been claimed, on the basis of slight differences in timing of their activity with respect to the atrial systoles. Because of the nature of their responses the baroreceptor endings in the heart or great vessels measure both rate of change in pressure and absolute pressure. The endings are, strictly speaking, stretch endings, since pressure rise without change in dimensions does not usually activate them. It has however been claimed that some endings in the arterial walls are excited by the presence of noradrenalin, which suggests that they may be arranged in series with the muscular elements of the tunica intima (Landgren, 1952).

8.2.2 *Thermoreceptors*

It was discovered by Blix (1882) that in man cutaneous thermal sensation is restricted to localized 'warm' and 'cold' spots scattered over the skin surface. Electrophysiological recordings in animals have since revealed the existence of individual afferent units that are uniquely sensitive to warming or to cooling stimuli (see the reviews by Hensel, 1973a,b) and it is thus possible to distinguish these from the polymodal nociceptors and low threshold mechanoreceptors which may also be sensitive to temperature changes, since the thermal sensitivity of such endings does not approach that of true thermoreceptors.

Typically, both warm and cold receptors show a static discharge pattern which is related to the resting level of skin temperature. In warm fibres in cats, the discharge frequency is greatest at about 45°C, diminishing rapidly on either side of this optimum. In cold fibres the static frequency maximum is set much lower – at about 28°C (see Fig. 8.16a). When warm receptors are gently heated, they respond with dynamic activity which adapts to a new static pattern (Fig. 8.16b), and when the stimulus is removed, or the fibre is cooled, there is a short period in which the activity is totally inhibited. Cold receptors operate in the opposite manner, increasing their activity when cooled, and decreasing when warmed, both effects showing rapidly adapting and static components (Fig. 8.16c). Impulse activity typically takes the form of irregular bursts of a few impulses. Cold receptors are also activated strongly at temperatures above 45°C, (Dodt and Zotterman, 1952b) an anomaly which is probably related to the subjective experience of 'paradoxical cold' at high skin temperatures.

Iggo (1959) has also described thermoreceptor units which are activated only at high temperatures (over 48°C) but these appear to be relatively uncommon.

Temperature spots are present over the whole skin surface, but in animals with thick hairy coats, they are particularly numerous around the nose, on the tongue, and, at least in some species, on the surfaces of the genitalia. Their receptive fields usually take the form of single punctate areas. Thermoreceptors are endings of small nerve fibres – myelinated Aδ and unmyelinated C fibres, the ratios of these two classes varying between species, and topographically within individuals. Warm receptors appear to be exclusively the terminals of slowly conducting C fibres; cold receptors in monkey are predominantly endings of Aδ fibres, although a small proportion are C fibre endings, whereas in cat the majority are C fibres and only the lingual receptors are supplied by Aδ fibres (Iggo, 1969; Hensel and Iggo, 1971; Darian-Smith, Johnson and Dykes, 1973).

Far more cold receptors than warm receptors have been reported in the literature on this subject, indicating either that in fact there are more cold than warm endings in mammals, or that the fibres from warm endings, being unmyelinated, are more difficult to find. It has been suggested that the negative response of 'cold' receptors to heating might in itself provide sufficient information to the central nervous system about temperature increase, but Darian-Smith *et al.* (1973) have shown that the negative response is non-

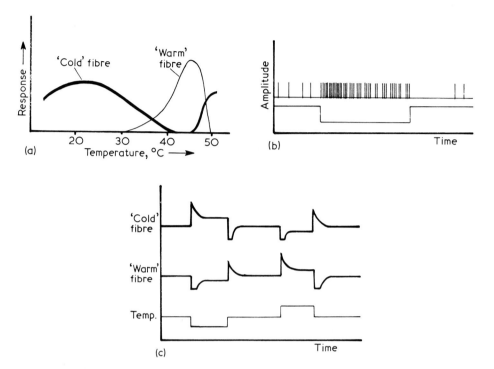

Fig. 8.16(a–c) *Characteristics of thermoreceptor responses*
(a) Static response amplitudes of 'cold' and 'warm' fibres at various temperatures, including the 'paradoxical cold' response at high temperatures. (After Hensel, 1973a.)
(b) Discharge pattern of a 'cold' afferent unit; note that the spikes occur in bursts in the slowly adapting part of the response.
(c) Diagram of the different responses of cold and warm endings to heating and cooling. (After Hensel, 1973a.)

discriminatory in temperature jumps above $3°C$ and so is unlikely to be of much value in this respect. It is also possible that since many other types of sensory ending alter their rates of activity when the temperature changes, these may also contribute thermal information. The most sensitive of such endings to thermal change are the low threshold mechanoreceptor terminals of C fibres; but their sensitivity appears to be too low to account for the observed temperature sense (Mountcastle, Lamotte and Carli, 1972).

While the physiology of thermoreceptors has been extensively explored, we know little about their structure, but since their parent nerve fibres are so fine it is unlikely that any of them are encapsulated. Hensel (1973a,b) has reported that cold spots contain fine branched unmyelinated terminals of Aδ fibres, and that on the hairy surface of the nose in cats these penetrate the basal lamina of the epidermis, invaginating the bases of the germinative layer of cells. The small terminal expansions of these endings contain mitochondria, microfilaments and microtubules. Electrophysiological evidence supports this suggestion that cold

433

detectors are superficially placed in the skin, but warm receptors may be more deeply situated (Bazzett and McGlone, 1930).

It is interesting that thermoreceptors may also be affected by certain chemicals – extracts from spices for example lower the thresholds of warm fibres and raise those of cold receptors, whereas menthol has the reverse effect, causing a sensation of cooling.

8.2.3 *Chemoreceptors*

Sensory endings which are sensitive to low concentrations of specific chemicals are present in the olfactory and gustatory epithelia of vertebrates. In addition to these, terminals in the walls of large arteries respond to changes in concentration of gases and other substances dissolved in the blood and, although their mode of action may be rather different, they are included under this heading. Other sensory endings which act as chemoreceptors may be present in the alimentary epithelium and in other situations, but their anatomy is at present unknown.

Olfactory receptors

These are present in the epithelium lining the postero-dorsal aspects of the nasal chamber, extending to the dorsal half of the nasal septum and the medial surfaces of the ethmo-turbinal bones (Allison, 1953; Moulton and Beidler, 1967). In many mammals and submammalian tetrapods, but not in man, a ventral diverticulum of this epithelium forms a distinct accessory olfactory area, the vomeronasal organ of Jacobson.

The main olfactory area is lined by the sensory epithelium containing the bipolar olfactory receptor cells (Figs. 8.17, 8.18a).. These are specialized sensory neurons in which the cell soma is placed peripherally rather than adjacent to the central nervous system. In addition to the sensory cells the epithelium contains non-sensory cells, differentiated and undifferentiated types of basal cells, and the duct and secretory cells of the glands of Bowman which are situated beneath the sensory epithelium. Lymphocytes, mast cells and macrophages are among the other temporary residents in this area. The epithelium varies in thickness, having a maximum of about ten layers of nuclei, the most apical row consisting of the pale oval nuclei of the supporting cells; nuclei of the other types of cells occupy the mid-epithelial and basal layers (Fig. 8.17). In young animals the pale, undifferentiated basal cells, 'blastema cells' (Andres, 1965) form a conspicuous layer at the base of the epithelium while the more densely-staining receptor cells are closely packed together in a wide band in the middle zone. In later life the 'blastema' cells are less numerous.

The sensory cells are flask-shaped, and have a single unbranched dendrite emerging from the apex of the soma, extending to the epithelial surface where it forms a slight expansion, the olfactory knob (Fig. 18a) upon which are situated clusters of olfactory cilia (Graziadei, 1972). From the base of the cell soma, a

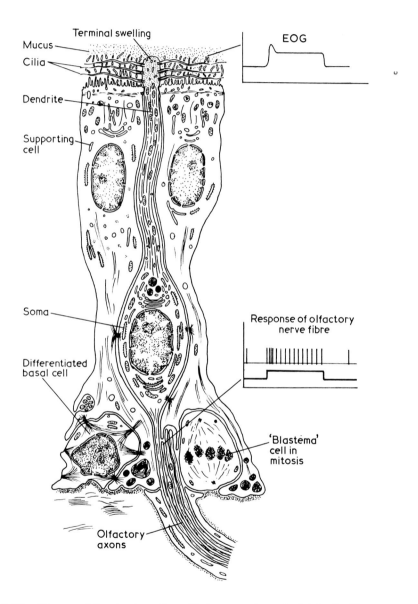

Fig. 8.17 Diagram of the structure of an olfactory receptor and related cells. The typical electrical responses of the surface regions (the EOG) and the deeper spike activity are shown on the right.

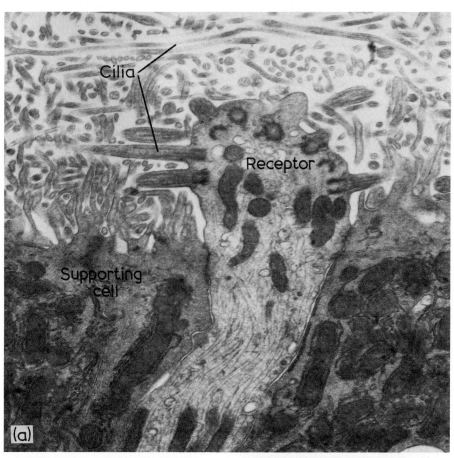

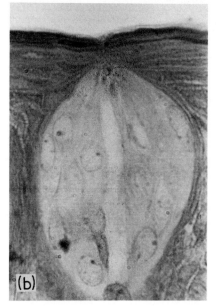

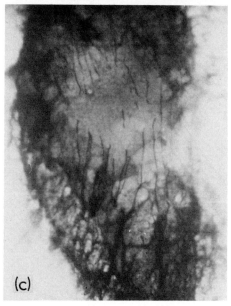

narrow (0.2 μm) axon emerges, and passes out of the epithelium base in company with other similar axons to form the fasciculi of the olfactory nerve. These fibres pass to the olfactory bulb where they synapse with the large mitral cells in olfactory glomeruli, many primary axons converging on a single secondary neuron.

The nuclei of the receptor cells are somewhat heterochromatic and crenated, and ultrastructurally the cytoplasm of the cell bodies contains much granular endoplasmic reticulum, numerous mitochondria and lysosomes, and an extensive golgi complex. The dendrites, about 2 μm in diameter, are filled with microtubules and abundant mitochondria, membranous cisternae and transport vesicles. The olfactory knob contains microfilaments, and pinocytotic and other vesicles; the bases of the cilia have a characteristic shape, their short (2 μm) proximal segments containing the '9 plus 2' configuration of microtubules being continuous with long narrow trailing distal segments supported by only a few microtubules. In lower vertebrates the cilia vary in their structural details, some species such as the lungfish *Neoceratodus* lacking olfactory cilia altogether, microvilli taking their place (Theissen, 1972). In birds both cilia and microvilli are present (Graziadei and Bannister, 1967), and in mammals the endings of the receptors in the vomeronasal organ possess microvilli rather than cilia (Kolnberger, 1971). These details indicate that cilia as such are not essential to chemoreceptor transduction, but represent one mechanism for the provision of a suitably expanded area of membrane surface.

Immediately basal to the olfactory knob the dendrite forms junctional complexes with adjacent supporting cells. Experiments with colloidal tracers have demonstrated unusual tight junctions with limited permeability and an interesting pattern of incomplete ridges demonstrable by freeze-fracture methods (Altner and Altner, 1974). A layer of mucus, secreted by the glands of Bowman, overlies the surface of the epithelium. The olfactory axons contain a few microtubules and occasional mitochondria. In the olfactory nerve they are grouped together in bundles of up to 20 or more within common Schwann cell sheaths.

The supporting cells are of interest in that they contain high concentrations of mitochondria and smooth endoplasmic reticulum, and are able to phago-cytose small extracellular particles. The undigested remnants of such engulfed material may contribute towards the formation of dense lipofuschin-like pigment bodies that accumulate at the bases of supporting cells with age, and are

Fig. 8.18 (a) An electron micrograph of an olfactory receptor ending of a mouse, in vertical section, showing the sensory cilia and microvilli of adjacent supporting cells. (x 30 000.)
(b) Light micrograph of taste bud of a pig, in vertical section showing the gustatory aperture and various types of cell within the sensory area. (Resin-embedded section, toluidine blue. (x 1200.)
(c) Vertical tangential section through part of a vibrissal follicle from mouse, showing parallel nerve endings. (Zinn and Morin method. x 80.)

responsible for the characteristic yellowish pigmentation of the olfactory mucosa (Dodson and Bannister, unpublished observations).

The basal cells of the epithelium are of two types, small well differentiated supportive elements and larger 'blastema' cells with embryonic characteristics (see p. 408). It is thought that the 'blastema' cells are capable of division throughout life and are responsible for the continual renewal of the population of receptor cells (Moulton, Çelebi and Fink, 1970; Graziadei, 1973). Physiological evidence indicates that sensory terminals of the Trigeminal nerve are present in the olfactory epithelium, but their structure is not known, nor is that of the endings of the 'nervus terminalis' which accompanies the olfactory nerve.

Electrophysiological recordings from olfactory receptors have demonstrated characteristics typical of sensory cells — the presence of a generator potential detectable in the mucus as a negative wave — the electro-olfactogram or E.O.G. (Ottoson, 1954, 1973), and impulse activity found in the olfactory nerves and (probably) the cell bodies. Relatively few intracellular studies have been achieved because of technical difficulties of recording from such small cells; but Gesteland, Lettvin and Pitts (1965) have shown that individual receptors respond differentially to a wide range of odours, and that single odours elicit a range of response in different cells, causing variations in discharge frequency, latency, rate of adaptation and the like. These findings suggest that each receptor has a variety of molecular receptor sites, and that these are scattered in different concentrations on the surfaces of different receptors. Odour discrimination would therefore appear to involve the the recognition of a pattern of discharge from many receptors, and such a mechanism might explain the enormous number of distinct odours the olfactory system is capable of detecting. What exactly is meant by a 'receptor site' is a matter of debate — but there is considerable evidence that molecular shape (Amoore, 1965) and the presence of certain chemical groups are of importance (Beets, 1971), pointing to an interaction not unlike that which occurs between an enzyme and a substrate, although perhaps less specific than is usual in such a system. Various other theories of olfaction have been suggested; these have invoked the molecular vibrations of odorants at infra-red frequencies (Wright, 1964), and the membrane-disrupting properties of lipid soluble odorants, which are particularly effective as smells (Davis, 1962).

The olfactory axons pass through the numerous foramina of the cribriform plate in small fasciculi, to enter the superficial layers of the olfactory bulb where they synapse in the olfactory glomeruli with the second order neurons, the mitral and tufted cells. Considerable convergence occurs at this stage, up to 26 000 primary axons synapsing with a single mitral cell (Allison and Warwick, 1949) and it is feasible, though not yet proved, that receptors with like chemical specificities are connected to the same mitral cells, so providing a means of discrimination between different odours.

From this point, the axons of the second order neurons pass to various destinations in the surrounding forebrain. Although too numerous to mention individually, the more important connections are made via the lateral olfactory tract with various parts of the olfactory cortex, including the ipsilateral prepyriform and perimygdaloid regions, olfactory tubercle, and amygdaloid nucleus (McLeod, 1971), the last two of these regions in turn being connected to the hypothalamus. More rostrally, the anterior olfactory nuclei are connected to the corresponding contralateral nuclei via the anterior commisure and also to inhibitory interneurons within the olfactory bulb, thus providing a means of centifugal and contralateral control of olfactory bulbar activity.

It is apparent that the olfactory system differs in some respects from those of other sensory modalities since the second order neurons are connected directly to the primary projection areas of the cortex without an intervening thalamic relay, a state of affairs perhaps reflecting the great antiquity of the olfactory forebrain centres. However, it has been shown (Powell, Cowan and Raisman, 1965) that third order olfactory neurons do in fact synapse in the ventromedial thalamus with neurons projecting, with those of the gustatory pathway, to the neocortex, a connection possibly related in man to the conscious perception of odours. The primary projection centres of the olfactory cortex have, in contrast, extensive connections to the limbic system and appear, amongst other functions, to be concerned with reproductive, aggressive and other appetitive aspects of behaviour.

In addition to these major connections, numerous short-range interactions occur within the olfactory bulb (see Pinching, 1972), and these have in recent years been explored by several groups of workers. It has been shown that mitral (and tufted) cells exert lateral inhibition on each other by means of inhibitory interneurons (the granule cells) which lack axons, but are able to convey their inhibitory influences in either direction along their dendritic processes (Rall, Shepherd, Reese and Brightman, 1966). Granule cells are excited by mitral cells at reciprocal synapses which also cause inhibition of the mitral cell which first caused the excitation. In this way the activity of individual mitral cells is considerably damped, providing yet another means of olfactory adaptation. As already implied, granule cells can also be excited by centrifugal and contralateral control, as can other small inhibitory interneurons situated peripherally between the glomeruli. It is obvious that the olfactory bulb possesses a wide range of possible activities which are only now beginning to be explored.

Gustatory receptors

In mammals, the sense of taste is distinct from the olfactory sense in its anatomical organisation and in its lower sensitivity and restricted range of discrimination. It is primarily concerned with feeding activities, and the receptor cells are scattered in groups – the taste buds – over the surface of the tongue, posterior pharynx, epiglottis, and, in some species such as rabbit, the palate. The receptors are spindle-shaped epithelial elements with which the afferent nerves form peripheral synaptic contacts (see the review by Moulton and Beidler, 1967).

Three cranial nerves supply the gustatory receptors, the lingual branch of the chorda tympani (VII) to the anterior tongue, the lingual branch of the glossopharyngeal nerve to the posterior tongue and the vagus nerve to the pharynx and other more posteriorly-placed receptors. Most work on gustation has centred on the tongue, and relatively little is known about the receptors in other sites.

On the tongue, many of the receptors are associated with raised papillae, the types and distribution of which vary greatly between species (Bradley, 1971). In man and other primates, two types of papillae bear taste buds – the fungiform papillae scattered over the anterior and middle tongue, and the more complex circumvallate papillae lying along the posterior lingual groove. In some species (e.g. rabbit) taste buds also line leaf-like (foliate) papillae at the sides of the tongue.

Each taste bud is surrounded by stratified squamous epithelium which leaves an apical taste pore through which substances can reach the sensory endings (Figs. 8.18, 8.19). More than forty fusiform cells may be present in a single taste bud, their apices converging on a cavity filled with dense material containing mucopolysaccharide (Scalzi, 1967). Unmyelinated branches of myelinated axons penetrate the taste bud basally and ramify amongst its cells.

Ultrastructurally several distinct types of cell have been described (Fig.8.19); some of these may represent developmental stages of fewer categories of cells, and Murray and Murray (1970), and Murray (1971), have distinguished at least five cell classes (I–V) in foliate taste buds of rabbits. Type I possesses numerous apical microvilli, secretory vesicles and a relatively dense cytoplasm replete with granular endoplasmic reticulum; these cells enwrap other types of cells and are probably supportive cells responsible for secreting the dense mucopolysaccharide of the apical cavity (Scalzi, 1967). Type II cells are paler, bear apical microvilli, contain many clear vesicles and are invaginated at many points by nerve fibres, but do not form synaptic junctions with them. Their functional significance is not clear. Type III cells bear only a few apical projections, contain a lucent cytoplasm, and show synaptic specialisations in relation to expanded nerve terminals which indent the cell surface; clear, rounded vesicles, 40–60 nm in diameter and a few dense-cored vesicles are present at these sites, and typical pre- and post-synaptic densities line the apposed membranes of gustatory cells and nerve endings at such junctional areas. The Type III cell therefore appears to be the gustatory receptor. Of the other cell types, basal cells (Type IV) are believed to be the origin of the other species of cell in the taste bud, while Type V cells, investing the perimeter of the bud, resemble the neighbouring keratinocytes of the stratified epithelium of the tongue.

The nerve fibres which penetrate the base of the taste bud are non-myelinated branches of myelinated afferent fibres, each unit supplying several taste buds

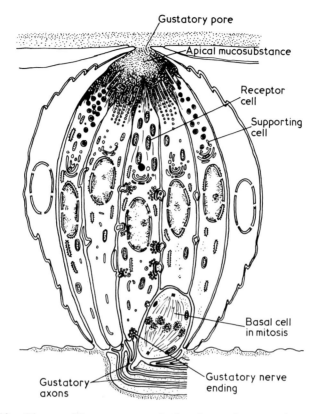

Fig. 8.19   Diagram of the arrangement of cells and synaptic contacts in a taste bud.

over a wide area; conversely, a single bud may be innervated by more than one afferent unit (Zalewski, 1969; Murray and Murray, 1970).

Taste quality is to some extent related to specific areas of tongue. In man, the tip is particularly sensitive to salty and to sweet substances, the sides to salty and sour stimuli, and the posterior aspect to bitter ones. In other mammals, similar sensitivities are present in separate lingual areas (Beidler, Fishman and Hardiman, 1955). Each afferent unit may respond to more than one of these four qualities of taste (Pfaffman, 1941; Beidler, 1971), and it seems likely that gustatory receptors with a wide variety of sensitivities are related to a single fibre. Moreover, recordings of receptor potentials have shown that individual receptors likewise respond to more than one taste 'quality' (Beidler, 1961; Sato, 1969). It is therefore likely that the perception of taste is related to the central analysis of a differential patterned response of many afferent units (Pfaffman, 1941). It is interesting that gustatory responses are greatly affected by temperature changes (Sato, 1971), thus perhaps providing extra possibilities for food discrimination.

The afferent gustatory fibres in the different cranial nerves (VII, IX and X) enter the brain stem where they pass to the nucleus of the tractus solitarius of the same side. The great majority of the taste fibres enter via the chorda tympani branch of VII nerve, and the IX nerve which project to the rostral and intermediate regions of the nucleus respectively, the fibres from the Xth nerve ending in the caudal part. Both gustatory and mechanoreceptor responses have been recorded in this nucleus. Second order neurons project to the ventromedial nucleus of the ventral nuclear group of the dorsal thalamus, most of the connections being ipsilateral, and projections pass from here to two distinct regions of the sensory cortex, namely the intra-oral projection region of the somatosensory Area I, and the anterior opercular-insular cortex immediately rostral to Somatic Sensory Area II. The first of these projections is somato-topically organized according to the area of tongue stimulated and receives cross and uncrossed fibres of mixed gustatory and mechanoreceptor function. The second is more completely gustatory, receives only ipsilateral connections, and is not somato-topically arranged. It has been suggested that the first of these areas is responsible for localization of stimulation and the second for fine qualitative discrimination (Burton and Benjamin, 1971).

Arterial chemoreceptors

Important chemoreceptors which form part of the reflex mechanism controlling ventilatory action are present in the walls of the major outflow arteries. These receptors monitor the levels of dissolved gases, pH and other parameters of arterial blood, and send their fibres to the medulla via two nerve trunks: those in the immediate vicinity of the heart – in the walls of the aorta and pulmonary vessels – are supplied by a branch of the vagus, and those of the carotid arteries by the glossopharyngeal nerve. The best known of these receptors are grouped around a vascular network arising at the carotid bifurcation and collectively form the carotid body. Much of what we know about arterial chemoreceptors stems from work on this structure, and most of the present account will be restricted to a consideration of its morphology and functions.

Early histological studies by de Castro (1926, 1928), and others, showed that small swellings of the adventitia of the carotid bifurcation are supplied by a rich plexus of capillaries and arterio-venous anastomoses connecting with the adjacent carotid vessel. Within these enlargements were clusters of large ovoid cells, in apposition to which were numerous nerve endings. These cells are the Type I glomus cells of De Kock (1951, 1954): other (Type II) cells with irregular profiles partially enclose the glomus cells and ensheath bundles of unmyelinated nerve fibres. Smaller bodies with a similar structure also occur along the walls of the other outflow arteries mentioned above.

Much work has been carried out on the fine structure of carotid bodies (see the reviews by Hess, 1968; Biscoe, 1971; Howe and Neil, 1972). The Type I glomus cell have been found to contain a pale rounded nucleus and a cytoplasm characterized by the presence of dense-cored vesicles about 80–100 nm in diameter. Fluorescence and electron microscope autoradiographic techniques have confirmed that these vesicles contain catecholamines (Chen and Yates, 1969) and Lever, Lewis and Boyd (1969) have reported that treatment with reserpine results in a depletion of their dense cores. Mitochondria are also numerous in these cells. Some investigators have reported two types of nerve ending associated with glomus cells, one of them apparently stemming from myelinated fibres of the glossopharyngeal nerve and terminating in an expanded bulb tightly packed with mitochondria and invaginating the surface of the glomus cell. No signs of synaptic specialization are present at this interface. The other type of nerve ending contains clear vesicles clustered against its terminal membrane where dense zones of cytoplasm indicate adhesion (Bock, Stockinger and Vyslonzil, 1970). This second ending therefore has at least some of the features of an efferent terminal, although other workers have disputed this interpretation. The Type II cells appear to be similar to Schwann cells in their relationship to the unmyelinated nerve fibres.

In addition to the structures described, other fine unmyelinated nerve endings are found close to the endothelial linings of the vascular supply to the carotid body and within the smooth muscle layer of its arterioles. The interpretation of the function of the various features of the organ has presented many problems, since the carotid bodies act in a complex manner. In addition to their chemoreceptor sensitivity the walls of the neighbouring carotid artery and particularly the carotid sinus contain stretch receptors responsive to vascular pressure. Some of the endings in the carotid body, in particular those close to the vascular system, are therefore in all probability mechanoreceptors. Other nerve endings are vasomotor terminals, since it is known that stimulation of nerves from the superior cervical ganglion causes changes in blood flow through the carotid body, and parasympathetic innervation is also probably involved in this control mechanism (see Howe and Neil, 1972). Another important source of innervation is found in the glossopharyngeal nerve itself, since stimulation of its trunk results in a decrease in the chemoreceptor sensitivity of the carotid body, apparently as a result of central nervous, efferent control. It is difficult however to exclude the possibility that this is an autonomic effect caused by sympathetic fibres that join the IXth nerve after it has left the brain. De Castro and Rubio (1968) sectioned the IXth nerve between its ganglion and the brain stem, in order to distinguish between the peripheral axons of the sensory neurons, which should survive such a lesion, and the motor fibres, which should not. They found no degeneration in the carotid body after this operation, but after sectioning the nerve distal to the ganglion, all endings degenerated, appearing to indicate that all the nerve terminals were sensory. Biscoe, Lall and Sampson (1970), however, repeated the first type of experiment over a longer time course, and found that up to 60% of endings on the Type I cells eventually degenerated. Since they considered all terminals on these cells to be of the same type, they suggested that all of these endings are motor, and that the chemoreceptor terminals end on the Type II cells without contacting the Type I (glomus) cells. This hypothesis may seem odd, in view of the presence of undegenerated endings on Type I cells; the results could be explained if there are two distinct categories of nerve endings on Type I cells one of them sensory and the other motor. However, it is likely in view of recent physiological evidence that the cytology of the chemoreceptor systems is even more complex than is suggested by the results of these degeneration experiments.

It is known from electrophysiological studies that all arterial chemoreceptors are highly sensitive to changes in the concentration of CO_2, O_2 and pH of the blood. When the partial pressure of CO_2 is raised, or that of O_2 is lowered, an initial dynamic response settles rapidly to a non-adapting increase in chemoreceptor activity. A similar response is observed to changes of pH in either direction, and appears to be independent of the level of CO_2. All of these responses show the typical hyperbolic relationship to stimulus level described for other types of receptor (see 8.2.2), and reach a plateau at a CO_2 concentration of about 24 mm Hg and an O_2 concentration of 150 mm Hg (Biscoe, Bradley and Purves, 1970).

Little is known about the transducer mechanisms responsible for initiating these responses. It has been suggested that the metabolic activity of the nerve terminals themselves might act as the reference level against which the availability of blood-borne oxygen is measured, hypoxic conditions causing a reduction in active transport of ions and so depolarization (see Biscoe, 1971). The finding of numerous mitochondria in the proposed sensory terminals associated with Type I cells (Bock *et al.*, 1970) makes this an attractive proposition; likewise the release of inhibitory catecholamines by the Type I cells, under possible control by the presumed efferent endings might be a cause of the decreased sensitivity of the receptor endings to chemoreceptor stimuli.

From this account it will be seen that the carotid body chemoreceptor endings are highly specific in their range of responses and may differ fundamentally from other chemoreceptors in the nature of their transducer mechanisms. However, it has also been reported that carotid sensory terminals may be sensitive to many other blood-borne substances and thus may possibly possess more general chemoreceptor sensitivity.

8.2.4 *Nociceptors*

Nociceptors are sensory endings which respond exclusively to noxious or potentially damaging stimuli. Such terminals are distributed widely in the body and are particularly numerous in dermal and subcutaneous connective tissues, which, because of their accessibility to investigation, have been the source of much of the information concerning the properties of nociceptors since the pioneering work of Zotterman (1933). A number of different types of terminal have been distinguished by their responsiveness to either one or several types of stimulus, but all of them appear to be endings of fine nerve fibres of the Aδ or C classes, and since such fibres are not directly associated with complex encapsulated end-organs, their structural identity should probably be sought among the 'free-ending' axons. In the skin nociceptor units supply groups of spot-like areas of one or a few millimetres diameter, and endings may be situated at varying depths in the dermis (Burgess and Perl, 1973).

Two distinct categories of nociceptor are known in mammals, one exclusively mechanoreceptive and the other responding to more than one form of stimulus (Iggo, 1960; Burgess and Perl, 1967, 1973). The first of these includes receptors with a wide range of thresholds, all of them much higher than other mechanoreceptors; in general their rate of adaptation to a maintained stimulus is related to their threshold level, those with the more rapidly adapting features requiring the strongest stimulus to elicit a response. Those with the highest thresholds also tend to be the slowest in conducting impulses.

The second group of nociceptors comprises firstly, those receptors which respond to extreme mechanical stimuli and either heating or cooling, and secondly the 'polymodal' receptors (Burgess and Perl, 1973) which react equally well to mechanical stimuli, to heating, and in the skin, also respond to irritant chemicals placed on the surface of the epidermis. The polymodal receptors have somewhat lower thresholds than the first type, show a characteristic prolonged discharge after intense stimulation, and approach the 'irritant' receptors of the respiratory tract and other visceral sites (see p. 430) in their responsiveness. It is likely that in the skin polymodal receptors are superficially placed and this may in part be responsible for their characteristic features. These categories apply primarily to cutaneous nociceptors, and it is not yet clear how far the different types described above are present in other parts of the body. Nociceptors resembling cutaneous polymodal receptors have been demonstrated in the connective tissues of muscles (Group III afferents, corresponding to Aδ cutaneous fibres), where they signal local deformation, excessive muscular contraction, temperature extremes and tissue damage which, in man, are associated with muscle pain (see Matthews, 1973). Dentinal afferents are also nociceptive, although it is possible that they are primarily high threshold mechanoreceptors (see Section 8.4.3).

Although the precise means of transduction in nociceptors has yet to be determined, it is known that changes in their chemical environment alter their reactions. Histamine, bradykinin and potassium ions which are released from damaged cells, greatly increase the sensitivity of cutaneous nociceptors when injected into the skin (see Keele and Armstrong, 1964), and quite low concentrations of these materials cause the sensation of itch in human subjects (Lewis, 1942; Bessou and Perl, 1969). It is likely that such influences are important when actual damage to tissues has occurred or when they are inflamed, although it is improbable that they are the usual means of stimulation in the case of rapid nociceptor reactions.

The central nervous connections of nociceptors will be described briefly in Section 8.3.1.

8.3 Receptor arrays

In the previous section, the individual classes of receptor terminal were considered in isolation. It is however important to consider how the activities of various receptors are related one to another, and how these are finally analyzed and integrated within the central nervous system; whilst a full account of the sensory pathways is beyond the scope of this chapter, three examples of topographically grouped receptor arrays will be briefly described.

8.3.1 *Cutaneous arrays*

The receptors in and immediately adjacent to the integument include mechano-receptors, thermoreceptors and nociceptors (Fig. 8.20). The mechanoreceptors include endings with a wide range of thresholds and adaptation rates, providing information about deformation of the skin surface, deflection of hairs, and vibrational stimuli amongst other mechanical factors. The absolute number of receptors present, and the numerical proportions of their varieties, vary over the body surface. In glabrous skin covering the flexor surfaces of the digits, paws,

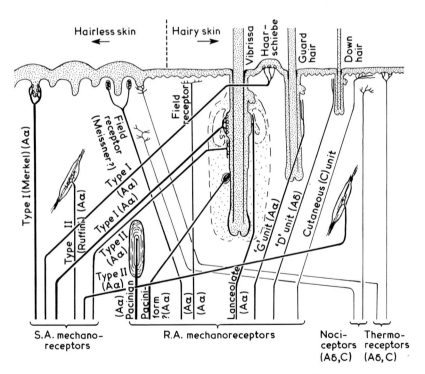

Fig. 8.20 Diagram summarizing the chief types of cutaneous afferent units innervating hairless and hairy skin. The slowly adapting (SA) mechanoreceptor units are shown on the left and the rapidly adapting (RA) ones on right. For details see p. 447 *et seq.*

hands and feet, and the snouts of some species of mammals, typical mechanoreceptive arrays include (1) rapidly adapting units with limited receptive fields sensitive to vibrations, probably corresponding to Meissner's endings; (2) high concentrations of slowly adapting (Type I S.A.) Merkel's disc terminals responding to both the amplitude and the rate of deformation of the overlying epithelium; (3) some slowly adapting (Type II S.A.) Ruffini endings capable of detecting steady stresses in the dermis; and (4) Pacinian endings present in the superficial fascia, sensitive to rapid single mechanical transients and to high frequency vibration (Talbot, Darian-Smith, Kornhuber and (Mountcastle, 1968).

In hairy skin, a similar spectrum of responses is found, with the difference that no Meissner endings are present, their place being taken by rapidly adapting 'field' receptors of unknown structure but similar patterns of response (the F1 units of Burgess and Perl, 1973). Pacinian endings are likewise rare or absent in hairy skin, and Type I S.A. endings are restricted to isolated touch spots or touch domes, and to the follicles of certain large hairs, as will be described later. Free endings of mechanoreceptive C fibres with low thresholds, requiring prolonged stimulation but which adapt relatively rapidly, lie between hairs, providing information about gentle, slowly moving mechanical stimuli. Hairy skin is of course especially remarkable for the large numbers of mechanoreceptive endings associated with the follicles of hairs, first demonstrated physiologically by Adrian (1931) and since studied extensively by several groups of research workers. The morphology of different types of hair varies between species, and it is not clear at present if a common pattern of hair innervation exists in all mammals.

In rabbits, at least four distinct hair types are recognized (see Iggo, 1966; Burgess and Perl, 1973); these include the fine *down hairs* which form the majority of the body cover, the longer and stouter *guard hairs*, large *tylotrich hairs* (Straile, 1960) typically positioned close to touch domes, and on the snout, *vibrissae*, which, being surrounded by cavernous vascular tissue are also known as *sinus hairs*. In other species, for example cats and dogs, vibrissae are present on other parts of the head, and smaller 'sinus hairs' have been described surrounding the foot pads (carpal hairs, see Nilsson, 1969a,b). In primates similar sinus hairs have been found on the fore-arm. All of these hairs are able to transmit the forces which bend their shafts to the sensory endings surrounding their follicles, to signal movements occurring at a distance from the actual skin surface including their velocity, energy content, and direction.

All hairs are innervated at least in part by rapidly adapting receptors. In general, the larger the hair, the higher the velocity threshold of the rapidly adapting response, the larger the afferent fibre (and thus the wider the dynamic range), and the fewer the number of follicles innervated by a single afferent unit (Brown and Iggo, 1967); down hair (D) endings begin to respond to movements at velocities below 0.5 mm/sec, guard hair terminals include a spectrum of more rapidly adapting endings (G2, intermediate and G1 types: Burgess and Perl,

1973) with thresholds, of 0.5—20 mm/sec, and tylotrich (T) terminals respond to yet higher velocities (Brown and Iggo, 1967). The smaller hairs are thus suited to detecting gentle, slow moving widespread stimuli, while the other hairs signal more rapid, localized movements.

Endings present in or around the follicles of sinus hairs (Figs. 8.3, 8.18) are more varied in their response patterns. In addition to the rapidly adapting units described above for smaller hairs, mechanoreceptors with high velocity thresholds have been shown in the vicinity of carpal hairs (Nilsson, 1969a,b) and of vibrissa (Gottschaldt et al., 1974). The responses of such endings are similar to those of Pacinian corpuscles, and indeed Andres (1966) has demonstrated histologically that paciniform endings are present around the vibrissae of rats, and Nilsson (1969a,b) has described Pacinian endings situated close to carpal hairs.

Slowly adapting units with response characteristics of Type I S.A. endings are also present around the follicles of tylotrichs and sinus hairs, and are believed to be related to Merkel's disc terminals present on the upper part of the follicle (Andres, 1966b; Smith, 1967; Nilsson, 1969a,b; Gottschaldt et al., 1974). Other slowly adapting responses similar to those of Type II S.A. endings have also been recorded from vibrissal afferents, but, although it has been suggested that one category of lanceolate terminals may be solely responsible, their origin is uncertain.

It is interesting that, with two exceptions, the mechanoreceptor afferents of skin are myelinated, the majority being the large nerve fibres of Class Aα which possess a wide dynamic range and are capable of rapidly signaling peripheral events to the central nervous system. Other mechanoreceptors are supplied by the low threshold C fibres and the high threshold C or Aδ nociceptive units. Thermoreceptor afferents likewise have relatively low conduction velocities; 'cool' endings corresponding to Aδ or C fibres, and 'warm' endings to C fibres.

The central pathways concerned with cutaneous sensation are both complex and incompletely explored, but the present account would be incomplete without some reference to this area of sensory organization.

Cutaneous afferents entering the spinal roots send information to the brain along a number of parallel pathways, some of which are specific to the sensory modality of the afferent fibre, and others being polymodal; in yet other cases a single type of afferent may activate a number of different pathways. It has been customary to divide the routes to the higher centres into those which pass through the medial lemniscus of the brain stem and those which are extra-lemniscal (for general review, see Brodal, 1969).

In the lemniscal pathways two major types of organization are known. Some larger primary mechanoreceptor fibres, on entering the cord branch to send a major collateral via the dorsal (posterior) funiculi to synapse in the dorsal column nuclei (gracile and cuneate) of the medulla oblongata. Second order neurons pass from these nuclei chiefly contralaterally via the medial lemniscus to the thalamus, terminating in the ventrobasal nuclei; the thalamic neurons, in turn, project to the sensory cortex, in particular to somatosensory areas I and II, to the motor cortex, and to various other regions of the forebrain. Throughout the length of this pathway, the peripheral organization of the sensory endings is reflected in the spatial arrangement of the central neurons with which they are connected, i.e. they are somatotopically organized in a kind of three dimensional map of the body surface. As already mentioned, afferents which send information along this pathway are characterized by their large (class Aα) fibres, and they include those of Type I and II S.A. mechanoreceptor and Pacinian units.

Secondly, many primary afferent units terminate directly in the grey matter close to their point of entry into the spinal cord; this category includes all of the mechanoreceptors, thermoreceptors and nociceptors with small fibres (Aδ and C), and also collaterals from the larger fibres already mentioned. These various afferents synapse in different laminae of the dorsal grey, the mechanoreceptors chiefly in laminae IV, V and VI (Rexed's terminology), nociceptors in laminae I and IV, and thermoreceptors in lamina IV (Brown, 1973; Wall, 1967, 1973). Mechanoreceptor information passes from the laminae of the dorsal grey along two routes. Some of the second order neurons carry impulses in the dorsal funiculi of the cord to the dorsal column nuclei of the medulla oblongata and thence via the median lemniscus to the contralateral ventrobasal thalamus and cerebral cortex; others are connected, via the spino-cervical tract, to the lateral cervical nucleus, which itself is connected (again via the medial lemniscus) to the ventrobasal thalamic nuclei.

Finally, extra-lemniscal routes are followed by signals arriving from nociceptors and thermoreceptors, the majority of which synapse in laminae I and IV of the dorsal grey with second order neurons, their axons being situated in the ventrolateral spino-thalamic tracts (contralateral and ipsilateral). Again, these axons terminate in the ventrobasal thalamus, but also convey information directly to the reticular formation, and the cerebellum, amongst other areas of the brain. Nociceptive and thermoreceptive pathways project from the thalamus to the somatosensory areas I and II, to the non-specific cortex, and to other forebrain regions.

Considerable variation in these different pathways occurs between species and it is not possible at present to provide a comprehensive picture to fit all mammals, nor to extrapolate satisfactorily from non-primate species to man. It does appear however that some synthesis of somatosensory information can occur before it reaches the cortical level of organization.

Lateral inhibition by adjacent sensory pathways provides the means of enhancing contrasts in the excitation of neighbouring areas of skin as in other sensory systems, a phenomenon which has been shown to occur at several levels of neural organization. The ability of the terminal branches of one type of primary afferent fibre to depress the excitation of other types at the presynaptic level in the spinal cord (presynaptic afferent depolarisation) is of particular interest, and presents the possibility that different modalities may compete with one another for access to major somatosensory pathways (see Schmidt, 1973). It is not yet clear how functionally important such interactions may be, but the hypothesis has generated much argument (see for instance the 'gate' theory of Melzak and Wall, 1965).

Another important type of interaction occurs between excitation arriving in the spinal cord from the periphery and efferent impulses descending to the cord from the brain. Such control systems apparently enable the higher centres of the brain to selectively either inhibit or facilitate sensory inflow, and to focus attention both on particular regions of the body and on particular modalities of sensation. For more details of this complex and rapidly expanding subject, the reader is referred to recent reviews, such as that by Schmidt (1973).

Cutaneous sensation of the head is conveyed along cranial axons particularly of the trigeminal nerve; although the precise central connections of these nerves differ in detail from those of the spinal roots, their general arrangement is similar. Central branches of the primary afferents, the cell bodies of which lie in the gasserian ganglion, pass in the trigeminal spinal tract to the trigeminal nuclei, and end there in a somatotropic manner. Second order neurons send axons to the contralateral ventral thalamus, alongside the medial lemniscus, and the final cortical representation is similar to that of the spinal sensory pathways. The general arrangement of the trigeminal system seems therefore to be closely similar to that of the other sensory pathways, although differing in detail (see Darian-Smith, 1973).

8.3.2 *Receptors in synovial joints*

Synovial joints are supplied by nerves derived from both cutaneous trunks and from branches running to adjacent muscles (Rudinger, 1857; Gardner, 1948, 1950), and these ramify extensively in the outer layers of the joint capsules. Of the few joints which have been investigated the nerve fibre spectra include the largest myelinated class $A\alpha$ fibres, as well as $A\delta$ and non-myelinated fibres.

Histologically, at least five sets of sensory terminals have been found in the joint capsule; these include (a) golgi endings similar to tendon organs situated in the ligaments of the joint, (b) Ruffini sprays situated in the superficial layers of the fibrous capsule, (c) paciniform terminals, similar to Pacinian endings but smaller and with fewer lamellae, placed in the deeper layers of the capsule and, in the temperomandibular joint, in the posterior fat pads (Skoglund, 1956; Freeman and Wyke, 1967a,b; Klineberg, Greenfield and Wyke, 1970); (d) 'free' endings of fine myelinated fibres; (e) unmyelinated 'free' terminals.

Two types of position detector and at least one type of velocity detector have been described electrophysiologically (Boyd and Roberts, 1953; Skoglund, 1956, 1973; Burgess and Clark, 1969). Of the position detectors, one has the activity expected of a golgi end organ — that is a highly stable non-adapting discharge pattern unaffected by the action of the surrounding muscles and conveyed to the central nervous system by rapidly conducting class Ib or $A\alpha$

fibres. The second type of position detector is similar to Type II S.A. cutaneous receptors, having a similar resting discharge, inconspicuous velocity response and highly regular static discharge; it seems likely that the numerous Ruffini endings of joint capsules are responsible for this type of discharge. In the knee joint of cats Ruffini endings are grouped in small clusters, with individual endings orientated in different directions around the posterior aspect of the capsule (Skoglund, 1956). It is not perhaps surprising that in the intact joint their responses are rather complex. In general, each ending responds only to positions within a small angle of movement, some showing maximum discharge at extreme flexion or extension, others being active in the middle of the range of movement. Complex tensions developed by the activity of the muscles bearing on the joint also alter the activity of these receptors, as again might be expected from their positions within the joint capsule.

Of the rapidly adapting velocity detector responses, at least one has been correlated with the paciniform ending; Burgess and Clark (1969) have also reported another, rather different, rapidly adapting response having some positional characteristics when strongly stimulated, and it is possible that other mechanoreceptor terminals are present amongst the free endings. In addition at least some of the smaller myelinated and unmyelinated fibres are almost certainly involved in the signalling of pain stemming from excessive joint stresses and other noxious stimuli.

It is possible to suggest that amongst the various receptors, the Golgi ligament endings may give the broad position and direction of movement of the joint surfaces, and that the Ruffini endings could report the small changes in stress accompanying slight movements, and so signal position, speed and direction with a high degree of discrimination. The velocity detectors may provide general information relating to movement, including high frequency vibrations.

The central connections of joint receptors are incompletely known, but it appears that the chief pathway to the somatosensory cortex is by way of post-synaptic connections through the dorsal funiculi and medial lemniscus system to the ventrobasal thalamus, from which fibres project to the contralateral sensory areas I and II and ipsilateral area II of the cerebral cortex (Gardner, Latimer and Stilwell, 1949; Skoglund, 1973). Some Ruffini endings are also connected directly to dorsal column nuclei via the dorsal funiculi. The activities of the thalamic and cortical neurons of this pathway have been explored by Mountcastle (1957), Mountcastle, Poggio and Werner (1963) and others, and individual neurons responding to a range of angular positions and directional movements of joints have been demonstrated. Other afferents pass to the direct and crossed spinocerebellar pathways of the cord, and to the spino-olivary and spinoreticular systems in association with other proprioceptive pathways.

In addition to the connections to the brain, reflex pathways exist within the spinal cord, although their precise significance is not yet entirely clear. Gardner (1950b), Eckholm, Eklund and Skoglund (1960) and others found that stimulation of joint nerves facilitated flexor activity and inhibited extensor movements in decerebrate cats, but it is possible that this was primarily a nociceptive response. The difficulties of identifying the effects of activity of individual receptors on reflex behaviour have so far prevented detailed exploration of this system, and similar difficulties also apply to the connections between the various joint receptors and the brain.

8.3.3 *The innervation of teeth*

It is useful to separate the nerves supplying teeth into two groups — those which end within the tooth itself, the intradental innervation, and those which terminate in the connective tissues surrounding the root — the periodental nerves. Mechanical factors acting on teeth may also be transmitted to the sensory endings of the surrounding bone, gingival epithelium, temperomandibular joint and even the ear apparatus (Anderson, Hannam and Matthews, 1970).

The intradental endings have been known in detail since the pioneering work of Fearnhead (1957), Sosa and Stella (1957), and Arwil (1958). Silver impregnation methods have shown a pattern of branching nerve endings of varying sizes, some terminating within the pulp, often around blood vessels, and others forming a plexus adjacent to the inner dentinal surface; from this plexus, fine fibres pass for some distance into the dentinal tubules, running parallel to the odontoblast processes. Electron microscopy of rodent and other mammalian teeth (see Frank, 1968) has confirmed the presence of such intradentinal nerve endings at the fine structural level, and have also shown that they are much commoner in mature animals than in immature (Corpron and Avery, 1973). The intradentinal endings are somewhat varicose, and are separated by about 20 nm from the adjacent odontoblast process which they invaginate intermittently. Junctional areas resembling rudimentary desmosomes exist between the membranes of two structures. It is interesting that within the endings, numerous mitochondria and membrane bound vesicles of various sizes are present, in addition to microtubles and microfilaments; in contrast the odontoblast processes possess few organelles, and show no evidence of presynaptic vesicles. More deeply within the pulp, unmyelinated fibres ensheathed by Schwann cells ramify around and between the odontoblast somata. Corpron and Avery (1973) have also demonstrated the presence of small myelinated fibres in mouse dentinal pulp.

The periodontal innervation is of a more complex nature, and endings similar to those seen in other connective tissues have been described. Fibres stemming from branches of the maxillary and mandibular nerves emerge from the alveolar bone and branch dorsally and ventrally amongst the collagen fibres of the alveolar ligament (Lewinsky and Stewart, 1937). Silver stained preparations (Rapp, Kirstine and Avery, 1956) have demonstrated nerve terminals which branch and spiral in complex patterns around and between the collagen bundles, these endings being variously described as spindle shaped, spiral, or as resembling

Meissner's cutaneous endings. Both coarse and fine nerve fibres have been described and measurements of their conduction velocities indicate that they are from 1 to 4 μm in diameter.

The physiological roles of intradental and periodontal terminals are not entirely clear. In human subjects, the only conscious sensation arising from stimulation of the intradental endings by a variety of stimuli – temperature changes, high osmotic strength solutions, mechanical forces and electrical stimulation – appears to be one of pain. There is evidence that in addition to such nociceptive responses, other more sensitive and purely mechanoreceptive responses may also occur: when teeth are loaded mechanically, the perceived threshold to such loading is lower in intact teeth than those from which the pulp has been removed, but when a metal cap is placed over the crown, so preventing local dentinal deformation, the threshold is again raised. This implies that the intradental terminals are involved in mechanoreceptor activity. In animals separate intradental fibres responding individually to hot or cold stimuli and to mechanical influences have been reported (B. Matthews, 1968) suggesting that not all fibres are nociceptors.

Another related problem concerns the site of sensory transduction within the tooth. Exposed dentine is sensitive to mechanical, osmotic, thermal and electrical stimulation, but the nerve endings, as far as is known, do not penetrate to the zone of maximum sensitivity – i.e. the enamel/dentinal junction. The thermal responses are also thought to occur too rapidly to be caused merely by the conduction of heat through the dentine to the more deeply placed sensory fibres. Brännström (1963) has proposed a theory of hydraulic flow, in which he claims that any stimulus affecting the volume of the fluid in the dentinal tubules such as mechanical deformation, heating, etc., causes the excitable cells at their bases to become electrically active; according to this view, the intradental endings are all high threshold mechanoreceptors. Some authors have suggested that the odontoblast rather than the nerve ending is the initial sensory cell, but both structural and pharmacological evidence indicates that odontoblasts play a predominantly passive role in the sensory process. It remains possible however that volume changes in the odontoblasts can cause distortion and stimulation of the closely associated nerve terminals.

The physiological behaviour of the periodontal innervation is rather better understood than that of their intradental counterparts. Rapidly adapting and slowly adapting mechanoreceptors, with directional sensitivity, have been shown to exist in the periodontal ligament (see Anderson *et al.*, 1970) providing information about the forces acting on the whole tooth during biting. Both slowly conducting and rapidly conducting fibres appear to be present, and some individual fibres may supply several teeth. The slowly adapting mechanoreceptors are similar in their responses to Types I and II S.A. cutaneous endings (see Above). Gross overloading of teeth is associated in man with pain, and it is likely that deformation of some of the fine nerve fibres of the periodontal tissues is responsible for this sensation. The physiological characteristics of the other receptor types are not known, but the corpuscular endings similar in structure to Meissner terminals may act as rapidly adapting mechanoreceptors. The periodontal fibres pass to the gasserian ganglion and thence to the trigeminal nucleus. Some of the fibres may be connected directly to the mesencephalic nucleus of the trigeminal nerve, the tooth rows being represented in a somatotopic manner within the nucleus. From this trigeminal nucleus axons pass to the ventrobasal thalamus, and the higher order neurons of this region project, in common with those subserving other forms of general sensation, to the somato-sensory cortex (see p. 449) motor cortex, reticular formation cerebellum, and other areas of the brain.

Acknowledgements

I wish to thank all those who have assisted in the preparation of this chapter, particularly Miss Christina Reigate for considerable secretarial help, Mrs. Hilary Dodson Mr. D. Ristow and Mr. R. Bilhous for histological assistance, Mr. K. Fitzpatrick for help with photomicrography and Dr W. Haman for advice.

I am also much indebted to Professor D. Barker for Fig. 8.14a, and to Dr D. Landon for Fig. 8.14b and c.

References

Aidal, M. N. (1969) The fine structure of the sensory endings of cat muscle spindles. *Journal of Ultrastructural Research*, 26, 332–354.

Adler, J. (1969) Chemoreceptors in bacteria. *Science* 166, 1588–1597

Adrian, E. D. (1931) The messages in sensory nerve fibres and their interpretation. *Proceedings of the Royal Society of London (Series B)*, 109, 1–18.

Allison, A. C. (1953) the morphology of the olfactory system in vertebrates. *Biological Reviews*, 28, 195–244.

Allison, A. C. and Warwick, R. T. (1949) Quantitative observations of the olfactory system of the rabbit. *Brain*, 72, 186–197.

Alnaes, E. (1967) Static and dynamic properties of Golgi tendon organs in the anterior tibial and soleus muscles of the cat. *Acta Physiologica scandinavica*, 70, 176–187.

Altner, H. and Altner, I. (1974) In *Transduction Mechanisms in Chemoreception*, (ed.) Poynder, T. M. pp. 59–70. Information Retrieval Ltd.: London.

Anraku, Y. (1968) Transport of sugars and amino acids in bacteria. *Journal of Biological Chemistry*, 243, 3123–3127.

Amoore, J. E. (1965) Psychophysics of odor. *Cold Spring Harbor Symposium on Quantitative Biology*, 30, 623–637.

Anderson, D. J., Hannam, A. G. and Matthews, B. (1970) Sensory mechanisms in mammalian teeth and their supporting structures. *Physiological Reviews*, 50, 171–195.

Andres, K. H. (1965) Differenzierung und Regeneration von Sinneszellen in der Regio olfactoria. *Naturwissenschaften*, 17, 500.

Andres, K. H. (1966a) Der Feinbau der Regio Olfactoria von Makrosmatikern. *Zeitschrift für Zellforschung und mikroskopische Anatomie*, 69, 140–154.

Andres, K. H. (1966b) Über die Feinstruktur der Rezeptoren an Sinushaaren. *Zeitschrift für Zellforschung und mikroskopische Anatomie*, 75, 339–365.

Andres, K. H. (1969) Zur Ultrastruktur verschiedener Mechanorezeptoren von köheren Wirbeltieren. *Anatomische Anzeiger*, 124, 551–565.

Arwill, T. (1968) In *Dentine and Pulp: their Structure and Relations*, (ed.) Symons, N. B. B. pp. 147–167. Livingstone: London.

Atema, J. (1973) Microtubule theory of sensory transduction. *Journal of Theoretical Biology*, 38, 181–190.

Barker, D., Stacey, M. J. and Adal, M. N. (1970) Fusimotor innervation in the cat. *Philosophical Transactions of the Royal Society (Series B)*, **258**, 315–346.

Bazett, H. C. and McGlone, B. (1930) Experiments on the mechanism of stimulation of end-organs for cold. *American Journal of Physiology*, **93**, 632.

Beets, M. G. J. (1971) In *Handbook of Sensory Physiology*, (ed.) Beidler, L. M., Vol.4, Part 1, Chapter 12, pp. 257–321. Springer: Berlin.

Beidler, L. M. (1961) Taste receptor stimulation. *Progress in Biophysics and Biophysical Chemistry*, **12**, 107–151. Pergamon: London.

Beidler, L. M. (1971) In *Handbook of Sensory Physiology*, (ed.) Beidler, L. M. Vol. 4, Part 2. Chapter 11, pp. 200–220. Springer: Berlin.

Beidler, L. M., Fishman, I. Y. and Hardiman, C. W. (1955) Species difference in taste responses. *American Journal of Physiology*, **181**, 235–239.

Beidler, L. M. and Smallman, R. L. (1965) Renewal of cells within taste buds. *Journal of Cell Biology*, **27**, 263–272.

Bessou, P., Burgess, P. R., Perl, E. R. and Taylor, C. B. (1971) Dynamic properties of mechanoreceptors with unmyelinated (C) fibres. *Journal of Neurophysiology*, **34**, 116–131.

Bessou, P. and Perl, E. R. (1969) Response of cutaneous sensory units with unmyelinated fibers to noxious stimuli. *Journal of Neurophysiology*, **32**, 1025–1043.

Biscoe, T. J. (1971) Carotid body: structure and function. *Physiological Reviews*, **51**, 437–495.

Biscoe, T. J., Bradley, G. W. and Purves, M. J. (1970) The relation between carotid body chemoreceptor discharge, carotid sinus pressure and carotid body venous flow. *Journal of Physiology (London)*, **208**, 99–120.

Biscoe, T. J., Lall, A. and Sampson, S. R. (1970) Electron microscopic and electrophysiological studies on the carotid body following intracranial section of the glossopharyngeal nerve. *Journal of Physiology (London)*, **208**, 133–152.

Blix, M. (1882–1883) Experimentala bidrag till lösning af frågan om hudnervernas specifika energi. I. *Uppsala läkareförhandlingar*, **18**, 87–102.

Bock, P., Stockinger, L. and Vyslonzil, E. (1970) The fine structure of the human carotid body. *Zeitschrift für Zellforschung und mikroskopische Anatomie*, **105**, 543–568.

Boyd, I. A. (1962) The structure and innervation of the nuclear bag muscle fibre system and the nuclear chain muscle fibre system in mammalian muscle spindles. *Philosophical transactions of the Royal Society, London (Series B)*, **245**, 81–136.

Boyd, I. A. and Roberts, T. D. M. (1953) Proprioceptive discharges from stretch-receptors in the knee joint of the cat. *Journal of Physiology (London)*, **122**, 38–58.

Bradley, W. H.(1963) Central localization of gustatory perception: an experimental study. *Journal of Comparative Neurology*, **121**, 417–423.

Brännström, M. (1963) In *Sensory Mechanisms in Dentine*, (ed.) Anderson, D. J. pp. 73–79. Pergamon: Oxford.

Brazier, M. A. B. (1957) Rise of neurophysiology in the 19th century. *Journal of Neurophysiology*, **20**, 212–226.

Breathnach, A. S. and Robins, J. (1970) Ultrastructural observations on Merkel cells in human foetal skin. *Journal of Anatomy*, **106**, 411.

Bridgeman, C. F. (1968) The structure of tendon organs in the cat: a proposed mechanism for responding to muscle tension. *Anatomical Record*, **162**, 209–220.

Brodal, A. (1969) *Neurological Anatomy in relation to Clinical Medicine*. Second Edition. University Press: Oxford.

Brown, A. G. (1973) In *Handbook of Sensory Physiology*, (ed.) Iggo, A. Vol. 2, pp. 315–338. Springer: Berlin.

Brown, A.G. and Iggo, A. (1962) The structure and function of cutaneous 'touch corpuscles' after nerve crush. *Journal of Physiology (London)*, **165**, 28–29.

Brown, A. G. and Iggo, A. (1967) A quantitative study of cutaneous receptors and afferent fibres in the cat and rabbit. *Journal of Physiology*, **193**, 707–733.

Burgess, P. R. and Clark, F. J. (1969) Characteristics of knee joint receptors in the cat. *Journal of Physiology (London)*, **203**, 317–335.

Burgess, P. R., English, K. B., Horch, K. W. and Stensaas, L. J. (1974) Patterning in the regeneration of type I cutaneous receptors. *Journal of Physiology*, **236**, 57–82.

Burgess, P. R. and Perl, E. R. (1967) Myelinated afferent fibres responding specifically to noxious stimulation of the skin. *Journal of Physiology (London)*, **190**, 541–562.

Burgess, P. R. and Perl, E. R. (1973) In *Handbook of Sensory Physiology*, Vol. **2**, (ed.) Iggo, A., Chapter 2, pp. 29–78. Springer: Berlin.

Burgess, P. R., Petit, D. and Warren, R. M. (1968) Receptor types in cat hairy skin supplied by myelinated fibers. *Journal of Neurophysiology*, **31**, 833–848.

Burton, H. and Benjamin, R. M. (1971) In *Handbook of Sensory Physiology*, (ed.) Beidler, L. M., Vol. **4**, Part 2, pp. 148–164.

Catton, W. T. (1970) Mechanoreceptor function. *Physiological Reviews*, **50**, 297–318.

Cauna, N. (1965) In *Advances in Biology of Skin*, (ed.) Montagna, W., Vol. **6** (Ageing), pp. 63–96. Pergamon: Oxford.

Cauna, N. (1966) In *Ciba Symposium:* Touch, Heat and Pain (eds.) Reuck, A. V. S. de, and Knight, J., pp. 117–127. Churchill: London.

Cauna, N. (1969) The fine morphology of the sensory receptor organs in the auricle of the rat. *Journal of Comparative Neurology*, **136**, 81–98.

Cauna, N., Hinderer, K. H. and Wentges, R. T. (1969) Sensory receptor organs of the human nasal respiratory mucosa. *American Journal of Anatomy*, **124**, 187–209.

Cauna, N. and Mannan, G. (1958) The structure of human digital Pacinian corpuscles (corpuscula lamellosa) and its functional significance. *Journal of Anatomy, London*, **92**, 1–20.

Cauna, N. and Ross, L. L. (1960) The fine structure of Meissner's touch corpuscles of human fingers. *Journal of Biophysical and Biochemical Cytology*, **8**, 467–482.

Chambers, M. R., Andres, K. H., Duering, M. von, and Iggo, A. (1972) The structure and function of the slowly adapting Type II receptor in hairy skin. *Quarterly Journal of Experimental Physiology*, **57**, 417–445.

Chen, I-Li and Yates, R. D. (1969) Electron microscopic radioautographic studies of the carotid body following injections of labelled biogenic amine precursors. *Journal of Cell Biology*, **42**, 794–803.

Chouchkov, C. N. (1971) Ultrastructure of Pacinian corpuscles in men and cats. *Zeitschrift für mikroskopische – anatomische Forschung*, **83**, 17–32.

Chouchkov, C. N. (1973) The fine structure of small encapsulated receptors in human digital glabrous skin. *Journal of Anatomy*, **114**, 25–33.

Corpron, R. E. and Avery, J. K. (1973) The ultrastructure of intradental nerves in developing mouse molars. *Anatomical Record*, **175**, 585–606.

Corvaja, N., Marinozzi, V. and Pompeiano, O. (1969) Muscle spindles in the lumbrical muscle of the adult cat. Electron microscopic observations and functional considerations. *Archives Italianes de Biologie*, **107**, 365–543.

Cunningham, F. O. and Fitzgerald, M. J. T. (1972) Encapsulated nerve endings in hairy skin. *Journal of Anatomy*, **112**, 93–97.

Darian-Smith, I. (1973) In *Handbook of Sensory Physiology*, (ed.) Iggo, A., Vol. **2**, pp. 271–314. Springer: Berlin.

Darian-Smith, I., Johnson, I. and Dykes, R. (1973) 'Cold' fiber population innervating palmar and digital skin of the monkey: responses to cooling pulses. *Journal of Neurophysiology*, **36**, 325–346.

Davies, J. T. (1971) In *Handbook of Sensory Physiology*, (ed.) Beidler, L. M., Vol. **4**, Part 1, Chapter 13, pp. 322–350. Springer: Berlin.

de Castro, F. (1926) Sur la structure et l'innervation de la glande intercarotidienne (glomus caroticum) de l'homme et des mammifères, et sur un nouveau système d'innervation autonome du nerf glossopharyngien. Études anatomiques et expérimentales. *Trabajos del Laboratorio de investigaciones biológicas de la Universidad de Madrid*, **24**, 365–432.

de Castro, F. (1928) Sur la structure et l'innervation du sinus carotidien de l'homme et des mammifères. Nouveaux faits sur l'innervation et la fonction du glomus caroticum. Études anatomiques et physiologiques. *Trabajos del Laboratorio de investigaciones biológicas de la Universidad de Madrid*, **25**, 331–380.

de Castro, F. and Rubio, M. (1968) In *Arterial Chemoreceptors*, (ed.) Torrance, R. W., pp.267–270. Blackwell: Oxford.

de Kock, L. L. (1951) Histology of the carotid body. *Nature (London)*, **167**, 611–612.

de Kock, L. L. (1954) The intraglomerular tissue of the carotid body. *Acta anatomica*, **21**, 101–116.

Diamond, J., Gray, J. A. B. and Inman, D. R. (1958) The relation between receptor potentials and the concentration of sodium ions. *Journal of Physiology (London),* **142,** 382–394.

Dijkstra, C.(1933) Die De – und Regeneration der sensiblen Endkörperchen des Entenschnabels (Grandry – und Herbst – Korperchen) nach Durchschneidung des Nerven, nach Fortnahme der ganzen Haut und nach Transplantation des Hautstückchens. *Zeitschrift für mikroskopische-anatomische Forschung,* **34,** 75–158.

Dodt, E. and Zotterman, Y. (1952) The discharge of specific cold fibres at high temperatures. (The paradoxical cold.) *Acta Physiologica Scandinavica,* **26,** 358–365.

Dogiel, A. S. (1903) Ueber die Nervenapparate in der Haut des Menschen. *Zeitschrift für Wissenschaftliche Zoologie,* **75,** 46–110.

Eccles, J. C. (1969) The inhibitory pathways of the central nervous system. *The Sherrington Lectures* IX. Charles C. Thomas: Springfield, Illinois.

Eckholm, J. Eklund, G. and Skoglund, S. (1960) On the reflex effects from the knee joint of the cat. *Acta Physiologica Scandinavica,* **50,** 167–174.

Fearnhead, R. W. (1957) Histological evidence for the innervation of human dentine. *Journal of Anatomy,* **91,** 267–277.

Fechner, G. T. (1860) *Elemente der Psychophysik. Breitkopf und Härtel: Leipzig.*

Fex, J. (1962) Auditory activity in centrifugal and centripetal fibers in cat, a study of a feedback system. *Acta physiologica Scandinavica,* Suppl. **189,** 1–68.

Fidone, S. J. and Sato, A. (1969) A study of chemoreceptor and baroreceptor A and C-fibres in the cat carotid nerve. *Journal of Physiology (London),* **205,** 527–548.

Fillenz, M. and Widdicombe, J. G. (1972) In *Handbook of Sensory Physiology,* (ed.) Neil, E., Vol. 3, Part 1, Chapter 3, pp. 81–112.

Fillenz, M. and Woods, R. I. (1970) In *Ciba symposium: Breathing (Hering-Breuer Centenary)* (ed.) Porter, R., pp. 101–109. Churchill: London.

Flock, Å. (1965) Transducing mechanisms in the lateral line canal organ receptors. *Cold Spring Harbor Symposium on Quantitative Biology,* **30,** 133–145.

Frank, R. M. (1968) Attachment sites between the odontoblast process and the intradental nerve fibre. *Archives of Oral Biology,* **13,** 833–834.

Freeman, M. A. R. and Wyke, B. (1967a) The innervation of the knee joint. An anatomical and histological study in the cat. *Journal of Anatomy,* **101,** 505–532.

Freeman, M. A. R. and Wyke, B. (1967b) The innervation of the ankle joint. An anatomical and histological study in the cat. *Acta anatomica,* **68,** 321–333.

Gardner, E. (1950a) Physiology of moveable joints. *Physiological Reviews,* **30,** 127–176.

Gardner, E. (1950b) Reflex muscular responses to stimulation of articular nerves in the cat. *American Journal of Physiology,* **161,** 133–141.

Gardner, E., Latimer, F. and Stilwell, D. (1949) Central connections for afferent fibres from the knee joint of the cat. *American Journal of Physiology,* **159,** 195–198.

Gesteland, R. C., Lettvin, J. Y. and Pitts, W. H. (1965) Chemical transmission in the nose of the frog. *Journal of Physiology (London),* **181,** 525–559.

Gegenbauer, C. (1851) Untersuchungen über die Tasthaare einiger Säugethiere. Zeitshrift für *wissenschaftliche Zoologie,* **3,** 13–26.

Golgi, C. (1880a) Sui nervi nei tendini dell'uomo e di altri vertebrati e di un nuovo organo nervoso terminale musculo-tendineo. *Memorie della R. Accademia delle Scienze di Torino:* Serie II, **38.**

Golgi, C. (1880b) Sui nervi dei tendini dell'uomo e di altri vertebrati e di un nuovo organo nervoso terminale musculo-tendineo. *Opera Omnia,* Ulrico Hoepli, Milano, 1870–83. Second edition (1903), **1,** 171–198.

Gottschaldt, K. M. and Lausmann, S. (1974) Mechanoreceptors and their properties in the beak skin of geese (*Anser anser*). *Brain Research,* **65,** 510–515.

Gottschaldt, K. M., Iggo, A. and Young, D. W. (1973) Functional chacteristics of mechanoreceptors in sinus hair follicles of the cat. *Journal of Physiology (London),* **235,** 287–315.

Granit, R. (1955) *Receptors and Sensory Perception. Yale University Press: New Haven.*

Granit, R. (1970) *The basis of motor control.* Academic Press: London.

Graziadei, P. P. C. (1971) in *Handbook of Sensory Physiology,* The chemical senses, (ed.) Beidler, L. M., Vol. 4, Part 1, Chapter 2, pp. 27–58. Springer: Berlin.

Graziadei, P. P. C. (1973) Cell dynamics in the olfactory mucosa. *Tissue and Cell,* **5,** 113–131.

Graziadei, P. P. C. and Bannister, L. H. (1967) Some observations on the fine structure of the olfactory epithelium in the Domestic Duck. *Zeitschift für Zellforschung und mikroskopische Anatomie,* 80, 220–228.

Grundfest, H. (1971) In *Handbook of Sensory Physiology,* (ed.) Loewenstein, W. R., Vol. 1, Chapter 4, pp. 135–165. Springer: Berlin.

Guth, L. (1973) In *Handbook of Sensory Physiology,* (ed.) Beidler, L. M., Vol. 4,Part 1, Chapter 4, pp. 63–74. Springer: Berlin.

Halata, Z. (1971) Ultrastructure of Grandry nerve endings in the beak skin of some aquatic birds. *Folia Morphologia,* 19, 225–232.

Hartline, H. K. and Ratliffe, F. (1957) Inhibitory interactions of receptor units in the eye of Limulus. *Journal of General Physiology,* 40, 357–376.

Hashimoto, K. (1972) The ultrastructure of the skin of human embryos. X. Merkel tactile cells in the finger and nail. *Journal of Anatomy,* 111, 99–120.

Hensel, H. (1973a) In *Handbook of Sensory Physiology, (ed.)* Iggo, A., Vol. 2, Chapter 3, pp. 79–110. Springer: Berlin.

Hensel, H. (1973b) Neural process in thermoregulation. *Physiological Reviews,* 53, 948–1017.

Hensel, H. (1974) Thermoreceptors. *Annual Review of Physiology,* 36, 233–249.

Hensel, H. and Iggo, A. (1971) Analysis of cutaneous warm and cold fibres in primates. *Pflügers Archiv,* 329,1–8.

Hess, A. (1968) In *Arterial Chemoreceptors,* (ed.) Torrance, R. W., pp. 51–56. Blackwell: Oxford.

Houk, J. and Henneman, E. (1967) Responses of Golgi tendon organs to active contractions of the soleus muscle of the cat. *Journal of Neurophysiology,* 30, 466–481.

Howe, A. and Neil, E. (1972) In *Handbook of Sensory Physiology,* (ed.) Neil, E., Vol. 3, Part 1, Chapter 2, pp. 48–80. Springer: Berlin.

Hubbard, S. J. (1958) A study of rapid mechanical events in a mechanoreceptor. *Journal of Physiology,* 141, 198–218.

Hubel, D. H. and Wiesel, T. N. (1961) Integrative action in the cat's lateral geniculate body. *Journal of Physiology,* 155, 385–398.

Hubel, D. H. and Wiesel, T. N. (1968) Receptive fields and functional architecture of monkey striate cortex. *Journal of Physiology,* 195, 215–243.

Hunt, C. C. (1961) On the nature of vibration receptors in the hind limb of the cat. *Journal of Physiology,* 155, 175–186.

Husmark, I. and Ottoson, D. (1971) Is the adaptation of the muscle spindle of ionic origin? *Acta Physiologica Scandinavica,* 81, 138–140.

Iggo, A. (1955) Tension receptors in the stomach and urinary bladder. *Journal of Physiology (London),* 128, 593–607.

Iggo, A. (1959) Cutaneous heat and cold receptors with slowly conducting (C) afferent fibres. *Quarterly Journal of experimental Physiology,* 44, 362–370.

Iggo, A. (1960) Cutaneous mechanoreceptors with afferent C fibres. *Journal of Physiology (London),* 152, 337–353.

Iggo, A. (1963) An electrophysiological analysis of afferent fibres in primate skin. *Acta Neurovegetativa,* 24, 225–240.

Iggo, A. (1966) In *Ciba Foundation Symposium: Touch, Heat and Pain,* (eds.) Reuck, A. V. S. and Knight, J., pp. 237–256. Churchill: London.

Iggo, A. (1969) Cutaneous thermoreceptors in primates and sub-primates. *Journal of Physiology,* 200, 403–430.

Iggo, A. and Muir A. R. (1969) The structure and function of a slowly adapting touch corpuscle in hairy skin. *Journal of Physiology,* 200, 763–796.

Jacobson, M. (1970) *Developmental Neurobiology.* Rinehart and Winston, Inc.: New York.

Jänig, W. (1971) Morphology of rapidly and slowly adapting mechanoreceptors in the hairless skin of the cat's hind foot. *Brain Research,* 28, 217–232.

Jänig, W., Schmidt, R. F. and Zimmermann, M. (1968) Single unit responses and the total afferent outflow from the cat's foot upon mechanical stimulation. *Experimental Brain Research,* 6, 100–115.

Jansen, J. K. S. and Rudjford, T. (1964) On the silent period and Golgi tendon organs of the soleus muscle of the cat. *Acta Physiologica Scandinavica,* 62, 364–379.

Kadanoff, D. (1925) Untersuchungen über die Regeneration der sensiblen Nervendigungen nach Vertauschung verschieden innervierten Hautstücke. *Archiv für Entwicklungs-mechanik der Organismen,* 106, 249–278.

Katz, B. (1950) Depolarisation of sensory terminals and the initiation of impulses in the muscle spindle. *Journal of Physiology (London)*, 111, 261–282.

Keele, C. A. and Armstrong, D. (1964) *Substances producing Pain and Itch.* Edward Arnold: London.

Kimura, K. and Beidler, L. M.(1961) Microelectrode study of taste receptors of rat and hamster. *Journal of Cellular and Comparative Physiology*, 58, 131–139.

Klineberg, I. J., Greenfield, B. E. and Wyke, B. D. (1970) Contributions to the reflex control of mastication from mechanoreceptors in the temperomandibular joint capsule. *The Dental Practitioner*, 21, 73–83.

Kolnberger, I. (1971) Vergleichende Untersuchungen am Riechepithel, inbesondere des Jacobsonschen Organs von Amphibien, Reptilien und Säugetieren. *Zeitschrift für Zellforschung und mikoskopische Anatomie*, 122, 53–67.

Krause, W. (1881) Die Nervendigung innerhalb der terminalen Körperchen. *Archiv für mikroskopische Anatomie*, 19, 53–136.

Kristensson, K. and Olsson, Y. (1973) Diffusion pathways and retrograde axonal transport of protein tracers in peripheral nerves. *Progress in Neurobiology*, 1, 85–109.

Lambertini, G. (1961) Nouvelles recherches sur les récepteurs nerveux de l'homme et du singe pratiquées a l'aide de la méthode de Ruffini. *Bulletin de l'Association des Anatomistes*, 47, 3–30.

Landgren, S. (1952) On the excitation mechanism of the carotid baroreceptors. *Acta Physiologica Scandinavica*, 26, 1–34.

Landon, D. N. (1966) In *Control and Innervation of Skeletal Muscle*, (ed.) Andrew, B. L., pp. 96–110. Thomson: Dundee.

Landon, D. N. (1972) The fine structure of the equatorial regions of developing muscle spindles in the rat. *Journal of Neurocytology*, 1, 189–210.

Leek, B. F. (1972) In *Handbook of Sensory Physiology*, (ed.) Neil, E., Vol. 3, Chapter 4, pp. 113–160.

Lever, J. D., Lewis, P. R. and Boyd, J. D. (1969) Observations on the fine structure and histochemistry of the carotid body in the cat and rabbit. *Journal of Anatomy*, 93, 478–490.

Lewinsky, W. and Stewart, D. (1937) A comparative study of innervation of the periodontal membrane. *Proceedings of the Royal Society for Medicine*, 30, 1355–1369.

Lewis, T. (1942). *Pain.* Macmillan: New York.

Lindblom, U. and Lund, L. (1966) The discharge from vibration-sensitive receptors in the monkey foot. *Experimental Neurology*, 15, 401–417.

Lipetz, L. E. (1971) In *Handbook of Sensory Physiology*, (ed.) Loewenstein, W. R., Vol. 1, Chapter 6, pp. 192–225. Springer: Berlin.

Loewenstein, W. R. (1971) In *Handbook of Sensory Physiology*, (ed.) Loewenstein, W. R., Vol. 1, Chapter 9, pp. 269–290. Springer: Berlin.

Loewenstein, W. R. and Mendelson, M. (1965) Components of receptor adaptation in a Pacinian corpuscle. *Journal of Physiology (London)*, 177, 377–397.

Lynn, B. (1969) The nature and location of certain phasic mechanoreceptors in the cat's foot. *Journal of Physiology (London)*, 201, 765–773.

Mackay, D. M. (1963) Psychophysics of perceived intensity: a theoretical basis for Fechner's and Steven's laws. *Science*, 139, 1213–1216.

Matthews, B. (1968) Hot sensitive and cold sensitive nerves in teeth. *Journal of Dental Research*, 47, 974P.

Matthews, B. H. C. (1933) Nerve endings in mammalian muscle. *Journal of Physiology (London)*, 78, 1–33.

Matthews, P. B. C. (1971) In *The Scientific Basis of Medicine Annual Reviews*, (eds.) Gilliland, I. and Francis, J., pp. 99–128. Athlone Press: London.

Matthews, P. B. C. (1973) *Mammalian muscle receptors and their central actions.* Edward Arnold: London.

MacLeod, P. (1971) In *Handbook of Sensory Physiology*, (ed.) Beidler, L. M., Vol. 4, Part 1, pp. 182–204. Springer: Berlin.

Meissner, G. (1853) *Beitrage zur Anatomie und Physiologie der Haut.* Leopold Voss: Leipzig.

Melzack, R. and Wall, P. D. (1965) Pain mechanisms: a new theory. *Science*, 150, 971–979.

Merkel, F. (1875) Tastkörperchen beiden Hausthieren und beim Menschen. *Archiv für mikroskopische Anatomie und Entwicklungsmechanik*, 11, 636–652.

Merrilees, N. C. R. (1962) In *Symposium on Muscle Receptors*, (ed.) Barker, D., pp. 199–206. Hong Kong University Press: Hong Kong.

Merton, P. A. (1953) Speculations on the servo-control of movement in the spinal cord. *Ciba Foundation Symposium,* pp. 247–260. Churchill: London.

Milburn, A. (1973) The early development of muscle spindles in the rat. *Journal of Cell Science,* **12**, 175–195.

Montagna, W. (1960) In *Advances in Biology of Skin,* (ed.) Montagna, W., Vol. 1, pp. 74–86. Pergamon: New York.

Moulton, D. G. and Beidler, L. M. (1967) Structure and function in the peripheral olfactory system. *Physiological Reviews,* **47**, 1–52.

Moulton, D. G., Celebi, G. and Fink, R. P. (1970) In *Ciba Foundation Symposium: Taste and Smell in Vertebrates,* (eds.) Wolstenholme, G. E. W. and Knight, J., pp. 227–250. Churchill: London.

Mountcastle, V. B. (1957) Modality and topographic properties of single neurons of cat's somatic sensory cortex. *Journal of Neurophysiology,* **20**, 408–434.

Mountcastle, V. B., LaMotte, R. H. and Carli, G. (1972) Detection thresholds for stimuli in humans and monkeys: comparison with threshold events in mechanoreceptive afferent nerve fibres innervating the monkey hand. *Journal of Neurophysiology,* **35**, 122–136.

Mountcastle, V. B., Poggio, G. F. and Werner, G. (1963) The relation of the thalamic cell response to peripheral stimuli varied over an intensive continuum. *Journal of Neurophysiology,* **26**, 807–834.

Munger, B. L. (1965) The intraepidermal innervation of the snout skin of the opossum. A light and electron microscope study, with observations on the nature of Merkel's *Tastzellen. Journal of Cell Biology,* **26**, 79–96.

Munger, B. L. (1971) In *Handbook of Sensory Physiology,* (ed.) Loewenstein, W. R., Vol. 1, Chapter 17, pp. 523–556. Springer: Berlin.

Murray, R. G. (1971) In *Handbook of Sensory Physiology*, (ed.) Beidler, L. M., Vol. 4, Part 1, Chapter 2, pp. 31–50. Springer: Berlin.

Murray, R. G. and Murray, A. (1970) In *Mechanisms of taste and smell in Vertebrates,* (eds.) Wolstenholme, G. E. W. and Knight, J., *Ciba Foundation.,* pp. 3–30. Churchill: London.

Nafstad, P. H. and Andersen, A. E. (1970) Ultrastructural investigation on the innervation of the Herbst corpuscle. *Zeitschrift für zellforschung und mikroskopische Anatomie,* **103**, 109–114.

Nillson, B. Y. (1969a) Structure and function of the tactile hair receptors on the cat's foreleg. *Acta Physiologica Scandinavica,* **77**, 396–416,

Nillson, B. Y. (1969b) Hair discs and Pacinian corpuscles functionally associated with the carpal tactile hairs in the cat. *Acta Physiologica Scandinavica,* **77**, 417–428.

Nishi, K., Oura, C. and Pallie, W. (1969) Fine structure of Pacinian corpuscles in the mesentery of the cat. *Journal of Cell Biology,* **43**, 539–552.

Nishi, K. and Sato, M. (1968) Depolarizing and hyperpolarizing receptor potentials in the non-myelinated nerve terminal in Pacinian corpuscles. *Journal of Physiology (London),* **199**, 383–396.

Oakley, B. (1967) Altered temperature and taste responses from crossregenerated sensory nerves in the rat's tongue. *Journal of Physiology (London),* **188**, 353–371.

Olmsted, J. H. D. (1920) The nerve as a formative influence in the development of taste-buds. *Journal of Comparative Neurology,* **31**, 465–468.

Ottoson, D. (1954) Sustained potentials evoked by olfactory stimulation. *Acta Physiologica Scandinavica,* **32**, 384–386.

Ottoson, D. (1964) The effect of sodium deficiency on the response of the isolated muscle spindle. *Journal of Physiology (London),* **171**, 109–118.

Ottoson, D. (1973) In *Handbook of Sensory Physiology*, (ed.) Beidler, L. M., Vol. 4, Part 1, Chapter 5, pp. 95–131. Springer: Berlin.

Ottoson, D. (1974) In *Transduction Mechanisms in Chemoreception,* (ed.) Poynder, T. M. pp. 231–240. Information Retrieval Ltd.: London.

Ottoson, D. and Shepherd, G. M. (1968) Changes of length within the frog muscle spindle during stretch as shown by stroboscopic photomicroscopy. *Nature,* **220**, 912–914.

Ozeki, M. and Sato, L. M. (1964) Initiation of impulses at the non-myelinated nerve terminal in Pacinian corpuscles. *Journal of Physiology (London),* **170**, 167–185.

Paintal, A. S. (1972) In *Handbook of Sensory Physiology,* (ed.) Neil, E., Vol. 3, Part 1, Chapter 1, pp. 1–45. Springer: Berlin.

Paintal, A. S. (1973) Vagal sensory receptors and their reflex effects. *Physiological Reviews,* 53, 159–227.

Patrizi, G. and Munger, B. L. (1965) The Ultrastructure and innervation of encapsulated nerve endings in the rat penis. *Journal of Ultrastructure Research,* 12, 500–515.

Pfaffman, C. (1941) Gustatory afferent impulses. *Journal of Cellular and Comparative Physiology,* 17, 243–258.

Pinching, A. J. (1972) Spatial aspects of the neuronal connections in the rat olfactory bulb. In *Olfaction and Taste,* 4, (ed.) Schneider, D., pp. 40–48. Wissenschaftliche Verlagsgesellschaft MBH: Stuttgart.

Pinkus, F. (1905) Über Hautsinnesorgane neben dem menschhen Haar (Haarschieben) und ihre vergleichend anatomische Bedeutung. *Archiv für mikroskopische Anatomie und Entwicklungsmechanik,* 65, 121–179.

Polaček, P. (1966) Receptors of the joints. Their structure, variability and classification. *Acta Facultatis medicae Universitatis brunensis.*

Polaček, P. and Halata, Z. (1970) Development of simple encapsulated corpuscles in the nasolabial region of the cat. Ultrastructural study. *Folia Morphologica,* 18, 359–368.

Polaček, P. and Malinowsky, L. (1971) Die Ultrastruktur der Genitalkörperchen in der Clitoris. *Zeitschift für mikroskopische-anatomische Forschung,* 84, 293–311.

Powell, T. P. S., Cowan, W. M. and Raisman, G. (1965) The central olfactory connexions. *Journal of Anatomy,* 99, 791–813.

Poynder, T. M. (1974) In *Transduction Mechanisms in Chemoreception.* (ed.) Poynder, T. M., pp. 241–250. Information Retrieval Ltd.: London.

Price, S. (1974) In *Transduction Mechanisms in Chemoreception,* (ed.) Poynder, T. M., pp. 177–188. Information Retrieval Ltd.: London.

Quilliam T. A. (1962) Growth, degrowth and regrowth in the Herbst corpuscle. *Anatomical Record,* 142, 322.

Quilliam, T. A. (1966) In *Ciba Foundation Symposium: Touch, Heat and Pain,* (eds.) Reuck, A. V. S. de, and Knight, J., pp. 86–112. Churchill: London.

Rall, W., Shepherd, G. M., Reese, T. S. and Brightman, M. W. (1966) Dendrodendritic synaptic pathway for inhibition in the olfactory bulb. *Experimental Neurology,* 14, 44–56.

Rapp, R., Kirstine, W. D. and Avery, J. K. (1956) A study of neural endings in the human gingiva and periodontal membrane. *Journal of the Canadian Dental Association,* 23, 637–643.

Rees, P. M. (1967) Observations on the fine structure and distribution of presumptive baroreceptor nerves at the carotid sinus. *Journal of Comparative Neurology,* 131, 517–547.

Retzius, G. (1892) Über die Nervendigungen an den Haaren. *Biologisches Untersuchungen,* 4, 45–48.

Rüdinger, N. (1857) *Die gelenknerven des menschlichen Körpers.* Verlag Ferdinand Enke: Erlangen.

Ruffini, A. (1894) Sur un nouvel organe nerveux terminal et sur la presence des corpuscules Golgi-Mazzoni dans le conjonctif sous-cutane de la pulpe des doigts de l'homme. *Archives italiennes de biologie,* 21, 249–265.

Ruffini, A. (1898) On the minute anatomy of the neuromuscular spindles of the cat, and on their physiological significance. *Journal of Physiology* (*London*), 23, 190–208.

Santini, M. (1969) New fibers of sympatic nature in the inner core region of Pacinian corpuscles. *Brain Research,* 16, 535–538.

Santini, M., Ibata, Y. and Pappas, G. D. (1971) The fine structure of the sympathetic axons within the Pacinian corpuscle. *Brain Research,* 33, 279–287.

Sassen, M. and Zimmermann, M. (1971) Capacity of cutaneous C fibre mechano-receptors to transmit information on stimulus intensity. *Proceedings of the International Union of Physiological Sciences,* 9, 493.

Sato, M. (1961) Response of Pacinian corpuscles to sinusoidal vibration. *Journal of Physiology (London),* 159, 391–409.

Sato, T. (1969) The response of frog taste cells (*Rana nigromaculata* and *Rana catesbeana*). Experientia *(Basel),* 25, 709–710.

461

Sato, M. (1971) In *Handbook of Sensory Physiology,* (ed.) Beidler, L. M., Vol. **4**, Part 2, pp. 116–147. Springer: Berlin.

Scalzi, H. A. (1967) The cytoarchitecture of gustatory receptors from the rabbit foliate papillae. *Zeitschrift für Zellforschung und mikroskopische Anatomie,* **80**, 413–435.

Schmidt, R. F. (1973) In *Handbook of Sensory Physiology,* (ed.) Iggo, A., Vol. **2**, Chapter 6, pp. 151–206. Springer: Berlin.

Schoultze, T. W. and Swett, J. E. (1972) The fine structure of the Golgi tendon organ. *Journal of Neurocytology,* **1**, 1–26.

Schoultze, T. W. and Swett, J. E. (1974) Ultrastructural organization of the sensory fibers innervating the Golgi tendon organ. *Anatomical Record,* **179**, 147–162.

Sherrington, C. S. (1894) On the anatomical constitution of nerves of skeletal muscles, with remarks on recurrent fibres in the ventral spinal nerve-root. *Journal of Physiology (London),* **17**, 211–258.

Sherrington, C. S. (1898) Decerebrate rigidity, and reflex coordination of movements. *Journal of Physiology (London),* **22**, 319–332.

Sherrington, C. S. (1909) On plastic tonus and proprioceptive reflexes. *Quarterly Journal of Experimental Physiology,* **2**, 109–156.

Shields, J. E., Dinovo, E. C., Henriksen, R. A., Kimbel, R. L. and Millar, P. G. (1967) The purification of amino acid composition of bovine rhodopsin. *Biochimica Biophysica Acta,* **147**, 238–251.

Sinclair, D (1967) *Cutaneous sensation.* Oxford University Press: London.

Skoglund, S (1956) Anatomical and physiological studies of knee joint innervation in the cat. *Acta Physiologica Scandinavica,* **36**, Suppl. **124**.

Skoglund, S. (1960) Properties of Pacinian corpuscles of ulnar and tibial location in cat and fowl. *Acta physiologica Scandinavica,* **50**, 385–386.

Skoglund, S. (1973) In *Handbook of Sensory Physiology,* (ed.) Iggo, A., Vol. **2**, Chapter 4, pp. 110–136.

Smith, K. R. (1967) The structure and function of *Haarscheibe. Journal of Comparative Neurology,* **131**, 459–474.

Smith, K. R. (1970) The ultrastructure of the human *Haarscheibe* and Merkel cell *Journal of Investigative Dermatology,* **54**, 150–159.

Smith, K. R. and Creech, B. J. (1967) Effects of pharmacological agents on the physiological responses of hair discs. *Experimental Neurology,* **19**, 477–482.

Smith, R. S. (1966) Properties of intrafusal muscle fibres. In *Muscular Afferents and Motor Control. Nobel Symposium I.* (ed.) Granit, R. pp. 69–80. Almqvist and Wiksell: Stockholm.

Sosa, J. M. and Stella, A. P. (1957) Investigaciónes sobre la fina inervación dentaria. *Anales de la Facultad de odontología. Universidad de la República oriental del Uruguay,* **3**, 81–125.

Spencer, P. S. and Schaumberg, H. H. (1973) An ultrastructural study of the inner core of the Pacinian corpuscle. *Journal of Neurocytology,* **2**, 217–235.

Stevens, S. S. (1967) Intensity functions in sensory systems. *International Journal of Neurology,* **6**, 202–209.

Stevens, S. S. (1971) In *Handbook of Sensory Physiology.* (ed.) Loewenstein, W. R., Chapter, 7, pp. 226–242.

Straile, W. E. (1960) Sensory hair follicles in mammalian skin: the tylotrich follicle. *American Journal of Anatomy,* **106**, 133–147.

Talbot, W. H., Darian-Smith, I., Kornhuber, H. H. and Mountcastle, V. B. (1968) The sense of flutter-vibration: comparison of the human capacity with response patterns of mechanoreceptive afferents from the monkey hand. *Journal of Neurophysiology,* **31**, 301–334.

Theisen, B. (1972) Ultrastructure of the olfactory epithelium in the Australian Lungfish *Neoceratodus forsteri. Acta Zoologica,* **53**, 205–218.

Tello, J F. (1917) Genesis de las terminaciones nerviosas motrices y sensitivas. *Trabajos del Laboratorio de investigaciones biológicas de la Universidad de Madrid,* **15**, 101–199.

Todd, J. K. (1964) Afferent impulses in the pudendal nerves of the cat. *Quarterly Journal of Experimental Physiology,* **49**, 258–267.

Tower, S. S. (1932) Atrophy and degeneration in the muscle spindle. *Brain,* **55**, 77–89.

von Frey, M. (1894) Beiträge zur Physiologie des Schmerzsinns. *Bericht Sächsische Akademie der Wissenschaften*, **46**, 185–196; 283–296.

von Frey, M. (1906) The distribution of afferent nerves in the skin. *Journal of the American medical Association*, **47**, 645–648.

Walker, B. E. (1960) Renewal of cell populations in the female mouse. *American Journal of Anatomy*, **107**, 95–105.

Wall, P. D. (1967) The laminar organisation of the dorsal horns and effects of descending impulses. *Journal of Physiology (London)*, **188**, 403–423.

Wall, P. D. (1973) In *Handbook of Sensory Physiology*. (ed.) Iggo, A., Vol. **2**, pp 253–270. Springer: Berlin.

Werner, G. and Mountcastle, V. B. (1965) Neural activity in mechanoreceptive cutaneous afferents: stimulus-response relations, Weber functions and information transmission. *Journal of Neurophysiology*, **28**, 359–397.

Weddell, G. and Miller, S. (1962) Cutaneous sensitivity. *Annual Review of Physiology*, **24**, 199–222.

Weddell, G., Palmer, E. and Pallie, W. (1955) Nerve endings in mammalian skin. *Biological Reviews*, **30**, 159–195.

Weismann, A. (1861) Ueber die Verbindung der Muskelfasern mit ihren Ansatzpunkten. *Zeitschrift für Rationale Medezin*, **12**, 126–144.

Whitear, M. (1960) An electron microscope study of the cornea in mice, with special reference to its innervation. *Journal of Anatomy (London)*, **94**, 387–409.

Wohlfart, G. and Henriksson, K. G. (1960) Observations on the distribution, number, and innervation of Golgi musculo-tendinous organs. *Acta Anatomica*, **41**, 192–204.

Wright, R. H. (1964) Odor and molecular vibration: the far infra-red spectra of some perfume chemicals. *Annals of the New York Academy of Science*, **166**, 552.

Zalewski, A. A. (1969) Combined effects of testosterone and motor, sensory, or gustatory nerve reinnervation on the regeneration of taste buds. *Experimental Neurology*, **24**, 285–297.

Zelená, J. (1957) The morphological influence of innervation on the ontogenic development of muscle spindle. *Journal of Embryology and Experimental Morphology*, **5**, 283–329.

Zelená, J. (1964) Development, degeneration and regeneration of receptor organs. *Progress in Brain Research*, **13**, 175–211.

Zotterman, Y. (1933) Studies on the peripheral nervous mechanism of pain. *Acta Medica Scandinavica*, **80**, 1064.

THE MOTOR END-PLATE: STRUCTURE*

Geraldine F. Gauthier

9.1 General Morphology of the Motor End-plate

A major function of the peripheral nervous system is to transmit signals, rapidly and without fail ... *efferent* messages going back to executive organs such as muscles and glands' (Katz, 1966). The structural relationship, therefore, between peripheral nerves and the skeletal musculature is a critical one; even primitive multicellular organisms possess neuromuscular associations which permit them to respond to their environment (see *Symposium on Invertebrate Neuromuscular Systems Amer. Zool.* **13**, No. 2, 1973). In the present chapter, this relationship as it occurs in the mammal will be emphasized, but reference will be made to other vertebrates and also some invertebrates, where important data have been obtained and where information concerning mammalian neuromuscular systems is limited. Comprehensive historical and comparative reviews can be found elesewhere (Couteaux, 1960; Zacks, 1964; Coërs, 1967; Csillik, 1967).

Morphological variation in the motor end-plates of vertebrate species is considerable, and so also is variation among the muscles of a given species (Cole, 1955; Cole, 1957). Caution must be exercised, therefore, when extrapolating information concerning structure or function from one neuromuscular system to another.

The terminals of a given motor nerve fibre, or axon, may be confined to a single muscle fibre, or they may be distributed among several muscle fibres. It is likely, however, that an individual mammalian muscle fibre recieves no more than one axon (Tiegs, 1953; Schwarzacher, 1957; Coërs, 1959). Each efferent axon, together with the muscle fibre supplied by its branches, comprises a motor unit. However, the muscle fibres involved are not grouped into circumscribed anatomical fascicles, but are scattered (Fig. 9.16) among muscle fibres from other motor units (Edström and Kugelberg, 1968).

Each axon loses its myelin sheath as it approaches the vicinity of a motor

---

*This chapter represents structural aspects of the motor end-plate as of July, 1973. Since that time, there have been significant new advances in the understanding of the structural basis of presynaptic and postsynaptic events in neuromuscular transmission. For recent reviews the reader is referred to:
The Peripheral Nervous System. (1974) Hubbard, J. I. (ed.), Plenum Press, London and New York.
Cholinergic Mechanisms. (1975) Waser, P. G. (ed.), Raven Press, New York.
The Synapse. (1976) Cold Spring Harbor Symposia on Quantitative Biology, **40**.

end-plate, and it may branch extensively before making actual contact with the muscle fibre. The motor end-plate is defined, in this presentation, as that area of a muscle fibre upon which the branches of a single axon terminate (Fig. 9.1). This is therefore primarily a light microscopic definition. At this site, numerous muscle nuclei are aggregated within an abundant superficial sarcoplasm, giving rise to the so-called muscle sole-plate. The entire complex may assume a variety of patterns. Two major configurations, namely, *en grappe* and *en plaque* terminations (Tchiriew, 1879) are recognized in vertebrate muscles, depending on whether the components of the end-plate form a discontinuous or a relatively compact pattern. However, structural variation is more extensive than can be encompassed by these two categories.

Each point of contact between a motor axon and a muscle fibre, defined here as the neuromuscular junction, is a discrete structural unit, which is best resolved at the ultrastructural level. It consists of the axonal ending, its accompanying Schwann cell, and a modification of the muscle fibre surface (Figs. 9.2 and 9.3). Beneath an extensive array of lamellae, which are more or less perpendicular to the surface, is an accumulation of sarcoplasm which is often rich in mitochondria (see below). So intimate is the relationship between axonal ending and muscle fibre that, prior to analysis with the electron microscope, some investigators believed that the axon actually penetrated the sarcolemma, giving rise to the view that the axon was in fact 'hypolemmal' (for example, see Boeke, 1911). This concept was discarded, however, when the complexity of the neuromuscular relationship was resolved by electron microscopy.

Ordinarily, the light-microscope composition of the motor end-plate is best analysed by histochemical procedures that take advantage of specific staining properties of the nerve terminals, or demonstrate sites of enzymic activity within the end-plate (see chapter by Hallpike in this volume). In addition, special optical systems, such as those used in phase-contrast or interference microscopy, enhance the identification of certain components (for example, see McMahon, Spitzer and Peper, 1972). Ultimately, however, our understanding of the structural configuration of the neuromuscular complex has been derived largely from observation with the electron microscope.

9.2 Ultrastructure of the mammalian neuromuscular junction

9.2.1 *Basic features*

With the earliest ultrastructural observations of the neuromuscular junction, it became apparent that the lamellar 'subneural apparatus', described by Couteaux using the light microscope, consisted of a series of infoldings of the muscle cell surface (Palade, 1954; Reger, 1954, 1955; Robertson, 1954). The axonal ending and the muscle fibre, furthermore, were described as 'separate' (Palade, 1954). The extensive invagination of the muscle fibre surface, accounts in part for the early belief based on light microscopy, that the position of the axon was 'hypolemmal'.

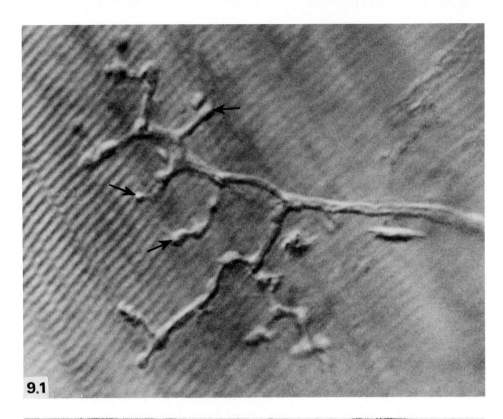

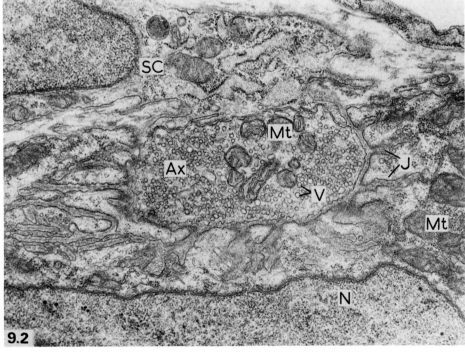

The most significant early contribution to the understanding of neuro-muscular ultrastructure was made by J. D. Robertson (1956) in an analysis of the reptilian neuromuscular junction. Most of the basic ultrastructural features were described in this work, and since that time, similar observations have been made in other classes of vertebrates, including mammals (Reger, 1958; Andersson-Cedergren, 1959; Zacks and Blumberg, 1961; Nickel, 1966; Düring, 1967. Padykula and Gauthier, 1970). In addition, certain unresolved aspects of Robertson's study have been elucidated. It is now clear, for example, that the various 'layers' or 'zones' of the 'synaptic membrane complex' reflect the composition of the membranous structures and their associated basal laminae. Also, structural features which Robertson considered to be 'interpretive' have become demonstrable realities with the advent of more effective methods of ultrastructural preservation. The surface relationships between axon and Schwann cell, for example, are comparable to Robertson's earlier diagrammatic interpretation.

The axonal ending is a specialized, more of less elliptical terminal portion of the motor neuron (Figs. 9.2 and 9.3), and it can be readily distinguished from the preterminal portion of the axon by the lack of neurofilaments and neurotubules. Instead, there is an abundance of vesicles and mitochondria as in the axonal endings of synapses in the central nervous system (Palay, 1956; Palay, 1958). The size of the vesicle varies, but the average diameter is probably close to 45 nm (Robertson, 1956; Andersson-Cedergren, 1959; Birks, Huxley and Katz, 1960). In addition, their shape appears to vary depending on the fixation procedure employed (Korneliussen, 1972b). These axonal vesicles (often called synaptic vesicles) lie in close proximity to, and often make contact with, the axolemma facing the muscle fibre (Fig. 9.3), lending support to the hypothesis that they are the morphological equivalents of the individual quantal units of acetylcholine which are released upon nerve stimulation (see DeRobertis, 1958). The actual amount of acetylcholine in a 'quantum', however, may be more than that which would be expected to be contained within a single vesicle (see Hall,

---

Fig. 9.1 Light micrograph of motor end-plate on a striated muscle fibre from the mudpuppy, *Necturus maculosus*. Photographed using Nomarski optics after treatment with collagenase to remove overlying connective tissue. Terminal branching of a single axon (extending from right) gives rise to several points of contact (arrows) between the axonal endings and the surface of the muscle fibre. Transverse striations of the muscle fibre are readily apparent. (x 1250: Reproduced from McMahan *et al.*, 1972.)

Fig. 9.2 Electron micrograph of neuromuscular junction from rat diaphragm fixed with osmium tetroxide alone. The axonal ending (Ax) is more or less elliptical and contains moderate numbers of vesicles (V) and a few mitochondria (Mt). It is located in a depression of the muscle fibre surface (primary synaptic cleft), which is further invaginated to form secondary synaptic clefts or junctional folds (J). Large mitochondria (Mt) are abundant in the junctional sarcoplasm, but only a few are included in this micrograph, together with a portion of the muscle nucleus (N). A Schwann cell (SC) forms a covering over the entire neuromuscular complex. (x 23 800: Reproduced from Gauthier, 1970.)

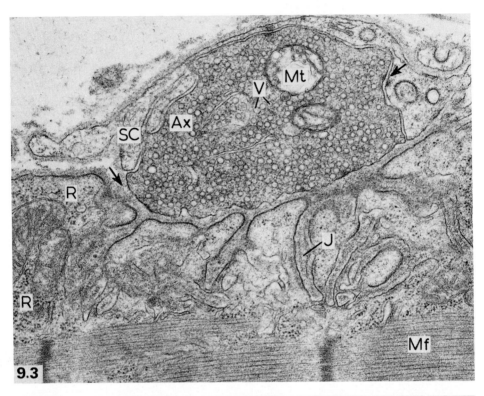

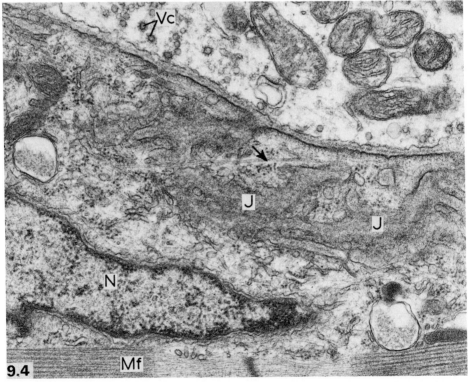

1972), and thus, one axonal vesicle does not necessarily equal one quantum. It is also possible that some vesicles are storage sites for trophic substances, and in addition, frequent structural continuities between vesicles (Fig. 9.3) suggest that they may form part of a tubular cytomembrane system (Düring, 1967). Another characteristic feature of the terminal axoplasm is the presence of fairly numerous mitonchondria and a few coated vesicles (Fig. 9.4). The mitochondria tend to be elliptical, and their cristae are aligned, for the most part, parallel to the long axis, as is generally true of neuronal mitochondria (see Peters, Palay and Webster, 1970). Coated vesicles are similar to those described in other tissues, where thay have been implicated in the process of protein absorption (Friend and Farquhar, 1967).

Specialization of the muscle fibre at the neuromuscular junction is extensive and complex. The surface is invaginated to form a shallow trough or primary synaptic cleft, in which the axonal ending is situated (Fig. 9.3). The sarcolemma is further invaginated to form numerous deeper secondary synaptic clefts or junctional folds (Figs. 9.3 and 9.5). On the basis of an impressive comprehensive analysis of serial sections carried out by Andersson-Cedergren in 1959, it is apparent that these folds are not simple tubular indentations. Rather, they are flattened in one plane perpendicular to the muscle fibre surface (Figs. 9.4 and 9.5). In addition, the folds become expanded abruptly as they leave the point of origin at the surface of the fibre, and they then branch (Figs. 9.6 and 9.10). They are arranged, furthermore, in a complex three-dimensional radiating pattern with respect to the axonal ending (Figs. 9.6 and 9.7), a pattern which has not yet been adequately described. It is difficult, therefore, to determine their configuration, especially on a quantitative basis, from one plane of section alone.

An additional specialization of the post-junctional membrane was observed recently in the earthworm. Rows of projections extend toward the nerve fibre, and they appear to reflect a hexagonal array in surface view (Rosenbluth, 1972).

Fig. 9.3   Neuromuscular junction from rat diaphragm fixed with gluraraldehyde and post-fixed with osmium tetroxide. The relationship between Schwann cell (SC) and axonal ending (Ax) is seen to advantage. The basal lamina of the former is fused with that of the muscle fibre at the entrance to the primary synaptic cleft (left arrow), but it does not enter the space between Schwann cell and axon. It forms a single layer, separating nerve fibre from muscle fibre at all points, and then enters the junctional folds, divides, and forms a covering over the inner surface of each invagination (J). Junctional attachments occur between Schwann cell and axon (right arrow). Tubular profiles are present in addition to the more common circular profiles (V) of axonal vesicles. The junctional sarcoplasm contains fairly numerous ribosomes (R), and part of a myofibril (Mf) is included just below the junctional sarcoplasm. Some fixation damage is apparent in one of the axonal mitochondria (Mt). (x 35 000.)

Fig. 9.4   Portion of axonal ending which contains a few coated vesicles (Vc). Underlying junctional folds tend to be sectioned parallel to their broad faces (e.g., at J), and therefore illustrate the flattened configuration of these invaginations in three dimensions. A microtubule (arrow) is evident in the junctional sarcoplasm. N – Mf – myofibril. (x 30 000.)

They have a spacing which suggests that they may represent receptor sites in the membrane. We have recently observed similar structures (Fig. 9.8) on the outer surface of the junctional sarcolemma in the diaphram of the rat (Gauthier, unpublished observations). The spacing is close to the estimated distance between acetylcholine receptors in the same muscle (see section 9.3.1).

Characteristic of the junctional sarcoplasm are aggregations of large mito-chondria with abundant cristae (Figs. 9.2 and 9.6). These mitochondria tend to be larger than those present in the terminal axoplasm, and their overall form is more variable. A Golgi complex is frequently observed in this region in a paranuclear position. Ribosomes, which are sparse in normal adult skeletal muscle fibres (Gauthier and Dunn, 1973), are moderately abundant in the junctional sarcoplasm (Figs. 9.3, 9.5, and 9.7), and they are frequently associated with profiles of rough-surfaced endoplasmic reticulum (Andersson-Cedergren, 1959; Padykula and Gauthier, 1970). These sites, furthermore, are basophilic (Gauthier, unpublished observations), which is consistent with the accumulation of ribosomes in this region. We have suggested that these ribosomes, together with cisternae of rough-surfaced endoplasmic reticulum, reflect mechanisms for the synthesis of specific junctional proteins such as acetylcholinesterase or a component of the acetylcholine receptor. They may be involved also in the synthesis of new surface membrane, which is so extensive in the region of the neuromuscular junction.

Small vesicle-like structures are present in the junctional sarcoplasm, and, like axonal vesicles, they are frequently closely associated with the plasma membrane, in this case the sarcolemma of the junctional folds (Fig. 9.8). Direct continuity between junctional folds and these subsurface caveolae suggest a role in conduction of the depolarization wave into the T system of the muscle fibre (Zacks and Saito, 1970). Coated vesicles (see above) occur in both the prejunctional axonal (Fig. 9.4) and postjunctional muscle cytoplasm (Fig. 9.5), amd these appear to be involved in macromolecular transport. Evidence of pinocytosis of horse-radish peroxidase has been linked to a 'feedback system' which might operate between the synaptic cleft and the axonal ending (Zacks and Saito, 1969).

Fig. 9.5   Portion of axonal ending illustrating several junctional folds, one of which (J) is sectioned parallel to its broad aspect. These invaginations are therefore not simple tubular extensions as the remaining profiles in this micrograph would suggest. Free ribosomes (R), cisternal rough-surfaced endoplasmic reticulum (ER), and a coated vesicle (arrow) are included in the junctional sarcoplasm adjacent to a myofibril (Mf). (x 38 500.)

Fig. 9.6   Neuromuscular junction sectioned parallel to the surface of the muscle fibre at the level of the junctional folds. The latter form a complex branching pattern which radiates from the region of an axonal ending (Ax). A second array of junctional folds extends from the upper right of the micrograph, but the axonal ending in this complex is not included. One section of a junctional fold (J) illustrates the manner in which the basal lamina lines each aspect of the inner surface. Numerous mitochondria (Mt), and a few ribosomes (R) are present in the junctional sarcoplasm. (x 16 500.)

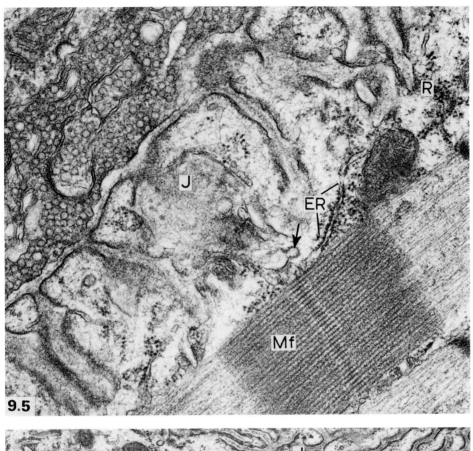

9.5

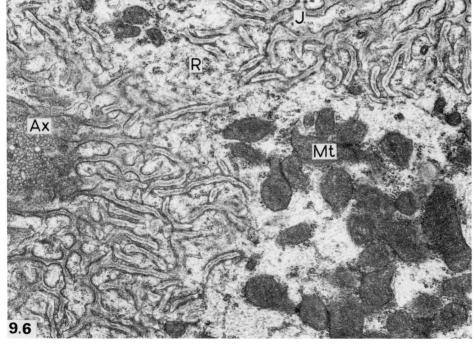

9.6

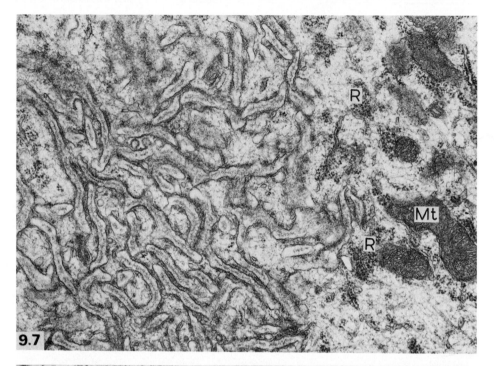

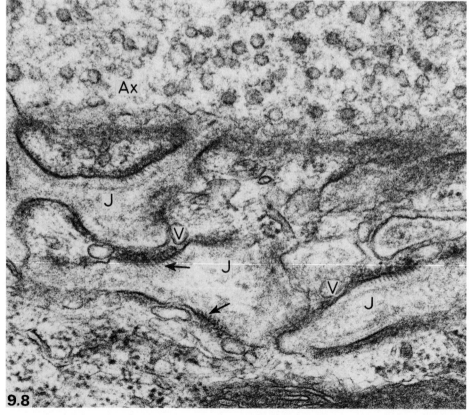

In the junctional sarcoplasm, microtubules (Figs. 9.4, 9.7, and 9.8) form an irregular meshwork (Padykula and Gauthier, 1970) of unknown significance, but it seems reasonable that they might contribute to the structural integrity of this region. Their function in support as well as in movement has been documented in other cellular systems (Tilney, 1971).

The plasma membranes of the axon and muscle fibre are, at all points, separate. Unlike most electrical synapses, however, which may have a 'gap' as small as 2 nm across, the primary synaptic cleft may be as wide as 60 nm. The basal lamina of the Schwann cell becomes fused with that of the muscle fibre at the entrance to the primary synaptic cleft (Fig. 9.3). This composite cell coating extends, as a single layer, into the space separating nerve fibre from muscle fibre (Figs. 9.2 and 9.3). It enters each junctional fold and divides shortly after the opening of the fold, giving rise thereby to a coating over the entire inner surface of the junctional fold (Figs. 9.3, 9.6, and 9.8). The basal lamina does not, on the other hand, enter the space between nerve fibre and Schwann cell (Birks, Huxley and Katz, 1960). Instead, the Schwann cell maintains a close association with the axonal ending, with no intervening cell coat, and discrete junctional attachments may occur between these two cells (Fig. 9.3). The Schwann cell forms a covering over the entire neuromuscular junction so that the axonal ending is actually enclosed, at all points, by the Schwann cell on one surface and by the muscle fibre of the other (Figs. 9.2 and 9.3).

9.2.2 Ultrastructural heterogeneity

Differences among neuromuscular junctions are apparent even within individual skeletal muscles. In the mammal, as well as in other vertebrates, variation in the size of the motor end-plate appears to be directly related to the size of the muscle fibre (Coërs, 1959; Coërs and Woolf, 1959; Anzenbacher and Zenker, 1963; Gruber, 1966; Nyström, 1968). Beyond this difference in size, however, reports of morphological variation among mammalian motor nerve endings have been concerned primarily with those special muscles which possess both twitch and tonic fibres, namely the extraocular and tympanic muscles (Zenker and Anzenbacher, 1964; Dietert, 1965; Mayr, Stockinger and Zenker, 1966; Pilar and Hess, 1966; Düring, 1967; Teräväinen, 1968c; Fernand and Hess, 1969). Ultrastructural differences between the nerve endings of these two types of

---

Fig. 9.7 Branching array of junctional folds sectioned parallel to the surface of the muscle fibre. Mitochondria (Mt), free ribosomes (R),and rough-surfaced endoplasmic reticulum are characteristic of the junctional sarcoplasm. A few microtubules are present as well. (x 26 000.)

Fig. 9.8 This micrograph shows the edge of axonal ending (Ax) and portions of three junctional folds (J). In addition to the basal lamina, which covers the inner surface of the folds, conspicuous rod-shaped profiles (arrows) are aligned in regular parallel rows along the sarcolemma. A few vesicles (V) are closely associated with the sarcoplasmic surface of the sarcolemma, and a single microtubule is evident in the sarcoplasm below. (x 65 000.)

fibres are comparable to those of amphibian twitch and tonic fibres (Birks, Huxley and Katz, 1960; Page, 1965). In pure twitch muscles, which comprise most of the mammalian skeletal musculature, it has been assumed that the motor end-plates of the various muscles of a given mammalian species are uniform in appearance (Coërs, 1967). On the other hand, Cole reported a definite lack of uniformity among end-plates in the rat. The 'widest variation in morphology' was exhibited by the diaphragm; that is, *en grappe* end-plates as well as 'all types *of terminaisons en plaque*' exist within this one muscle (Cole, 1957). Recent observations with the electron microscope have established that neuromuscular junctions vary in their ultrastructure (Ogata, Hondo and Seito, 1967; Murata and Ogata, 1969; Duchen, 1971), even within a single muscle (Padykula and Gauthier, 1970; Fardeau, 1973; Korneliussen and Waerhaug, 1973).

In the diaphragm of the rat, three types of neuromuscular junctions can be distinguished by their ultrastructural characteristics (Padykula and Gauthier, 1970). The three types of junctions are associated with three types of muscle fibres, namely, red, white and intermediate fibres, which can be identified most conveniently by using Z-line width as a criterion, although other criteria are valid as well (Gauthier, 1970, 1971). Because of the branching nature of the nerve terminal with respect to the muscle fibre which it serves, interpertation of the plane of section is difficult at the ultrastructural level. For this reason, comparison of the overall configuration of neruomuscular junctions in ultrathin sections can be misleading. Nevertheless, certain distinguishing ultrastructural features can be observed consistently in favourably orientated sections. As described in the previous section, the terminal can be distinguished from the preterminal portion of the axon by the absence of neurofilaments and neurotubules. In addition, approximate transverse sections through the terminal can be recognized by the presence of a complete primary synaptic cleft, which recieves only the terminal portion of the axon. In such sections of a red fibre (Fig. 9.9), the axonal ending is more or less elliptical in profile, and it contains moderate numbers of axonal vesicles; junctional folds are relatively short and sparse. In contrast, the axonal endings on the white fibre (Fig. 9.10) tend to be broader, and axonal vesicles are abundant and closely packed; junctional folds are longer, more numerous, and more closely spaced than in the red fibre. In

---

Fig. 9.9   Red muscle fibre (RF), rat diaphragm. The axonal ending (Ax) is elliptical and contains moderate numbers of vesicles. Junctional folds are relatively short and sparse. Compare with Fig. 9.10, which illustrates a white fibre at the same magnification. (x 17 500: Reproduced from Padykula and Gauthier, 1970.)

Fig. 9.10   White muscle fibre (WF), rat diaphragm. The axonal ending (Ax) is more elongated than in the red fibre. Axonal vesicles are closely packed, and junctional folds (J) are long, closely spaced, and highly branched. Compare with Fig. 9.9 which illustrates a red fibre at the same magnification. Note that the Z lines (Z) are only about half as wide in the white fibre as those in the red fibre, a useful criterion for the ultrastructural identification of these two fibre types. (x 17 500: Reproduced from Gauthier, 1970.)

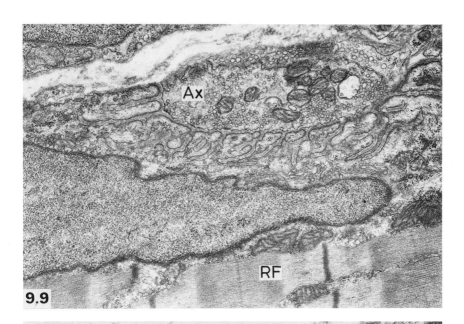

9.9

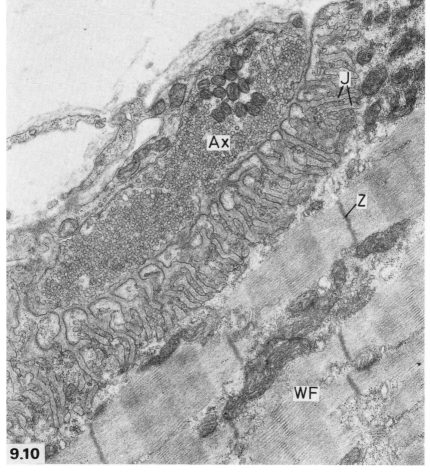

9.10

addition, branching of junctional folds is extensive (Fig. 9.10), and thus the overall postjunctional surface area is greater in the white than in the red fibre. Although the closeness of packing of axonal vesicles may vary with the method of fixation, the appearance ascribed to the differences in fibre type is consistent for any given fixative (for example in Figs. 9.9 and 9.10). The significance of these structural differences has not been established, but quantitatively at least, the number of axonal vesicles may be related to impulse transmission or to transport of trophic substances. The amount of sarcoplasmic surface area at the site of contact with the axon may also be related to neuromuscular transmission; in particular, the vast postjunctional surface area in the white fibre suggests a greater availability of receptors for acetylcholine (see also Section 9.3.1).

9.2.3 Development of the neuromuscular relationship

Interpretation of the sequence of events involved in the formation of the neuromuscular junction differs, not only according to the muscle or species examined, but also according to the procedure used to identify the junction. Thus, while histochemical localization of acetylcholinesterase suggests that end-plate formation occurs at very early stages in the embryo, this enzymic activity is not necessarily associated with the subneural apparatus. That is, true postjunctional activity arises only after contact with the motor neuron has been established; before this time, activity is believed to be either prejunctional or to be associated with the muscle fibre outside the junctional region (Zelená and Szentagothai, 1957; Csillik, 1960; Mumenthaler and Engel, 1961; Csillik, 1967; Filogamo and Gabella, 1967; Teräväinen, 1968a). Morphological manifestations of end-plate formation, likewise become apparent only after neuromuscular contact has been established (Couteaux, 1941; 1960).

The morphological events that occur during differentiation have not been fully explored, but in general, it is agreed that the presence of a motor neuron, or its equivalent (see below), is a required stimulus for initiating formation of the neuromuscular junction. In addition, the muscle fibre must have differentiated, probably to the stage at which nuclei have acquired a peripheral location (Couteaux, 1941); nuclei then become aggregated at the muscle sole-plate, and the subneural apparatus begins to form. These observations have been extended and, for the most part, confirmed at the ultrastructural level.

Even with the electron microscope, it is difficult to recognize the cellular elements which contribute to the neuromuscular relationship during early development, especially before the formation of myotubes. As a result, conflicting views remain concerning the exact sequence of events that take place during differentation. Thus, if simple contact between two cells is used as a criterion for identification, then it may be assumed that the neuromuscular junction is formed early, in the myotube stage of muscle development (Kelly and Zacks, 1969b). If, on the other hand, a recognizable sole-plate or subneural apparatus is the criterion, then it is clear that the existence of a muscle fibre with peripheral nuclei is necessary for formation of the neuromuscular junction, as suggested by Couteaux (1941, 1960).

That both nerve fibre and muscle fibre are well-differentiated before neuromuscular junctions are formed is confirmed at the ultrastructural level; the nerve terminal already possesses moderately abundant vesicles, and the muscle cell has developed beyond the myotube stage (Hirano, 1967; Teräväinen, 1969b; Lentz, 1969). According to Kelly and Zacks (1969b), peripheral migration of muscle nuclei coincides with the accumulation of sole-plate nuclei in intercostal muscles of the rat. However, the possibility that peripheral nuclei are present before aggregation cannot be excluded without examining material from close time intervals, especially immediately before and after birth, the time at which muscle fibres pass beyond the myotube stage in the rat intercostal muscles. On the basis of their observations Kelly and Zacks (1969a, 1969b) suggested that sole-plate nuclei arise, not by mitosis, as previously believed, but by the fusion of undifferentiated cells with the muscle fibre. Although not fully documented, this hypothesis is consistent with the view that once a muscle cell has differentiated its nuclei are no longer capable of mitosis (Holtzer, 1970).

Once apposition is established between an axonal ending and a muscle fibre, ultrastructural manifestations of the neuromuscular junctions become evident. The sarcolemma and subjacent sarcoplasm first exhibit localized densities, the muscle cell surface then becoming indented to form a shallow primary synaptic cleft, which recieves the axonal ending. Schwann cell cytoplasm partially surrounds the axon, but is not present at the surface which faces the muscle fibre, and the axonal ending and muscle fibre are separated only by an intervening basal lamina (see Section 9.2.1), which initially lies closer to the muscle fibre than to the axon (Lentz, 1969). Indentations of the muscle fibre surface then occur between local densities. These extend inward and give rise thereby to small secondary synaptic clefts, or junctional folds (Fig. 9.11), which eventually elongate to form the more complex array characteristic of the adult neuromuscular junction. It has been suggested that junctional folds are formed by an outward growth of elevations along the surface of the muscle fibre rather than by infolding of the spaces between (Lentz, 1969). The Schwann cell remains close to the surface of the axonal ending which faces away from the junction, and thus forms a covering over the entire complex. These ultrastructural observations have been made in a number of mammalian skeletal muscles (Bleckschmidt and Daikoku, 1966; Teräväinen, 1968b; Kelly and Zacks, 1969b), as well as in avian muscles (Hirano, 1967), and they have been confirmed in an analysis of muscle regeneration in the newt, *Triturus viridescens* (Lentz, 1969). In the last study, it was demonstrated that not only the morphological characteristics of the neuromuscular junction but also the ultrastructural localization of acetylcholinesterase becomes apparent only after the axonal ending has become apposed to the muscle fibre. This confirms earlier observations with the light microscope.

9.3 Ultrastructural and cytochemical manifestations of molecular configuration at the receptor site

9.3.1 *Molecular composition*

The chemical and structural composition of the receptor for acetylcholine is only partially understood (De Robertis, 1971; Hall, 1972; O'Brien, Eldefrawi and Eldefrawi, 1972). Recent experimental data have provided important information, which collectively suggest that the receptor site is a mosaic of separate molecules, each associated with a specific aspect of neuromuscular transmission. Using the techniques of ultrastructural cytochemistry, acetylcholinesterase has been localized at the neuromuscular junction (Barrnett, 1962; Davis and Koelle, 1967; Csillik and Knyihár, 1968), and it is likely that most of the enzymic activity is associated with the postjunctional membrane (Salpeter, 1967, 1969; Salpeter, Plattner and Rogers, 1972). However, these procedures alone do not yield information concerning the spatial relationship of the cholinestrases to other components of the membrane. Through imaginative use of specific radioactive inhibitors, Barnard and his associates have devised methods whereby individual molecules can be localized and quantitated by autoradiography. Radioactive d-isopropylfluorophosphate (DFP), an inhibitor of cholinesterase, can be used to identify this group of enzymes (Salpeter, 1967; Rogers, Darzynkiewicz, Salpeter, Ostrowski and Barnard, 1969; Rogers and Barnard, 1969). In addition, acetylcholinesterase can be distinguished from other cholinesterases by using pyridine-2-aldoxime (2-PAM), which removes the DFP block preferentially from this cholinestrase. The radioactive neurotoxin, α-bungarotoxin (BuTX) binds specifically and irreversibly to the cholinergic receptor, and thus can be used to differentiate this receptor from the enzymic component. Such investigations suggest that there are equal numbers of cholinergic receptors and cholinesterase sites at a given neuromuscular junction (Barnard, Wieckowski and Chiu, 1971), and furthermore prior saturation with either DFP or BuTX does not alter the number of sites subsequently bound by the other, indicating that the two sites are seperate. A third component has been identified by means of another radioactive neurotoxin, histrionicotoxin (HTX), which specifically blocks ionic conductance at the postjunctional membrane (Albuquerque, Barnard, Chiu, Lapa, Dolly, Jansson, Daly, and Witkop, 1973). In addition, acetylcholinesterase can be selectively removed from the neuromuscular junction without adversely affecting the electrical properties of the junctional membrane (Hall and Kelly, 1971). It appears, therefore, that at least three molecular entities are present at the receptor site, and that they do not coincide but contribute to a mosaic pattern, consisting of (1) a receptor which binds acetylcholine, (2) a component (possibly equivalent to the so-called ionophore) which alters ionic permeability, and (3) an acetylcholinesterase which hydrolyses the acetylcholine released by the axonal ending.

It is possible to localize end-plates cytochemically by taking advantage of their enzymic activity and to measure the number of molecules of acetyl-cholinesterase by autoradiography in the same material. In this way, the molecular composition can be related to the number of end-plates present. Accordingly, it has been calculated that there are about 3×10^7 to 9×10^7 cholinesterase sites and the same number of receptors per end-plate in skeletal muscles of the mouse; and the exact number depends on the particular muscle examined (Rogers *et al.*, 1969; Barnard *et al.*, 1971). Other investigators have estimated that approximately 5×10^7 (Miledi and Potter, 1971) or 4×10^7 receptors (Fambrough and Hartzell, 1972) are present at each end-plate in the rat diaphragm. By evaluating the approximate membrane surface area provided by the infolding of the junctional sarcolemma, it is concluded that the centre-to-centre spacing of receptors is about 10 nm (Fambrough, Hartzell, Powell, Rash and Joseph, 1974).

The size of the receptor is not known, nor has any visible structure been equated with the receptor. However, in the body wall muscle of the earthworm (Rosenbluth, 1972), in an insect flight-muscle (Rosenbluth, 1973) and in the diaphragm of the rat (Gauthier, unpublished observations), a regular array of rod-like profiles is evident in certain planes of section through the junctional sarcolemma (Fig. 9.8). Preliminary measurements indicate that the distance between consecutive projections is about 15 nm in the rat diaphragm. In the earthworn muscle, the distance is about 16 nm. Both values are compatible with the estimated spacing of receptors. It is likely, if these structures do in fact represent receptor sites, that the discrepancy between the measured spacing (15 or 16 nm) and the estimated inter-receptor distance (10 nm) reflects the variation in total surface area per end-plate used to calculate spacing within the junctional membrane (see Section 9.2.2). Unless the surface area and the total number of receptors are calculated for the same type of motor end-plate, the estimated value for spacing may be misleading.

The number of cholinergic sites per motor end-plate is directly proportional to the diameter of the muscle fibre (Barnard, Wieckowski and Rymaszenska, 1970; Barnard, Rymaszenska and Wieckowski, 1971), and since there is a 1:1 ratio of receptors to cholinergic sites (Barnard, Wieckowski and Chiu, 1971), it may be assumed that the number of receptors is also proportional to fibre diameter. Also, large muscle fibres exhibit a greater junctional surface area than do small muscle fibres (Padykula and Gauthier, 1970), and therefore receptor density or spacing could be constant despite variation in the total number of receptors per end-plate.

9.3.2 *Distribution of receptors*

Inasmuch as events involved in neuromuscular transmission take place at sites other than the neuromuscular junction, extrajunctional receptors will be considered briefly. Evidence of sensitivity to acetylcholine outside the junctional region has come primarily from the physiological literature. In contrast to the

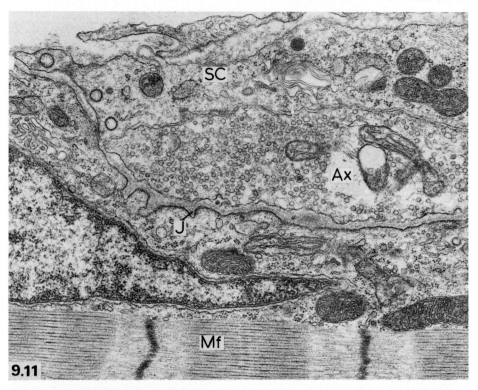

9.11

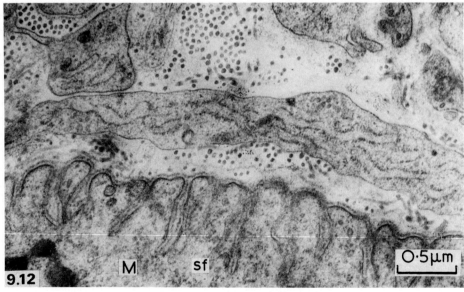

9.12

situation in normal adult muscle, where sensitivity to acetylcholine is confined to the neuromuscular junction, both denervated and newborn muscle fibres exhibit sensitivity alc ng their entire surfaces (Ginetsinskii and Shamarina, 1942; Axelsson and Thesleff, 1959; Miledi, 1960; Diamond and Miledi, 1962; Fambrough, 1970; Fambrough and Rash, 1971; Lømo and Rosenthal, 1972). In these physiological states, the binding of α-bungarotoxin to the receptor site is extended beyond the neuromuscular junction to the entire muscle fibre surface (Miledi and Potter, 1971; Berg, Kelly, Sargent, Williamson and Hall, 1972; Hartzell and Fambrough, 1972; Vogel, Sytkowski and Nirenberg, 1972). Increased sensitivity to acetylcholine apparently reflects a proliferation of new receptors, and ultrastructural manifestations of receptor synthesis have been observed in our laboratory. Whereas ribosomes and rough-surfaced endoplasmic reticulum are abundant in the normal adult muscle fibre only at the neuromuscular junction (Padykula and Gauthier, 1970), they are accumulated in massive numbers in the entire subsarcolemmal sarcoplasm following denervation and also at birth (Gauthier and Dunn, 1973; Gauthier and Schaeffer, 1974). We have suggested that this concentration of protein synthetic machinery at the cell surface is involved in the formation of new receptors.

It is probable, moreover, that important differences exist between junctional and extrajunctional receptor sites. Electrophysiological measurements at the neuromuscular junction differ from those at receptor sites outside the junctional region (see Thesleff, 1973), and the capacity to bind α-bungarotoxin differs according to the region of the muscle fibre examined (Berg et al., 1972). In addition, there appear to be at least three different forms of acetyl-cholinesterase, and their relative proportions vary depending on whether they are associated with junctional or extrajunctional sites (Hall, 1973).

9.4 Recent functional interpretations of neuromusclar unltrastructure

9.4.1 Response to experimental alteration

A number of points concerning the functional significance of ultrastructural features at the neuromuscular junction have been presented above in relation to the individual cytological components being discussed. The following is a

Fig. 9.11 Neuromuscular junction during postnatal development, rat diaphragm. The axonal ending (Ax) has come into close contact with the muscle fibre (Mf), and is separated from it by a distinct basal lamina. A few very short junctional folds (J) extend into the junctional sarcoplasm from the primary synaptic cleft. The entire complex is covered by a Schwann Cell (SC). (× 22 500: From H. A. Padykula and G. F. Gauthier, unpublished observations.)

Fig. 9.12 Neuromuscular junction following denervation (15 days), rat diaphragm. The axonal ending has degenerated and is no longer evident, but junctional folds (sf) are present. Connective tissue cells lie directly above but are clearly separated from the surface of the muscle fibre (Mf) by intervening connective tissue. (Reproduced from Miledi and Slater, 1968.)

consideration of some broader aspects of structural-functional relationships, especially as viewed in the light of recent experimental findings.

Neuronal integrity and maintenance of the junctional relationship

The neuromuscular complex is largely dependent on an intact nerve fibre. This becomes evident following denervation. After section of the nerve to a mammalian muscle (Reger, 1957, 1959; Miledi and Slater, 1968; Nickel and Waser, 1968; Miledi and Slater, 1970), the axonal endings degenerate, Schwann cells become interposed between axon and muscle fibre, and axonal fragments are enclosed within these intervening Schwann cells. The Schwann cells actually replace the axon, but eventually they become less closely associated with the muscle fibre. Junctional folds are retained for remarkably long periods of time following denervation (Fig. 9.12); in some fibres, they may persist for several months. Cholinesterase activity likewise may persist at these sites after denervation (Csillik and Knyihár, 1968). In the newt, on the other hand (Lentz, 1972), junctional folds are disrupted, and are almost completely absent as early as seven days following denervation. This loss of junctional folds can be prevented *in vitro* by the presence of a sensory ganglion, which presumably supplies a trophic substance equivalent to that present in an intact motor neuron. However, the participation of the muscle fibre itself cannot be overlooked, for the junctional folds do survive in some denervated muscles (see above). It has been reported, moreover, that, during spontaneous reinnervation of the denervated rat diaphragm, axon terminals make contact with 'preserved subneural apparatuses' (Lüllmann-Rauch, 1971).

Disruption of the neuromuscular junction correlates, in time, with loss of electrical activity. Both the morphological and the physiological events, furthermore, are inversely related to the length of the nerve stump remaining after section (Miledi and Slater, 1970; Harris and Thesleff, 1972). A relatively long stump, for example, delays loss of miniature end-plate potentials as well as degeneration of the axonal ending. It has been suggested, moreover, that the early persistence of miniature end-plate potentials following denervation is related to the presence of the Schwann cell, which is apparently capable of releasing acetylcholine (Miledi and Slater, 1968, 1970; Miledi and Stefani, 1970). Axonal fragments engulfed by the Schwann cell have been implicated as a direct source of acetylcholine (Lentz, 1972). On the other hand, there is evidence that the Schwann cell possesses a mechanism for synthesis of acetylcholine, and this is supported by the fact that compounds which block protein synthesis are able to suppress acetylcholine release (Bevan, Miledi and Grampp, 1973).

Analysis of tissue culture systems further demonstrates the importance of the neuronal element in control of the neuromuscular junction. In the newt, for example, even a sensory ganglion is capable of preserving the subneural apparatus, as described above (Lentz, 1972). In the mammal, explants of fetal spinal cord send out axons, which eventually make contact with adult as well as fetal skeletal muscle fragments. These contacts consist of morphologically and functionally well-defined motor end-plates in which acetylcholinesterase activity can be localized (Peterson and Crain, 1970, 1972). Using highly purified systems of nerve and skeletal muscle cells *in vitro* it has been demonstrated that, in the absence of all other structural components, such as satellite cells, Schwann cells, and even the basal lamina of the muscle fibre, a functional neuromuscular association can develop (Fischbach, 1972).

That the neuron provides a trophic factor for the control of neuromuscular structure and function is suggested by the effectiveness, under some circumstances, of ganglion cells in maintaining junctional folds, by the importance of nerve stump length, and by the apparent involvement of the Schwann cell in neuronal function following denervation. This suggestion is supported by experiments using colchicine. The drug induces a supersensitivity to acetylcholine, similar to that produced by denervation, but without altering impulse transmission in skeletal muscles of the rat (Hofmann and Thesleff, 1972; Thesleff, 1974). In the newt, treatment with colchicine results in disruption of the neuromuscular junction, and this includes the loss of axonal microtubules and disappearance of junctional folds (Hsu and Lentz, 1972). This, together with the absence of change in impulse transmission in the rat further implicates a trophic substance in maintenance of the integrity of the neuromuscular junction.

Neuronal stimulation and the role of axonal vesicles

Recent studies on the ultrastructural effects of stimulation on nerve-muscle preparations have provided new insights into the function of axonal vesicles during neuromuscular transmission (see also Section 9.2.1). After stimulation with black widow spider venom (Clark, Hurlbut and Mauro, 1972) or following direct electrical stimulation (Ceccarelli, Hurlbut and Mauro, 1972; Korneliussen, 1972a; Ceccarelli, Hurlbut and Mauro, 1973; Heuser and Reese, 1973), the vesicle population in the axonal ending becomes severely depleted (Fig. 9.13), and distortion of the axonal plasma membrane facing the muscle fibre suggests that there has been extensive coalescence between the membranes of these recently depleted vesicles and the axonal membrane. Presumably, the vesicles have become fused at the surface in conjunction with the release of acetylcholine by exocytosis. Although detectable vesicle loss does not necessarily accompany depletion of acetylcholine, especially at low frequencies of stimulation of relatively short duration, this may reflect rapidity of recovery rather than failure to become depleted (Ceccarelli, Hurlbut and Mauro, 1973). When such preparations are exposed to horseradish peroxidase, this electron-opaque tracer becomes enclosed within axonal vesicles, but only after stimulation of the nerve (Figs. 9.14 and 9.15). This has been interpreted as a mechanism for recovering previously discharged vesicles (Holtzman, Freeman and Kashner, 1971; Ceccarelli, Hurlbut and Mauro. 1972, 1973; Heuser and

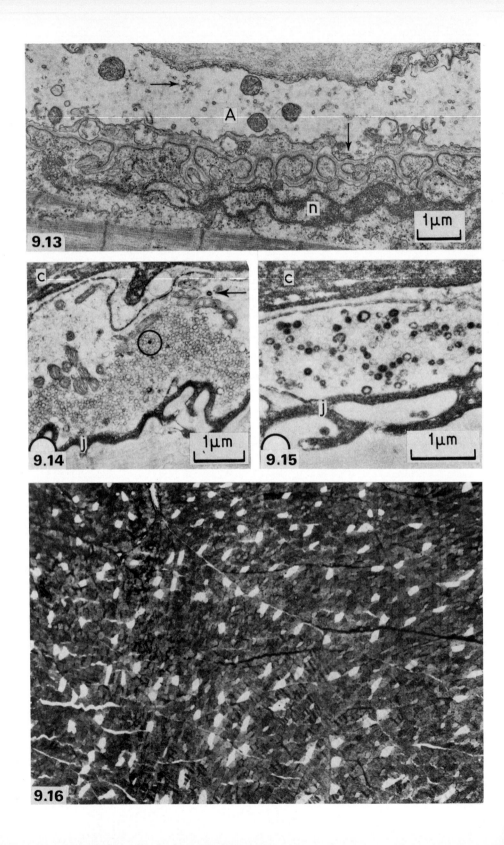

9.13

9.14

9.15

9.16

Reese, 1973; Holtzman, Teichberg, Abrahams, Citkowitz, Crain, Kawai and Peterson, 1973). In this way vesicle membranes that fuse with the axonal membrane during exocytosis can be re-utilized by endocytosis.

There is general agreement regarding the basic concept of axonal vesicle discharge and formation, but opinion varies concerning the exact mechanisms involved. Thus, perioxidase-filled vesicles may represent true synaptic vesicles re-formed directly from axonal membrane contributed by discharging vesicles (Ceccarelli, Hurlbut and Mauro, 1973). On the other hand, some investigators view uptake by coated vesicles as a necessary preliminary phase, after which ingested material is transferred to a cisternal membrane system, and then finally to definitive synaptic vesicles (Heuser and Reese, 1973), although coated vesicles have the capacity to absorb protein even without stimulation (Section 9.2.1 and Fig. 9.14). It has been suggested, in addition, that the vesicles which ultimately contain ingested material, regardless of the mechanism of formation, are not functional synaptic vesicles, but rather are destined for degradation by lysosomal activity (Holtzman *et al.*, 1973). Overall, these experiments have given support to the vesicle hypothesis of acetylcholine release, and they have, in addition, provided an explanation for the constancy of the vesicle population, namely through a balance of discharge, coalescence, and re-utilization of the vesicle membrane.

9.4.2 *Implications of ultrastructural heterogeneity*

Ultrastructural differences among neuromuscular junctions (see Section 9.2.2) represent but one aspect of a pattern of heterogeneity generally exhibited by

---

Fig. 9.13   Neuromuscular junction (n) from the frog, *Rana pipiens*. Electrical stimulation for 7 hours at 2 per second. The axonal ending (A) is almost completely depleted of vesicles except at arrows. (Reproduced from Ceccarelli *et al.*, 1972.)

Fig. 9.14   Frog neuromuscular junction exposed to horseradish peroxidase. Unstimulated. Reaction product, which demonstrates the site of peroxidase activity, is present in intercellular spaces, including the junctional folds (j), but is, for the most part, absent from vesicles except in areas marked (synaptic vesicle circled; coated vesicle at arrow). (Reproduced from Ceccarelli *et al.*, 1973.)

Fig. 9.15   Frog neuromuscular junction exposed to horseradish peroxidase. Stimulated for 2 hours at 2 per second. Not only the junctional folds (j), but also many of the axonal (synaptic) vesicles are now filled with reaction product. Compare with control preparation in Fig. 9.14. (Reproduced from Ceccarelli *et al.*, 1973.)

Fig. 9.16   Low magnification light micrograph of cat gastrocnecius muscle, transverse section. Glycogen is stained by the PAS reaction, and thus most of the muscle fibres appear dark in the micrograph. A single motor neuron has been stimulated, and the muscle fibres supplied by it are depleted of their glycogen (PAS-negative). This histochemical endpoint serves as a 'map' indicating the distribution of a single motor unit. The illustration shows only part of an 'FF' motor unit (see text), and all the component muscle fibres are large white fibres. Note also that these PAS-negative fibres are scattered among various fascicles throughout the field along with PAS-positive fibres. They do not, therefore, form a circumscribed anatomical unit. (x 22: Reproduced by courtesy of R. E. Burke and P. Tsairis.)

mammalian skeletal muscle fibres (see Gauthier, 1970 and 1971). The cytological variation among muscle fibres is clearly related to differences in the source of innervation, and this is well-illustrated in experiments with cross-innervation. Many of the physiological and biochemical properties (Buller, Eccles and Eccles, 1960; Close, 1965; Prewitt and Salafsky, 1967; Buller, Mommaerts and Seraydarian, 1969; Mommaerts, Buller, and Seraydarian, 1969; Samaha, Guth and Albers, 1970), as well as the histological pattern (Dubowitz, 1967; Romanul and van der Meulen, 1967; Robbins, Karpati and Engel, 1969; Guth, Samaha and Albers, 1970; Prewitt and Salafsky, 1970), can be altered and, to some extent, actually reversed by switching the nerve supplies of a fast and a slow muscle. It is not altogether surprising, therefore, that neuromuscular junctions differ in their ultrastructural appearance (Padykula and Gauthier, 1970).

The contractile properties of individual mammalian skeletal muscle fibres have not been established. Certain physiological properties, such as speed of contraction, have been associated with specific ultrastructural or cytochemical features, but such correlations are based largely on extrapolation from measurements made on whole mammalian muscles or on isolated fibres from other vertebtate classes. Thus, while twitch and tonic fibres can be isolated, characterized physiologically, and examined with the electron microscope, the small-diameter fibres which comprises mammalian muscles cannot be examined so readily. Furthermore, most mammalian muscles consist entirely of twitch fibres, and therefore observations made on amphibian material cannot be applied to the mammal (see above). Perhaps the most fruitful approach to the problem is that used in the correlated histochemical and physiological analysis introduced by Kugelberg and Edström and extended by Burke and his associates. These studies have established that the pattern of cytological heterogeneity among muscle fibres reflects the composition and arrangement of the motor unit.

When a single motor nerve fibre is stimulated, glycogen is depleted from those muscle fibres which are innervated by it (Kugelberg and Edström, 1968). Glycogen can be localized in sections of stimulated muscles by the periodic acid-Schiff (PAS) procedure, and its absence from individual fibres can be used as a cytochemical end-point for neuronal stimulation (Fig. 9.16). In this way, the muscle fibres served by a given motor neuron can be identified, and, in addition, the corresponding physiological properties of the motor unit can be measured directly. It has been demonstrated, in the tibialis anterior of the rat, that the muscle fibres comprising a single motor unit are scattered among fibres representing other motor units, and that all the fibres of a single motor unit are of one type based on histochemical classification (Edström and Kugelberg, 1968). At least three clearly distinguishable types of motor units have been localized in the gastrocnemius of the cat, and the physiological properties have been analysed extensively by direct recording from the motor neuron (Burke, Levine, Zajac, Tsairis and Engel, 1971; Burke and Tsairis, 1974; Burke, Levine, Tsairis and Zajac, 1973). On the basis of their physiological characteristics, these motor units have been designated 'FF' (fast-fatigue), 'FR' (fatigue-resistant), and 'S' (slow). In addition, the various cytochemical features and cross-sectional dimensions of the muscle fibres in these motor units suggest that each corresponds to one of three types (Burke *et al.*, 1973; Burke and Tsairis, 1974), which have been designated white, intermediate, and red, respectively, according to criteria used in our laboratory (Gauthier and Padykula, 1966; Gauthier, 1969, 1971). In Fig. 9.16, for example, all stimulated (PAS-negative) muscle fibres are large white fibres, which correspond to 'FF' motor units.

These findings, together with ultrastructural observations of neuromuscular junctions, indicate that the well-established differences among skeletal muscle fibres correspond to differences in the motor neurons serving them. The morpholigical differences, moreover, are consistent with the suggestion that a single motor unit is composed of a single type of muscle fibre. These studies offer, therefore, another example of the role of the motor neuron in the integrated functioning of the neuromuscular complex, and ultimately in the co-ordinated activity of the skeletal musculature as a whole.

9.5 Summary and conclusion

A precise and complex association between two very different cell types, namely a motor neuron and a muscle fibre, is essential to the normal functioning of the skeletal musculature. This relationship gives rise to the neuromuscular junction, which involves characteristic regional specialization of the two cells. In the above presentation, the neuromuscular junction has been described primarily as it appears in mammalian twitch fibres. The terminal portion of the neuron, or axonal ending is more or less elliptical and contains an abundance of synaptic or axonal vesicles, which have been implicated in the release of discrete units of acetylcholine upon stimulation; mitochondria are also aggregated at the nerve terminal. This specialized ending is located in a primary depression of the muscle fibre surface, which is secondarily invaginated to form an elaborate array of branching junctional folds. The underlying junctional sarcoplasm is characterized by abundant large mitochondria and free ribosomes as well as by the presence of rough-surfaced endoplasmic reticulum and a Golgi apparatus. The entire neuromuscular complex is covered by a Schwann cell. The basal lamina of the Schwann cell fuses with that of the muscle fibre and extends between the axonal ending and the muscle fibre. It enters each junctional fold, but does not enter the space between the axonal ending and the Schwann cell. The nerve terminal, therefore, is enclosed by a Schwann cell on one surface and a muscle fibre on the other. However, the nerve fibre and muscle fibre are clearly separated from each other by a distinct cell coating, that is, the basal lamina. The neuromuscular junction, therefore, differs from the electrical synapses of the central nervous system, where only a gap junction separates two cell components. Recent studies of denervated and stimulated neuromuscular systems have underlined the importance of the motor neuron in maintaining integrity of the neuromuscular relationship.The muscle fibre, however, exhibits some degree of autonomy, since the junctional folds can persist even after denervation.

Some facets of the chemical as well as the ultrastructural composition of the neuromuscular junction are beginning to be understood. This problem has been approached recently through enzyme cytochemistry and autoradiography, which have permitted chemical analysis of intact ultrastructural relationships. By using specific radioactive inhibitors, it has been possible to localize and quantitate three molecular components of the receptor site. Acetylcholinesterase, an acetylcholine receptor, and also a component involved in ionic permeability have been demonstrated selectively, and the data suggest that the three entities are arranged in a mosaic pattern. The ultrastructural appearance of the postjunctional membrane suggests, furthermore, that a series of precisely arranged densities might reflect the spatial configuration of molecules at the receptor site.

Finally, quantitative as well as qualitative ultrastructural differences among skeletal muscle fibres and their neuromuscular junctions appear to reflect the composition and functional activity of different motor units. In general, mammalian twitch muscles are composed of at least three types of fibres, which can be recognized at both the light and electron microscopic levels. Physiological properties of individual motor units have also been classified into three groups, and their characteristics can be correlated with the three types of muscle fibres. Specifically, 'slow', 'fatigue-resistant', and 'fast-fatigue' motor units appear to correspond to 'red', 'intermediate', and 'white' muscle fibres, respectively. Ultrastructural differences, moreover, among the axonal endings which serve these fibre types are consistent with the view that a given motor unit is composed of only one type of muscle fibre. These observations lend support to the emerging concept that the total contractile activity of a mammalian twitch muscle represents the integrated functioning of at least three different types of motor units, each consisting of a single type of nerve fibre, muscle fibre and neuromuscular junction.

Acknowledgements

The author wishes to acknowledge Richard V. T. Stearns for his skill in preparing the photographic illustrations and Ann W. Hobbs for her assistance in the ultrastructural procedures.

Investigations from this Laboratory, which are included in this publication, were supported by grants from the United States Public Health Service (HD-01026) and from the Muscular Dystrophy Associations of America, Inc.

References

Albuquerque, E. X., Barnard, E. A., Chiu, T. H., Lapa, A. J., Dolly, J. O., Jansson, S.-E., Daly, J. and Witkop, B. (1973) Acetycholine receptor and ion conductance modulator sites at the murine neuromuscular junction: Evidence from specific toxin reactions. *Proceedings of the National Academy of Sciences U.S.A.*, **70**, 949–953.

Andersson-Cedergreen, E. (1959) Ultrastructure of motor end-plate and sarcoplasmic components of mouse skeletal muscle fiber as revealed by three-dimensional reconstruction from serial sections. *Journal of Ultrastructural Research*, Suppl. 1, 1–191.

Anzenbacher, H. and Zenker, W. (1963) Über die Grossenbeziehung der Muskelfasern zu ihren motorischen Endplatten und Nerven. *Zeitschrift für Zellforschung und mikroskopische Anatomie*, 60, 860–871.

Axelsson, J. and Thesleff, S. (1959) A study of supersensitivity in denervated mammalian skeletal muscle. *Journal of Physiology, London*, 147, 178–193.

Barnard, E. A., Wieckowski, J. and Rymaszewska, T. (1970) The numbers of molecules of the cholinesterases at individual motor end plates in various muscle types. *Journal of Cell Biology*, 47, 13a.

Barnard, E. A., Rymaszewska, T. and Wieckowski, J. (1971) Cholinesterases at individual neuromuscular junctions. In *Cholinergic Ligand Interactions*, pp. 175–200. Academic Press: New York.

Barnard, E. A., Wieckowski, J. and Chiu, T. H. (1971) Cholinergic receptor molecules and cholinesterase molecules at skeletal muscle junctions. *Nature*, 234, 207–209.

Barrnett, R. J. (1962) The fine structural localization of acetylcholinesterase at the myoneural junction. *Journal of Cell Biology*, 12, 247–262.

Berg, D. K., Kelly, R. B., Sargent, P. B., Williamson, P. and Hall, Z. W. (1972) Binding of α-bungarotoxin to acetylcholine receptors in mammalian muscle. *Proceedings of the National Academy of Sciences, U.S.A.*, 69, 147–151.

Bevan, S., Miledi, R. and Grampp, W. (1973) Induced transmitter release from Schwann cells and its suppression by actinomycin D. *Nature New Biology*, 241, 85–86.

Birks, R., Huxley, H. E. and Katz, B. (1960) The fine structure of the neuromuscular junction of the frog. *Journal of Physiology, (London)*, 150, 134–144.

Blechschmidt, E. and Daikoku, S. (1966) Die Entstehung der motorischen Innervation in der menschlichen Zungenmuskulatur: Elektronenmikroskopie der embryonalen Endplatte. *Acta anatomica*, 63, 179–198.

Boeke, J. (1911) Beiträge zur Kenntnis der motorischen Nervenendigungen. *International Monatsschrift für Anatomie und Physiologie*, 28, 377–457.

Buller, A. J., Eccles, J. C. and Eccles. R. M. (1960) Interactions between motoneurones and muscles in respect of the characteristic speeds of their responses. *Journal of Physiology, (London)*, 150, 417–439.

Buller, A. J., Mommaerts, W. F. H. M. and Seraydarian, K. (1969) Enzymic properties of myosin in fast and slow twitch muscles of the cat following cross-innervation *Journal of Physiology, (London)*, 205, 581–597.

Burke, R. E., Levine, D. N., Tsairis, P. and Zajac, F. E. (1973) Physiological types and histochemical profiles in motor units of the cat gastrocnemius. *Journal of Physiology*, 234, 723–748.

Burke, R. E., Levine, D. N. and Zajac, F. E., III. (1971) Mammalian motor units: Physiological-histochemical correlation in three types in cat gastrocnemius. *Science*, 174, 709–712.

Burke, R. E. and Tsairis, P. (1974) The correlation of physiological properties with histochemical characteristics in single muscle units. *Annals of the New York Academy of Sciences*, 228, 145–159.

Ceccarelli, B., Hurlbut, W. P. and Mauro, A. (1972) Depletion of vesicles from frog neuromuscular junctions by prolonged tetanic stimulation. *Journal of Cell Biology*, 54, 30–38.

Ceccarelli, B., Hurlbut, W. P. and Mauro, A. (1973) Turnover of transmitter and synaptic vesicles at the frog neuromuscular junction. *Journal of Cell Biology*, 57, 499–524.

Clarke, A. W., Hurlbut, W. P. and Mauro, A. (1972) Changes in the fine structure of the neuromuscular junction of the frog caused by black widow spider venom. *Journal of Cell Biology*, 52, 1–14.

Close, R. (1969) Dynamic properties of fast and slow skeletal muscles of the rat after nerve cross-union. *Journal of Physiology, (London)*, 204, 331–346.

Coërs, C. (1959) Structural organization of the motor nerve endings in mammalian muscle spindles and other striated muscle fibres. *American Journal of Physical Medicine*, 38, 166–175.

Coërs, C. and Woolf, A. T. (1959) *The Innervation of Muscle: A Biopsy Study*. Blackwell Scientific: Oxford.

Coërs, C. (1967) Structure and organization of the myoneural junction. *Internation Review of Cytology*, 22, 239–267.

Cole, W. V. (1955) Motor endings in the striated muscle of vertebrates. *Journal of Comparative Neurology*, 102, 671–715.

Cole, W. V. (1957) Structural variations of nerve endings in the striated muscles of the rat. *Journal of Comparative Neurology*, 108, 445–463.

Couteaux, R. (1941) Recherches sur l'histogenèse du muscle strié des mammifères et la formation des plaques motrices. *Bulletin Biologique*, 75, 101–239.

Coteaux, R. (1960) Motor end-plate structure, In *Structure and Function of Muscle*, (ed.) G. H. Bourne, Vol. 1 pp. 337–380. Academic Press: New York.

Csillik, B. (1960) Contributions to the development of the myoneural synapses: Ontogenetic aspects of the subneural apparatus. *Zeitschrift für Zellforschung und mikroskopische Anatomie*, 52, 150–162.

Csillik, B. (1967) *Functional Structure of the Post-synaptic Membrane in the Myoneural Junction*. Akadémiai Kiadó: Budapest.

Csillik, B. and Knyihár, E. (1968) On the effect of motor nerve degeneration on the fine-structural localization of esterases in the mammalian motor end-plate. *Journal of Cell Science*, 3, 529–538.

Davis, R. and Koelle, G. B. (1967) Electron microscopic localization of acetylcholinesterase and nonspecific cholinesterase at the neuromuscular junction by the gold-thiocholine and gold-thiolacetic acid methods. *Journal of Cell Biology*, 34, 157–172.

De Robertis, E. (1958) Submicroscopic morphology and function of the synapse. *Experimental Cell Research*, Suppl. 5, 347–369.

De Robertis, E. (1971) Molecular biology of synaptic receptors. *Science*, 171, 963–971

Diamond, J. and Miledi, R. (1962) A study of foetal and newborn rat muscle fibres. *Journal of Physiology, (London)*, 162, 393–408.

Dietert, S. E. (1965) The demonstration of different types of muscle fibres in human extraocular muscle by electron microscopy and cholinesterase staining. *Investigative Ophthalmology*, 4, 51–63.

Dubowitz, V. (1967) Cross-innervated mammalian skeletal muscle: Histochemical, physiological and biochemical observations. *Journal of Physiology, (London)*, 193, 481–496.

Duchen, L. W. (1971) An electron microscopic comparison of motor end-plates of slow and fast skeletal muscle fibres of the mouse. *Journal of Neurological Sciences*, 14, 37–45.

Düring, M. v. (1967) Uber die Feinstruktur der motorischen Endplatte von höheren Wirbeltieren. *Zeitschrift für Zellforschung und mikroskopische Anatomie*, 81, 74–90.

Edström, L. and Kugelberg, E. (1968) Histochemical composition, distribution of fibres and fatiguability of single motor units: Anterior tibial muscle of the rat. *Journal of Neurology, Neurosurgery and Psychiatry*, 31, 424–433.

Fambrough, D. M. (1970) Acetylcholine sensitivity of muscle fiber membranes: Mechanism of regulation by motoneurons. *Science*, 168, 372–373.

Fambrough, D. M. and Rash, J. E. (1971) Development of acetylcholine sensitivity during myogenesis. *Developmental Biology*, 26, 55–68.

Fambrough, D. M. and Hartzell, H. C. (1972) Acetylcholine receptors: Number and distribution at neuromuscular junctions in rat diaphragm. *Science*, 176, 189–191.

Fambrough, D. M., Hartzell, H. C., Powell, J. A., Rash, J. E. and Joseph, N. (1974) On the differentiation and organization of the surface membrane of a post-synaptic cell – the skeletal muscle fiber. In *Synaptic Transmission and Neuronal Interaction* (ed.) M. L. V. Bennett. Raven Press: New York. 285–314.

Fardeau, M. (1973) Caractéristiques cytochimiques et ultrastructurales des différents types de fibres musculaires Squelettiques extra-fusales (chez l'Homme et quelques Mammifères). *Annales D'Anatomie Pathologique (Paris)*, 18, 7–34.

Fernand, V. S. V. and Hess, A. (1969) The occurence, structure and innervation of slow and twitch muscle fibres in the tensor tympani and stapedius of the cat. *Journal of Physiology, (London)*, 200, 547–554.

Filogamo, G. and Gabella, G. (1967) The development of neuromuscular correlations, in vertebrates. *Archives de Biologie (Liège)*, 78, 9–60.

Fischbach, G. G. (1972) Synapse formation between dissociated nerve and muscle cells in low density cell cultures. *Developmental Biology,* 28, 407–429.

Friend, D. S. and Farquhar, M. G. (1967) Functions of coated vesicles during protein absorption in the rat vas deferens. *Journal of Cell Biology,* 35, 357–376.

Gauthier, G. F. (1969) On the relationship of ultrastructural and cytochemical features to color in mammalian skeletal muscle. *Zeitschrift für Zellforschung und mikroskopische Anatomie,* 95, 462–482.

Gauthier, G. F. (1970) The ultrastructure of three fiber types in mammalian skeletal muscle. In *The Physiology and Biochemistry of Muscle as a Food,* Vol. 2 (eds) E. J. Briskey, R. G. Cassens and B. B. Marsh, pp. 103–130. The University of Wisconsin Press: Madison.

Gauthier, G. F. (1971) The structural and cytochemical hetero-geneity of mammalian skeletal muscle fibers. In *Contractility of Muscle Cells and Related Processes* (ed.) R. J. Podolsky, pp. 131–150. Prentice-Hall: Englewood Cliffs.

Gauthier, G. F. and Padykula, H. A. (1966) Cytological studies of fiber types in skeletal muscle. A comparative study of the mammalian diaphragm. *Journal of Cell Biology,* 28, 333–354.

Gauthier, G. F. and Dunn, R. A. (1973) Ultrastructural and cytochemical features of mammalian skeletal muscle fibres following denervation. *Journal of Cell Science,* 12, 525–547.

Gauthier, G. F. and Schaeffer, S. F. (1974) Ultrastructural and cytochemical manifestations of protein synthesis in the peripheral sarcoplasm of denervated and newborn skeletal muscle fibres. *Journal of Cell Science,* 143, 113–137.

Ginetsinskii, A. G. and Shamarina, N. M. (1942) The tonomotor phenomenon in denervated muscle. *Uspekhi Sovremennoi Biologii* 15, 283–294. Translation number RTS 1710, Department of Scientific and Industrial Research, Lending Library Unit, London.

Gruber. H. (1966) Die Grössenbeziehung von Muskelfaservolumen und Fläche der motorischen Endplatte bei verschiedenen Skeletmuskeln der Ratte. *Acta anatomica.* 64, 628–633.

Guth, L., Samaha, F. J. and Albers, R. W. (1970) The neural regulation of some phenotypic differences between the fiber types of mammalian skeletal muscle. *Experimental Neurology,* 26, 126–135.

Hall, Z. W. (1972) Release of neurotransmitters and their interaction with receptors. *Annual Review of Biochemistry,* 41, 925–952.

Hall, Z. W. (1973) Multiple forms of acetylcholinesterase and their distribution in endplate and non-endplate regions of rat diaphragm muscle. *Journal of Nuerobiology,* 4, 343–361.

Hall, Z. W. and Kelly, R. B.(1971) Enzymatic detachment of endplate acetylcholinesterase from muscle. *Nature New Biology,* 232, 62.

Harris, J. B. and Thesleff, S. (1972) Nerve stump length and membrane changes in denervated skeletal muscle. *Nature New Biology,* 236, 60–61.

Hartzell, H. C. and Fambrough, D. M. (1972) Acetycholine receptors: Distribution and extrajunctional density in rat diaphragm after denervation correlated with acetylcholine sensitivity. *Journal of General Physiology,* 60, 248–262.

Heuser, J. E. and Reese, T. S. (1973) Evidence for recycling of synaptic vesicle membrane during transmitter release at the frog neuromuscular junction. *Journal of Cell Biology,* 57, 315–344.

Hirano, H. (1967) Ultrastructural study on the morphogenesis of the neuromuscular junction in the skeletal muscle of the chick. *Zeitschrift für Zellforschung und mikroskopische Anatomie,* 79, 198–208.

Hofmann, W. W. abd Thesleff, S. (1972) Studies on the trophic influence of nerve on skeletal muscle. *European Journal of Pharmacology,* 20, 256–260.

Holtzer, H. (1970) Proliferative and quantel cell cycles in the differentiation of muscle, cartilage, and red blood cells. In *Control Mechanisms in the Expression of Cellular Phenotypes,* Symposia of the International Society for Cell Biology, (ed.) H. A. Padykula, Vol 9 pp. 69–88. Academic Press: New York.

Holtzman, E., Freeman, A. R. and Kashner, L. A. (1971) Stimulation-dependent alterations in peroxidase uptake at lobster neuromuscular junctions. *Science,* 173, 733–736.

Holtzman, E., Teichberg, S., Abrahams, S. J., Citkowitz, E., Crain, S. M., Kawai, N. and Peterson, E. R. (1973) Notes on synaptic vesicles and related structures, endoplasmic reticulum, lysosomes and peroxisomes in nervous tissue and the adrenal medulla. *Journal of Histochemistry and Cytochemistry*, **21**, 349–385.

Hsu, L. and Lentz, T. L. (1972) Effect of colchicine on the fine structure of the neuromuscular junction. *Zeitschrift für Zellforschung und mikroskopische Anatomie*, **135**, 439–448.

Katz, B. (1966) *Nerve, Muscle, and Synapse* (ed.) Wald, G: McGraw-Hill: New York.

Kelly, A. M. and Zacks, S. I. (1969a) The histogenesis of rat intercostal muscle. *Journal of Cell Biology*, **42**, 135–153.

Kelly, A. M. and Zacks, S. I. (1969b) The fine structure of motor endplate morphogenesis. *Journal of Cell Biology*, **42**, 154–169.

Korneliussen, H. (1972a) Ultrastructure of normal and stimulated motor endplates, with comments on the origin and fate of synaptic vesicles. *Zeitschrift für Zellforschung und mikroskopische Anatomie*, **130**, 28–57.

Korneliussen, H. (1972b) Elongated profiles of synaptic vesicles in motor endplates. Morphological effects of fixative variations. *Journal of Neurocytology*, **1**, 279–296.

Korneliussen, H. and Waerhaug, O. (1973) Three morphological types of motor nerve terminals in the rat diaphragm, and their possible innervation of different muscle fiber types. *Zeitschrift für Anatomie und Entwicklungsgeschichte*, **140**, 73–84.

Kugelberg, E. and Edström, L. (1968) Differential histochemical effects of muscle contractions on phosphorylase and glycogen in various types of fibres: Relation to fatigue. *Journal of Neurology, Neurosurgery and Psychiatry*, **31**, 415–423.

Lentz, T. L. (1969) Development of the neuromuscular junction. I. Cytological and cytochemical studies on the neuromuscular junction of differentiating muscle in the regenerating limb of the newt *Triturus*. *Journal of Cell Biology*, **42**, 431–443.

Lentz, T. L. (1972) Development of the neuromuscular junction. III. Degeneration of motor end plates after denervation and maintenance in vitro by nerve explants. *Journal of Cell Biology*, **55**, 93–103.

Lømo, T. and Rosenthal, J. (1972) Control of ACh sensitivity by muscle activity in the rat. *Journal of Physiology, (London)*, **221**, 493–513.

Lüllmann-Rauch, R. (1971) The regeneration of neuromuscular junctions during spontaneous re-innervation of the rat diaphragm. *Zeitschrift für Zellforschung und mikroskopische Anatomie*, **121**, 593–603.

Mayr, R., Stockinger, L. and Zenker, W. (1966) elektronenmikroskopische Untersuchungen an unterschiedlich innervierten Muskelfasern der äusseren Augenmuskulatur des Rhesusaffen. *Zeitschrift für Zellforschung und mikroskopische Anatomie*, **75**, 434–452.

McMahan, U. J., Spitzer, N. C. and Peper, K. (1972) Visual identification of nerve terminals in living isolated skeletal muscle. *Proceedings of the Royal Society of London (Series B)*, **181**, 421–430.

Miledi, R. (1960) The acetylcholine sensitivity of frog muscle fibres after complete or partial denervation. *Journal of Physiology, (London)*, **151**, 1–23.

Miledi, R. and Slater, C. R. (1968) Electrophysiology and electron-microscopy of rat neuromuscular junctions after nerve degeneration. *Proceedings of the Royal Society of London (Series B)*, **169**, 289–306.

Miledi, R. and Slater, C. R. (1970) On the degeneration of rat neuromuscular junctions after nerve section. *Journal of Physiology, (London)*, **207**, 507–528.

Miledi, R. and Stefani, E. (1970) Miniature potentials in denervated slow muscle fibres of the frog. *Journal of Physiology (London)*, **209**, 179–186.

Miledi, R. and Potter, L. T. (1971) Acetylcholine receptors in muscle fibres. *Nature*, **233**, 599–603.

Mommaerts, W. F. H. M., Buller, A. J. and Seraydarian, K. (1969) The modification of some biochemical properties of muscle by cross-innervation. *Proceedings of the National Academy of Sciences, U.S.A.* **64**, 128–133.

Mumenthaler, M. and Engel, W. K. (1961) Cytological localization of cholinesterase in developing chick embryo skeletal muscle. *Acta anatomica*, **47**, 274–299.

Murata, F. and Ogata, T. (1969) The ultrastructure of neuromuscular junctions of human red, white and intermediate striated muscle fibers. *Tohoku Journal of Experimental Medicine*, **99**, 289–301.

Nickel, E. (1966) Die Ultrastruktur der motorischen Endplatte. *Bulletin der Schweizerischen Akademie der medizinischen Wissenschaften*, 22, 433–442.

Nickel, E. and Waser, P. G. (1968) Elektronenmikroskipische Untersuchungen am Diaphragma der Maus nach einseitiger Phrenikotomie. I. Die degenerierende motorische Endplatte. *Zeitschrift für Zellforschung und mikroskopische Anatomie*, 88, 278–296.

Nyström, B. (1968) Postnatal development of motor nerve terminals in 'slow-red' and 'fast-white' cat muscles. *Acta Neurologica Scandinavica*, 44, 363–383.

O'Brien, R. D., Eldefrawi, M. E. and Eldefrawi, A. T. (1972) Isolation of acetycholine receptors. *Annual Review of Pharmacology*, 12, 19–34.

Ogata, T., Hondo, T. and Seito, T. (1967) An electron microscopic study on differences in the fine structures of motor endplate in red, white and intermediate muscle fibers of rat intercostal muscle. A preliminary study. *Acta Medicinae Okayama*, 21, 327–338.

Padykula, H. A. and Gauthier, G. F. (1970) The ultrastructure of the neuromuscular junctions of mammalian red, white, and intermediate skeletal muscle fibers. *Journal of Cell Biology*, 46, 27–41.

Page, S. G. (1965) A comparison of the fine structures of frog slow and twitch muscle fibres. *Journal of Cell biology*, 26, 477–497.

Palade, G. E. (1954) Electron microscope observations of interneuronal and neuromuscular synapses. *Anatomical Record*, 118, 335–336.

Palay, S. L. (1965) Synapses in the central nervous system. *Journal of Biophysical and Biochemical Cytology*, 2, Supplement 193–201.

Palay, S. L. (1958) The morphology of synapses in the central nervous system. *Experimental Cell Research*, Suppl. 5, 275–293.

Peters, A., Palay, S. L., Webster, H. De F. (1970) *The Fine Structure of The Nervous System*. Harper & Row: New York.

Peterson, E. R. and Crain, S. M. (1970) Innervation in cultures of fetal rodent skeletal muscle by organotypic explants of spinal cord from different animals. *Zeitschrift für Zellforschung und mikroskopische Anatomie*, 106, 1–21.

Peterson, E. R. and Crain, S. M. (1972) Regeneration and innervation of adult mammalian skeletal muscle coupled with fetal rodent spinal cord. *Experimental Neurology*, 36, 136–159.

Pilar, G. and Hess, A. (1966) Differences in internal structure and nerve terminals of the slow and twitch muscle fibers in the cat superior oblique. *Anatomical Record*, 154, 243–252.

Prewitt, M. A. and Salafsky, B. (1967) Effect of cross innervation on biochemical characteristics of skeletal muscles. *American Journal of Physiology*, 213, 295–300.

Prewitt, M. A. and Salafsky, B. (1970) Enzymic and histochemical changes in fast and slow twitch muscles after cross innervation. *American Journal of Physiology*, 218, 69–74.

Reger, J. F. (1954) Electron microscopy of the motor end-plate in intercostal muscle of the rat, *Anatomical Record*, 118, 344.

Reger, J. F. (1955) Electron microscopy of the motor end-plate in rat intercostal muscle. *Anatomical Record*, 122, 1–15.

Reger, J. F. (1957) The ultrastructure of normal and denervated neuromuscular synapses in mouse gastrocnemius muscle. *Experimental Cell Research*, 12, 662–665.

Reger, J. F. (1958) The fine structure of neuromuscular synapses of gastrocnemii from mouse and frog. *Anatomical Record*, 130, 7–23.

Reger, J. F. (1969) Studies on the fine structure of normal and denervated neuromuscular junctions from mouse gastrocnemius. *Journal of Ultrastructure Research*, 2, 269–282.

Robbins, N., Karpati, G. and Engel, W. K. (1969) Histochemical and contractile properties in the cross-innervated guinea pig soleus muscle. *Archives of Neurology*, 20, 318–329.

Robertson, J. D. (1954) Electron microscope observations on a reptilian nyoneural junction. *Anatomical Record*, 118, 346.

Robertson, J. D. (1956) The ultrastructure of a reptilian myoneural junction. *Journal of Biophysical and Biochemical Cytology*, 2, 381–393.

Rogers, A. W. and Barnard, E. A. (1969) Quantitative studies on enzymes in structures in striated muscles by labeled inhibitor methods. II. Confirmation of radioautographic measurements by liquid-scintillation counting. *Journal of Cell Biology*, 41, 686–695.

Rogers, A. W., Darzynkiewicz, Z., Salpeter, M. M., Ostrowski, K. and Barnard, E. A. (1969) Quantitative studies on enzymes in structures in striated muscles by labeled inhibitor methods. I. The number of acetylcholinesterase molecules and of other DFP-reactive sites at motor endplates, measured by radioautography. *Journal of Cell Biology,* **41,** 665–685.

Romanul, F. C. A. and Van der Meulen, J. P. (1967) Slow and fast muscles after cross innervation. Enzymatic and physiological changes. *Archives of Neurology,* **17,** 387–402.

Rosenbluth, J. (1972) Myoneural junctions of two ultrastructurally distinct types in earthworm body wall muscle. *Journal of Cell Biology,* **54,** 566–579.

Rosenbluth, J. (1973) Membrane specialization at an insect myoneural junction. *Journal of Cell Biology,* 143–149.

Salpeter, M. M. (1967) Electron microscope radioautography as a quantitative tool in enzyme cytochemistry. I. The distribution of acetylcholinesterase at motor end plates of a vertebrate twitch muscle. *Journal of Cell Biology,* **32,** 379–389.

Salpeter, M. M. (1969) Electron microscope radioautography as a quatitative tool in enzyme cytochemistry. II. The distribution of DFP-reactive sites at motor endplates of a vertebrate twitch muscle. *Journal of Cell Biology,* **42,** 122–134.

Salpeter, M. M., Plattner, H. and Rogers, A. W. (1972) Quantitative assay of esterases in end plates of mouse diaphragm by electron microscope autoradiography. *Journal of Histochemistry and Cytochemistry,* **20,** 1059–1068.

Samaha, F. J., Guth, L. and Albers, R. W. (1970) The neural regulation of gene expression in the muscle cell. *Experimental Neurology,* **27,** 276–282.

Schwarzacher, H. G. (1957) Zur Lage der motorischen Endplatten in den Skelettmuskeln. *Acta anatomica,* **30,** 758–774.

Tchiriew, S. (1879) Sur les terminaisons nerveuses dans les muscles striés. *Archives de Physiologie, Paris* **2,** 89–116.

Teräväinen, H. (1968a) Carboxylic esterases in developing myoneural junctions of rat striated muscle. *Histochemie* **12,** 307–315.

Teräväinen, H. (1968b) Development of the myoneural junction in the rat. *Zeitschrift für Zellforschung und mikroskopische Anatomie,* **87,** 249–265.

Teräväinen, H. (1968c) Electron microscopic and histochemical observations on different types of nerve endings in the extraocular muscles of the rat. *Zeitschrift für Zellforschung und mikroskopische Anatomie,* **90,** 372–388.

Thesleff, S. (1974) Physiological effects of denervation of muscle. *Annals of the New York Academy of Sciences,* **228,** 89–104.

Tiegs, O. W. (1953) Innervation of voluntary muscle. *Physiological Reviews,* **33,** 90–144.

Tilney, L. G. (1971) Origin and continuity of microtubules. In *Origin and Continuity of Cell Organelles,* pp. 222–260. Springer-Verlag: New York.

Vogel, Z., Sytkowski, A. J. and Nirenberg, M. W. (1972) Acetylcholine receptors of muscle grown in vitro. *Proceedings of the National Academy of Sciences U.S.A.,* **69,** 3180–3184.

Zacks, S. I. (1964) *The Motor Endplate.* W. B. Saunders: Philadelphia.

Zacks, S. I. and Blumberg, J. M. (1961) Observations on the fine structure and cytochemistry of mouse and human inter-costal neuromuscular junctions. *Journal of Biophysical and Biochemical Cytology,* **10,** 517–528.

Zacks, S. I. and Saito, A. (1969) Uptake of exogenous horse-radish peroxidase by coated vesicles in mouse neuromuscular junctions. *Journal of Histochemistry and Cytochemistry,* **17,** 161–170.

Zacks, S. I. and Saito, A. (1970) Direct connections between the T system and the subneural apparatus in mouse neuromuscular junctions demonstrated by lanthanum. *Journal of Histochemisty and Cytochemistry,* **18,** 302–304.

Zelená, J. and Szentágothai, J. (1957) Verlagerung der Lokalisation spezifischer Cholinesterase während der Entwicklung der Muskelinnervation. *Acta histochemica, Jena,* **3,** 284–296.

Zenker, W. and Anzenbacher, H. (1964) On the different forms of myo-neural junction in two types of muscle fiber from the external ocular muscles of the Rhesus monkey. *Journal of Cellular and Comparative Physiology,* **63,** 273–285.

10 THE MOTOR END-PLATE: FUNCTION

A.J. Buller

10.1 Introduction

The characteristic activity of the neuron is the initiation and propagation of the nerve impulse, the characteristic activity of muscle is contraction. The motor end-plate, the junctional region of a motor nerve terminal and a muscle fibre, is designed so that nerve impulses passing down the motor nerve may bring about a contractile response in the muscle. As has been clearly stated in other parts of this volume the propagation of a nerve impulse depends upon the spread of local currents ahead of the region of active nerve. These local currents flowing outward through the inactive nerve membrane produce a degree of depolarization which, when sufficiently intense, results in those permeability changes which are characteristic of the nerve impulse. It is also known that the contractile activity of skeletal muscle is, under normal conditions, initiated by a sufficiently intense depolarization of the muscle cell's membrane. This depolarization produces an increase in the calcium ion concentration within the sarcoplasm, which brings about the interaction between the primary contractile proteins and results in muscle shortening and/or tension development. At the end of the depolarization, calcium ions are removed from the environment of the contractile proteins and the muscle reverts to a state of rest.

Since the nerve impulse is preceded along its nerve fibre by a region of depolarization it might be imagined that when an excitatory motor nerve terminal came into very close approximation with a muscle fibre the local currents generated by the nerve impulse would penetrate not only the nerve membrane but also that of the muscle fibre, thereby producing sufficient depolarization to trigger the contractile machinery. However, such is not the case. The structural discontinuity between the nerve and muscle fibres, together with the typically very much larger diameter of the latter, renders the junctional region a most unsuitable situation for direct electrical communication from nerve to muscle. It may be noted in passing however that the converse is not necessarily true. There are a number of references in the literature (for example Brown and Matthews, 1960) which strongly suggest that under certain conditions the action potentials of large diameter, skeletal muscle fibres may initiate impulses in small intramuscular nerve fibres.

If forward transmission from nerve to muscle does not occur as a direct result of electrical events how is it achieved? There is now overwhelming evidence that neuro-muscular transmission is achieved by a chemical mediator, and that the sequence of events at an excitor neuromuscular synapse is first, the propagation of the nerve impulse into the terminal nervous elements of the myo-neural junction; second, the release from the nerve terminals of a quantity of chemical transmitter; third, the diffusion of the transmitter across the synaptic cleft to that specialized part of the muscle fibre membrane underlying the nerve terminals, and fourth, a resultant depolarization of that membrane which either directly or indirectly results in muscle contraction.

It is the purpose of this chapter to review briefly current knowledge concerning the mechanisms underlying the sequence of events outlined above. Much of what will emerge originates from the work of Bernard Katz and his colleagues, who have dominated this field of investigation for over twenty years. Nevertheless, as so often occurs in research, the trail blazed by one worker attracts many others, and it is hoped that their contributions are also made apparent. Readers requiring a recent but more detailed review of this field are referred to that by Hubbard (1973).

10.2 Types of myoneural junctions

It has been indicated in the previous chapter that the morphology of motor end-plates can show considerable variation. This is also true of their physiology. Terminations of post-ganglionic fibres belonging to the autonomic nervous system may come into proximity with either cardiac or smooth muscle cells, and by the liberation of chemical transmitters modify the intrinsic activity of those cells. However, in these cases specialized junctional areas are not typically seen and the term motor end-plate is not used. However, even if consideration is confined to the junctional regions which occur between motor nerves and skeletal muscle there is wide variation in both form and function.

In some invertebrates skeletal muscle may be supplied not only by excitatory motor nerve fibres which when active cause depolarization of the muscle fibres they innervate thereby producing contraction, but also by less numerous inhibitory motor nerve fibres. When these inhibitory fibres are active alone they may produce a small hyperpolarization of the muscle fibre membrane, but no mechanical response. However when contraction is occurring in response to activity in the excitatory fibres activation of the inhibitory motor fibres decreases the extent of muscle fibre depolarization and thereby reduces the strength of contraction. Such interaction between excitatory and inhibitory motor nerve fibres innervating skeletal muscle has been studied most extensively in the crab (see for example Hoyle 1957). However definite end-plate structures are typically absent from crustacean muscles, so that sub-vertebrate skeletal muscle will not be further considered in this review.

The motor innervation of vertebrate skeletal muscle is invariably excitatory, and the neuromuscular junctions clearly discernable. Nevertheless vertebrate muscle is certainly not homogeneous, and two broad groups of muscle fibres may be identified, the slow fibres and the twitch fibres. Single slow muscle fibres recieve many motor nerve terminals along their entire length. In some slow muscle fibres all of the junctional regions are supplied by the same motor neuron, whilst in other slow muscle fibres different junctions may be innervated by different motor neurons. In either case a nerve impulse reaching a single nerve ending gives rise, via a chemical transmitter, to a localized, non-propagated depolarization of the muscle fibre membrane. this depolarization in turn produces a contractile response which is confined to the region immediately surrounding the nerve ending (Kuffler and Vaughan Williams, 1953 a,b). Contractile activity occurring under an increasing number of myoneural junctions along the length of a single muscle fibre increases the isometric force developed by the fibre.

In contrast, a single twitch muscle fibre is typically innervated at only one junctional region, though very long muscle fibres may show two widely separated nerve endings, both being supplied by the same motorneuron. Under normal conditions a single motor nerve impulse reaching the nerve terminal innervating a twitch muscle fibre causes a release of chemical transmitter that results in a depolarization of the underlying junctional membrane, but, unlike the situation in slow muscle, this depolarization initiates in the adjacent muscle fibre membrane a propagated electrical wave (the muscle action potential) which, travelling outwards in both directions from the junctional region is responsible for turning on the underlying contractile machinery as it passes. The contraction following a single motor nerve impulse is known as the twitch response.

While the sequence of transmitter release and muscle depolarization are qualitatively similar in slow and twitch muscle fibres the reason why no propagated action potential occurs in the former is not understood. It has been stated in the previous chapter that recent ultrastructural studies have tentatively identified ion channels, possibly the macromolecule which forms the sodium channel. Miledi, Stefani, and Steinbach (1971) have suggested that the motor axons innervating slow muscle release a substance (independent of the chemical transmitter) which represses the production of sodium channels by the muscle fibres thereby preventing the initiation of an action potential. This hypothesis, which has recieved some recent support from experiments on slow muscle fibres poisoned by botulinum toxin (Miledi and Spitzer, 1974), suggests that the neuromuscular junction may subserve 'trophic' functions which are independent of neuromuscular transmission, a topic to which a return will be made in Section 10.6.

Within the vertebrate kingdom there are, between species, many minor differences to be found both in the organization of slow fibres and twitch fibres, and Chapter 9 draws attention to some of the morphological differences which may be observed between end-plates of the different types of twitch muscle found within the same mammal.

In closing this section it may be noted that while slow muscle fibres are widely distributed in the frog (Kuffler and Vaughan Williams, 1953b), in the mammal they have only been identified in some of the muscles innervated by cranial nerves. The limb muscles of mammals consist entirely of twitch fibres.

10.3 Chemical transmission

The first experimental evidence that neuromuscular transmission at the vertebrate motor end-plate was due to the release of a chemical substance was provided by the classical experiments of Dale and his colleagues (see Dale, Feldberg and Vogt, 1936). In a series of experiments they demonstrated that stimulation of the motor nerve supplying a skeletal muscle which was being perfused with eserinized Locke solution led to the appearance of acetycholine (ACh) in the perfusate leaving the muscle. It was necessary to add eserine to the perfusing fluid in order to avoid the destruction of ACh, which is normally rapidly hydrolysed by cholinesterase (AChE) following its release. Many control experiments were necessary to substantiate the suggestion that the ACh was released from the nerve terminals and not the contracting muscle; they included curarization of the animal which prevented muscle contraction but not the appearance of ACh in the perfusate, and the direct stimulation of chronically denervated muscle which failed to produce any ACh. In a separate series of experiments (Brown, Dale and Feldberg, 1936) it was demonstrated that a small rapid intra-arterial injection of ACh very close to the end-plate region of a muscle produced a contraction similar to, but not identical with, the twitch response of that muscle.

10.3.1 General

These experiments strongly suggested ACh as the chemical transmitter at the vertebrate skeletal muscle end-plate, and acted as an incentive to the study of chemical transmission at synapses within the central nervous system. Since that time much effort has been made to elucidate the nature of the various central nervous system neurotransmitters, and many chemical candidates have been suggested. Whilst by no means all of these suggestions have been favourably received, it is now agreed that to qualify for serious consideration as a chemical transmitter a proposed substance must satisfy certain criteria. These requirements include:

    1. That it can be manufactured by the pre-synaptic cell,

    2. That its release, in a quantity sufficient to produce the normally observed post-synaptic effects, can be provoked by a nerve impulse in the presynaptic fibre,

    3. That its direct application to the post-synaptic cell can mimic the effect of pre-synaptic activity, and

    4. That a mechanism exists to remove the transmitter from the environment once it has completed its action.

Many further requirements are argued by some workers, including the identity of interaction between other drugs and the artificially prepared candidate and the interaction of the same drugs with the naturally released transmitter.

The experiments of Dale *et al.*, gave the first indications that the second and third conditions stated above might be met by ACh as the neuromuscular junction. Furthermore, the fourth condition seemed to be satisfied since it was necessary to add eserine to the fluid perfusing the muscle in order to prevent the destruction of ACh. The great volume of work that has been undertaken on vertebrate neuromuscular transmission since the 1930's has been concerned with the detailed examination of whether ACh completely satisfies the criteria set out above, and with the study of both the mechanism by which it is released from the pre-synaptic membrane and its action on the postsynaptic membrane. It is of some interest that the study of the neuromuscular junction has, at each stage, preceded the elucidation of the mechanisms of synaptic action within the central nervous system.

10.3.2 *Transmitter manufacture*

It is now universally accepted that ACh may be synthesized in both the cell body and the axon of the vertebrate motorneuron, but that manufacture is most active at the motor nerve terminals. It is this part of the motor-neuron that the essential enzyme choline-acetyltransferase (ChAc) is in highest concentration. It is also generally conceded, though on indirect evidence, that the major part of the ACh contained within the motor nerve terminals is concentrated inside the numerous vesicles, to which extensive reference has been made in Chapter 9. Hence there are three questions to be answered, how is the ACh synthesized, how are the vesicles formed and how does the Ach become concentrated within these structures?

The enzyme ChAc is present in the axoplasm. The substance acetyl-CoA is a product of the numerous mitochondria found in motor nerve terminals. Choline is the other factor which must be reacted with acetyl-CoA, under the catalylic influence of ChAc, in order to produce cytoplasmic ACh. Choline is obtained from outside the nerve terminals and is transported across the membrane by an active process that can be blocked by the hemicholinium group of drugs. Once inside the nerve endings choline is converted to ACh by the reaction outlined above, the level of intracellular choline thereby being kept low.

The cytoplasmic ACh so formed is however at risk, since esterases also exist in the axoplasm. It is possibly to protect the ACh from destruction that the vesicular packaging is necessary.

Our understanding of the life cycle of a vesicle owes much to the studies of Heuser (see Heuser and Reese, 1972). The formation of a vesicle is believed to occur as follows. An area of the surface membrane of a nerve terminal becomes invaginated and fractures into the cytoplasm (endocytosis). Such fractures always occur at regions of the membrane which are some distance from the sites of ACh release. The detached surface membrane then forms a 'complex' vesicle, so named because, unlike the synaptic vesicle, it is surrounded by an additional outer shell. The nature of this shell is not known. Complex vesicles fuse to form cisternae from which the synaptic vesicles are derived by a process of budding. It is at this stage that the vesicles accumulate ACh from the surrounding cytoplasm, but the method by which this is achieved is not yet clear. If it is assumed that each 50 nm vesicle concentrates ACh within itself to an isosmotic level it would come to contain some thousands of molecules of ACh. Once the vesicle discharges its contents into the synaptic cleft the vesicular membrane fuses with the surface membrane of the nerve terminal and the cycle is repeated.

It is apparent that, at rest, the motor nerve terminal contains the biochemical machinery to manufacture ACh, a relatively low contration of cytoplasmic ACh and a large number of vesicles each containing some thousands of molecules of ACh. However, it appears that, at any instant, not all of these vesicles have an equal probability of releasing their contents into the synaptic cleft. This is probably saying no more than that some vesicles are lying close to release sites on the surface membrane, towards which they may be rapidly moved by Brownian motion, while others are more distant. Nevertheless it has become customary to describe the total population of vesicles as the 'releasable store' and to divide this into 'available' store (for rapid release) and 'depot' store.

10.4 Transmitter release

The early experiments of Dale and his colleagues on ACh release from the motor nerve terminals of the cat have already been alluded to. Since that time more accurate estimates of the amount of acetylcholine released at each end-plate per nerve impulse have been made, for example by Krnjević and Mitchell (1961) using the rat diaphragm. Their calculations yielded a figure of approximately 5×10^6 molecules. From the figure quoted above for the ACh content of a single vesicle it is immediately apparent that a single nerve impulse must cause the discharge of many vesicles. However, even the most accurate measurements from this type of perfusion experiment cannot provide the detailed information desirable for a complete understanding of the mechanism of transmitter release.

It is at times like this that the wise physiologist pays heed to the old adage attributed to A. V. Hill, 'If you want to solve a problem in biology, first choose the most suitable preparation'. Readers of Chapter 9 will already have been impressed by the morphological complexity of the mammalian end-plate. In contrast the structure of some amphibian neuromuscular junctions is relatively simple. In particular the myoneural junctions on the under surface of the sartorius muscle of the frog offer access to relatively long lengths ($>100 \ \mu m$) of terminal, unmyelinated nerve axon lying in their synaptic grooves. The recent application of Normanski interference microscopy to this preparation (McMahan, Spitzer and Pepper, 1972) has made possible even closer control of the experimental situation. Much of what will now be reported concerning the events of neuromuscular transmission were first demonstrated using this biological preparation. However, it is perhaps wise to pause briefly and enquire if it is proper to use knowledge acquired from the study of one vertebrate preparation (the frog satorius) to extrapolate to another (mammalian) preparation. Katz (1969), in his lucid Sherrington Lecture, drew attention to the fact that the neuromuscular junction of the frog is not strictly speaking an end-plate, which term should be reserved for the compact plate-like structures seen for example in mammals and lizards. However there are undoubtedly great similarities between the events occurring at the frog neuromuscular junction and the mammalian end-plate. Where direct functional comparisons have proved experimentally possible no fundamental differences have been observed. This fact, coupled with the much simpler structure of the frog motor endings, makes the latter preparation the one of choice for the experimentalist. Addtionally the frog neuromuscular junction is often referred to an an end-plate. This common practice will be followed in the remainder of the present chapter.

10.4.1 *Quantal release*

At the present time there is no technique which allows the direct observation of transmitter release from a nerve terminal. However advantage can be taken of the fact that the end-plate region of a normally innervated skeletal muscle fibre is exquisitely sensitive to ACh. Before motor innervation occurs (Diamond and Miledi, 1962), or some time after the motor nerve has been cut (Axelsson and Thesleff, 1957) every part of the entire length of a vertebrate muscle fibre responds to the local application of ACh by a local depolarization. Following innervation or re-innervation the major part of the muscle fibre effectively loses all sensitivity to ACh, but the end-plate region retains, or even increases, its responsiveness to focal application of the drug. While there are minor differences between the responsiveness of the extrajunctional regions of different types of innervated muscle fibres (e.g. between fast-twitch and slow-twitch), and there is also a tendency for all myotendious junctions to retain some sensitivity to ACh these responses are attributed to extrinsic ACh receptors which respond somewhat differently from those at the end-plate. The maximum sensitivity which is exhibited by every innervated fibre at its motor end-plate is attributed to intrinsic ACh receptors. Recent experiments, in which the ionophoretic application of ACh chloride from a micropipette placed on the surface of a muscle fibre has been performed under direct observation using Normanski optics (Peper and McMahan 1972), have demonstrated that the region of maximum sensitivity to ACh lies within the grooves of the post-synaptic membrane which contain the terminal motor axons. Moving the tip of the micropipette only 10 μm laterally from a groove, while retaining it on the surface of the muscle fibre, greatly reduced the depolarization resulting from a pulse of ACh.

Using the ionophoresis technique to apply very localized doses to ACh to the post-synaptic membrane, detailed studies have been made both of the absolute sensitivity of the post-synaptic membrane (Miledi, 1961), and also of the changes produced in the response to ACh following the prior application of additional drugs (e.g. del Castillo and Katz, 1957). In the latter case it has been shown that prior application of curarine decreases the depolarization produced by ACh (presumably by a process of competative inhibition) while the application of cholinesterase inhibitors, such as eserine, neostigmine or edrophonium, greatly potentiates the effects of ACh. Cholinesterase (AChE), which has the capability of splitting ACh into choline and acetic acid, is known to be present in high concentration immediately below the postsynaptic membrane where its presence may be demonstrated by a well-established histochemical technique (Couteax, 1955). These studies of the responsiveness of the post-synaptic membrane to ACh, whether applied alone or in the presence of another drug, invite a comparison with the responses produced by the release of the natural neuromuscular transmitter.

Since the observation of Fatt and Katz (1950, 1952) it has been shown that even when a skeletal muscle fibre is mechanically completely at rest there are still small, infrequent (1–3/second) depolarizations occurring on the post-synaptic side of the end-plate. Such potentials are limited to the immediate vicinity of each myoneural junction and cannot be recorded from elesewhere along the length of the muscle fibre. Each transient depolarization is known as a miniature end-plate potential (min EPP). That these potentials are predominantly due to the presence of the motor nerve terminals is apparent from their almost complete disappearance following degeneration of the motor nerve (Birks, Katz and Miledi, 1960). The very rare minEPPs (Schwann minEPPs) which may still occur following nerve section are assumed to come from the terminal Schwann cells which may invade the synaptic grooves after the disintegration of the motor axons. Recording with an intracellular microelectrode positioned at the end-plate region Fatt and Katz noted that the great majority of the miniature potentials from normally innervated muscle were of a very similar amplitude, and that the occasional exceptions tended to be either twice or more rarely three times as large. They also noted that the application of curarine reduced the size of the spontaneous potentials, while prostigmine increased both their size and duration. It was also observed that the application of botulinum toxin, which is known to reduce the release of ACh from nerve terminals (Brooks, 1956) caused a reduction in the frequency of miniature end-plate potentials. More recently Boroff, del Castillo, Evoy and Steinhardt (1974) have suggested that Type A botulinum toxin acts by preventing the concentration of axoplasmic ACh within the nerve terminal vesicles (see Section 10.3.2).

Miledi's (1961) ionophoretic studies have demonstrated that in order to produce a postsynaptic depolarization comparable in amplitude and duration to a single miniature end-plate potential approximately 10^5 molecules of ACh have to be applied to an end-plate gutter. Smaller depolarizations could be produced with lesser amounts of ACh, but only recently have potential fluctuations attributable to the action of single molecules of ACh been reported (Katz and Miledi, 1972). These authors suggest that the 'shot' depolarization of the post-synaptic membrane caused by a single molecule of ACh is approximately a thousand times smaller than a single minEPP, though they stress the many assumptions and approximations used in reaching this conclusion.

These two series of experiments on the minEPP and ionophoretic application of ACh strongly support both the hypothesis that ACh is the natural transmitter (since the pharmacological effects of curarine and prostigmine are similar in the two cases) and the suggestion that the natural transmitter is commonly released in multimolecular amounts. It was suggested in 10.3.2 that each vesicle might well accumulate several thousand molecules of ACh, and it seems very probable that each miniature end-plate potential results from the chance emptying of a single vesicle into the synaptic cleft. It is clear that there is still considerable uncertainty about the number of molecules of ACh contained in a single quantal packet. Miledi's ionophoretic studies (1961) (which are likely to give an over-estimate) suggest 10^5, Krnjević and Mitchell's collection studies suggest approximately 5×10^4, consideration of the dimensions of the vesicles and their internal concentration of ACh suggest perhaps 10^4 while the studies of Katz and Miledi (1972) on the post-synaptic responses to single molecules of ACh suggest that only 10^3 reacting molecules are necessary to produce a minEPP. Although the evidence connecting the vesicles with the minEPPs is indirect it is sufficiently convincing for Eccles (1973) to have written 'If electronmicroscopy hadn't revealed the existance of vesicles ... the prepackaging of transmitter would still have to be postulated with the additional proviso that for some reason you couldn't see the packages!' The assumption that vesicular release can occur does not preclude the chance liberation of individual molecules of ACh from the axoplasm of the nerve terminals. However all the evidence suggests that any such loss could represent only a very small fraction of the total spontaneous ACh release.

Since the packets of ACh released appeared to be similar in size Katz chose to call them quanta, a decision he defends in his 1969 monograph. It has been generally agreed that, to a first approximation, the spontaneous quantal release is a random process, there being at any instant a low probability of any one of the many vesicle contained within the terminal nerve arborization liberating its contents into the synaptic cleft. The occasional appearance of spontaneous postsynaptic dipolarizations having double, or, less frequently, treble the size of unitary minEPPs has been explained by assuming the simultaneous release of two or three quanta, the frequency of such events being approximately matched by Poisson theory. Slow changes in the probability of release have been observed, together with 'bursts' of miniature end-plate potentials, but the physiological significance, if any, of such occurrences is not known. Recently the goodness of fit between the minEPP pattern and a Poisson process has been examined in detail by Hubbard and Jones (1973) and by Cohen, Kita and van der Kloot (1974). Both groups agree that the fit of their experimental data by a single Poisson model is unsatisfactory. Hubbard and Jones explain their departure from simple Poisson expectation by assuming that there are only a finite number of sites from which the release of ACh quanta can occur. Cohen, Kita and van der Kloot, who also used external minEPP recording (see below), examined a number of alternate mathematical systems in an attempt to match their data and obtained the best fit with a branching Poisson model. Such a model would infer that quantal release from a single site would temporarily render that site more likely to discharge further vesicles, but this expectation has not yet been experimentally verified (but see Barrett, Barrett, Martin and Rahaminoff, 1974). It is not yet clearly established whether vesicles can discharge their ACh from any part of the terminal nerve membrane or whether there are a limited number of specialized release sites, the latter view seems to be gaining ground, both from electron microscopical and physiological studies.

10.4.2 *Multiquantal release*

The mean rate of quantal release may be greatly increased by depolarizing the terminal nerve axon (del Castillo and Katz, 1954). This observation suggested that a nerve impulse invading the axon might also release ACh, and such has proved to be the case. However in order to investigate in detail the effects of physiological activity in the nerve terminals different techniques have had to be used. A microelectrode inserted into a muscle fibre at its motor end-plate records all the depolarizations which occur anywhere within the territory of that myoneural junction. This is because the relatively high impedance of the muscle cell permits any potential change produced at one site to spread over several hundreds of micrometres with only small decrement (hence the similar sizes of the unitary depolarizations; for further explanation see Katz, 1966). A method that has now been extensively used by Katz and Miledi (1965a,b,c) involves the use of extracellular recording microelectrodes placed as close as possible to the terminal nerve axons. By using two such electrodes separated by a conduction distance of approximately 50 μm it can be shown that the nerve action potential is propagated to the most distant parts of the terminal arborization. The conduction velocity of the small diameter nonmyelinated nerve terminals is about 40 cms^{-1} (at 24°C) as compared with a velocity of approximately 30 ms^{-1} for the large diameter myelinated parent axon. The use of extracellular microelectrodes greatly increases the spatial resolution of recording, restricting pickup to a distance of only some 10 μm from the electrode. By recording from active sites of the nerve membrane, not only may the nerve impulse be recorded but also, following the release of ACh, the potential change occurring as a result of current flow into the post-synaptic membrane.

Under normal conditions the arrival of a single motor nerve impulse at a vertebrate neuromuscular junction is followed by a muscle potential which, in turn, produces muscle contraction. This sequence of events provides two problems of an investigator using microelectrodes. In the first place the initiation of an action potential complicates the recording of the end-plate potential, and secondly the inevitable movement caused by the contracting muscle is likely to displace, if not break, the microelectrode. In order to overcome these problems, curare, which has been known to block neuromuscular transmission since the time of Claude Bernard, is often introduced into the solution bothing the preparation. As has been stated above curarine (a purified curare) has the pharmacological effect of reducing the depolarizing effect of ACh on the post-synaptic membrane, whilst, in low concentration, having a negligible effect on both its manufacture and pre-synaptic release. By reducing the post-synaptic response to ACh the initiation of an action potential and the resultant muscle contraction may both be avoided.

It is now universally agreed that the depolarization of the nerve membrane which occurs during its action potential greatly increases the probability of quantal release of ACh into the synaptic cleft, and that the resultant post-synaptic depolarization, the end-plate potential (EPP), is caused by the approximately simultaneous release of ACh from many synaptic vesicles. However in order for ACh release to occur following a nerve impulse calcium ions must be present in the fluid surrounding the nerve terminal. Also magnesium ions, which have an antagonistic action to that of Ca^{2+} and therefore an inhibiting effect on ACh release, must not be present in excess. Indeed it is possible to decrease the amount of ACh released following a single nerve impulse either by decreasing (Ca^{2+}), increasing (Mg^{2+}) or a combination of both. It is a point of some interest that whereas there must be calcium present in the extracellular fluid if ACh is to be released following a nerve action potential, external calcium does not appear to be necessary for the production of minEPPs. This may be explained by supposing that the low concentration of free calcium ions within the axoplasm is adequate to permit the infrequent release of single quanta, but that an external store of calcium is necessary for multiquantal release. The studies of Katz and Miledi (1965a,b,c) have done much to clarify the mode of calcium action. By ingenious experiments involving the focal ionophoresis of Ca^{2+} they have demonstrated that the external ions must be present during the depolarization if transmitter release is to occur, and also that it is the depolarization of the presynaptic membrane that is important rather than the nerve action potential *per se*. The latter point was demonstrated by blocking nervous transmission with tetrodotoxin (TTX) which specifically impairs sodium ion channels, and applying to the nerve terminal depolarising pulses which, in the presence of external calcium, proved adequate to cause the release of ACh. A further observation made during this important series of experiments was a delay between the depolarization of the nerve terminal (whether produced by an action potential or artificially) and the depolarization of the postsynaptic membrane which signalled the effective action of the released ACh. Even at a single recording site this delay could vary between 0.5

and 2.5 ms. Putting all these observations together it seems likely that, under normal conditions, an action potential invading the end-plate produces a transient opening of calcium channels in the nerve membrane that must be independent of the sodium channels. Calcium ions move into the axoplasm along the concentration gradient and then react either with the inside of the nerve membrane, or with the vesicles, or both, thereby increasing the probability of quantal release. The variable delay before release suggests that some specific configuration has to be achieved. While the exact stochiometry is not known it seems that two to four calcium ions must enter for each quantum of ACh released.

If the number of quanta released per nerve impulse is greatly reduced either by lowering the external (Ca^{2+}) or raising external (Mg^{2+}) so that any resultant EPP is small, the distribution of the number of quanta released per impulse (including failures, when the impulse fails to achieve any release) may be satisfactorily fitted by a Poisson distribution (Boyd and Martin, 1956). However, as with spontaneous quantal release (10.4.1 above) the goodness of fit is more apparent than real. If EPPs resulting from the release of many quanta are examined it is said that binomial rather than Poisson statistics apply (Rahamimoff quoted by Hubbard, 1973).

10.5 Postsynaptic events

The sensitivity of the end-plate postsynaptic membrane to ACh, to which frequent reference has been made above, is due to the presence in that membrane of intrinsic acetylcholine receptors. The nature of these receptors is not known but they are probably proteolipid, and they are believed to lie adjacent to the molecules of the enzyme cholinesterase (AChE). By the use of αBungarotoxin (αBgt), which is believed to bind specifically to ACh receptors, the number of receptors at a single frog neuromuscular junction has been estimated as 10^9 (Miledi and Potter 1971). It is the combination of a molecule of ACh with one of the ACh receptors that is the fundamental event in initiating post-synaptic activity.

10.5.1 *Miniature end-plate potentials*

The release of the contents of a single vesicle into the synaptic cleft places some thousands of molecules of acetylcholine approximately 50 nm away from the postsynaptic membrane. Some of the molecules escape from the cleft by diffusion, some come directly into contact with AChE molecules and are immediately inactivated, whilst the remainder initially combine with ACh receptors and only subsequently either become split by AChE or escape by diffusion (Katz and Miledi, 1973). It is with this last group of ACh molecules that we are now concerned. The ACh/receptor combination is probably a reversible two step reaction, the second stage leading to a conformational change in the receptor that opens ion channels. The analysis of 'ACh noise' or 'shot effects' (the individual depolarizations produced by single ACh/receptor combinations, Katz and Miledi, 1973) suggests that individual ion gates are opened for 1–1.5 ms, and that during this time there is an inward current due to a net influx of ions. The work of Takeuchi and Takeuchi (1960) has shown that during ACh/receptor combination the permeability to both sodium ions and potassium ions at the end-plate is raised rapidly and simultaneously to about the same extent. At the resting end-plate the equilibrium potential for sodium is approximately +50 mV and that for potassium approximately −95 mV. During ACh/receptor combination the resultant permeability changes briefly alter the equilibrium potential towards −15 mM. The elemental conductance change, each due to the interaction between a single molecule of ACh and an ACh receptor, occur in parallel and sum linearly. However, the resultant potential change across the membrane is not the sum of the elemental potential changes but a non-linear (hyperbolic) summation of the individual events (see Martin, 1955). The extent of the individual depolarizations has been estimated to be 0.3 μV, while the amplitude of a single miniature end-plate potential recorded under comparable conditions is approximately 0.4 mV (Katz and Miledi, 1972). Because of the non-linear addition of potential changes mentioned above this suggests that something in excess of 1000 ion gates are opened as a result of the release of a single quantum of ACh.

Compared with the current pulse which causes it, (the miniature end-plate current or minEPC), the minEPP has a slower rising phase and a slower decline, having a total duration of approximately 20 ms. This slower time course is determined by the membrane time constant.

10.5.2 *End-plate potential*

The end-plate potential is the potential change across the post-synaptic membrane resulting from the multiquantal release of ACh which follows the invasion of the motor nerve terminals by an action potential. As in the previous section where it was shown that the minEPP is the summed result of many individual ACh/receptor events, so the EPP is the summed result of many quantal releases. While the permeability changes of the end-plate membrane occur in parallel the individual potential changes resulting from these alterations of conductance do not sum linearly, and each succeeding minEPP exerts a smaller depolarization effect the closer the end-plate membrane approaches its equilibrium potential of −15 mV. While the existance of a potential at the end-plate clearly discernable from the muscle action potential has been known for many years (Eccles and O'Connor, 1939) the intracellular investigation of the EPP awaited the work of Fatt and Katz (1951). These authors measured both the time course of the EPP, which is similar to that of the minEPP described above, and the decrement with distance from the end-plate. They observed that the EPP spread, decrementally, some 1–2 mm from the end-plate region. When the EPP was not reduced in amplitude by the use of curarine the electric response at the end-plate following nerve stimulation showed an initial large (40 mV) brief end-plate step, followed by a spike potential which showed only a small overshoot and a pronounced hump on its descending phase. If the potential change at the end-plate was recorded following direct stimulation of the muscle fibre instead of following indirect stimulation of the motor nerve it much more closely resembled that of a normal muscle action potential, including a considerably larger overshoot. These observation, together with additional evidence obtained later, suggest that the synchronous release of many quanta of ACh produces a depolarization of the post-synaptic end-plate membrane (the EPP) which is sufficiently intense to activate depolarization dependent sodium and potassium ion channels which are separate and distinct from the ion channels associated with the ACh receptors. The end-plate region then attempts to contain both a 40 mV amplitude end-plate potential, the time course of which is determined by the opening of the ACh sensitive ion channels, and an action potential that is determined by sequential changes in the depolarization dependent sodium and potassium channels. The complex potential recorded at the active end-plate is the resultant of the concomitant events.

10.5.3 *Muscle action potential*

An active end-plate potential can only occupy that length of post-synaptic membrane that contains both intrinsic ACh receptors and is subjected to a sufficient dose of ACh. However, by local current spread the active end-plate region can critically depolarize the adjacent muscle fibre membrane, thereby initiating a normal muscle action potential. The permeability changes which give rise to the muscle potential, together with its method of propagation, are analagous to those described elesewhere in this volume for the nerve action potential. The much slower conduction velocity of muscle fibres, compared with nerve fibres, in spite of their large diameter, is due to the different values of membrane constants, and in particular the large value of the muscle's transverse membrane capacity.

10.6 Non transmitter action between nerve and muscle

Brief reference has already been made to the posibility that the motor end-plate may play a role in communication between nerve and muscle which is independent of acetylcholine. It has been known for many years that a skeletal muscle deprived of its motor innervation undergoes changes which include a diffuse hypersensitivity of the muscle fibre membrane to ACh, the appearance of spontaneous fibrillation potentials, slowing of the mechanical twitch speed and wasting. Such changes have often been attributed to the abscence of 'trophic' (unidentified) factors which, under conditions of normal innervation, pass from the motor nerve to the muscle. The observations of Buller, Eccles and Eccles

(1960) that a skeletal muscle's motorneuron determined its speed of contraction appeared to lend further support to the concept of neural 'trophic' factors. While, at this time, the existance of one or more 'trophic' factors cannot be ruled out (Miledi and Spitzer, 1974) there is as yet no positive indentification of any 'chemical messenger' other than ACh. On the other hand there is increasing evidence that the pattern and/or the total number of motor nerve impulses reaching a muscle can exert considerable influence on such characteristics as the ACh sensitivity of its muscle fibres (Lømo and Rosenthal, 1972) and the contractile proteins it manufactures (Stréter, Gergely, Salmons and Romanul, 1973). Only further work will determine whether ACh is the sole messenger at the vertebrate neuromuscular junction, or whether it is but one part of a more complicated system of neuromuscular interactions.

10.7 Summary and conclusions

This brief statement of the physiology of the neuromuscular junction is far from complete. The description of events has intentionally been kept essentially qualitative. The reader requiring more quantitative data is referred to the original papers which have been quoted. Many questions remain unanswered. For example, by what method is the ACh concentrated within the vesicles; where does Ca^{2+} act in order to bring about vesicular discharge; how many sites exist for the discharge of presynaptic vesicles and where are they situated; what is the exact configuration and nature of the post-synaptic ACh receptor. These and many other problems will be solved only by the continuation of the considerable effort that has been made to understand the functioning of the neuromuscular junction over the last twenty-five years, and by the elaboration of new methods to facilitate our study of this subtle structure.

References

Axelsson, J. and Thesleff, S. (1957) A study of supersensitivity in denervated mammalian skeletal muscle. *Journal of Physiology,* 149, 178—193.
Barrett, Ellen F., Barrett, J. N., Martin, A. R. and Rahamimoff, R. (1974) A note on the interaction of spontaneous and evoked release at the frog neuromuscular junction. *Journal of Physiology,* 237, 453—463.
Birks, R., Katz, B. and Miledi, R. (1960) Physiological and structural changes at the amphibian myoneural junction in the course of nerve degeneration. *Journal of Physiology,* 150, 145—168.
Boroff, D. A., del Castillo, J., Evoy, W. H. and Steinhardt, R. A. (1974) Observations on the action of type A botulinum toxin on frog neuromuscular junctions. *Journal of Physiology,* 240, 227—253.
Boyd, I. A. and Martin, A. R. (1956) The end-plate potential in mammalian muscle. *Journal of Physiology,* 132, 74—91.
Brooks, V. B. (1956) An intracellular study of the action of repetitive nerve volleys and of botulinum toxin on miniature end-plate potentials. *Journal of Physiology,* 134, 264—277.
Brooks, G. L., Dale, H. H. and Feldberg, W. (1936) Reactions of the normal mammalian muscle to acetylcholine and eserine. *Journal of Physiology,* 87, 394—424.

Brown, M. C. and Matthews, P. B. C. (1960) The effect on a muscle twitch of the back-response of its motor nerve fibres. *Journal of Physiology,* **150**, 332–346.

Buller, A. J., Eccles, J. C. and Eccles Rosamund, M. (1960) Interactions between motorneurones and muscles in respect of the characteristic speeds of their responses. *Journal of Physiology,* **150**, 417–439.

Cohen, Ira., Kita, H. and van der Kloot, W. (1974) The stochastic properties of spontaneous quantal release of transmitter at the frog neuromuscular junction. *Journal of Physiology,* **236**, 341–361.

Couteaux, R. (1955) Localization of cholinesterases at neuromuscular junctions. *International Review of Cytology,* **4**, 335–375.

Dale, H. H., Feldberg, W. and Vogt, M. (1936) Release of acetylcholine at voluntary motor nerve endings. *Journal of Physiology,* **86**, 353–380.

del Castillo, J. and Katz, B. *Proceedings of the Royal Society of London Series B,* **146**, 357–361.

Diamond, J. and Miledi, R. (1962) A study of foetal and new-born rat muscle fibres. *Journal of Physiology,* **162**, 393–408.

Eccles, J. C. (1973) The understanding of the brain. McGraw-Hill: New York.

Eccles, J. C. and O'Connor, W. J. (1939) Responses which nerve impulses evoke in mammalian striated muscles. *Journal of Physiology,* **97**, 44–102.

Fatt, P. and Katz, B. (1950) Some observations on biological noise. *Nature,* **166**, 597–598.

Fatt, P. and Katz, B. (1951) Analysis of the end-plate potential recorded with an intracellular electrode. *Journal of Physiology,* **115**, 320–370.

Fatt, P. and Katz, B. (1952) Spontaneous subthreshold activity at motor nerve endings. *Journal of Physiology,* **117**, 109–128.

Heuser, J. E. and Reese, T. S. (1973) Evidence for the recycling of synaptic vesicle membrane during transmitter release at the frog neuromuscular junction. *Journal of Cell Biology,* **57**, 315–344.

Hoyle, G. (1957) Comparative physiology of the nervous control of muscular contraction. Cambridge Monographs in Experimental Biology No. 8, Cambridge University Press.

Hubbard, J. I. (1973) Microphysiology of Vertebrate Neuromuscular transmission. *Physiological Reviews,* **53**, 674–723.

Hubbard, J. I. and Jones, S. F. (1973) Spontaneous quantal transmitter release: a statistical analysis and some implications. *Journal of Physiology,* **232**, 1–21.

Katz, B. (1956) Nerve, muscle and synapse. McGraw-Hill: New York.

Katz, B. (1969) The release of neural transmitter substances. The Sherrington lectures X Liverpool University Press.

Katz, B. and Miledi, R. (1965a) Propagation of electric activity in motor nerve terminals. *Proceedings of the Royal Society of London (Series B),* **161**, 453–482.

Katz, B, and Miledi, R. (1965b) The measurement of synaptic delay, and the time course of acetylcholine release at the neuromuscular junction. *Proceedings of the Royal Society of London Series B,* **161**, 483–495.

Katz, B. and Miledi, R. (1965c) The effect of calcium on acetylcholine release from motor nerve terminals. *Proceedings of the Royal Society of London (Series B),* **161**, 496–503.

Katz, B. and Miledi, R. (1972) The statistical nature of the acetylcholine potential and its molecular components. *Journal of Physiology,* **224**, 665–699.

Katz, B. and Miledi, R. (1973) The binding of acetylcholine to receptors and its removal from the synaptic cleft. *Journal of Physiology,* **231**, 549–574.

Krnjević, K, and Mitchell, J. F. (1961) The release of acetylcholine in the isolated rat diaphragm. *Journal of Physiology,* **155**, 246–262.

Kuffler, S. W. and Vaughan Williams, E. M. (1953a) Small-nerve junctional potentials. The distribution of small motor nerves to frog skeletal muscle and the membrane characteristics of the fibres they innervate. *Journal of Physiology,* **121**, 289–317.

Kuffler, S. W. and Vaughan Williams, E. M. (1953b) Properties of the 'slow' skeletal muscle fibres of the frog. *Journal of Physiology,* **121**, 318–340.

Lømo, T. and Rosenthal, J. (1972) Control of ACh sensitivity by muscle activity in the rat. *Journal of Physiology,* **221**, 493–513.

Martin, A. R. (1955) A study of the statistical composition of the end-plate potential. *Journal of Physiology,* **130**, 114–122.

McMahan, U. J., Spitzer, N. C. and Peper, K. (1972) Visual identification of nerve terminals in living isolated skeletal muscle. *Proceedings of the Royal Society of London (Series B),* **181**, 421–430.

Miledi, R. (1961) From nerve to muscle. *Discovery,* **22**, 442–450.

Miledi, R., Stefani, E. and Steinbach, A. B. (1971) Induction of the action potential mechanism in slow muscle fibres of the frog. *Journal of Physiology,* **217**, 737–754.

Miledi, R. and Potter, L. T. (1971) Acetylcholine receptors in muscle fibres. *Nature,* **233**, 599–603.

Miledi, R. and Spitzer, N. C. (1974) Absence of action potentials in frog slow muscle fibres paralysed by Botulinum toxin. *Journal of Physiology,* **241**, 183–199.

Peper, K, and McMahan, V. J. (1972) Distribution of acetylcholine receptors in the vicinity of nerve terminals on skeletal muscle of the frog. *Proceedings of the Royal Society of London (Series B),* **181**, 431–440.

Stréter, F. A., Gergely, J., Salmons, S. and Romanul, F. (1973) Synthesis by fast muscle of myosin light chains characteristic of slow muscle in response to long-term stimulation. *Nature New Biology,* **241**, 17.

Takeuchi, A. and Takeuchi, N. (1960) On the permeability of end-plate membrane during the action of transmitter. *Journal of Physiology,* **154**, 52–67.

11 THE CHEMISTRY AND STRUCTURE OF MYELIN

N.A. Gregson

11.1 Introduction

The myelin sheath of the myelinated nerve fibre occupies a central position in the theory of saltatory conduction, the now generally accepted theory which describes and explains the observed phenomena of nerve impulse conduction in this type of fibre (Lillie, 1925; Huxley and Stampfli, 1949; Frankenhauser, 1952; Hodgkin, 1964). The role of the sheath is to provide a high capacitance insulator, an important but essentially passive role. Its significance in the integrated behaviour of the nervous system is, however, recognisable in those pathologies involving demyelination or dysmyelination.

The myelin sheath has been recognized as a morphological entity in the mammalian nervous system since the nineteenth century (Virchow, 1854) and reasonable deductions had been made concerning its gross composition and structure by 1940 (Schmitt and Bear, 1939). The much more detailed knowledge added since has not required major alterations to these early conclusions.

For some time the myelin sheath was the source of much of the information used in discussing the structural generalities of biological membranes (Robertson, 1959), but of late it has fallen out of favour in this respect (Stoeckinius and Engleman, 1969; Singer, 1971), since it is now considered that in fulfilling its uniquely passive role it has become a 'minimal membrane'.

Myelin, although it may be considered to represent a membrane having few active functional attributes, in fact represents a high degree of specialization, and is found only in the vertebrates above the level of the jawless fishes. Thus its appearance, in evolution, was concomitant with that of the more advanced vertebrate nervous system. It represents a problem in ontogeny — the regulated production of a specialized membraneous organelle by one cell type which complements the functional activities of another cell type; and also in phylogeny, viz. the evolutionary emergence and significance of such a specialized structure.

It is intended here to examine the myelin sheath primarily from the point of view of its possible molecular structure, and how this may correlate with its postulated physiological role in the nerve fibre and its experimentally observed properties and activities.

Before attempting to discuss what is known of the composition and fine structure of myelin it is necessary to make some remarks about its gross structure. The myelin sheath is segmented, the segments terminating at the nodes of Ranvier, with the bulk of each segment consisting of the compacted multilamellar structure generally considered to be typical of myelin. The compacted membrane extends between the specialized paranodal regions, and is interrupted by one or more discontinuities, the Schmidt—Lantermann incisures (Fig. 11.1). Thus, although compacted membrane provides the bulk of the sheath segment and presumably contributes the most to the bulk chemical data, these more specialized regions must not be neglected in the interpretation of results obtained by biochemical techniques. This caveat is of particular importance when dealing with metabolic data obtained from isolated myelin since the fate of these specialized regions during subcellular fractionation is unknown and there is no a priori reason to assume that the composition or structure of the myelin membrane is uniform through these regions.

Finally it is necessary to state that in producing this review, information has been drawn from work on central nervous system myelin as well as from that dealing with myelin of the peripheral nervous system, since in many areas the amount of information available on central nervous system derived myelin is considerably more extensive. Consequently it must be emphasized that great care is necessary when comparing peripheral and central myelin in view of their known differences in ultrastructure and composition, and their differing reactivities in pathological states, either experimentally induced or of natural occurrence.

11.1.1 *The physiological role of the myelin sheath*

The membrane theory of nerve conduction leads to the conclusion that conduction velocity should be a function of the axon diameter, as is indeed observed to be the case (Erlanger and Gasser, 1937). However, conduction velocity in myelinated vertebrate nerves is much higher than in non-myelinated nerves of similar or greater fibre diameter. Lillie (1925) proposed that conduction in myelinated fibres should be described as saltatory; i.e. the activity jumps from one node to the next without the active participation of the intermediate myelinated lengths of axon. According to this hypothesis the myelinated internodes behave like sections of co-axial cable and the nodes as generator segments. Over the myelinated internode ionic flow between the external medium and the axon is restricted and passive, 'current flow' occurring only between adjacent nodes. Thus, the potential developed at a node shows a diminishing decay along the adjacent internodes but ensures sufficient potential to activate the next node, most of the longitudinal current, or ionic flow, passing outside of the myelin sheath (Huxley and Stampfli, 1949). The myelinated axon shows some modifications in that there appears to be a contraction of ionic channels at the nodal region, resulting in a net influx of some 300 000 sodium ions per unit area over the duration of the action potential compared to 20 000

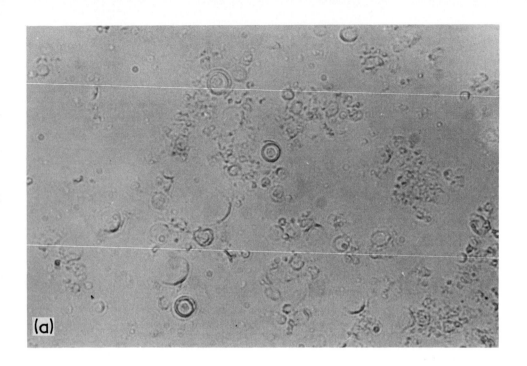

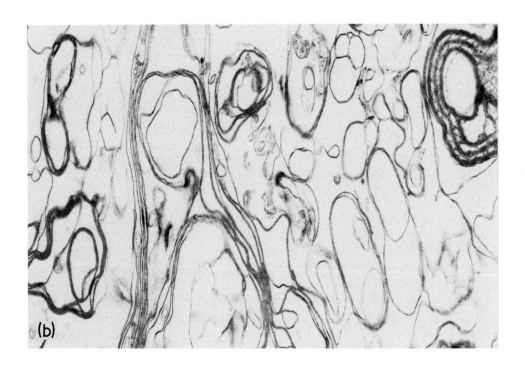

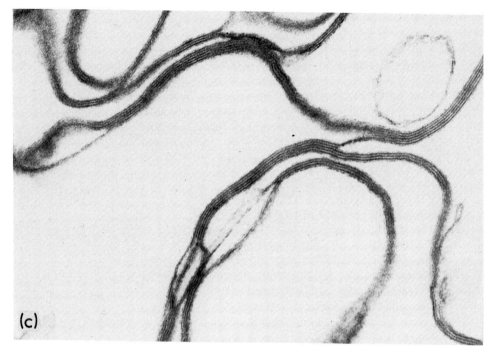

Fig. 11.1 *Appearance of isolated myelin*
(a) Fresh myelin fraction isolated from rabbit brain, suspended in distilled water, conventional light microscopy (× 850). Predominantly spherical vesicles, a few reasonably thick walled. (b) and (c) Myelin fraction fixed in glutaraldehyde. Electron microscopic appearance of sectioned material. (b) (× 22 500), appearance of concatenate of vesicles (c) (× 89 250), regions of compact myelin sheath showing some regions of normal electron microscope morphology and splitting of lamellae at the intraperiod line.

sodium ions per unit area in the non-myelinated axon (Hodgkin, 1964). Nonetheless the quantity of sodium ions passing into the axon during the passage of an impulse is less in the myelinated fibre than in non-myelinated fibre of similar diameter, and it is considered that this will result in a reduction in the energy flux. A suggested further consequence of myelination is that it restricts the interaction between adjacent fibres. Mutual interaction certainly can occur between non-myelinated fibres (Katz and Schmitt, 1940) and there is some indication of a similar phenomenon in myelinated nerve trunks (Rosenbluth, 1943).

There is evidence therefore to suggest that myelination increases conduction velocity and optimizes energy expenditure. Rushton (1951) pointed out that conduction velocity should be dependent upon the overall external diameter of the fibre-(D) and the dimensions of axon diameter (d) and internodal length (l) relative to the value of D. Numerous theoretical treatments since Rushton's paper have come to the same conclusion, i.e. for any given fibre the conduction velocity will be maximal when the ratio d/D lies between 0.6 and 0.7 (e.g. Hodgkin, 1964; Pickard, 1969; Smith and Koles, 1970). The internodal length, l, shows a relationship to D and to d, but nonetheless should have some optimum value to ensure the fastest conduction velocity with the greatest saving in the rate of energy expenditure. The morphological data from peripheral nerve fibres, relating the axon and total fibre diameters, shows considerable disagreement as to whether or not the value of d/D tends towards a constant value and as to its precise numerical value, (see Williams and Wendell-Smith, 1971). Undoubtedly, some of the discrepancies between the reported observations can be attributed to variations in both preparative techniques and the neglect of correction factors necessary in making the relevant measurements (Wendell-Smith and Williams, 1959; Williams and Wendell-Smith, 1971). However, the results of Williams and Wendell-Smith (1971) clearly indicate that the relationship d/D as a function of d varies with the nerve bundle studied and type of fibre it contains. Thus, although there may be a tendency for the value of d/D to reach a constant value of around 0.6 in the mature sural and gastrocnemius medalis nerves of the rabbit the same is not true for the dorsal and ventral roots, where d/D increases with the increasing values of D and approaches a constant of about 0.7. It would appear that the theory as it stands at present offers a reasonable generalized statement of the relationships between axon diameter, myelin sheath thickness and conduction velocity, but the published evidence suggests that although selection pressure may be directed towards maximising conduction velocity, this occurs within the restraints imposed by other mechanisms operating in the handling of information by the whole nervous system, a point stressed by Rushton but overlooked by many subsequent workers. The indicated relationships between axon diameter and the amount of myelin produced by the Schwann cell are also of general interest in connection with ideas concerning the mechanism of control of myelin synthesis during development. This point will be referred to later.

11.1.2 *The properties of the myelin sheath related to its suggested physiological role*

The properties of the sheath relative to its suggested physiological role in saltatory conduction can be considered in terms of (a) its overt structural form, and (b) its structural relationships as demonstrated indirectly by its electrical properties.

A basic requirement of the theory of saltatory conduction is that ionic current should pass from one node to the next external to the intervening internode. Thus, it is necessary that the gap of 15–50 nm between the inner aspect of the myelin sheath and the axolemma should not be open to the general extracellular fluid space. Ultrastructurally this space appears to be isolated by the presence of junctions between the paranodal loops and the axolemma (see

Table 11.1 Electrical characteristics of nerve

	Capacitance μF cm^{-2}		Resistance ohms cm^2	
	Internode	Node	Internode	Node
Tasaki (1965)	0.005	3.7	1×10^5	8−20
Huxley (1964)	0.0025	−	1.6×10^5	10−20

Chapter 1), which appear morphologically to be tight junctions (Robertson, 1960). The only other path open to ionic flow which has a morphological basis is the Schmitt−Lanterman incisure (see Chapter 1). Under normal *in vivo* conditions the incisure provides only a narrow spiral leading from the external mesaxon to the inner mesaxon (Hall and Williams, 1970). This space can be increased by a variety of physical and chemical insults to the fibre (Hall and Williams, 1970; Williams and Hall, 1971a). Expansion of the extracellular compartment of the incisures occurs largely by an extension of the separation of the intraperiod line into the adjacent regions of the internode and is within limits reversible (Hall and Williams, 1970). Generally there are between 12 and 20 incisures within an internode of 370 to 850 μm (Hiscoe, 1947). Thus, morphologically there may be two distinct types of spiral channel offering possible continuity between the extracellular compartment outside the internode and that between the myelin and the axolemma. Use has been made of electron dense tracers, lanthanum, ferritin and peroxidase, to demonstrate the extent of diffusional continuity, and it is concluded that the paranodal loops do restrict the diffusion of such markers from the nodal region (Hall and Williams, 1971). The results of such studies are discussed more fully in Chapter 1, but the results obtained using tracer molecules should be regarded with caution, for although they may indeed indicated diffusion channels they may also be even stronger indicators of non-specific binding sites, (e.g. Doggenweiler and Frank, 1965; Matter, Orci and Rouiller, 1969).

Singer (1968) has suggested, on the basis of autoradiographic studies, that free amino acids may be transported across the myelin sheath from the extracellular space to the axon. However, given the difficulty of precise localization inherent in electron microscopic autoradiographs, the exact route of this suggested transport system is difficult to define.

The electrical characteristics, of capacitance and resistance of a material or system are structurally dependent. Values for the internodal capacitance and resistance have been obtained for frog myelinated fibres (Huxley and Stampfli, 1949; Tasaki, 1955), and are within the range of 0.005 to 0.01 μF cm^{-2} and 0.1 to 0.16 megohms cm^2 respectively, (Table 11.1). These values when substituted into the model equations give predicted conduction velocities in agreement with those observed experimentally (Hodgkin, 1964; Pickard, 1969). Tasaki (1955)

517

Table 11.2 Calculations of capacitance and resistance of myelin unit lamella: Frog sciatic (1).

Fibre diameter	$12-15\ \mu$		
d/D	0.6	0.7	0.8
Sheath thickness	2.7	2.025	1.35 μm
Average no. lamella (2)	318	238	126
Capacitance $\mu F\ cm^{-2}$	1.47	1.19	0.63
Dielectric constant (3)	17.5	14.14	7.48
Resistance ohm cm^2	318	420	794

(1) Using internodal values of capacitance and resistance from Tasaki (1955), and with the assumption that the internode is only myelin sheath.
(2) Lamella thickness taken as 8.5 nm.
(3) Calculated from $C = D/411.d$. Where C is the capacitance in e.s.u. and d is the lamella thickness.

found that the progressive lysis of the internodal sheath with saponin initially produced a progressively increasing capacitance and falling resistance, in a manner compatible with a simple reduction of sheath thickness, indicating that the observed electrical characteristics were principally determined by the sheath.

It has been suggested that the myelin membrane has specialized characteristics which adapt it to its role as an insulator. The resistance and capacitance values found for the sheath reflect, (i) the thickness of the sheath and its compact nature, and (ii) the resistance and capacitance intrinsic to the single membrane unit of which the sheath is constructed. The values intrinsic to the single mambrane unit can be calculated, but the calculated values depend on the assessment of sheath thickness. Tasaki (1955) used a value of d/D of between 0.7–0.8 and calculated the dielectric constant of the myelin lamella to be in the range of 6–10 e.s.u. The calculated values for capacitance, dielectric constant and resistance for myelin lemellae are given in Table 11.2, as a function of various values of d/D. A comparison of the calculated data for the myelin lamella with values found for a variety of other cell membranes (Table 11.3) indicates that the capacitance is unlikely to be very different and, that therefore, the overall dielectric constant is also likely to be familiar. Since capacitance is largely dependent upon the organization and the nature of the molecules providing the structure, these observations might suggest that there is no major constitutive or structural divergence between myelin and other cell membranes. The resistance of myelin is, however, somewhat lower than that recorded for most other cell membranes, e.g. resting squid axon, erythrocyte, and resting Nitella, although higher than the values reported for the nodal axon membrane (Table 11.1) and the muscle sarcolemma (Table 11.3). This is rather surprising, since one might have suspected that the intrinsic myelin resistance would be higher than that of ordinary cell membranes if it has evolved as an 'insulator'. It is of interest to note that Tasaki (1955) found that the internodal resistance was

Table 11.3 Capacitance and resistance characteristics of cell membranes

Membrane	Capacitance μF cm^{-2}	Resistance ohm cm^2	Reference
Squid axon			
resting	1.1	1.5×10^3	Cole & Hodgkin, 1939
excited	1.1	25	Cole & Curtis, 1941
Erythrocyte, human	0.80		Fricke, 1931
ox, lysed	0.90	100	Schwann & Carstensen, 1957
Muscle, resting	1.5	40	Cole & Curtis, 1936
Pleuropneumonia-like			
organisms	1.3–1.4	–	Schwann & Morowitz, 1962
Rat liver mitochondria	0.5–0.6	–	Paully, Packer & Schwann: 1960
Guinea pig heart mitochondria			
unswollen	1.1	–	Paully & Packer: 1960
swollen	1.3	–	
Nitella			
resting	0.94	2.5×10^5	Cole & Curtis, 1937
active	0.80	5×10^2	Cole & Curtis, 1938

increased by immersion in hypertonic NaCl, or a reduction in temperature, and was decreased by 0.5% cocaine-Ringer, without any concomitant alteration in capacitance. It is possible that these results indicate the presence of a low resistance pathway through the sheath. The Schmitt–Lanterman incisure is known to be readily influenced by alterations in the external medium (Hall and Williams, 1970 and Chapter 1) and may provide the suggested low resistance pathway across the sheath.

The most common model system in use at the present time for the study of the behaviour of biological membranes is the black lipid membrane (BLM) prepared from purified phospholipid or lipid mixtures (Bangham, 1968). The observed capacitance for the phospholipid BLM ranges from 0.3 to 0.6 μF cm^{-2}, and Taylor and Haydon (1966) found a relationship between alkyl chain length and capacitance, indicating that in these model systems the capacitance was derived almost entirely from the hydrocarbon layer. Hanai, Haydon and Taylor (1965) showed that the capacitance could be increased by the inclusion of cholesterol and suggested that the addition of conducting polar pores parallel to the capacitance would cause the overall membrane capacitance to approach 1 μF cm^{-2}, a value closer to that of biological membranes. The resistance of the BLM system is more variable than the capacitance. The resistance found for the unmodified BLM is in the range of 10^8 to 10^9 ohm cm^2 and thus, the electrical properties of this type of model system may only resemble those of biological membranes as their structural homogeneity is reduced. The capacitance of two adhering BLMs is strictly additive, 0.19 μF cm^{-2} (Badzhinyan and Chailakhyan, 1971). Using a value for the single membrane thickness (d) of 6.0 to 9.0 nm, and a capacitance of 0.36 μF cm^{-2} then $e = 2.5$ to 3.7. For the double BLM with $d = 120$ to 180 nm then $e = 2.6$ to 3.8 indicating that the interacting polar regions do not generate a new capacitive layer and that the overall capacitance is still derived predominantly from the alkyl chains. The resistance, however, is not additive and actually decreases (Badzhinyan, Dunin-Barkovsky, Kovalev and Chailakhyan, 1971; viz 1.2×10^8 ohm cm^2 for the area of contact and 5.4×10^8 ohm cm^2 for the single BLM). Unfortunately nothing is known about the electrical impedance of biological membranes when they are brought into close contact, but if they were to behave like the BLM then this could possibly explain the rather low resistance calculated for the single myelin lamella. Alternatively the Schwann cell membrane may have a low inherent resistance, and this may necessitate the production of a series of compacted layers of membrane in order to produce a layer of high resistance.

Summary of Section 11.1

The suggested role of the myelin sheath is to achieve rapid impulse conduction at lower axon diameters and at lower rates of energy expenditure. The electrical resistance and capacitance of the sheath do not suggest that the membrane *per se* possesses any unique properties relating to its suggested physiological role, rather it is the compacted structure of the sheath which is significant.

11.2 The composition of myelin

The macrostructure of the myelin sheath is the consequence of the association of a number of different molecular species, the whole structure being readily dissociable by the action of organic solvents and a number of detergents, indicating that the different molecular species are associated by forces not involving direct covalent linkage. A knowledge of the chemical composition is essential before the molecular structure can be resolved.

11.2.1 *The gross composition of myelin*

The gross composition of myelin was deduced quite early, Schmitt, Bear and Palmer (1941) calculating from X-ray diffraction data that the weight ratio of lipid to protein in the myelin sheath was 4:1, with a minimum of 30% bound water.

The estimation of water content is difficult, and generally involves the measurement of some structural dependent parameter, such as X-ray diffraction spacing, as a function of hydration of the tissue. Schmitt, Bear and Palmer (1941) noted an irreversible change in X-ray diffraction spacing on drying peripheral nerve, and estimated the minimal amount of bound water to be 30% of the wet wt., from comparisons with lipid-water systems with varying water contents. Finean (1957) recorded weight loss and X-ray diffraction changes during slow drying of frog sciatic nerve, and concluded that the myelin contained some 40–50% water. He noted the presence of a smaller, apparently tightly bound, water fraction of 0.2 g/g dry wt., but he considered this pool to be too small to represent the total water of any major component, but rather to represent the tightly bound water associated with generally distributed hydrophilic groups. Later work (Finean, Coleman, Green and Limbrick, 1966) again utilizing X-ray diffraction with controlled drying, but using isolated central myelin, suggested a minimum water content of 30–40% of wet wt., the removal of this water causing irreversible changes in X-ray spacing. By comparison the bound water content determined for the red blood cell membrane was between 10–20%.

Ladbrooke, Jenkinson, Kamat and Chapman (1968), using differential scanning calorimetry (DSC), suggested that in isolated brain myelin there is approximately 0.25 g bound water per 1 g dry myelin. This water did not show normal ice formation at $0°C$, and no thermal transitions of the myelin lipids appeared until this fraction of water began to be removed. Gent, Grant and Tucker (1970), examined the high frequency dielectric dispersion characteristics of suspensions of crude brain myelin and concluded from the dielectric characteristics that bound water existed to the extent of 1 g per g dry wt.

Using tritium oxide and ^{14}C-glycerol, the estimate of the bound water fraction in isolated myelin is 28.5% of the wet wt. (Gregson, unpublished observations).

It seems from these results that the water associated with the myelin may be considered to occur in two pools, since the results, depending upon the criteria used for determining the critical point, indicate a pool of either 0.5 to 1.0 g/g dry wt. or a pool of not less than 0.25 g/g. The smaller pool may be presumed to represent the water tightly bound to ionic groups, carbohydrate residues, and peptide bonds, while the larger will include the secondarily adsorbed water.

The dry mass of central myelin appears to consist entirely of lipid and protein, and estimates of their proportions, based upon the analysis of isolated myelin, suggest that the protein accounts for between 20–30% of the total dry weight (Table 11.4). The analytical results available for peripheral nerve are rather limited but in general suggest the presence of a higher proportion of protein than is found in central myelin of the same species.

Estimation of the total protein content of myelin is not simple and three principal methods have been employed, viz. direct gravimetric analysis following lipid extraction (O'Brien, 1965; Wolfgram and Kotorii, 1968; Winder and Gent, 1970); colorimetric determination by the method of Lowry, Rosebrough, Farr

Table 11.4   Protein   content   of   CNS   and   PNS
myelin

	Protein content, g/100 g dry wt.	
	Bovine	Squirrel/Monkey
Brain	23.8 (1)	–
	24.8 (2)	
Spinal cord	25.3 (3)	20 (5)
Optic nerve	23.7 (1)	
Peripheral nerve	24.1 (4)	30 (5)
	28.0 (3)	
	19.0 (6)	

(1) MacBrinn and O'Brien, 1969
(2) Norton and Autilio, 1966
(3) Uyemura, Tobari, Hirano and Tsukada, 1972
(4) O'Brien, Sampson and Stern, 1967
(5) Horrocks, 1967
(6) Greenfield et al., 1973

and Randall (1951), (Norton and Autilio, 1966); and amino acid content (Hulcher, 1963; Wolfgram and Kotorii, 1968). The colorimetric assay suffers from not having the appropriate reference standard, i.e., the myelin proteins themselves, but the use of bovine serum albumin does not appear to introduce an excessively large error, (Lowry et al., 1951; Gent, Gregson, Lovelidge and Winder, 1973). The method using amino acid analysis is open to the problems and uncertainties of loss during hydrolysis as well as the requirement for expensive equipment. The gravimetric procedure is the most direct and should be the most suitable, but because of the nature of the proteins it is difficult to preclude some loss due to solubility in the organic solvents when there is concomitant total extraction of lipid. Some use has been made of ultraviolet absorbtion (Laatsch, Kies, Gordon and Alvord, 1962; Gent Gregson, Gammack and Raper, 1964; Cuzner, Davidson and Gregson, 1965b) but this method has been found to overestimate the protein because of absorbtion in the 210–220 nm region by lipids, and the considerable turbidity and forward scatter error (Gent, et al., 1973). However, the three major methods of estimation appear to agree reasonably well and are further supported by total nitrogen analyses (Wolfgram and Kotorii, 1968; Gent et al., 1973).

11.2.2 The isolation of myelin

More exact analyses of the myelin lipids and proteins have only really become feasible since the development of techniques for the isolation of reasonably large amounts of 'purified' myelin (Laatsch, Kies, Gordon and Alvord, 1962; Davison and Gregson, 1962; Hulcher, 1963; Autilio, Norton and Terry, 1964; Eichberg, Whittaker and Dawson, 1964). Several methods are now commonly used for the isolation of myelin, but the differences between the individual methods are quite small and all rely on the common observation that reasonably compacted myelin has a low flotation density and is found not to sediment in sucrose solutions of concentrations greater than twenty per cent (w/v).

The methods of isolation of central myelin have recently been reviewed (Spohn and Davison, 1972a). In general the methods involve the preparation of tissue suspensions in a 0.32 M sucrose solution and subsequent centrifugation against either 0.656 M (20.5% w/v) or 0.8 M (24.9% w/v) sucrose solutions. The myelin is isolated either by layering the crude particulate fraction containing myelin suspended in 0.32 M sucrose over the dense sucrose and sedimenting the non-myelin particles through the interface leaving the myelin at the interface (Autilio, Norton and Terry, 1964), or by suspending the crude fraction in the denser sucrose and floating the myelin up to the interface (Laatsch, Kies, Gordon and Alvord, 1962). Some authors have used linear gradients of sucrose for the isolation of myelin, and Thompson, Goodwin and Cummings (1967) described the isolation of myelin on linear gradients of caesium chloride. This method appears to yield a myelin fraction comparable to that obtained by the use of sucrose gradients and has been used for the further characterization of the myelin fraction (Morell, Greenfield, Costantino-Ceccarini and Wisniewski, 1972; Greenfield, Brostoff, Eylar and Morell, 1973).

Myelin has been isolated from suspensions of peripheral nerve tissue using the zonal rotor (London, 1972). Using this technique a single band of myelin was obtained from ox intradural root tissue which equilibrated at 15.2% (w/v) sucrose, whereas ox spinal cord produced three bands of myelin at 11%, 14% and 16% (w/v) sucrose. A similar result was obtained with brain suspensions by Day, McMillan, Mickey and Appel (1971). These methods for the isolation of myelin were developed using suspensions of central nervous system and they have been applied either directly or with slight modification to peripheral nervous tissue with reasonable success.

The major practical difficulty in working with the peripheral nervous tissue is that of obtaining an adequate suspension of the tissue. The presence of large amounts of collagen render normal homogenization procedures inefficient and result in a low yield of myelin (Horrocks, 1967). The collagen can be avoided by the use of intradural roots (O'Brien, Sampson and Stern, 1967; London, 1972), or reduced by initially stripping off the perineurium (e.g. Evans and Finean, 1965; Adams, Abdulla, Turner and Bayliss, 1968), the pre-incubation of slices of peripheral nerve in glycine-triethylamine buffer at pH 6.0 has been used to assist in the dispersion of the collagen (Adams et al., 1968). More recently the grinding of tissue frozen in liquid nitrogen has been found to produce a good tissue dispersion from which the myelin can be isolated by the usual procedures (Brostoff, Burnett, Lampert and Eylar, 1972; Greenfield, Brostoff, Eylar and Morell, 1973). The yield of myelin from sciatic nerve by this procedure is 3 to 5 g dry wt./100 g wt. of nerve (Greenfield et al., 1973).

The final stages in the purification of myelin fractions involve treating the isolated myelin with a large volume of water, to give a hypotonic 'shock' to the myelin and thus release trapped axonal contents. The myelin is then isolated from this aqueous suspension either by sedimentation (O'Brien, *et al.*, 1967) or by isolating again on a sucrose gradient (Horrocks, 1967). These procedures yield a final myelin fraction identifiable as such by electron microscopy and containing low levels of activity of enzymes usually associated with other cellular structures (Evans and Finean, 1965; Adams *et al.*, 1968; London, 1972).

11.2.3 *Properties of isolated myelin*

The flotation density of myelin has been determined in linear gradients of sucrose or caesium chloride, and has been found to differ in these two solutes. In sucrose gradients central myelin has been found to equilibrate at a mean density of $1.08 \, \text{g cm}^{-3}$ (rat, $-$ Norton, 1971b; and in the mouse, $-$ Gregson and Oxberry, 1972). Using zonal centrifugation Day *et al.*, (1971) and London (1972) have recorded much lower flotation densities, of 1.04 to $1.064 \, \text{g cm}^{-3}$, for myelinated axonal fragments. Rather shorter centrifugation times were used in these experiments and they do not relate to water shocked myelin. The flotation density of myelin in gradients of caesium chloride is greater than in sucrose gradients, giving a tight band of material at a density of $1.11 \, \text{g cm}^{-3}$ (Thompson, Goodwin and Cummings, 1967; Kornguth, Walberg, Anderson, Scott and Kubinski, 1967). The reasons for these differences are not known, although several explanations can be offered, e.g. effect of the differing solutes on the hydration of myelin (Norton, 1971a) and the fact that since the myelin particles are vesicular their flotation density will be an average of three compartments, the particle wall, the entrapped fluid interior and the hydration layer, and their fractional volumes, the density of the entrapped fluid depending on the permeability of the vesicle wall to the secondary solute.

Morphology

All published micrographs of isolated myelin, from both the peripheral and central nervous systems, indicate that the myelin has undergone breakage and resealing to produce spherical vesicles, and there is commonly extensive splitting of the intraperiod line and the formation of complex multivesicular forms (Fig. 11.1). However, some areas of compact myelin remain in which it is possible to distinguish the period and intraperiod lines. Examination in plane polarized light indicates the vesicles to have kept their birefringence (Fig. 11.1). Isolated myelin also shows the typical major X-ray diffraction pattern (Finean *et al.*, 1966). These results suggest that the molecular arrangement has not been greatly changed.

While it is not possible, to recognize in these preparations any fragments which, on morphological grounds, could be said to represent the incisural or paranodal regions, it is of interest to note that a 'myelin-like' fraction has been obtained from central and peripheral tissue (Agrawal, Banik, Bone, Davison, Mitchell and Spohn, 1970; London, 1972; Morell, Greenfield, Costantino-Ceccarini and Wisniewski, 1972), which is membrane material and has some similarity of composition with myelin.

11.2.4 *Protein composition of myelin*

Since the constituent proteins of membranes are characterized by an almost total insolubility in aqueous systems, the analysis and the investigation of their properties is rendered very difficult. The techniques which have been applied to the complete resolution of such protein mixture have involved the use of detergents, or solvents such as phenol, coupled with acrylamide gel disc electrophoresis. Using these techniques it is possible to show that the membranes of different organelles are characterized by different patterns of protein components (e.g. Cotman and Mahler, 1967; Agrawal, Banik *et al.*, 1970; Agrawal *et al.*, 1972; Gurd, Mahler and Moore, 1972). However, such procedures dissociate the protein and lipid, and since these proteins normally function in association with lipid, isolation in this fashion renders functional studies either impossible, or at least very difficult.

Before discussing peripheral nerve myelin, the protein composition of central myelin will be described since this has been more intensely investigated, and provides a basis for comparison with peripheral myelin.

Before the use of phenol or sodium dodecylsulphate to give complete solubilization of the myelin proteins prior to acrylamide gel electrophoresis, the proteins of myelin had been fractionated by differential solvent extraction and fractionation. Using these methods, three major proteins had been described in central myelin, viz. proteolipid protein, soluble in chloroform methanol (Folch and Lees, 1951); basic protein extractable by dilute mineral acid (Laatsch, Kies, Gordon and Alvord, 1962), and the Wolfgram protein extractable by acidified chloroform methanol (Wolfgram, 1966). The estimation of these protein fractions by extraction methods is restricted since the resolution is limited by the production of protein fractions, which may themselves contain one or more components, e.g. the basic protein fraction from rat central myelin contains two proteins. Eng, Chao, Gerstl, Pratt and Tavaststjerna (1968) devised a combined salt-detergent extraction procedure which indicated the proportions of basic, proteolipid and Wolfgram proteins to be 28:52:20 in human central myelin, and 29:54:17 in bovine myelin. Gonzalez-Sastre (1970) devised a fractionation procedure using chloroform-methanol-salt, which yielded three comparable fractions in the proportions of 26:63:10 in bovine central myelin. The proportions of the proteins of peripheral myelin have also been estimated in terms of these fractions by Eng *et al.*, (1968) who concluded that they occur in the proportions 21:23:55, basic : proteolipid : Wolfgram protein (Table 11.5).

These fractionation procedures have now been superseded by techniques

Table 11.5 Protein composition of myelin

Method of fractionation	Source of myelin	mg/100 dry wt. Protein content	Per cent protein composition				References
			Basic protein	Folch Lees proteolipid	Wolfgram protein	Minor components	
Salt-detergent	Bovine cerebral	22	29	54	17	–	Eng et al. 1968
	Bovine sciatic	19	21	23	55	–	Eng et al. 1968
Acrylamide electrophoresis phenol/acid system	Bovine cerebral	22 (1)	37.4 (2)	37.6	–	24	Mehl & Wolfgram 1969
	Optic nerve	18	50.6	30.4	–	19	Mehl & Wolfgram 1969
	Spinal cord	13	38.8	21.0 18.2	–	22	Mehl & Wolfgram 1969
	Spinal root	–	20.5	49.5	–	30	Mehl & Wolfgram 1969
Acrylamide electrophoresis SDS system	Mouse brain	–	31 10	28	15	16	Greenfield et al., 1972
	Rabbit sciatic	–	18 26	56	–	–	Brostoff et al., 1972
	Rabbit sciatic	18	8.5 13.7 8.7	53.1	–	–	Greenfield et al., 1973
	Bovine spinal root	19	15 7 11	54	–	–	Greenfield et al., 1973
	Guinea pig sciatic	2	16.3 8.5	47.6	–	–	

(1) Protein content from Wolfgram and Kotorii 1968 and 1968a
(2) For electrophoretic systems the proteins are indicated in order of decreasing mobility, highest mobility being on the left.

involving the solubilization of the total protein in phenol-acid or SDS followed by acrylamide gel electrophoresis. In both of these solvent systems central and peripheral myelin have been found to contain more than three proteins. The major identifiable proteins in these systems are shown diagramatically in Fig. 11.2: the nomenclature used is a compromise between the systems used by several authors. It is seen that the analysis of peripheral myelin proteins by a

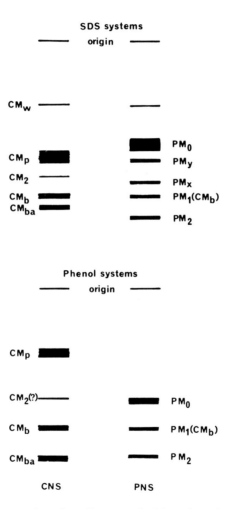

Fig. 11.2 *The major proteins of myelin, as resolved by polyacrylamide electrophoresis.* The major proteins of central and peripheral nerve myelin are shown as resolved in both the sodium dodecyl sulphate and phenol containing systems. The rather more variable high molecular weight proteins are not shown. The nomenclature is a compromise between that used by several previous authors. The central myelin proteins Cm_W, Cm_P and Cm_b correspond to the Wolfgram, proteolipid apoprotein and basic protein respectively. The protein Cm_{ba} corresponds to the small molecular weight basic protein of rat and mouse. The mobilities are approximately to scale.

fractionation procedure devised for central myelin is misleading since only the basic protein occurs in both.

The value of the electrophoretic methods depends upon the complete solubilization of the protein. The phenol-formic acid-water system of Thorun and Mehl (1968) and SDS appear to satisfy this requirement. Both of these protein solvent systems are considered to destroy the tertiary and secondary structure of proteins, and the electrophoretic separation has been shown to relate directly to the proteins' molecular weight (Thorun and Mehl, 1968; Shapiro, Vinuela and Maizel, 1967; Shapiro and Maizel, 1969; Weber and Osborn, 1969).

The charge density of proteins in these systems is by implication fairly constant. In SDS the amount of detergent bound to any particular protein depends on a number of factors (Pitt-Rivers and Impiombato, 1968), but even basic proteins run anodically in SDS systems and the mobility appears to relate to molecular weight. With regard to membrane proteins, it has been assumed that the same molecular weight-mobility relationship holds as is true for water soluble proteins, but in view of the specialized properties of these proteins such assumptions may well be ill founded.

In the phenol systems the myelin proteins are all catonic, (Cotman and Mahler, 1967; Mehl and Wolfgram, 1969; Mehl and Halaris, 1970) whereas in SDS they are all anionic (Greenfield, Norton and Morell, 1971; Agrawal et al., 1972, Morell, et al., 1972). Although the net charge of the proteins is opposite in these two systems the relative mobilities of the proteins is of the same order, supporting the view that the separation is primarily in terms of molecular weight. The only major difference is CMw (Wolfgram protein) which does not appear to be resolved in the phenol-formic acid-water system.

The molecular weights of the major proteins of central myelin have been estimated by acrylamide electrophoresis and slightly different values are obtained in the phenol-acid-water system compared with the SDS system. Thorun and Mehl (1968) using the phenol system estimated the molecular weight of CMp to be 34 000, and that of CMb to average 25 000 in ox and guinea pig brain myelin. In SDS the molecular weight of CMp from rat central myelin has been estimated to be 24 760 and that of the two basic proteins CMb and CMba to be 16 700 and 13 400 respectively (Agrawal et al., 1972). These values are to be compared with the value of 18 400 for bovine CMb estimated from its primary structure (Eylar, 1972). Agrawal et al. (1972) have also given the molecular weights of CMw and CM_2 estimated by acrylamide electrophoresis as 51 300 and 20 500 respectively.

The examination of the proteins of peripheral myelin by acrylamide electrophoresis in either the phenol system (Wolfgram and Kotorii, 1968; Mehl and Wolfgram, 1969; Csjetey, Hallpike, Adams and Bayliss, 1972) or the SDS system (Brostoff et al., 1972; Greenfield et al., 1973) indicate that they differ from those of central myelin. Up to the present time a maximum of five major proteins have been recognized to be present in peripheral myelin (Fig. 11.2), and of these only the fast running component, PM_1, is also found in central myelin, i.e. CMb, the encephalitogenic protein (Greenfield *et al.*, 1973). The conclusion that the remaining proteins of peripheral myelin differ from those of central myelin is further supported by a comparison of their amino acid compositions (Wolfgram and Kotorii, 1968; Eng *et al.*, 1968; Brostoff *et al.*, 1972; Greenfield *et al.*, 1973). In examining myelin isolated from various regions of the peripheral nervous system it has been noted that while the qualitative pattern of protein components is constant, the proportions of the individual proteins may vary widely (Greenfield *et al.*, 1973).

Both central and peripheral myelin when examined by acrylamide electrophoresis also contain a number of high molecular weight proteins, the exact number and proportions of which vary with the precise methods used in isolating the myelin, and with the manner of treating the samples for electrophoresis, and thus it has not been possible to ascribe these to myelin *per se*.

Examination of central myelin during development indicates that the proportions of the individual proteins varies with age (Morell *et al.*, 1972) (see Table 11.12) supporting the view that myelin undergoes a process of 'maturation'.

11.2.5 *Lipid composition of myelin*

The lipid composition of central myelin has been reported for a number of vertebrate species and has been extensively reviewed (Mokrasch, 1969; Davison, 1970 and Norton, 1971a). Some representative results for central myelin are given in Table 11.6, and for peripheral myelin in Table 11.7. The data on peripheral myelin is unfortunately much less extensive.

In agreement with the general experience relating to the lipid composition of biological membranes, myelin does not exhibit any qualitatively unique composition. However, the various lipids are present in characteristic proportions differing from those of other membranes and organelles both of brain and other tissues (see Eichberg, Whittaker and Dawson, 1964; Cuzner, Davison and Gregson, 1965b; O'Brien, 1967; Hamberger and Svennerholm, 1971). Furthermore, the lipid composition of central myelin differs from that of oligodendroglial plasma membrane (Davison, Cuzner, Banik and Oxberry, 1966; Hamberger and Svennerholm, 1971; Poduslo and Norton, 1972). Unfortunately, the biological significance of the various lipids present is not understood, and thus, although a considerable amount of compositional data is available, its relevance is obscure and only rather general comments can be made at present.

The proportions of cholesterol, total phospholipid and glycolipid in myelin are unique, there being a much greater proportion of cholesterol and glycolipid than is found in other membranes of neural origin. The cholesterol accounts for about forty moles per cent of the total lipid, a very high proportion when compared to other membranes.

Table 11.6 Lipid composition of CNS myelin

Lipid	Man (1)	Squirrel monkey (2) Spinal cord	Ox (3)	Rat (4)	Rabbit (3)	Guinea Pig (5)	Pigeon (3)	Frog (3)	Dogfish (3)
					moles %				
Cholesterol	40.4	44.6	46.2	42.8	42.4	40.5	47.9	42.33	37.0
Galactocerebroside	15.7	22.3	16.7	14.2	12.4	20.35	18.6	8.6	8.0
Sulphatide	3.5		3.1	2.9	3.2		2.8		4.8
Total phospholipid	38.9	33.2	32.7	40.2	41.0	39.2		49.1	50.2
Choline phospholipid	8.4	6.5	7.2	10.5	7.6	10.1	7.8	19.2	12.3
Serine phospholipid	5.3	5.9	6.7	6.3	6.2	5.0	2.8	3.7	4.2
Enthanolamine phospholipid	11.8	14.8	12.6	18.0	14.7	13.5	13.8	19.6	22.2
Sphingomyelin	4.4	6.0	6.2	3.5	6.8	4.9	2.5	4.6	7.4
Phosphoinositide	—	—	—	1.8	1.1	1.1	—	1.1	1.3
Other phospholipid	9.0	—	—	1.1	3.1	—	2.7	.9	3.3

(1) O'Brien and Sampson, 1965
(2) Horrocks, 1967
(3) Norton and Autilio, 1966
(4) Cuzner, Davison and Gregson, 1965
(5) Eichberg, Whittaker and Dawson, 1964

Table 11.7   Lipid composition of peripheral myelin

Lipid class	Bovine spinal root (1)	Squirrel monkey brachial plexus (2)
	Lipid moles %	
Cholesterol	40.1	42.80
Galactocerebroside	10.20	18.20
Sulphatide	1.30	
Total phospholipid	47.60	39.03
Choline phospholipid	10.00	5.34
Serine phospholipid	6.90	7.44*
Ethanolamine phospholipid	12.50	15.20
Sphingomyelin	12.90	11.05
Uncharacterised	5.30	—

(1) O'Brien, Sampson and Stern, 1967
(2) Horrocks, 1967
*includes P.I.

Glycolipids are common components of plasma membranes and have strong antigenic properties (Hakomori, 1971), but their concentration in myelin is extremely high. The major glycolipid components are the relatively simple galactocerebroside, and its sulphate ester, sulphatide. In the central myelin of mammals glycolipid accounts for approximately twenty moles per cent of the total lipid, but in peripheral myelin the proportion is lower. Myelin from the dogfish and frog central nervous system also contains a lower proportion of glycolipid (Table 11.6), and more closely resembles mammalian peripheral myelin.

The other major glycolipid present is ganglioside, which has been found in central myelin of mammals in small amounts, 50 μg of N-acetylneuraminic acid/100 mg dry wt. of myelin (Suzuki, Poduslo and Norton, 1967; Suzuki, Poduslo and Poduslo, 1968; Suzuki, 1970). Suzuki et al. (1968) found that in myelin from the brain of the rat and ox, 90% of the myelin ganglioside is present as the monosialoganglioside GM_1, but Hamberger and Svennerholm (1971), and Avrova, Chenykaeva and Obukhova (1973) find GM_1 and GD_{1a} to be the principal gangliosides of rabbit and rat brain myelin. This pattern of gangliosides is quite distinct from that found in other brain subcellular fractions. In an investigation of the gangliosides of human central myelin Ledeen, Yu and Eng (1973) have reported the presence of the ganglioside, sialosylgalactosylceramide, and that it accounted for 15% of the total lipid bound sialic acid of the myelin fraction. Its fatty acid and long chain base composition lead the authors to suggest a metabolic relationship to cerebroside and sulphatide. The virtual absence of this ganglioside from grey matter and its concentration in white matter suggest that it may be unique to myelin. There are no reliable data on the ganglioside content of peripheral myelin, but it is certain that in the peripheral nerve as a whole it is very low (Langley, 1971). Small amounts of acylgalacto-sylceramides and monogalactosyl diglyceride have also been reported in central and peripheral neural tissues (Norton and Brotz, 1963; Steim, 1967; Tamai, Taketomi and Yamakawa, 1967; Kishimoto, Wajda and Radin, 1968; Inoue, Deshmukh and Pieringer, 1971; Singh, 1973). The presence of galactosyl diglyceride has been associated with myelination in the central nervous system (Inoue *et al.*, 1971) and it has been reported to be present in peripheral myelin (Singh, 1973).

The phospholipid content of myelin is characterized by a higher proportion of ethanolamine phospholipid than of choline containing phospholipid, the reverse being found in other membrane fractions. The ethanolamine phospho-lipid of myelin is present primarily as the plasmalogen whereas none of the choline phospholipid is in this form. The ratio of ethanolamine phospholipid to lecithin is much lower in peripheral myelin, and the mole fraction of sphingomyelin is higher (Table 11.7). The acidic phospholipids, containing serine and polyphosphoinositide, are not present in large amounts, accounting for only some fifteen to twenty moles per cent of the total phospholipid. However, the polyphosphoinositides are of considerable interest since the di- and tri-phosphoinositides may be almost exclusively confined to myelin (Eichberg and Dawson, 1965; Norton and Autilio, 1966; Eichberg and Hauser, 1969; Sheltawy and Dawson, 1966), and appear to show a high rate of phosphate turnover (Jungalwala and Dawson, 1971). Furthermore the distribution of the molecular species of phosphatidylinositol in the subcellular fractions from ox brain indicates that myelin contains a characteristic proportion of the mono, di- and trienoic species with the other fractions containing more of the tetraenoic phosphatides (Luthra and Sheltawy, 1972).

The distribution of fatty acids within the lipid classes provides further support for the concept of a discrete distribution of the lipids within myelin. The phosphatides tend to contain predominantly the C_{16} and C_{18} acids, while the sphingolipids contain the C_{24} acids (Fig. 11.3). It is to be noted that greater differences are found between the central and peripheral myelin of any individual species than between the central myelins of different species (Fig. 11.3).

Summary of Section 11.2

The composition of myelin from the peripheral and central nervous systems is sufficiently similar to allow for its isolation from these sources by similar methods. The major constituents are water, protein and lipid, the bound water essential for structural integrity accounting for at least 20% of the wet wt. The protein content varies between 20–30% of the dry wt., and peripheral myelin may contain more protein on a dry weight basis than central myelin. The remaining 70–80% of the myelin dry mass appears to be solely lipid in nature.

Peripheral and central myelin differ markedly in terms of protein constituents, the only protein species apparently common to both being the basic encephalito-genic protein. Similarly peripheral and central myelin differ in lipid composition, peripheral myelin having lower concentrations of galactocerebroside and higher concentrations of choline phosphatide and sphingomyelin. The composition of myelin thus appears to be system specific, showing much smaller variation between species.

11.3 Structural studies of myelin

11.3.1 *Electron microscopy*

Electron microscopy, unlike X-ray diffraction, has the distinct advantage of providing a direct pictorial representation of structure but has the very real disadvantage that specimens require considerable chemical modification prior to examination. However the image of the myelin sheath provided by the electron microscope does contain certain consistent features which are independent of the processing to which the specimen has been submitted. The type of image which is most familiar is that obtained from thin sections of tissue fixed with glutaraldehyde and osmium textroxide, dehydrated, resin embedded and stained with heavy metal salts (Fig. 11.1), in which the sheath typically appears to be a lamellar structure. The lamellae are delineated by electron dense bands, separated by electron lucent intervals, alternate dense bands having unequal electron density. This lamellar structure is also visible in both negatively stained (Whittaker, 1963), and freeze etched preparations (Bischoff and Moor, 1967a,b; Branton, 1967). The denser of the two lines, the major dense or period line, is continuous with the apposed intracellular surfaces of the satellite cell plasma membrane during myelination, and at the Schmidt—Lanterman incisures and the paranodal regions in the mature sheath, whereas the intraperiod line is continuous with the apposed extracellular surfaces of the same membrane. Karlsson (1966) in a careful comparison of thin sections of rat sciatic and optic nerves found the repeat distance, from centre to centre of adjacent period lines, was 11.9 ± 0.7 nm in peripheral and 10.7 ± 0.5 nm in central myelin, the larger repeat distance in peripheral myelin agreeing with the X-ray diffraction findings (vide infra). Karlsson also found that the periodicity was more difficult to measure in the thicker sheaths of increasing lamellar irregularity.

Bischoff and Moor (1967b), who used the freeze etch technique give a figure of 18.5 nm for the period repeat distance of myelin from the mouse sciatic nerve, and 160 nm for that from the lumbar spinal cord (Bischoff and Moor, 1967a), but they give no details as to how the measurements were made. The values are considerably larger than those seen in fixed tissue, as might be expected since fixation is known to reduce the repeat distance (Fernandez-Moran and Finean, 1957), and correspond to the value obtained by X-ray diffraction from fresh mammalian tissues (see Table 11.8). Their findings were

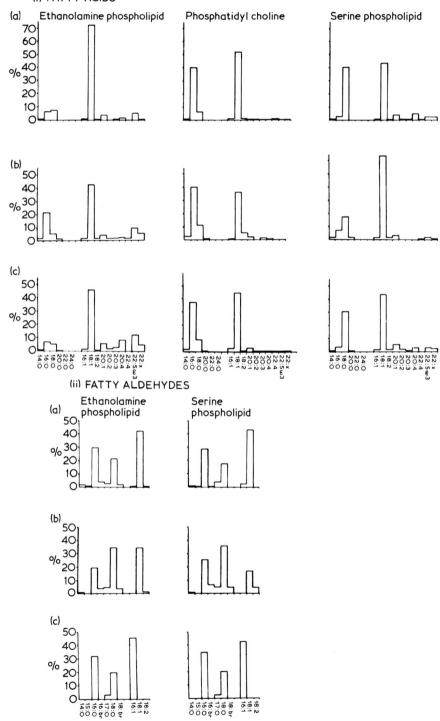

(i) FATTY ACIDS

(a) Ethanolamine phospholipid | Phosphatidyl choline | Serine phospholipid

(ii) FATTY ALDEHYDES

(a) Ethanolamine phospholipid | Serine phospholipid

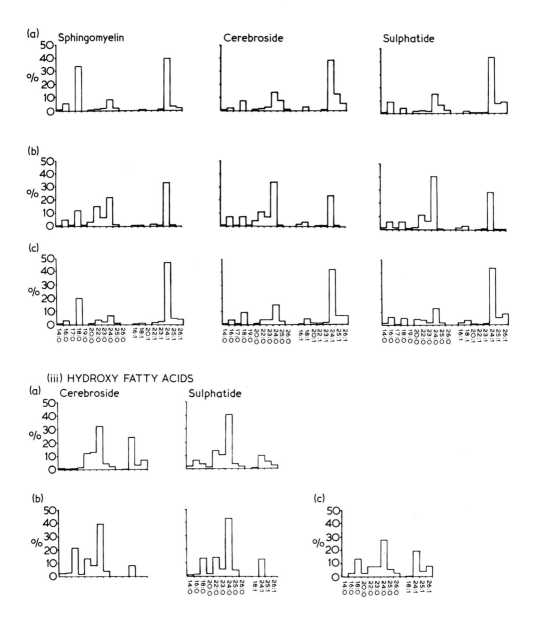

Fig. 11.3 *The fatty acid and aldehyde composition of the major lipids of myelin from the central and peripheral nervous systems.* The histograms represent the percentage composition for lipids from (a) human brain myelin; (b) bovine peripheral nerve; (c) bovine brain myelin, and are drawn from the work of (a) O'Brien and Sampson, 1965b; (b) O'Brien, Sampson and Stern, 1967; (c) MacBrinn and O'Brien, 1969. The histograms give the per cent distribution of fatty acids and aldehydes classified according to chain length, i.e. the number of carbon atoms and the degree of unsaturation. e.g. 16:0 is palmitic acid and 16:1 is palmitoleic acid. x represents acids of uncertain high order of unsaturation, and Br indicates aldehydes having a branched chain.

Table 11.8 Dimensions of radial repeating unit

| Species | Radial repeat distance (nm) in fresh tissue | |
	P.N.	C.N.S.
Dog/cat	18.4 (1)	
Chicken	18.2 (2)	
Dove/duck/hen	18.3 (3)	
Man/monkey/sheep		
Rabbit/guinea pig	18.5 (3)	
(Weak diffraction in fish)	18.4 (2)	18.2–18.3
Frog/toad	17.1 (1,2,3)	
Rat	17.6 (2)	
Frog		15.4–15.3 (2)
Chicken		15.5 (2)
Rabbit		15.6 (4)
Ox		15.7 (2)
Rat		15.9 (2)
Fish	15.9 (2)	15.6 (2)
	16.1 (3)	

(1) Schmitt, Bear and Palmer, 1941
(2) Worthington and Blaurock, 1969
(3) Hogland and Ringertz, 1961
(4) Caspar and Kirschner, 1971

somewhat unexpected since it has been reported that freezing produces an expansion of the myelin period (Elkes and Finean, 1953a; Finean, 1953).

The difference in electron density between the period and the intraperiod line suggests an asymmetry in the single membrane which constitutes the repeating unit of the myelin sheath. This asymmetry is further emphasized by the fact that the intraperiod line, in contrast to the period line, is readily 'split' into two lines by physical insult, both *in vitro* (Fernandez-Moran and Finean, 1957), and *in vivo* (Hall and Williams, 1970), and by variations in fixation and staining technique (Revel and Hamilton, 1969). It has been suggested that the intraperiod line is normally double *in vivo*, becoming condensed by the action of the fixative osmium tetroxide (Revel and Hamilton, 1969), but other experiments suggest that splitting of the intra-period line is initiated by any mild physical insult (Hall and Williams, 1970). In the study by Bischoff and Moor (1967a,b) using the freeze fracture technique it is the period line which appears to be split, rather than the intraperiod line. These particular studies provide additional support for the view that the myelin membrane is asymmetric since they show two types of membrane fracture face, a 'smooth' finely granular surface, and a 'rough', course granular surface, the latter being said to correspond to the period line face, and the 'smooth' surface to that of the intra-period line (Fig. 11.4). Branton (1967) who employed the same technique, but used tadpole and neonate mice in contrast to the young adult animals used by Bischoff and Moor, concluded that the myelin membrane fracture surface was solely of the 'smooth' type. Bischoff and Moor found that although the two types of surface alternated in the myelin sheath, the sheaths usually appeared to fracture so as to show surfaces all of one type, or all of the other. A particulate type of structure has also been reported for myelin examined by negative contrast at low temperatures (Fernandez-Moran, 1967).

Branton has proposed that the fracture plane of a membrane lies within its hydrophobic core, implying the assumption of a lipid bilayer within the structure, and that any particulate structure revealed indicates penetration of the lipid by protein. More recent evidence suggests that the plane of fracture is not consistent but may lie at either surface, as well as within the thickness of the membrane (Hereward and Northcote, 1973). In addition to the uncertainty concerning the precise plane of fracture in frozen material it is unclear whether or not displacement of material occurs due to either ice crystal growth or phase transitions, with concomitant initiation of new equilibrium structures (Zingsheim, 1972).

In conclusion the electron microscopic appearance of myelin provides no direct support for the view that its structure differs fundamentally from that of other cellular membranes, and its unequal affinity for various electron dense stains suggests a comparable asymmetry of structure to that seen in other cell membranes. The dimensional differences observed between peripheral and central myelin sheaths are of considerable interest when coupled with the overall similarity of their structure, and the differences in their protein and lipid compositions.

11.3.2 *Polarized light studies*

Investigations into the birefringent properties of the myelin sheath were amongst the earlier structural studies undertaken, and their results have been reviewed by Schmidt (1936), Schmidt and Bear (1939), and Bear (1971). The effects of nerve fibres upon plane polarized light were examined using illumination both perpendicular and parallel to the long axis of the fibres, the latter by the use of frozen section. In summary the observations indicated that the sheath behaved as though composed of a series of positive elements with their optical axes arranged radially, suggesting that the elements are arranged randomly about every radial direction, with some non-randomness along the radii (Schmidt, 1936). It was concluded from solvent extraction and immersion experiments that the birefringence of myelin is the sum of two components, a strong positive contribution from the lipid, and a second weaker, negative contribution from protein components. The immersion experiments also indicated that the protein contribution was due to 'form birefringence', the molecules being anisodiametric with their long axes oriented in planes parallel to the surface of the sheath. The optically indicated predominance of the lipid component of the sheath was

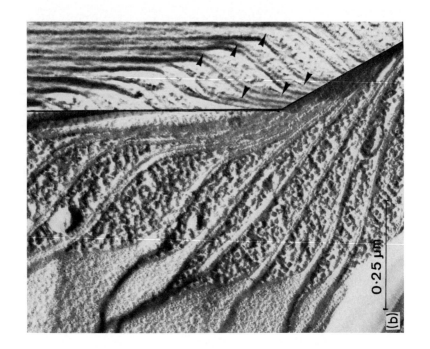

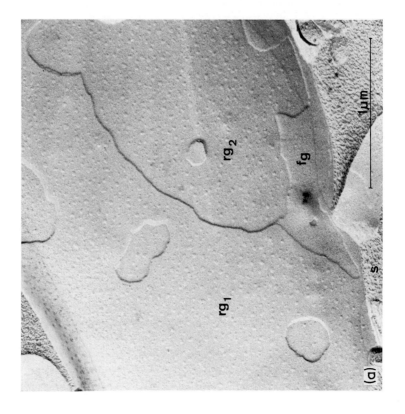

shown to vary continuously with the fibre diameter, apparently disappearing at fibre diameters of less than 2 μm, the lower limit of size for myelinated axons (Schmidt and Bear, 1937). It is perhaps somewhat surprising that the birefringence of the sheath varies in this curvilinear fashion with thickness if it is assumed that it has the same composition and structure throughout in all sheaths independent of thickness. Although the broader features of the structure revealed by the optical studies are compatible with the structure postulated from the electron microscopic and X-ray diffraction evidence, some of the optical experiments require repetition in conjunction with ultrastructural studies. This is particularly necessary with regard to the immersion and extraction studies, since these procedures are now recognized to produce significant alterations in the structure of the sheath.

11.3.3 X-diffraction studies of myelin

The X-ray diffraction patterns obtained from fresh nerves from a wide variety of sources have certain features in common. The series of equally spaced equatorial reflections obtained from the small angle diffraction of myelin indicate a period repeat structure of from 15.4 to 18.5 nm, depending upon the source of the nerve studied. Furthermore, the intensity of the even order spacings, 2 and 4, is greater than that of the odd orders 1, 3 and 5 (particularly in central myelin), indicating that there is a division of the large repeat into a smaller unit of 7.7–9.5 nm. The large unit is arranged radially (Schmidt and Bear, 1939). The wide angle diffractions (Boehm, 1933; Schmidt and Bear, 1939; Bear, 1971) are (i) a radially diffuse, tangentially unorientated halo at 0.33 nm spacing ascribable to water; (ii) a moderately diffuse, meridionally accentuated ring, with a spacing of 0.48 nm; and (iii) an equatorial spot at a spacing of 1.7 nm.

The diffuse meridional diffraction at 0.48 nm is considered to represent hydrocarbon chain spacings in a tangential plane, the diffuseness and meridional accentuation being considered to indicate a lack of crystallinity in the hydrocarbon phase (Schmidt and Bear, 1939). However it has been pointed out by Bear (1971) that proteins also show diffuse diffraction at 0.4 to 0.5 nm so that a small contribution from protein cannot be excluded (Palmer, Schmidt and Chargaff, 1941). Schmidt, Bear and Palmer (1941) also observed a weak diffuse, meridionally accentuated reflection at 0.94 nm in fresh nerve but they were unable to determine its origin. Blaurock and Wilkins (1969) also mention a diffuse equatorial orientated diffraction of 1.2 nm from frog sciatic nerve, which they

---

Fig. 11.4 *Freeze fracture appearance of myelin in the peripheral nerve of the adult mouse.* (a) Surface views of myelin lamellae showing rough granular (rg) and fine granular (fg) surfaces in alternating fashion. (b) Section through a Schmidt-Lanterman incisure, the rough granular surface can be seen at the obliquely fractured period line at the edge of the incisure. (Reproduced from Bischoff and Moor, 1967a, by courtesy of A. Bischoff and the editors of Z f. Zellforschung.)

assumed to arise from the myelin sheath, possibly from protein orientated in the plane of the membrane. One may speculate that this may correspond to the form dependent protein birefringence found in the earlier optical studies. The phosphate groups, which are considered to provide strong reflections in the radial direction, do not appear to give rise to any obvious reflections in the tangential plane.

The more recent studies of nerves of central and peripheral origin from a variety of vertebrate species, are of some interest, since they suggest some grouping of the values for the dimension of the major repeating unit (Table 11.8). In general the spacing obtained from peripheral nerves is quite distinct from that from central myelin, and the relative intensities of the first five orders also differ (Blaurock and Worthington, 1969). Furthermore rat peripheral nerve appears to differ from those of other mammalian species investigated. (Table 11.8).

The interpretation of the small angle diffraction pattern of fresh nerve in terms of a one dimensional electron density distribution normal to the surface of the sheath has been attempted by a number of workers (Finean and Burge, 1963; Moody, 1963; Worthington and Blaurock, 1969a; Caspar and Kirschner, 1971). The principal difficulty in determining a structure is that of assigning the correct relative phases to the structure factors. There is no simple independent solution of this problem. Its resolution has been attempted by (a) taking advantage of the property of myelin to swell in solutions of low ionic strength (Finean and Burge, 1963; Worthington, 1972). (b) the use of models having structural features assumed to be shared by myelin (Worthington and King, 1971); (c) the comparison of homologous structures, i.e. central and peripheral myelin (Caspar and Kirschner, 1971), and (d) the use of heavy metal labelling (Akers and Parsons, 1970; Harker, 1972). The methods (a), (b) and (c) have tended to produce similar solutions, partly because they contain the assumption of a centrosymmetric hydrocarbon layer, although in the finally proposed myelin structure the hydrocarbon layer appears to be slightly asymmetric, due either to an asymmetric distribution of cholesterol (Kirschner and Caspar, 1972) or to protein penetration (Blaurock, 1972, 1973). The method of Caspar and Kirschner (1971) relies on the assumption that central and peripheral myelin have the same structure, differing only in their fatty acid composition, but the compositional differences are in fact more extensive than this (*vide supra*), and the choice of two structural solutions giving the greatest correspondence between the two myelins may not be justified.

The absolute densities of the membrane profile have been obtained from studies of myelin swelling in sucrose solutions (Worthington and Blaurock, 1969a). The use of this system to resolve the phase problem has been criticized on the grounds that it involves the assumption that the average electron density of the myelin was less than that of the fluid which entered between the myelin lamellae, and it has been stated that the choice between the structures was 'not that definite,' (Harker, 1972). Recently McIntosh and Worthington (1973) have attempted to meet this criticism by using glycerol instead of sucrose in their swelling experiments, but in view of the ready diffusion of glycerol through cell membranes it is questionable whether it really only equilibriates with the fluid space. A further criticism of the use of swelling experiments is that the mechanism of the swelling is not understood, it certainly is not related to osmotic phenomena but may arise from changes in electrostatic binding (*vide infra*). That it is certainly not a simple 'swelling' is indicated by the fact that reversal of the swelling leads to a contracted structure which slowly reverts to the normal pattern (Worthington and Blaurock, 1969b), thus the major criticism of this approach is that a structural change has occurred; whether this is reversible is irrelevant.

The method of heavy atom labelling used by Akers and Parsons, while of interest, is obviously open to a variety of interpretations (see Harker, 1972). This method relies on the assumption that the binding of even a small amount of heavy metal will not disturb the structure to such an extent as to drastically alter the relative phases, but will change them in a continuous manner. Part of the difficulty inherent in this approach lies in deciding how many types of binding site exist. Akers and Parsons assume two are present whereas Harker proposes only one. It is of interest however that in both cases the structures chosen are quite different from those proposed by other workers.

In most of these studies the lipid bilayer of the Davson-Danielli hypothesis is assumed to be the relatively symmetrical centre of the structure, but the electron density of this layer in myelin is not known with sufficient accuracy to exclude its penetration by protein. Kirschner and Caspar (1972) suggest that up to 10% of the volume of the hydrocarbon layer could be protein, implying that up to one third of the total protein could be present in this region.

Several points must be made about the X-ray diffraction observations and their interpretation. Firstly the structure derived is an average of the real structure and thus the diagramatic representation of the various interpretations represents an average picture, and does not reflect the total extensive structure. Secondly, the method will not reveal structure units in the plane of the membrane if they have separations greater than 300 Å, even if they are arranged in a regular fashion. As myelin is composed of many different components, lipid and protein, the possibility of large structural arrays must not be overlooked. Thirdly whatever structural model of the membrane is put forward it must be compatible with the observed X-ray diffraction pattern.

Summary of Section 11.3

The investigations of myelin ultrastructure by the techniques of electron microscopy, polarized light birefringence and X-ray diffraction all indicate the occurence of a radial repeat structure with an overall orientation of the constituent molecules in the radial direction. Peripheral and central myelin appear to be homologous structures differing in the dimensions of the radially repeating unit. The radially repeating unit of structure has continuity with the plasma membrane of the parent cell and demonstrates some asymmetry corresponding to the internal and external faces of the membrane. The small angle X-ray diffraction pattern of myelin can be interpreted in terms of a structure closely resembling the Danielli-Davson hypothetical membrane structure.

11.4 Short range interactions

The heterogeneity of the constituents of membranes has naturally directed attention toward examining interactions between these individual constituents. The methods applied mainly provide information about the physical state of the lipid molecules and their interactions. Up to the present only a small amount of work has been performed directly upon myelin, but a number of reviews exist giving the results of investigations into biological membranes in general (Chapman, 1968; Ladbrooke and Chapman, 1969; Chapman and Dodd, 1971; Chapman, 1972).

Most interest has been shown in the state of (a) the membrane associated water, (the results of differential scanning calorimetry (DSC) pertinent to this have been mentioned above; these in general indicate the presence of a consistent fraction of 'bound' water having an average structure differing from that of the bulk water), and (b) the hydrocarbon chains of the lipids. With regard to the latter, calorimetry of wet myelin fails to demonstrate any endotherm attributable to fatty acid chain melting (Ladbrooke et al., 1968).No endotherm attributable to chain melting is detectable until the water content of the myelin preparation falls below 20%, and with further dehydration the endotherm becomes progressively larger. The temperature of the transition is $35°C$ at 15% water content, rising to the limiting temperature of $55°C$ at 3% water content. Examination of the isolated lipid and lipid fractions indicates that the $35°C$ transition is attributable to a cholesterol transition, and that at $55°C$ to the phospholipid mesomorphic transition. Hydrated mixtures of cholesterol-phospholipid, show progressively smaller fatty acid transitions as the molar ratios approach 1:1 (Ladbrooke and Chapman, 1969). It has therefore been proposed that the absence of transitions in wet myelin can be explained by an admixture of cholesterol and phospholipid (Ladbrooke, et al., 1968). Similar behaviour can be demonstrated for sphingomyelin-cholesterol and cerebroside-cholesterol mixtures (Oldfield and Chapman, 1972). The effect of drying myelin is to produce a separation of the lipid phases, a conclusion arrived at during the early X-ray studies of dried myelin (Schmitt and Palmer, 1940).

Proton magnetic resonance spectoscopy (PMR) of the model lipid systems suggests that the effect of cholesterol is to place the fatty acid chains in a state intermediate to that of a transition, in that at temperatures below their transition point they appear to be relatively more mobile, whereas at temperatures above the transition point they do not achieve the full mobility found with the pure phospholipid (Chapman and Dodd, 1971); melting of the hydrocarbon chain however, does not appear to take place. The cholesterol, on the other hand, appears to be constrained (Chapman and Dodd, 1971). Similar changes in the PMR spectra are obtained from experimental cerebroside-cholesterol mixtures (Oldfield and Chapman, 1972). In wet myelin, ultra-sonically dispersed in deuterium oxide or myelin lipid at 65°C, a similar restriction of the hydrocarbon chain motion is observed (Jenkinson et al., 1969), and lyophilized myelin shows a sharp spectral transition between 23°C and 40°C in agreement with the DSC results (Lecar, Ehrenstein and Stillman, 1971). Thus, it appears that the mixing of cholesterol with amphipathic lipids in the hydrated state results in a limited 'melting' of the hydrocarbon chain that is relatively insensitive to temperature. The interaction between the cholesterol and the hydrocarbon chain may be greater at the polar interface, becoming progressively less toward the methyl end of the fatty acid. The overall consequence of this interaction is to reduce the crystallinity of the hydrocarbon chains at the lower temperature, compatible with the postulated random packing of fatty acid chains suggested by the early X-ray diffraction studies (Schmitt and Bear, 1939). Since similar behaviour is exhibited both by the total myelin lipid fraction and myelin itself, it has been suggested that the lipid of the myelin membrane is organized as in the purely lipid system. However, similar behaviour is exhibited by the erythrocyte membrane, which contains far less cholesterol than myelin, but the erythrocyte membrane lipids do not give the same PMR spectrum as the intact membrane (Chapman and Dodd, 1971). There is therefore a possibility that in membranes the observed phenomena may not necessarily arise from interactions involving cholesterol. The presence of a critical amount of bound water in myelin, as well as the influence of water on the structural properties of pure lipid system, indicates that dipole interactions of the polar groups of the lipids, and possibly of proteins, are of considerable importance in determining the properties of lipid alkyl chain interactions. In this respect water must be considered to be an important structural element in the myelin membrane.

The PMR spectra of myelin possess sharp resonance peaks attributable to choline methyls and sugar rings, suggesting that these groups are predominantly in a free state (Jenkinson, et al., 1969); and a lipoprotein complex has been obtained from myelin following succinylation, the PMR spectrum of which indicates that the lipid-protein binding involves the polar groups of the lipid rather than the hydrophobic regions (Joffe and Block, 1972). It has been suggested that such complexes may occur naturally in native myelin.

A further interesting observation made in the calorimetric studies was the absence of any endotherm attributable to a bulk protein denaturation in either wet or dry myelin (Ladbrooke et al., 1968). Although basic protein is thought not to have an H-bonded secondary structure, the proteolipid protein is believed to have some α-helix content (Folch Pi and Stoffyn, 1972). However, it has been found that a globular protein such as haemoglobin does not show any denaturation endotherm until a certain minimal hydration has been achieved of about 1.5 molecules of water/residue (personal unpublished observations). It may then follow that if the bulk of the protein in the membrane is not hydrated, a denaturation endotherm may not be evident. It has been noted that the 2:3 cyclic AMP phosphodiesterase can be thermally inactivated (personal unpublished observations) suggesting that the thermal denaturation of some protein is possible.

Once again, the methods used provide only an average picture of the structural characteristics of myelin. Calorimetry can provide quantitative information which could help to determine the proportion of the components involved in any transition, provided that reliable values for the heats of transition have been established. Accurate quantitation of PMR is also difficult, particularly since it is not known what proportion of the chemical groups present may be contributing to the signals detected.

Summary of Section 11.4

The techniques of differential scanning calorimetry and proton magnetic resonance when applied to myelin both indicate the significance of a critical proportion of water in maintaining its structure, and the fact that the lipid alkyl chains are not in a crystalline state but are nonetheless restrained so that sharp 'melting' is not observed as the temperature is increased. The experimental findings have been interpreted in terms of a cholesterol fatty acid interaction, by analogy with model systems of pure lipid, but this explanation ignores the role of the proteins in such interactions, which may be just as significant.

11.5 Modification of structure

A variety of experimental procedures will modify the structure of myelin, and structural changes induced by mild treatment with solutions of various ionic compositions and osmolarity have, for example, been used in techniques designed to resolve its structure (*vide supra*).

Basically such experimental procedures involve (a) the modification of the interactions within the sheath by changing the pH or ionic strength of the suspending medium or changes in temperature; (b) the preferential extraction of individual components or classes of components and (c) the use of enzymes to modify or partially degrade constituent molecular species.

11.5.1 *Influence of ionic composition of suspending medium: swelling phenomena and the influence of temperature*

Observations concerning the relationship between swelling of myelin sheath and changes in the composition of the suspending medium were first made some years ago (Finean and Millington, 1957). Early interpretations were expressed in terms of osmotic effects, although such explanations took no account of the fact that sucrose solutions, even when hypertonic, fail to reverse the swelling induced by water, and may indeed even initiate such swelling.

A slightly more systematic investigation of the phenomenon, suggested that the swelling of the sheath, is a consequence of the separation of the lamellae at the intra-period line (Robertson, 1958), a phenomenon more easily explained in terms of electrostatic effects. With decreasing ionic strength an increase in period separation occurs at strengths below 0.08 (Worthington and Blaurock, 1969b). In dilutions of Ringer's solution swelling occurs at dilutions of 0.3, equivalent to an ionic strength of 0.05. In such experiments swelling is signalled by a change in the X-ray diffraction pattern, and the soaking of nerve fibres in sucrose solutions of 0.24 M also results in changes to the diffraction indicative of swelling (Worthington and Blaurock, 1969b). Swelling by immersion in water for periods of time up to 30 h increased the period repeat distance of frog sciatic nerve from 17.1 nm to a maximum of 28 nm, and immersion in water, followed by hypertonic sucrose produced a periodicity of up to 42.6 nm. The increase in periodic spacing is accompanied by changes in the relative intensity of the diffraction orders and in their definition. The swelling can be reversed, as indicated by changes in both its electron microscopic appearance and X-ray diffraction pattern (Robertson, 1958; Worthington and Blaurock, 1969b), by increasing the ionic strength of the bathing medium. The published data is not sufficiently systematic to enable one to tell whether or not there is any particular specificity in this reaction, except with respect to Ca^{++} ions, which will reverse the swelling, even at concentrations as low as 2 mM (ionic strength 0.003). If the swelling process is an electrostatic repulsion originating in the fixed charges at the surfaces of the lamellae, then the greater effectiveness of Ca^{++} ions in reducing this separation is to be expected, as Ca^{++} has earlier been found to be very effective in condensing lipid systems (Schmitt and Palmer, 1940). Although it has been stated on the basis of the X-ray diffraction observations that the swelling is 'reversed' by increasing the ionic strength, it is not a direct reversal but shows hysteresis.

Following swelling and subsequent treatment with a solution of a higher ionic strength the new period for frog sciatic nerve myelin is 16.4–16.8 nm. On prolonged standing the 'subnormal' pattern slowly reverts to a pattern close to that of fresh nerve (Worthington and Blaurock, 1969b). Hall and Williams (1970) in their study of the incisures, noted that intraperiod line splitting was observed in solutions of 0.07 M NaCl, and that this began at the incisures and gradually advanced into the inter-incisural regions of compact myelin, suggesting that the double layer ions equilibriate with the external fluid by lateral diffusion along the lamellae, rather than radially across the sheath. This proposition would be compatible with the sheath's suggested high resistance. Hall and Williams further noted a degree of irreversible change in the periodicity of the compacted myelin following such treatment, i.e. a collapse to a smaller repeating unit, in which no obvious distinction between period and intraperiod line could be found.

The fact that the passage of myelin from a low ionic strength to a higher solution induces a new diffraction pattern may now be taken to indicate that some change in the structure of the membranes has occurred. It is possible that by removing or reducing the electrostatic shielding, the charged groups have undergone some reorientation, or participate in a wider reorganization of the two dimensional ionic lattice consequent upon the establishment of a new equilibrium. It is not possible to be certain whether such a change has occurred on the reduction of the ionic strength or its subsequent increase. The changes in the X-ray pattern accompanying swelling have been interpreted solely in terms of an increase in the fluid space, but again this appears to be much a matter of personal choice.

All of these experiments were presumably conducted at approximately pH 7.0. No systematic study of the effects of pH has been carried out, which is unfortunate since it might throw some light on the nature of the response of the myelin to a change in its ionic environment and the kinds of chemical groups involved.

The binding of small amounts of osmium, brought about be exposing nerves to osmium tetroxide vapour, results in a slight degree of shrinkage of the sheath (Akers and Parsons, 1970; McIntosh and Worthington, 1973). Treatment with the solutions normally used for electron microscopic fixation results in much more obvious changes (Fernandez-Moran and Finean, 1957), and subsequent dehydration produces further shrinkage. Although these facts are well known they lack a convincing explanation. A comparison of these results with those obtained from lipid extracted nerve by Napolitano, LeBaron and Scaletti (1967) (*vide infra*) indicates the complexity of the reactions inherent in the treatments involved in the preparation of material for electron microscopy.

The effect of temperature changes upon myelin structure, as indicated by X-ray diffraction, was first undertaken by Schmidt, Bear and Clark, (1935) and Schmidt, Bear and Palmer (1941). Their initial experiments indicated a change with rise in temperature (Schmitt, Bear and Clark, 1935), but later experiments in which care was taken to prevent longitudinal contraction of the nerve during heating, failed to demonstrate any marked change in the diffraction pattern at temperatures of up to 70°C, (Schmitt, Bear and Palmer, 1941). Finean has made a more systematic study of the effects of temperature change upon myelin structure, as indicated by its X-ray diffraction pattern (Elkes and Finean, 1953a), and has found that the normal pattern is abolished at temperatures below 0°C and that a reduction of temperature to −180°C was associated with the appearance of an increasingly strong reflection at 6.1–6.3 nm. Unlike Schmitt, Bear and Palmer (1941), Elkes and Finean found that when the temperature was raised to about 55°C the diffraction lines became more diffuse, and that between 58°C and 60°C a new pattern appeared consisting of a diffuse band at 7.55 nm together with a broad weak band at 4.1 nm.

11.5.2 *Extraction studies*

The major component of the myelin sheath is water (*vide supra*) and its removal leads to marked structural alterations which are irreversible (Schmitt and Palmer, 1940). The major period shrinks and a number of new diffraction lines appear, characteristic of the X-ray diffraction pattern of the nerve lipids. The variations in the diffraction pattern of dried nerve with change in temperature are similar to those observed for the total lipid extract (Elkes and Finean, 1953a), the first appearance of the dry diffraction pattern occurring at a water concentration of 30–40% (Finean, Coleman, Green and Limbrick, 1966) with the most pronounced new line to occurring at 6.3 nm (Schmitt and Palmer, 1940; Elkes and Finean, 1953a). Following rehydration of dried nerves a new diffraction pattern appears, having a fundamental period of 8–9 nm (Schmitt, Bear and Palmer, 1941).

The electron microscopic appearance of dried myelin reveals considerable compaction, with many areas of laminar structure resembling lipid, and the available evidence suggests that the main consequence of the removal of water from myelin is a dissociation of the lipid and protein components, with the appearance of a discrete lipid phase (Schmitt and Palmer, 1940; Finean, 1953).

Organic solvents will obviously remove lipid from the myelin sheath, and the amount and type of lipid removed is to some extent dependent upon the solvent employed. Acetone extraction of fresh nerve, in the cold, removes 30% of the cholesterol, and preserves the periodicity with a slight increase in spacing (Fernandez-Moran and Finean, 1957; Elkes and Finean, 1953b). Electron microscopy suggests that a separation has occurred at the intraperiod line, and regions of a collapsed phase, possibly lipid, are to be found. Most other organic solvents have more severe effects upon myelin structure (Fernandez-Moran and Finean, 1957; Elkes and Finean, 1953b; Finean and Burge, 1963; Rumsby and Finean, 1966a,b). This structure destroying effect can be correlated with a combination of extensive lipid extraction and protein denaturation, and in the case of chloroform-methanol mixtures the additional extraction of proteolipid protein (Finean and Burge, 1963). However, even after extraction of up to 98% of the lipid from glutaraldehyde fixed nerve, and subsequent treatment with osmium in a non-polar solvent (CCl_4), the electron microscopic image of the sheath is largely preserved (Napolitano, LeBaron and Scaletti, 1967). The lamellar appearance, with distinct period and intraperiod lines, remains intact, although the perodicity is 17 nm, a higher value than that usually found in electron micrographs. Treatment of the lipid extracted material with the more usual aqueous buffered osmium tetroxide solutions resulted in a loss of structure. It is presumed that cross linking of the protein with glutaraldehyde stabilizes the myelin structure, but this does not rule out some rearrangements of its constituents. In addition these experiments indicate that the electron opaque osmium, lead and uranyl ions used as 'stains' may be bound principally by the protein.

The myelin specific basic protein can be extracted from central myelin by exposure to low pH (below pH 3.0), and it is reported that following such treatment the myelin has a collapsed structure in which the intraperiod line is no longer distinguishable (Dickinson, Jones, Aparicio, and Lumsden, 1970). This has been interpreted to indicate that the basic protein is localized to the intraperiod line, although alternative electron microscopic histochemical evidence has been advanced in favour of the localization of basic protein to the period line (Adams, Bayliss, Hallpike and Turner, 1971).

11.5.3 *Action of enzymes*

The actions of the phospholipases A and C on myelin have been investigated to some extent. Phospholipase A_2 injected intraneurally in the living mouse produces a rapid and extensive 'lysis' of the myelin, indistinguishable from that produced by its product lysolecithin (Hall and Gregson, 1971). It was concluded that the structural effects are brought about by lysolecithin, which is an effective detergent and will completely solubilize the myelin (*vide infra* and Gent, Gregson, Gammack and Raper, 1964). Phospholipase C produces some further splitting and fragmentation of myelin under *in vitro* conditions, the fragments remaining vesicular in form (McIlwain and Rapport, 1971). Some 64% of the lipid phosphorous is lost under these conditions, and large amorphous globules, presumably of lipid, appeared in the membrane walls of the vesicles. In other membranes treated with phospholiphase C similar globules have been shown to consist largely of diglycerides and cholesterol but the remaining membrane appearance was little changed (see Finean and Coleman, 1970).

Summary of Section 11.5

Changes in the ionic strength and nature of the suspending media greatly change the period spacing of myelin, providing further support for the idea that the compaction of myelin is dependent upon dipole interaction. Concomitant changes occur in the X-ray diffraction pattern, suggesting that the orientation and interaction of the polar regions have a general effect on the membrane structure. Both careful lipid extraction and phospholipase C treatment suggest that the normal electron dense lines seen in the electron microscope after osmium treatment and staining may be dependent on groups other than the phosphates of the phospholipids.

11.6 Myelin proteins and their properties

It is a central tenet in modern biology that only proteins display sufficient specificity of interaction to be the major determinants of structure. In membranes this is emphasized by the observation that the characteristic features of their lipid composition concern the relative concentrations of the constituent lipids rather than differences in kind. The individual lipids of a membrane may thus be considered to be analogous to amino acids in a protein, although due to variations in fatty acid composition the number of lipid species is much greater, their assembly in a membrane being dependent upon the properties of the proteins, the genetically more directly determined characteristic components. The protein-lipid interaction shows some versatility, since some change in fatty acid composition can occur as a consequence of changes in dietary fatty acid intake and temperature. The nature of membrane proteins is such that the extraction and purification procedures employed are likely to cause them to undergo significant configurational changes making the investigation of their properties difficult. Nonetheless a number of proteins primarily derived from central myelin have been isolated and studied.

11.6.1 *Proteolipid protein*

Probably the most familiar myelin protein is the proteolipid protein originally isolated in chloroform-methanol extracts of brain by Folch and Lees (1951). It was the unusual solubility of this protein in a medium of low dielectric constant which first attracted attention, and it is now recognized that while the major proteolipid protein extracted from white matter is derived from myelin, a protein of similar solubility can be extracted from both other brain subcellular fractions (Lapetina, Soto and De Robertis, 1968), and other non-neural tissues (Murakami, Sekine and Funahashi, 1962). The myelin proteolipid protein appears to be quite distinct from the other proteolipid proteins so far isolated.Whikehart and Lees (1973) found two N-terminal amino acids, glycine and glutamic in the ratio of 6:1.4, whereas non myelin proteolipid proteins have aspartic acid as the major N-terminal acid. The C-terminal acids of myelin proteolipid protein are phenylalanine and glycine, with phenylalanine the major acid. Gagnon, Finch, Wood and Moscarello (1971) report only glycine as the N-terminal acid in a preparation of proteolipid protein from human myelin.

The proteolipid protein in initial chloroform methanol extracts appears to be in association with lipid (LeBaron, 1969; Folch-Pi and Stoffyn, 1972), and in particular with polyphosphoinositide. It is however possible to obtain the apoprotein free of lipid by dialysis against acidified chloroform methanol (Tennenbaum and Folch-Pi, 1966; Stoffyn and Folch-Pi, 1972). Alternatively the protein can be freed from lipid by the substitution of detergent (Eng *et al.*, 1968; Nguyen Le, Nicot and Alfsen, 1971). When prepared as the lipid free apoprotein it is soluble in both lipid solvents and aqueous media (Tennenbaum and Folch-Pi, 1966; Folch-Pi and Stoffyn, 1972). Gagnon *et al.* (1971) have also obtained aprotein fraction from human myelin which, on the basis of its composition, appears to be proteolipid protein apoprotein; it is free of associated lipid but is not soluble in aqueous systems.

The proteolipid apoprotein appears to have certain fairly characteristic features, having amino acid composition distinctive from that of other myelin proteins (Table 11.9). It is characterized by a low content of polar amino acids and a high proportion of aromatic acids, when compared with other myelin proteins, serum lipoproteins or a typical globular protein (Table 11.10), and although it can in general be said to contain a high proportion of non-polar amino acids, this feature is particularly noticeable in the aromatic amino acid fraction. The most unusual feature of the composition of the apoprotein is that it contains a large amount of fatty acid apparently covalently bound, some 2 to 3% of bound fatty acid by weight (approximately 9 millimoles per 100 g) with the greater proportion, more than 80% being palmitic (16:0) and oleic (18:1) acids. Folch-Pi and Stoffyn (1972) record a low carbohydrate content, less than 0.1%, as galactose, but Gagnon et al. (1971) in their preparations find fucose and hexosamine in concentrations of 3 and 13 millimoles/100 g respectively (equivalent to 2.8 g/100 g protein).

The phosphorous content in pure apoprotein preparations appears to be very low. On the basis of the amino acid composition, taking a methionine content of 1 residue, the minimum polypeptide molecular weight has been calculated to be 12 500 (Folch-Pi, 1959), but the molecular weight of the apoprotein as determined by a number of experimental methods has been found to be much higher. When associated with SDS, or dissolved in a phenol-acid system the apoprotein has a molecular weight of between 20 000 and 30 000 when determined by acrylamide gel electrophoresis (Agrawal et al., 1972) or gel chromatography (Nguyen Le et al., 1971). The water soluble apoprotein prepared by the dialysis method appears to be in an aggregated state, having sedimentation values of 62s and 95s at pH 5.0 and 7.0 respectively. The apoprotein even when denatured can still be dissociated by the action of phenol-acetic or 98% formic acid systems to produce smaller units (having sedimentation values of 0.95 and 1.25s (Gagnon et al., 1971)). The proteolipid protein prepared by the method of Folch, Webster and Lees (1959) in organic solvent also appears to be predominantly in an aggregated form, having a molecular weight of between 7.2×10^4 (number average weight, determined by osmotic pressure method) and 2.9×10^6 (weight average weight, determined by light scattering) (Zand, 1968). Furthermore, the indications from the results of light scattering and viscosity measurements of chloroform-methanol solutions of proteolipid protein, are that the protein aggregates are asymmetric and show strong solvent interaction (Zand, 1968). Thus, although the lipid free apoprotein is capable of solution in organic solvents (with the addition of some 2–3% of water, Folch-Pi and Stoffyn, 1972), as well as in aqueous systems, it is apparent that in both systems it exists in a micellar form, behaving in a manner analogous to that of lecithin in benzene or aqueous systems, and it is suggested that the individual subunits may aggregate in such a way that each aggregate presents either a hydrophilic or a hydrophobic face to the bulk phase. In addition it appears probable, on the basis of circular dichroism and rotary dispersion measurements, that the apoprotein has an α-helical content of some 60% in an organic solvent, and 30–40% when in aqueous systems (Sherman and Folch-Pi,

Table 11.9   Amino acid composition of myelin proteins

| | Rabbit Sciatic | | | Bovine root (1) | | | | Bovin CNS | | Human |
	P_0(1)	P_1(1)	P_2(2)	P_0	P_2	CM_W(3)		CM_b(2)	CM_p(4)	CM_p(5)
Lysine	7.1	7.4	10.8	7.9	12.1	6.4		7.6	4.3	4.4
Histidine	2.3	4.8	1.9	2.5	2.1	2.1		5.9	1.9	2.3
Arginine	6.3	9.9	5.9	6.3	6.1	5.4		10.6	2.6	1.8
Aspartic acid	8.3	7.2	8.3	7.2	9.3	9.1		5.5	4.2	4.8
Threonine	5.6	5.9	8.8	5.2	7.5	4.8		4.1	8.5	8.4
Serine	7.9	9.5	6.9	8.2	7.6	5.4		11.2	8.5	6.3
Glutamic acid	10.7	6.8	10.3	9.3	9.9	12.0		5.9	6.0	7.2
Proline	5.3	6.8	3.8	5.1	4.4	4.3		7.1	2.8	2.8
Glycine	9.1	13.4	10.8	8.9	10.2	7.4		14.7	10.3	11.2
Alanine	7.8	8.1	6.7	7.1	6.1	7.8		8.2	12.5	12.0
½ cystine	–	–	–	1.3	–	0.9		0	4.0	4.2
Valine	8.6	3.3	5.9	8.0	6.0	5.4		1.8	6.9	6.6
Methionine	1.0	0.9	1.6	1.5	1.6	2.0		1.2	1.9	1.6
Isoleucine	3.9	2.0	4.2	3.7	3.6	4.0		1.8	4.9	4.4
Leucine	8.3	6.1	7.3	8.3	7.6	8.9		5.9	11.1	11.7
Tyrosine	3.8	2.3	1.9	2.8	2.1	2.7		2.4	4.6	4.9
Plenylalanine	4.0	4.4	4.3	5.6	3.9	3.9		4.7	7.9	8.0
Tryptophan	0.6	0.5	0.9	+	+	–		0.6	–	1.3

(1) Greenfield, Brostoff, Eylar and Morell, 1973
(2) Brostoff, Burnett, Lampert and Eylar, 1972
(3) Wolfgram, 1966
(4) Tenenbaum and Folch-Pi, 1966
(5) Gagnon, Finch, Wood and Moscarrello, 1971

TABLE 11.10 Comparison of amino acid composition of a number of globular proteins with myelin proteins

(Amino acid content as moles %)

Amino acids	CM_P (1)	PM_{po} (2)	CM_w (3)	Human haemoglobin (4)		Human serum lipoprotein (5)			Rabbit (4) actin	Human (6) cyt.b_5
				α chain	β chain	Lp_a	LDL	HDL		
Lys + Hist + Arg	8.7	16.7	13.9	18.4	14.7	12.4	13.2	16.3	12.8	15.2
Asp + Glu	10.2	16.5	21.1	11.8	16.1	21.7	22.9	25.5	25.6	25.2
Thre + Ser	17.0	13.4	10.2	13.6	7.4	14.6	14.5	11.6	13.6	13.7
Tryp + Phe + Tyr	12.5	8.4	6.6	7.5	8.1	7.9	8.7	8	8.4	8.0
Leu + Ile + Val + Ala	35.4	27.1	26.1	36.7	33.0	27.1	29.2	28.2	20.7	27.3
Gly	10.3	8.9	7.4	4.8	8.4	7.5	5.2	4.4	7.9	5.0
Pro	2.8	5.1	4.3	5.0	4.7	5.4	4.0	4.4	5.2	3.6
Cys + Met	5.9	2.8	2.9	2.0	1.9	3.4	2.3	1.5	4.9	2.2

(1) Tenenbaum and Folch-Pi, 1966
(2) Greenfield, Brostoff, Eylar and Morell, 1973
(3) Wolfgram, 1966
(4) Tristram and Smith, 1963
(5) Ehnholm, Simons and Garoff, 1971
(6) Ozols, 1972

1970; Folch-Pi and Stoffyn, 1972), the helical content being reversible, with transference from one solvent to the other. The X-ray powder diagram of proteolipid proteins shows no reflection indicative of any particular secondary structure (Zand, 1968).

The studies just described indicate that the proteolipid apoprotein shows strong protein-protein interaction. It is not yet clear whether this property is a consequence of the removal of the lipid, or some particular fraction of it, or whether similar protein-protein interactions are exerted in its native biological structure. The major part of the lipid in chloroform-methanol extracts is not strongly associated with the protein, but a proportion, including the polyphosphoinsitides and phosphatidyl serine in particular, is more strongly associated. It is not clear, however, whether or not this binding reflects a natural biological association or arises as a secondary consequence of the dissociation of its natural structure, but there is evidence to suggest that such lipid-protein complexes may be artefacts of the dissolution process (Dawson, 1965). It has been demonstrated that the apoprotein, in aqueous dispersion, will interact with anionic lipids and that such aggregates will bind large amounts of neutral and zwiterionic lipids (Braun and Radin, 1969). These apoprotein-anionic lipid complexes appear to involve ionic interactions primarily between the basic residues, since succinylation of the protein markedly reduces the amount of phosphatidyl serine which will interact with it (Braun and Radin, 1969). The apoprotein-anionic lipid complexes, even in the absence of Ca^{++} ions, are obviously of high molecular weight, whereas when complexed with SDS, which can be regarded as an analogue of the anionic lipids, their molecular weight is much reduced. This finding may reflect a difference in micelle size between SDS and the anionic lipids. It also indicates that there cannot be extensive intermolecular disulphide bridging, despite the reasonably high cysteine/cystine content. Braun and Radin (1969) found that the apoprotein would bind about 1.2 μmoles of phosphionositide/mg of protein. Since the concentration of anionic lipid in myelin is approximately 130 μmoles/g myelin, and 30% of the total protein is proteolipid protein, there are approximately 2 μmoles of anionic lipid available/mg of proteolipid protein, sufficient to permit the formation of such a complex.

Some knowledge of the primary structure of proteolipid apoproteins would be of considerable interest, but these proteins appear to be resistant to the action of trypsin, papain and erepsin, and show only limited susceptibility to attack by pronase (Folch-Pi and Stoffyn, 1972). The reason for this resistance to proteolytic enzymes is not understood, but it is unaffected by the presence or absence of lipids.

Comparative data relating to interspecies differences in brain or myelin proteolipid protein is limited, but it is known that amino acid compositions of human and bovine proteolipid protein fractions are very similar (Table 11.9).

Spinal cord yields only small amounts of chloroform methanol soluble protein (Amaducci, Pazzagli and Pessina, 1962), the protein content of cord myelin being reported to be only 13% (Wolfgram and Korii, 1968). The total amino acid composition differs significantly from cerebral myelin (Wolfgram and Kotorii, 1968) and following electrophoresis in phenol-formic acid-water the protein corresponding to proteolipid protein (CM_p) is said to be replaced by one of slower mobility (Mehl and Wolfgram, 1969). Peripheral nerve also contains only small amounts of chloroform methanol soluble protein (Folch, Lees and Carr, 1958; Wolfgram and Rose, 1961). On acrylamide electrophoresis peripheral myelin does not show a protein corresponding to CMp (see Fig. 11.2), the major protein PMo which may be analogous to CMp, is extractable into chloroform-methanol following acid extraction of the myelin (Greenfield et al., 1973). This protein shows other differences from the proteolipid apoprotein in that it seems to be susceptible to tryptic hydrolysis (Csejtey et al., 1972) and its amino acid composition is quite different (Table 11.9).

The protein fraction PM_3 of peripheral myelin, accounting for some 6–13% of the total protein is soluble in chloroform-methanol (Greenfield et al., 1973) but this is a minor component of peripheral myelin and no data is available at present concerning its amino acid composition or other properties. Finally the Wolfgram protein (CMw, Fig. 11.2), extractable into acidified chloroform-methanol is a minor component of central myelin, its amino acid composition resembling that of peripheral PMo (Table 11.9).

Thus, a question remains as to whether or not the properties of brain proteolipid apoprotein are significant reflections of its biological function, or whether homologous structures have evolved having marked differences in molecular association and structure.

11.6.2 *Myelin basic proteins*

Both central and peripheral myelin contain protein which is extractable into dilute mineral acid. The basic protein from central myelin was recognized to be the antigen responsible for inducing the autoimmune disease, experimental allergic encephalomyelitis (EAE) (Laatsch, Kies, Gordon and Alvord, 1962). This observation stimulated intensive investigation into the preparation, purification and properties of the protein, and since the protein's properties are reasonably uncomplicated, these investigations have been successful. The central basic protein, CM_B is also found in peripheral myelin (PM_1) and to date, this appears to be the only myelin common to both the central and peripheral myelins (Greenfield et al., 1973; Brostoff and Eylar, 1972). This protein is the first membrane protein for which the primary structure has been established (Carnegie, 1971; Eylar, Brostoff, Hashim, Caccam and Burnett, 1971). In aqueous solutions the purified protein shows no regular secondary structure (Palmer and Dawson, 1969a; Oshiro and Eylar, 1970) and diffusion and viscosity measurements indicate that the molecule is highly asymmetric with an axial ratio of around 10:1 (Palmer and Dawson, 1969a; Eylar and Thompson, 1969), however it is not known whether the molecule has these same structural

554

characteristics when in situ in the myelin, but it should be remembered that an isometric protein element was deduced from the polarized light studies (*vide supra*).

The primary structure of the protein is compatible with its observed properties (Table 11.11). The polar and non-polar residues are distributed apparently randomly throughout the amino acid sequence, with several clusters of basic and acidic residues, possibly giving rise to strong centres of electrostatic repulsion. The three consecutive proline residues 99–101 (Bovine CM_B) are inferred to provide a hinge region in the molecule, by analogy with a similar sequence found in the hinge region of rabbit IgG (Smyth and Utsumi, 1967). Adjacent to this region, residue 98, lies a threonine residue susceptible to glycosylation by the polypeptide N-acetylgalactosaminyl transferase obtained from bovine submaxillary glands (Hagopian, Westall, Whitehead and Eylar, 1971), emphasizing the similarities between this region in the basic protein and the hinge region in rabbit IgG. A further characteristic of the myelin protein is the presence of a methylated arginine at position 107 which has been suggested to support the bend in the configuration (Brostoff and Eylar, 1971). This methylated arginine has been found in the protein from human, monkey, bovine, rabbit, guinea pig, rat, chicken and turtle brain (Brostoff and Eylar, 1971). Although the molecule appears to be bent, it is of interest that there are no disulphide linkages to fix such a configuration. The even distribution of polar and non-polar residues suggests that stabilization is produced by interaction of the polar groups with their aqueous environment, as has been postulated for globular proteins, leaving the central groove to be filled by the non-polar residues. Although this is a plausible proposal for the configuration in aqueous solution, it need not correspond to that adopted when associated in the membrane, and since the proposed configuration is not stabilized by covalent linkage, it is obvious that the molecule may be capable of undergoing considerable configurational change.

The amino acid sequence of this protein is highly conservative, only some 10% of the residues differing between the bovine, human and rabbit proteins (Table 11.11). Furthermore, certain parts of the sequence appear to be very similar even in such distant vertebrates as the turtle (Brostoff and Eylar, 1971) and urodele amphibians (Martenson, Deibler, Kies, Levine and Alvord Jr., 1972). The only major evolutionary divergence from this pattern appears to have occurred in the rodents. Gene duplication and deletion has occurred in the ancestors of the Myomorpha and Sciuromorpha, leading to the presence of a second basic protein, CMba, which in the rat has the segment corresponding to the residues 117–156 of bovine CMb missing (Martenson, Deibler, Kies, McKneally, Shapira and Kibler, 1972). This raises an interesting question concerning the regulation of these two genes, since although the two proteins are present in the central myelin of the Myomorpha and Sciuromorpha, only the large protein, PM_1 has been found in the peripheral myelin of the rat (Greenfield *et al.*, 1973). If it is assumed that in the central myelin the two proteins can

Table 11.11 Amino acid sequence variations in myelin encephalitogenic protein

										10		
Bovine	N–Ac.Ala	Ser	Ala	Gln	Lys	Arg	Pro	Ser	Gln	Arg	Ser	Lys
Human										His	Gly	
Monkey												
Rabbit										His	Gly	
Guinea pig										His	Gly	
Rabbit PM₁												

				30								
Bovine	Phe	Leu	Pro	Arg	His	Arg	Asp	Thr	Gly	Ile	Leu	Asp
Human												
Monkey												
Rabbit												
Guinea pig												
Rabbit PM₁												

								60				
Bovine	Arg	Gly	Ser	Gly	Lys	Asp	Gly	His	His	Ala	Ala	Arg
Human							Ser			Pro		
Monkey							Ser					
Rabbit							( )	( )				
Guinea pig							Ser					
Rabbit PM₁							( )	( )				

		80										90
Bovine	Arg	Pro	Gly	Asp	Glu	Asn	Pro	Val	Val	His	Phe	Phe
Human		Thr										
Monkey		Thr										
Rabbit												
Guinea pig		Ser										
Rabbit PM₁												

			Me			110						
Bovine	Lys	Gly	Arg	Gly	Leu	Ser	Leu	Ser	Arg	Phe	Ser	Trp
Human												
Monkey												
Rabbit					(Leu	Ser	Val	Thr)				
Guinea pig												
Rabbit PM₁					(Leu	Ser	Val	Thr)				

										140		
Bovine	Ala	Ser	Asp	Tyr	Lys	Ser	Ala	His	Lys	Gly	Leu	Lys
Human											Phe	
Monkey												
Rabbit		Ala										
Guinea pig												
Rabbit PM₁		Ala										

				160								
Bovine	Gly	Gly	Arg	Asp	Ser	Arg	Ser	Gly	Ser	Pro	Met	Ala
Human												
Monkey												
Rabbit												
Guinea pig												
Rabbit PM₁												

							20						
Tyr	Leu	Ala	Ser	Ala	Ser	Thr	Met	Asp	His	Ala	Arg	His	Gly
			Thr										
			Thr										
			Thr										
	40										50		
Ser	Leu	Gly	Arg	Phe	Phe	Gly	Ser	Asp	Arg	Gly	Ala	Pro	Lys
	Ile						Gly				Val		
	Ile					Ser	Gly			Ala			
	Ile												
					70								
Thr	Thr	His	Tyr	Gly	Ser	Leu	Pro	Gln	Lys	Ala	Gln	Gly	His
	Ala									Ser	( )		
	Ala									Ser			
										Ser	( )		
										Ser			
										Ser	( )		
									100				
Lys	Asn	Ile	Val	Thr	Pro	Arg	Thr	Pro	Pro	Pro	Ser	Gln	Gly
		120											130
Gly	Ala	Glu	Gly	Gln	Lys	Pro	Gly	Phe	Gly	Try	Gly	Gly	Arg
					Arg								
							150						
Gly	His	Asp	Ala	Gln	Gly	Thr	Leu	Ser	Lys	Ile	Phe	Lys	Leu
	Val												
	Ala								Arg	Leu			
									Arg	Leu			
170													
Arg	Arg-COOH												

occur simultaneously in the same sheath, then either the duplicated gene is controlled independently or in peripheral myelin the modified protein is a poor 'fit'. It will be necessary to examine the peripheral myelin from these rodents very closely to be certain that the smaller protein is absent. Such observations would be of particular interest in light of the smaller repeat distance found in rat peripheral myelin (see Table 11.8).

Several groups of workers have investigated the formation of binary complexes between myelin basic protein and lipids, and basic protein has been found to readily produce insoluble complexes with acidic lipids (Palmer and Dawson, 1969b; Mateu *et al.*, 1973; London and Vosseberg, 1973). With triphosphoinositide, low proportions of lipid to protein give rise to insoluble complexes, but at higher ratios and low ionic strength the complexes remain soluble, presumably owing to the micellar stability of triphosphoinositide (Palmer and Dawson, 1969b). Changes in the optical rotary dispersion measurement of the protein in such complexes indicate either an increase in the complexity of the structure of the protein, or, as seems more likely, they may reflect the micellar nature of the complex. London and Vosseberg (1973) suggest that sulphatide may be the natural lipid associated with basic protein, since they found this lipid to give complexes more readily than did phosphatidyl serine. The insoluble complexes formed between basic protein and a total acidic lipid fraction have been examined by X-ray diffraction (Mateu *et al.*, 1973), and found to be predominantly lamellar in nature, having a periodicity of 15.4 nm. The structure assigned to this lamellar repeat is an asymmetric one with sulphatide bound to one face of the protein layer and acidic phospholipids to the other, but there is no comment concerning the configuration of the protein. London and Vosseberg (1973) investigated the structure of such complexes by an indirect method, i.e. by examining the tryptic digestion of the protein when complexed with lipid. The middle region of the protein, from residue 20 through to 113 appears to be less accessible to trypsin when complexed with sulphatide and the acidic lipid fraction, but more open to degradation when complexed with phosphatidyl serine. The protection involves six peptide linkages out of a total of fourteen, and includes the hinge region; if the molecule remains bent then one half appears to be strongly associated with the lipid. Considering the nature of the protein the formation of binary complexes with anionic lipids is perhaps not surprising, and the complexes certainly involve electrostatic interaction since the complex with triphosphoinositide, at a ratio of approximately 0.25 μmoles lipid per mg protein, possesses zero electrophoretic mobility (Palmer and Dawson, 1969b). Mateu *et al.* (1973) postulate a structure involving only ionic interaction between lipid and protein, a classic Dannielli-Davson type of structure, whereas the results of London and Vosseberg (1973) suggest a somewhat different interaction with sulphatide, although whether the difference is one of magnitude or of kind is not known.

The antigenic behaviour of CMb and the extent of the immune response of different species to the various regions of the protein are undoubtedly related to the way in which the protein is associated in the myelin sheath. The importance of this point is emphasized by the observation that the monkey when immunized against intact sciatic nerve myelin does not develop EAE, but that when purified PM_1 protein (Brostoff, Carter, Reuter and Eylar, 1972) or PM_2 (Brostoff, Burnett et al., 1972) are used lesions are produced in the central nervous system. One explanation for this difference is that the relevant antigenic segments are not exposed to the immunizing process when intact myelin is used. Some information is available about the relevant segments of the protein in which various experimental animals are sensitive. For example, the guinea pig and the rabbit are sensitive to the segment in the region of residues 114–122 in bovine CMb, including the single tryptophan residue, whereas the monkey is insensitive to this segment (Eylar, 1972). The rabbit and monkey are sensitive to the region 44 to 88, (Shapiro, Chou, McKneally, Urban and Kibler, 1971), and the rat is presumed to be sensitive to regions other than that between residues 117 to 156 (Martenson, et al., 1972). part of this variation in antigenic susceptibility may reflect the sequence possibilities amongst the animals total repertoire of proteins, for example the sequence 98–101 of CMb is found in IgG of the rabbit. It may also reflect variations in the accessibility of different regions of the protein molecule in situ in the myelin sheath. This question is obviously of considerable importance in arriving at an understanding of the development of EAE and its peripheral variant, EAN. The differences observed, i.e. that rabbit central myelin will induce EAE in the monkey whereas peripheral myelin produces EAN, and that purified PM_1 will produce both EAN and EAE, indicate that different segments of the protein molecule are involved in the two conditions and that different segments of the protein are accessible in the two kinds of myelin during the immunization process. The monkey is not sensitive to the tryptophan region 114–122, whereas the guinea pig is, (Eylar, 1972) and rabbit peripheral myelin will produce EAE in guinea pig (Waksman and Adams, 1956). The monkey on the other hand is sensitive to the segment from residue 45 to 90 (Kibler, Re, McKneally and Shapiro, 1972). Thus from the view-point of accessibility these findings suggest that in peripheral myelin the segment 114 to 122 is available as an immunogen but that the 45 to 90 region is not. This is compatible with the suggested close involvement of the region from residue 20 to residue 113 with lipid. The other question that needs to raised is why, if the sensitizing segment is obscured in intact myelin as far as the immunizing process is concerned, is it accessible in vivo in the sensitized animal? A suggested answer is that the arrangement of the protein and the lipid within the myelin differs widely in different species. This might be verified by testing the monkey against monkey peripheral myelin and PM_1. If this suggestion is correct, it would seem strange that the primary structure of the basic protein exhibits such a high degree of conservatism.

The peripheral myelin of all species so far examined contains a second smaller molecular weight basic protein PM_2, the amino acid composition of which differs markedly from CMb/PM_1 (Table 11.9; Brostoff, Burnett, et al., 1972;

Greenfield *et al.*, 1973). From investigations of its antigenicity it is apparent that it shares some parts of its residue sequence with PM_1 (Brostoff, Burnett, *et al.*, 1972; Eylar, 1972), and the protein contains the triproline sequence and the glycosylation site (Eylan, 1972). Unlike PM_1 it has some secondary structure, ORD and CD spectra indicate a possible 50% β-structure (Eylar, 1972). When associated with acidic lipids the resulting complex lamellar phase has a periodicity of approximately 180 Å (Mateu *et al.*, 1973). The proportions of PM_1 and PM_2 present in peripheral myelin vary according to the region examined, suggesting the possibility that there are either different types of myelin sheath or that the two proteins perform similar structural functions in different regions of the sheath, their proportions varying in amount relative to the frequency of paranodes or incisures, or of some other structural feature of the sheath.

11.6.3 *Enzymes associated with myelin*

Myelin fractions as normally prepared, appear to contain small amounts of many enzymes usually assigned to other subcellular fractions, and these small amounts of enzyme activity are therefore considered to reflect contamination of the fraction. There appear to be only three enzymes which are likely to have a genuine association with myelin, and of these only the 2:3 cyclic AMP phosphodiesterase has been studied extensively.

The leucine aminopeptidase was reconized by Adams, Davison and Gregson to be a possible myelin enzyme, in 1963 but only some 17% of the total activity was recovered in a central myelin fraction. A similar situation appears to pertain in the peripheral nervous system, only some 13–23% of the L-leucyl-β-Naphthylamidase activity of whole nerve homogenate being recoverable in the myelin fraction (Hallpike, 1972), although London (1972) reports a complete absence of β-Naphthylamidase activity from peripheral myelin. The total activity detectable in peripheral nerve increases some days after nerve crush or section, and the proportion recovered in the myelin fraction decreases (Hallpike, 1972).

Recently Eto and Suzuki (1973a) have reported the almost exclusive localization of a cholesterolester esterase in central myelin. This enzyme has a pH optimum of 7.2, was activated by sodium taurocholate, and could be clearly distinguished from a microsomal esterase having a pH optimum of 6.0. Some 70–80% of the whole brain activity was recovered in the myelin fraction, and in the brains of the murine mutants, 'quaking' and 'jimpy', the activity was markedly depressed when compared to that of the microsomal enzyme. During the development of the spinal cord and brain of the rat the activity of the enzyme follows closely the progress of myelination, rising sharply from negligible values at 5–10 days post partum, and reaching adult levels at around 30 days in the cord, with a continued slow increase in the brain (Eto and Suzuki, 1973b).

The 2–3'cyclic AMP 3'-phosphohydrolase activity of brain, noted by

560

Drummond, Iyer and Keith (1962) in acetone preparations of ox brain, has subsequently been associated with the myelin fraction (Kurihara and Tsukada, 1967; Olafson, Drummond and Lee, 1969). More than 60% of the enzyme activity could be recoved in the myelin fraction from the central nervous system (Kurihara and Tsukada, 1967), the activity being much reduced in murine mutants showing marked inhibition of myelination (Kurihara, Nussbaum and Mandel, 1969). There is evidence that this enzyme may also occur in the oligodendroglia (Poduslo and Norton, 1972; Zanetta, Benda, Gombos and Morgan, 1972). Cyclic nucleotides are considered to be produced during the degradation of RNA, but the brain enzyme shows a marked preference for the adenosine $- 2'-3'$ cyclic nucleotide (Drummond et al., 1962), and will hydrolyse tetra and octa-adenosyl nucleotide, having $2'-3'$ cyclic adenosine as the terminal group, without degradating the oligonucleotide (Olafson, Drummond and Lee, 1969). The ezyme activity is not specifically associated with the myelin fraction from peripheral nerve, but rather appears to be associated with the membrane fraction also enriched with the $5'$-nucleotidase activity (London, 1972). The activity in spinal cord myelin being some twenty times greater than that found in peripheral myelin (London, 1972). Thus, although the enzyme is present in central myelin, its significance is rather obscure; its Km is reported variously as between 1.9×10^{-3} M (Olafson et al., 1969) to 0.38×10^{-3} M (Kurihara and Takahashi, 1973), and RNA is a minor constituent of myelin (Norton, 1971a). It remains to be shown whether or not this particular enzyme activity has any special significance in the structure or synthesis of the myelin sheath.

11.6.4 Glycoproteins associated with myelin

Considerable interest is at present directed towards determining the significance of glycoproteins in membranes, particularly with respect to recognition functions related to differentiation and cellular interaction. The recent reports of glycoproteins in both central and peripheral myelin are thus of interest. Quarles, Everly and Brady, (1973) have reported evidence indicating the occurrence of a major periodic acid-Schiff positive protein fraction in rat brain myelin; this can be isotopically labelled following the intracerebral injection of radio labelled fucose, glucosamine or N-acetylmannosamine. This protein does not correspond to any of the major protein fractions recognized in myelin, occurring in the high molecular weight fraction with an apparent molecular weight of approx. 110 000. A similar protein is found in the myelin of normal mice and that of the myelin deficient mutant 'quaking', although in the latter it may behave as if it has a slightly higher molecular weight (Matthieu, Brady and Quarles, 1974). The amount of the major glycoprotein/mg of total myelin protein is about the same, or slightly reduced in myelin from the mutant compared to the normal, whereas the amounts of the minor glycoprotein constituents is increased. If the major glycoprotein is associated with the oligodendroglial plasma membrane at the region of its transition into myelin or the external or internal layers, as has been suggested by these authors, the thinness of the sheaths in the mutant would lead these regions to be present in greater concentration than in the normal, and it therefore might be expected that higher concentrations of the glycoprotein would be found in both the mutant and the immature animals. If, on the other hand, this material is associated with the process of compaction smaller amounts of glycoprotein would be expected since the myelin is poorly compacted in these animals. Finally it is possible that the glycoprotein is abnormal in the mutant and that this is the cause of poor compaction Everly, Brady and Quarles (1973) have further reported that the major protein of rat sciatic nerve myelin (presumably PMo) is also a glycoprotein; and a second protein, of lower molecular weight was also labelled following the injection of radio labelled fucose.

The occurrence of glycoproteins in myelin increases the similarity between this membrane and the cell plasma-membrane, but it is not known at present whether these particular glycoproteins are unique to myelin or whether they also occur in the plasma-membrane of the parent cell.

11.7 Lipoprotein complexes isolated from myelin

It has been recognized for many years that there exists the possibility of isolating complexes of lipid and protein from myelin which may reflect their natural association in the native membrane. The membrane is an extensive structure, and since the constituent molecules are not held together by covalent bonds, it must be recognized that the process of dissociation or dispension of such a structure may induce the formation of new molecular associations. This possibility is increased if, during the dispersion, the protein components are exposed to environmental conditions likely to induce conformational change. The proteolipid protein complexes were the earliest of such complexes to be investigated (Folch-Pi and Lees, 1951), containing anionic lipids and sphingo-myelin, as judged by dialysis (Folch-Pi and Stoffyn, 1972), and they appear to exist in the form of large micellar aggregates (Zand, 1968; Folch-Pi and Stoffyn, 1972). Recombination experiments have demonstrated that proteolipid apopro-tein will form binary complexes with anionic lipids that are insoluble in aqueous media (Braun and Radin, 1969), and it has been suggested that such complexes constitute the self-assembly component of myelin. However purified basic protein will also form insoluble complexes with anionic lipids (Palmer and Dawson, 1969b; London and Vosseberg, 1973; Meteu et al., 1973), although it has been suggested that basic protein shows a greater affinity for sulphatide (London and Vosseberg, 1973). The phosphatidopeptides isolated from whole brain are also complexes of acidic polyphosphoinositides with protein (LeBaron and Folch-Pi, 1956; LeBaron, 1969) and evidence has been presented which shows that triphosphoinsitide in the presence of Ca^{2+} ions will form complexes with many common proteins such as, for example, serum albumin (Dawson, 1965). Since these myelin proteins have no recognized activity (they are not known to have any specific associated enzymatic activity for example), it is not possible to examine the consequences of purification or recombination with lipids, as is possible with membrane bound enzymes.

Detergents, both synthetic and naturally occurring, are widely used for the dispersion of membranes in aqueous media. There is no good general theory to explain the action of detergents on membranes, and indeed it seems highly probable that not all detergents interact with membranes in the same way, but nevertheless the common result of their action is the production of binary complexes of detergent-protein and detergent-lipid and less commonly of ternary complexes of protein-lipid-detergent. As has been noted already SDS will dissolve myelin to produce binary complexes of protein-SDS and lipid-SDS, although at low concentrations ternary complexes exist (Nguyen-Le, Nicot and Alfsen, 1971). Soller and Koenig (1970) describe the formation of water soluble complexes from myelin by treatment with Triton X-100. Two types of ternary complex were distinguishable, varying in their ratios of protein to lipid, both being anionic at pH 9.0. Following dialysis some material came out of solution, and after glutaraldehyde-O_sO_4 fixation this appeared to have the form of membraneous vesicles.

The ability of the naturally occurring detergent, l-acyl-lysophosphatidyl choline (LPC) to clear whole brain homogenates has long been recognized (Webster, 1957; Gent, 1959). It has further been shown that it will completely solubilize central myelin, both *in vitro* (Gent, Gregson, Gammack and Raper, 1964), and *in vivo* (Hall and Gregson, 1971; Hall, 1972; Gregson and Hall, 1973). The ability of LPC to solubilize membranes is dependent on the chemical composition of the membrane as well as its source (Gottfried and Rapport, 1963; McIlwain, Graf and Rapport, 1971). The mechanism whereby LPC solubilizes the membrane is not known, but there is evidence from NMR studies that it is bound to the membrane components, principally via the alkyl residues, and that this binding does not release the binding of the intrinsic lipids (Chapman *et al.*, 1968). A close examination of the solubilization of myelin reveals that it exhibits a strict stoichiometry under specified conditions (Gent *et al.*, 1964), and that it is a two stage process in which discrete components are released at each of the stages (Gent, Gregson, Lovelidge and Winder, 1971a).

The complexes formed by the action of LPC on central myelin can be resolved electrophoretically (Gent and Gregson, 1966), by molecular sieve chromatography (Gent *et al.*, 1971b), and, most successfully by isopycnic centrifugation (Gent *et al.*, 1971c). Isopycnic centrifugation reveals that all of the complexes have a density greater than lipid-LPC mixtures and less than that of pure myelin. They fall into two broad groups (Fig. 11.5), the highest density group, centred at a buoyant density of 1.044 g cm^{-3}, consists of the components released predominantly in the first stage of the solubilization, and a lower density group centred at 1.023 g cm^{-3} representing the products of the second stage of solubilization. The actual number of components is dependent upon the source of the myelin (Fig. 11.5), five components being recognizable in

563

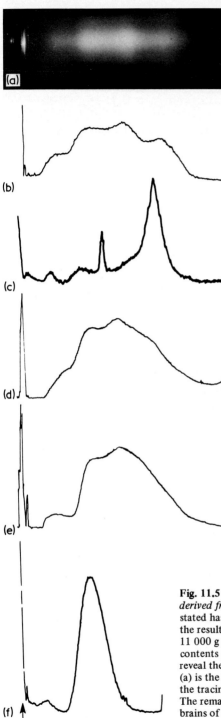

Meniscus   Increasing density

Fig. 11.5 *Isopycnic separation of lipoprotein complexes derived from myelin.* Myelin from the brains of the species stated has been solubilized with lysophosphatidylcholine and the resulting complexes separated by centrifugation at 11 000 g for 16 h. on a 5 to 20% sucrose gradient. The tube contents are photographed under indirect illumination to reveal the components by scattered light. The photograph (a) is the preparation from normal mouse brain myelin and the tracing (b) is the densitometer recording of the negative. The remaining traces are of similar preparations from the brains of (c) the mutant mouse 'quaking'; (d) rat; (e) rabbit; (f) dogfish. (Data from Bradbrook and Gregson, 1973 and unpublished results of Gent, Gregson and Lovelidge.)

the rat and the mouse, two in the dogfish and three in the rabbit (Gent *et al.*, 1971c). Myelin isolated from the central nervous system of the mutant mouse 'quaking' differs both qualitatively and quantitatively from that of normal animals (Bradbrook and Gregson, 1973). Furthermore, if the normal lipid-protein association of the myelin is first disrupted by freeze-drying (see Section 11.5.2), only a single group of components of low density are found after solubilization (Lovelidge, 1972). The low density components contain predominantly proteolipid protein, and the 2:3 cyclic AMP phosphodiesterase activity, whereas the high density group components account for the basic protein (Gent *et al.*, 1971c). The galactocerebroside is distributed throughout three major fractions (Gregson, Kennedy and Leibowitz, 1971) and the complement fixing activity of myelin with anti-galactocerebroside sera is recovered following isopycnic centrifugation in a single peak which corresponds to the major peak of galactocerebroside (Gregson, Kennedy and Leibowitz, 1971, 1974). The two subsidiary peaks of galactocerebroside do not appear to display complement fixing activity, although they can be detected by immuno-diffusion against anticerebroside sera (Gregson, Kennedy and Leibowitz, 1974). This is of considerable interest since it is known that the antigenic activity of galactocerebroside is greatly influenced by other lipid constituents (Rapport, Cavanna and Graf, 1967).

Joffe (1971) has recently described the isolation of lipoprotein complex from succinylated myelin. The complex is extracted following partial lipid extraction with ether: ethanol mixtures, and is unusual in that the lipid bound in the complex appears from an NMR investigation to be bound by the polar head groups (Joffe and Block, 1972).

The suggestion is frequently made that the lipoprotein complexes which have been isolated may represent the self assembly units of the myelin sheath. From the information available and discussed in Section 11.8, it is becoming apparent, however, that this need not, and is indeed unlikely, to be the case. It appears very probable that the sheath elements initially assembled may become modified either during the process of assembly, or subsequently.

11.8 The synthesis and metabolism of myelin

In considering the function of the myelin sheath it is appropriate and necessary to ask why should it have the form of a compacted spiral of membrane. The compaction may be related to the achievement of a sufficiently high reactance, radially and longitudinally, but the fact that it is in the form of a spiral would appear to be related to the mechanism of its synthesis and growth, since the spiral form permits the existance of continuous cytoplasmic connections through the thickness of the sheath, that may be concerned with further metabolic interaction after the period of growth. Peripheral and central sheaths have very similar morphology, the main difference between them being that peripherally a single internodal segment of myelin is produced by, and remains associated with, a single Schwann cell, whereas each myelin producing oligodendrocyte in the central nervous system forms many segments of myelin around a number of different axons. The continued association of the oligodendroglia with the myelin sheaths in the mature central nervous system, is an assumption and has proved difficult to demonstrate morphologically. (Peters and Vaughn, 1970). The growth of the myelin sheath thus presents a problem in topology – how is the spiral formed? Furthermore, since it has continuity with the plasma membrane of the myelin-producing cell, it also presents a metabolic problem, i.e. what are the spatial and temporal characteristics of the synthesis and assembly of its components? Is the process one of differentiation of a plasma membrane or is the myelin an independently produced and discrete cell organelle? Once produced how labile a structure is it, that is, is there a continued long term flux of constituents both into and out of it?

11.8.1 *The synthesis and growth of the myelin sheath*

The electron microscopic demonstration that the myelin sheath was a spiral of membrane, continuous with the plasma membrane of the satellite cell (Geren, 1954; Robertson, 1958) naturally led to the postulation of a single theory of myelin formation involving the wrapping of a cell process around the axon, and the continued extension of this process to form a spiral (Bunge, 1968). In the initial stages of myelination it is easy to visualize the mechanics of spiral formation as the progress of a tongue of the cell around the axon, but once a reasonable thickness of sheath has been produced more complex explanations would appear to be required. The need for an increase in the inner circumference of the sheath to allow for increasing axon diameter during growth, the appearance of bizarre forms of sheath, particularly in the central nervous system, and the fact that one oligodendrocyte produces myelin at several internodes on a number of different fibres, all place restrictions on the possible physical explanations of the mechanisms by which myelin sheath grows. Further complexities are introduced by the fact that as longitudinal growth of the axon occurs, the internodal lengths also increase, since the number of internodes is fixed at the time of onset of myelination (Vizoso and Young, 1948). Longitudinal growth cannot be achieved simply by the laying down of additional paranodal 'loops', since the size of the paranodal region is insufficient to account for the observed increment in internodal length (see the data of Williams and Wendell-Smith, 1971).

The rate of growth of the myelin membrane in the peripheral nervous system is initially very rapid (Webster, 1971, 1972), but appears to settle to a steady rate which in the rabbit has been calculated to be of the order of 1.1 to 1.6 x 10^5 μm^2/day (Williams and Wendell-Smith, 1971). Using a density of 1.11 g cm^{-3} and an 18 nm period this would correspond to the net synthesis of some 21 to 34 x 10^{-12} g of myelin per Schwann cell/day. The figures of Webster (1971) indicate that the rate of synthesis in the rat is much lower.

It is generally considered that the mesaxon, which appears to be continuous along the whole internode, provides the most likely growth zone for the myelin sheath, the mesaxon either moving around the perimeter of the cell as growth occurs, or remaining stationary while the spiral slips as new membrane is added. In peripheral nerve fibres the nucleus would be swept around the axon if the mesaxon were to move as growth occurred; such rotation of the nucleus has been reported to occur in myelinating fibres in tissue culture (Murray, 1965) but was not observed in the myelinating fibres of the frog tadpole tail (Speidel, 1964). The question of nuclear rotation needs to be answered by the observation of the behaviour of myelinating fibres *in vivo*, as the low packing density of the tissue elements in culture may allow movements to occur which would be impossible *in vivo*

. Slippage of the myelin spiral has been invoked as the mechanism by which the inner circumference of the sheath adjusts to the radial growth of the axon during development. No data are available, however, concerning the shear characteristics between the myelin lamellae. In the central nervous system movement of the mesaxon appears to be impossible because of the involvement of each oligodendroglial cell with many internodes. Furthermore, Peters (1964) has analyzed the relative positions of the external and internal mesaxons in optic nerve fibres and finds that they have a tendency to lie in the same quadrant of the sheath. This observation is rather surprising, since the spiral, as seen in tranverse section, may be considered to represent the history of the movement of a point (the external mesaxon) around the axon, leading to an expectation that there would be a random relationship between the relative positions of the mesaxons. The explanation suggested by Peters for his findings of a non random relationship was that the synthesis of the sheath occurs in bursts, involving units of one complete revolution of the mesaxon, and that this requires that the time spent on one such excursion is relatively much shorter than the interval spent at rest. Peters further comments on the finding that a 'radial component' (see Chapter 1) is frequently seen in that region of the sheath in which the external and internal mesaxons lie, and he suggests that the radial component may represent a 'transporting region'. It is not clear, however, how real a structure the 'radial component' is, since it is only seen in some electron micrographs.

If the myelin sheath is indeed produced more rapidly in the early stages of development, it may indicate that the mechanism by which this initial growth is achieved differs in some way from that which follows. In the early stages of myelination the sheath is frequently seen to consist of an uncompacted cytoplasmic spiral (Peters and Vaughn, 1970). In the peripheral nerve a radial series of bands of cytoplasm are frequently seen in the quadrant in which the external mesaxon lies, compaction at the cytoplasmic interface only occurring as an arc around the remaining 2/3 of the sheath (Webster, 1971). This form of partial compaction has also been observed in central nervous tissue (Caley, 1967). If it is assumed that net growth will only occur where the membrane has direct contact with cytoplasm, such ribs of cytoplasm and membrane existing only in early sheaths could provide additional growth points. Careful examination of micrographs of early myelinating fibres shows that the Schwann cell processes often appear as a series of reversed loops around the axon, and that the external mesaxon does not provide a simple spiral (see for example Figs. 2 to 4 in Webster, 1971). It can easily be seen that growth and fusion of the ends of such processes would produce a spiral. It is of interest that abnormal concentric lamellae have been observed in material from oligodendrogliomata (Robertson and Vogel, 1962), a geometrical arrangement that could readily arise from the fusion of cell processes encircling an axon but not from a spiralling motion.

Whatever the growth mechanism may be it would seem unlikely that it will differ in essentials between the central and peripheral nervous systems, since the final form is almost identical. Further, it would seem unlikely that rapid growth of the membrane could occur in regions not in direct contact with cytoplasm, suggesting that the possible growth zones are the external and internal mesaxons, the paranodal loops and the Schmidt—Lanterman incisures, the latter two sites probably providing the regions of longitudinal growth. The growth of the sheath at such zones can be envisaged as involving the insertion of lipoprotein units into the existing membrane structure. Potentially, the most useful experimental method for locating the growth zones is undoubtedly autoradiography, but the small dimensions involved have made this a difficult undertaking.

While the problem of the mechanism of growth is obviously a considerable one, other biologically intriguing questions concern the factors which govern whether or not a particular axon is to be myelinated, and the nature of the signal which initiates myelination? Axon diameter is usually considered to be the deciding factor in whether or not an axon will be myelinated. In the peripheral nervous system, axons below 2 μm in diameter tend not to myelinate, but in the central nervous system myelinated axons of 0.6 to 0.7 μm diameter can be found (Fleischhauer and Wartenberg, 1967). In the peripheral nervous system Schwann cells initially encircle bundles of many axons, but as the Schwann cell number increases they enclose fewer and fewer fibres, the large axons gradually become separated from the remainder until they are completely segregated within a single Schwann cell (Peters and Vaughn, 1970). All the available evidence indicates that it is the characteristics of the axon which determine whether or not the satellite cell will produce myelin (see for example Hillarp and Olivercrona, 1946).

It is unlikely that it will be possible to decide from morphological studies alone whether myelin is synthesized as such or by a differentiation of invaginated plasma membrane. Lamellar compaction has been considered by some workers to indicate a final differentiation step of the myelin membrane (see Davison, 1970), and to be the morphological correlate of the changing chemical composition of myelin during early development (Cuzner and Davison, 1968; Morell et al., 1972).

The compositional studies on myelin fractions isolated from young animals are complicated by the fact that these fractions are heterogeneous (Cuzner and

TABLE 11.12   Protein composition of mouse myelin, changes during growth

Age (days)	Relative concentration of protein, %					
	CM_2	CM_b	CM_{ba}	CM_P	CM_w	High mol. wt.
9	2.5	8.6	10.2	7.0	12.3	59.4
15	4.3	9.5	12.7	12.0	14.3	47.2
20	4.5	9.8	14.3	13.4	15.2	42.8
25	6.8	11.8	15.4	21.4	14.8	29.8
45	7.5	12.7	16.6	23.2	15	25
60	7.5	12.0	17.0	23.2	15.0	26.3
300	10	12.7	18.6	28.2	14.1	16.4

Data taken from Morell et al., 1972

Davison, 1968; Eng and Noble, 1968; Benjamin, Miller and McKhann, 1973). However even when care is taken to prepare homogeneous fractions of myelin from the brains of developing animals the chemical composition varies with the age of the animal (Cuzner and Davison, 1968; Eng and Noble, 1968; Eng, Chao, et al., 1968; Morell et al., 1972; Norton and Poduslo, 1973). The compositional changes during development involve both the protein, particularly the proteo-lipid protein (Table 11.12), and the lipid components galactocerebroside, and the choline and ethanolamine phospholipids. There have as yet been no parallel studies on the developing peripheral nervous system, but the analysis of whole nerve suggests that a similar situation exists (Oxberry, 1971).

The myelin isolated from the brains of young developing animals can be subfractionated by what appears to be a form of rate sedimentation separation through discontinuous density gradients (Cuzner and Davison, 1968; Benjamin, Miller and McKhann, 1973). The fractionation is related to composition and the relative proportions of the subfractions appear to change with age in a way that is consistent with the change in composition of the total myelin fraction. Davison and co-workers have drawn attention to a fraction dubbed 'myelin-like' which can be isolated from the initial myelin fraction from the brains of young animals (Agrawal, et al., 1970). This material is membraneous and has a higher protein content than myelin, agreeing with its observed higher flotation density on CsCl gradients (Morell et al., 1972), and a similar fraction has been isolated from ox intradural spinal roots (London, 1972). The galactocerebroside content of this material is lower than that in myelin, there is a higher proportion of lecithin than ethanolamine phospholipid, the proteins are principally of high molecular weight (Agrawal, et al., 1970; Morell et al., 1972), and the fraction contains both $2'-3'$ cyclic AMP $3'$-phosphohydrolase and Na^+-K^+-ATPase (Banik and Davison, 1969; Agrawal et al., 1970). This 'myelin-like' fraction was suggested to represent an intermediate transition stage between the oligodendro-glial membrane and myelin (Davison, et al., 1966), with the implication that the plasma membrane becomes differentiated to form myelin. This fraction can be isolated from the adult as well as from the immature nervous system, and thus whatever cellular components may contribute this fraction it does not appear to represent the membrane specifically associated with the first formed myelin. If this fraction represents the mesaxon membrane considered to be the postulated growth zone, the amount recoverable should increase with growth, as more fibres become myelinated and as the mesaxon increases with increasing internodal length (although decreasing as a proportion of the total myelin fraction). There is, unfortunately, some conflict of evidence as to whether the absolute amount of this fraction indeed increases with growth of the brain (Agrawal, *et al.*, 1970; Morell *et al.*, 1972; Benjamin, Miller and McKhann, 1973). The amount of the fraction isolated from the adult rat and mouse brain has been reported as being between 1/3 and 1/9 of the amount of myelin (Agrawal *et al.*, 1970; Morell *et al.*, 1972), whereas in ox peripheral nerve a similar fraction accounts for between 0.5 to 2.0 μg of protein/g wet wt. of tissue and the myelin for 12.5 to 20 μg protein/g (London, 1972). These quantities appear to be rather high for the fraction to represent the growth zone of the external mesaxon, which in mature fibres is short and may not be visible at all in the central nervous system, and it is possible that this fraction may include membranes from the Schmidt—Lanterman incisures and paranodal regions. However it is equally possible that the 'myelin-like' fraction may have no connection at all with either myelin or myelination. The myelin fraction used in biochemical studies is operationally defined and the presence of a second type of membrane within the initial fraction does not necessarily mean that it has any direct morphological connection with myelin.

If one accepts the evidence for change in the composition of myelin during development there remain the problems of whether this change relates to all of the segments of the sheath, and whether or not the composition changes in an uniform and active fashion, or whether only the average composition alters as a consequence of further growth.

11.8.2 *Metabolism and synthesis*

The injection of a radio-labelled precursor into experimental animals, either systemically or locally, leads to the incorporation of that precursor into the appropriate components of the myelin sheath. The amount and time of such incorporation varies with the age of the animal, and combines contributions from both the turnover and the net synthesis of the structure and its component parts. The two processes are difficult to distinguish but in the young animal net synthesis of myelin obviously predominates, and thus more precursor is incorporated during the period of active myelination in the central nervous system (Fig. 11.6). This observation relates to that period of growth at which the maximum number of tracts are being myelinated, and not to a period of increased rate of synthesis per internode.

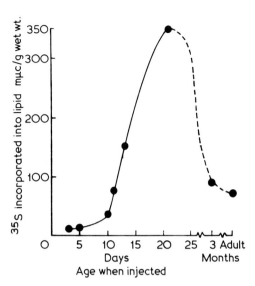

Fig. 11.6 *The incorporation of $^{35}S-SO_4$ into the lipid of rat brain as a function of age.* Rats were given carrier free $^{35}S-SO_4{}^{2-}$ at the ages indicated, 10 μci/25 g body weight and killed after 48 h. The radioactivity in the whole brain lipid fraction is recorded. (Reproduced from Davison and Gregson, 1966, by courtesy of the Biochemical Journal.)

The synthesis and incorporation of myelin lipids has been the most closely studied, and because of their variety, the most complex aspect of myelin metabolism. The case of cholesterol incorporation into the myelin sheath serves as a good example.

Neural tissue can sysnthesize cholesterol from glucose and acetate (Smith, 1969; Kandutsch and Saucier, 1969), and cholesterol can be incorporated from the plasma pool into both the central and peripheral nervous systems (Davison and Wajda, 1959; Clarenburg, Chaikoff and Morris, 1963; Simon, 1966; Spohn and Davison, 1972b). The uptake of plasma cholesterol is low and Clarenburg *et al.* (1963) estimated that over a period of sixteen days during myelination in the rabbit only 8% of the accumulated brain cholesterol was derived from the plasma. The bulk of the tissue cholesterol accumulated is thus synthesized by the tissue itself. The maximal synthesis of cholesterol from acetate in the mouse brain occurs prior to the period of maximal myelination, the rate limiting step being the activity of β-hydroxy-β-methyl glutaryl CoA reductase, the activity of this enzyme declining from 5 days post partum (Kandutsch and Saucier, 1969). It is not known whether or not the synthetic activity declines concurrently in all cell types, but the maximal rate of cholesterol accumulation occurs before the initiation of myelination, and even when myelination starts, cholesterol is primarily accumulated in non-myelin structures (Cuzner, 1968; Davison, 1970). The major site of cholesterol synthesis is the microsomal fraction (Ramsey, Jones, Rios and Nicholas, 1972) from which it is transferred, possibly directly to

571

the myelin (Banik and Davison, 1971). A further indication that cholesterol synthesis does not occur *in situ* in the sheath has been provided by studies using inhibitors of cholesterol synthesis. Following the administration of such inhibitors to young animals, the metabolic intermediates 7- and 24-dehydro-cholesterol accumulate in the sheath (Scott and Barber, 1964; Smith, Hasinoff and Fumagalli, 1970; Rawlins and Uzman, 1970; Banik and Davison, 1971), and disappear following withdrawal of inhibitor (Banik and Davison, 1971) although the reductases involved are localized in the microsomal fraction (Banik and Davison, 1971; Hinse and Shah, 1971). Cholesterol is the major lipid of the myelin sheath on a molar basis, and interference with its synthesis in turn depresses myelin synthesis. Thus desmosterol and 7-dehydrocholesterol are found in the sheath following the administration of AY 9944 or 20:25-diazo-cholesterol to suckling rats, and although the lipid composition is otherwise unchanged the total amount of myelin recoverable from the brain is much reduced (Smith, Hasinoff and Fumagalli, 1970). In addition, the in vitro incorporation of ^{14}C from glucose into all of the lipids and proteins of the myelin is also diminished under these circumstances, providing further evidence of an overall reduction in myelin synthesis. The peripheral effect of such inhibitors is to reduce both the sheath thickness and the total number of myelinated fibres, suggesting that both the initiation and further synthesis of myelin are inhibited (Rawlins and Uzman, 1970). Following drug withdrawal ^{14}C-labelled cholesterol intermediates are slowly replaced by ^{14}C-cholesterol (Fumagalli, Smith, Urna and Paoletti, 1969), suggesting the possibility that such intermediates impart some instability to the structure of the sheath; the finding of debris-laden macrophages within the nerve also suggests that active demyelina-tion may occur. Alternatively the slow replacement of the cholesterol intermediates by cholesterol may be an indication of a normally occurring turnover and recycling of the myelin constituents, for although there is evidence of a long term persistence of cholesterol in the sheath (Cuzner, Davison and Gregson, 1966) this can be explained either in terms of the stability of the structure or of the recycling of constituents within a closed pool. Metabolic stability was envisaged simply to be the consequence of the sequestration of constituents deeply placed within the structure of the sheath. By studying the release of cholesterol ester during Wallerian degeneration Simon, Wade, DeLarco and Baker (1969) found that the myelin cholesterol deposited late during myelination is the first to be removed during degeneration, and vice versa, a result compatible with the concept that there is a compartmentation of cholesterol within the sheath during myelination. A similar conclusion regarding other lipid constituents has been arrived at from studies of myelin degradation in the central nervous system in chronic triethyl-tin poisoning (Smith, 1973).

Small amounts of cholesterol ester occur normally in the developing nervous system (Adams and Davison, 1959; Clarenburg *et al.*, 1963), these increase with age and show a further transient rise during the period of maximal myelination (Eto and Suzuki, 1972a), possibly reflecting the remodelling of fibre tracts, some degenerating fibres being a normal feature of developing tissue. The brain cholesterol ester does not derive from the plasma, as it has a different fatty acid pattern to that of the plasma esters, and appears to be produced in situ by an esterifying system not requiring CoA or lecithin-cholesterol transacylase (Eto and Suzuki, 1972b). Cholesterol esterases also occur in brain tissue, their activity increasing up to the peak period of myelination (Eto and Suzuki, 1972b). A discrete cholesterol esterase is associated with myelin (Eto and Suzuki, 1973a) and, as might be expected, the detectable activity of this enzyme increases with myelination (Eto and Suzuki, 1973b). This finding suggests in turn that cholesterol ester would not be found in myelin except in very small amounts.

In summary these investigations into aspects of cholesterol metabolism related to myelination indicate (a) that the constituent cholesterol is not synthesized by the myelin sheath but is transferred to it from elsewhere; (b) that interference with the synthesis of a constituent part of the myelin membrane will affect the synthesis of the whole sheath; and (c) that there is some evidence of metabolic compartmentation. Examination of the synthesis and incorporation of other myelin constituents tends to support these general findings.

Most of the precursor studies carried out on myelination indicate that the lipid constituents are synthesized by components of the microsomal fraction (Miller and Dawson, 1972a), but they do not reveal how this material is transferred to the myelin sheath. Free lipid is not transferred as such in biological systems, but is associated with protein, and there is evidence for the existence of a specific sulphatide transport protein (Herschkowitz, *et al.*, 1968a b; Pleasure and Prockop, 1972). Furthermore a high molecular weight component of the supernatant fraction is necessary for the *in vitro* transfer of phospholipid from brain microsomes to mitochondria (Miller and Dawson, 1972b), although in this system there is no transfer to myelin, which is in fact inhibitory to the microsomal-mitochondrial exchange. Exchange of cholesterol and 7-dehydro-cholesterol between microsomes and myelin has been reported, but in these experiments the requirement for a supernatant factor was not tested (Banik and Davison, 1971). Soluble lipoproteins containing phospholipid have been identified in fractions of mammalian brain and these are readily and rapidly labelled by precursors (Robertson, 1960; Benjamin and McKahn, 1973a). The sulphatide carrier liprotein systems of brain (Herschkowitz, *et al.*, 1968a,b; 1969), and of peripheral nerve (Pleasure and Prockop, 1972) have been the most studied. In *in vitro* conditions this system accepts sulphatide from the microsomal fraction, the site of galactocerebroside sulphation (Herschkowitz, *et al.*, 1968a), and will then transfer it to myelin (Pleasure and Prockop, 1972). Following the inhibition of protein synthesis by puromycin and cycloheximide, the incorporation of sulphatide into myelin is initially unaffected but after 90 min it progressively diminishes (Pleasure and Prockop, 1972). This delayed effect is considered to be due to a slow reduction in the availability of the lipoprotein, since although sulphatide synthesis remains unaltered, transfer of sulphatide from the microsomal fraction to lipoprotein is quickly reduced (Herschkowitz *et al.*, 1969; Pleasure and Prockop, 1972). While none of these experiments provide definitive proof of the involvement of specific transport lipoproteins in the synthesis of myelin they appear to give support to such an hypothesis. It is of interest to note that tissue from adult animals was used in the experiments of Miller and Dawson (1972b), in which they failed to demonstrate the transference of phospholipid from microsomes to myelin, whereas the studies on sulphatide transfer described above employed tissue from immature, actively myelinating animals.

In vitro studies indicate that the amino acid incorporation into proteolipid protein reaches a maximum at around the eighth day of post natal life in the rat (Mokrasch and Manner, 1963). Proteolipid protein synthesis during development thus appears to resemble lipid synthesis, in that it is at a maximum in advance of the period of maximal myelination, the incorporation of amino acid into proteolipid and basic protein decreasing rapidly from fifteen days onwards (Smith, 1969; Rawlins and Smith, 1971). Further correlation of studies of protein and lipid deposition is undoubtedly required, in view of the marked change in the protein composition of myelin during myelination.

Experimental studies concerned with the metabolic turnover of the myelin sheath are difficult to interpret, but all of such studies indicate that myelin turnover is slow relative to that of other tissue components. This is particularly well shown in studies concerned with the persistance of isotope incorporated during myelination (Davison, Dobbing, Morgan and Payling Wright, 1959; Davison and Gregson, 1962; Smith and Eng, 1965; Cuzner, Davison and Gregson, 1965a; Jungalwala and Dawson, 1971). These published accounts differ concerning the rate of turnover of the individual lipids, and whereas Smith and co-workers (Smith, 1967) found that the choline, inositol and serine lipids turned over more rapidly than the other lipids, the results of Davison and his co-workers indicated that there was no statistically significant difference in the turnover rates of any of the constituent lipids (Cuzner, Davison and Gregson, 1965a, 1966). This disparity may have arisen in part from the methods used to present the results of this kind of experiment, and also from the fact that the rat is the experimental animal most commonly used, since in this animal growth of the brain, and thus net myelin synthesis, continues throughout adult life, albeit at a slow rate (e.g. Rawlins and Smith, 1971; Eto and Suzuki, 1973b). The results of these experiments are expressed in terms of either specific activity of concentration within a whole organ, the latter being considered to provide an automatic correction for the accretion of new material during growth. If such an allowance is to be made when expressing the results in terms of specific activity a correction factor must be applied. The choice of such a factor is not a simple matter however, and it may be necessary to provide a different correction factor for each lipid at each stage, because the composition of myelin changes during maturation, and in the mature animal myelin accretion accounts for an increasing proportion of the total incremental growth of the brain.

An apparent contradiction to the concept of a slow rate of lipid turnover is the common finding that in both *in vivo* and *in vitro* systems myelin from mature adult animals shows incorporation of radioactive precursor, but this increment is of a more transient nature than that observed in young animals (Davison and Gregson, 1966; Jungalwala and Dawson, 1971). In an analysis of the turnover of myelin sulphatide in the adult rat for example (Davison and Gregson, 1966), the results were interpreted in terms of a two pool system. The labile pool had a half life of approximately two and a half days, involved the largest fraction of ^{35}S-SO$_4$ incorporated, but represented only 0.2% of the total myelin sulphatide (Davison and Gregson, 1966). This two pool system appears to fit the observed data well but could still be a simplification (see for example the treatment of serum cholesterol as a three pool system by Goodman, Noble and Dell, 1973). Comparison of the specific activities of the microsomal and precursor pools with that of the myelin lipids led Jungalwala and Dawson (1971) to suggest that in the adult rat there is a large, labile pool of the myelin lipids. Such simple comparisons of data in terms of specific activity at fixed time intervals presupposes, firstly, a uniform metabolic pool within each subcellular fraction, and secondly, a rapid equilibration of the precursor pool with all structures involved. However, with the possible exception of the phosphoinositides and phosphatidic acid, the maximum uptake of label shows a delay and the amount of material incorporated over a given time interval is thus related to the integral of the specific activity of the precursor (see Davison and Gregson, 1966). This is a consequence of the system being an open one, the precursor having more than a single fate, the observed incorporation being the product of all of the processes of synthesis, transfer and incorporation into the myelin structure. The observation that in the rat a small amount of material is incorporated into a pool having a slow turnover rate may be explained by either the continuous accretion of myelin or its recycling, and there is some evidence to support a recycling of cholesterol (Rawlins, Hedley-White, Villegers and Uzman, 1970; Spohn and Davison, 1972b). The analytical complications of such recycling can be overcome by the use of suitably labelled precursors such as Gaunidino-^{14}C-arginine (Aschenbrenner, Druyom, Albin and Rabinowitz, 1970) and 2-^{3}H-glycerol (Benjamin and McKhann, 1973b).

Myelin lipids and proteins will both become labelled when central and peripheral nervous tissues from adult animals are incubated with labelled precursor *in vitro* (Mokrasch and Manner, 1963; Smith, 1969; Rawlins and Smith, 1971), and the pattern of uptake of ^{14}C from glucose and acetate into the individual lipids agrees with the order of turnover found *in vivo* (Smith, 1969). The observed uptake obviously reflects both synthesis and incorporation into myelin, and the apparent variation in the turnover of the individual myelin lipids may be a reflection of their differing rates of synthesis. The rate of lecithin synthesis by neural tissue in the adult is clearly quite rapid (Ansell and Spanner, 1972), and is certainly faster than that of sulphatide synthesis (Smith, 1969). The monoesterified phosphate of myelin triphosphoinositide also undergoes rapid turnover; it disappears *post mortem* (Dawson and Eichberg, 1965) and is rapidly labelled both *in vivo* and *in vitro* (Eichberg and Dawson, 1965), and the di- and tri-phosphoinositide phosphomonoesterases being found in the supernatant fraction. *In vivo* and *in vitro* myelin phosphoinositide shows rapid uptake of label from acetate, glucose and glycerol (Smith, 1967, 1969; Jungalwala and Dawson, 1971), and it is considered that the high metabolic turnover indicates a functional role for this group of lipids which have been implicated in the regulation of ion permeability in a number of other cell membranes, including the axon membrane (Hawthorne, 1972). It has been suggested that the phosphoinositides may occur at the paranodal region where they may be involved in some process of ion regulation, possibly of Ca^{2+}.

In the rat the synthesis of lipid proceeds at a higher rate than that of protein during development, but from six months onwards the level of synthesis remain reasonably constant (Rawlins and Smith, 1971). The level of *in vitro* incorporation of leucine into the myelin proteins of thirty-five day old rats indicates that the synthesis and incorporation of proteolipid protein is greater than that of basic protein (Smith and Hasinoff, 1971), but this finding is somewhat at variance with conclusions derived from *in vivo* studies (Wood and King, 1971; Sammeck, Martenson and Brady, 1971). The turnover time determined by Sammeck, Martenson and Brady (1971) for the basic protein in the adult, is presumably an overestimate since they used immature animals. From the known properties of proteolipid and basic protein it would be expected that the basic proteins would be the more likely to undergo metabolic turnover since they are more susceptible to endogenous proteolytic degradation, (Sammeck and Brady, 1972), and it is possible that the low level of basic protein synthesis found *in vitro* can be attributed to an abnormally high rate of degradation of the newly synthesized material.

It is apparent that the synthesis and further metabolism of myelin is a complex process. Myelin has been found to lack both synthetic capacity and the principal catabolic systems, so that highly purified myelin for example, can be incubated *in vitro* without any apparent loss of basic protein (Sammeck and Brady, 1972). Lipids do not appear to exist *in vitro* without associated protein, and there is strong evidence for the involvement of soluble lipoprotein being involved in the process by which preformed lipid is incorporated into myelin (*vide supra*). Once synthesized the myelin isolated from tissues appears to represent at least two distinct metabolic compartments, certainly with respect to its lipid constituents. A number of different metabolic systems can be envisaged that may explain these observations. The original proposal of Cuzner, Davison and Gregson (1965a) was that myelin could be considered to turn over in unitary fashion within the context of a lipoprotein membrane structure. This suggestion has not been found to be compatible with all subsequent experimental observations, and alternative hypotheses are necessary. In Fig. 11.7 several suggested mechanisms are shown diagramatically. Fig. 11.7a illustrates the early hypothesis, Fig. 11.7b the system of individual component turnover, and Fig. 11.7c includes the suggestion of a membrane precursor that is converted into myelin by a process of differentiation. It is not possible to decide which, if any, of these suggestions is the most plausible at the present time, although suggestion 11.7a has the advantage that it is testable since it should be possible to demonstrate the presence of water soluble lipoproteins having both protein and lipid components in common with myelin.

11.9 Abnormalities of myelin synthesis and metabolism in disease

There are a number of naturally occurring diseases in man and other mammals, in which faulty myelination or demylination is a feature of the pathology. In the vast majority of these diseases the myelin abnormalities are secondary consequences of the disease process and form part of a complex pathology. The differences between the central and peripheral nervous system, particularly in relation to the satellite cells, is frequently underlined by the finding that many of the diseases are restricted to one or the other system, only a few involving both. In addition to these naturally occurring diseases many experimental systems have been discovered that involve changes in myelin stability. One might imagine that it would be possible to recognize diseases involving predominantly either the synthesis and turnover of myelin, or its excessive destruction, however, such a clear cut distinction has not been found and most pathologies appear to lie somewhere between these two extremes.

It is possible however to recognize some conditions in which a partial failure or depression of myelination has occurred. Thus the administration of hypocholesterolaemic drugs, which block the synthesis of cholesterol, slow the rate of myelin synthesis and may even inhibit its initiation (*vide supra*). The effect is seen both in peripheral and central nervous tissues, and the myelin which is produced is of virtually normal composition and active demyelination is not a conspicuous feature. Undernutrition, as well as retarding brain growth, leads to a reduced synthesis of myelin (Dobbing, 1964; Benton, Moser, Dodge and Carr, 1966; Dickerson, Dobbing and McCance, 1967), as does vitamin B_6 deficiency (Kuntz and Kanfer, 1973), phenylketonuria (Shah, Peterson and McKean, 1972a), experimental hyperphenylalaninaemia (Shah, Peterson, and McKean, 1972b), and neonatal thyroidectomy (Balazs, Brooksbank, Davison, Eayrs and Wilson, 1969). In these conditions the myelin deficiency can be reversed by dietary correction or hormonal therapy, as is appropriate. Although the effects of undernutrition and thyroid deficiency on myelination could be due to a generalized reduction of metabolism and growth, there may also be a more specific metabolic effect. Fatty acid synthesis for example is effected by both pyridoxine deficiency and thyroidectomy (Kurtz and Kanfer, 1973; Volpe and Kishimoto, 1972) but is unaffected in undernutrition. The nature of the inhibition of myelination in phenylketonuria must be more specific. In animals with hyperphenylalaninaemia the incorporation of ^{14}C from glucose into the total lipid fraction is reduced (Shah, Peterson and McKean, 1970), and the synthesis of cholesterol from mevalonate in brain tissue is inhibited by 30–60%,

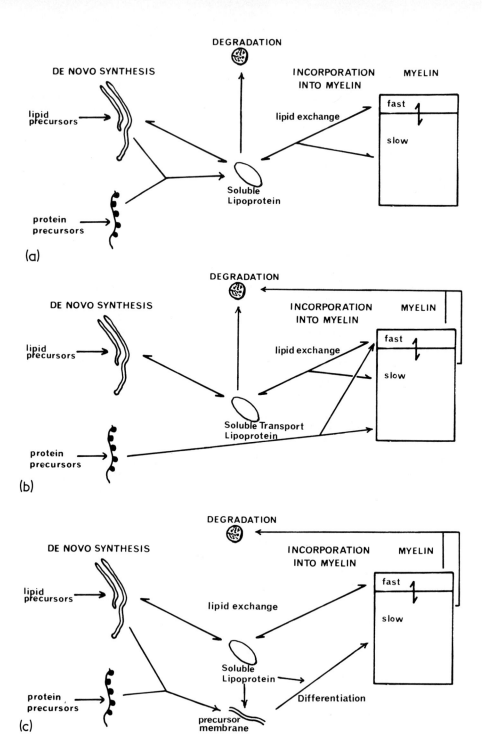

although the activity of the liver is unaffected (Shah, Peterson and McKean, 1968). The experiments with inhibitors of cholesterol synthesis suggest that, certainly in the early stages of development, the syntheses of the various myelin constituents must be closely integrated, since inhibition of cholesterol synthesis is accompanied by inhibition of the synthesis of both myelin protein and total lipid (Smith, Hasinoff and Fumagalli, 1970).

There are a number of other diseases or conditions in which a partial failure of myelination is one feature of the pathology. These include the genetically determined lipidoses, the murine mutants 'quaking', 'jimpy' and 'm.s.d.', 'border disease' of sheep, 'swayback', and the various congenital hypomyelinogeneses of pigs and cattle. These diseases have a variety of differing aetiologies and the animals affected show numerous chemical and structural abnormalities in their myelin.

In the 'quaking mouse', and certain of the human lipidoses that have been investigated, not only is production of myelin limited, but that formed has an abnormal composition. The lipid compositions of myelin from metachromatic leucodystrophy, GM_1-gangliosidosis, Tay-Sachs and Niemann Pick diseases have been investigated and all have been found to be abnormal (Table 11.13). The primary abnormality in this group of diseases involves catabolism, there being a defect in one of the enzymes responsible for the degradation of a particular lipid. The lipids involved are in all cases sphingolipids, and with the exception of Niemann Pick disease, the enzymes are specifically concerned with the degradation of the various glycosphingolipids (see Brady, 1972). Neurons, oligodendroglia and Schwann cells are found to possess large numbers of laminated bodies, containing large amounts of the undegraded lipid, and in metachromatic leucodystrophy in the peripheral nervous system, laminated inclusions are found in the paranodal loops of myelin and in the axon. Most of the myelin sheaths appear structurally normal apart from a few scattered abnormal regions of increased electron density and smaller lamellar periodicity (Webster, 1962). It is presumed that the presence of large amounts of these particular lipids either disturbs the normal pattern of synthetic activity of the cell or upsets the usual associations between lipid and protein in the formed myelin sheath. Which ever explanation may apply, it is clear that in the diseases investigated to date, the changes in myelin composition are many and diverse.

The murine mutants are characterized by a failure of myelination, although in

---

Fig. 11.7 *Hypothetical systems of turnover and synthesis of the myelin sheath. De novo* synthesis refers to the synthesis of the individual constituents at the appropriate sites in the satellite cell, with myelin represented by the box on the right. They myelin sheath is represented as having two metabolic compartments, the lesser having a faster exchange rate than the larger. The major distinctions between the three systems are that (a) represents the incorporation and exchange of whole lipoprotein subunits; (b) the separate incorporation of lipid and protein components, the lipid being transfered on 'transport' lipoproteins; and (c) the production of a 'precursor' membrane which differentiates into myelin by the insertion of lipids and proteins.

Table 11.13   Composition of CNS myelin in human diseases

	Normal	Spongy degeneration (1)		Tay Sachs (2)	GM$_1$ (2) gangliosidosis
Yield mg dry wt.					
per 100 g wet	1007.2	121.2		–	–
CM insol (%)	12.5	20.2		9.3	8.9
Proteolipid					
protein (%)	21.2	15.6		26.0	21.2
Total lipid (%)	67.2	66.3		63.8	68.0
Upper phase					
solid (%)	1.1	2.2		3.0	3.6
		patient (a)	patient (b)		Lipid, wt %
Cholesterol	23.5	30.9	63	52.4	44.5
Total phospholipid	45.3	44.2	29	36.2	35.4
Ethanolainine					
phospholipid	14.6	14.3	7.8	9.1	7.9
Phosphatidyl					
choline	13.8	13.2	10.9	14.5	12.3
Sphingomyelin	7.7	6.6	5.0	5.6	7.0
Inosital					
phospholipid	0.9	1.3	0.6	1.7	1.7
Serine phospholipid	8.4	8.7	4.8	5.2	6.5
Total galactolipid	26.2	15.9	8.9	13.2	12.9
Cerebroside	17.1	9.8	5.0	10.3	9.5
Sulphatide	4.8	3.1	1.6	3.9	2.9
NANA					
μg/100 mg myelin	40.2	–	–	284	234

(1) Kamoshita, Rapin, Suzuki and Suzuki, 1968
(2) Suzuki, Suzuki and Kamoshita, 1969
(3) Suzuki, Tucker, Rorke and Suzuki, 1970

'jimpy' and 'm.s.d.' there is also active demyelination (Sidman and Hayes, 1965; Meier and MacPike, 1970), a similar pathology being seen in sheep with border disease (Cancilla and Barlow, 1970). Border disease is apparently produced by a transmissable agent (Shaw, Winkler and Terlecki, 1967) as is one of the variants of cerebrospinal hypomyelinogenesis of pigs (Brooksbank, 1955; Emerson and Delez, 1965). In the congenital tremors of piglet type A III, the condition more closely resembles that of the 'quaking' mouse (although it is sex linked as are 'jimpy' and 'm.s.d.' Patterson, Sweasey and Harding, 1972); in this condition there may be a deficiency of oligodendrocytes (Blakemore, 1974), whereas in type A IV the process is one of active demylination (Patterson, Sweasey, Brush and Harding, 1973). The condition 'quaking' is produced in mice by an autosomal recessive gene and is characterized by a graded deficiency of myelin

Schilder's disease (3)	Normal (4)	SSLE (4)	Metachromatic (5) leucodystrophy	Normal (6)	Refsum's (6) disease
70.5	–	–	–	–	–
14.0					
	30	21.3	36.8	21	28.1
22.1					
61.6	70.0	73.7	63.2	79	71.9
2.0	–	–	–	–	–
32.5	27.7	43.7	21.2	25.2	25.8
46.7	43.1	36.6	36.1	39.9	36.2
12.9	15.6	9.7	8.1	15.4	7.2
14.4	11.2	10.4	10.7	12.5	10.4
7.2	7.9	8.8	7.1	5.7	7.2
1.3	0.6	1.4	3.1	–	–
6.8	4.8	4.6	3.8	6.3	11.4
17.5	–	–	–	–	–
12.5	22.7	18.8	9.0	20.8	18.1
3.3	3.8	2.8	28.4	5.2	6.6
111	–	–	–	–	–

(4) Norton, Poduslo and Suzuki, 1966
(5) Norton and Poduslo, 1966; cited in Norton, 1971a
(6) MacBrinn and O'Brian, 1968

within the nervous system, the deficit being most severe centrally (Samorajski, Friede and Beimer, 1970; Berger, 1971). Unlike the mutations 'jimpy' and 'm.s.d.' the affected animals reach maturity and the females will produce and rear young. The myelin isolated from the brain shows marked differences from the normal in lipid composition (Singh, Spritz and Geyer, 1971; Gregson and Oxberry, 1972; Baumann, Bourre, Jacque and Harpin, 1973), and is deficient in proteolipid protein (Greenfield, Norton and Morell, 1971; Gregson and Oxberry, 1972) (Table 11.14). The change in composition thus involves both lipid and protein and is further manifested as an alteration in the pattern of lipoprotein complexes produced on solubilization with lysophosphatidyl choline (Bradbrook and Gregson, 1973). The nature of the defect is not known, but attention has been drawn to the similarity between the myelin composition of the 'quaking'

Table 11.14   The composition of myelin from the
CNS of the mutant mouse 'quaking'

	Normal	Mutant
Protein mg/100 mg dry wt. (1)	31.5	36.1
CMb (% total protein) (2)	18.7	10.0
CMba	18.6	7.1
CMp	24.1	7.6
Lipid (moles %) (3)		
Cholesterol	37.6	43.9
Galactocerebroside	21.1	14.8
Sulphatide	6.2	7.7
Total phospholipid	31.0	32.7
Ethanolamine phospholipid	16.8	9.9
Phosphatidyl choline	12.0	14.8
Inositol & serine phospholipid	3.7	6.1
Sphingomyelin	2.6	1.8

(1) Singh *et al.*, 1971
(2) Greenfield, Norton and Morell, 1971
(3) Gregson and Oxberry, 1972

mouse and that of myelin from young developing animals, and this has naturally
led to a suggestion that the mutation may involve failure of a regulatory system
necessary for normal ontogeny. Low levels of cerebroside are found in these
animals, particularly of those containing the nonhydroxy fatty acids (Baumann
et al., 1968; Gregson and Oxberry, 1972); and Baumann *et al.* (1973) have
suggested the possibility that fatty acid synthesis is impaired. The deficiency of
cerebroside is less apparent in non-neural tissues (Kishimoto, 1971), and
although fatty acid synthesis in the brain is depressed after the onset of
myelination, it is normal up to twelve days post natal (Kandutsch and Saucier,
1972). Glycosphinyolipid synthesis is reduced in both the 'jimpy' and 'quaking'
mutants (Neskovic, Nussbaum and Mandel, 1969), and while cerebroside
synthesis in the 'jimpy' mutant is normal up to 7—10 days post natal it fails to
increase to the same extent as in normal animals with the onset of myelination
(Druse and Hogan, 1972). Furthermore sterol synthesis is relatively reduced in
all three types of murine mutant, the relative deficit increasing with the onset of
myelination. In the 'quaking' mouse however, which is long lived, the relative
rate of sterol synthesis is found to increase as myelination finishes (Kandutsch
and Saucier, 1969, 1972). These observations suggest a failure of the further
induction of the synthetic systems associated with the major phase of myelin
production.

Damage to the nervous system is commonly followed by demyelination,
generally involving the process known as Wallerian degeneration (see Chapter
14). Crush injury to a mouse peripheral nerve evokes a rapid response, i.e. within
minutes, up to 5—20 mm distal to the lesion, and involves dilation of the

Schmidt—Lanterman incisures and withdrawal of the paranodal myelin from the node. There is collapse of the normal myelin period repeat to 4 nm in the sheath adjacent to the distended incisures, and this change may represent the onset of myelin degradation (Williams and Hall, 1971a). This response of the Schwann cells to injury can be seen to extend for several internodes distal to the crush. Within 24 h the activity of acid proteinases and other lytic enzymes increases and obvious myelin degradation begins (Hallpike, 1972). The evidence available indicates that the response to injury is similar in the central nervous system, but that it develops rather more slowly (Bignami and Eng, 1973). The rapid response of the satellite cell is obviously initiated by a signal from the damaged axon, of either a positive or negative kind, and this may perhaps be related to the interaction between Schwann cell and axon responsible for initiating myelination. Demyelination may also result from metabolic insult, or deficiency. Inhibition of respiration by cyanide (Ibrahim, Briscoe, Bayliss and Adams, 1963; Hall, 1972a), copper deficiency (Howell, 1970), chronic triethyltin intoxication (Smith, 1973), and the inhibition of protein synthesis by diptheria toxin will all lead to demyelination. Such findings would seem to support the idea that the myelin sheath must to a certain extent be 'maintained' by the metabolic activity of the satellite cell in the normal adult animal. However, evidence is available which shows that the sheath can be damaged directly, without there being any obvious damage to the remainder of the satellite cell (Hall and Gregson, 1971; Hall, 1972b; Gregson and Hall, 1973).

The most important disease, in human terms, directly affecting the myelin sheath, is multiple sclerosis. The pathology of this disease is one of primary segmental demyelination, occurring focally throughout the central nervous system, with a tendency for lesions to appear in certain regions preferentially, for example the optic nerves and the sub-ependymal corpus callosum. The disease commonly develops at a time when it is believed that most myelination has ceased, and must thus be ascribed to a defect of myelin maintenance, rather than of its synthesis. It is a chronic disease characterized by intermittent acute episodes, and at present its aetiology is unknown.

There is evidence for the existence of a genetic link in the aetiology of multiple sclerosis, and the involvement of both dietary and transmissable agents has also been proposed. It is not known whether there is any basic abnormality of myelin chemistry, a suggestion which has been made on the basis of lipid analyses of apparently normal white matter (Cummings, 1953; Gerstl, Kahnke, Smith, Tavaststjerna and Hayman, 1961; Baker, Thompson and Zilkha, 1963) in which the cerebroside content of such normal white matter was found to be reduced, in agreement with a low recovery of myelin (Gerstl, Eng, Tavaststjerna, Smith and Kruse, 1970). Fatty acid abnormality has also been suggested as a possible factor in the myelin instability of multiple sclerosis (Thompson, 1972), and there is some evidence that such a fatty acid abnormality may not be restricted to the central nervous system and is in fact a general systemic alteration involving both the serum phospholipids and the phospholipids of red cells and platelet membranes (Baker, Thompson and Zilkha, 1964; Gul, Smith, Thompson, Wright and Zilkha, 1970). The concept of a general disturbance of fatty acid balance in patients having multiple sclerosis accords with the suggestion that the geographical distribution of the disease may be related to the nature of the dietary fat (Swank, 1950; Sinclair, 1956). One objection to such a dietary explanation is that, for an individual, the specific risk of development of the disease is unchanged by migration to a geographical area of differing risk (Acheson, 1972). Change in the dietary fat of rats has little effect upon the fatty acid composition of myelin (Rathbone, 1965), but it has been suggested that the disturbance of the fatty acid balance may become significant under conditions of stress and lead to an increase in the turnover of myelin (Thompson, 1972). There have also been reports of the finding of abnormalities in the serum lecithin-cholesterol acyl transferase activity in multiple sclerosis patients, an important enzyme in the system of fatty acid exchange in the blood, although the observed differences appear mainly to concern the lipoprotein substrate (DeMedio, Amaducci, Borri, Gaita and Porcellati, 1972). The relevance of this finding to brain fatty acid metabolism is nor clear, since lecithin-cholesterol acyl transferase activity does not appear to be present in normal brain tissue (Eto and Suzuki, 1971a), and although there is indirect evidence of such enzyme activity in the brains of patients with Schilder's disease, GM_1-gangliosidosis and Tay Sach's disease (Eto and Suzuki, 1971b), this may be related to the occurrence of active demyelination in these diseases.

If, as has been suggested, a fatty acid imbalance affects myelin stability when myelin metabolism has been disturbed, the question remains, as to the factor responsible for the initial disturbance of myelin metabolism? The involvement of immune mechanisms in multiple sclerosis seems fairly certain, the elevated levels of immunoglobin in the C.S.F. (Tourtellotte, 1970), and the demonstration of synthesis of immunoglobulin by cultured cells derived from the C.S.F. (Cohen and Bannister, 1967), indicating the presence of immunologically competent cells within the central nervous system. This finding is not, however, unique to multiple sclerosis, elevated C.S.F. immunoglobulins also being found in neurosyphilis, and the perivenular cuffing found in acute multiple sclerosis is a feature common to a range of allergic and viral encephalopathies, and also to experimental allergic encephalomyelitis (EAE). In EAE the condition is one of auto-immunity, involving delayed hypersensitivity, rather than an immuno-globulin action, the autoimmune reaction being induced by sensitization to myelin basic protein. The evidence adduced for or against the presence of antimyelin antibodies in the C.S.F. and serum of multiple sclerosis patients is contradictory, and tests involving the demonstration of myelinolytic activity in tissue culture which appear to demonstrate the action of antimyelin antibodies (Lumsden, 1972), may in fact represent actions directed against other components of the test system, such as the astrocytes or oligodendroglia. Similar myelinolytic activity has been found to be present in sera from patients with other diseases affecting the central nervous system and thus again this property does not appear to be specific to multiple sclerosis. It may be concluded that while immunological involvement in this condition is, in general, probably a secondary feature, it may be an important factor in the acute exacerbations of the disease.

Currently the most favoured explanation for the combination of the geographical distribution, risk and immunological features of multiple sclerosis invokes a transmissable agent of the 'slow' virus type, but it is true to say that multiple sclerosis remains an enigma. The mechanism of the demyelination process is not known, i.e. whether it involves the satellite cell or other brain cells directly or only through the action of the immune system, either immuno-globulin or cells, or whether the risk of occurrence of demyelination is intrinsic to the myelin or induced, possibly as a consequence of viral infection.

In conclusion it can be seen that the viability of the myelin sheath, as demonstrated by investigations of disease processes involving amyelination and demyelination, is susceptible to errors of composition, alterations to satellite cell metabolism, and the direct action of lytic materials. The critical degree of variation necessary for the loss of viability of myelin is not known however.

Variations in composition of peripheral nerve myelin, such as the substitution of phytanic acid for the normal fatty acid constituents of lecithin, are considered to induce physical instability in the membrane, leading to subsequent demyelination (MacBrinn and O'Brien, 1968). Similarly the slight variation in long chain fatty acid content observed in several diseases has been invoked as the chemical basis for the disease process. Such ideas rest heavily on the acceptance of a lipid bilayer structure for the myelin membrane (O'Brien, 1967). At the present time however, the information we have concerning membrane structure is inadequate to permit the complete acceptance of such basically simple concepts as these but investigation of pathological processes will undoubtedly assist the formulation of more exact ideas concerning membrane structure, and these may in turn provide a clearer understanding of the disease process.

11.10 Current hypotheses of membrane structure and their relevance to myelin

All hypotheses of membrane structure proposed to date are no more than generalized sketch maps, based at best on data which represents an average of the real structure, and at the worst on observations which are merely the indirect consequences of that structure. The range of proposed structures extends from the original Danielli-Davson hypothesis characterized by an extensive lipid bilayer as the major structural determinant, through structures having smaller and less extensive regions of bilayer, to pure micellar and lipoprotein structures. In addition structures have been proposed which can undergo transitions from one extreme form to the other as a consequence of variations in the immediate milieu of the membrane or its metabolic avtivity. Thus, so far as can be seen, no possibility appears to have been overlooked. The very fact that such a plethora of models have been proposed suggests that none are very satisfactory, and that all need to be examined more rigorously.

Studies of myelin once furnished much of the data used in discussions of membrane structure, but as pointed out in the introduction, myelin has since come to be considered to be a highly specialized structure and therefore less relevant to discussions of membrane structure in general; as Singer (1971) states 'the structure of myelin, while interesting in its own right, is of uncertain relevance to the structure of cell membranes'. Indeed it is now considered that there may not be a single basic structure for cell membranes and that considerable structural variation may occur. Myelin, the most lipid rich of cell membranes so far studied, may represent an atypical extreme condition.

Just how different is myelin from other membranes? The structurally dependent properties of myelin do not appear to differ markedly from those of other membranes; its membrane capacitance is the same (Table 11.2); the X-ray diffraction pattern is of the same kind as that of other membranes and does not exclude some penetration of the central region of the membrane by protein (Kirschner and Caspar, 1972). its electron microscopic appearance is similar in thin section and can be preserved even after the extraction of the lipid (Napolitano *et al.*, 1967); and the alkyl chains of the lipid moieties do not appear to be crystalline but show some disorder (Schmidt and Bear, 1939; Ladbrooke *et al.*, 1968). Other properties indirectly related to structure, such as the susceptibility of its phospholipid to phospholipase *c* activity, are also similar to those of other membranes (McIlwain and Rapport, 1971). The membrane contains glycolipid, perhaps in rather higher concentration than most plasma membranes, and this is antigenic and accessible for reaction with specific antibody (Rapport, Graf, Autilio and Norton, 1964; Gregson, Kennedy and Leibowitz, 1974). The major fraction of the membrane protein is not extractable into aqueous media, and even when dissolved in non-aqueous media appears to be in an aggregated or micellar state (Folch Pi and Stoffyn, 1972). Finally a proportion of the protein appears to contain some α-helical configuration, but no β-keratin configuration has so far been detected (Folch Pi and Stoffyn, 1972).

The primary hypothesis of membrane structure, from which all subsequent models appear to be derived, is that of Dannielli and Davson (see Stoeckinius and Engleman, 1969; Hendler, 1971; Singer, 1971). Whichever particular hypothesis has been favoured by the numerous authors who have discussed membrane structure, the myelin membrane has been considered to represent an extreme form the membrane structure proposed by Dannielli and Davson, the essential feature of the Danielli-Davson hypothesis being the existence of a 'more or less' extensive lipid bilayer which forms the major structural determinant. This arrangement of lipid molecules is considered to be the one that they will most naturally take up when they are exposed to aqueous systems, and therefore represents the thermodynamically most probable structure. Even if this particular structural arrangement does occur in biological membranes, the question remains as to how this molecular association can be controlled, since control of molecular association is the hallmark of a biological system. Proteins are considered to be the principal controlling agents in biological systems, as only these molecules possess a sufficient diversity of specific molecular affinities, and this fact alone may suggest some specificity of interaction between the proteins and lipids of the membrane. The occurrence of such interactions is in general not in dispute, what is not known are their nature and their degrees of specificity.

Protein interactions in the membrane may range from the purely ionic to the purely hydrophobic. The release of protein following alterations to the bulk phase pH, ionic strength, dielectric constant or ionic composition in part support the idea of ionic interaction, and the release of basic protein from myelin by a change in pH provides indirect evidence in favour of an ionic binding of this protein within the membrane. On the other hand, the current view of membrane proteins as globular amphipathic molecules, macromolecular analogues of lipids (Green, 1972; Colacicco, 1972), suggests a significant role for hydrophobic interactions. The proposal that membrane proteins 'float' in a lipid matrix (see Singer, 1971) allows for this form of protein interaction, and appears to fit very well the case of rhodopsin in the retinal rod disc membrane (Vanderkooi, 1972) and of cytochrome b_5 in the microsomal membrane (Strittmatter, Rogers and Spatz, 1972). The evidence for the amphipathic nature of cytochrome b_5 and its associated reductase is reasonably well established (Strittmatter *et al.*, 1972), but with proteolipid apoprotein, while it possesses the relevant properties and contains covalently bound fatty acid, resists proteolytic cleavage which renders confirmation of such an amphipathic structure difficult (*vide supra*). In a discussion of the binding between serum albumin and amphipathic substances, Tanford (1972), concluded that both hydrophobic and ionic interactions contributed to such binding, the hydrophobic binding being less specific. Such a combination of binding forces would be more compatible with the situation found in membranes.

In the Danielli-Davson hypothesis, as it is usually stated, the lipid bilayer is regarded as being not only extensive but also homogeneous in the surface plane. It is becoming ever more apparent, however, that in mixed lipid systems segregation of the various lipid species occurs at temperatures intermediate to the range of transition temperatures of the individual lipids (Chapman, 1973), and there is evidence of cluster formation and phase segregation in lecithin mixtures (Phillips, Ladbrooke and Chapman, 1970; Phillips, Hauser and Paltauf, 1972). With the added variation of the polar head groups the possible degree of heterogeneity of the lipid phases is likely to be high, and the addition of protein showing specificity of binding to both polar and acyl regions to such a system should obviously assist the process of phase separation. Observations relating the activity of bacterial membrane enzymes to fatty acid composition (e.g. Overath, Schairer, Hill and Lamnek-Hirsch, 1971) demonstrate the occurrence of temperature dependent phase transitions in membrane activity. Furthermore the transition temperatures of different activities can differ both from one another and from the observed range of transition temperatures for the membrane lipids (Wakil and Esfahani, 1972), the transition temperature of the enzyme activities nonetheless being dependent on the acyl portion of the associated phospholipid (Esfahani, Crowfoot and Wakil, 1972).

It is thus clear that there is a strong possibility that the lipid within the surface plane of the membrane is structurally heterogeneous, and include coexisting but segregated zones of both liquid-crystalline and crystalline lipid. The dimensions of these various clusters may be relatively small, and as a consequence the 'unit cell' of the membrane could be quite large and therefore difficult to detect by X-ray diffraction.

One aspect of membrane structure which has not been considered is its asymetry normal to the surface. Different proteins and different regions of proteins, are present at the two surfaces, and such a differential distribution of protein may obviously lead to a differential distribition of lipid polar groups. There is some evidence, albeit of an indirect nature, relating to such an asymmetric arrangement of lipid in cell membranes (Bretscher, 1972), and an asymmetric arrangement of cholesterol has been suggested to occur in myelin (Caspar and Kirschner, 1971).

Since it may be concluded that there is no good reason to believe that the membrane structure of myelin will differ radically from that of other membranes, it follows that all of the above considerations must apply to any hypothesis of myelin structure. It may also be concluded that there is no valid reason to reject myelin as a suitable model for investigations into the general structure of membranes, indeed with its apparent paucity of protein species and the opportunities it provides for comparisons between homologous structures it should continue to be an extremely fruitful subject for further investigation.

References

Acheson, E. D. (1972) In *Multiple Sclerosis, a re-appraisal*, by McAlpine, D., Lumsden, C. E. and Acheson, E. D. The epidemiology of multiple sclerosis. pp. 3–80. Churchill Livingstone: London.

Adams, C. W. M. and Davison, A. N. (1959) The occurrence of esterified cholesterol in the developing nervous system. *Journal of Neurochemistry*, 4, 282–289.

Adams, C. W. M., Davison, A. N. and Gregson, N. A. (1963) Enzyme inactivity of myelin: histochemical and biochemical evidence. *Journal of Neurochemistry*, 10, 383–395.

Adams, C. W. M., Abdulla, Y. H., Turner, D. R. and Bayliss, O. B. (1968) Subcellular preparation of peripheral nerve myelin. *Nature (London)*, 220, 171–173.

Adams, C. W. M., Bayliss, O. B., Hallpike, J. F. and Turner, D. R. (1971) Histochemistry of myelin XII Anionic staining of myelin basic proteins for histology, electrophoresis and electron microscopy. *Journal of Neurochemistry*, 18, 389–394.

Agrawal, H. C., Banik, N. L., Bone, A. H., Davison, A. N., Mitchell, R. F. and Spohn, M. (1970) The identity of a myelin-like fraction isolated from developing brain. *Biochemical Journal*, 120, 635–642.

Agrawal, H. C., Burton, R. M., Fishman, M. A., Mitchell, R. F. and Prenskey, A. L. (1972) Partial characterization of a new myelin protein component. *Journal of Neurochemistry*, 19, 2083–2090.

Akers, C. K. and Parsons, D. F. (1970) X-ray diffraction of myelin membrane II. Determination of phase angles of frog sciatic nerve by heavy atom labelling and calculation of electron density distribution of the membrane. *Biophysical Journal,* **10,** 116–136.

Amaducci, L., Pazzagli, A. and Pessina, G. (1962) The relation of proteolipids and phosphatidopeptides to tissue elements in the bovine nervous system. *Journal of Neurochemistry,* **9,** 509–518.

Ansell, G. B. and Spanner, S. (1972) In *Current Trends in the Biochemistry of Lipids,* (ed.) Ganguly, J. and Smellie, R. M. S. The metabolism of phosphatidycholine in brain tissue. 151–159. Academic Press: London.

Aschenbrenner, V., Drieyan, R., Albin, R. and Rabinowitz, M. (1970) Haem *a,* cytochrome *c* and total protein turnover in mitochondria from rat, heart and liver. *Biochemical Journal,* **119,** 157–160.

Autilio, L. A., Norton, W. T. and Terry, R. D. (1964) The preparation and some properties of purified myelin from the central nervous system. *Journal of Neurochemistry,* **11,** 17–28.

Avrova, N. F., Chenykaeva, E. Yu, and Obukhova, E. L. (1973) Ganglioside composition and content of rat-brain subcellular fractions. *Journal of Neurochemistry,* **20,** 979–1004.

Badzhinyan, S. A. and Chailakhyan, L. M. (1971) Measurement of the electrical capacitance of the region of contact of two bimolecular phospholipid membranes. *Biofizika,* **16,** 1141–1143.

Badzhinyan, S. A., Durin-Barkovsky, V. L., Kovalev, S. A. and Chailakhyan, L. M. (1971) Electrical resistance of the region of adhesion of two bimolecular phospholid membranes. *Biofizika,* **16,** 1019–1024.

Baker, R. W. R., Thompson, R. H. S. and Zilkha, K. J. (1963) Fatty acid composition of brain lecithins in multiple sclerosis. *Lancet,* **i,** 26–27.

Baker, R. W. R., Thompson, R. H. S. and Zilkha, K. J. (1964) Serum fatty acids in multiple sclerosis. *Journal of Neurology, Neurosurgery and Psychiatry,* **27,** 408–414.

Balazs, R., Brooksbank, B. W. L., Davison, A. N., Eayrs, J. T. and Wilson, D. A. (1969) The effect of neonatal thyroidectomy on myelination in the rat brain. *Brain Research,* **15,** 219–232.

Bangham, A. D. (1968) In *Progress in Biophysics and Molecular Biology,* (eds) Butler, J. A. V. and Noble, D. Vol. **18,** Membrane models with phospholipids. 29–95. Pergamon Press: Oxford.

Banik, N. L. and Davison, A. N. (1969) Enzyme activity and composition of myelin and subcellular fractions in the developing rat brain. *Biochemical Journal* **115,** 1051–1062.

Banik, N. L. and Davison, A. N. (1971) Exchange of sterols between myelin and other membranes of developing rat brain. *Biochemical Journal,* **122,** 751–758.

Baumann, N. A., Jacque, C. M., Pollet, S. A. and Harpin, M. L. (1968) Fatty acid and lipid composition of the brain of a myelin deficient mutant, the 'Quaking' mouse. *European Journal of Biochemistry,* **4,** 340–344.

Baumann, N. A., Bourre, J. M., Jacque, C. M. and Harpin, M. L. (1973) Lipid composition of quaking mouse myelin: comparison with normal mouse myelin in the adult and during development. *Journal of Neurochemistry,* **20,** 753–760.

Bear, R. S. (1971) In *Neuroscience Research Program Bulletin,* Vol. 9, No. 4, 507–510.

Benjamins, J. A. and McKhann, G. M. (1973a) Properties and metabolism of soluble lipoproteins containing choline and ethanolamine phospholipids in rat brain. *Journal of Neurochemistry,* **20,** 1121–1129.

Benjamins, J. A. and McKhann, G. M. (1973b) [2-³H] glycerol as a precursor of phospholipids in rat brain and evidence for lack of recycling. *Journal of Neurochemistry,* **20,** 1111–1120.

Benjamins, J. A., Miller, K. and McKhann, G. M. (1973) Myelin subfractions in developing rat brain; characterization and sulphatide metabolism. *Journal of Neurochemistry,* **20,** 1589–1603.

Benton, J. W., Moser, H. W., Dodge, P. R. and Carr, S. (1966) Modification of the schedule of myelination in the rat by early nutritional deprivation. *Pediatrics,* **38,** 801–807.

Berger, B. (1971) Quelques aspects ultrastructuraux de la substance blanche chez la souris 'quaking'. *Brain Research,* **25,** 35–53.

Bignami, A. and Eng, L. F. (1973) Biochemical studies of myelin in Wallerian degeneration of rat optic nerve. *Journal of Neurochemistry*, **20**, 165–173.

Bischoff, A. and Moor, H. (1967a) Ultrastructural differences between the myelin sheaths of peripheral nerve fibres and CNS white matter. *Zeitschrift für Zellforschung*, **81**, 303–310.

Bischoff, A. and Moor, H. (1967b) The ultrastructure of the 'difference factor' in the myelin. *Zeitschrift für Zellforschung*, **81**, 571–580.

Blakemore, W. F. (1974) Pig congenital tremors, type AIII an EM study. *Research in Veterinary Science*. In press.

Blaurock, A. E. (1972) Locating protein in membranes. *Nature (London)*, **240**, 556–557.

Blaurock, A. E. (1973) X-ray diffraction pattern from a bilayer with protein outside. *Biophysical Journal*, **13**, 281–289.

Blaurock, A. E. and Wilkins, M. H. F. (1969) Structure of frog photoreceptor membranes. *Nature (London)*, **223**, 906–909.

Balurock, A. E. and Worthington, C. R. (1969) Low angle X-ray diffraction patterns from a variety of myelinated nerves. *Biochemica Biophysica Acta*, **173**, 419–426.

Boehm, V. G. (1933) Das Rontgendiagram der Nerven. *Kolloid Zeitschrift*, **82**, 22–26.

Bradbrook, I. D. and Gregson, N. A. (1973) A comparison of lipoproteins derived from the CNS and myelin of the normal and the mutant 'quaking' mouse. In *Protides of the Biological Fluids*. (ed.) Peeters, H. Vol. **21**, pp. 237–240. Pergamon Press: Oxford.

Brady, R. O. (1972) Genetics of abnormal lipid metabolism. In *Current Topics in Biochemistry*, (1971) N.I.H. Lecture series (eds.) Anfinsen, G. B., Goldberger, R. F. and Schechter, A. N. pp. 1–48. Academic Press: New York.

Branton, D. (1967) Fracture faces of frozen myelin. *Experimental Cell Research*, **45**, 703–707.

Braun, P. E. and Radin, N. S. (1969) Interaction of lipids with a membrane structural protein from myelin. *Biochemistry Journal*, **8**, 4310–4318.

Bretscher, M. S. (1972) Asymmetrical lipid bilayer structure for biological membranes. *Nature New Biology*, **236**, 11–12.

Brooksbank, N. H. (1955) Trembles in piglets. *Veterinary Record*, **67**, 576–577.

Brostoff, S. and Eylar, E. H. (1971) Localization of methylated arginine in the A protein from myelin. *Proceedings of National Academy of Science, U.S.A.*, **68**, 765–769.

Brostoff, S., Burnett, P., Lampert, P. and Eylar, E. H. (1972) Isolation and characterization of a protein from sciatic nerve myelin responsible for Experimental Allergic Neuritis, *Nature (New Biology)*, **235**, 210–212.

Brostoff, S. W., Carter, H., Reuter, W. and Eylar, E. H. (1972) Chemical and immunologic properties of peripheral nerve myelin and myelin proteins. *Federation Proceedings*, **31**, 843.

Brostoff, S. W. and Eylar, E. H. (1972) The proposed amino acid sequence of the P_1 protein of rabbit sciatic nerve myelin. *Archives of Biochemistry and Biophysics*, **153**, 590–598.

Bunge, R. P. (1968) Glial cells and the central myelin sheath. *Physiological Reviews*, **48**, 197–251.

Caley, D. W. (1967) Ultrastructural differences between central and peripheral myelin sheath formation in the rat. *Anatomical Record*, **157**, 223A.

Cancilla, P. A. and Barlow, R. M. (1968) An electron microscope study of the spinal cord in Border Disease of Lambs. *Research in Veterinary Science*, **9**, 88–90.

Carnegie, P. R. (1971) Amino acid sequence of the encephalitogenic basic protein from human myelin. *Biochemical Journal*, **123**, 57–67.

Caspar, D. L. D. and Kirschner, D. A. (1971) Myelin membrane structure at 10Å resolution. *Nature New Biology*, **231**, 46–52.

Chapman, D. (1968) Recent physical studies of phospholipids and natural membranes. In *Biological Membranes*, (ed.) Chapman, D. pp. 125–202, Academic Press: London.

Chapman, D., Kamat, V. B., de Grier, J. and Penkett, S. A. (1966) Nuclear magnetic resonance studies of erythrocyte membranes. *Journal of Molecular Biology*, **31**, 101–114.

Chapman, D. and Dodd, G. H. (1971) Physiochemical probes of membrane structure. In *Structure and Function of Biological Membranes*, (ed.) Rothfield, L. I. pp. 13–81. Academic Press: London.

Chapman, D. (1973) Some recent studies of lipids, lipid-cholesterol and membrane systems.

In *Biological Membranes*, (eds.) Chapman, D. and Wallach, D. F. H. Vol. 2, pp. 91–144. Academic Press: London.

Clarenburg, R., Chaikoff, I. L. and Morris, M. D. (1963) Incorporation of injected cholesterol into the myelinating brain of the 17 day old rabbit. *Journal of Neurochemistry*, 10, 135–143.

Cohen, S. and Bannister, R. (1967) Immunoglobulin synthesis within the central nervous system in disseminated sclerosis. *Lancet*, i, 366–367.

Colacicco, G. (1972) Surface behaviour of membrane proteins. *Annals of New York Academy of Sciences*, 195, 224–261.

Cole, K. S. and Curtis, H. J. (1936) Electrical impedance of nerve and muscle. *Cold Spring Harbour Symposia*, 56, 351–358.

Cole, K. S. and Curtis, H. J. (1937) Transverse electric impedance of Nitella. *Journal of General Physiology*, 21, 189–201.

Cole, K. S. and Curtis, H. J. (1938) Electric impedance of Nitella during activity. *Journal of General Physiology*, 22, 37–64.

Cole, K. S. and Hodgkin, A. L. (1939) Membrane and protoplasm resistance in squid giant axon. *Journal of General Physiology*, 22, 671–687.

Cole, K. S. and Curtis, H. J. (1941) Membrane potential of squid giant axon during current flow. *Journal of General Physiology*, 24, 551–563.

Cotman, C. W. and Mahler, H. R. (1967) Resolution of insoluble proteins in rat brain subcellular fractions. *Archives of Biochemistry and Biophysics*, 120, 384–396.

Csejtey, J., Hallpike, J. F., Adams, C. W. M. and Bayliss, O. B. (1972) Histochemistry of myelin; XIV peripheral nerve myelin proteins: electrophoretic and histochemical correlations. *Journal of Neurochemistry*, 19, 1931–1936.

Cummings, J. N. (1953) The cerebral lipids in disseminated sclerosis and in amaurotic familial idiocy. *Brain*, 76, 551–562.

Cuzner, M. L., Davison, A. N. and Gregson, N. A. (1965) The chemical composition of vertebrate myelin and microsomes. *Journal of Neurochemistry*, 12, 469–481.

Cuzner, M. L., Davison, A. N. and Gregson, N. A. (1966) Turnover of brain mitochondrial membrane lipids. *Biochemical Journal*, 101, 618–626.

Cuzner, M. L. and Davison, A. N. (1968) The lipid composition of rat brain myelin and subcellular fraction during development. *Biochemical Journal*, 106, 29–34.

Davison, A. N., Dobbing, J., Morgan, R. S. and Payling Wright, G. (1959) The persistance of 4-^{14}C-cholesterol in the mammalian central nervous system. *Lancet*, i, 658–660.

Davison, A. N. and Wajda, M. (1959) Persistence of cholesterol [4-^{14}C] in the central nervous system. *Nature* (London), 183, 1606.

Davison, A. N. abd Gregson, N. A. (1962) The physiological role of cerebron sulphuric acid (sulphatide) in the brain. *Biochemical Journal*, 85, 558–567.

Davison, A. N., Cuzner, M. L., Banik, N. L. and Oxberry, J. M. (1966) Myelinogenesis in the rat brain. *Nature* (London), 212, 1373–1374.

Davison, A. N. (1970) In *Myelination*, (eds.) Davison, A. N. and Peters, A. pp. 80–143. Charles C. Thomas: Springfield, Illinois.

Dawson, R. M. C. (1965) 'Phosphatido-peptide' like complexes formed by the interaction of calcium triphosphoinositide with protein. *Biochemical Journal*, 97, 134–138.

Dawson, R. M. C. and Eichberg, J. (1965) Diphosphoinositide and triphosphoinositide in animal tissues, extraction, estimation and changes post mortem. *Biochemical Journal*, 96, 634–643.

Day, E. D., McMillan, P. N., Mickey, D. D. and Appel, S. H. (1971) Zonal centrifuge profiles of rat brain homogenates. *Analytical Biochemistry*, 39, 29–45.

DeMedio, G. E., Amaducci, L., Borri, P., Craiti, A. and Porcellati, G. (1972) Plasma lecithin-cholesterol-acyl-tranferase activity in multiple sclerosis. *Lancet*, i, 1233.

Dickerson, J. T. W., Dobbing, J. and McCance. R. A. (1967) The effect of undernutrition in the post natal development of the brain and cord in pigs. *Proceedings of the Royal Society of London (Series B)*, 166, 396–407.

Dickinson, J. P., Jones, K. M., Aparicio, S. R. and Lumsden, C. E. (1970) Localization of the encephalitogenic basic protein in the intraperiod line of lamellar myelin. *Nature (London)*, 227, 1133–1134.

Dobbing, J. (1964) The influence of early nutrition on the development and myelination of the brain. *Proceedings of the Royal Society of London (Series B)*, 159, 503–509.

Doggenweiler, C. F. and Frank, S. (1965) Staining properties of Lanthanum on cell membranes. *Proceedings of the National Academy of Science, U.S.A.,* **53**, 425–430.

Drummond, G. I., Iyer, N. T. and Keith, J. (1962) Hydrolysis of ribonucleoside 2'-3'-cyclic phosphates by a diesterase from brain. *Journal of Biological Chemistry,* **237**, 3535–3537.

Druse, M. J. and Hogan, E. L. (1972) Metabolism *in vivo* of brain galactolipids: the jimpy mutant. *Journal of Neurochemistry,* **19**, 2435–2441.

Ehnholm, C., Simons, K. and Garoff, H. (1971) Subunit structure of the Lp(a) lipoprotein. In *Protides of the Biological Fluids,* (ed.) Peeters, H. Vol. 19, pp. 191–196. Pergamon Press: Oxford.

Eichberg, J., Whittaker, V. P. and Dawson, R. M. C. (1964) Distribution of lipids in subcellular particles in guinea pig brain. *Biochemical Journal,* **92**, 91–100.

Eichberg, J. and Dawson, R. M. C. (1965) Polyphosphoinositides in myelin. *Biochemical Journal,* **96**, 644–650.

Eichberg, J. and Hauser, G. (1969) Polyphosphoinositide biosynthesis in developing rat brain homogenates. *Annals New York Academy of Science,* **165**, 784–789.

Elkes, J. and Finean, J. B. (1953a) X-ray diffraction studies on the effect of temperature on the structure of myelin in the sciatic nerve of the frog. *Experimental Cell Research,* **4**, 69–81.

Elkes, J. and Finean, J. B. (1953b) Effects of solvents on the structure of myelin in the sciatic nerve of the frog. *Experimental Cell Research,* **4**, 82–95.

Emerson, J. L. and Delez, A. C. (1965) Cerebellar hypoplasia, hypomyelinogenesis and congenital tremors of pigs, associated with prenatal Hog cholera vaccination of sows. *Journal of American Veterinary Medicine Association,* **147**, 47–54.

Eng, L. F., Chao, F. C., Gerstl, B., Pratt, D. and Tavastjerna, M. G. (1968) The maturation of human white matter myelin. Fractionation of the myelin membrane proteins. *Biochemistry,* **7**, 4455–4456.

Eng, L. F. and Noble, E. P. (1968) The maturation of rat brain myelin. *Lipids,* **3**, 157–162.

Erlanger, J. and Gasser, H. S. (1937) In *Electrical signs of nervous activity.* Philadelphia: University of Pennsylvania.

Esfahani, M., Crowfoot, P. D. and Wakil, S. J. (1972) Molecular organisation of lipids in the *E. coli* membranes. II Effect of phopholipids on succinic-ubiquinone reductase activity. *Journal of Biological Chemistry,* **247**, 7251–7256.

Eto, Y. and Suzuki, K. (1971a) Cholesterol metabolism in the brain: properties and subcellular distribution of cholesterol esterifying enzymes and cholesterol ester hydrolases in adult rat brain. *Biochimica Biophysics Acta,* **239**, 293–311.

Eto, T. and Suzuki, K. (1971b) Fatty acid composition of cholesterol esters in brains of patients with Schilder's disease, GM_1-gangliosidosis and Tay sachs disease and its possible relationship to the β-position fatty acids of lecithin. *Journal of Neurochemistry,* **18**, 1007–1016.

Eto, Y. and Suzuki, K. (1972a) Cholesterol esters in developing rat brain: concentration and fatty acid composition. *Journal of Neurochemistry,* **19**, 109–115.

Eto Y. and Suzuki, K. (1972b) Cholesterol esters in developing rat brain enzymes of cholesterol ester metabolism. *Journal of Neurochemistry,* **19**, 117–121.

Eto Y. and Suzuki, K. (1973a) Cholesterol ester metabolism in rat brain a cholesterol ester hydrolase specifically localised in the myelin sheath. *Journal of Biological Chemistry,* **248**, 1986–1991.

Eto, Y. and Suzuki, K. (1973b) Developmental changes of cholesterol ester hydrolases localized in myelin and microsomes of rat brain. *Journal of Neurochemistry,* **20**, 1475–1477.

Evans, M. J. and Finean, J. B. (1965) The lipid composition of myelin from brain and peripheral nerve. *Journal of Neurochemistry,* **12**, 729–737.

Everly, J. L., Brady, R. O. and Quarles, R. H. (1973) Evidence that the major protein in rat sciatic nerve myelin is a glycoprotein. *Journal of Neurochemistry,* **21**, 329–334.

Eylar, E. H. and Thompson, M. (1969) Allergic encephalomyelitis: the physico-chemical properties of the basic protein encephalitogen from bovine spinal cord. *Archives of Biochemistry and Biophysics,* **129**, 468–479.

Eylar, E. H., Brostoff, S., Hashim, G., Caccam, J. and Burnett, P. (1971) Basic P1 protein of the myelin membrane. The complete amino acid sequence. *Journal of Biological Chemistry,* 246, 5770–5784.

Eylar, E. H. (1972) The structure and immunologic properties of basic proteins of myelin. *Annals of the New York Academy of Science,* 195, 481–491.

Fernandez-Moran, H. (1967) In *The Neurosciences,* a study program, (eds.) Quarton, G. C., Melnechuck, T. and Schmitt, F. O. pp. 281–304. Rockefeller University Press: New York.

Fernandez-Moran, H. and Finean, J. B. (1957) Electron microscope and low angle X-ray diffraction studies of the nerve myelin sheath. *Journal of Biophysical and Biochemical Cytology,* 3, 725–748.

Finean, J. B. (1953) Further observations on the structure of myelin. *Experimental Cell Research,* 5, 202–215.

Finean, J. B. (1957) The role of water in the structure of peripheral nerve myelin. *Journal of Biophysical and Biochemical Cytology,* 3, 95–102.

Finean, J. B. and Millington, P. F. (1957) Effects of ionic strength of immersion medium on the structure of peripheral nerve myelin. *Journal of Biochemical and Biophysical Cytology,* 3, 89–94.

Finean, J. B. and Burge, R. E. (1963) The determination of the Fourier transform of the myelin layer from a study of swelling phenomena. *Journal of Molecular Biology,* 7, 672–682.

Finean, J. B., Coleman, R., Green, W. G. and Limbrick, A. R. (1966) Low angle X-ray diffraction and EM studies of isolated cell membranes. *Journal of Cell Sciences,* 1, 287–296.

Finean, J. B. and Coleman, R. (1970) Integration of structural and biochemical approaches in the study of cell membranes. In *Membranes, Structure and Function,* (eds.) Villanueva, J. R. and Ponz, F. pp. 9–16. Academic Press: London.

Fleischhauer, K. and Wartenberg, H. (1967) Elecktron mikroskopische Untersuchumgen uber das wachtum der Nervenfasern und uber das aufreten von marscheiden im corpus callosum der katze. *Zeitschrift Zellforschung Mikroskopic Anatomi,* 83, 568–581.

Folch-Pi, J. and Lees, M. (1951) Proteolipids, a new type of tissue lipoproteins. Their isolation from brain. *Journal of Biological Chemistry,* 191, 807–817.

Folch-Pi, J., Lees, M. and Carr, S. (1958) Studies of the chemical composition of the nervous system. *Experimental Cell Research,* Suppl. 5, 58–71.

Folch, J. (1959) Etudes récentes sur la chimie du cerveau et leur rapport avec la structure de la gaine myelinique. *Exposés Annuels de Biochimie Médicale,* 21, 81–95.

Folch-Pi, J., Webster, G. R. and Lees, M. (1959) The preparation of proteolipids. *Federation Proceedings,* 18, 898.

Folch-Pi, J. (1963) In *Brain Lipids and Lipoproteins and the Leucodystrophies,* (eds.) Folch-Pi, J. and Bauer, H. J. pp. 18–30. Elsevier: Amsterdam.

Folch-Pi, J. and Stoffyn, P. J. (1972) Proteolipids from membrane systems. *Annals New York Academy of Science,* 195, 86–107.

Frankenhauser, B. (1952) Saltatory conduction in myelinated nerve fibres. *Journal of Physiology,* 118, 107–112.

Fricke, H. (1931) Electrical conductivity and capacity of disperse systems. *Physics,* 1, 106–115.

Fumagalli, R., Smith, M. E., Urna, G. and Paoletti, R. (1969) The effect of hypocholesteremic agents on myelinogenesis. *Journal of Neuchemistry,* 16, 1329–1339.

Gagnon, J., Finch, R. R., Wood, D. D. and Moscarello, M. A. (1971) Isolation of a highly purified myelin protein. *Biochemistry,* 10, 4756–4763.

Gent, W. L. G. (1959) Boundary electrophoresis of brain homogenates cleared by the action of lysolecithin. *Biochemical Journal,* 73, 6.

Gent, W. L. G., Grant, E. H. and Tucker, S. W. (1970) Evidence from dielectric studies for the presence of bound water in myelin. *Biopolymers,* 9, 124–126.

Gent, W. L. G., Gregson, N. A., Gammack, D. B. and Raper, J. H. (1964) The lipid protein unit in myelin *Nature (London),* 204, 553–555.

Gent, W. L. G. and Gregson, N. A. (1966) Inhomogeneity of lysolecithin – solubilized membrane systems. *Biochemical Journal,* 98, 27–28P.

Gent, W. L. G., Gregson, N. A., Lovelidge, Carol, A. and Winder, A. F. (1971a) Interaction of lysophosphatidyl choline with central nervous system myelin. *Biochemical Journal,* **122,** 64–65P.

Gent, W. L. G., Gregson, N. A., Lovelidge, Carol, A. and Winder, A. F. (1971b) Resolution of protein components in lysophosphatidyl choline solubilized rat brain myelin. *Biochemical Journal,* **122,** 64P.

Gent, W. L. G., Gergson, N. A., Lovelidge, Carol, A. and Winder, A. F. (1971c) Separation of lipid-protein complexes of rat brain myelin by isopycnic centrifugation. *Biochemical Journal,* **122,** 63P.

Gent, W. L. G., Gregson, N. A., Lovelidge, Carol, A. and Winder, A. F. (1973) Ultraviolet absorption characteristics of myelin from the central nervous system. *Journal of Neurochemistry,* **21,** 697–702.

Geren, B. B. (1954) The formation from the Schwann cell surface of myelin in the peripheral nerves of chick embryos. *Experimental Cell Research,* **7,** 558–562.

Gerstl, B., Eng, L. F., Tavaststjerna, M., Smith, J. K. and Kruse, S. L. (1970) Lipids and proteins in multiple sclerosis white matter. *Journal of Neurochemistry,* **17,** 677–689.

Gerstl, B., Kahnke, M. J., Smith, J. K., Tavestsjerna, M. G. and Hayman, R. B. (1961) Brain lipids in multiple sclerosis and other diseases. *Brain,* **84,** 310–319.

Gonzalez-Sastre, F. (1970) The protein composition of isolated myelin. *Journal of Neurochemistry,* **17,** 1049–1056.

Goodman, D. W. S., Noble, R. P. and Dell, R. B. (1973) Three pool model of the long term turnover of plasma cholesterol in man. *Journal of Lipid Research,* **14,** 178–188.

Gottfried, E. L. and Rapport, M. M. (1963) The biochemistry of plasmalogens: II hemolytic activity of some plasmalogen derivatives, *Journal of Lipid Research,* **4,** 57–62.

Green, D. E. (1972) Membrane proteins – a perspective. *Annals of New York Academy Science,* **195,** 180–195.

Greenfield, S., Brostoff, S., Eylar, E. H. and Morell, P. (1973) Protein composition of myelin of the peripheral nervous system. *Journal of Neurochemistry,* **20,** 1207–1216.

Greenfield, S. Norton, W. T. and Morell, P. (1971) Quaking mouse: isolation and characterization of myelin protein. *Journal of Neurochemistry,* **18,** 2119–2128.

Gregson, N. A. and Hall, S. M. (1973) A quantitative analysis of the effects of the intraneural injection of lysophosphatidyl choline. *Journal of Cell Science,* **13,** 257–277.

Gregson, N. A., Kennedy, Mary, C. and Leibowitz, S. (1971) Immunological reactions with lysolecithin-solubilized myelin. *Immunology,* **20,** 501–512.

Gregson, N. A., Kennedy, M. and Leibowitz, S. (1974) The specificity of anti-galactocerebroside antibody and its reaction with lysolecithin-solubilized myelin. *Immunology,* **26,** 743–757.

Gregson, N. A. and Oxberry, J. M. (1972) The composition of myelin from the mutant mouse 'quaking'. *Journal of Neurochemistry,* **19,** 1065–1071.

Gul, S., Smith, A. D., Thompson, R. H. S., Wright, H. P. and Zilkha, K. J. (1970) Fatty acid composition of phospholipids from platelets and erythrocytes in multiple sclerosis. *Journal of Neurology, Neurosurgery and Psychiatry,* **33,** 506–510.

Gurd, R. S., Mahler, H. R. and Moore, W. J. (1972) Differences in protein patterns on polyacrylamide gel electrophoresis of neuronal membranes from mice of different strains. *Journal of Neurochemistry,* **19,** 553–556.

Hagopian, A., Westall, F. C., Whitehead, J. S. and Eylar, E. N. (1971) Glycosylation of the A_1 protein from myelin by a polypeptide N-acetylgalactosaminyltransferase. *Journal of Biological Chemistry,* **246,** 2519–2523.

Hakomori, S. I. (1971) Glycolipid changes associated with maligment transformation. In *The Dynamic Structure of Cell Membranes,* (eds.) Hölzl Wallach, D. F. and Fischer, H. pp. 65–96. Springer Verlag: Amsterdam.

Hall, S. M. (1972a) The effects of injection of patassium cyanide into the sciatic nerve of the adult mouse: *in vivo* and electron microscopic studies. *Journal of Neurocytology,* **1,** 233–254.

Hall, S. M. (1972b) The effect of injections of lysophosphatidyl choline into white matter of the adult mouse spinal cord. *Journal of Cell Science,* **10,** 535–546.

Hall, S. M. and Gregson, N. A. (1971) The *in vivo* and ultra structural effects of injection of lysophosphatidyl choline into myelinated peripheral nerve fibres of the adult mouse. *Journal of Cell Science,* **9,** 769–789.

Hall, S. M. and Williams, P. L. (1970) Studies on the 'incisures' of Schmidt and Lanterman. *Journal of Cell Science*, 6, 767–792.

Hall, S. M. and Williams, P. L. (1971) The distribution of electron-dense tracers in peripheral nerve fibres. *Journal of Cell Science*, 8, 541–555.

Hallpike, J. F. (1972) Enzyme and protein changes in myelin breakdown and multiple sclerosis. *Progress in Histochemistry and Cytochemistry*, 3, 179–218.

Hamberger, A. and Svennerholm, L. (1971) Composition of gangliosides and phospholipids of neuronal and glial cell enriched fractions. *Journal of Neurochemistry*, 18, 1821–1830.

Hanai, T., Haydon, D. A. and Taylor, J. (1965) The influence of lipid composition and of some adsorbed proteins on the capacitance of black hydrocarbon membranes. *Journal of Theoretical Biology*, 9, 422–432.

Harker, D. (1972) Myelin membrane structure as revealed by X-ray diffraction. *Biophysical Journal*, 12, 1285–1295.

Hawthorne, J. N. (1972) Inositol lipid metabolism and the cell membrane. In *Current Trends in the Biochemistry of Lipids*, (eds.) Ganguly, J. and Smellie, R. M. S. pp. 383–393. Academic Press: London.

Hendler, R. W. (1971) Biological membrane ultrastructure. *Physiological Reviews*, 51, 66–97.

Hereward, R. V. and Northcote, D. H. (1973) Fracture planes of the plasmalemma of some higher plants revealed by freeze etch. *Journal of Cell Science*, 13, 621–635.

Herschkowitz, N., McKhann, G. M., Saxena, S. and Shooter, E. M. (1968a) Studies of water soluble lipoproteins in rat brain. *Journal of Neurochemistry*, 15, 161–168.

Herschkowitz, N., McKhann, G. M., Saxena, S. and Shooter, E. M. (1968b) Characterisation of sulphatide-containing lipoproteins in rat brain. *Journal of Neurochemistry*, 15, 1181–1188.

Herschkowitz, N., McKhann, G. M., Saxena, S., Shooter, E. M. and Herdon, R. (1969) Synthesis of sulphatide-containing lipoproteins in rat brain. *Journal of Neurochemistry*, 16, 1049–1057.

Hillorp, N. A. and Olivecrona, H. (1946) Role played by axons and Schwann cells in degree of myelination of peripheral nerve fibres. *Acta Anatomica*, 2, 17–32.

Hinse, C. H. and Shah, S. N. (1971) Desmosterol reductase activity of rat brain during development. *Journal of Neurochemistry*, 18, 1989–1998.

Hiscoe, H. B. (1947) Distribution of nodes and incisures in normal and regenerated nerve fibres. *Anatomical record*, 99, 447–475.

Hodgkin. A. L. (1964) In *The conduction of the nerve impulse*. Charles C. Thomas: Springfield, Illinois.

Höglund, G. and Ringertz, H. (1961) X-ray diffraction studies on peripheral nerve myelin. *Acta Physiologica Scandanavica*, 51, 290–295.

Horrocks, L. A. (1967) Composition of myelin from peripheral and central nervous systems of the squirrel and monkey. *Journal of Lipid Research*, 8, 569–576.

Howell, J.Mc. (1970) Diseases affecting myelination in domestic animals. In *Myelination*, (eds.) Davison, A. N. and Peters, A. pp. 199–228. Charles C. Thomas: Springfield, Illinois.

Hulcher, F. H. (1963) Physical and chemical properties of myelin. *Archives of Biochemistry and Biophysics*, 100, 237–244.

Huxley, A. F. and Stampfli, R. (1949) Evidence for saltatory conduction in peripheral myelinated nerve fibres. *Journal of Physiology*, 108, 315–339.

Ibrahim, M. Z. M., Briscoe, P. B. Jr., Bayliss, O. B. and Adams, C. W. M. (1963) The relationship between enzyme activity and neuroglia in the prodromal and demyelinating stages of cyanide encephalopathy in the rat. *Journal of Neurology Neurosurgery Psychiatry*, 26, 479–486.

Inoue, T., Oeshmukh, D. S. and Pieringer, R. A. (1971) The association of galactosyl diglycerides of brain with myelination. *Journal of Biological Chemistry*, 246, 5688–5694.

Jenkinson, T. J., Kamat, V. B. and Chapman, D. (1969) Physical studies of myelin. II Proton magnetic resonance and infrared spectroscopy. *Biochemica et Biophysica Acta*, 183, 427–433.

Joffe, S. (1971) Isolation and some properties of a succinylated protein-lipid complex derived from calf brain myelin. *Archives Biochemistry and Biophysics*, 146, 46–53.

Joffe, S. and Block, R. E. (1972) Nuclear magnetic resonance studies suggestive of a lipid population tightly bound to myelin structural proteins. *Brain Research,* **46**, 381–390.

Jungalwala, F. B. and Dawson, R. M. C. (1971) The turnover of myelin phospholipids in the adult and developing rat brain. *Biochemical Journal,* **123**, 683–693.

Kamoshita, S., Rapin, I., Suzuki, K. and Suzuki, K. (1968) Spongy degeneration of the brain: a chemical study of two cases including isolation and characterisation of myelin. *Neurology,* **18**, 975–985.

Kandutsch, A. A. and Saucier, S. E. (1969) Regulation of sterol synthesis in developing brains of normal and jimpy mice. *Archives Biochemistry and Biophysics,* **135**, 201–208.

Kandutsch, A. A. and Saucier, S. E. (1972) Sterol synthesis and fatty acid synthesis in developing brains of 3 myelin-deficient mouse metants. *Biochemica et Biophysica Acta,* **260**, 26–34.

Karlsson, U. (1966) Comparison of the myelin period of peripheral and central origin by electron microscopy. *Journal of Ultrastructural Research,* **15**, 451–468.

Katz, B. and Schmitt, F. O. (1940) Electric interaction between two adjacent nerve fibres. *Journal of Physiology,* **97**, 471–488.

Kibler, R. F., Re, P. K., McKneally, S. and Shapiro, R. (1972) Biological activity of an encephalitogenic fragment in the monkey. *Journal of Biological Chemistry,* **247**, 969–972.

Kirschner, D. A. and Caspar, D. D. (1972) Comparative diffraction studies on myelin membranes. *Annals of the New York Academy of Science,* **195**, 309–320.

Kishimoto, Y. (1971) Abnormality in sphingolipid fatty acids from sciatic nerve and brain of quaking mice. *Journal of Neurochemistry,* **18**, 1365–1368.

Kishimoto, Y., Wajda, M. and Radin, N. S. (1968) 6-acyl galactosyl ceramides of pig brain: structure and fatty acid composition. *Journal of lipid Research,* **9**, 27–33.

Kornguth, S. E., Walberg Anderson, J., Scott, G. and Kubinski, H. (1967) Fractionation of subcellular elements from rat central nervous tissue in a caesium chloride gradient. *Experimental Cell Research,* **45**, 656–670.

Kurihara, T., Nussbaum, J. L. and Mandel, P. (1969) 2',3'-cyclic nucleotide 3'-phosphohydrolase in the brain of the jimpy mouse, a mutant with deficient myelin. *Brain Research,* **13**, 401–403.

Kurihara T. and Takahashi, Y. (1973) Potentiometric and colorimetric methods for the assay of 2'-3'-cyclic nucleotide 3'-phosphohydrolase. *Journal of Neurochemistry,* **20**, 719–727.

Kurihara, T. and Tsukada, Y. (1967) The regional and subcellular distribution of 2'-3'-cyclic nucleotide 3'-phosphohydrolase in the central nervous system. *Journal of Neurochemistry,* **14**, 1167–1174.

Kurtz, D. J. and Kanfer, J. N. (1973) Composition of myelin lipids and synthesis of 3-ketodihydrosphingosine in the vitamin B_6-deficient developing rat. *Journal of Neurochemistry,* **20**, 963–968.

Laatsch, B. A., Kier, M. W., Gordon, S. and Alvord, E. C. (1962) The encephalomyelitic activity of myelin isolated by ultracentrifugation. *Journal of Experimental Medicine,* **115**, 777–788.

Ladbrooke, B. D., Jenkinson, T. J., Kamat, V. B. and Chapman, D. (1968) Physical studies of myelin I Thermal analysis. *Biochemica et Biophysica Acta,* **164**, 101–108.

Ladbrooke, B. D. and Chapman, D. (1969) Thermal analysis of lipids, proteins and biological membranes, a review and summary of some recent studies. *Chemistry and Physics of Lipids,* **3**, 304–356.

Langley, O. K. (1971) Sialic acid and membrane contact relationships in peripheral nerve. *Experimental Cell Research,* **68**, 97–105.

Lapetina, E. G., Soto, E. F. and DeRobertis, E. (1968) Lipids and proteolipids in isolated subcellular membranes of rat brain cortex. *Journal of Neurochemistry,* **15**, 437–445.

LeBaron, F. N. (1969) The lipid-protein complexes of myelin. In *Structural and functional aspects of lipoproteins in living systems,* (eds.) Tria, E. and Scanu, A. M. pp. 201–226. Academic Press: London.

LeBaron, F. N. and Folch-Pi, J. (1956) The isolation from brain tissue of a trypsin-resistant protein fraction containing combined inositol, and its relation to neurakeratin. *Journal of Neurochemistry,* **1**, 101–108.

Lecar, H., Ehrenstein, G. and Stillman, I. (1971) Detection of molecular motion in lyophilised myelin by nuclear megnetic resonance. *Biophysical Journal*, 11, 140–145.

Ledeen, R. W., Yu, R. K. and Eng, L. F. (1973) Gangliosides of human myelin: sialosylgalactosylceramide (G7) as a major component. *Journal of Neurochemistry*, 21, 829–839.

Lillie, K. S. (1925) Factors affecting transmission and recovery in the passive iron wire model. *Journal of General Physiology*, 7, 463–507.

London, Y. (1972) Preparations of purified myelin from ox-intradural spinal roots by rate isopycnic zonal centrifugation. *Biochimica et Biophysica Acta*, 282, 195–204.

London, Y. and Vosseberg, F. G. A. (1973) Specific interaction of central nervous system myelin basic proteins with lipids. Specific regions of the protein sequence Protected from the proteolytic action of trypsin. *Biochimica et Biophysica Acta*, 478, 478–490.

Lovelidge, C. A. (1972) Protein components of central-nervous system myelin. Ph.D. Thesis, University of London.

Lowry, O. K., Rosebrough, N. J., Farr, A. L. and Randall, R. N. 1951) Protein measurement with the Folin phenol reagent. *Journal of Biological Chemistry*, 193, 265–275.

Lumsden, C. E. (1972) The clinical pathology of multiple sclerosis. In *Multiple Sclerosis, a re-appraisal*, by McAlpine, D., Lumsden, C. E. and Acheson, E. D. Churchill Livingstone: London.

Luthra, M. G. and Sheltawy, A. (1972) The distribution of molecular species of phosphatidylinositol in ox brain and its subcellular fractions. *Biochemical Journal*, 128, 587–595.

MacBrinn, M. C. and O'Brien, J. S. (1968) Lipid composition of the nervous system in Refsums disease. *Journal of Lipid Research*, 9, 552–561.

MacBrinn, M. C. and O'Brien, J. S. (1969) Lipid composition of optic nerve myelin. *Journal of Neurochemistry*, 16, 7–12.

McIlwain, D. L., Graf, L. and Rapport, M. M. (1971) Membrane fragments from myelin treated with different detergents. *Journal of Neurochemistry*, 18, 2255–2264.

McIlwain, D. L. and Rapport, M. M. (1971) The effects of phospholipase c (Clostridium perfringens) on purified myelin. *Biochimica et Biophysica Acta*, 239, 71–80.

McIntosh, T. J. and Worthington, C. R. (1973) The choice between the positive and negative structures for nerve myelin. *Biophysical Journal*, 13, 498–500.

Martenson, R. E., Deibler, G. E., Kies, M. W., Levine, S. and Alvord, E. C. (1972) Myelin basic proteins of mammalian and submammalian vertebrates: encephalitogenic activities in guinea pigs and rats. *Journal of Immunology*, 109, 262–270.

Martenson, R. E., Deibler, G. E., Kies, M. W., McKneally, S. S., Shapiro, R. and Kibler, R. F. (1972) Differences between the two myelin basic proteins of rat central nervous system. *Biochimica et Biophysica Acta*, 263, 193–203.

Mateu, L., Luzzati, V., London, Y., Gould, R. M., Vosseberg, F. G. A. and Olive, J. (1973) X-ray diffraction and electron microscope study of the interactions of myelin components. The structure of a lamellar phase with a 150 to 180 A repeat distance containing basic proteins and acidic lipids. *Journal of Molecular Biology*, 75, 697–709.

Matter, A., Oria, L, and Rouiller, C. (1969) A study on the permeability barriers between Disses space and the bile canaliculus. *Journal of Ultrastructural Research*, Suppl. 11.

Matthieu, J. M., Brady, R. O. and Quarles, R. H. (1974) Anomalies of myelin associated glycoproteins in 'quaking' mice. *Journal of Neurochemistry*, 22, 291–296.

Mehl, E. and Halaris, A. (1970) Stoichiometric relation of protein components in cerebral myelin from different species. *Journal of Neurochemistry*, 17, 659–668.

Mehl, E. and Wolfgram, F. (1969) Myelin types with different protein components. *Journal of Neurochemistry*, 16, 1091–1097.

Meier, H. and MacPike, A. D. (1970) A neurological mutation (m.s.d.) of the mouse causing a deficiency of myelin synthesis. *Experimental Brain Research*, 10, 512–525.

Miller, E. K. and Dawson, R. M. C. (1972a) Can mitochondria and synaptosomes of guinea pig brain synthesize phopholipids? *Biochemical Journal*, 126, 805–821.

Miller E. K. and Dawson, R. M. C. (1972b) Exchange of phospholipds between brain membranes *in vitro*. *Biochemical Journal*, 126, 823–835.

Mokrasch, L. C. (1969) Myelin. In *Handbook of Neurochemistry*, Vol. 1 Chemical architecture of the nervous system, (ed.) Lajtha, A. pp. 171–193. Plenum Press: New York.

Mokrasch, L. C. and Manner, P. (1963) Incorporation of ^{14}C-amino acids and ^{14}C palmitate into proteolipids of rat brains *in vitro*. *Journal of Neurochemistry*, **10**, 541–548.

Moody, M. F. (1963) X-ray diffraction pattern of nerve myelin: a method for determining the phases. *Science*, **142**, 1173–1174.

Morell, P., Greenfield, S., Costantino-Ceccarini, E. and Wisniewski, H. (1972) Changes in the protein composition of mouse brain myelin during development. *Journal of Neurochemistry*, **19**, 2545–2554.

Murakami, M., Sekine, H. and Funahashi, S. (1962) Proteolipid from beef heart muscle. Application of organic dialysis to preparation of proteolipid. *Journal of Biochemistry*, **51**, 431–435.

Murray, M. R. (1965) Nervous tissue *in vitro*. In *Cells and Tissues in Culture*, (ed.) Willmer, E. N. Vol. 2, pp. 373. Academic Press: New York.

Nepolitano, L., LeBaron, F. and Scalletti, J. (1967) Preservation of myelin lamellar structure in the absence of lipid. *Journal of Cell Biology*, **34**, 817–826.

Neskovic, N., Nussbaum, J. C. and Mandel, P. (1969) Etude de la galactosylsphingosine transferase du cerveau de souris mutante. *Compte rendu d'Academie des Sciences*, **269**, 1125–1128.

Nguyen-Le, T., Nicot, C. and Alfsen, A. (1971) A new method of preparation for the apoprotein moiety from Folch-Pi proteolipid. In *Protides of Biological Fluids*, (ed.) Peeters, H. Vol. **19**, pp. 217–220. Pergamon Press: Oxford.

Norton, W. T. (1971a) The Myelin Sheath. In *The Cellular and Molecular Basis of Neurologic Disease*, (eds.) Shy, G. M., Goldensohn, E. S. and Appel, S. M. Lea and Ferbiger: Philadelphia.

Norton, W. T. (1971b) Recent developments in the investigation of purified myelin. In *Advances in Experimental Medicine and Biology*, Vol. **13**, Chemistry of Brain Development, (eds.) Paoletti, R. and Davison, A. N. pp. 327–337. Plenum Press: New York.

Norton, W. T. and Autilio, L. A. (1966) The lipid composition of purified bovine brain myelin. *Journal of Neurochemistry*, **13**, 213–222.

Norton, W. T. and Brotz, M. (1963) New galactolipids of brain: a monalkyl-monoacyl glyceryl galactoside and cerebroside fatty acid esters. *Biochemical and Biophysical Research Communications*, **12**, 198–203.

Norton, W. T. and Poduslo, S. E. (1966) Metachromatic leucodystrophy: chemically abnormal myelin and cerebralbiopsy studies of three siblings. In *Variation in the chemical composition of the nervous system*, (ed.) Ansell, G. B. p. 82. Pergamon Press: Oxford.

Norton, W. T. and Puduslo, S. E. (1973) Myelination in rat brain: changes in myelin composition during brain maturation. *Journal of Neurochemistry*, **21**, 759–773.

Norton, W. T., Poduslo, S. E. and Suzuki, K. (1966) Subacute sclerosing leukoencephalitis. II Chemical studies including abnormal myelin and an abnormal ganglioside pattern. *Journal of Neuropathology and Experimental Neurology*, **25** 582–597.

O'Brien, J. S. (1965) The stability of the myelin membrane. *Science*, **147**, 1099–1107.

O'Brien, J. S. (1967) Cell membranes-composition; structure: function. *Journal of Theoretical Biology*, **15**, 307–324.

O'Brien, J. S. and Sampson, E. L. (1965) Metachromatic leucodystrophy – myelin analysis. *Science*, **150**, 1613–1614.

O'Brien, J. S. and Sampson, E. L. (1965b) Fatty acid and fatty aldehyde composition of the major brain lipids in normal human gray matter, white matter and myelin. *Lipid Research*, **6**, 545–551.

O'Brien, J. S., Sampson, E. L. and Stern, M. B. (1967) Lipid composition of myelin from the peripheral nervous system. *Journal of Neurochemistry*, **14**, 357–365.

Olafson, R. W., Drummond, G. J. and Lee, J. F. (1969) Studies on 2'-3'-cyclic nucleotide-3'-phosphohydrolase from brain. *Canadian Journal of Biochemistry*, **47**, 961–966.

Oldfield, E. and Chapman, D. (1972) Molecular dynamics of cerebroside-cholesterol and sphingomyelin-cholesterol interaction: implications for myelin membrane structure. *FEBS letters*, **21**, 303–306.

Oshiro, Y. and Eylar, E. H. (1970) Allergic encephalomyelitis: a comparison of the encephalitogenic A1 protein from human and bovine brain. *Archives of Biochemistry and Biophysics*, **138**, 606–613.

Overath, P., Schairer, H. U., Hill, F. F. and Lamnek-Hirsch, I. (1971) Structure and function of hydrocarbon chains in bacterial phopholipids. In *The dynamic structure of cell membranes*, (eds.) Hölzl Wallach, D. F. and Fischer, H. pp. 149–164. Springer Verlag: Amsterdam.

Oxberry, J. M. (1972) Biochemical changes during development of the peripheral nervous system. M.Phil thesis, University of London.

Ozols, J. (1972) Cytochrome b_5 from a normal human liver. *Journal of Biological Chemistry*, **247**, 2242–2245.

Palmer, F. B. and Dawson, R. M. C. (1969a) The isolation and properties of experimental allergic encephalitogenic protein. *Biochemical Journal*, **111**, 629–636.

Palmer, F. B. and Dawson, R. M. C. (1969b) Complex-formation between triphospho-inositide and experimental allergic encepgalitogenic protein. *Biochemical Journal*, **111**, 637–646.

Palmer, K. J., Schmitt, F. O. and Chargaff, E. (1941) X-ray diffraction studies of certain lipid-protein complexes. *Journal of Cellular and Comparative Physiology*, **18**, 43–47.

Patterson, D. S. P., Sweasey, D., Brush, P. J. and Harding, J. D. (1973) Neurochemistry of the spinal cord in British saddleback piglets affected with congenital tremor, Type A-IV, a second form of hereditary cerebrospinal hypomyelinogenesis. *Journal of Neurochemistry*, **21**, 397–406.

Patterson, D. S. P., Sweasey, D. and Harding, J. D. J. (1972) Lipid deficiency in the central nervous system of landrace piglets affected with congenital tremor A III, a form of cerebrospinal hypomyelinogenesis. *Journal of Neurochemistry*, **19**, 2791–2800.

Pauly, H., Packer, L. and Schwan, H. P. (1960) Electrical properties of mitrochondrial membranes. *Journal of Biophysical Biochemical Cytology*, **7**, 589–601.

Pauly, H. and Packer, L. (1960) Relationship of conductance and membrane capacity to mitrochondrial volume. *Journal of Biophysical Biochemical Cytology*, **7**, 603–612.

Peters, A. (1964) Further observations on the structure of myelin sheaths in the central nervous system. *Journal of Cell Biology*, **20**, 281–296.

Peters, A. and Vaughn, J. E. (1970) Morphology and Development of the myelin sheath. In *Myelination*, (eds.) Davison, A. N. and Peters, A. pp. 3–79. Charles C. Thomas: Springfield, Illinois.

Phillips, M. C., Ladbrooke, B. D. and Chapman, D. (1970) Molecular interactions in mixed lecithin systems. *Biochemica et Biophysica Acta*, **196**, 35–44.

Phillips, M. C., Hauser, H. and Paltauf, F. (1972) The inter- and intra-molecular mixing of hydrocarbon chains in lecithin-water systems. *Chemistry and Physics of Lipids*, **8**, 127–128.

Pickard, W. F. (1969) Estimating the velocity of propagation along myelinated and unmyelinated fibres. *Mathematical Biosciences*, **5**, 305–319.

Pitt-Rivers, R. and Impiombato, F. S. A. (1968) The binding of sodium dodecyl sulphate to various proteins. *Biochemical Journal*, **109**, 825–830.

Pleasure, D. E. and Prockop, D. J. (1972) Myelin synthesis in peripheral nerve in vitro: sulphatide incoporation requires a transport lipoprotein. *Journal of Neurochemistry*, **19**, 283–296.

Poduslo, S. E. and Norton, W. T. (1972) Isolation and some chemical properties of oligodendroglia from calf brain. *Journal of Neurochemistry*, **19**, 727–736.

Quarles, R. H., Everly, J. L. and Brady, R. O. (1973) Evidence for the close association of a glycoprotein with myelin in rat brain. *Journal of Neurochemistry*, **21**, 1177–1191.

Ramsey, R. B., Jones, J. P., Rios, A. and Nicholas, A. J. (1972) The biosynthesis of cholesterol and other sterols by brain tissue. *Journal of Neurochemistry*, **19**, 101–107

Rapport, M. M., Cavanna, R. and Graf, L. (1967) Immunochemical studies of organ and tumour lipids XVI The existence of two complement-fixing systems involving cerebroside. *Journal of Neurochemistry*, **14**, 9–18.

Rapport, M. M., Graf, L., Autilio, L. A. and Norton, W. A. (1964) Immunochemical studies of organ and tumor lipids XIV Galactocerebroside determinants in the myelin sheath of the central nervous system. *Journal of Neurochemistry*, **11**, 855–864.

Rathbone, L. (1965) The effect of diet on the fatty acid composition of serum, brain, brain mitochondria and myelin in the rat. *Biochemical Journal*, **97**, 620–628.

Rawlins, F. A., Hedley-White, E. T., Villegas, G. and Uzman, B. G. (1970) Reutilization of cholesterol-1,2-³H in the regeneration of peripheral nerve. An autoradiographic study. *Laboratory Investigation,* **22,** 237–240.

Rawlins, F. A. and Smith, M. E. (1971) Myelin synthesis *in vitro:* a comparative study of central and peripheral nervous tissue. *Journal of Neurochemistry,* **18,** 1861–1870.

Rawlins, F. A. and Uzman, B. G. (1970) Retardation of peripheral nerve myelination in mice treated with inhibitors of cholesterol biosynthesis. *Journal of Cell Biology,* **46,** 505–517.

Revel, J. P. and Hamilton, D. W. (1969) The double nature of the intermediate dense line in peripheral nerve myelin. *Anatomical Record,* **163,** 7–15.

Robertson, D. M. (1960) The electrophoretic distribution of the lipoproteins of the supernatant fraction of rat whole brain. *Journal of Neurochemistry,* **6,** 105–111.

Robertson, D. M. and Vogel, F. S. (1962) Concentric lamination of glial processes in oligodendrogliomas. *Journal of Cell Biology,* **15,**313–334.

Robertson, J. D. (1958) Structural alterations in nerve fibres produced by hypotonic and hypertonic solutions. *Journal of Biophysical Biochemical Cytology,* **4,** 349–364.

Robertson, J. D. (1959) The ultrastructure of cell membranes and their derivatives. *Biochemical Society Symposia,* No. 16 pp. 1–43. Cambridge University Press.

Robertson, J. D. (1960) The molecular structure and contact relationshin of cell membranes. *Progress in Biophysics and Biophysical Chemistry*, Butler, J. A. W. and Katz, B. Vol. **10** pp. 343–418. Pergamon Press: Oxford.

Rosenbluth, A. (1943) The interaction of myelinated fibres in mammalian nerve trunks. *American Journal of Physiology,* **140,** 656–670.

Rumsby, M. G. and Finean, J. B. (1966a) The action of organic solvents on the myelin sheath of peripheral nerve tissues-I. *Journal of Neurochemistry,* **13,** 1501–1507.

Rumsby, M. G. and Finean, J. B. (1966b) The action of organic solvents on the myelin sheath of peripheral nerve tissue-II. *Journal of Neurochemistry,* **13,** 1509–1511.

Rushton, W. A. H. (1951) A theory of the effects of fibre size in medullated nerve. *Journal of Physiology,* **115,** 101–122.

Sammeck, R. and Brady, R. O. (1972) Studies of the catabolism of myelin basic proteins of the rat *in situ* and *in vitro. Brain Research,* **42,** 441–453.

Sammeck, R., Martenson, R. E. and Brady, R. O. (1971) Studies of the metabolism of myelin basic protein in various regions of the central nervous system of immature and adult rats. *Brain Research,* **34,** 241–254.

Samorajski, T., Friede, R. L. and Reimer, P. R. (1970) Hypomyelination in the quaking mouse. A model for the analysis of disturbed myelin formation. *Journal of Neuropathology, Experimental Neurology,* **29,** 507–523.

Saunders, L. (1966) Molecular aggregation in aqueous dispersions of phosphatidyl and lysophosphatidyl cholines. *Biochimica Biophysica Acta,* **125,** 70–74.

Schmidt, W. S. (1936) Doppelbrechung und freinbau der marksheide der nervenfasern. *Zeitschrift für Zellforschung Mikroskopi Anatomie,* **23,** 657–676.

Schmitt, F. O. and Bear, R. S. (1937) The optical properties of vertebrate nerve axons as related to fibre size. *Journal of Cellular and Comparative Physiology,* **9,** 261–273.

Schmitt, F. O. and Bear, R. S. (1939) The ultrastructure of the nerve axon sheath. *Biological Reviews,* **14,** 27–50.

Schmitt, F. O., Bear, R. S. and Clark, G. L. (1935) X-ray diffraction studies on nerve. *Radiology,* **25,** 131–151.

Schmitt, F. O., Bear, R. S. and Palmer, K. J. (1941) X-ray diffraction studies on the structure of the nerve myelin sheath. *Journal of Cellular and Comparative Physiology,* **18,** 31–42.

Schmitt, F. O. and Palmer, K. J. (1940) X-ray diffraction studies of lipide and lipide-protein studies. *Cold Spring Harbour Symposium,* **8,** 94–99.

Schwann, H. P. and Carstensen, E. L. (1957) Dielectric properties of the membrane of lysed erythrocytes. *Science,* **125,** 985–986.

Schwann, H. P. and Morowitz, H. J. (1962) Electrical properties of the membranes of the pleuropneumonia like organism A5969. *Biophysics Journal,* **2,** 395–407.

Scott, T. G. and Barber, V. C. (1964) An enzyme histochemical and biochemical study of the effect of an inhibitor of cholesterol synthesis on myelinating mouse brain. *Journal of Neurochemistry,* **11,** 423–429.

Shah, N., Peterson, N. A. and McKean, C. M. (1968) Inhibition of in vitro sterol biosynthesis by phenylalanine. *Biochemica et Biophysica Acta*, 164, 604–606.

Shah, S. N., Peterson, N. A. and McKean, C. M. (1970) Cerebral lipid metabolism in experimental hyperphenylalaninaemia: Incorporation of 14-C labelled glucose into total lipids. *Journal of Neurochemistry*, 17, 279–284.

Shah, S. N., Peterson, N. A. and McKean, C. M. (1972a) Lipid composition of human cerebral white matter and myelin in phenylketonuria. *Journal of Neurochemistry*, 19, 2369–2376.

Shah, S. N., Peterson, N. A. and McKean, C. M. (1972b) Impaired myelin formation in experimental hyperphenylalaninaemia. *Journal of Neurochemistry*, 19, 479–485.

Shapira, R., Chou, C. H., McKneally, S. S., Urban, E. and Kibler, R. F. (1971) Biological activity and synthesis of an encephalitogenic determinant. *Science*, 173, 736–738.

Shapira, R., McKneally, S. S., Chou, F. and Kibler, R. F. (1971) Encephalitogenic fragment of myelin basic protein: amino acid sequence of bovine, rabbit, guinea pig, monkey and human fragment. *Journal of Biological Chemistry*, 246, 4630–4640.

Shapiro, A. L. and Maizel, J. V. (1969) Molecular weight estimation of polypeptides by SDS polyacrylamide gel electrophoresis. *Analytical Biochemistry*, 29, 505–514.

Shapiro, A. L., Vinuela, E. and Maizel, J. V. (1967) Molecular weight estimation of polypeptide chains by electrophoresis in SDS polyacrylamide gels. *Biochemical Biophysical Research Communications*, 28, 815–820.

Shaw, I. G., Winkler, C. E. and Terlecki, S. (1967) Experimental reproduction of hypomyelinogenesis congenital of lambs. *The Veterinary Record*, 81, 115–116.

Sheltawy, A. and Dawson, R. M. C. (1966) The polyphosphoinositides and other lipids of peripheral nerves. *Biochemical Journal*, 100, 12–18.

Sherman, G. and Folch-Pi, J. (1970) Rotary dispersion and circular dichroism of brain proteolipid protein. *Journal of Neurochemistry*, 17, 597–605.

Sidman, R. K. and Hayes, R. (1965) Jimpy: a mouse with inherited sudanophilic leukodystrophy. *Journal of Neuropathology and Experimental Neurology*, 24, 173.

Simon, G. (1966) Cholesterol ester in degenerating nerve: origin of cholesterol moiety. *Lipids*, 1, 369–370.

Simon, R. G., Wade, R. R., DeLarco, J. E. and Baker, M. L. (1969) Wallerian degeneration: a sequential process. *Journal of Neurochemistry*, 16, 1435–1438.

Sinclair, H. M. (1956) Deficiency of essential fatty acids and atherosclerosis, etc. *Lancet*, i, 381–383.

Singer, M. (1968) Penetration of labelled amino acids into the peripheral nerve fibre from surrounding body fluids. In *Growth of the Nervous System*, (eds.) Wolstenholme, O. and O'Connor, M. Ciba Foundation Symposium, pp. 200–215. Churchill: London.

Singer, S. J. (1971) The molecular organisation of biological membranes. In *Structure and Function of Biological Membranes*, (ed.) Rothfield, L. I. pp. 145–222. Academic Press: London.

Singh, H. (1973) Glycolipids of peripheral nerve: isolation and characterization of glycolipids from rabbit sciatic nerve. *Journal of Lipid Research*, 14, 41–49.

Singh, H., Spritz, N. and Geyer, B. (1971) Studies of brain myelin in the 'quaking mouse'. *Journal of Lipid Research*. 12, 473–481.

Smith, M. E. (1967) The metabolism of myelin lipids. *Advances in Lipid Research*, 5, 241–278.

Smith, M. E. (1969) An *in vitro* system for the study of myelin synthesis. *Journal of Neurochemistry*, 16, 83–92.

Smith, M. E. (1973) Studies on the mechanism of demyelination: triethyltin-induced demyelination. *Journal of Neurochemistry*, 21, 357–372.

Smith, M. E. and Eng, L. F. (1965) The turnover of lipid components of myelin. *Journal of the American Oil Chemists Society*, 42, 1013–1018.

Smith, M. E. and Hasinoff, C. M. (1971) Biosynthesis of myelin proteins in vitro. *Journal of Neurochemistry*, 18, 739–747.

Smith, M. E., Hasinoff, C. M. and Fumagalli, R. (1970) Inhibitors of cholesterol synthesis and myelin formation. *Lipids*, 5, 665–671.

Smith, R. S. and Koles, Z. J. (1970) Myelinated nerve fibres: computed effect of myelin thickness on conduction velocity. *American Journal of Physiology*, 219, 1256–1258.

Smyth, D. S. and Utsumi, S. (1967) Structure at the hinge region in rabbit immuno-globulin-G. *Nature* (London), 216, 332–335.

Soller, M. and Koenig, H. (1970) Lipoprotein subunit of myelin: Isolation, characterisation, in vitro formation of myelin membranes. *Transaction of American Neurological Association*, 95, 309–312.

Speidel, C. C. (1964) *In vivo* studies of myelinated nerve fibres. *International Review of Cytology*, 16, 173–231.

Spohn, M. and Davison, A. N. (1972a) Separation of myelin fragments from the central nervous system. In *Research methods in Neurochemistry*, (eds.) Marks, N. and Rodnight, R. Vol. 1, pp. 33–44. Plenum Press: London.

Spohn, M. and Davison, A. N. (1972b) Cholesterol metabolism in myelin and other subcellular fractions of rat brain. *Journal of Lipid Research*, 13, 563–570.

Steim, J. M. (1967) Monogalactosyl diglyceride: a new neurolipid. *Biochimica Biophysica Acta*, 144, 118–126.

Stoeckinius, W. and Engelman, D. M. (1969) Current models for the structure of biological membranes. *Journal of Cell Biology*, 42, 613–646.

Stoffyn, P. and Folch-Pi, J. (1971) On the type of linkage binding fatty acids present in brain white matter proteolipid apoprotein. *Biochemical Biophysical Research Communications*, 44, 157–161.

Strittmatter, P., Rogers, M. J. and Spatz, L. (1972) The binding of cytochrome b_5 to liver microsomes. *Journal of Biological Chemistry*, 247, 7188–7194.

Suzuki, K. (1970) Formation and turnover of myelin ganglioside. *Journal of Neurochemistry*, 17, 209–213.

Suzuki, K., Poduslo, J. F. and Poduslo, S. E. (1968) Further evidence for a specific ganglioside fraction closely associated with myelin. *Biochimica et Biophysica Acta*, 152, 576–585.

Suzuki, K., Poduslo, S. E. and Norton, W. T. (1967) Gangliosides in the myelin fraction of developing rats. *Biochimica et Biophysica Acta*, 144, 375–381.

Suzuki, K., Suzuki, K. and Kamoshita, S. (1969) Chemical pathology of GM_1-gangliosidosis (generalised gangliosidosis). *Journal of Neuropathology and Experimental Neurology*, 28, 25–73.

Suzuki, Y., Tucker, S. H., Rorke, K. B. and Suzuki, K. (1970) Ultrastructural and biochemical studies of Schilders disease. *Journal of Neuropathology and Experimental Neurology*, 29, 405–419.

Swank, R. L. (1950) Multiple sclerosis: a correlation of its incidence with dietary fat. *American Journal of the Medical Sciences*, 220, 421–430.

Tamai, Y., Taketoni, T. and Yamakawa, T. (1967) New glycolipids in bovine brain. *Japanese Journal of Experimental Medicine*, 37, 79–81.

Tanford, C. (1972) Hydrophobic free energy micelle formation and the association of proteins with Amphiphiles. *Journal of Molecular biology*, 67, 59–74.

Tasaki, I. (1955) New measurements of the capacity and the resistance of the myelin sheath and the nodal membrane of the isolated frog nerve fibre. *American Journal of Physiology*, 181, 639–650.

Taylor, J. L. and Haydon, D. A. (1966) Stabilization of thin films of liquid hydrocarbons by alkyl chain interaction. *Discussions of the Faraday Society*, 42, 51–59.

Tenenbaum, D. and Folch-Pi, J. (1966) The preparation and characterization of water-soluble proteolipid protein from bovine brain white matter. *Biochimica et Biophysica Acta*, 115, 141–147.

Thompson, E. J., Goodwin, H. and Cummings, J. N. (1967) Caesium chloride in the preparation of membrane fractions from human cerebral tissue. *Nature* (London), 215, 168–169.

Thompson, R. H. S. (1972) Fatty acid metabolism in multiple sclerosis. In *Current trends in the Biochemistry of Lipids*, (eds.) Ganguly, J. and Smellie, R. M. S. pp. 103–112. Academic Press: London and New York.

Thorun, W. and Mehl, E. (1968) Determination of molecular weights of microgram quantities of protein components from biological membranes and other complex mixtures: gell electrophoresis across linear gradients of acrylamide. *Biochimica et Biophysica Acta*, 160, 132–134.

Tourtellotte, W. W. (1970) On cerebrospinal fluid immunoglobulin-G (IgG) notients in multiple sclerosis and other diseases. *Journal of Neurological Science,* 10, 279–304.

Tristam, G. R. and Smith, R. H. (1963) The amino acid composition of some purified proteins. *Advances in Protein Chemistry,* 18, 227–318.

Uyemura, K., Tobari, C., Hirano, S. and Tsukada, T. (1972) Comparative studies on the myelin proteins of bovine peripheral nerve and spinal cord. *Journal of Neurochemistry,* 19, 2607–2614.

Vanderkooi, J. (1972) Molecular architecture of biological membranes. *Annals New York Academy of Sciences,* 195, 6–15.

Virchow, R. (1854) Ueber das aurgebreitete vorkommen einser dem Nervenmark analogen substanz in den tierische Geweben. *Archiv fur pathologische Anatomie und Physiologie und fur Klinische Medicin,* 6, 562–572.

Vizoso, A. D. and Toung, J. Z. (1948) Internode length and fibre diameter in developing and regenerating nerves. *Journal of Anatomy,* 82, 110–134.

Volpe, J. J. and Kishimoto, Y. (1972) Fatty acid synthetase of brain: development influence of nutritional and hormonal factors and comparison with liver enzyme. *Journal of Neurochemistry,* 19, 737–753.

Wakil, S. J. and Esfahani, M. (1972) The role of lipids in the structure and function of *E. coli* membrane. In *Current Trends in the Biochemistry of Lipids,* (eds.) Ganguly, J. and Smellie, R. M. S. pp. 395–405. Academic Press: London.

Waksman, B. and Adams, R. J. (1956) A comparative study of experimental allergic neuritis in the rabbit, guinea pig and mouse. *Journal of Neuropathology and Experimental Neurology,* 15, 293–332.

Weber, K. and Osborn, M. (1969) The reliability of molecular weight determinations by dodecyl sulfate-polyacrylamide gel electrophoresis.*Journal of Biological Chemistry,* 244, 4406–4416.

Webster, G. R. (1957) Clearing action of lysolecithin on brain homogenates. *Nature (London),* 180, 660–661.

Webster, H. de F. (1962) Schwann cell alterations in metachromatic leucodystrophy, preliminary phase and electron microscopic observations. *Journal of Neuropathology and Experimental Neurology,* 21, 534–554.

Webster, H. de F. (1971) The geometry of peripheral myelin sheaths during their formation and growth in rat sciatic nerves. *Journal of Cell Biology,* 48, 348–367.

Webster, H. de F. (1972) Structural aspects of myelin. *Neurosciences Research Programme Bulletin,* 9, No. 4 470–477.

Wendell-Smith, C. P. and Williams, P. L. (1959) The use of teased preparations and frozen sections in quantitative studies of mammalian peripheral nerve. *Quarterly Journal of Microscopic Science,* 100, 499–508.

Whikehart, D. R. and Lees, M. B. (1973) Amino- and carboxyl-terminal amino acids of proteolipid proteins. *Journal of Neurochemistry,* 20, 1303–1316.

Whittaker, V. P. (1963) The separation of subcellular structures from brain tissue. *Biochemical Society Symposia,* 23, 109–126.

Williams, P. L. and Hall, S. M. (1971a) Prolonged *in vivo* observations of normal peripheral nerve fibres and their acute reactions to crush and deliberate trauma. *Journal of Anatomy,* 108, 397–408.

Williams, P. L. and Wendell-Smith, C. P. (1960) The use of fixed and stained sections in quantitative studies of peripheral nerve. *Quarterly Journal of Microscopic Science,* 101, 43–54.

Williams, P. L. and Wendell-Smith, C. P. (1971) Some additional parametric variations between peripheral nerve fibre populations. *Journal of Anatomy,* 109, 515–526.

Winder, A. F. and Gent, W. L. G. (1970) Gravimetric estimation of myelin proteins. *Journal of Neurochemistry,* 17, 1695–1696.

Wolfgram, F. (1966) A new Proteolipid fraction of the nervous system I. Isolation and amino acid analyses. *Journal of Neurochemistry,* 13, 461–470.

Wolfgram, F. and Kotorii, K. (1968) The composition of the myelin proteins of the central nervous system. *Journal of Neurochemistry.* 15, 1281–1290.

Wolfgram, F. and Rose, A. S. (1961) A study of some component proteins of central and peripheral nerve myelin. *Journal of Neurochemistry,* 8, 161–168.

Wood, J. G. and King, N. (1971) Turnover of basic proteins of rat brain. *Nature (London)*, **229**, 56–57.

Worthington, C. R. (1972) X-ray studies on nerve and photoreceptors. *Annals of New York Academy of Sciences*, **195**, 293–308.

Worthington, C. R. and Blaurock, A. E. (1969a) Electron density model for nerve myelin. *Nature (London)*, **218**, 87–88.

Worthington, C. R. and Blaurock, A. E. (1969b) A low angle X-ray diffraction study of the swelling behaviour of peripheral nerve myelin. *Biochimica et Biophysica Acta*, **173**, 427–435.

Worthington, C. R. and King, G. I. (1971) Electron density profiles of nerve myelin. *Nature (London)*, **234**, 143–145.

Zand, R. (1968) Solution properties and structure of brain proteolipids. *Biopolymers*, **6**, 939–953.

Zanetta, J. P., Benda, P., Gombos, G. and Morgan, I. G. (1972) The presence of 2'3' cyclic AMP 3'-phosphohydrolase in glial cells in tissue culture. *Journal of Neurochemistry*, **19**, 881–884.

Zingsheim, H. P. (1972) Membrane structure and electron microscopy: the significance of physical problems and techniques (freeze etching). *Biochimica et Biophysica Acta*, **265**, 339–366.

12 HISTOCHEMISTRY OF PERIPHERAL NERVES AND NERVE TERMINALS

J.F. Hallpike

List of abbreviations

ACH — acetylcholine, AChE — acetylcholinersterseae, ADP — adenosine-diphosphate, AMP— adenosine monophosphate, ATCh — acetylthiocholine, ATP — adenosine triphosphate, BAH — Baker's acid Haematin, BTCh — butyrylthiocholine, CHAc — choline acetyltransferase, C/M — chloroform: methanol, 2:1 v/v, CNS — central nervous system, DFP — diisopropylfluoro-phosphonate, DMAB — p-dimethylaminobenzaldehyde, DNA — desoxyribo-nucleic acid, EAE — experimental allergic encephalitis, EBA — Evans blue-albumin, FA — fatty acids, FFA — free fatty acids, GERL — Golgi endoplasmic reticulum, GHA — gold hydroxamic acid, GLD — globoid cell leucodystrophy, LDH — lactate dehydrogenase, LNAase — L-leucyl-β-naphthylamidase, MAO — monoamine oxidase, MLD — metachromatic leucodystrophy, MS — multiple sclerosis, NA — noradrenaline, NADH — reduced nicotinamide adenine dinucleotide, NsE — non-specific esterase, OTAN — osmium tetroxide α-naphthylamine, PAN — Perchloric acid naphthoquinone, PAS — periodic acid Schiff, PASD — periodic acid silver diamine, PMS — phenazine methosulphate, PNS — peripheral nervous system, PP$_i$ase — inorganic pyrophosphatase, PTAH — phosphotungstic acid haematoxylin, SB — sudan black, SBB — sudan black B, TDP — trypsin digestible protein, TOCP — triorthocresyl phosphate, TRP — trypsin resistant protein, TRPR — trypsin resistant protein residue, WD — Wallerian degeneration.

12.1 Introduction

The peripheral nerve has been intensively studied by histochemical techniques. Such investigations have served to bridge the gap between morphological and biochemical observations and, moreover, the localization of enzyme activity in axons and nerve terminals has added a new dimension to concepts of their function. Recent progress in the cytochemistry of the nervous system has been closely linked to advances in histochemical technique at both the light and electron microscopic levels. This is especially the case in the peripheral nervous system where subcellular fractionation and cell isolation methods, applied widely to the brain, have so far enjoyed only limited success. In the present account emphasis is laid on those aspects of the function and pathology of the peripheral nerve in which histochemical analysis has proved a useful tool. Prefixative artefacts, fixation effects and difficulties in the quantitation of results are all recognized limitations to histochemical techniques, and while the refined microchemical methods evolved in certain laboratories have had their impact their application remains largely restricted to central nervous tissue and cell cultures. Information obtained from slide-histochemistry thus continues to require correlation with biochemical and ultrastructural data.

12.2 The normal nerve

12.2.1 *The neuron*

Detailed descriptions of the anatomical components of the peripheral nerve are given in other chapters in this volume, and various aspects of neuronal ultrastructure, enzyme localization and metabolism have been comprehensively described and reviewed elesewhere (Palay and Palade, 1955; Adams, 1965a; Novikoff, 1967a; de-Thé, 1968; Giacobini, 1969). Of particular relevance to the function of the nerve fibre is the protein-synthesizing ability of the neuron. Nissl substance, abundant in chromophilic neurons, contains ribosomal and polysomal ribonucleic acid (RNA). Much of the evidence relating to nucleolar synthesis of RNA, the appearance of RNA in the perinuclear region and its subsequent incorporation into cytoplasmic Nissl material resulted from the classical micro-analytical studies of Caspersson, Lowry, Hydén and their co-workers (see Adams, 1965 for references). Autoradiography with ^{3}H-labelled aminoacids has been successfully employed to demonstrate the rapidity of protein synthesis in neurons when compared with that occurring in the neuropil, white matter and unmyelinated tracts (Leblond and Amano, 1962; Prescott, 1962; Altman, 1963). Nuclear desoxyribonucleic acid (DNA) can be demonstrated both qualitatively and quantitatively by means of the Feulgen reaction; Einerson's gallocyanin-chrome alum method and methyl green-pyronin stain both DNA and RNA, and selective display of RNA or DNA with these methods can be obtained by employing ribonuclease digestion procedures. A periodic acid-silver diamine method provides relatively, selective staining of DNA, and this technique can conveniently be combined with oil red O (PASDORO) for the simultaneous demonstration of DNA and lipid in neural material (Bayliss, Adams and Hallpike, 1970).

Neurons in general display a high level of oxidative enzyme activity, and the subcellular distribution of Krebs cycle, glycolytic and pentose-shunt oxido-reductases has been reviewed by Adams (1965b); Freide (1966); and Roodyn (1967). False localization of dehydrogenase activity in histochemical prepar-ations may arise as a result of diffusion of either the enzyme or the reaction product, and coenzyme activity can prevent detection of some specific dehydrogenases. This last difficulty can sometimes be avoided by the use of phenazine methosulphate (PMS) as the intermediate electron acceptor (see Glenner, 1965), and brief tissue fixation has been advocated as a means to improve the localization of some oxidative enzymes through better preservation

606

of the organelles within which they are contained (Novikoff, 1959). In general, however, unfixed cryostat sections are to be preferred.

Nucleoside phosphatase (ATPase, ADPase, AMPase) activities at neutral pH are demonstrable in many neural cell membranes (Goldfischer, Essner and Novikoff, 1964; Novikoff, 1967a). The function of these enzymes in the cell membrane remains uncertain; inhibition studies indicate that nucleoside phosphatases displayed histochemically differ from biochemically characterized transport ATPases (Novikoff *et al.*, 1961). Creatine kinase, required for generation of ATP, has recently been quantified in isolated neurons (Krasnov, 1973). Acid phosphomonoesterase activity in normal neurons is sequestered in lysosomes in conjunction with other acid hydrolases, cathepsin, β-glucuronidase, arylsulphatases, galactosidases (de Duve and Wattiaux, 1966; Koenig, 1969). As a group, these enzymes share two features: uniform sedimentability in density-gradient centrifugation and structure-linked latency. Disruption of the lysosomal organelle leads to release of enzymes and accounts for the increase in acid phosphatase activity encountered after freeze-thawing, osmotic shock, ultrasonification, detergent lysis and on cell death. Although lysosomes can be visualized in neurons by virtue of some non-enzymatic properties, i.e. acridine orange fluorescence, osmiophilia, periodic acid-Schiff (PAS) staining (Koenig, 1962, 1969), the most widely used histochemical method for demonstrating lysosomes and related autophagic vacuoles is the acid phosphatase reaction. Acid phosphatase activity within lysosomes is particulate and best demonstrated against β-glycerophosphate after brief formalin fixation and infiltration of the tissue with gum-sucrose to prevent osmotic damage to the organelle (Holt, 1959; Bitensky, 1963; Novikoff, 1967b). Application of the Gomori β-glycerophsophate technique cannot, however, be relied on to display all intracellular acid phosphatase activity (Hallpike and Adams, unpublished observations).

Naphthol AS-TR acid phosphatase (Barka and Anderson, 1962) in neural tissue for example is readily inhibited by formalin. Moreover, biochemical (Neil and Horner, 1964) and electrophoretic (Barron *et al.*, 1964) studies suggest that although aldehyde fixation may be accepted as a requirement for displaying β-glycerophosphatase in lysosomes, especially at the level of ultrastructure, other species of acid phosphatase present in the cytoplasm can only be satisfactorily demonstrated biochemically or in unfixed cryostat material against naphthol substrates. Nucleoside phosphatases and thiamine pyrophosphatase are present in the Golgi lamellae of mammalian neurons (Novikoff and Goldfischer, 1961; Goldfischer, 1964), and the thiamine pyrophosphatase technique has been effectively employed to demonstrate the morphology of the neuronal Golgi apparatus (Shanthaveerappa and Bourne, 1965). Acid phosphatase is located in the Golgi apparatus and the endoplasmic reticulum (GERL complex). The ultrastructural disposition of these phosphatases within the GERL complex of small neurons has been extensively studied by Novikoff and his co-workers (Novikoff, 1967a,b) who have linked these enzymes to the biosynthesis of protein, intracellular vesicles and lysosomes.

Histochemical evidence of increased protein synthesis during the chromatolytic reaction in neurons that follows axon section has been fully reviewed by Lieberman (1971). Lysosomal cathepsin D is some twenty-five times more abundant in the neuronal cell body than in the neuropil (Hirsch and Parks, 1973), and increased lysosomal activity in the neuronal perikaryon is a characteristic part of the early response to axon section (Nandy, 1968; Means and Barron, 1972). Accumulations of mitochondria and increased pentose shunt, i.e. glucose-6-phosphate dehydrogenase, activity have also been found in chromatolytic neurons (Lieberman, 1971). Conversely, acetylcholinesterase (AChE) activity in the neuron is reduced following nerve section denoting loss of enzyme from the axon and perikaryon. The lipid pigment lipofuscin occurs widely in neuronal cells and increases in amount with age; its histochemical features have been reviewed by Adams (1965b). It seems likely that this pigment represents incomplete degradation of intracellular lipid within phagosomes since it is consistently associated with both β-glycerophosphatase and catheptic activity. It may be relevant in this connection that peroxisomes, which are thought to have a role in lipid catabolism, are infrequent in neurons by comparison with Schwann cells (Citkowitz and Holtzman, 1973). Selective deficiencies of specific lysosomal enzymes occur on a genetic basis and are now thought to be implicated in the pathogenesis of neuronal storage diseases (see Section 12.5).

12.2.2 *The axon*

Present concepts of axonal function embrace much more than the propagation of the bioelectric nerve impulse. The observations of Weiss and his co-workers laid the foundations of evidence for the concept of a broad traffic of protein, enzymes, energy sources and chemical neurotransmitters from the cell perikaryon along the axon to its distal or central termination. The absence of any accepted ultrastructural basis for protein synthesis in the mature axon, namely Nissl material or ribosomes, gave added weight to the idea of complete axonal dependence on its continuity with the neuronal cell body. Evidence is now emerging, however, of a limited axonal protein-synthesizing capacity (Koenig, 1969 and Chapter 1), the rate of acetylcholinesterase regeneration in peripheral nerve after irreversible inactivation with organo-phosphorus inhibitors for example suggests the existence of local production of the enzyme (Koenig and Koelle, 1960; Clouet and Waelsch, 1961). Microspectrophotometric analysis and autoradiographic studies of the giant axon of the fish Mauthner neuron have shown both that RNA is present in these axons, and that incorporation of labelled amino acids into axonal protein occurs *in situ* (Edström, 1966; Edström and Edström, 1968). Other studies (Koenig, 1965; Hartmann, Lin and Shively, 1968) have demonstrated that RNA is also present in mammalian nerve fibres.

Acetylcholinesterase (AChE) activity is found in the GERL complex of the neuron and in a proximo-distal gradient down the peripheral nerve (Lubińska *et al.*, 1963). High levels of such specific cholinesterase activity characterize cholinergic fibres. No clear cut differences in AChE activity are found between sensory and motor nerves, and in histochemical studies of mixed peripheral nerves there appears to be a marked nodal distribution of enzyme activity. Some two thirds of the AChE in peripheral nerve is probably of axonal origin, whereas non-specific (butyryl) cholinesterase activity resides largely in the Schwann cells and connective tissue elements (Sawyer, 1946; Cavanagh, Thompson and Webster, 1954). The introduction of acetylthiocholine as a histochemical substrate for cholinesterases (Koelle and Friedenwald, 1949) led to improved demonstration of enzyme activity as a result of speedier hydrolysis of the synthetic substrate and thus shorter incubation times. Koelle and Friedenwald's thiocholine method was later modified by the addition of ferricyanide to the medium to allow direct visualization of sites of enzymic action and eliminate the ammonium sulphide precipitation stage. In the now widely used Karnovsky and Roots (1964) technique, released thiocholine reduces the ferricyanide and the resulting ferrocyanide combines with Cu^{2+} to form insoluble copper ferrocyanide (Hatchett's Brown). The cytochemistry of the cholinesterases has been reviewed by Adams (1965). The histochemical distribution of cholinesterases in mixed, motor and sensory peripheral nerve trunks, and in sympathetic fibres, has been examined using the direct-colouring thiocholine-ferricyanide method (Adams, Grant and Bayliss, 1967; Grant, Bayliss and Adams, 1967). Mere selection of acetylthiocholine (ATCh) or butyrylthiocholine (BTCh) as substrates does not in general provide sufficient grounds to allow distinction between true and non-specific cholinesterases, and certain cholinesterase inhibitors, iso-OMPA (10^{-6} M) in the case of BChE, and 62 C 47 (10^{-5} M) in the case of AChE, are usually employed in parallel incubations. In addition di-isopropylfluorophosphonate (DFP), a variable inhibitor of BChE, and eserine can also be used to suppress both AChE and BChE activities. Application of the thiocholine-ferricyanide method with BChE and AChE inhibitors has shown that myelinated and unmyelinated fibres in motor and mixed (rat sciatic) nerve possess both true and some pseudo-cholinesterase activity (Adams, Grant and Bayliss, 1967). An intact perineurium impedes penetration of the ferricyanide ion and serves to explain the indifferent cholinesterase staining of whole nerve preparations obtained when using the Karnovsky and Root's technique, and it has also been established that both ferricyanide and substrate fail to enter the myelin sheath (Grant, Bayliss and Adams, 1967). The validity of the finding of cholinesterase localization at nodes of Ranvier (Fig. 12.1) has been questioned. Sulphated mucopolysaccharides are present in nodal gap substance which surrounds the axolemma at this site giving rise to the possibility of cation binding, including copper and thiocholine, and thus artefactual localization of AChE activity (Langley and Landon, 1968). Further evidence from blockading and inhibitor studies (Adams, Bayliss and Grant, 1968, 1969) appears to support the validity of the indentification of AChE at the nodes and it has been suggested that the enzyme at this site may have a role in the mechanism of

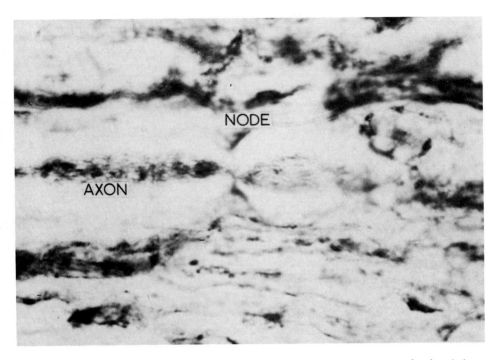

Fig. 12.1 Acetylcholinesterase at the node of Ranvier and in the axon of rat's sciatic nerve. Karnovsky-Roots' method, 18h incubation. (x 1330.)

saltatory conduction (Gerebtzoff, 1963, 1964). AChE probably occurs in two main locations within the axon: one fraction is bound to membrane of the endoplasmic reticulum and is capable of migration along the axon, and the other is bound to axonal surface membrane (Niemierko and Lubinska, 1967). The principle representatives of the acetylcholine system, choline acetyltransferase (ChAc), acetylcholine and acetylcholinesterase, have now been identified ultrastructurally within the cholinergic nerve cell (Kása, 1971). Motor neurons stain heavily for ChAc and distinct populations of boutons have been identified which are either ChAc positive or negative (Burt, 1971).

Acid phosphomonoesterases, active at about pH 5, have been extensively studied in both the normal and degenerating peripheral nerve. Acid phosphatase activity may be demonstrated histochemically against β-glycerophosphate using Gomori's (1950) lead capture technique, or by means of naphthylphosphate substrates (Burstone, 1958) employing simultaneous diazo coupling (Barka and Anderson, 1963). The electron-dense reaction product obtained in Gomori-type reactions has permitted the use of this method to demonstrate acid phosphatase activity at the ultrastructural level in aldehyde-fixed tissue (Novikoff and Essner, 1962; Novikoff, 1967b).

Earlier biochemical studies of acid phosphatase in nerve suggested that the principle sources might be the Schwann cell or invading inflammatory cells

(Heinzen, 1947; McCaman and Robins, 1959), and little or no β-glycerophosphatase activity is discernable by histochemical means in undamaged axons (Gould and Holt, 1961; Holtzman and Novikoff, 1965). However, in Wallerian degeneration, there is histochemical evidence of increased acid phosphatase activity in the axon (Bubis and Wolman, 1965; Hallpike and Adams, 1969). The appearance of acid phosphatase located ultrastructurally within lysosomes in axons undergoing degeneration (Holtzman and Novikoff, 1965) is consistent with results of a combined histochemical and biochemical study of transected nerve (Hallpike, Adams and Bayliss, 1970b) in which very early changes in acid phosphatase levels were associated with concomitant increases in other enzymes of probable lysosomal origin. Comparison of the distribution of acid phosphatase in normal and degenerating rat sciatic nerve revealed that the principal sites of enzyme activity are the axon, and the Schwann cell in the paranodal regions.

The histochemical demonstration of proteolytic activity in peripheral nerve using a silver-gelatin autogram technique was described by Adams and Tuqan (1961a,b). Two proteases have been characterized by this method, an acid cathepsin (pH optimum 3.5) and a neutral protease (pH 7.4). The acid protease conforms to a lysosomal distribution in both histochemical and subcellular fractionation studies while the neutral protease is probably confined to axons and myelin (Hallpike, 1972), but in the usual type of autogram preparations cytochemical localization is limited by the low resolution of the method. Recent modifications (Fratello, 1968; Penn, Gledhill and Darzynkiewicz, 1972) of the silver-gelatin process and immunochemical visualization (Poole, Dingle and Barret, 1972) of cathepsin have not yet been systematically applied to nerve. Biochemical studies (Marks and Lajtha, 1963; Porcellati, 1965; Marks, Datta and Lajtha, 1970) indicate that the principal neural protease is cathepsin D, of lysosomal origin (de Duve *et al.*, 1955). The sulphydryl-dependent neutral protease occurring in axons (Orrego, 1971) may be responsible for degrading axonal protein, but the relationship of this group of hydrolases to nerve function is largely unknown. However, protease and peptidase activity may be responsible for the local generation of amino acids and a correlation has been claimed between nerve impulse transmission and endopeptidase activity (Gabrielesco, Stoenesco and Bordeianu, 1966).

While a number of specific ATPases have been identified biochemically in the peripheral nerve (Porcellati, 1969), the available histochemical techniques largely demonstrate non-specific ATPase activity in tissues (see Moss, 1974). Three classes of enzyme hydrolysing ATP may be recognized using the Wachstein and Meisel (1957) and Padykula and Herman (1955a,b) methods (see Adams, 1967). Non-specific alkaline phosphatase, a polyphosphatase and mitochondrial ATPase may be distinguished on the basis of their inhibition by sulphydryl agents and metallic ions, but it is doubtful whether membrane-bound sodium or potassium activated ATPases can be convincingly demonstrated histochemically (Torack, 1965). Histochemical studies at the light microscope level indicate that ATPase is distributed within the axon and outer Schwann sheath but there is no evidence of activity within the myelin sheath (Adams, Davison and Gregson, 1963).

Oxido-reductase activity in peripheral nerve occurs in axonal mitochondria, at nodes of Ranvier and in the cells of the neural sheath. The biochemical distribution and relative activities of Krebs cycle, glycolytic and pentose-shunt enzymes have been reviewed elsewhere (Porcellati, 1969), and the histochemistry of NAD and NADP-linked dehydrogenases has been extensively studied in brain cells (Adams, 1965b; Friede, 1966). The distribution of NADH-dehydrogenase in rat sciatic nerve is shown in Fig. 12.2. The activity of this enzyme is localized predominantly in the axons and as halos in the enzymatically active cytoplasm

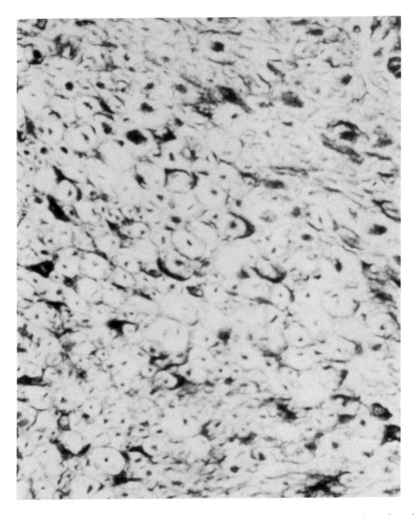

Fig. 12.2 NADH-dehydrogenase activity in rat sciatic nerve proximal to a three day old crush lesion. Transverse section. (x 380.)

of the Schwann cell. A proximo-distal gradient of oxido-reductase activity exists in the sciatic nerve and this is linked to the inferred axonal transport of these enzymes.

Non-specific esterases have been studied in the central and peripheral nervous systems (Barron, Bernsohn and Mitzen, 1972). Simple or substituted naphthyl acetates are employed as histochemical substrates with simultaneous coupling azo dye methods (see Barka and Anderson, 1963). A different principle underlies the indoxyl acetate technique developed by Holt and Withers (1958). Hydrolysis of these substrates cannot confidently be ascribed to aliesterase activity unless possible effects of cholinesterases have been excluded, preferably by eserine (10^{-5} M) or diethyl-p-nitrophenyl phosphate (E 600; 10^{-7} M) which inhibit both AChE and BChE. Such E 600 resistant esterase activity is inconspicuous in normal peripheral nerve but occurs during Wallerian degeneration (Gould and Holt, 1961; Bubis and Wolman, 1965), and in reactive Schwann cells during the evolution of diphtheritic lesions. 5'nucleotidase has been localized histochemically within the axon of the normal nerve (Wolfgram amd Rose, 1960), but it is difficult to differentiate this enzyme from alkaline phosphatase. Topographic histochemical studies of 5'nucleotidase in mouse brain have shown that this enzyme is widely distributed in neurones and axons with intriguing regional variations (Scott, 1967). Inorganic pyrophosphatase (PP$_i$ase) appears to be responsible for driving many biosynthetic reactions to completion (Kornberg, 1962). The localization of this enzyme in a wide range of tissues was surveyed by Korhonen (1966) and more recently in peripheral nerve by Hallpike and McArdle (1974). The enzyme is present in axons, satellite cells and myelin; there is an increase in activity during regeneration of peripheral nerve (Fig. 12.3) and it seems likely that PP$_i$ase may be useful as a histochemical marker for protein synthesis.

Interruption of axonal continuity leads to Wallerian degeneration in the nerve distal to the injury. Regeneration of nerve always occurs from the proximal segment and, while there may be a very limited capacity to synthesize protein within the axon, it is clear that axonal function and structure are critically dependent upon a continuous flow of materials in a proximo-distal direction from the nerve cell body (see Baronedes, 1969). In addition evidence is now appearing of the existence of a retrograde axonal transport system (Kristensson and Olsson, 1973) but the functional implications of this finding are not yet clear. Considerable information on axonal flow in peripheral nerve has been obtained from the study of catecholamines in adrenergic nerve fibres by histochemical methods based on the Eränkö principle of formaldehyde-induced monoamine fluoresence. The distribution of noradrenaline (NA) in adrenergic neurons, sympathetic ganglia, axon networks and storage vesicles found by fluorescence methods (Falck et al., 1962) was reviewed by Norberg (1967). It is now well established that dense cord NA-storage vesicles are synthesized in the perikarya of noradrenergic neurons and subsequently pass along the axons to the terminal sites of transmitter release (Dahlström, 1971; Banks and Mayor, 1972).

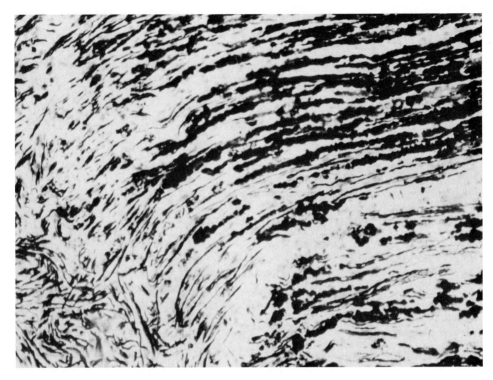

Fig. 12.3 PP$_i$ase activity in regenerating axons and in the Schwann sheaths in the proximal stump of rat sciatic nerve 80 days after neurotomy. (x 360.)

Catecholamine (NA) accumulates only on the proximal side of a nerve constriction, and such an accumulation is prevented by treatment with reserpine, which depletes vesicles of NA, and by colchicine. The axonal transport of monoamine oxidase (MAO) and other enzymes involved in catecholamine metabolism has also been demonstrated (Wooten and Coyle, 1973; Dairman, Geffen and Marchelle, 1973). The ultrastructural basis of axoplasmic flow is not yet established although the neurotubule system has been strongly implicated (Weiss and Mayr, 1971; Shelansky, 1973). Proteins linked to organelles, i.e. microsomal dopamine-β-hydroxylase, appear to be more rapidly transported than soluble proteins (Sjöstrand and Karlsson, 1969). Antimitotic agents such as colchicine and vinblastine disrupt the microtubule system and among other effects interfere with axoplasmic flow, but the effects of these agents are by no means uniform, and, in contrast to NA, mitochondrial transport is not blocked by colchicine (Banks and Mayor, 1972).

The effects of constricting ligatures around nerves, on nerve development and myelination have been studied by Friede (1972) using autoradiographic methods. Such interference leads to retardation of axon growth and a reduction in the thickness of myelin distal to the ligature. These effects may be the consequences of impaired axoplasmic flow and it will be of value to determine whether disturbances of axon flow are of importance in the pathogenesis of diseases of nerve and muscle. In some preliminary studies of this problem Bradley and Williams (1973) were unable to find any clear correlation between rates of axon flow and the severity of lesions produced by tri-ortho cresyl phosphate, acrylamide and vinblastine.

12.2.3 Nerve terminals

The preparation of synaptosomes by means of density gradient centrifugation has been widely applied to the study of the sequestration and release of neurotransmitters from presynaptic nerve terminals in brain tissue (Whittaker, 1969a; de Robertis and Arnaiz, 1969). In the peripheral nervous system attention has chiefly been devoted to NA, ACh and AChE in the nerve terminal and synaptic junction regions since other known transmitters (serotonin, dopamine, γ-aminobutyric acid) appear to be confined to the central nervous system and certain non-nervous stores such as mast cells, chromaffin tissue and blood platelets. In peripheral nerve, therefore, the requirement is to distinguish adrenergic from cholinergic fibres. This may be accomplished by fluorescence microscopy and cholinesterase histochemistry linked, where possible, with parallel biochemical and ultrastructural observations.

The concentration of NA in the nerve terminals of peripheral adrenergic neurones greatly exceeds that in the cell body (see Livett, 1973). While relatively little catecholamine is demonstrable in normal adrenergic axons fluorescence accumulates proximal to nerve section or constriction (Dahlström, 1971) providing evidence of passage of amines from the perikaryon along the axon to terminal storage vesicles. With electron microscopy the terminal varicosities of non-myelinated adrenergic fibres are found to contain dense-cored vesicles, neurotubules, neurofilaments and mitochondria. Large (70 nm diameter) dense-core vesicles occur in the cell bodies and axons whereas smaller (45 nm diameter) vesicles predominate in the nerve terminals. Both species of dense-core vesicles contain NA and dopamine β-hydroxylase (Bloom, 1970; Geffen and Livett, 1971). Use of highly specific immunofluorescent methods, based on the production of antisera to individual enzymes involved in catecholamine biosynthesis, to map adrenergic pathways in the central nervous system has recently been reviewed (Livett, 1973).

Knowledge of the detailed morphology of cholinergic nerve terminals has been obtained from histochemical, ultrastructural and subcellular fractionation studies. The characterization of ACh containing vesicles has largely depended on the application of density-gradient separation techniques (see Whittaker, 1969b; Cooper, Bloom and Roth, 1970) but for the most part such information relates strictly to brain. Two forms of ACh are recognized: cytoplasmic ACh, present in axoplasm and the cell body, is readily labelled with radioactive precursors (Marchbanks, 1967), while vesicle-bound ACh is refractory to labelling, presumably reflecting an effective compartmentalization of pre-formed ACh in the nerve terminals. The subcellular distribution of choline acetylase corresponds to that of ACh; some of the enzyme appears in the supernatant and a further proportion is bound to membrane and organelles. It appears that a requirement for the bioelectric function of ACh in excitable membranes is the means for its speedy local removal. Thus, at sites of neurotransmission AChE histochemistry can also be used to provide indirect evidence of ACh localization. Electron histochemical studies of AChE activity in peripheral nerve (Schlaepfer and Torack, 1966; Brzin, 1966; Nachmansohn, 1971) clearly reveal cholinesterase in the axolemmal membrane of unmyelinated fibres. The patchy staining of myelinated fibres (see Adams, Grant and Bayliss, 1967) may be improved with Triton X-100 suggesting that poor substrate penetration inhibits visualization of enzyme activity in the thicker fibres. The permeability characteristics of the nerve fibre may also provide an explanation for the apparent discrepancy between the neuromuscular blocking effect of relaxant drugs and cholinesterase inhibitors, and for the fact that such agents have little or no effect on axonal conduction. Cholinesterase staining is intense at the external membrane of the nerve terminal but synaptic vesicles are unstained (see Whittaker, 1969a). Consideration of the ultrastructural localization of AChE suggests that it is formed within the endoplasmic reticulum and is subsequently incorporated into the axolemma and nerve-ending membrane (Brzin, Tennison and Duffy, 1966). This is not inconsistent with the results of nerve ligation experiments referred to previously (12.2.3) from which it was concluded that some AChE migrated along the axon while a further proportion was 'fixed' to the surface membrane.

12.2.4 *The myelin sheath*

The wrapping process (Geren, 1954; Robertson, 1955) by which the myelin sheath of the peripheral nerve is thought to be derived from Schwann cell plasma membrane is now generally accepted but it fails to account adequately for either longitudinal or radial growth of the nerve sheath during subsequent development (see Hirano and Dembitzer, 1967). Current molecular models of myelin membrane (Finean, 1965; Vandenheuvel, 1965; Handler, 1971) are based on the results of polarization, X-ray diffraction, electron-microscopic, solvent-extraction and chemical studies. Changes occurring during myelination, namely compaction of lamellae and alterations in lipid and protein composition, have been reviewed recently (Davison, 1970 and Chapter 11). Isotope experiments (Waelsch *et al.*, 1940; Davison *et al.*, 1958, 1959) had indicated a very low turnover of myelin lipids, but more recent studies of phospholipid (Smith and Eng, 1965; Smith, 1967) and protein (Davison, 1970; Vrba and Cannon, 1970; Smith and Hasinoff, 1971) turnover in myelin have led to some recasting of previous views concerning the supposed metabolic inertness of the myelin sheath. Certain myelin constituents do appear to undergo continuous replacement and, while such activity may be limited, this may nevertheless be vital to the survival and stability of the sheath under normal circumstances.

Myelin lipids

The systematic study of brain lipids has its origin in the work of Thudichum during the latter part of the last century, and until recently, biochemical evidence concerning myelin lipids was largely based on comparative analyses of white and grey matter. In the last decade however differential centrifugation procedures have been developed for the selective isolation of myelin from brain. Myelin obtained by these methods is subject to preparative artefact due either to contamination, or to loss of its more loosely bound constituents. The advantage of an histochemical approach is that tissue can be examined without disrupting its normal cellular relationships; and moreover, small areas can be conveniently be selected for analysis. The limitations of the method lie in the relatively restricted range and variable specificity of the available histochemical techniques, and the difficulty of quantitating results obtained with slide methods. If, however, serial sections are alternately stained for microscopy and eluted for either chromatography or isotope counting, a picture may be obtained of both the distribution and amounts of the lipids present.

That which follows is intended to provide an outline of the essential histochemical features of the lipids of the normal myelin sheath. Such a survey must necessarily be brief and reference should also be made to such wider reviews that include the theoretical and technical aspects of this topic (Adams and Davison, 1965; Adams, 1969; Bayliss, 1972; Adams and Bayliss, 1974). The identification of lipids in tissue sections depends in the first instance upon the physical and surface properties of the lipid concerned. Phospholipids (phosphoglycerides and phosphosphingosides) contain polar hydrophilic groupings which render the molecules miscible with water. Other polar lipids (i.e. cerebroside, sulphatide) show less hydrophilia, and unconjugated sterols (cholesterol), and the simple ester lipids (not usually present in myelin), are strongly hydrophobic owing to their apolar configuration. The most widely used stain for lipids is the Sudan dye Oil Red O (Lillie and Ashburn, 1943; Cain, 1950). The organotropic properties of this dye enable it to penetrate liquid hydrophobic lipid droplets, although those remaining in a crystalline state at room temperature, i.e. cholesterol (M.P. 145°), are poorly stained. Sudan Black B (SBB) has a much wider affinity for lipids than the red Sudan dyes staining all classes of lipid present in a liquid state. While SBB is valuable as a general screening test for lipids it has the disadvantage that cholesterol crystals are unstained and some phosphoglycerides and free fatty acids (FFA) are lost from tissue sections through the action of the dye solvents. Preliminary bromination can be employed to overcome these drawbacks; cholesterol appears to be converted to sudanophilic bromo-derivatives and, in tissues thus modified, the SBB technique can be used to stain almost all classes of lipid including free cholesterol (Bayliss and Adams, 1972). Phospholipids in myelin exhibit a blue-grey staining with SBB while hydrophobic lipids appear black; in addition, myelin phospholipids show bronze dichroism in polarized light (Diezel, 1958). Chromatographic analysis of SBB (Lansink, 1968) has demonstrated the presence of two principal constituents, an organotropic dye, and a basic dye capable of reacting with phospholipids and causing a metachromatic shift.

The use of Nile Blue sulphate for the histochemical indentification of lipids has been critically assessed by Dunnigan (1968a,b). Phospholipids are stained blue by the oxazine (absorption peak for densitometry 630 nm), whereas triglycerides and cholesterol esters are stained red by the oxazone component of this dye (540 nm). Free FA appear magenta due to staining by both oxazine and oxazone dye constituents. Cholesterol is not stained with Nile Blue sulphate, Identification of phospholipids is facilitated by previous extraction with cold anhydrous acetone to remove apolar lipids from the section (Adams and Bayliss, 1968e; Elleder and Lojda, 1973), but appreciable loss of myelin phospholipids may occur following acetone extraction of sections of unfixed brain (Urbanova and Adams, 1970). The general lipid nature of any material examined can be confirmed by extraction with chloroform-methanol (C/M, 2:1 v/v) for 1 to 18 h at room temperature, but removal of certain protein-bound lipids may require acidified C/M (LeBaron and Folch, 1956), or the application of enzyme digestion methods (see Adams and Bayliss, 1962).

Early histochemical studies of the myelin sheath made extensive use of polarized light (Göthlin, 1913; Schmidt, 1936). The conclusion drawn from these observations, that there exists an orderly (liquid crystalline) layered arrangement of lipids and protein within the sheath, has been borne out by later X-ray diffraction studies (Schmitt and Bear, 1939; Finean and Robertson, 1958). It must be emphasized however that birefringence is not a physical property peculiar to lipids, and that polarization optics have a strictly limited role in the identification of particular lipids in tissue sections (see Weller, 1967).

The perchloric acid-naphthoquinone (PAN) technique (Adams, 1961) now appears to be the method of choice for the demonstration of cholesterol in myelin (Fig. 12.4). Although the PAN reaction also stains cholesterol esters these are not present in the normal sheath, except transiently during myelination (Adams and Davison, 1959; El-Eishi, 1967). Free cholesterol can theoretically be distinguished from esterified cholesterol by pretreating sections with digitonin, but the practical value of this step has been questioned (see Adams, 1969). Mordant-haematoxylin methods have been used in the staining of phospholipids since the introduction of Weigert's original technique in 1885. Baker's acid haematin method has been found mainly to stain choline-containing phospholipids, a strong reaction usually indicating the presence of either lecithin or sphingomyelin, and has been adapted to stain sphingomyelin selectively (Adams, 1965c). This modified method relies on the fact that the ester bonds of phosphoglycerides (i.e. lecithin) are susceptible to alkaline hydrolysis whereas

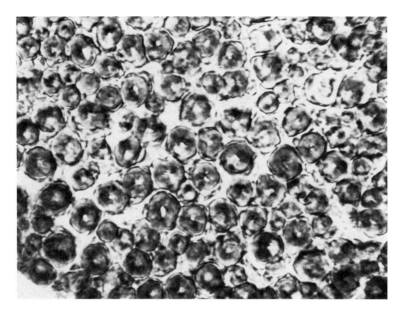

Fig. 12.4   Rat sciatic nerve to show the presence of cholesterol in myelin. (× 1380: Reproduced by kind permission of Professor C. W. M. Adams. PAN.)

phosphosphingosides (sphingomyelin) resist such treatment. Thus, immersion of sections in 2N NaOH for 1h effectively permits staining only of sphingomyelin with BAH (NaOH-BAH method). On the other hand the gold hydroxamic acid (GHA) reaction (Adams *et al.*, 1963) allows highly selective demonstration of the phosphoglycerides in myelin in a stable red-purple colour (Fig. 12.5). The specificity of the periodic acid-Schiff (PAS) method for the hexose groupings in glycolipids (cerebroside, protein-bound ganglioside) is greatly enhanced by blockading procedures designed to eliminate other chemical configurations capable of conferring PAS positivity (Adams and Bayliss, 1963; Adams *et al.*, 1963). Using the modified PAS technique cerebroside is localized to myelin and can be extracted with lipid solvents.

Myelin proteins

There are general accounts of myelin proteins in a number of recent reviews devoted to the chemical composition of nerve (Porcellati, 1969; Shooter and Einstein, 1971) and to the demyelinating process (Adams and Leibowitz, 1969; Hallpike, 1972). Two main classes of peripheral nerve myelin protein have been distinguished on histochemical grounds. One protein class contains abundant tryptophan, and is resistant to both acid extraction and tryptic digestion. The other class is basic, trypanophilic, and is very much more susceptible to acid extraction and proteolysis (Adams and Bayliss, 1968a). Significant differences

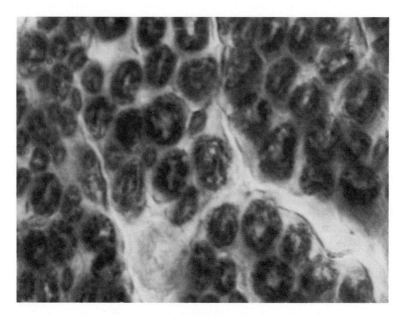

Fig. 12.5   Rat sciatic nerve to show localization of phosphoglyceride in myelin. (× 1650: Reproduced by kind permission of Professor C. W. M. Adams. GHA.)

between central and peripheral myelin proteins are now recognized. In the central nervous system, the trypsin-resistant myelin protein (TRP) is soluble in c/m and appears to correspond to Folch and Lees (1951) proteolipid. The TRP of peripheral myelin, however, is insoluble in c/m and is analogous, therefore, to the neurokeratin of nerve or the trypsin-resistant protein residue (TRPR) of brain myelin remaining after c/m extraction (see Hallpike, 1972). Biochemical studies and amino acid analyses also indicate that the amount of proteolipid in peripheral myelin is small in comparison with that in the brain (Eng *et al.*, 1968; Wolfgram and Kotorii, 1968). This TRP protein is recognized histochemically, therefore, by staining for tryptophan (Adams, 1957) after c/m extraction and tryptic digestion (Fig. 12.6). Biochemically, the term neurokeratin is applied to an insoluble and indigestible residue of neural proteins (Block, 1951), and a higher phosphoinositide content appears to distinguish neurokeratin derived from central nervous white matter from its counterpart in the peripheral nerve (Le Baron and Folch, 1956). While neurokeratin cannot be precisely located in cytochemical models of myelin, protein resisting both lipid extraction and proteolysis is found mainly at the major dense line (Finean, 1963). The neurokeratin network seen in many histological preparations of peripheral nerve is an artefact which may be avoided with suitable methods of tissue preparation (Wolfgram and Rose, 1960; Adams *et al.*, 1963). Nevertheless the notion that neurokeratin represents a TR group of myelin proteins has been of value, despite uncertainties of terminology, particularly in the histochemical study of myelin

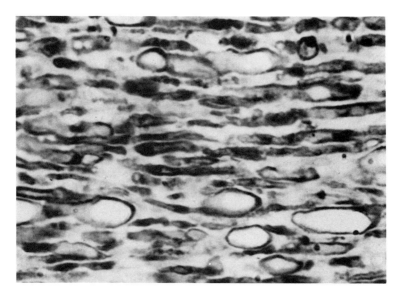

Fig. 12.6   Rat sciatic nerve, 5 days after nerve section. Tryptophan-containing trypsin-resistant myelin protein, DMAB. (x 450: Reproduced by courtesy of the editor of the *Histochemical Journal*.)

breakdown. Recently, however, correlative electrophoretic, biochemical and histochemical studies (Wolfgram and Kotorii, 1968; Csejtey *et al.*, 1972) have indicated that the major protein component of peripheral myelin, which is c/m insoluble, rich in tryptophan and indentifiable with neurokeratin, is in fact susceptible to proteolysis (Fig. 12.7). Such findings emphasize that conclusions based solely on histochemical findings can be misleading. It also appears that the value of trypsin-sensitivity may have been overplayed in the histochemical identification of different classes of myelin protein. The major protein component of peripheral myelin shows a degree of trypsin-sensitivity inter-mediates between that of the extreme resistance of Folch and Lees' proteolipid, and the relative lability of the basic myelin proteins. A second class of acidic proteolipid (Wolfgram, 1966) found in brain was not detected histochemically in peripheral myelin (Csejtey *et al.*, 1972).

The presence of a trypsin-digestible protein (TDP) in myelin was inferred from electron microscope and X-ray diffraction studies of the effects of trypsin on the nerve sheath (Fernández-Morán and Finean, 1957). Histochemical studies (Wolman and Hestrin-Lerner, 1960; Tuqan and Adams, 1961) also suggested the presence in myelin of a TDP, removal of which caused a diminution in the staining of the sheath for lipids. This TDP was subsequently shown to be acid extractable and to contain more basic aromatic amino acids, but less tryptophan, than either neurokeratin or proteolipid (Adams and Bayliss, 1968a) The basic properties of TDP are made use of in the histochemical methods used to display

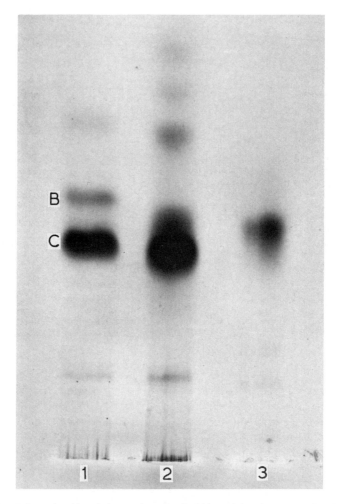

Fig. 12.7   Polyacrylamide gel electrophoresis of rabbit peripheral nerve myelin: 1, control; 2, after incubation in buffer for 21h; 3, after incubation in buffer and trypsin for 21h. B — basic protein, C — principal protein component of peripheral myelin.

this class of myelin protein. Anionic dyes, for example, Trypan Blue, Phosphotungstic acid Haematoxylin (PTAH), Fast Green, can be used to stain the basic TDP in unfixed cryostat sections (Hallpike and Adams, 1969; Adams *et al.*, 1971). The trypanophilia of myelin is abolished by previous tryptic digestion or acid extraction and substantially reduced by deamination and tissue fixation (Adams and Bayliss, 1968a). All these manoeuvres appear to leave the neurokeratin or TRP of peripheral nerve intact and provide strong histochemical grounds for distinguishing a trypanophilic basic myelin protein. This basic protein is demonstrated in cryostat sections of nerve after staining in 0.1% Trypan Blue at pH 5.0 (Fig. 12.8). In combined electrophoretic and histo-

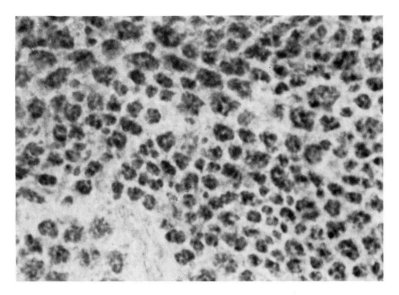

Fig. 12.8   Trypanophilia of myelin proteins. Rat sciatic nerve. Transverse, unfixed cryostat section. Tyrpan blue, pH 5.0. (x 680.)

chemical studies (Csejtey *et al.*, 1972) histochemical stains were applied to myelin proteins separated in polycrylamide 'micro-gels'. Here, both the principal protein component of periphral myelin and the more rapidly moving basic proteins stain with Trypan Blue. Thus, it seems that Trypan Blue can only be employed to stain basic proteins selectively if applied to unfixed tissue sections.

Histochemically characterized TDP also appears to correspond well with the basic protein isolated biochemically from white matter of myelin. A water soluble and encephalitogenic basic protein was isolated from brain and spinal cord by Kies *et al.* (1961) and by Einstein *et al.* (1962), and it has been shown that this encephalitogenic protein is present in myelin fractions, is susceptible to the action of trypsin and can be extracted by acid (for references see Hallpike, 1972). Interest in this protein stems from the fact that the antigen responsible for the production of experimental allergic encephalomyelitis (EAE) resides in the basic (A1) protein or in small peptide derivatives resulting from its tryptic digestion (Eylar, 1972). Basic protein constitutes 30 per cent of total myelin protein in adult brain and some 20 per cent in peripheral nerve (Eng *et al.*, 1968), and there are differences in the electrophoretic mobilities and amino acid compositions of basic protein from brain or spinal cord on the one hand, and peripheral nerve on the other (Wolfgram and Kotorii, 1968; Bencina *et al.*, 1969). These differences are in part species-dependent, but they may also reflect the glial and Schwann cell origins of central and peripheral myelin respectively.

Some lipid staining persists in peripheral nerve myelin following extraction with chloroform-methanol (Adams and Bayliss, 1969b). This residual lipid can, however, be removed with acidified c/m and may be bound to the TRP or neurokeratin in peripheral myelin. Although the presence of glycoprotein in myelin has been disputed in the past (see Margolis, 1968; Adams and Bayliss, 1968d) there is recent electroporetic and histochemical evidence that the major protein component of peripheral nerve myelin is PAS positive whereas no comparable staining of proteolipid, basic or 'Wolfgram' protein is found in central myelin (Wood and Dawson, 1973). Amino acid analyses of peripheral myelin proteins (Wolfgram and Kotorii, 1968; Eng et al., 1968; Wood and Dawson, 1973) suggest that there is more basic protein in peripheral myelin than can be accounted for by the acid-extractable or fast-migrating electrophoretic fractions, and Wood and Dawson suggest that the protein moiety of the glycoprotein in peripheral myelin may be a trypsin-sensitive basic protein. If confirmed, these findings may go a long way towards explaining the susceptibility of the whole range of peripheral nerve myelin proteins to proteolysis (Csejtey et al., 1972), and the discrepancies found between the electrophoretic and histochemical changes in myelin proteins during Wallerian degeneration (Adams et al., 1972).

Lipid-protein relationships

The limitations of present operational definitions of the different classes of myelin proteins have added considerably to the difficulty of combining chemical and ultrastructural data in a composite picture. For instance, while c/m extraction of white matter fails to yield basic protein, similar extracts of myelin isolated on ion-free sucrose gradients contain both basic protein and proteolipid, and basic proteins can be precipitated by the addition of electrolytes to such extracts leaving proteolipid in the organic phase (Gonzalez-Sastre, 1970). Complexes comprising protein, polysaccharides, cerebroside, cholesterol and phospholipids have been identified in detergent extracts of central white matter but were not obtainable from peripheral nerve (Wolman, 1962). The stability of proteolipids is also influenced by the pH and ionic strength of the medium. Destruction of protein-lipid linkages has been shown to be proportional to the concentration of the salts of certain monovalent cations (Webster and Folch, 1961). It is likely that the protein moiety obtained in these experiments is of the nature of TRPR, differing from peripheral nerve neurokeratin by virtue of its higher inositide content. The effects of solvent extractions and enzyme digestion on the histochemical properties of myelin have been examined in some detail (Wolman and Hestrin-Lerner, 1960; Adams and Bayliss, 1968b,c). Trypsin removes most lipids and basic protein from unfixed myelin; however, this loss of lipid cannot be attributed solely to enzymic action on lipid-protein associations since certain lipids are readily extracted from unfixed tissue by water or buffers alone (see Adams, 1965c). When applied to fixed tissue, trypsin removes substantially less myelin protein and lipid. Acetone extraction abolishes the reaction for cholesterol although the results of histochemical tests for other lipid and protein constituents of myelin remain unchanged (Adams and Bayliss, 1968c). Histochemical reactions for lipid are negative following extraction of proteolipid from central myelin, but in the peripheral nerve such treatment fails to remove all myelin lipid, some of which presumably remaining bound to c/m-insoluble neurokeratin. These histochemical results certainly suggest that myelin lipids are attached partly to basic protein (TDP), and partly to proteolipid or, in the case of peripheral nerve, to neurokeratin. The site of neurokeratin and basic protein within peripheral myelin has not yet been satisfactorily established, but there is some evidence (Wolman, 1971; Adams *et al.*, 1971) that TRP is located mainly at the intraperiod line, and basic protein at the period or major dense line, the lipids of the sheath being interposed between the electron-dense protein layers. Hence, lipid-protein attachments may contribute in considerable measure to the radial stability of the myelin lamellae.

Myelin enzymes

In the past, histochemical evidence of enzyme activity in myelin has been conflicting, and early indications (Tewari and Bourne, 1960; Wolfgram and Rose, 1960) of a wide range of oxidative and hydrolytic enzymes in myelin were not confirmed in later histochemical and biochemical studies (Adams *et al.*, 1963). This enzyme inactivity of myelin appeared to be consistent with the results of isotope studies (see Davison, 1970) which indicated that the principal constituents of the mature sheath were remarkably stable. Identification of enzymes in myelin is rendered difficult for several reasons. In histochemistry, low enzyme activity frequently necessitates prolonged incubation, and this may result in the diffusion and false localization of lipid-soluble reaction products. Prolonged incubation also increases the liklihood of artefacts arising as a result of the affinity of myelin for capture reagents in Gomori-type reactions. Furthermore, myelin preparations used in biochemical studies are required to meet certain standards of purity (Norton, 1971) with the result that enzymes which are not tightly bound to myelin may be washed out during the preparative procedures. Conversely, contamination of myelin by other subcellular fraction cannot be excluded unless fairly rigorous criteria of purity have been met.

In spite of these difficulties a number of enzymes do appear to be associated with myelin. The presence of a neutral proteinase in central nervous myelin has been established with reasonable certainty (Marks and Lajtha, 1963; Riekkinen and Clausen, 1969), and subcellular fractionation studies of peripheral nerve indicate that a neutral proteinase is also present in peripheral myelin (Hallpike, 1971). Other studies have confirmed that some aminopeptidase activity resides in myelin fractions of both brain (Adams, Davison and Gregson, 1963; Hasinoff and Smith, 1968; Porcellati, 1969), and peripheral nerve (Adams *et al.*, 1968; Hallpike, 1972). The histochemical detection of neutral and acid endopeptidase activity in nerve by means of the silver-gelatin autogram technique (Adams and

Tuqan, 1961a,b), and its modifications (Fratello, 1968), has recently been discussed in the context of Wallerian degeneration and myelin breakdown (Hallpike, Adams and Bayliss, 1970b). Histochemical, solvent extraction and subcellular fractionation studies are in accord in indicating that an appreciable proportion of the total neutral protease activity of nerve residues in myelin (see also Section 12.3.2). The acidic neural protease present in brain and peripheral nerve has however been shown to be of lysosomal origin and unassociated with myelin (Marks and Lajtha, 1963; Hallpike, 1971). The simultaneous coupling method of Burstone and Folk (1956) for L-leucyl-β-naphthylamidase (LNAase) has proved an unsatisfactory method for detecting low levels of activity of this group of enzymes in brain and nerve (Adams and Glenner, 1962). The discrepancy between good biochemical evidence of LNAase activity in myelin, obtained by a post-coupling method, and negative histochemistry led to the conclusion that there must be inhibition of enzyme by the diazotate in the incubation medium. More recently, however, it has been shown that instability of the diazo salt at pH 7.0 or above is responsible for failure to demonstrate LNAase histochemically in nerve (Hallpike, 1972). Reduction of the pH of the incubation medium enhances the stability of the diazo salt and permits prolongation of incubation (Figs. 12.9, 12.14).

Alkaline phosphatase in peripheral nerve is found mainly in the walls of capillaries, at nodes of Ranvier and at the Schmidt–Lanterman incisures (Pinner, Davison and Campbell, 1964).

However small amounts of alkaline phosphatase are also found in myelin (Adams, Davison and Gregson, 1963) together with small amounts of Mg^{2+} dependent and Na^+ and K^+ activated ATPases (Whittaker, 1966). Further data concerning the metabolic activity of myelin have been obtained from modifications of the usual preparative procedures designed to stablilize membranes and reduce 'wash-out' of labile enzymes. Thus the use of polyvinylpyrrolidine (PVP) has led to the isolation of glycolytic enzymes from myelin and the suggestion that up to 25 per cent of total glycolytic activity of a brain homogenate may reside in the myelin fraction (Miani, Cavallotti and Caniglia, 1969). Similarly, substitution of 0.01 M $CaCl_2$ or 0.05 M buffer for H_2O during osmotic shock and subsequent washings enhances enzyme recovery, i.e. non-specific esterase (NsE), from myelin (Mitzen, Barron and Koeppen, 1971). Because of the technical difficulties in preparing myelin from peripheral nerve, opportunities to compare histochemical findings with biochemical data are fewer in peripheral nerve than in brain; moreover, observations on central nervous myelin are not necessarily applicable to peripheral nerve. A 2′,3′-cyclic nucleotide-3′-phosphohydrolase has recently been found in brain myelin (Kurihara and Tsukada, 1967; Olafson, Drummond and Lee, 1969). While attempts to develop a histochemical method for this enzyme have not yet been successful, it is known to be also present in peripheral myelin and can be employed as a marker for myelin in peripheral nerve fractionation studies (Hallpike, 1971). Inorganic pyrophosphatase (PP$_i$ase) can also be demonstrated histochemically in myelin as well as in regenerating axons (Fig. 12.3).

12.2.5 *Cells and blood vessels*

The Schwann cell in peripheral nerve is enzymically more active than the corresponding cell, the oligodendrocyte, in the central nervous system (Adams, Davison and Gregson, 1963). The principal function of the Schwann cell appears to be the formation and maintenance of myelin; however, a further role in providing metabolic support for the axon has also been postulated (Williams and Landon, 1964; Singer, 1968), but the evidence for the existence of a metabolic unit comprising neurone and satellite cells in the peripheral nervous system is, as yet, less convincing than in the brain (see Hydén, 1967).

A wide range of phosphohydrolases, 5′nucleotidase and PP$_i$ase have been reported in the Schwann cell (Adams, 1965b). In transverse sections of normal nerve, oxidative enzyme activity is observed in Schwann cell cytoplasm in the form of a crescent or halo around the myelin (Fig. 12.2). Acid phosphatase activity in normal Schwann cells increases with age and is largely confined to the perinuclear region of the cells associated with large myelinated fibres (Weller and Herzog, 1970). Such perinuclear acid phosphatase activity occurs partly within lysosomes and, more diffusely, in association with lamellar bodies. These perinuclear bodies appear to correspond to the Reich or π-granules (Noback, 1953; Tomonaga and Sluga, 1970), which stain metachromatically with toluidine blue and are considered to be remnants of lysosomal autophagy as they contain indigestible products of lipid metabolism. Lysosomal activation, characterized by the appearance of particulate acid phosphatase activity, is encountered in the paranodal regions of both small and large diameter fibres during myelin breakdown (Weller and Mellick, 1966; Weller and Nester, 1972), and the concentrations of mitochondria in the paranodal regions (Williams and Landon, 1963) support the view that this part of the sheath is a site of relatively high metabolic activity. Butyrylcholinesterase (pseudocholinesterase) activity also occurs in Schwann cells and has been used as an index of Schwann cell proliferative activity during nerve degeneration (Cavanagh, Thompson and Webster, 1954).

Information concerning the presence in peripheral nerve of mast cells, known to be rich in herapin and various biogenic amines (5-hydroxytryptamine, histamine, dopamine), has been reviewed by Olsson (1968). Mast cells stain metachromatically with toluidine blue and are found in the epineurium, perneurium and endoneurium. The chromotrophic substance responsible for the metachromasia is believed to be a sulphomucopolysaccharide, most probably herapin (Schubert and Hammerman, 1956; Olsson, 1968). Mast cell metachromasia persists after c/m extraction whereas that attributable to Reich cells is extinguished by such treatment (Noback, 1953; Schnabel and Sir, 1962).

Monoamines present in peripheral nerve mast cells have been extensively studied by formaldehyde gas-induced fluorescence techniques together with the degranulation process resulting from injury, or the injection of histamine liberator (compound 48/80) either intraperitoneally or into the nerve trunk (Olsson, 1967, 1968).

The now classical experiments by Ehrlich (1885) established that trypan blue injected intravenously fails to enter brain tissue, although all other organs are stained. The concept of a blood-brain barrier, susceptible to injury, which stemmed from these experiments has been extrapolated to the state of vascular permeability existing in the peripheral nerve (Waksman, 1961; Mellick and Cavanagh, 1967). Epineurial blood vessels anastomose with vessels between the perinuclear cell layers, and these in turn communicate with the endoneurial vascular plexus which appears to be surrounded by a much larger extracellular space than pertains in the central nervous system. Protein tracer studies using Evans blue albumin (EBA), fluorescein isothiocyanate labelled albumin (FLA) and horseradish peroxidase have been employed to demonstrate the state of the blood-nerve barrier in both undamaged and injured nerves (Olsson, 1971; Olsson, Kristensson and Klatzo, 1971). While certain species differences are apparent a broad distinction emerges between the permeability of epineurial blood vessels and the endoneurial circulation to protein tracers. Thus, labelled proteins rapidly appear in the connective tissue around epineurial vessels, although they do not pass into the extracellular space of the endoneurium. Despite the limited data in this field, it seems that vascular permeability in spinal nerve roots considerably exceeds that found in either the spinal cord or the peripheral nerve trunks (Olsson, 1968).

12.3 Wallerian degeneration

12.3.1 *Introduction*

Axon degeneration is the primary event in Wallerian degeneration (Vial, 1958), and the associated breakdown of myelin may be due to either local conformational changes (Young, 1945), or to autolysis and phagocytic activity (Gutmann and Holubář, 1950). During the first week after peripheral nerve transection, physical fragmentation of the sheath proceeds in the distal segment of nerve without any accompanying chemical (Johnson, *et al.*, 1950) or histochemical (Noback and Montagna, 1952) alteration of myelin lipids. Subsequently cholesterol ester accumulates in the degenerating nerve and the concentration of myelin lipids diminishes (Rossiter, 1955). More up to date studies of myelin lipids (Berry, Cevallos and Wade, 1965; Domonkos and Heiner, 1968) have confirmed that there is no characteristic early lipid change in the first few days of Wallerian degeneration (WD), but by the end of the first week loss of cerebroside and phosphatidyl enthanolamine exceeds that of other lipids. In view of the finding of marked cerebroside loss in brain tissue affected by multiple sclerosis (Gerstl *et al.*, 1970) it may well be that cerebroside can be readily dislocated from the sheath. Lysophosphatides are not usually detected in significant amounts before the end of the second week of Wallerian degeneration, but the recent findings (Webster, 1973) of increased phospholipase A activity as early as 2 days after nerve section suggests that a possible pathogenic role may exist for lysophosphatides in early myelin breakdown. Cholesterol ester is not found in normal myelin except transiently during development (Adams and Davison, 1959), and it has been established by labelling experiments that at least 85 per cent of the cholesterol of cholesterol ester appearing in degenerating nerve is derived from myelin (Simon, 1966).

Fragmentation of myelin can be observed one day after peripheral nerve section (Terry and Harkin, 1959; Glimstedt and Wohlfart, 1960; Webster, 1962a). The changes seen include increased myelin periodicity, lamellar separation and splitting at the intraperiod lines, and these commence mainly at nodes of Ranvier (Ballin and Thomas, 1969). The incisures of Schmidt–Lanterman also dilate rapidly after nerve injury leading to splitting of the intraperiod lines of adjacent myelin lamellae (Williams and Hall, 1971). Taken collectively, such findings are hard to reconcile with the report by Friede and Martinez (1970) that the early changes in myelin during Wallerian degeneration can be attributed simply to shrinkage of the axon. Evidence of marked breakdown of myelin between 1 and 4 days after nerve section has been provided by Wolman (1968), the degradation of the axon and myelin occuring initially within the Schwann cells (Holtzman and Novikoff, 1965). It appears that the early increase in DNA (Logan, Mannell and Rossiter, 1952) found in nerves undergoing Wallerian degeneration is due mainly to Schwann cell proliferation (Oderfeld-Nowak and Niemierko, 1969). Similarly, increased incorporation of labelled precursors into lipids in degenerating nerve, at a time when the total amount of these lipids is decreasing, has been attributed to the activity of Schwann cells and phagocytic elements (Berry and Coourad, 1967). Neither invasion of the degenerating nerve by blood-borne macrophages nor the proliferation of endoneurial cells are conspicuous until the second week after nerve section (Abercrombie and Johnson, 1946; Joseph, 1950; Thomas, 1970), although it is clear that limited entry of haematogenous cells into peripheral nerve does occur during the first week of degeneration (Olsson and Sjöstrand, 1969; Asbury, 1970). Mast cell degranulation occurs at sites of peripheral nerve damage (Olsson, 1967, 1968) and release of biogenic amines stored within these cells may alter local vascular permeability and the blood-nerve barrier (see Section 12.3.5). It has also been suggested that herapin, similarly derived from mast cells, plays some part in promoting loss of lipid from the degenerating nerve sheath. Certain neurotoxic substances, for instance tri-orthocresyl phosphate (TOCP), isoniazid, acrylamide, cause a Wallerian-type degeneration of the distal portions of longer axons through what is thought to be a primary action on metabolism within the neuronal cell body (Cavanagh, 1969; Gilliatt, 1969).

12.3.2 *Enzyme changes*

It is of value in Wallerian degeneration to distinguish between enzyme activity of axonal origin and that arising from the nerve sheath or connective tissue elements. Enzyme changes in the axon after nerve section or crush reflect the immediate effects of interrupting axoplasmic flow as well as the ensuing degeneration. The initial changes in Schwann cells, together with the formation of ellipsoids and digestion chambers, are reactive in nature and are concerned with dispersal of the myelin and axonal debris.

Ultrastructural studies in Wallerian degeneration have shown swelling of mitochondria (Vial, 1958), focal accumulation of mitochondria in the paranodal axoplasm (Webster, 1962a), and the appearance of lysosomes (Holtzman and Novikoff, 1965). Widening of the nodes of Ranvier with simultaneous fragmentation of the axons and loosening of myelin lamellae have been described in the distal segment within the first 24 h of Wallerian degeneration (Terry and Harkin, 1959; Glimstedt and Wohlfart, 1960; Barton, 1962). Williams and Hall (1971) have described a process of axonal shutdown with formation of ellipsoids and breakdown of axon and myelin occurring solely within Schwann cells until the fifth day of nerve degeneration. Ultrastructural changes occurring in the proximal stump in Wallerian degeneration have been described by Morris, Hudson and Weddell (1972a,b); the Schwann cells appeared to be primarily responsible for the removal of myelin debris, and no cells identifiable as endoneurial or haematogenous macrophages were found to contain membrane fragments or lipid.

The enzymes dehydrogenases and acetylcholinesterase have been the most extensively studied histochemical indicators of axonal reaction in Wallerian degeneration. In spite of earlier reports of a fall in both oxidative enzyme (Houten and Friede, 1964) and AChE activity (Sawyer, 1946; Snell, 1957) in nerve distal to the point of injury, it is now clear that there is an initial increase in the activity of both of these enzymes immediately proximal and distal to the site of section or crush (Fig. 12.10). The increased oxidative enzyme activity in the proximal part of the distal stump was noted by Kreutzberg (1964), and it was established that this change could not be due to local synthesis of enzyme as no increased uptake of radiolabelled precursors was found autoradiographically (Kreutzberg, 1967). The accumulation proximal to the lesion of enzymes known to be associated with the axon can be readily attributed to damming-back of axonal flow. However, in order to account for increased activity of such axonal enzymes immediately distal to the injury it has been necessary to suggest that translocation of enzyme occurs within the degenerating segment (Lubińska *et al.*, 1964; Lubińska, 1964), or that there is an obstruction to retrograde axonal

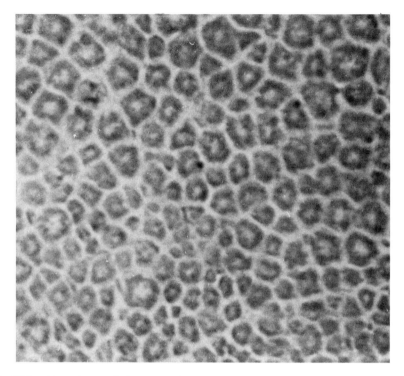

Fig. 12.9   Normal rat sciatic nerve. Transverse section to show staining for naphthyl-amidase activity in myelin. LNAase at pH 6.5. (x 550: Reproduced by courtesy of the editors of *Progress in Histochemistry and Cytochemistry*.)

transport (Kristensson and Olsson, 1973). Local increases in lactate dehydro-genase (LDH) and NADH-dehydrogenase activity found in single nerve fibres following crush are accompanied by striking morphological changes in damaged axon terminals (Morgan-Hughes and Engel, 1968). This raises the possibility that, adjacent to trauma, increased histochemical staining may sometimes reflect increased permeability of damaged membrane to low molecular weight sub-strates and capture agents. Axonal transport in adrenergic fibres of enzymes (MAO, dopamine-β-hydroxylase) concerned with monoamine metabolism and the effects of constriction or crush have already been referred to (Section 12.2.3).

   Pseudocholinesterase (BChE) shows its greatest rise in the second week of Wallerian degeneration, *pari passu* with the period of greatest cellular prolifer-ation, and represents activity within the Schwann cell and endoneurium (Cavanagh and Webster, 1955). Similarly, staining for ATPases and 5'-nucleotidase is strongest at this time in Schwann cells and macrophages (Wolfgram and Rose, 1960). In normal peripheral nerve, histochemically demonstrable alkaline phosphatase activity is confined to vascular endothelium, although small amounts can be detected biochemically in myelin membrane (Adams, Davison and Gregson, 1963). Alkaline phosphatase activity in the distal stump has been reported to decline during the first two weeks of Wallerian degeneration (Samorajski, 1957; Pinner and Campbell, 1965), but it is of interest that activation of capillary alkaline phosphatase is said to occur during experimental cerebral oedema (Emmenegger and Ruge, 1968) and might also, therefore, be expected to increase in the early stage of nerve degeneration. Inorganic pyrophasphatase (PP_i ase) activity in Wallerian degeneration has been observed over a three month period (Hallpike and McArdle, 1974) and is localized to regenerating axons, myelin and cell nuclei (Fig. 12.3). Phospholipase activity (A_1 and A_2) increases markedly in early Wallerian degeneration (Webster, 1973), and although the pathogenic significance of such activity has not yet been established, intraneural injection of very small (6-10 μg) amounts of 1-acyl lysophosphatidylcholine is reported to produce selective demyelination in mouse sciatic nerve (Hall and Gregson, 1971). Non-specific esterases (NsE) are widely distributed in brain and peripheral nerve, and enzymes with different inhibitor characteristics have been isolated from central and peripheral myelin (Barron, Bernsohn and Mitzen, 1972). Esterases active against 1-naphthyl acetate, naphthol-AS-acetate and 5-bromo-indoxyl acetate become more active during Wallerian degeneration (Gould and Holt, 1961; Bubis and Wolman, 1965). While such activity appears to be associated with phagocytosis, the NsE comprise a heterogeneous group of enzymes, and the problem of identifying the origin and significance of increased esterase activity in Wallerian degeneration requires the use of zymograms and the application of specific inhibitors (eserine, diethyl-p-nitrophenylphosphate − E600).

Increased acid phosphate activity has frequently been observed in Wallerian degeneration (Bodian, 1947; Heinzen, 1947; Hollinger, Rossiter and Upmalis, 1952; McCaman and Robins, 1958a,b; Wolfgram amd Rose, 1960; Gould and Holt, 1961; Anderson and Song, 1962; Bubis and Wolman, 1965; Weller and Mellick, 1966). Electron histochemical observations (Holtzman and Novikoff, 1965) indicate that the early increase in acid phosphatase activity after nerve section could be attributed to lysosomal proliferation in degenerating axons. In our own histochemical studies, acid β-glycerophosphatase and azo-naphthol phosphatase activity were found to increase in axons, Schwann cells and macrophages (Fig. 12.11) in the first two weeks after nerve section (Hallpike, Adams and Bayliss, 1970b). Acid phosphatase was also estimated biochemically in whole nerve homogenates (Fig. 12.12) and subcellular fractions in Wallerian degeneration. During the first week a three-fold increase in activity occurred but there was no significant recovery of the enzyme from myelin fractions (Hallpike, 1972). In the segment of nerve proximal to the section or crush a marked increase in acid phosphatase activity is found in the stump, with a lesser but significant increase in the more proximal apparently undamaged, nerve (Samorajski, 1957).

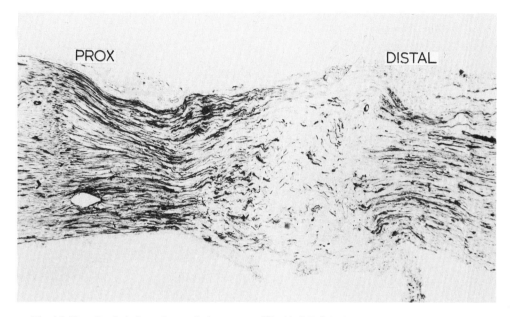

Fig. 12.10   Crush lesion of rat sciatic nerve at 48h. NADH-dehydrogenase activity proximal and distal to the lesion. (× 56.)

It was suggested by Gutmann and Holubář (1950) that some of the early changes occurring in the nerve sheath after neurotomy might be due to the local release of proteolytic enzymes. Porcellati and Thompson (1957) found an increase in amino acids in peripheral nerve undergoing Wallerian degeneration and increased peptidase activity in this situation was reported by McCaman and Robins (1959b). Subsequent studies (Porcellati and Curti, 1960; Adams and Tuqan, 1961) confirmed an increase in the activity of a neutral protease in nerve during the first week of degeneration, and increased protease activity can be detected histochemically in silver-gelatin autograms from the third day onwards (Hallpike and Adams, 1969a,b; Hallpike, Adams and Bayliss, 1970b). In early Wallerian degeneration protease activity is mainly distributed along nerve fibres but later such activity becomes concentrated in the regions at which myelin is breaking down within ellipsoids and digestion chambers (Fig. 12.13). Much of this observed protease activity is due to the enzyme with an acid pH optimum (pH 3.5 in histochemical incubations) which is considered to be largely of lysosomal origin (Marks and Lajtha, 1963, 1965). There is good correlation between the histochemical and subcellular distribution of this acid protease and that of acid phosphatase. Biochemical assays on whole nerve homogenates show a parallel increase in both neutral and acid proteases, and acid phosphatase, during the first week after nerve section (Fig. 12.12). In the first few days of Wallerian degeneration the regions of most conspicuous morphological damage,

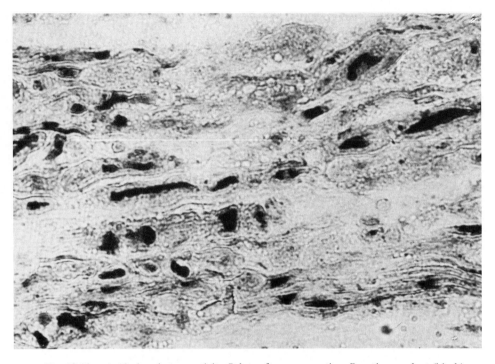

Fig. 12.11 Acid phosphatase activity 7 days after nerve section. Reaction product (black) seen mainly in degenerating axons. β-glycerophosphatase. (x 522: Reproduced by courtesy of the editors of *Progress in Histochemistry and Cytochemistry*.)

namely the axon and nodal areas, are also the sites of early lysosomal activity (Weller and Mellick, 1966; Ballin and Thomas, 1969) The implications of *in vivo* proteolysis in the pathogenesis of myelin breakdown and demyelinating disorders have been argued principally by Adams and his co-workers, and by Porcellati and by Gabrielescu (see Section 12.4). Further histochemical and biochemical evidence pointing towards active proteolysis during early Wallerian degeneration has recently been reviewed (Hallpike, 1972) Subcellular fraction-ation studies of both brain (Riekkinen and Clausen, and Arstila, 1970) and peripheral nerve (Hallpike, 1972) indicated that some neutral protease activity is associated with myelin membrane, and will survive repeated washing and water-shocking (Table 12.1). Conversely, acid protease, in common with acid phosphatase, is almost entirely lost from the myelin fraction during sucrose washing. Subcellular fractionation of peripheral nerve undergoing Wallerian degeneration reveals a marked increase in recovery of lysosomal enzymes (acid protease, acid phosphatase, β–glucuronidase) from the supernatant fraction. However, myelin thus isolated may be expected to retain many normal characteristics and to be unrepresentative of material subject to pathological change. Data on protease activity in nerve proximal to a section or crush is limited; Porcellati (1966) found that acid protease activity increased almost

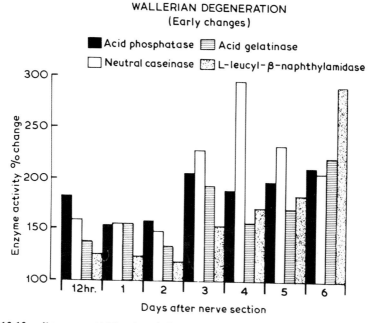

Fig. 12.12 Enzyme activities in whole nerve homogenates during the first week of Wallerian degeneration. 100% − control nerve value. (Reproduced by courtesy of the editors of *Progress in Histochemistry and Cytochemistry*.)

two-fold in the first week, whereas neutral protease remained essentially unaltered.

Early histochemical studies of aminopeptidase (LNAase) acitivity in peripheral nerve, (Adams and Glenner, 1962) employed the simultaneous coupling method of Burstone and Folk (1956). No significant reaction was obtained in myelin, axons or Schwann cells with this technique and it seemed likely that inhibition of the enzyme had resulted from the presence of diazonate in the incubation mediun (Section 12.2.4). With modifications (see Sylvén, 1968), which included lowering of the pH of the reaction to 6.5, and the use of copper chelation to diminish the solubility of the final reaction product, it has been possible to demonstrate LNAase activity in the myelin of normal nerve (Fig. 12.9), and in axons and Schwann sheaths of nerve undergoing Wallerian degeneration (Fig. 12.14). Histochemical and biochemical studies of LNAase in Wallerian degeneration have been reviewed elsewhere (Hallpike, 1972). It appears that a proportion (some 13 per cent) of LNAase in normal nerve is associated with the myelin fraction. During degeneration the specific activity of the enzyme in myelin shows little change but total recovery from myelin falls to 1–2 per cent. The fact that LNAase activity shows a later rise than acid phosphatase and acid protease (Fig. 12.12) suggests that at least a part of this increase derives from the release of enzyme from breaking down myelin.

Table 12.1[1]

Whole nerve activity	n-moles tyrosine/mg Protein/hour
Acid protease (pH 3.5)	3.6 (S.E.M. 0.54)
Neutral protease (pH 7.4)	1.1 (S.E.M. 0.18)

	pH	% Recovery
Sucrose-washed myelin	3.5	3.0(5)*
	7.4	15.5(5)
Water-shocked myelin	3.5	0.5(5)
	7.4	18.3(5)

*Figures in brackets denote number of experiments
[1] From Hallpike (1972), by permission of the Editors, Progr. Histochem. Cytochem.

12.3.3 *Protein changes*

As discussed in Section 12.2.4 peripheral nerve myelin contains three major classes of protein: (a) neurokeratin + some proteolipid, (b) acidic or Wolfgram protein, (c) basic protein. There is little proteolipid in peripheral nerve myelin as most of the trypsin-resistant, tryptophan-rich protein resists extraction with unacidified c/m and corresponds, therefore, to neurokeratin. It has been suggested (Mehl and Halaris, 1970) that a 1:1 molar ratio of proteolipid to basic protein pertains in central myelin, but in nerve, however, a higher proportion of proteolipid is of the Wolfgram rather than the Folch Lees' type (Wolfgram and Kotorii, 1968; Eng *et al.*, 1968). In polyacrylamide electrophoresis of myelin proteins dissolved in phenol/formic acid, a single major protein component can be resolved, together with basic proteins (Csejtey *et al.*, 1972). The basic proteins can be detected histochemically by staining with anionic dyes (Trypan Blue or PTAH) under suitable conditions, through their sensitivity to typsin, and by immunofluorescent techniques (Kornguth and Anderson, 1965).

It has been postulated (Adams and Tuqan, 1961) that the early physical disintegration of the myelin sheath in the first week of Wallerian degeneration is due to the disruption of lipid-protein bonds, and Tuqan and Adams (1961) have shown that proteolytic enzymes cause *in vitro* myelin breakdown with release of lipid bound to a trypsin-digestible myelin protein. In later histochemical studies (Hallpike, Adams and Bayliss, 1970d) evidence was obtained of selective damage to the basic TDP of myelin after 24 h of Wallerian degeneration (Fig. 12.15), and such a loss of basic protein may be reproduced *in vitro* by extracts of generating nerve, rich in neural protease (Hallpike, Adams and Bayliss, 1970c). Basic, trypanophilic, protein is also absent from multiple sclerosis (MS) plaques and a zone deficient in basic protein staining frequently surrounds acute lesions (Hallpike and Adams, 1970; Adams, Hallpike and Bayliss, 1971). In a combined biochemical and histochemical study (Einstein *et al.*, 1972) acid proteinase activity in and around MS plaques was found to correlate well with the absence or reduction of basic protein determined electrophoretically. These observations, taken collectively, suggest that loss of the basic protein could be an initial biochemical event in the demyelinating process.

In further microdensitometric and electrophoretic studies of Wallerian degeneration, a substantial early loss of basic protein has been found together with a somewhat slower but progressive loss of the major protein component of

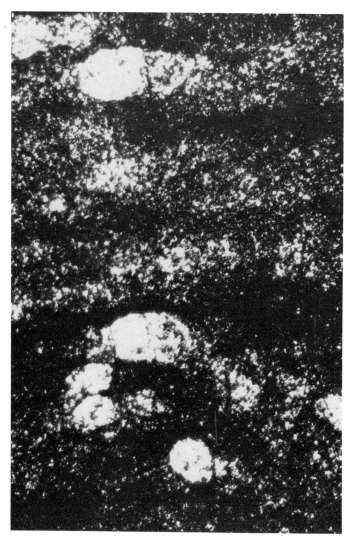

Fig. 12.13 Protease activity (Translucency = digestion of gelatin) 14 days after nerve section. Activity concentrated in 'digestion chambers'. Silver-gelatin autogram, pH 3.5. (x 340.)

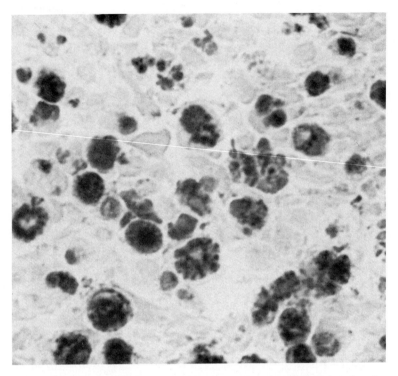

Fig. 12.14   Rat sciatic nerve, 7 days after neurotomy. Strong axonal and periaxonal reaction, LNAase, pH 6.5, (x 550.)

peripheral nerve myelin (Adams *et al.*, 1972). Whole nerve electrophoresis (Fig. 12.16) demonstrates this early loss of the slower moving basic protein (B) and progressive degradation of the major component (C). Microdensitometry using Trypan Blue and DMAB as histochemical markers for basic groupings and neurokeratin respectively, (Fig. 12.17) confirms the earlier and more complete loss of the basic myelin protein in tissue sections during the first week of nerve degeneration, and the PAS and modified PAS methods disclose an early loss of cerebroside from degenerating myelin which appears to parallel the decline in the DMAB-positive major protein component. Phosphoglycerides (GHA method) in myelin show little early change, however, and certain discrepancies between the histochemical and electrophoretic findings are apparent. The latter indicate a greater fall in the major protein component than is suggested by micro-densitrometric comparisons of Trypan Blue and DMAB staining. It may be concluded therefore, that basic protein is degraded more rapidly than neuro-

Fig. 12.15   Basic, trypanophilic, protein in myelin of normal rat sciatic nerve and marked loss of trypanophilia 1 day after nerve section. Trypan blue (pH 5.0). (x 285: Reproduced by courtesy of the editor of the *Histochemical Journal.*)

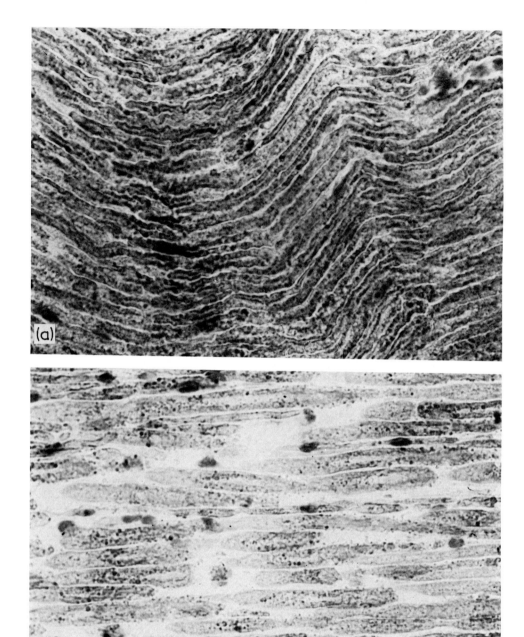

(a)

(b)

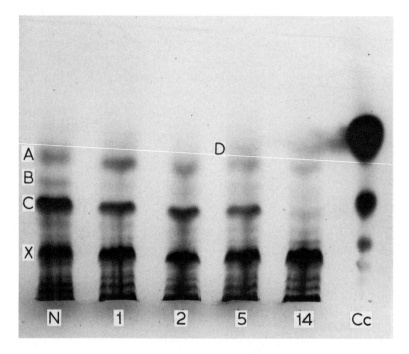

Fig. 12.16 Polyacrylamide gel electrophoresis of whole rat sciatic nerve undergoing Wallerian degeneration. A and B – fast and slow moving basic proteins; C – principal protein component of peripheral myelin; X – non-myelin proteins; D – fast moving band (? breakdown product) appearing at 5th day. N – control nerve, 1 – 1 day after nerve section, 2 – 2 days, 5 – 5 days, 14 – 14 days after section. Cc – cytochrome marker. (Reproduced by courtesy of the editor of the *Journal of Neurochemistry*.)

keratin in early Wallerain degeneration, and that the neurokeratin of peripheral myelin is susceptible to *in vitro* tryptic digestion (Csejtey *et al.*, 1972). These conclusions are in accord with the observation (Lees, Messinger and Burnham, 1967) that, under certain conditions, brain proteolipid can be degraded by trypsin. Thus, the clear distinction previously drawn between trypsin-resistant and trypsin-sensitive proteins can no longer be considered valid.

12.3.4 *Lipid changes*

Histochemical studies have established that there are two phases in the breakdown of myelin lipids during nerve degeneration (Noback and Montagna, 1952; Adams, 1962 and 1965a). During the initial phases the myelin sheath undergoes physical fragmentation, recognizable microscopically, but this is not accompanied by any detectable chemical alteration to the lipids. Subsequently during the second week of degeneration, as shown by Rossiter and his co-workers, the levels of lipid-bound phosphorus, sphingomyelin and cerebroside all fall dramatically, while esterified cholesterol content increases. Reduction of osmium tetroxide (OsO_4) to black osmium dioxide (OsO_2) has been widely employed to detect unsaturated bonds in lipids in tissue sections. When a polar oxident, i.e. $K_4Cr_2O_7$ (Marchi, 1886) or $KClO_3$ (Swank and Davenport, 1935) is added to OsO_4 such agents readily penetrate hydrophilic unsaturated lipids and are oxidized in perference to OsO_4. Thus, Marchi-type reagents selectively blacken hydrophobic unsaturated lipids and are employed to demonstrate such lipids in tissue sections (see Adams, 1958; Adams, Abdulla and Bayliss, 1967). Normal nerve fails to stain by the Marchi method presumably because of the effective masking of hydrophobic elements by phospholipids in the intact sheath. The positive Marchi reaction obtained during myelin breakdown is largely due to the appearance of esterified cholesterol and develops strongly in the second week of Wallerian degeneration. Unreduced osmium held within hydrophilic unsaturated lipids in the Marchi reaction may subsequently be displayed by its orange-brown chelate or complex with α-naphthylamine. This is the basis of the OTAN method (Adams, 1959) which distinguishes hydrophobic cholesterol ester (OTAN-black) from unsaturated phospholipids, phospho-glycerides and sphingomyelin, (orange-brown) in degenerating nerve. The specificity of the OTAN reaction has, however, been questioned and the application of these lipid histochemical techniques has recently been discussed in detail elsewhere (Adams and Bayliss, 1974). Some lipid histochemical staining reactions in Wallerian degeneration are illustrated in Fig. 12.18. In the first 5 or 6 days after nerve section myelin shows a virtually normal staining pattern with SB, BSB, Nile blue sulphate, oil red O, OTAN, but after this initial phase of 'physical disruption', the loss of phospholipid and accumulation of cholesterol ester greatly modifies the appearances seen with both histophysical and histochemical methods.

The chemical and cellular mechanisms responsible for the fate of cholesterol and its esters in degenerating nerve are still far from clear. Initially, cholesterol may be 'unscreened' through loss of phospholipids or basic protein or dislocated from its normal locus in myelin membrane. Degradative enzymes (see Section 12.3.2) probably play an important part in the early disruption of myelin and are likely to exert their main effects within phagosomal systems involving Schwann cells or macrophages. Both cholesterol and fatty acid radicals accumulate in degenerating myelin and are probably most easily disposed of as cholesterol ester. However, the marked decrease in cholesterol esterase activity found during the first week of Wallerian degeneration (Mezei, 1970) may contribute to the subsequent build-up of ester in the nerve at later stages in the degenerative process. Histochemical evidence concerning the appearance of cholesterol esters in Schwann cells and macrophages has been reviewed by Adams (1965a), and there is nothing to suggest that cholesterol esterification is a primary event in demyelination processes. The esters may be transported to blood vessels within phagosomes or broken down *in situ* by lysosomal esterases (Werb and Cohn, 1972). It has not yet been established whether a recycling mechanism exists for the local incorporation of such regenerated cholesterol into

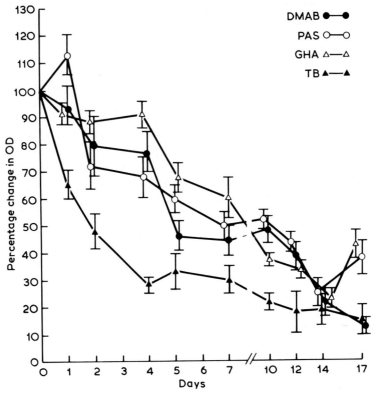

Fig. 12.17 Mircrodensitometric analysis of changes in trypanophilia (TB, protein basic groups, DMAB for tryptophan, PAS for cerebroside, GHA for phosphoglycerides) in rat sciatic nerve undergoing Wallerian degeneration. (Reproduced by courtesy of the editor of the *Journal of Neurochemistry*.)

fresh myelin. Mast cells contain herapin as well as certain biogenic amines, histamines, 5-HT, and in the sectioned peripheral nerve mast cell proliferation is a conspicuous early feature. This proliferation in conjunction with an increased endoneurial vascular permeability to circulating histamine liberators and other mast cell degranulating agents, could result in a considerable outpouring of lipid-mobilizing factors (phospholipase and lipoprotein lipase activators) with access to myelin (Olsson, 1968).

12.3.5 *Vascular permeability*

It has been established that in normal peripheral nerve the perineurium acts as a diffusion barrier serving to isolate the nerve interior or endoneurium from the general extracellular space (Olsson and Kristensson, 1973). A fluorescent Evans blue albumin (EBA) mixture injected around a nerve trunk is prevented from entering the endoneurium by intact perineurium. However, following prolonged nerve ischaemia or trauma, fluorescent protein tracers pass freely in either direction across the perineurial barrier (Lundberg *et al.*, 1973). Recent observations on the anatomy and ultrastructure of vasa nervorum have been summarized by Olsson, Kristensson and Klatzo (1971). The nutrient artery forms a plexus of epineurial vessels which, in turn, communicates with the endoneurial capillary plexus. Although there are considerable species variations (Olsson, 1971) it appears that a large extracellular space exists within the endoneurium and in this respect the peripheral nerve differs from the central nervous system, where glial cells closely invest the capillaries and the extracellular space appears to be small. The endoneurial capillaries are normally impermeable to proteins by virtue of tight endothelial cell junctions Olsson and Reese, 1969, 1971) while epineurial vessels allow passage of protein across their walls. In Wallerian degeneration leakage of intravenously injected fluorescent protein tracers occurs into the endoneurial space of the distal segment (Olsson, 1966). Similar findings have been reported in studies using radio-iodinated albumin in which increased endoneurial vascular permeability in the distal segment was observed from twenty-four hours after a nerve crush (Mellick and Cavanagh, 1968).

12.4 Demyelination

In demyelinating diseases the axon is characteristically spared, the pathological process being centred on the myelin sheath or myelin-supporting cell. Thus, distal to a demyelinating lesion both the axon and the sheath appear normal distinguishing this process from Wallerian degeneration. The first description of segmental demyelination in peripheral nerve was provided by Gombault (1880), who observed degeneration and regeneration of myelin unaccompanied by axonal damage in guinea-pigs suffering from chronic lead intoxication. Electron-microscopic observations in lead neuropathy (Lampert and Schochet, 1968) suggest that the loss of myelin in this condition results from an initial proliferation of Schwann cells, followed by degeneration. Diphtheria toxin is thought to interfere with ATP production (Kato and Pappenheimer, 1960) and protein synthesis (Matheson and Cavanagh, 1967) within the Schwann cell, and this agent has now been extensively employed to produce experimental demyelination in peripheral nerve. In susceptible species, rabbit, hen, guinea-pig, parenteral injection of an underneutralized toxin/antitoxin mixture induces a generalized demyelinating peripheral neuropathy (Waksman, Adams and Mansmann, 1957; McDonald, 1963; Morgan-Hughes, 1965). Ultrastructural features of the diphtheritic lesion in peripheral nerve include initial focal alterations in the lamellar pattern of myelin at the nodal region coinciding with the onset of clinical weakness (Webster, 1964). Ultrastructural and electron-histochemical studies of diphtheritic neuropathy in the chicken (Weller, 1965; Weller and Mellick, 1966) demonstrated an accumulation of acid phosphatase-positive dense bodies, identified as lysosomes, in juxta-axonal Schwann cell

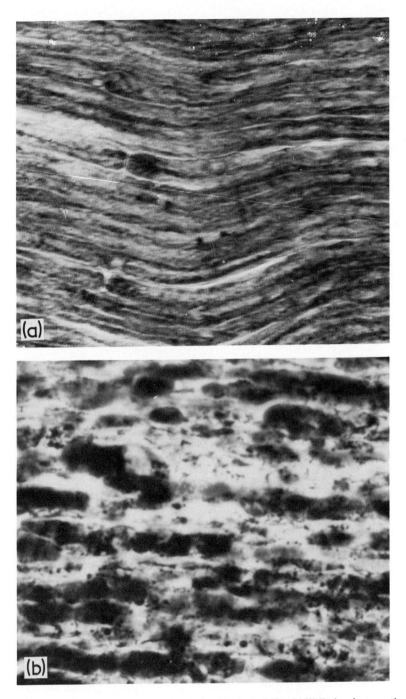

Fig. 12.18 (a) Normal rat sciatic nerve, Sudan Black. (x 360); (b) Wallerian degeneration, 12 days, Sudan Black, (x 360); (c) normal nerve viewed in polarized light, (x 104); nerve undergoing Wallerian degeneration (24 days) showing anisotropic lipid accumulations and loss of normal sheath birefringence. (x 104.)

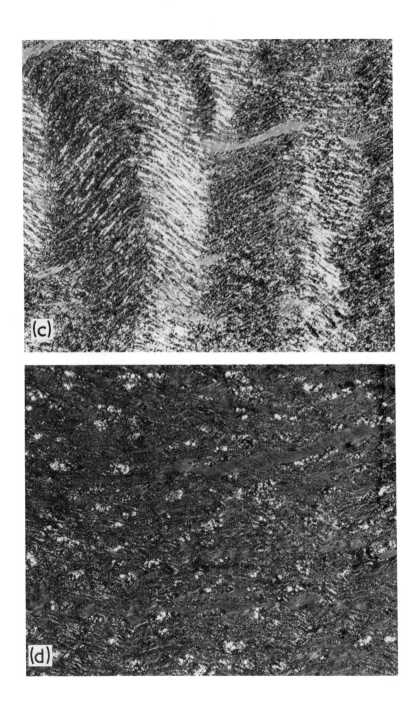

Table 12.2[2]

Days after injection*	0	3	4	5	6	7	12	16	20
Acid protease (pH 3.5)	29[1] (16−50) n9	60.55	105.85	50	60	80	75	40	48
Neutral protease (pH 7.4)	13.5 (8−19) n8	14	19	18	16.5	12	17	12	28

*2.5 Lf units diphtheria toxin in saline with 0.1% trypan blue
[1] Results expressed as m-u moles tyrosine liberated/mg protein/hour
[2] From Hallpike (1972), by permission of the editors, *Progr. Histochem. Cytochem.*

cytoplasm before the onset of myelin breakdown. Although the peripheral nervous system of the rat is resistant to the effect of parenterally administered diphtheria toxin, localized demyelination can, nevertheless, be produced by direct intraneural micro-injection of toxin (Jacobs, 1967). Employing this technique, increased protease activity can be detected histochemically in rat sciatic nerve before paralysis becomes clinically evident (Hallpike, 1972). Biochemical determinations of protease activity (Table 12.2) in diphtheritic neuropathy show that during the first week after intraneural injection of toxin there is an initial increase in activity of the acid protease (pH 3.5) with a later and less conspicuous rise in neutral protease activity. Acid phosphatase activity is prominent in Schwann cells (Fig. 12.19) and, at the ultrastructural level, such activity is discerned in lysosomes within the juxta-axonal Schwann cell cytoplasm (Fig. 12.20). This parallel increase in acid phosphatase and acid protease activity in early diphtheritic neuropathy suggests a common lysosomal source. These findings (Table 12.2) differ from those in Wallerian degeneration (Fig. 12.12) in that in the demyelination lesion there is no early rise in neutral protease activity, suggesting that axons are the principal source of the neutral protease in early Wallerian degeneration (Marks, Datta and Lajtha, 1970); subsequent release of such protease from disintegrating myelin may account for the increased recovery of this enzyme once the diphtheritic neuropathy has become well established. Two patterns of demyelination have been reported, affecting small and large diameter myelinated fibres respectively, on the basis of histochemical and ultrastructural studies of diphtheritic lesions in rat sciatic nerve (Weller and Nester, 1972). In the smaller fibres breakdown of myelin appears to be initiated by lysosomal enzymes whereas in large diameter fibres initial widening of the nodal gap and detachment of paranodal myelin end-loops is not preceded by local lysosomal activation. In human hypertrophic neuropathy, often representing the outcome of repeated episodes of demyelination

Fig. 12.19 Acid phosphatase activity in diphtheritic neuropathy. Longitudinal (a) and transverse sections (b). Naphthol AS-TR phosphate substrate. Ilford 404 filter. (x 360.)

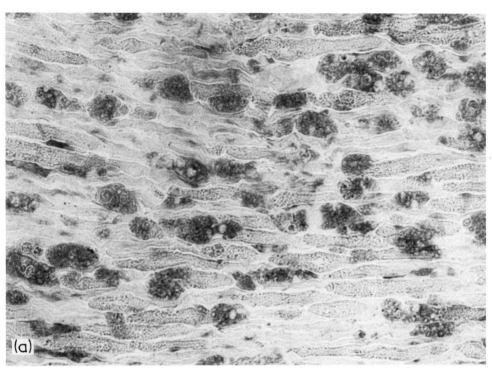

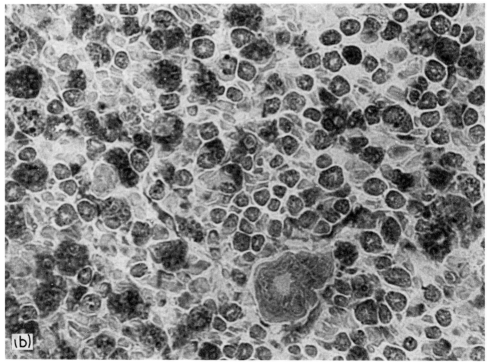

and remyelination (Thomas and Lascelles, 1967), acid phosphatase activity is prominent in lysosomes in the perinuclear regions of the Schwann cell (Weller and Herzog, 1970). It has been suggested (Wolman, 1968) that myelin breakdown follows one of two distinctive patterns: 'centripetal' where lysosomal enzymes originate in the Schwann cell to produce a demyelinating lesion and 'centrifugal' where the inital change occurs in the axon, and enzymes damage the sheath from within outwards. Such a simplistic view offers a possible explanation of the process of myelin breakdown in Wallerian degeneration.

There now appears to be good evidence that activation of the Schwann cell lysosomal apparatus with release of hydrolases (see Brunk and Ericsson, 1973) may be an important early pathogenic event in the demyelination process, and that the basic protein component of peripheral myelin is vulnerable to proteolysis (Hallpike, Adams and Bayliss, 1970c; Fig. 12.14). The relevance of these experimental observations in peripheral nerve to human demyelination diseases involving the central nervous system has recently been reviewed (Adams, 1972; Hallpike, 1972). Increased lysosomal activity has been detected histochemically and biochemically at the edges of 'active' multiple sclerosis lesions (Einstein et al., 1972) and has been correlated with loss of basic protein in and around such plaques (Hallpike, Adams and Bayliss, 1970d; Riekkinen et al., 1971; Einstein et al., 1972). Activation of lysosomal neuroproteases has also been described in experimental allergic encephalitis (Kerekas, Feszt and Kovacs, 1965; Gabrielescu, 1969; Dienssner and Schmidt, 1972). It must be admitted, however, that a clear cause-and-effect relationship between these enzyme changes and the initiation of myelin breakdown has not been proved, least of all in the case of multiple sclerosis in which lesions are almost invariably well established by the time observations can be made.

12.5 Storage disorders

Storage diseases have now been shown to be largely due to deficiencies of specific lysosomal enzymes resulting in faulty catabolism and accumulation of the stored products of metabolism within membraneous lysosomal bodies (Resibois et al., 1970). The sphingolipidoses are characterized by the accumulation, in different organs, of distinctive complex lipids each containing ceramide (sphingosone-amide-link-C_{22} or C_{24} FA) as a common moiety (Brady, 1972), while in the mucopolysaccharidoses, dermatan and herapin sulphate are the principal substances stored or excreted (Suzuki, 1972). The clinical diagnosis of these disorders has traditionally been made on the basis of inheritance and evidence of predominantly neural, neuro-visceral, visceral or skeletal involvement. However with the increasing application of sensitive biochemical screening procedures and direct enzyme assays, accurate diagnosis is now possible where either the clinical syndrome is incompletely developed, or where suspicion rests solely on the presence of a genetic risk. While proof of involvement of peripheral nerves in neuro-vesceral lipidoses is limited to a few disorders, their number is

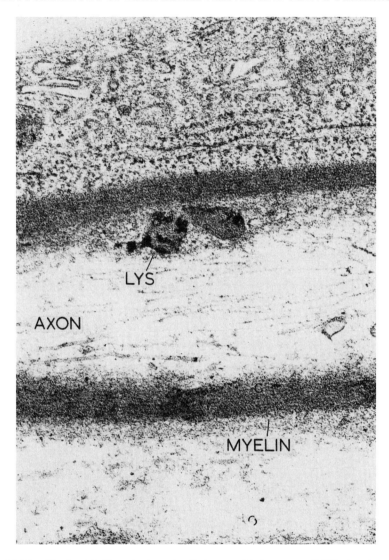

Fig. 12.20 Myelinated fibre, $1-2\,\mu$m in diameter, with lysosomes (LYS) showing acid phosphatase activity situated in the para-axonal Schwann cytoplasm. Twenty days after intraneural injection of diphtheria toxin. (x 42 000: Reproduced by courtesy of Dr R. O. Weller and the editor of *Brain*.)

increasing with the more frequent employment of histochemical and electron microscopic techniques.

12.5.1 *Metachromatic leucodystrophy*

The finding of metachromatic material in peripheral nerves of children suffering from metachromatic leucodystrophy (MLD) and recognition of the value of

649

nerve biopsy in the diagnosis of this condition by Thieffry and Lyon (1959) have been confirmed in numerous subsequent reports (Norman, Urich and Tingey, 1960; Hagberg, Sourander and Thoren, 1962; Webster, 1962b; Dayan, 1967; Olsson and Sourander, 1969). Chemically, the stored substance is sulphatide (ceramide galactose-3-sulphate) and the responsible metabolic defect is a deficiency of arylsulphatase A, one of three sulphuric acid esterases present in mammalian tissues (see Brady, 1972). The sulphatide or sulphatide-lipid complex stains brown with cresyl violet (Hirsch and Peiffer, 1957) or pink-red with toluidine blue. This material is also SB, PAS positive and birefringent in polarized light (see Adams, 1965d). Metachromatic accumulations are found principally in the perinuclear regions of Schwann cells, in phagocytes and within endoneurial and perinuclear capillaries. Myelin itself does not stain meta-chromatically but appears to undergo increased turnover, and the lipid deposits in Schwann cells and elsewhere may be regarded as abnormal myelin breakdown products (Dayan, 1967). The presence of extensive segmental demyelination in MLD has been correlated with the marked slowing in peripheral nerve conduction frequently found in this condition (Fullerton, 1964).

12.5.2 *Krabbe leucodystrophy*

Together with sulphatide lipidosis (MLD), Krabbe's disease or globoid cell leucodystrophy (GLD) comprise the two best recognized heredodegenerative diseases affecting white matter of the nervous system. The stored material is ceramide galactoside (galactocerebroside) resulting from absence or deficiency of the enzyme β-galactosidase (see Brady, Johnson and Uhlendorf, 1971). Involvement of peripheral nerves in GLD is now known to be a frequent occurrence (Allen and de Veyra, 1967; Sourander and Olsson, 1968; Hagberg *et al.*, 1969), and there is evidence (Lake, 1968) of segmental demyelination. The lipid deposits found in Schwann cells and endoneurial macrophages stain with the modified PAS technique (Adams, Bayliss and Ibrahim, 1963) and contain cerebroside. Although extensive myelin breakdown is present, histochemical studies (Hagberg *et al.*, 1969) have failed to reveal the presence of cholesterol esters, characteristic of Wallerian degeneration, supporting the view that the changes in nerve are directly related to a metabolic defect in myelin or Schwann cell metabolism.

12.5.3 *Fabry's disease*

Deposition of ceramide trihexoside within arterial smooth muscle, myocardium, kidneys, bone marrow and the reticulo-endothelial system is now recognized to be the principal pathological finding in this distinctive clinical syndrome. The underlying biochemical defect is an α-galactosidase deficiency (see Brady, 1972). The histochemical features of the stored lipid in Fabry's disease have been described by Lehner and Adams (1968) and these indicate the presence of a cerebroside-like material. Kocen and Thomas (1970) in their report of a peripheral nerve biopsy in this condition stress the loss of small myelinated fibres, the absence of any evidence of segmental demyelination and the presence of PAS, SB and PAN positive birefringent lipid in perinuclear cells and within the vasa nervorum. No lipid inclusions were found in Schwann cells or axons.

12.5.4 *Tangier disease*

This very rare disorder is characterized by a severe deficiency or absence from the plasma of the normal alpha or high density lipoprotein (HDL), and is associated with a low concentration of plasma cholesterol and accumulation of cholesterol esters in body organs (Fredrickson, Gotto and Levy, 1972). Peripheral nerve involvement in this disease is now well documented (Engel *et al.*, 1967; Kocen *et al.*, 1967) and the nerve biopsy findings in two cases of Tangier disease have recently been reported (Kocen *et al.*, 1973). The principal features were loss of smaller myelinated and unmyelinated fibres, deposition of lipid within Schwann cells and excessive endoneurial collagenization. Histochemical studies revealed Sudan III, SB and Schultz positive intrafascicular lipid droplets indicating the probable presence of esterified cholesterol. The finding of lipid within Schwann cells and excessive endoneurial collagenization. Histosegmental demyelination was not observed and the nerve degeneration appeared to follow a pattern of primary axonal loss.

12.5.5 *Normal myelin breakdown, xanthomata, amyloid*

In Tay-Sachs disease (GM$_2$ gangliosidosis) and the generalized (GM$_1$) gangliosidoses, sphingolipid accumulates in neurones within the central nervous system. Histochemically, it is possible to recognize both this stored material and the products of Wallerian breakdown of normal myelin found in glial and phagocytic cells (see Adams, 1965d). Where peripheral nerve involvement has been described in Tay-Sachs disease (Kristensson, Olsson and Sourander, 1967) the changes were almost certainly secondary to neuronal and axonal change with nothing to suggest a Schwann cell disorder. Thus, in disease processes which primarily affect the neurone, Wallerian degeneration may be expected to occur with the consequent appearance of cholesterol esters within nerve, and the changes described in 13.3.4. In biliary cirrhosis with cutaneous xanthomata, a mild sensory neuropathy may develop associated with the presence of widespread epi- and endoneurial cholesterol deposits (Thomas and Walker, 1965). Involvement of the peripheral nervous system is also a conspicuous feature in certain forms of familial amyloidosis (Andrade, 1952; Coimbra and Andrade, 1971a,b; Zalin *et al.*, 1974). The histochemical features of amyloid material have recently been discussed by Wolman (1971); these include positive reactions with congo red, PAS, methyl violet metachromasia, toluidine blue dichroism in polarized light, thioflavine dye fluorescence, DMAB staining for tryptophan and negative results with collagen stains. The amyloid deposits are mainly endoneurial, leading secondarily to Wallerian change but are also found in endo- and perineurial blood vessels.

References

Abercrombie, M. and Johnson, M. L. (1946) Quantitative histology of Wallerian degeneration. I. *Journal of Anatomy*, 80, 37–50.

Adams, C. W. M. (1957) A p-Dimethylaminobenzaldehyde-nitrite method for the histochemical demonstration of tryptophane and related compounds. *Journal of Clinical Pathology*, 10, 56–62.

Adams, C. W. M. (1958) Histochemical mechanisms of the Marchi reaction for degenerating myelin. *Journal of Neurochemistry*, 2, 178–186.

Adams, C. W. M. (1959) A histochemical method for the simultaneous demonstration of normal and degenerating myelin. *Journal of Pathology and Bacteriology*, 77, 648–650.

Adams, C. W. M. (1961) A perchloric acid-naphthoquinone method for the histochemical localization of cholesterol. *Nature (London)*, 192, 331–332.

Adams, C. W. M. (1962) In *Neurochemistry*, (eds.) Elliott, K. A. C., Page, I. H. and Quastel, J. H. 2nd edition p. 85–112, Charles C. Thomas: Springfield, Illinois.

Adams, C. W. M. (1965a) *Neurochemistry*. Elsevier: Amsterdam.

Adams, C. W. M. (1965b) Histochemistry of the cells in the nervous system. In *Neurohistochemistry*. (ed.) Adams, C. W. M. Chapter 8, Elsevier: Amsterdam.

Adams, C. W. M. (1965c) Histochemistry of lipids. In *Neurohistochemistry*. (ed.) Adams, C. W. M. pp. 6–66. Elsevier: Amsterdam.

Adams, C. W. M. (1965d) Cerebral storage disease. In *Neurohistochemistry*. (ed.) Adams, C. W. M. p. 488–517, Elsevier: Amsterdam.

Adams, C. W. M. (1967) *Vascular histochemistry*. Lloyd Duke: London.

Adams, C. W. M. (1969) Lipid Histochemistry, *Advances in Lipid Research*, 7, 1–62.

Adams, C. W. M. (1972) Research on Multiple Sclerosis. Charles C. Thomas: Springfield, Illinois.

Adams, C. W. M., Abdulla, Y. H. and Bayliss, O. B. (1967) Osmium tetroxide as a histochemical and histological reagent. *Histochemie*, 9, 68–77.

Adams, C. W. M., Abdulla, Y. H., Turner, D. R. and Bayliss, O. B. (1968) Subcellular preparation of peripheral nerve myelin. *Nature (London)*, 220, 171–173.

Adams, C. W. M. and Bayliss, O. B. (1962) The release of protein, lipid and polysaccharide components of the arterial elastica by proteolytic enzymes and lipid solvents. *Journal of Histochemistry and Cytochemistry*, 10, 222–226.

Adams, C. W. M. and Bayliss, O. B. (1963) Histochemical observations on the localization and origin of sphingomyelin, cerebroside and cholesterol in the normal and atherosclerotic human artery. *Journal of Pathology and Bacteriology*, 85, 113–119.

Adams, C. W. M. and Bayliss, O. B. (1968a) Histochemistry of Myelin V. Trypsin-digestible and trypsin-resistant proteins. *Journal of Histochemistry and Cytochemistry*, 16, 110–114.

Adams, C. W. M. and Bayliss, O. B. (1968b) Histochemistry of myelin. VI. Solvent action of acetone on brain and other lipid-rich tissues. *Journal of histochemistry and Cytochemistry*, 16, 115–118.

Adams, C. W. M. and Bayliss, O. B. (1968c) Histochemistry of myelin. VII. Analysis of lipid-protein relationships and the absence of acid mucopolysaccharide. *Journal of Histochemistry and Cytochemistry*, 16, 119–127.

Adams, C. W. M. and Bayliss, O. B. (1968d) Myelin carbohydrates. *Journal of Histochemistry and Cytochemistry*, 16, 486–487.

Adams, C. W. M. and Bayliss, O. B. (1968e) Reappraisal of osmium tetroxide and OTAN histochemical reactions. *Histochemie*, 16, 162–166.

Adams, C. W. M. and Bayliss, O. B. (1974) *Lipid Histochemistry in Techniques of Biochemical and Biophysical Morphology*, (ed.) Glick, D. and Rosenbaum, H. Vol. 2, pp. 99–155, Interscience: New York.

Adams, C. W. M., Bayliss, O. B. and Grant, R. T. (1968) Cholinesterases in peripheral nervous system. III. Validity of localization around the node of Ranvier. *Histochemical Journal*, 1, 68–77.

Adams C. W. M., Bayliss, O. B. and Grant, R. T. (1969) Copper binding and cholinesterase activity around the node of Ranvier. *Journal of Histochemistry and Cytochemistry*, 17, 125–127.

Adams, C. W. M., Bayliss, O. B. and Ibrahim, M. Z. M. (1963) Modification to histochemical methods for phosphoglyceride and cerebroside. *Journal of Histochemistry and Cytochemistry*, 11, 560–561.

Adams, C. W. M., Bayliss, O. B., Hallpike, J. F. and Turner, D. R. (1971) Histochemistry of Myelin. XII. Anionic staining of myelin basic proteins for histology, electrophoresis and electronmicroscopy. *Journal of Neurochemistry*, 18, 389–394.

Adams, C. W. M., Csejtey, J., Hallpike, J. F. and Bayliss, O. B. (1972) Histochemistry of Myelin. XV. Changes in the myelin proteins of the peripheral nerve undergoing Wallerian degeneration – Electrophoretic and microdensitometric observations. *Journal of Neurochemistry*, 19, 2043–2048.

Adams, C. W. M. and Davison, A. N. (1959) The occurrence of esterified cholesterol in the developing nervous system. *Journal of Neurochemistry*, 4, 282–289.

Adams, C. W. M. and Davison, A. N. (1965) The Myelin Sheath. In *Neurohistochemistry*, (ed.) Adams, C. W. M. p. 332–400, Elsevier: London.

Adams, C. W. M., Davison, A. N. and Gregson, N. A. (1963) Enzyme inactivity of myelin: histochemical and biochemical evidence. *Journal of Neurochemistry*, 10, 383–395.

Adams, C. W. M. and Glenner, G. C. (1962) Histochemistry of Myelin, IV. Aminopeptidase activity in CNS and PNS. *Journal of Neurochemistry*, 9, 233–239.

Adams, C. W. M., Grant, R. T. and Bayliss, O. B. (1967) Cholinesterases in peripheral nervous system. I. Mixed, motor and sensory trunks. *Brain Research*, 5, 366–376.

Adams, C. W. M., Hallpike, J. F. and Bayliss, O. B. (1971) Histochemistry of Myelin. XIII. Digestion of basic protein outside acute plaques of multiple sclerosis. *Journal of Neurochemistry*, 18, 1479–1483.

Adams, C. W. M. and Leibowitz, S. (1969) The general pathology of demyelinating diseases. In *The Structure and Function of Nervous Tissue*. Vol. III, (ed.) Bourne, G. H. Chapter 8, Academic Press: New York.

Adams, C. W. M. and Tuqan, N. A. (1961a) Histochemistry of Myelin II. Proteins, lipid-protein dissociation and proteinase activity in Wallerian degeneration. *Journal of Neurochemistry*, 6, 334–341.

Adams, C. W. M. and Tuqan, N. A. (1961b) The histochemical demonstration of protease by a gelatin-silver film substrate. *Journal of Histochemistry and Cytochemistry*, 9, 469–472.

Allen, N. and de Veyra, E. (1967) Microchemical and histochemical observation in a case of Krabbe's leucodystrophy. *Journal of Neuropathology and Experimental Neurology*, 26, 456–474.

Altman, J. (1963) Regional utilization of leucine-H^3 by normal rat brain: microdensitometric evaluation of autoradiograms. *Journal of Histochemisty and Cytochemistry*, 11, 741–750.

Anderson, P. J. and Song, S. K. (1962) Acid phosphatase in the nervous system. *Journal of Neuropathology and Experimental Neurology*, 21, 263–283.

Andrade, C. (1952) *A peculiar form of peripheral neuropathy*, Brain, 75, 408–427.

Asbury, A. K. (1970) The histogenesis of phagocytes during Wallerian degeneration: radioautographic observation. *Proceedings VIth International Congress of Neuropathology*, 666–682. Masson: Paris.

Ballin, R. H. M. and Thomas, P. K. (1969) Changes at the node of Ranvier during Wallerian degeneration: an electronmicroscopic study. *Acta Neuropathologica (Berlin)*, 14, 237–249.

Banks, P. and Mayor, D. (1972) Intraaxonal transport in noradrenergic neurons in the sympathetic nervous system. *Biochemical Society Symposia*, 36, 133–149.

Barka, T. and Anderson, P. J. (1962) Histochemical methods for acid phosphatase using hexazonium pararosaniline as coupler. *Journal of Histochemistry and Cytochemistry*, 10, 741–753.

Barka, T. and Anderson, P. J. (1963) *Histochemistry: Theory, Practice and Bibliography*. p. 120, Hoeber and Row: New York.

Barron, K. D., Bernsohn J. and Hess, A. R. (1964) Zymograms of neural acid phosphatases. Implications for slide histochemistry. *Journal of Histochemistry and Cytochemistry*, **12**, 42–44.

Barron, K. D., Bernsohn, J. and Mitzen, E. (1972) Nonspecific esterases of human peripheral nerve and centrum ovale. *Journal of Neuropathology and Experimental Neurology*, **31**, 562–582.

Baronedes, S. H. (1967) Axoplasmic transport. *Neurosciences Research Program Bulletin*, **5**, 307–419.

Barton, A. A. (1962) An electron microscope study of degeneration and regeneration of nerve. *Brain*, **85**, 799–812.

Bayliss, O. B. (1972) Lipid histochemistry. Validity of techniques. M.Phil. Thesis (University of London).

Bayliss, O. B. and Adams, C. W. M. (1972) Bromine-Sudan Black: a general stain for lipids including free cholesterol. *Histochemical Journal*, **4**, 505–515.

Bayliss, O. B., Adams, C. W. M. and Hallpike, J. F. (1970) The PASDORO method for simultaneously demonstrating DNA and lipids in the brain. *Histochemical Journal*, **2**, 87–89.

Beck, C. S., Hasinoff, C. W. and Smith, M. E. (1968) L-alanyl-β-naphthylamidase in rat spinal cord myelin. *Journal of Neurochemistry*, **15**, 1297–1301.

Bencina, B., Carnegie, P. R., McPherson, T. A. and Robson, G. (1969) Encephalitogenic basic protein from sciatic nerve. *FEBS Letters*, **4**, 9–12.

Berry, J. F., Cevallos, W. H. and Wade, R. R. (1964) Lipid class and fatty acid composition of intact peripheral nerve during Wallerian degeneration. *Journal of American Oil Chemists' Society*, **42**, 492–500.

Berry, J. F. and Coonrad, J. D. 1967) Hydrolysis of nucleoside diphosphate esters in peripheral nerve during Wallerian degeneration. *Journal of Neurochemistry*, **14**, 245–255.

Bitensky, L. (1963) The reversible activation of lysosomes in normal cells and the effects of pathological conditions. *CIBA Symposium on Lysosomes*. p. 362–383, Churchill: London.

Block, R. J. (1951) A comparative study on two samples of neurokeratin. *Archives of Biochemistry*, **31**, 266–272.

Bloom, F. E. (1970) The fine structural localization of biogenic monoamines in nervous tissue. *International Review of Neurobiology*, **13**, 27–66.

Bodian, D. (1947) Nucleic acid in nerve-cell regeneration. *Society of Experimental Biology Symposia*, **1**, 163–178.

Bradley, W. G. and Williams, M. H. (1973) Axoplasmic flow in axonal neuropathies. *Brain*, **96**, 235–246.

Brady, R. O. (1972) Lipidoses. In *Handbook of Neurochemistry*, (ed.) Lajtha, A., Chapter 3, Plenum Press: New York.

Brady, R. O., Johnson, W. G. and Uhlendorf, B. W. (1971) Identification of heterozygous carriers of lipid storage diseases. *American Journal of Medicine*, **51**, 423–431.

Brunk, U. T. and Ericsson, J. L. E. (1973) Cytochemical evidence for the leakage of acid phosphatase through ultrastructurally intact lysosomal membranes. In *Fixation in Histochemistry*, (ed.) Stoward, P. J. p. 137–149, Chapman and Hall: London.

Brzin, M. (1966) The localization of acetylcholinesterase in axonal membranes of frog nerve fibres. *Proceedings of the National Academy of Science (Washington)*, **56**, 1560–1563.

Brzin, M., Tennyson, V. M. and Duffy, P. (1966) Acetylcholinesterase in frog sympathetic and dorsal root ganglia. A study by electron microscope, cytochemistry and microgasometric analysis with the magnetic diver. *Journal of Cell Biology*, **31**, 215–242.

Bubis, J. J. and Wolman, M. (1965) Hydrolytic enzymes in Wallerian degeneration. *Israel Journal of Medical Science*, **1**, 410–414.

Burstone, M. S. and Folk, J. E. (1956) Histochemical demonstration of aminopeptidase. *Journal of Histochemistry and Cytochemistry*, **4**, 217–226.

Burt, A. M. (1971) The histochemical localization of choline acetyltransferase. In *Histochemistry of Nervous Transmission, Progress in Brain Research*, **34**, 327–335.

Cain, A. J. (1950) The histochemistry of lipids in animals. *Biological Reviews*, **25**, 73–112.

Cavanagh, J. B. (1969) Toxic substances and the nervous system. *British Medical Bulletin*, **25**, 268–273.

Cavanagh, J. B., Thompson, R. H. S. and Webster, G. R. (1954) The localization of pseudo-cholinesterase activity in nervous tissue. *Quarterly Journal of Experimental Physiology*, **39**, 185–197.

Cavanagh, J. B. and Webster, G. R. (1955) On the changes in Ali-Esterase and Pseudo-cholinesterase activity of chicken sciatic nerve during Wallerian degeneration and their correlation with cellular proliferation. *Quarterly Journal of Experimental Physiology*, **40**, 12–23.

Citkowitz, E. and Holtzman, E. (1973) Peroxisomes in Dorsal Root Ganglia. *Journal of Histochemistry and Cytochemistry*, **21**, 34–41.

Clouet, D. H. and Welsch, H. (1961) Amino acid protein metabolism of the brain. VIII. The recovery of cholinesterase in the nervous system of the frog after inhibition. *Journal of Neurochemistry*, **8**, 201–215.

Coimbra, A. and Andrade, C. (1971a) Familial amyloid polyneuropathy: an electron microscope study of the peripheral nerve in five cases: I. Interstitial changes. *Brain*, **94**, 199–206.

Coimbra, A. and Andrade, C. (1971b) Familial amyloid polyneuropathy: an electron microscope study of the peripheral nerve in five cases. II. Nerve Fibre Changes. *Brain*, **94**, 207–212.

Cooper, J. R., Bloom, F. E. and Roth, R. H. (1970) *The biochemical basis of Pharmacology*. Oxford University Press: New York.

Csejtey, J., Hallpike, J. F., Adams, C. W. M. and Bayliss, O. B. (1972) Histochemistry of Myelin. XIV. Peripheral nerve myelin proteins: electrophoretic and histochemical correlation. *Journal of Neurochemistry*, **19**, 1931–1935.

Dahlström, A. (1971) Effects of vinblastine and colchicine on monoamine containing neurons of the rat, with special regard to the axoplasmic transport of amine granules. *Acta Neuropathologica (Berlin)*, Suppl. V, 226–237.

Dairman, W., Geffen, L. and Marchelle, M. (1973) Axoplasmic transport of aromatic L-amino acid decarboxylase (EC 4.1.1.26) and Dopamine-β-hydroxylase (EC 1.14.2.1) in rat sciatic nerve. *Journal of Neurochemistry*, **20**, 1617–1623.

Davison, A. N. (1970) The biochemistry of the myelin sheath. In *Myelination*, (ed.) Davison, A. N. and Peters, A. 80–161, C. C. Thomas: Springfield, Illinois.

Davison, A. N., Dobbing, J., Morgan, R. S. and Payling Wright, G. (1958) The deposition and disposal of $(4 - {}^{14}C)$ cholesterol in the brain of growing chickens. *Journal of Neurochemistry*, **3**, 89–94.

Davison, A. N., Morgan, R. S., Wajda, M. and Payling Wright, G. (1959) Metabolism of myelin lipids: incorporation of $(3 - {}^{14}C)$ serine in brain lipids of the developing rabbit and their persistence in the central nervous system. *Journal of Neurochemistry*, **4**, 360–365.

Dayan, A. D. (1967) Peripheral neuropathy of metachromatic leucodystrophy: observations on segmental demyelination and remyelination and the intracellular distribution of sulphatide. *Journal of Neurology, Neurosurgery and Psychiatry*, **30**, 311–318.

De Duve, C., Pressman, B. C., Gianetto, R., Wattiaux, R. and Appelmans, F. (1955) Tissue fractionation studies; intracellular distribution patterns of enzymes in rat-liver tissues. *Biochemical Journal*, **60**, 604–617.

De Duve, C. and Wattiaux, R. (1966) Function of lysosomes. *Annual Review of Physiology* **28**, 435–492.

Diessner, H. and Schmidt, R. M. (1972) Verhalten der proteolytischen Enzyme des Hirns bei der experimentellen allergischen Enzephalomyelitis. *Wien Zeitschrift Nervenheilkunde*, **30**, 213–221.

Diezel, P. B. (1958) Die metachromasie mit verchiedenen Farbstoffen im Mischlicht und im polarisierten Licht. *Acta Histochemica* (Jena), Suppl. I, 134–139.

Domonkos, J. and Heiner, L. (1968) Decomposition of phospholipids during Wallerian degeneration. *Journal of Neurochemistry*, **15**, 87–91.

Dunnigan, M. G. (1968a) Chromatographic separation and photometric analysis of the components of Nile blue sulphate. *Stain Technology*, **43**, 243–248.

Dunnigan, M. G. (1968b) The use of Nile blue sulphate in the histochemical identification of phospholipids. *Stain Technology*, **43**, 249–256.

Edström, A. (1966) Amino acid incorporation in isolated Mauthner nerve fibre components. *Journal of Neurochemistry*, **13**, 315–321.

Edström, A. and Edström, J-E. (1968) Identification and properties of RNA from Mauthner nerve fibre components of the goldfish. In *Macromolecules and the function of the Neuron*. (ed.) Lodin, Z. and Rose, S. P. R. p. 103–110. Excerpta Medica: Amsterdam.

Ehrlich, P. (1885) Das Sauerstufbedürfnis des Organismus. In *Eine Farbenanalytische Studie*. Berlin.

Einstein, E. R., Csejtey, J., Dalal, K. B., Adams, C. W. M., Bayliss, O. B. and Hallpike, J. F. (1972) Proteolytic activity and basic protein loss in and around multiple sclerosis plaques: combined biochemical and histochemical observations. *Journal of Neurochemistry*, 19, 653–662.

Einstein, E. R., Robertson, D. M., DiCaprio, J. M. and Moore, W. (1962) The isolation from bovine spinal cord of a homogeneous protein with encephalitogenic activity. *Journal of Neurochemistry*, 9, 353–361.

Elleder, M. and Lojda, Z. (1973) Studies in Lipid Histochemistry. XI. New, Rapid, Simple and Selective Methods for the Demonstration of Phospholipids. *Histochemie*, 36, 149–166.

El-Eishi, H. I. (1967) Biochemical and histochemical studies on myelination in the chick embryo spinal cord. *Journal of Neurochemistry*, 14, 405–412.

Emmenegger, H. and Ruge, W. M. (1968) The actions of Hydergine on the brain. *Pharmacology*, 1, 65–78.

Eng, L. F., Chao, F. C., Gerstl, B., Pratt, D. and Tavaststjerna, M. G. (1968) The maturation of human white matter myelin. Fractionation of the myelin membrane proteins. *Biochemistry*, 7, 4455–4465.

Engel, W. K., Dorman, J. D., Levy, R. I. and Fredrickson, D. S. (1967) Neuropathy of Tangier Disease. *Archives of Neurology (Chicago)*, 17, 1–9.

Eylar, E. H. (1972) Experimental allergic encephelomyelitis and multiple sclerosis. In *Multiple Sclerosis, Immunology, Virology and Ultrastructure*, (ed.) Wolfgram, F., Ellison, G. W., Stevens, J. G. and Andrews, J. M. Chapter 23, Academic Press: New York.

Falck, B., Hillarp, N.-Å., Thieme, G. and Torp, A. (1962) Fluorescence of catecholamines and related compounds condensed with formaldehyde. *Journal of Histochemistry and Cytochemistry*, 10, 348–354.

Fernández-Morán, H. and Finean, J. B. (1957) Electron microscope and low-angle X-ray diffraction studies of the nerve myelin sheath. *Journal of Biophysical and Biochemical Cytology*, 3, 725–748.

Finean, J. B. (1963) The nature and stability of lipid-protein-polysaccharide association in nerve myelin. In *Brain Lipids and Lipoproteins, and the Leucodystrophics*, p. 57–63. Elsevier: Amsterdam.

Finean, J. B. (1965) Molecular parameters in the nerve myelin sheath. *Annals of the New York Academy of Sciences*, 122, 51–56.

Finean, J. B. and Robertson, J. D. (1958) Lipids and the structure of myelin. *British Medical Bulletin*, 14, 267–273.

Folch, J. and Lees, M. (1951) Proteolipids, a new type of tissue lipoprotein: their isolation from brain. *Journal of Biological Chemistry*, 191, 807–817.

Fratello, B. (1968) Enhanced interpretation of tissue protease activity by use of photographic color film as a substrate. *Stain Technology*, 43, 125–128.

Fredrickson, D. S., Gotton, A. M. Jr. and Levy, R. I. (1972) Familial lipoprotein deficiency (abeta lipoproteinaemia, hypobetalipoproteinaemia, Tangier Disease). In *The Metabolic Basis of Inherited Disease*, 3rd Edition pp. 513–544, (ed.) Stanbury J. B., Wyngaarden, J. B. and Fredrickson, D. S. McGraw-Hill: New York.

Friede, R. L. (1966) *Topographic Brain Chemistry*. Academic Press: New York.

Friede, R. L. (1972) Control of Myelin Formation by Axon Caliber (with a model of the control mechanism). *Journal of Camparative Neurology*, 144, 233–252.

Friede, R. L. and Martinez, A. J. (1970) Analysis of axon-sheath relationships in early Wallerian degeneration. *Brain Research*, 19, 199–212.

Fullerton, P. M. (1964) Peripheral nerve conduction in metachromatic leucodystrophy (sulphatide lipidosis). *Journal of Neurology, Neurosurgery, and Psychiatry*, 27, 100–105.

Gabrielesco, E. (1969) Contributions to enzyme histochemistry of the experimental demyelination. *Review Roumanian Physiology*, 6, 45–54.

Gabrielesco, E., Stoenesco, L. and Bordeianu, A. (1966) Histochemical modifications of endopeptidase activity in the peripheral nerve during stimulation and recovery. *Annals of Histochemistry*, 11, 289–301.

Geffen, L. B. and Livett, B. G. (1971) Synaptic vesicles in sympathetic neurons. *Physiological Reviews*, 51, 98–157.

Gerebtzoff, M. A. (1963) Contribution histochemique à la théorie de la conduction saltatoire dans les fibre myélinisees périphériques et centrales. *Acta Neurologica et Phychiatrica Belgica*, 65, 7–21.

Gerebtzoff, M. A. (1964) Histoenzymologie de l'etranglement de Ranvier dans la fibre myelinisée périphérique normale et en dégénéresence. *Annals of Histochemistry*, 9, 209–216.

Geren, B. B. (1954) The formation from the Schwann cell surface of myelin in the peripheral nerves of chick embryos. *Experimental Cell Research*, 7, 558–562.

Gerstl, B., Eng. L. F., Tavaststjerna, M., Smith, J. K. and Kruse, S. L. (1970) Lipids and proteins in multiple sclerosis white matter. *Journal of Neurochemistry*, 17, 677–689.

Giacobini, E. (1969) Chemistry of isolated invertebrate neurons. In *Handbook of Neurochemistry*. (ed.) Lajtha, A. Vol. 2, Chapter 10, Plenum Press: New York.

Gilliatt, R. W. (1969) Experimental peripheral neuropathy. Lectures on the Scientific Basis of Medicine. British Postgraduate Medical Federation, pp. 202–219.

Glenner, G. C. (1965) Enzyme histochemistry. In *Neurohistochemistry*. (ed.) Adams, C. W. M. Chapter 4, Elsevier: Amsterdam.

Glimstedt, G. and Wohlfart, G. (1960–1961) Electron microscopic observations on Wallerian degeneration in peripheral nerves. *Acta Morphologica Neerlando-Scandinavica*, pp. 135–196.

Grant, R. T., Bayliss, O. B. and Adams, C. W. M. (1967) Cholinesterases in peripheral nervous system. II. The motor, sensory and sympathetic nerves in the rabbit ear perichondrium and rat cremasteric muscle. *Brain Research*, 6, 457–474.

Goldfischer, S. (1964) The Golgi apparatus and the endoplasmic reticulum in neurons of the rabbit. *Journal of Neuropathology and Experimental Neurology*, 23, 36–45.

Goldfischer, S., Essner, E. and Novikoff, A. B. (1964) The localization of phosphatase activities at the level of ultrastructure. *Journal of Histochemistry and Cytochemistry*, 12, 72–95.

Gombault, A. (1880–1881) Contribution a l'étude anatomique de la névrite parenchymateuse subaigue ou chronique. Névrite segmentaire péri-axile (suite). *Archives of Neurology (Paris)*, 1, 177–190.

Gomori, G. (1950) An improved histochemical technique for acid phosphatase. *Stain Technology*, 25, 81–85.

Gonzalez-Sastre, F. (1970) The protein composition of isolated myelin. *Journal of Neurochemistry*, 17, 1049–1056.

Gothlin, G F. (1913) Die doppelbrechenden Eigenschaften des Nervengewebes. *Kungliga Svenska ventenskapsakademiens handlingar*, 51, No. 1.

Gould, R. P. and Holt, S. J. (1961) Observations on acid phosphatase and esterases in the rat sciatic nerve undergoing Wallerian degeneration. *Proceedings of the Anatomical Society (Gt. Britain and Ireland)*, pp. 45–48.

Gutmann, E. and Holubář, J. (1950) The degeneration of peripheral nerve fibres. *Journal of Neurology, Neurosurgery and Psychiatry*, 13, 89–105.

Hagberg, B., Kollberg, H., Sourander, P. and Akessen, H. O. (1969) Infantile globoid cell leucodystrophy. *Neuropädiatrie*, 1, 74–88.

Hagberg, B., Sourander, P. and Thoren, L. (1962) Peripheral nerve changes in the diagnosis of metachromatic leucodystrophy. *Acta Paediatria supplement*, 135, 63–71.

Hall, S. M. and Gregson, N. A. (1971) The *in vivo* and ultrastructural effects of injection of lysophosphetidyl choline into myelinated peripheral nerve fibres of the adult mouse. *Journal of Cell Science*, 9, 769–789.

Hallpike, J. F. (1971) Proteolytic activity and basic protein loss in experimental myelin breakdown and multiple sclerosis. M.D. Thesis, London University.

Hallpike, J. F. (1972) Enzyme and protein changes in myelin breakdown and multiple sclerosis. *Progress in Histochemistry and Cytochemistry*, 3, 179–215.

Hallpike, J. F. and Adams, C. W. M. (1969a) Proteolytic enzymes in myelin breakdown. *Neuropatologie Polska*, 7, 225–231.

Hallpike, J. F. and Adams, C. W. M. (1969b) Proteolysis and myelin breakdown: a review of recent histochemical and biochemical studies. *Histochemical Journal*, **1**, 559–578.

Hallpike, J. F. and Adams, C. W. M. (1970) Proteolysis and the local pathogenesis of the multiple sclerosis lesion: histochemical and biochemical studies. *Proceedings VIth Congress of Neuropathology Masson, Paris*, pp. 487–488.

Hallpike, J. F., Adams, C. W. M. and Bayliss, O. B. (1970a) Proteolytic activity around multiple sclerosis plaques. *Histochemical Journal*, **2**, 199–208.

Hallpike, J. F., Adams, C. W. M. and Bayliss, O. B. (1970b) Histochemistry of myelin IX. Neutral and acid proteinases in early Wallerian degeneration. *Histochemical Journal*, **2**, 209–218.

Hallpike, J. F., Adams, C. W. M. and Bayliss, O. B. (1970c) Histochemistry of myelin. X. Proteolysis of normal myelin and release of lipid by extracts of degenerating nerve. *Histochemical Journal*, **2**, 315–321.

Hallpike, J. F., Adams, C. W. M. and Bayliss, O. B. (1970d) Histochemistry of myelin. XI. Loss of basic proteins in early myelin breakdown and multiple sclerosis plaques. *Histochemical Journal*, **2**, 323–328.

Hallpike, J. F. and McArdle, B. (1974) Inorganic pyrophosphatase (PP_iase) activity in nerve regeneration. *Excerpta Medica, Int. Congr. Ser.*, **334**, 39.

Hartmann, H. A., Lin, J. and Shively, M. C. (1968) RNA of nerve cell bodies and axons after beta-iminodiproprionitrile. *Acta Neuropathologica*, **11**, 275–281.

Heinzen, B. (1947) Acid phosphatase activity in transected sciatic nerves. *Anatomical Record*, **98**, 193–205.

Hendler, R. W. (1971) Biological membrane ultrastructure. *Physiological Reviews*, **51**, 66–97.

Hirano, A. and Dembitzer, H. M. (1967) A structural analysis of the myelin sheath in the central nervous system. *Journal of Cell Biology*, **34**, 555–567.

Hirsch, H. E. and Parks, M. E. (1973) The quantitative histochemistry of acid proteinase in the nervous system: localization in neurons. *Journal of Neurochemistry*, **21**, 453–458.

Hirsch, T. von, and Peiffer, J. (1955) Über Histologische Methoden in der differential diagnose von Leukodystrophien und Lipoidosen. *Archive fur Psychatrie und Nervenkrankheiten*, **194**, 88–104.

Hollinger, D. M., Rossiter, R. J. and Upmalis, H. (1952) Chemical studies of peripheral nerve during Wallerian degeneration. 4.Phosphatases. *Biochemical Journal*, **52**, 652–659.

Holt, S. J. (1959) Factors governing the validity of staining methods for enzymes and their bearing upon the Gomori Acid Phosphatase technique. *Experimental Cell Research*, Suppl. 7, 1–27.

Holt, S. J. and Withers, R. F. (1958) Studies on enzyme cytochemistry. V. An appraisal of indigogenic reaction for esterase localization. *Proceedings of the Royal Society of London (Series B)*, **148**, 520–532.

Holtzmann, E. and Novikoff, A. B. (1965) Lysosomes in the rat sciatic nerve following crush. *Journal of Cell Biology*, **27**, 651–669.

Houten, van, W. H. and Friede, R. L. (1964) A histochemical study of Wallerian degeneration. *Journal of Neuropathology and Experimental Neurology*, **23**, 165–166.

Hydén, H. (1967) Dynamic aspects of the Neuron-Glia relationship – A study with micro-chemical methods. In *The Neuron*, (ed.) Hydén, H. Chapter 4. Elsevier: Amsterdam.

Jacobs, J. M. (1967) Experimental diphtheritic neuropathy in the rat. *British Journal of Experimental Pathology*, **48**, 204–216.

Johnson, A. C., McNabb, A. R. and Rossiter, R. J. (1950) Chemistry of Wallerian Degeneration. *Archives of Neurology and Psychiatry*, **64**, 105–121.

Joseph, J. (1950) Further studies in changes of nuclear population in degenerating nonmyelinated and finely myelinated nerves. *Acta Anatomica (Basel)*, **9**, 279–288.

Karnovsky, M. J. and Roots, L. (1964) A 'direct-coloring' thiocholine method for cholinesterase. *Journal of Histochemistry and Cytochemistry*, **12**, 214–221.

Kása, P. (1971) Ultrastructural localization of choline acetyltransferase and acetylcholinesterase in central peripheral nervous tissue. In *Histochemistry of Nervous Transmission, Progress in Brain Research*, **34**, 337–344.

Kato, I. and Pappenheimer, A. M. (1960) An early effect of diphtheria toxin on the metabolism of mammalian cells growing in culture. *Journal of Experimental Medicine*, **112**, 329–349.

Kerekes, M. F., Feszt, T. and Kovacs, A. (1965) Catheptic activity in the cerebral tissue of the rabbit during allergic encephalomyelitis. *Experientia, Basel,* 21, 42–43.

Kies, M. W., Murphy, J. B. and Alford, E. C. (1961) Studies on the encephalitogenic factor in guinea pig central nervous system. In *Chemical Pathology of the Nervous System,* (ed.) Folch-Pi, J. pp. 197–204, Pergamon Press: Oxford.

Kocen, R. S., King, R. H. M., Thomas, P. K. and Haas, L. F. (1973) Nerve biopsy findings in two cases of Tangier Disease. *Acta Neuropathologica (Berlin),* 26, 317–327.

Kocen, R. S., Lloyd, J. K., Lascelles, P. T., Fosbrooke, A. S. and Williams, D. (1967) Familial alpha-lipoprotein deficiency (Tangier Disease) with neurological abnormalities. *Lancet,* i, 1341–1345.

Kocen, R. S. and Thomas, P. K. (1970) Peripheral nerve involvement in Fabry's disease. *Archives of Neurology,* 22, 81–88.

Koelle, G. B. and Friedenwald, J. S. (1949) A histochemical method for localizing cholinesterase activity. *Proceedings of the Society for Experimental Biology,* (New York), 70, 617–622.

Koenig, E. (1965) Synthetic mechanisms in the axon. II. RNA in myelin-free axons of the cat. *Journal of Neurochemistry,* 12, 357–361.

Koenig, E. (1969) Nucleic acid and protein metabolism of the axon. In *Handbook of Neurochemistry,* (ed.) Lajtha, A. Vol. II, Plenum Press: New York.

Koenig, E. and Koelle, G. B. (1960) Acetylcholinesterase regeneration in peripheral nerve after irreversible inactivation. *Science,* 132, 1249–1250.

Koenig, H. (1962) Histological distribution of brain gangliosides; lysosomes as glycoprotein granules. *Nature (London),* 195, 782–784.

Koenig, H. (1969) 'Lysosomes'. In *Handbook of Neurochemistry,* (ed.) Lajtha, A. Vol. II, Chapter 12, Plenum Press: New York.

Korhonen, L. K. (1966) Studies on the histochemical demonstration of inorganic pyrophosphatase activity. *Annals Academiae Scientiarum Fennicae,* 124, 5–65.

Kornberg, A. (1962) On the metabolic significance of phosphorolytic and pyrophosphorolytic reactions. In *Horizon in Biochemistry,* (ed.) Kasha, M. and Pullman, B. Academic Press, New York.

Kornguth, S. E. and Anderson, J. W. (1965) Localization of a basic protein in the myelin of various species with the aid of fluorenscence and electronmicroscopy. *Journal of Cell Biology,* 26, 157–166.

Krasnov, I. B. (1973) Flurimetric determination of creatine kinase activity in isolated single neurons. *Journal of Histochemistry and Cytochemistry,* 21, 568–571.

Kreutzberg, G. (1964) Das Verhalten oxydativer Enzyme in peripheren Nerven bei der sekundären Degeneration. *Archiv für Psychiatrie und Nervenkrankheiten,* 206, 281–292.

Kristensson, K. and Olsson, Y. (1973) Diffusion pathways and retrograde axonal transport of protein tracers in peripheral nerves. *Progress in Neurobiology,* 1, 85–109.

Kristensson, K., Olsson, Y. and Sourander, P. (1967) Peripheral nerve changes in Tay-Sachs and Batten-Spielmeyer-Vogt Disease. *Acta Pathologia et Microbiologica Scandinavica,* 70, 630–632.

Kurihara, T. and Tsukada, Y. (1967) The regional and subcellular distribution of 2',3'-cyclic nucleatide 3'-phosphohydrolase in the central nervous system. *Journal of Neurochemistry,* 14, 1167–1174.

Lake, B. P. (1968) Segmental demyelination of peripheral nerves in Krabbe's Disease. *Nature (London),* 217, 171–172.

Lampert, P. W. and Schochet, S. S. (1968) Demyelination and remyelination in Lead Neuropathy. *Journal of Neuropathology and Experimental Neurology,* 27, 527–545.

Langley, O. K. and Landon, D. N. (1968) A light and electron histochemical approach to the node of Ranvier and myelin of peripheral nerve fibres. *Journal of Histochemistry and Cytochemistry,* 15, 722–731.

Lansink, A. G. W. (1968) Thin layer chromatography and histochemistry of Sudan black. *Histochemie,* 16, 68–84.

LeBaron, F. N. and Folch, J. (1956) The isolation from brain tissue of a trypsin-resistant protein fraction containing combined inositol and its relation to neurokeratin. *Journal of Neurochemistry,* 1, 101–108.

LeBlond, C. P. and Amano, M. (1962) Synthetic processes in the cell nucleus. IV. Synthetic activity in the nucleolus as compared to that in the rest of the cell. *Journal of Histochemistry and Cytochemistry,* **10**, 162–174.

Lees, M. B., Messinger, B. F. and Burnham, J. D. (1967) Tryptic hydrolysis of brain proteolipid. *Biochemical and Biophysical Research Communications,* **28**, 185–190.

Lehner, T. and Adams, C. W. M. (1968) Lipid histochemistry of Fabry's Disease. *Journal of Pathology and Bacteriology,* **95**, 411–415.

Lieberman, A. R. (1971) The axon reaction: a review of the principal features of perikaryal responses to axon injury. *International Review of Neurobiology,* **14**, 49–124.

Lillie, R. D. and Ashburn, L. L. (1943) Supersaturated solution of fat stain in dilute isopropanol for demonstration of acute, fatty degeneration not shown by Herzheimer's technique. *Archives of Pathology,* **36**, 432–435.

Livett, B. G. (1973) Histochemical visualization of peripheral and central adrenergic neurones. *British Medical Bulletin,* **29**, 93–99.

Logan, J. E., Mannell, W. A. and Rossiter, R. J. (1952) Chemical studies of peripheral nerve during Wallerian degeneration. 3.Nucleic acids and other protein-bound phospherous compounds. *Biochemical Journal,* **51**, 482–487.

Lubińska, L. (1964) Axoplasmic streaming in regenerating and in normal nerve fibres. *Progress in Brain Research,* **13**, 1–71.

Lubińska, L., Niemierko, S., Oderfeld-Nowak, B. and Szwarc, L. (1963) The distribution of acetylcholinesterase in peripheral nerves. *Journal of Neurochemistry,* **10**, 25–41.

Lubińska, L., Niemierko, S., Oderfeld-Nowak, B. and Szwarc, L. (1964) Behaviour of acetylcholinesterase in isolated nerve segments. *Journal of Neurochemistry,* **11**, 493–503.

Lundberg, G., Nordborg, C., Rydevik, B. and Olssen, Y. (1973) The effect of ischaemia on the permeability of perineurium to protein tracers in rabbit tibial nerves. *Acta Neurologica Scandinavica,* **49**, 287–294.

McCamen, R. E. and Robins, E. (1959a) Quantitative biochemical studies of Wallerian degeneration in the peripheral and central nervous systems. I. Chemical constituents. *Journal of Neurochemistry,* **5**, 18–31.

McCamen, R. E. and Robins, E. (1959b) Quantitative biochemical studies of Wallerian degeneration in the peripheral and central nervous systems. II. Twelve enzymes. *Journal of Neurochemistry,* **5**, 32–42.

McDonald, W. I. (1963) The effects of experimental demyelination on conduction in peripheral nerve: a histological and electrophysical study. *Brain,* **86**, 481–500.

Marchbanks, R. M. (1967) Compartmentation of acetylcholine in synaptosomes. *Biochemical Pharmacology,* **16**, 921–923.

Marchi, V. (1886) Sulle Degenerazioni Consecutive All' Estirtazione Totale E Parziale Del Cervelletto. *Rivista Sperimentale di Freniatria e Medicina Legale Della Alienazioni Mentali,* **12**, 50–56.

Margolis, R. U. (1968) Glycoproteins in Myelin. *Journal of Histochemistry and Cytochemistry,* **16**, 486.

Marks, N. and Lajtha, A. (1963) Protein breakdown in the brain: subcellular distribution and properties of neutral and acid proteinases. *Biochemical Journal,* **89**, 438–447.

Marks, N. and Lajtha, A. (1965) Separation of acid and neutral proteinases of brain. *Biochemical Journal,* **97**, 74–83.

Marks, N., Datta, R. K. and Lajtha, A. (1970) Distribution of amino acids and of exo- and endopeptidases along vertebrate and invertebrate nerves. *Journal of Neurochemistry,* **17**, 53–63.

Matheson, D. F. and Cavanagh, J. B. (1967) Protein synthesis in peripheral nerve and susceptibility to diphtheritic neuropathy. *Nature (London),* **214**, 721–722.

Means, E. D. and Barron, K. D. (1972) Histochemical and histological studies of axon reaction in feline motorneurons. *Journal of Neuropathology and Experimental Neurology,* **31**, 221–246.

Mehl, E. and Halaris, A. (1970) Stoichometric relation of protein components in cerebral myelin from different species. *Journal of Neurochemistry,* **17**, 659–668.

Mellick, R. and Cavanagh, J. B. (1967) Longitudinal movement of radio-iodinated albumin within extravascular spaces of peripheral nerves following three systems of experimental trauma. *Journal of Neurology, Neurosurgery and Psychiatry,* **30**, 458–463.

Mellick, R. S. and Cavanagh, J. B. (1968) Changes in blood vessel permeability during degeneration and regeneration in peripheral nerves. *Brain,* 91, 141—160.

Mezei, C. (1970) Cholesterol esters and hydrolytic cholesterol esterase during Wallerian degeneration. *Journal of Neurochemistry,* 17, 1163—1170.

Miani, N., Cavallotti, C. and Caniglia, A. (1969) Synthesis of adenosine triphosphate by myelin of spinal nerves of rabbit. *Journal of Neurochemistry,* 16, 249—260.

Mitzen, E., Barron, K. D. and Koeppen, A. (1971) Absorption of enzymes to myelin of human central nervous system. *Journal of Histochemistry and Cytochemistry,* 19, 718.

Morgan-Hughes, J. A. (1965) Diphtheritic polyneuropathy in the guinea pig. Cambridge University, M.D. Thesis.

Morgan-Hughes, J. A. and Engel, W. K. (1968) Structural and histochemical changes in the axons following nerve crush. *Archives of Neurology,* 19, 598—612.

Morris, J. H., Hudson, A. R. and Weddell, G. (1972) A study of degeneration and regeneration in the divided rat sciatic nerve based on electron microscopy. I. The traumatic degeneration of myelin in the proximal stump of the divided nerve. *Zeitschrift für Zellforschung,* 124, 76—102.

Morris, J. H., Hudson, A. R. and Weddell, G. (1972) A study of degeneration and regeneration in the divided rat sciatic nerve based on electron microscopy. II. The development of the 'regenerating unit'. *Zeitschrift für Zellforschung,* 124, 103—130.

Moss, D. W. (1974) Multiple forms of alkaline phosphatase: some topics of current interest. *Histochemical Journal,* 6, 353—360.

Nachmansohn, D. (1971) Proteins in Bioelectricity. Acetylcholine-Esterase and Receptor. In *Principles of Receptor Physiology,* (ed.) Loewenstein, W. R. 18—102. Springer-Verlag: Berlin.

Nandy, K. (1968) Histochemical study on chromatolytic neurons. *Archives of Neurology,* 18, 425—434.

Neil, M. W. and Horner, M. W. (1964) Studies on acid hydrolases in adult and foetal tissues. *Biochemical Journal,* 92, 217—224.

Niemierko, S. and Lubińska, L. (1967) Two fractions of axonal acetylcholinesterase exhibiting different behaviour in severed nerves. *Journal of Neurochemistry,* 14, 761—769.

Noback, C. R. (1953) The protagon (π) granules of Reich. *Journal of Comparative Neurology,* 99, 91—101.

Noback, C. R. and Montagna, W. (1952) Histochemical studies of the myelin sheath and its fragmentation products during Wallerian (secondary) degeneration. I. Lipids. *Journal of Comparative Neurology,* 97, 211—232.

Norberg, K. A. (1967) Transmitter histochemistry of the sympathetic adrenergic nervous system. *Brain Research,* 5, 125—170.

Norman, R. M., Urich, H. and Tingey, A. H. (1960) Metachromatic Leuco-encephalopathy: A form of Lipidosis. *Brain,* 83, 369—380.

Norton, W. T. (1971) Recent Developments in the Investigation of Purified Myelin. In *Chemistry and Brain Development,* (ed.) Paoletti, R. and Davison, A. N. 327—337, Plenum Press: New York.

Novikoff, A. B. (1959) Enzyme Cytochemistry: pitfalls in the current use of tetrazolium techniques. *Journal of Histochemistry and Cytochemistry,* 7, 301—302.

Novikoff, A. B. (1967a) Enzyme Localization and Ultrastructure of Neurons. In *The Neuron,* (ed.) Hydén, H. Chapter 6. Elsevier: Amsterdam.

Novikoff, A. B. (1967b) Lysosomes in nerve cells. In *The Neuron,* (ed.) Hydén, H. Chapter 7. Elsevier: Amsterdam.

Novikoff, A. B., Drucker, I., Shin, W-Y. and Goldfischer, S. (1961) Further studies of the apparent adenosine-triphosphatase activity of cell membranes in formal-calcium-fixed tissues. *Journal of Histochemistry and Cytochemistry,* 9, 934—951.

Novikoff, A. B. and Essner, E. (1962) Pathological changes in cytoplasmic organelles. *Federation Proceedings,* 21, 1130—1142.

Novikoff, A. B. and Goldfischer, S. (1961) Nucleosidediphosphatase activity in the Golgi apparatus and its usefulness for cytological studies. *Proceedings of the National Academy of Science,* 47, 802—810.

Olafson, R. W., Drummond, G. I. and Lee, J. F. (1969) Studies on 2′,3′,-cyclic nucleotide-3′-phosphohydrolase from brain. *Canadian Journal of Biochemistry,* **47,** 961–966.

Olderfeld-Nowak, B. and Niemierko, S. (1969) Synthesis of nucleic acids in the Schwann cells as the early cellular response to nerve injury. *Journal of Neurochemistry,* **16,** 235–248.

Olsson, Y. (1966) Studies on Vascular Permeability in Peripheral Nerves. I. Distribution of circulating fluorescent serum albumin in normal, crushed and sectioned rat sciatic nerve. *Acta Neuropathologica,* **7,** 1–15.

Olsson, Y. (1967) Degranulation of mast cells in peripheral nerve injuries. *Acta Neurologica Scandinavica,* **43,** 365–374.

Olsson, Y. (1968) Mast Cells in the Nervous System. *International Review of Cytology,* **24,** 27–70.

Olsson, Y. (1971) Studies on vascular permeability in peripheral nerves. IV. Distribution of intravenously injected protein tracers in the peripheral nervous system of various species. *Acta Neuropathologica (Berlin),* **17,** 114–126.

Olsson, Y. and Kristensson, K. (1973) The perineurium as a diffusion barrier to protein tracers following trauma to nerves. *Acta Neuropathologica (Berlin),* **23,** 105–111.

Olsson, Y., Kristensson, K. and Klatzo, I. (1971) Permeability of blood vessels and connective tissue sheaths in the peripheral nervous system to exogenous proteins. *Acta Neuropathologica (Berlin),* Supplement V, 61–69.

Olsson, Y. and Reese, T. S. (1969) Inaccessibility of the endoneurium of mouse sciatic nerve to exogenous protein. *Anatomical Record,* **163,** 318–319.

Olsson, Y. and Reese, T. S. (1971) Permeability of vasa nervorum and perineurium in mouse sciatic nerve studied by fluorescence and electron microscopy. *Journal of Neuropathology and Experimental Neurology,* **30,** 195–221.

Olsson, Y. and Sjöstrand, J. (1969) Origin of macrophages in Wallerian degeneration of nerves demonstrated autoradiographically. *Experimental Neurology,* **23,** 102–112.

Olsson, Y. and Sourander, P. (1969) The reliability of the diagnosis of metachromatic leucodystrophy by peripheral nerve biopsy. *Acta Paediatrica Scandinavica,* **58,** 15–24.

Orrego, F. (1971) Protein degradation in squid giant axons. *Journal of Neurochemistry,* **18,** 2244–2254.

Padykula, H. A. and Herman, E. (1955a) Factors affecting the activity of adenosine triphosphatase and other phosphatases as measured by histochemical techniques. *Journal of Histochemistry and Cytochemistry,* **3,** 161–169.

Padykula, H. A. and Herman, E. (1955b) The specificity of the histochemical method for adenosine triphosphatase. *Journal of Histochemistry and Cytochemistry,* **3,** 170–195.

Palay, S. L. and Palade, G. E. (1955) The fine structure of neurons. *Journal of Biophysical and Biochemical Cytology,* **1,** 69–88.

Penn, A., Gledhill, B. L. and Darzynkiewicz, Z. (1972) Modification of the gelatin substrate procedure for demonstration of acrosomal proteolytic activity. *Journal of Histochemistry and Cytochemistry,* **20,** 499–506.

Pinner, B. and Campbell, J. B. (1965) Alkaline phosphatase activity of incisures and nodes during degeneration and regeneration of peripheral nerve fibres. *Experimental Neurology,* **12,** 159–172.

Pinner, B., Davison, J. F. and Campbell, J. B. (1964) Alkaline phosphatase in peripheral nerves. *Science,* **145,** 936–938.

Poole, A. R., Dingle, J. T. and Barrett, A. J. (1972) The immunocytochemical demonstration of cathepsin D. *Journal of Histochemistry and Cytochemistry,* **20,** 261–265.

Porcellati, G. (1965) Biochemical aspects of protein metabolism during nerve degeneration and regeneration. In *Protides of the Biological Fluids,* (ed.) Peeters, H. p. 115–126. Elsevier: Amsterdam.

Porcellati, G. (1969) Peripheral Nerve. In *Handbook of Neurochemistry,* (ed.) Lajtha, A. Chapter 16, Plenum Press: New York.

Porcellati, G. and Curti, B. (1960) Proteinase activity of peripheral nerves during Wallerian degeneration. *Journal of Neurochemistry,* **5,** 277–282.

Porcellati, G. and Thompson, R. H. S. (1957) Effects of nerve section on the free amino acids of nervous tissue. *Journal of Neurochemistry,* **1,** 340–347.

Prescott, D. M. (1962) Synthetic processes in the cell nucleus. II. Nucleic acid and protein metabolism in the macronuclei of two ciliated protozoa. *Journal of Histochemistry and Cytochemistry*, **10**, 145–153.

Resibois, A., Tondeur, M., Mockel, S. and Dustin, P. (1970) Lysosomes and storage diseases. *International Review of Experimental Pathology*, **9**, 93–149.

Riekkinen, P. J. and Clausen, J. (1969) Proteinase activity of myelin. *Brain Research*, **15**, 413–430.

Riekkinen, P. J., Clausen, J. and Arstila, A. U. (1970) Further studies on neutral proteinase activity of central nervous system myelin. *Brain Research*, **19**, 213–227.

Riekkinen, P. J., Palo, J., Arstila, A. U., Savolainen, H. J., Rinne, U. K., Kivalo, E. K. and Frey, H. (1971) Protein composition of multiple sclerotic myelin. *Archives of Neurology*, **24**, 545–549.

Robertis, E. de and Arnaiz, G. R. de L. (1969) Structural components of the synaptic region. In *Handbook of Neurochemistry*, (ed.) Lajtha, A. Vol. 2, Chapter 15, Plenum Press: New York.

Robertson, J. D. (1955) The ultrastructure of adult vertebrate peripheral nerve fibres in relation to myelinogenesis. *Journal of Biophysical and Biochemical Cytology*, **1**, 271–278.

Roodyn, D. B. (1967) The Mitochondrion. In *Enzyme Cytology*, (ed.) Roodyn, D. B. p. 103–180. Academic Press: London.

Rossiter, R. J. (1955) Biochemistry of demyelination. In *Neurochemistry*, 1st Ed. 696–714, (ed.) Elliott, K. A. C., Page, I. H. and Quastel, J. H. C. C. Thomas: Springfield, Illinois.

Samorajski, T. (1957) Changes in phosphatase activity following transection of the sciatic nerve. *Journal of Histochemistry and Cytochemistry*, **5**, 15–32.

Sawyer, C. H. (1946) Cholinesterases in degenerating and regenerating peripheral nerves. *American Journal of Physiology*, **146**, 246–253.

Schlaepfer, W. W. and Torack, R. M. (1966) The ultrastructural localization of cholinesterase activity in the sciatic nerve of the rat. *Journal of Histochemistry and Cytochemistry*, **14**, 369–378.

Schmidt, W. J. (1936) Doppelbrechung und Feinbau der Markscheide der Nervenfasern. *Zeitschrift für Zellforschung und Mikroskopische Anatomie*, **23**, 657–676.

Schmitt, F. O. and Bear, R. S. (1939) The ultrastructure of the nerve axon sheath. *Biological Reviews*, **14**, 27–50.

Schnabel, R. and Sir, G. (1962) Histochemische untersuchnugen über die π-Granula (Reich) der peripheren markhaltigen Nervenfasern. *Zeitschrift für Zellforschung*, **56**, 1–19.

Schubert, M. and Hamerman, D. (1956) Metachromasia: chemical theory and histochemical use. *Journal of Hisotchemistry and Cytochemistry*, **4**, 159–189.

Scott, T. G. (1967) The distribution of 5′ Nucleotidase in the brain of the mouse. *Journal of Comparative Neurology*, **129**, 97–114.

Shanthaveerappa, T. R. and Bourne, G. H. (1965) The thiaminepyrophosphatase technique as an indicator of the morphology of the Golgi apparatus in the neurons. *Zeitschrift für Zellforschung*, **68**, 699–710.

Shelansky, M. L. (1973) Chemistry of the filaments and tubules of brain. *Journal of Histochemistry and Cytochemistry*, **21**, 529–539.

Shooter, E. M. and Einstein, E. R. (1971) Proteins of the Nervous System. *Annual Review of Biochemistry*, **40**, 635–652.

Simon, G. (1966) Cholesterol ester in degenerating nerve: origin of cholesterol moiety. *Lipids*, **1**, 369–370.

Singer, M. (1968) Penetration of labelled amino acids into the peripheral nerve fibre from surrounding body fluids. In *Growth of the Nervous System*, (ed.) Wolstenholme, G. E. W. and O'Conner, M. 200–215, Churchill: London.

Sjöstrand, J. and Karlsson, J. O. (1969) Axoplasmic transport in the optic nerve and tract of the rabbit: a biochemical and radioautographic study. *Journal of Neurochemistry*, **16**, 833–844.

Smith, M. E. (1967) The metabolism of myelin lipids. *Advances in Lipid Research*, **5**, 241–278.

Smith, M. E. and Eng, L. F. (1965) The turnover of the lipid components of myelin. *Journal of the American Oil Chemists' Society*, **42**, 1013–1018.

Smith, M. E. and Hasinoff, C. M. (1971) Biosynthesis of myelin proteins in vitro. *Journal of Neurochemistry*, **18**, 739–747.

Snell, R. S. (1957) Histochemical appearance of cholinesterase in the normal sciatic nerve and the changes which occur after nerve section. *Nature,* 180, 378–379.

Sourander, P. and Olsson, Y. (1968) Peripheral neuropathy in globoid cell leucodystrophy (Morbus Krabbe). *Acta Neuropathologica,* 11, 69–81.

Suzuki, K. (1972) Neurochemical aspects of mucopolysaccharidoses. In *Handbook of Neurochemistry,* (ed.) Lajtha, A. Vol. 7, Chapter 2, Plenum Press: New York.

Swank, R. L. and Davenport, H. A. (1935) Chlorate-Osmic Formalin Method for staining Degenerating Myelin. *Stain Technology,* 10, 87–90.

Sylvén, B. (1968) Studies on the Histochemical 'Leucine Aminopeptidase' reaction. VI. The selective demonstration of cathespin B activity by means of the naphthylamide reaction. *Histochemie,* 15, 150–159.

Terry, R. D. and Harkin, J. C. (1959) Wallerian degeneration and regeneration of peripheral nerves. In *The Biology of Myelin,* (ed.) Korey, S. R. pp. 303–320. Cassell: London.

Tewari, H. and Bourne, G. H. (1960) Neurokeratin network of the peripheral nerve fibre myelin sheath as a centre of metabolic activity. *Nature (London),* 186, 645–646.

Thé de, G. (1968) Ultrastructural cytochemistry of the cellular membranes. In *Ultrastructure in Biological Systems* (ed.) Dalton, A. J. and Haguenan, F. Vol. 4, 121–150. Academic Press: New York.

Thieffry, S. and Lyon, G. (1959) Diagnostic d'un cas de leucodystrophie métachromatique (type Scholz) par la biopsie d'un nerf périphérique. *Revue Neurologique,* 100, 452–456.

Thomas, P. K. (1970) The cellular response to nerve injury. 3. The effects of repeated crush injuries. *Journal of Anatomy,* 106, 463–470.

Thomas, P. K. and Lascelles, R. G. (1967) Hypertrophic neuropathy. *Quarterly Journal of Medicine,* 36, 223–238.

Thomas, P. K. and Walker, J. G. (1965) Xanthomatous neuropathy in primary biliary cirrhosis. *Brain,* 88, 1079–1088.

Tomonaga, M. and Sluga, E. (1970) Zur Ultrastruktur der π-Granula. *Acta neuropathologica (Berlin),* 15, 56–69.

Torack, R. M. (1965) Electron histochemistry of the nervous system. In *Neurohistochemistry,* (ed.) Adams, C. W. M. 161–188. Elsevier: Amsterdam.

Tuqan, N. A. and Adams, C. W. M. (1961) Histochemistry of Myelin I, Proteins and lipid-protein complexes in the normal sheath. *Journal of Neurochemistry,* 6, 327–333.

Urbanova, D. and Adams, C. W. M. (1970) Extraction of lipids from tissue sections with acetone: further qualitative and quantitative observations. *Histochemical Journal,* 2, 1–9.

Vandenheuvel, F. A. (1965) Study of biological structure at the molecular level with stereomodel projection. II. The structure of myelin in relation to other membrane systems. *Journal of American Oil Chemists' Society,* 42, 481–492.

Vial, J. D. (1958) The early changes in the axoplasm during Wallerian degeneration. *Journal of Biophysical and Biochemical Cytology,* 4, 551–555.

Vrba, R. and Cannon, W. (1970) Assimilation of glucose in rat brain and metabolic activities of various groups of brain proteins. In *Protein Metabolism of the Nervous System,* (ed.) Lajtha, A. p. 219–237, Plenum Press: New York.

Wachstein, M. and Meisel, E. (1957) Histochemistry of hepatic phosphatases at a physiologic pH. *American Journal of Clinical Pathology,* 27, 13–23.

Waelsch, H., Sperry, W. M. and Stoyanoff, V. A. (1940) Lipid metabolism in brain during myelination. *Journal of Biological Chemistry,* 135, 297–302.

Waksman, B. H. (1961) Experimental study of diphtheritic polyneuritis in the rabbit and guinea pig. III. The blood nerve barrier in the rabbit. *Journal of Neuropathology and Experimental Neurology,* 20, 35–77.

Waksman, B. H., Adams, R. D. and Mansmann, H. C. (1957) Experimental study of diphtheritic polyneuritis in the rabbit and guinea pig. *Journal of Experimental Medicine,* 105, 591–614.

Webster, G. R. (1973) Phospholipase A activities in normal and sectioned rat sciatic nerve. *Journal of Neurochemistry,* 21, 873–876.

Webster, G. R. and Folch, J. (1961) Some studies on the properties of proteolipids. *Biochimica et Biophysica Acta,* 49, 399–401.

Webster, H. de F. (1962a) Transient focal accumulation of axonal mitochondria during the early stages of Wallerian degeneration. *Journal of Cell Biology,* 12, 361–377.

Webster, H. de F. (1962b) Schwann cell alteration in metachromatic leucodystrophy: preliminary phase and electron microscopic observations. *Journal of Neuropathology and Experimental Neurology*, **21**, 534–541.

Webster, H. de F. (1964) Some ultrastructural features of segmental demyelination and myelin regeneration in peripheral nerve. *Progress in Brain Research*, **13**, 151–174.

Weiss, P. A. and May, R. R. (1971) Neuronal organelles in neuroplasmic ('axonal') flow. *Acta Neuropathologica (Berlin)*, Suppl. 5, 198–206.

Weller, R. O. (1965) Diphtheritic neuropathy in the chicken: an electron microscope study. *Journal of Pathology and Bacteriology*, **89**, 591–598.

Weller, R. O. (1967) Cytochemistry of lipids in atherosclerosis. *Journal of Pathology and Bacteriology*, **94**, 171–182.

Weller, R. O. and Herzog, I. (1970) Schwann cell lysosomes in hypertrophic neuropathy and in normal human nerves. *Brain*, **93**, 347–356.

Weller, R. O. and Mellick, R. S. (1966) Acid phosphatase and lysomal activity in diptheritic neuropathy and Wallerian degeneration. *British Journal of Experimental Pathology*, **47**, 425–434.

Weller, R. O. and Nester, B. (1972) Early changes at the node of Ranvier in Segmental Demyelination. Histochemical and electron microscopical observations. *Brain*, **95**, 665–674.

Werb, Z. and Cohn, Z. A. (1972) Cholesterol metabolism in the macrphage. III. Ingestion and intracellular fate of cholesterol and cholesterol esters. *Journal of Experimental Medicine*, **135**, 21–44.

Whittaker, V. P. (1966) Some properties of synaptic membrane isolated from the central nervous system. *Annals of the New York Academy of Sciences*, **137**, 982–998.

Whittaker, V. P. (1969a) The subcellular fractionation of nervous tissue. In *The Structure and Function of Nervous Tissue*, (ed.) Bourn, G. H. Vol. III, Chapter 1. Academic Press: New York.

Whittaker, V. P. (1969b) The Synaptosome. In *Handbook of Neurochemistry*, (ed.) Lajtha, A. Vol. II, Chapter 14. Plenum Press: New York.

Williams, P. L. and Hall, S. M. (1971) Chronic Wallerian degeneration – an in vivo and ultrastructural study. *Journal of Anatomy*, **109**, 487–503.

Williams, P. L. and Landon, D. N. (1963) Paranodal apparatus of peripheral myelinated nerve fibres of mammals. *Nature (London)*, **198**, 670–673.

Williams, P. L. and Landon, D. N. (1964) The energy source of the nerve fibre. *New Scientist*, No. 374, 166–169.

Wolfgram, F. (1966) A new proteolipid fraction of the nervous system. I. Isolation and aminoacid analysis. *Journal of Neurochemistry*, **13**, 461–470.

Wolfgram, F. and Kotorii, K. (1968) The composition of the myelin proteins of the peripheral nervous system. *Journal of Neurochemistry*, **15**, 1291–1295.

Wolfgram, F. and Rose, A. S. (1960) The histochemistry of neurokeratin in normal and degenerating sciatic nerve. *Neurology* (Mineap.), **10**, 365–371.

Wolman, M. (1968) Histochemistry of Demyelination and Myelination. *Journal of Histochemistry and Cytochemistry*, **16**, 803–807.

Wolman, M. (1962) Extraction of complexes from central and peripheral myelin of man. *Journal of Neurochemistry*, **9**, 59–62.

Wolman, M. (1971) Distribution of various protein fractions in central and peripheral myelin. *Experimental Neurology*, **30**, 309–323.

Wolman, M. (1971) Amyloid, Its nature and molecular structure. *Laboratory Investigation*, **25**, 104–110.

Wolman, M. and Hestrin-Lerner, S. (1960) A histochemical contribution to the study of molecular morphology of the myelin sheath. *Journal of Neurochemistry*, **5**, 114–120.

Wood, J. G. and Dawson, R. M. C. (1973) A major myelin glycoprotein of sciatic nerve. *Journal of Neurochemistry*, **21**, 717–719.

Wooten, G. F. and Coyle, J. T. (1973) Axonal transport of catecholamine synthesizing and metabolizing enzymes. *Journal of Neurochemistry*, **20**, 1361–1371.

Young, J. Z. (1948) Growth and differentiation of nerve fibres. *Symposia of the Society for Experimental Biology*, **2**, 57–74.

Zalin, A., Darby, A., Vaughan, S. and Raftery, E. B. (1974) Primary neuropathic amyloidosis in three brothers. *British Medical Journal*, i, 65–66.

13 PATHOLOGY OF THE PERIPHERAL NERVE

G. Allt

13.1 Introduction

The study of the pathology of peripheral nerves illuminates not only human disease processes, but also fundamental properties of the peripheral nerve. This approach is especially pertinent to studies of the axon-Schwann cell relationship. It is now apparent that normal function of the peripheral nerve fibre is greatly dependent on the continuing morphological integrity of this cellular relationship.

The advantages of *experimental* neuropathology in promoting our understanding of both pathogenic mechanisms and normal cellular functions and relationships are self-evident. The control of variables which is feasible in experimental studies permits the performance of correspondingly more precise investigations, while many studies are quite impossible in any form in human neuropathology. Similarly, experimental animal neuropathologies that are putative models of human diseases, e.g. experimental allergic neuritis for the Guillain–Barré syndrome, acquire much of their value from the degree of experimentation which they permit.

In this chapter it will be possible to deal only briefly with selected aspects of peripheral nerve pathology. Two examples of segmental demyelination will be discussed: experimental allergic neuritis and experimental diphtheritic neuropathy. They belong to the class of neuropathies in which the lesion and cellular response are confined for the most part to the Schwann cell, the axon being spared. In contrast, Wallerian degeneration will be described in which the primary cytological event is a disruption of the axon which in turn has effects upon the axon-Schwann cell relationship. Discussion of these phenomena will be largely devoted to findings obtained by electron microscopy and more recent light microscope studies. However, some pertinent data from immunological, biochemical and electrophysiological studies will also be discussed. It is my view that only by such a synthesis can experimental neuropathology realize its potential value. Limitations of space preclude discussion of the many other neuropathies, including the mixed neuropathies in which axonal degeneration and segmental demyelination occur to a comparable degree (see Bradley and Jennekens, 1971), for example uraemic neuropathy. For further information concerning the wide variety of pathological processes affecting the peripheral nervous system, the reader is referred to the bibliography and particularly to a new monograph largely devoted to peripheral nerve pathology (Dyck, Thomas and Lambert, 1975).

Segmental demyelination was first described by Gombault (1880) in guinea-pigs which were given repeated small doses of white lead. The epithet 'segmental' arises from the arrangement of Schwann cells as a longitudinal series along an axon, each cell supporting a segment of myelin. Since the disease process may affect single Schwann cells and not their neighbours, segmental loss of myelin can occur.

13.2 Experimental allergic neuritis – introduction

Experimental allergic neuritis (EAN) is a paralytic, demyelinating disease of the peripheral nervous system, first described by Waksman and Adams in 1955. Induction of EAN is by intradermal injection of homogenized peripheral nerve (of homologous or heterologous origin), or peripheral nerve myelin fractions together with Freund's adjuvant. Its aetiology is autoimmune and the myelin is the specific target of the immune response. Waksman and Adams, and Arnason, Asbury, Åström and Adams (1968), have proposed EAN as a model for the demyelinating condition seen in man, the Guillain–Barré syndrome (idiopathic polyneuritis).

Several aspects of EAN will be briefly reviewed. Where there is a paucity of relevant experimental data, evidence will be drawn from the studies of EAE (experimental allergic encephalomyelitis), the central nervous system analogue of EAN.

EAN has been chosen for discussion since, like diphtheritic neuropathy, it represents a relatively 'pure' example of a demyelinating disease, with little axonal involvement. Unlike diphtheritic neuropathy however, in which there is apparently a disturbance of Schwann cell metabolism that results in demyelination, the Schwann cell in EAN apparently plays a 'passive' role, demyelination being produced by immunocompetent cells.

13.3 Signs of EAN

EAN is a paralytic condition (Fig. 13.1) characterized by obvious locomotor disturbances (see Waksman and Adams (1955) and Allt, Evans and Evans (1971a)). The signs exhibited by EAN-affected rabbits are summarized in Table 13.1, and for convenience are graded on a three point scale. Early and mild cases of the disease (denoted by +) show only a few of the diagnostic features listed in Section A (Table 13.1). More marked cases (++) are characterized by an exaggeration of these features. Severe cases (+++) also show some of the additional signs of functional disturbance listed in Section B (Table 13.1).

In the studies of Waksman and Adams (1955) and ourselves (1971a), the average time of onset of signs in rabbits was 14–16 days following inoculation, with a range of 7–29 days. Irrespective of the severity of the final paralysis the

667

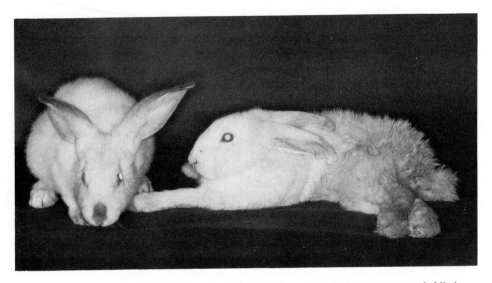

Fig. 13.1 Normal rabbit (left) and rabbit (right) showing EAN signs: note extended limbs, low slung posture, dishevelled appearance and evidence around hind quarters of incontinence.

signs usually reached their maximum expression within 3 days, and their average duration was 11 days with a range of 2–35 days.

Mild cases of EAN invariably showed recovery with a complete return to normal behaviour, but in severe cases death was common. Details of the physical signs of EAN in the guinea-pig are given by Cragg and Thomas (1964a), Hall (1967a), Ballin and Thomas (1968) and Waksman and Adams (1956), and in the mouse by Waksman and Adams. Waksman and Adams (1956), and Allt, Evans and Evans found that in the rabbit there was a good correlation between disease severity of EAN as indicated by functional signs and histopathological lesions; in the mouse and the guinea-pig however lesions of the peripheral nervous system did not correlate well with the signs.

13.4 Histology of EAN

13.4.1 *Light microscopy*

Waksman and Adams (1955) in the first description of EAN gave the definitive account of its histopathology as seen with the light microscope. The cardinal features were (a) segmental demyelination and (b) infiltration of endoneurial tissue by mononuclear leucocytes and smaller numbers of lymphocytes and polymorphonuclear leucocytes.

The relative distribution of lesions in rabbits suffering from EAN was investigated: in most animals dorsal spinal roots and spinal ganglia were found to

Table 13.1

A. *+ & ++ (Early/mild cases) diagnostic features:*
1. Dragging of one or both hind limbs.
2. Sliding of limbs into splayed position.
3. Ataxia, especially evident when running.
4. Poor 'displacement reflex'.
5. Poor 'withdrawal reflex'.
6. Low slung posture.
7. Unsteady and erratic in hopping.
8. Jumping too high or insufficiently high over obstacles.

B. *+++ (Late/severe cases) additional diagnostic features:*
1. Great difficulty in walking.
2. Flailing of limbs.
3. Musculature of limbs and trunk weak, offering little resistance.
4. Permanently extended flaccid limbs.
5. Total limb paralysis.
6. Extended flat posture.
7. Loss of appetite.
8. Loss of weight.
9. Incontinence.
10. Laboured breathing.

---

be selective sites containing the most lesions. Ventral roots and peripheral nerves by contrast had fewer lesions. In the most severely affected animals all dorsal roots examined, at all levels of the spinal cord from the cervical to the sacral regions were found to be involved; in mildly affected animals sparsely scattered lesions were seen in a few of the roots. The junction of dorsal root and spinal ganglion was found to be especially vulnerable. A similar distribution of lesions was found in EAN-affected mice i.e. spinal ganglia and roots were most affected, but the damage was invariably less severe (Waksman and Adams, 1956). In the guinea-pig the lesions were more widely distributed throughout the peripheral nervous system.

Within EAN lesions the cellular infiltrate was either focal, as in Fig. 13.4, or diffuse, and occurred most frequently around intraneural veins. In the vicinity of the cellular infiltrate the myelin sheaths were disorganized and macrophages were seen to contain irregular-shaped masses, or droplets of lipid, representing portions of disintegrated myelin sheaths. The Schwann cells appeared to retain their viability but some axons were observed to have degenerated. It was not possible to determine whether cellular infiltration preceded demyelination or vice versa, but the considerable infiltration of lymphocytes and mononuclear leucocytes observed was considered to be in excess of that which might be expected to occur as a secondary response to myelin degeneration. It was therefore inferred that this cellular infiltration represented a non-infectious type of inflammatory reaction of a similar kind to that seen in the allergic reactions of delayed tuberculin hypersensitivity. The cellular infiltrate formed foci some

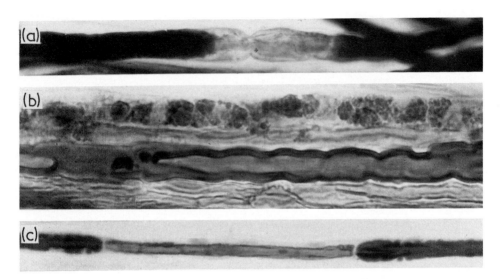

Fig. 13.2   Teased osmicated nerve fibres from EAN-affected rabbits showing: (a) Nodal widening (x 430). (b) Myelin sheath degraded into droplets (x 955). (c) Remyelination: short, intercalated segment. (x 375). (Reproduced from Allt, Evans and Evans, (1971a), by courtesy of *Brain Research*.)

50–200 μm in length; these occasionally involved the whole width of the nerve but more usually were narrow and extended across not more than 10–15 nerve fibres with their longitudinal axis parallel to that of the nerve fibres. No pathological changes were observed in the brains and spinal cords of rabbits affected by EAN. A similar situation was found in the mouse, but the guinea-pig commonly showed involvement of the central nervous system (*vide infra*).

Cragg and Thomas (1964a), Sherwin (1966) and Allt, Evans and Evans (1971a) examined individual teased, osmium-stained peripheral nerve fibres. This technique is especially useful for indentifying segmental myelin loss (Fig. 13.2) and for following the distribution and extent of lesions along individual fibres. Cragg and Thomas considered that the minimum detectable change was a widening of the nodal gap, other fibres showed more extensive paranodal myelin loss, and in more severely affected fibres there were considerable lengths of denuded axons. Such denuded segments usually corresponded to the length of one internode and sometimes to two or three successive internodes. Allt, Evans and Evans, and Hall (1967a) – employing longitudinal sections – were of the opinion that the initial lesion could occur either at the paranode or within the internode. Cragg and Thomas, and Allt, Evans and Evans both found evidence of remyelination (Fig. 13.2) in animals which had recovered from EAN. Such remyelination typically consisted of short, intercalated segments of thin myelin. As in diphtheritic neuropathy such internodes were never less than 15 μm in length.

13.4.2 *Electron microscopy*

Ballin and Thomas (1968) investigated the fine structure of demyelination in EAN in dorsal roots, dorsal root ganglia, sural nerves and peroneal nerves of guinea-pigs. Cells similar to monocytes in appearance, and containing myelin debris, were frequently observed within the endoneurial connective tissue space and also inside Schwann cell basement membranes when the associated axons were demyelinated (as in Fig. 13.4). The authors considered, however, that demyelination began without the direct involvement of mononuclear cells in myelin breakdown. In contrast Lampert (1969) reported that in EAN in rats of the Lewis strain, demyelination was observed to occur only in the presence of a mononuclear cell which has insinuated its processes between myelin lamellae, as shown in Fig. 13.3 (*vide infra*). Schröder and Krücke (1970) and Allt, Evans and Evans (1971a) found that early myelin breakdown in EAN in rabbits occurred in both ways, that is both with, and apparently without, immediate contact of mononuclear cells with myelin sheaths. Schröder and Krücke observed that the further breakdown of myelin debris took place in proliferating Schwann cells as well as within the infiltrating mononuclear cells.

Åström, Webster and Arnason (1968) and Lampert (1969) described ultrastructural evidence indicating changes in neural vascular permeability and the migration of mononuclear cells across vascular endothelial barriers. Plasma proteins had leaked from endoneurial vessels, a finding confirmed by Schröder and Krücke and ourselves, and mononuclear cells were found both between, and within, endothelial cells of venules. The earliest stage of the myelin breakdown process observed by Lampert was the penetration of the basement membrane of the Schwann cell by a cytoplasmic process of a mononuclear cell and its insertion into the mesaxon of the Schwann cell. Subsequent stages were seen in which the penetrating cytoplasmic process enveloped the myelin sheath and separated it from its supporting Schwann cell cytoplasm. The myelin lamellae in contact with the mononuclear process then underwent focal dissolution into vesicular profiles. Subsequently layers of myelin consisting of varying numbers of lamellae were stripped off by further mononuclear cell processes which penetrated the myelin sheath at the focal areas of dissolution. This process continued until the whole internodal segment of myelin had been removed.

Lysosomal enzymes, demonstrated biochemically, have been shown to be involved in myelin degradation (Molnár, Riekkinen, Rinne and Frey, 1974). Among the enzymes studied acid proteinase and acid phosphatase were the first to show an increase. Initially, increase in proteinase activity correlated well with clinical signs but later increases in enzyme activity were not accompanied by further changes in signs. Generally, increased activities of lysosomal enzymes were associated with myelin breakdown.

Ultrastructural changes at the node of Ranvier in EAN in the guinea-pig were described by Ballin and Thomas (1968). The earliest of these changes consisted of retraction of paranodal myelin loops and Schwann cell nodal processes, and these were replaced by Schwann cell cytoplasm which filled the nodal gap. The

671

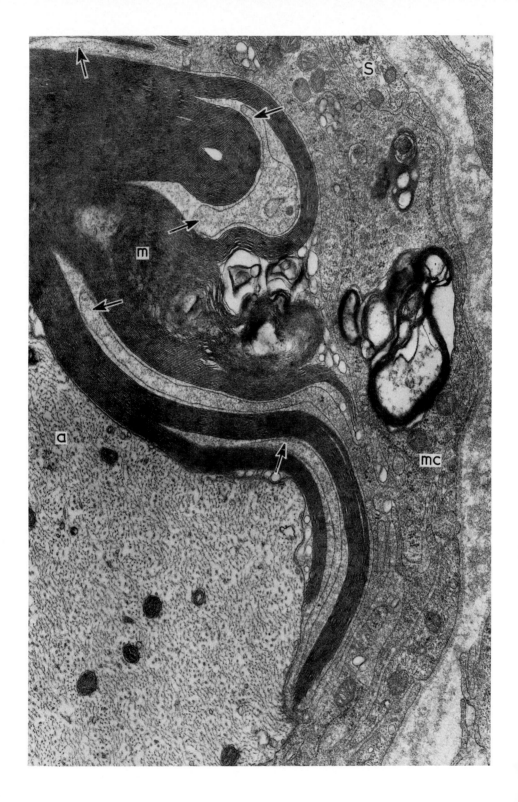

detached terminal myelin loops subsequently broke down into membraneous vesicles. Nodes which were more severely involved showed a widening of the nodal gap, the axon within the gap being covered by a cuff of Schwann cell cytoplasm or, less frequently, left denuded apart from a Schwann cell basement membrane. The Schwann cell cytoplasm within such nodal gaps frequently contained dense bodies, possibly of a lysosomal nature. When nodal widening progressed to segmental demyelination with breakdown of internodal myelin the process apparently occurred rapidly since intermediate stages were not observed. Such degenerating internodal myelin assumed the form of multiple small ovoids or spheres. Subsequent stages of demyelination were represented by totally demyelinated axons surrounded either by Schwann cell cytoplasm, or simply by Schwann cell basement membrane.

More recently I have described the degradation of the node of Ranvier in EAN in the rabbit (Allt, 1975). In contrast to the changes in the guinea-pig, breakdown of paranodal myelin was produced by the direct involvement of macrophages which inserted cytoplasmic processes between myelin terminal loops and between the myelin sheath and paranodal axolemma. Myelin lamellae were separated from each other in this way and underwent vesicular disorganization in contact with macrophage cytoplasmic processes.

The studies of Ballin and Thomas; Lampert; Schröder and Krücke, and ourselves emphasize first the survival of the Schwann cell despite demyelination, second the infrequency of Wallerian-type degeneration, and third the relatively normal appearance of the demyelinated axons (except for an irregular shape in transverse section, as in Fig. 13.4, and occasional intra-axonal lamellar bodies).

Wiśniewski, Prineas and Raine (1969) investigated the fine structure of peripheral nerves in rabbits with EAE. The lesions found were apparently indistinguishable from those seen in EAN, suggesting a close similarity between the two conditions. An attempt was also made to identify the infiltrating cells whose appearance within the nerves preceded demyelination. The following cell types were identified, small lymphocytes, large mononuclear cells, macrophages, plasma cells and polymorphonuclear leucocytes.

Fluorescence microscopy studies in the normal rat employing labelled albumen (Olsson, 1968) have demonstrated that capillaries in the dorsal and ventral spinal roots and dorsal root ganglia are more permeable to serum albumen than blood vessels in the sciatic nerve. A striking feature of the histopathology of EAN is the selective vulnerability of dorsal spinal roots and spinal ganglia, to segmental demyelination.

Waksman (1961) and ourselves (1971a) have suggested that a greater permeability of vessels of spinal roots and ganglia to cellular or humoral pathogenic agents in EAN might account for the greater susceptibility of these

---

Fig. 13.3   EAN: a splitting-off of layers of myelin (m) lamellae by cytoplasmic processes (arrows). Processes probably belong to a mononuclear cell (mc) which has invaded the Schwann cell (S). Axon (a). (x 27 500.)

sites. Olsson (1971) has described the presence of fenestrae in vascular endothelial cells in rhesus monkey dorsal root ganglia and an absence in endoneurial vessels of peripheral nerves, and it is known that fenestrated vessels allow the extravasation of circulating protein tracers (see Olsson). Correlations between ultrastructural characteristics and the permeability properties of blood vessels of the peripheral nervous system require further investigation, with particular reference to variations between different sites, and different species.

Allt (1972a) described the involvement of the perineurium in EAN. Serum protein was observed within the endoneurial space of nerves at the site of demyelinating lesions (as described above), the extravasated protein being especially abundant around blood vessels; some protein was also observed between the cellular laminae of the perineurium. Uptake of protein from the endoneurial space was inferred and a mechanism was proposed for the macropinocytotic transport of protein across the perineurium. This process was considered to be a homeostatic mechanism by the perineurium to restore the composition of the endoneurial fluid.

Ballin and Thomas (1969a) and Allt (1972b) described remyelination following EAN in guinea-pigs and rabbits respectively. Early remyelination was observed by Allt 20–32 days after antigen injection (Fig. 13.5), and it was evident that remyelination and the axon-Schwann cell relationships associated with this process frequently did not conform to descriptions of myelination in ontogeny (Geren, 1954). Of the axons which had been demyelinated, 71% were invaginated within a single Schwann cell, and the remyelination associated with this cellular relationship was in accordance with the spiral myelin concept (Fig. 13.6a). However 29% of demyelinated axons were each initially enveloped by several Schwann cell processes (Fig. 13.6b), and the associated mechanism of early remyelination (Fig. 13.6c and d) was by 'tunication' (apposition of Schwann cell processes), resulting in a transient irregular distribution of myelin around the axon circumference. The asymmetry of myelin deposition and the concomitant presence of multiple mesaxons were observed only during early remyelination, and were not seen when the myelin sheath consisted of more than 5–6 lamellae. Remyelination by tunication has also been observed in the peripheral nervous system in EAE (Raine, Wiśniewski and Prineas, 1969).

Whether one, or more, Schwann cell processes enveloped an axon, additional more loosely associated Schwann cell processes (Fig. 13.6e) were frequently

---

Fig. 13.4   EAN: a completely demyelinated axon (a) with irregular profile. A macrophage (m) has invaded the Schwann cell (S) basement membrane. Myelin debris (asterisks) within macrophage. Arrows indicate apposition of Schwann cell and macrophage. (x 11 000.)
Inset: Mononuclear cell infiltrate in perivascular situation. H. & E. Blood vessels (v). (x 300: Reproduced from Robinson, Allt and Evans, (1972), by courtesy of *Acta neuropathologica (Berlin)*.)

Fig. 13.5   EAN: incipient remyelination (1 lamella). Arrows indicate internal and external mesaxons. Note 'active' Schwann cell (S) cytoplasm. Axon (a). (x 13 750: Reproduced from Robinson, Allt and Evans (1972), by courtesy of *Acta neuropathologica (Berlin)*.)

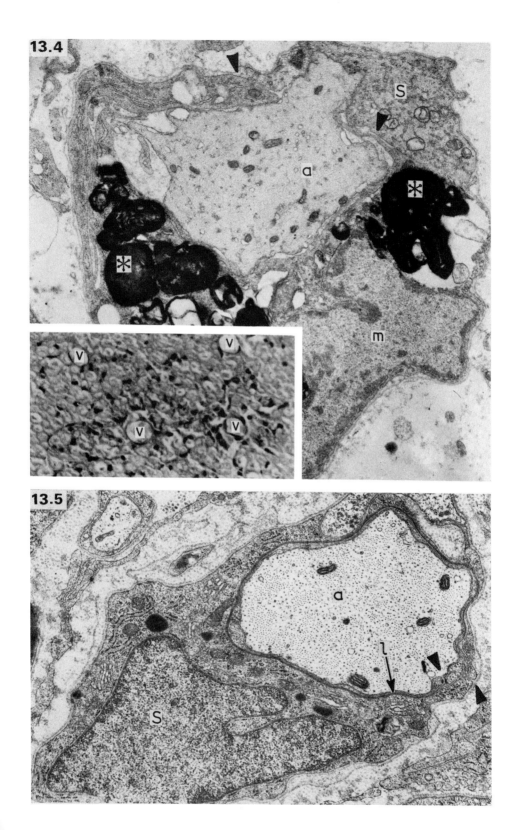

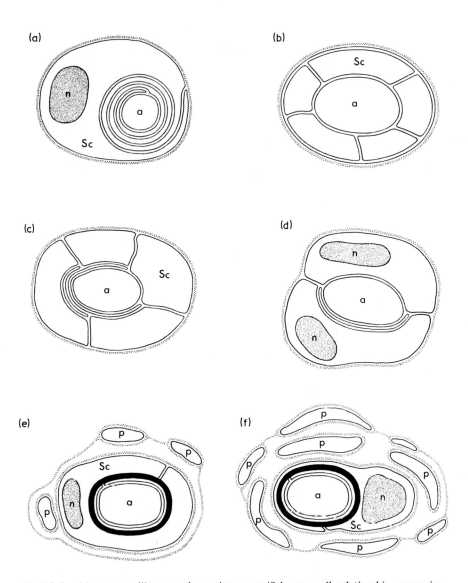

Fig. 13.6 Diagram to illustrate the various axon/Schwann cell relationships occurring during remyelination after segmental demyelination. (a) One axon/one Schwann cell with incipient spiral myelin formation; membrane layers are not yet compacted into myelin lamellae. (b) Five Schwann cell processes envelop an axon. (c) Four Schwann cell processes envelop an axon with incipient myelination by tunication; membrane layers are not yet compacted into myelin lamellae. (d) Two separate Schwann cells envelop an axon, one Schwann cell having formed uncompacted myelin lamellae by tunication. (e) A myelinating fibre has three Schwann cell processes (p) loosely associated and lying within the 'old' basement membrane of the Schwann cell. (f) A myelinating fibre is surrounded by a concentric array of Schwann cell processes (p) resembling 'onion bulbs' of hypertrophic neuropathy. Axon (a): Schwann cell nucleus (n); Schwann cell cytoplasm (Sc). (Reproduced from Allt, (1972b), by courtesy of *Acta neuropathologica (Berlin)*.)

present (in 82% of axons). These 'supernumerary' processes were frequently seen within the confines of the 'old' basement membrane of the original Schwann cell. Occasionally such processes were numerous and assumed the elaborate concentric array (Fig. 13.6f) characteristic of the 'onion bulbs' in hypertrophic neuropathy (Thomas and Lascelles, 1967; Weller, 1967). 'Supernumerary' Schwann cell processes and 'onion bulb' configurations have been observed in EAN by other authors (Ballin and Thomas, 1969a; Schröder and Krücke, 1970) and in peripheral nervous system involvement in EAE (Raine, Wiśniewski and Prineas, 1969).

The multiple Schwann cell processes associated either closely or more loosely with a single axon are likely to result in part from the Schwann cell proliferation which accompanies segmental demyelination in EAN (Asbury and Arnason, 1968). The number of Schwann cells produced is probably in excess of those required for remyelination, even allowing for the decreased internodal length associated with remyelination. The emergence of a one axon/one Schwann cell relationship in later stages of remyelination by tunication would support the view that the excess Schwann cell population is largely eliminated.

It is apparent that segmental demyelination and subsequent remyelination result in a considerable disturbance of the axon-Schwann cell relationship. Loss of the myelin sheath is not simply followed by reconstitution of the sheath leaving the original axon-Schwann cell relationship intact. It is clear that a new relationship is established in remyelination by spiral myelin, since mesaxons are lost in complete segmental demyelination and are presumably reformed by reinvagination of the axon by the original Schwann cell or its progeny. In remyelination by tunication several Schwann cells or Schwann cell processes come to envelop an axon and disturb the usual one axon/one Schwann cell relationship.

An examination of early remyelination after segmental demyelination serves to promote a deeper understanding of the axon-Schwann cell relationship. Recent evidence indicates that even incipient remyelination may also be of functional importance. Computer studies of conduction in myelinated nerve fibres (Koles and Rasminsky, 1972) indicate that the addition of a few myelin lamellae to a demyelinated fibre would restore saltatory conduction to a fibre whose safety factor (Tasaki, 1953) was minimally below one.

The appearances of regenerated nodes of Ranvier following EAN were described by Ballin and Thomas (1969a) who found that the majority of nodes conformed to the structure of normal nodes. In some instances however atypical nodal structures were observed: the gap between adjacent Schwann cells was reduced to about 20 nm and processes extended out laterally from the Schwann cells at the paranode. Occasionally such processes formed a 'collar' extending over the paranode of the adjacent Schwann cell, covering the site of the node. The processes were interpreted to be modified myelin terminal loops. A further feature of interest was the presence of a Schwann cell in a gap between two myelinated internodal segments only slightly greater than the length of the

Schwann cell nucleus; it was considered unlikely that a Schwann cell could ever form an intercalated myelin internode over such a short length.

As Ballin and Thomas point out the effect of these atypical nodes of Ranvier on conduction velocity is difficult to predict due to our present lack of understanding of the functional significance of the various morphological specializations of the Schwann cell at the node of Ranvier. The authors suggest however that the abnormal nodes of Ranvier may contribute to the incomplete restoration of normal conduction velocity associated with recovery from EAN.

13.5 Immune response in EAN

It is now generally accepted that EAN has an autoimmune aetiology (Åström and Waksman, 1962). The precise nature of the immune response elicited by the neural antigen and the role of that response in the aetiological mechanism of EAN is less clear. Elucidation of this mechanism would clearly be of considerable theoretical and practical importance. Two examples of pertinent experimental evidence will be briefly discussed.

13.5.1 *Passive transfer*

The successful passive transfer of EAN and EAE to normal recipients by means of intravenous injection of sensitized lymphoid cells from EAN/EAE animals (Åström and Waksman, 1962; Paterson, 1966) is considered evidence, *par excellence*, for the pathogenesis to be of a cell-mediated, delayed hypersensitivity type. Failure of passive transfer using serum (Kabat, Wolf and Bezer, 1948; Hurst, 1955) from sensitized animals indicates an absence of any role for circulating (humoral) antibodies in the aetiological mechanism. Such a failure might however be accounted for by either the antibody-containing serum being excluded from the neural target tissue of the normal recipient by the blood-nerve or blood-brain barrier, or by an excessive dilution of the serum antibodies despite the use of large quantities of serum (Chase, 1959). In an attempt to overcome these difficulties Allt, Evans and Evans (1971b) employed a technique of direct intraneural micro-injection, thus circumventing the blood-nerve barrier. Even so demyelination characteristic of EAN did not occur. Similarly passive transfer using EAE serum was unsuccessful even after the disruption of the blood-brain barrier by heat lesions (Levine and Hoenig, 1968). In contrast Arnason and Chelmicka-Szorc (1972) have described successful passive transfer of EAN by direct injection of sensitized lymphocytes into sciatic nerve.

Paterson (1966) reported that serum taken from EAE rats and injected intravenously into rats over a period of 19 days after encephalitogenic sensitization *prevented* the development of EAE signs. The suppressive effect was ascribed to the presence of protective (enhancing) antibodies in the sera. Salvin and Liauw (1968) and Lehrich and Arnason (1971) also have put forward evidence in favour of a protective role for humoral antibodies in EAN and EAE.

13.5.2 *Tissue culture studies*

Tissue culture studies employing mouse or rat dorsal root ganglia have provided a method for *in vitro* assay of EAN serum antibodies. Such cultures are first allowed to myelinate and subsequently the nutrient medium is replaced with one containing EAN serum. The results obtained have varied. Yonezawa and his co-workers (Yonezawa and Ishihara, 1967; Yonezawa, Ishihara and Matsuyama, 1968) reported that EAN sera were capable of inducing demyelination in cultures of spinal ganglia. In contrast, Arnason, Winkler and Hadler (1969) found that EAN-sensitized lymph node cells induced demyelination in cultures of rat trigeminal ganglia (supporting a cell-mediated aetiology), but that sera had either very weak activity or, more commonly, no demyelinating activity at all.

Since tissue culture experiments provide the best evidence for a complement-dependent serum factor being implicated in the aetiology of EAN and EAE, certain reservations about the significance of these findings must be considered; for example, the *in vitro* studies described have used sera from animals sensitized with preparations of whole peripheral nerve and thus may be detecting cytotoxic activity of antibodies produced in response to antigens other than those present within myelin basic protein. The studies of Gregson, Kennedy and Leibowitz (1971) suggest that the antibodies are elicited by galactocerebroside.

The two examples of experimental evidence described above demonstrate that the pathogenesis of EAN/EAE is largely cell-mediated. There is as yet little evidence in favour of a primary role for circulating antibodies in the development of EAN and EAE despite some suggestions to the contrary, and the possibility of humoral antibodies having a protective function requires further examination.

13.6 EAN/EAE induction process and identity of the antigen

The production of an encephalomyelitis by repeated injections of normal brain was first accomplished by Hurst (1932) in rabbits and subsequently by Rivers, Sprunt and Berry (1933) in monkeys. The efficiency of induction of EAE was later improved by the additional use of Freund's adjuvant (Freund and McDermott, 1942) which increased the antigenic activity of the inoculated brain. Initial attempts to produce a peripheral nervous system analogue of EAE were unsuccessful (Morgan, 1947; Kabat, Wolf and Bezer, 1948) until Waksman and Adams (1955) described EAN in rabbits. Waksman and Adams (1956) found spinal ganglia lesions in 92% of rabbits, 68% of guinea-pigs and 59% of mice challenged with peripheral nervous system 'antigens'. They further demonstrated that the peripheral nerve tissue used as 'antigen' to induce EAN may be of homologous or heterologous origin. Peripheral nerves from a variety of mammalian sources (guinea-pig, rabbit, dog, bovine and human) all produced similar signs and histopathology of EAN, when used as 'antigens' in rabbits (Waksman and Adams, 1955). More recently a chronic form of EAN has been described in rabbits, monkeys and guinea-pigs (Sherwin, 1966; Wiśniewski, Brostoff, Carter and Eylar, 1974; Pollard, King and Thomas, 1975). This form of EAN occurred spontaneously in a small number of animals in response to a single injection of antigen and more frequently following repeated injections.

It has been found that the route of injection of 'antigen' is of importance in the induction of EAE and EAN. Waksman and Morrison (1951) for example found that injection of encephalitogenic emulsion intradermally into the foot pad or the abdominal wall of the rabbit induced EAE, but that induction failed where injection was by subcutaneous or intraperitoneal route. Excision of the injection site as early as one hour after intradermal inoculation of the emulsion did not prevent the appearance of EAE (Freund and Lipton, 1955). This was attributed to the rapid distribution of antigen to the lymph nodes.

Investigations throughout the last two decades have progressively refined our knowledge about the localization of the encephalitogenic antigen which induces EAE, and to a lesser extent about the 'neuritogenic' antigen which induces EAN. A myelin fraction isolated from homogenized brain by ultracentrifugation and free from gross contamination with other cellular elements was shown to have a high encephalitogenic activity by Kies and her co-workers (Laatsch, Kies, Gordon and Alvord, 1962). An encephalitogenic protein was isolated from CNS myelin (Kies, Murphy and Alvord, 1960; Kies, Thompson and Ellsworth, 1965), and subsequently a polypeptide digest of myelin basic protein was demonstrated to have a high activity in producing EAE (Carnegie, McPherson and Robson, 1970). Eylar, Caccam, Jackson, Westall and Robinson (1970) have synthesized a highly active encephalitogenic peptide whose structure resembles the encephalitogenic antigenic determinant isolated from myelin. This active portion is a sequence of only nine amino-acid residues. Kibler, Shapira, McKneally, Jenkins, Selden and Chou (1969) propose that there are at least two encephalitogenic sites on the myelin basic protein. The nature of the EAN antigen has received less attention, but recently Eylar and his co-workers (Brostoff, Burnett, Lampert and Eylar, 1972) have isolated a basic protein from rabbit sciatic nerve which is 'neuritogenic' and which contains peptide regions with similar or identical amino acid composition to those of the encephalitogenic basic protein.

Robinson, Allt and Evans (1972) investigated the capacity of 'myelin-free' Schwann cells to induce EAN. Human fetal peripheral nerve and human adult abdominal vagus nerve, both containing little or no myelin, failed to induce EAN when injected intradermally (together with Freund's adjuvant) into rabbits. Thus Schwann cell plasma membrane, from which myelin is apparently derived (Geren, 1954) lacks the capacity to induce EAN. We proposed two alternative hypothoses to account for this paradox, either (a) the antigen is present in both myelin and Schwann cell plasma membrane but is protected in the plasma membrane by sialic acid, or (b) the antigenic determinant is formed *de novo* during myelination from molecular components which are present within the Schwann cell plasma membrane. Despite the use of large doses of 'antigen' the possibility cannot be excluded that insufficient Schwann cell plasma membrane was present to produce an autoimmune response. It should be recalled however that in EAN the Schwann cells survive, despite demyelination, also indicating that Schwann cell plasma membranes do not contain an effective antigen and so are spared from immune attack.

13.7 Suppression of EAN

Considerations of space do not allow a discussion of the very interesting findings concerning the suppression of EAE by:

(a) Cytotoxic drugs, such as methotrexate, 6-mercaptopurine, nitrogen mustard and the related cyclophosphamide (Hoyer, Good and Condie, 1962; Brandriss, 1963; Calne and Liebowitz, 1963; Paterson and Drobish, 1969; Paterson and Hanson, 1969; Lisak, Falk, Heinze, Kies and Alvord, 1970).

(b) Multiple injections of EAE antigen (Waksman, 1959; Paterson, 1966) including the reversal of established EAE (Eylar, Jackson, Rothenberg and Brostoff, 1972; Levine, Sowinski and Kies, 1972).

(c) Multiple injections of a synthetic polypeptide (Teitelbaum, Meshorer, Hirschfeld, Arnon and Sela, 1971; Teitelbaum, Webb, Meshorer, Arnon and Sela, 1972).

(d) Anti-lymphocyte serum (Leibowitz, Lessof and Kennedy, 1968).

(e) Protective (enhancing) antibodies (Paterson and Harwin, 1963; Paterson, 1966).

(f) X-irradiation (Scheinberg, Lee and Taylor, 1967).

(g) Steroids, including the reversal of the disease (Elliott, Gibbons and Greig, 1973).

(h) L-asparaginase (Khan and Levine, 1974).

Relatively few investigations have been concerned specifically with the suppression of EAN. Heitman and Mannweiler (1957) found that corticosteroid treatment of EAN was effective in controlling or preventing the disease only when administered prior to the development of signs of paralysis. It is considered that corticosteroids suppress cell-mediated immune responses almost entirely by their non-specific anti-inflammatory action at the periphery, and not by their action on the central immune mechanisms (Turk, 1969). The obvious disadvantage of corticosteroid treatment is that it suppresses the activity of the reticuloendothelial system and immune response, and the resulting impaired surveillance mechanism renders the animal more vulnerable to pathogenic agents.

Lehrich and Arnason (1971) suppressed the development of EAN in rats by prior intraperitoneal immunization with homogenized nerve in saline. The mechanism of suppression was interpreted in terms of protective (enhancing) antibodies being raised by the inoculated nerve and blocking antigenic sites on the myelin basic protein of the recipient rat. Allt, Evans, Evans and Targett (1971) demonstrated a suppression of EAN by the use of a concurrent infection with trypanosome parasites (*Trypanosoma brucei*), and we related our findings to recent studies on immunosuppression by parasitic protozoa. In *Trypanosoma brucei* infection, it has been demonstrated that B-cell (thymus-independent, lymphocyte) function is impaired, as indicated by the lack of antibody production, while T-cell (thymus-derived, lymphocyte) and macrophage functions are apparently unaffected (Murray, Jennings, Murray and Urquhart, 1974).

13.8 Experimental diphtheritic neuropathy – introduction

Diphtheritic neuropathy, like EAN, is characterized by an axon-sparing, segmental demyelination resulting in paralysis. It can be induced systemically by parenteral injection of the toxin produced by *Corynbacterium diphtheriae* (Waksman, Adams and Mansmann, 1957), locally by the direct injection of diphtheria toxin into the peripheral nerve (Cavanagh and Jacobs, 1964), or *in vitro* by the addition of toxin to cultures of myelinated dorsal root ganglia (Peterson and Murray, 1965). Human diphtheritic neuropathy (Fisher and Adams, 1956) possesses essentially the same characteristic features of pathology and patho-physiology as have been described experimentally. Demyelination produced by diphtheria toxin has been shown to be independent of the immune response and to be non-inflammatory (Waksman, Adams and Mansmann, 1957).

Experimental diphtheritic neuropathy is of considerable value as a model for demyelinating diseases in general, especially when induced locally, since it is highly reproducible, and with low doses of toxin produces little or no axonal damage. Recently McDonald and Sears (1970a) and Wiśniewski and Raine (1971) have demonstrated that focal demyelination in the central nervous system can be induced by localized injection of diphtheria toxin into the spinal cord and brain.

13.9 Signs of diphtheritic neuropathy

Waksman, Adams and Mansmann (1957) described the signs of functional disturbance associated with systemically-induced diphtheritic neuropathy. In the rabbit the signs of illness associated with the acute effects of toxin (thinness, apathy, poor coat) lasted about a week, and were followed by a sign-free interval of days or even weeks before the appearance of a mild to moderate weakness of all four limbs, accompanied by uncertainty of movement and gait (ataxia). At no time was there complete paralysis or loss of sphincter control. The signs thus resembled those of mild EAN but never became as gross as those of severe EAN.

In the guinea-pig the sign-free interval was frequently absent, the mild illness merging imperceptibly with the onset of weakness. The salient features consisted of a progressive weakness of the trunk and extremities progressing to complete paralysis, although sphincter control was retained. Death usually resulted from respiratory paralysis. The greater severity of signs in the guinea-pig compared with the rabbit could be correlated with the more extensive distribution of lesions in the guinea-pig.

Signs of functional disturbance in systemically-induced diphtheritic neuropathy have also been described by McDonald (1963a) in cats, by Cavanagh and

Jacobs (1964) in hens and by Morgan-Hughes (1968) in guinea-pigs, and in animals given local intraneural injections of toxin by Jacobs, Cavanagh and Mellick (1966) in hens, by Jacobs (1967) in rats, by Bradley and Jennekens (1971) in rabbits, and by Hallpike (1972) in rats.

McDonald reported a good correlation between the clinical signs and the severity of the histological damage in the cat. Webster (1964) described the earliest histological changes to be focal alterations in the lamellar pattern of myelin at the nodes of Ranvier and at Schmidt–Lanterman clefts, changes which occurred only at the onset of clinical weakness, 5–8 days after the injection of toxin into the guinea-pig. However, Cavanagh and Jacobs (1964), Weller (1965), and Morgan-Hughes (1968) found evidence of myelin breakdown before the onset of paralysis in both the hen and the guinea-pig.

13.10 Histology of diphtheritic neuropathy

13.10.1 *Light microscopy*

The breakdown of myelin following diphtheritic intoxication has been described using light microscopy by several authors (Fisher and Adams, 1956; Waksman, Adams and Mansmann, 1957; Webster, Spiro, Waksman and Adams, 1961; McDonald, 1963a; Cavanagh and Jacobs, 1964; Peterson and Murray, 1965; Jacobs, 1967; Morgan-Hughes, 1968; Bradley and Jennekens, 1971). In cultures of rat dorsal root ganglia, Peterson and Murray observed that nodal widening was followed by a fragmentation of myelin into ovoids which subsequently underwent further degradation to small spheres and granules. The process was seen to continue until all of the myelin had been completely resorbed within the cytoplasm of the Schwann cell. Thus breakdown of the myelin began paranodally, and the central portion of the sheath adjacent to the Schwann cell nucleus was the last to be effected. Histological descriptions of diphtheritic neuropathy *in vivo* differ in two respects: (a) nodal widening may not necessarily be followed by a complete segmental loss of myelin, since damage to myelin is restricted to the paranode in larger fibres at lower toxin dose levels, whilst in small fibres there is involvement and breakdown of the whole internode *ab initio* (Cavanagh and Jacobs, 1964; Jacobs, Cavanagh and Mellick, 1966; Jacobs, 1967); and (b), whilst most of the digestion of myelin takes place within the Schwann cells, some is also seen to occur in macrophages, and this has been confirmed by electron microscopy (Webster *et al.*, 1961; Webster, 1964; Weller, 1965; Allt, 1968).

As Waksman, Adams and Mansmann (1957) noted in the rabbit and the guinea-pig, isolated segments of myelin may be affected producing a patchy segmental breakdown of myelin. Fisher and Adams (1956) observed that myelin loss may involve part of an internode, a whole internode, or several successive internodes. McDonald (1963a) suggested that a region of myelin damage which involved only a part of an internode frequently stopped at a Schmidt–

Lanterman incisure. The reports of Bradley and Jennekens (1971), and Wiśniewski and Raine (1971) of an *increase* in the number of Schmidt–Lanterman clefts in the early phase of myelin disorganization is open to another interpretation. It is equally likely to reflect an increased prominence of pathologically widened incisures, as seen in Wallerian degeneration (see below and Chapter 1), especially since Bradley and Jennekens also describe a concomitant swelling of myelin sheaths and an increase in the size of Schmidt–Lanterman clefts.

Light microscopic studies of both human (Fisher and Adams, 1956) and experimental, systemic diphtheritic neuropathy (Waksman, Adams and Mansmann, 1957; Cavanagh and Jacobs, 1964) have in general revealed little or no involvement of axons in the histopathology. However, extensive axonal degeneration can be induced when a high dose of toxin (beyond that which can be administered systemically) is given by intraneural injection. This specific situation was investigated by Bradley and Jennekens (1971) who considered that the axonal changes resulted from a direct effect of toxin on the axons, and was not secondary to the Schwann cell damage or vascular changes. The authors interpreted their findings to be another example of axonal involvement occurring in a demyelinating neuropathy when the disease process is sufficiently severe. Similarly Fullerton (1966) has described lead neuropathy as being a segmental demyelinating condition with relative sparing of axons following moderate intoxication, but mainly a process of axonal degeneration in high dose intoxications. Morgan-Hughes (1968) observed extensive axonal involvement in systemic diphtheritic neuropathy in two guinea-pigs which showed especially severe paralysis, and Peterson and Murray (1965) noted that with high levels of diphtheria toxin damage can be induced *in vitro*.

The distribution of lesions in systemically-induced diphtheritic neuropathy varies in different species (Waksman, Adams and Mansmann, 1957). In the rabbit the disease was limited to the sensory ganglia and adjacent portions of spinal roots and nerves, whilst in the guinea-pig, roots and ganglia were little effected, but peripheral nerves were extensively involved. The distribution of lesions in man (Fisher and Adams, 1956) resembled that seen in the rabbit. In the cat the dorsal roots, dorsal root ganglia and adjacent spinal nerves were found to be particularly vulnerable (McDonald, 1963a), whilst peripheral nerves showed little involvement.

Hopkins and Morgan-Hughes (1969) reported that in systemically-induced diphtheritic neuropathy demyelination was more severe in the plantar nerves of the sole of the hind foot than in nerves from the dorsum of the foot, thigh and leg. This they attributed to a combined effect of toxin and local pressure, since similar lesions did not occur in response to either pressure or toxin alone. There was no histological evidence of an inflammatory reponse in either experimental diphtheritic neuropathy (Waksman, Adams and Mansmann, 1957) or human diphtheritic neuropathy (Fisher and Adams, 1956). In none of the species were there perivascular lesions, in contrast to EAN.

In human diphtheritic neuropathy and experimental, systemically-induced, diphtheritic neuropathy the central nervous system is completely free of lesions. The sparing of the central nervous system, and of parts of the peripheral nervous system, in the guinea-pig, rabbit and human was attributed by Fisher and Adams (1956), and Waksman, Adams and Mansmann (1957), to the presence of a blood-brain barrier to the toxin, and to a similar local blood-nerve barrier in the areas of the peripheral nervous system free from lesions. Waksman (1961) substantiated this suggestion by means of intravenous and subcutaneous injections of labelled proteins, together with various dyes (e.g. trypan blue), into guinea-pigs and rabbits. The nervous system was subsequently examined for evidence of the injected materials, and it was found, for example, that the parenchyma of rabbit peripheral nerves was free of the diphtheria toxin, human serum albumin and trypan blue previously injected intravenously, whilst spinal roots and ganglia showed uptake of these materials in correlation with the distribution of lesions in diphtheritic neuropathy.

Light microscope studies have emphasized that nodal widening (which may progress to complete segmental demyelination) is a prominent feature in diphtheritic neuropathy. Several parameters influencing the extent of nodal widening, and further myelin loss, in response to diphtheritic intoxication have been quantified by Cavanagh and Jacobs (1964), Jacobs, Cavanagh and Mellick (1966), Jacobs (1967) and Allt and Cavanagh (1969) in the sciatic nerves of the rat and hen. The extent of nodal widening is both time and dose dependent. Increasing dose levels of diphtheria toxin produce wider nodal gaps, and wider nodal gaps also occur with increasing time, until regeneration begins. There is a selective toxicity to fibres of different diameters, small fibres being more susceptible to the effect of toxin than larger fibres. Thus initially myelin lysis is restricted to small fibres, this is followed by nodal widening in large fibres, by which time complete internodal breakdown of myelin has occurred in small fibres. The age of the animal also determines the extent of neuropathic effects and in a young animal nodal widening occurs earlier and more rapidly than in an older animal. There is a delay period between the time of inoculation and the onset of observable changes in the myelin sheath, and this delay period is also dose dependent, being shorter at high dose levels than at low dose levels.

As Jacobs, Cavanagh and Mellick (1966) point out, diphtheria toxin has a profound effect on the Schwann cell as shown by the partial or complete breakdown of the myelin sheath, yet the cell retains its capacity to divide, there being a striking increase in nuclear population during the first 15 days after inoculation into the sciatic nerve of the hen: Gallus domesticus. Proliferation of Schwann cells following diphtheritic intoxication has also been noted by Fisher and Adams (1956) in human diphtheritic neuropathy, by Majno, Waksman and Karnovsky (1960) in the rabbit and guinea-pig, and by Jacobs (1967) in the rat. However, as Bradley and Jennekens (1971) described, an absence of Schwann cell proliferation and Schwann cell death can result from high doses of toxin.

At the light miscoscope level of analysis several authors have demonstrated various stages of remyelination following segmental demyelination induced by diphtheritic intoxication (McDonald, 1963a; Cavanagh and Jacobs, 1964; Fullerton, Gilliatt, Lascelles and Morgan-Hughes, 1965; Peterson and Murray, 1965; Morgan-Hughes, 1965, 1968; Jacobs, Cavanagh and Mellick, 1966; Jacobs, 1967). Cavanagh and his co-workers reported that in the hen at 21 days after inoculation distinct evidence of new myelin was found around small fibres, whilst in the young rat new myelin was found in relation to a high proportion of fibres by the fifteenth day. Beyond 22 days remyelination had progressed so rapidly in the rat that it was often difficult to distinguish remyelinating fibres from those that had not been damaged. By 47 days the damaged fibres of the immature animal appeared to have almost regained their original diameter. In contrast, in the adult rat the first signs of remyelination were seen in a few fibres at 31 days, at 47 days approximately 50% of damaged fibres were beginning to remyelinate, and at 56 days new myelin was seen around all but those fibres in which recent myelin loss had occurred. Remyelination in the adult rat is thus a slow process as even by 113 days the damaged fibres were far from their original diameter. Peterson and Murray (1965) were able to induce remyelination in rat dorsal root ganglia cultures by withdrawing diphtheria toxin during the early phase of demyelination. Those segments which had begun to degenerate continued the full cycle of demyelination before the same Schwann cell remyelinated its appropriate segment of the axon.

It was established by Vizoso (1950) that in peripheral nerves the internodal length normally increases with the diameter of the fibre, (Fig. 13.12a) and it is thought that the origin of this relationship can be ascribed to the fact that the largest fibres are the first to myelinate, and thus have the longest internodes, since they are subjected to the lengthening effect of growth for the longest time. Vizoso also demonstrated that the slope of the line expressing this relationship is related to the growth of the part of the body in which the nerve lies. Thus the tibial and ulnar nerves grow much more in absolute length than the facial nerve and their internodal lengths increase with diameter faster than do the internodes of the facial nerve. However, Vizoso encountered occasional exceptions to these principles in the form of very short internodes, occurring between internodes of normal length for the diameter of that particular fibre. He attributed the presence of these short internodes to previous episodes of local demyelination with subsequent remyelination.

Short internodes were observed as long ago as 1881 by Rénaut, and designated 'short intercalated segments'. Lubińska (1958) found some short internodes in normal laboratory cats and ascribed their origin to a local myelin breakdown which had occurred earlier. She noted that sometimes a short internode occurred singly but more often there was a succession of such internodes, which together had the same length as a normal internode of the same fibre. In the latter situation it would appear that a whole internodal segment of myelin had been broken down and replaced by several, short, intercalated segments. Lascelles and Thomas (1966) similarly found short internodes together with normal internodes on the same fibre as a consistent feature of sural nerves of man over 65 years of age. Short, intercalated internodes have been described in animals which had recovered from diphtheritic neuropathy by several authors (Fullerton *et al.*, 1965 (Fig, 13.12c); Morgan-Hughes, 1965, 1968; Jacobs and Cavanagh, 1969). It can be anticipated therefore that in remyelination following diphtheritic neuropathy the normal linear relationship of increase in internodal length with fibre diameter will no longer obtain.

Jacobs and Cavanagh (1969) investigated remyelination quantitatively in diphtheritic neuropathy in the adult hen and the rat. They reported the surprising finding that in remyelination in the hen, internodal length to some extent retained its relationship with axon diameter (Fig. 13.12d and e) although the regression coefficient was only one-half to one-third that of the normal nerve. They also found that for a given fibre size the internodal length was markedly less than for a normal nerve, the largest fibres, for example, had internodal lengths of only 1000 μm compared with at least 2000 μm in the normal. In the rat, however, the findings agreed with earlier studies of regeneration after Wallerian degeneration (*vide infra*), in that the internodal lengths were of approximately uniform size and bore no consistent relationship to axon diameter. In view of such differences between species, the authors drew attention to the need for a reassessment of the concept of the Schwann cell having a basic length of '300 μm or perhaps a little less' (Hiscoe, 1947) or 'about 230 μm' (Young, 1950). This basic length was approximately the same in both development and regeneration, for different nerves in both mammals and fish, and represented the initial cell length which was subsequently subjected to elongation during growth.

Mellick (1969) has described an increased vascular permeability in peripheral nerves during diphtheritic neuropathy and has related this to the metabolic demands of remyelination. Using labelled albumin (I^{131}) he demonstrated that the maximal permeability increase occurred during the recovery and remyelination phase, and that even 150 days after the onset of the neuropathy there was still a significantly elevated vascular permeability.

13.10.2 *Electron microscopy*

In diphtheritic neuropathy in the rat, I observed (1968) that splits usually occurred in myelin at the intraperiod line and were apparent as early as 3 days after intraneural injection of toxin, a situation reminiscent of the effects of hypotonic solutions on myelin (Robertson, 1958b). Webster *et al.* (1961) observed a loss of the intraperiod line and a variation in the period between dense lines (most frequently near Schmidt—Lanterman incisures and myelin terminal loops) in diphtheritic neuropathy in the guinea-pig. Similar changes were described in myelin in EAN by Allt, Evans and Evans (1971a) who also observed a separation of myelin lamellae at the intraperiod line, usually sparing

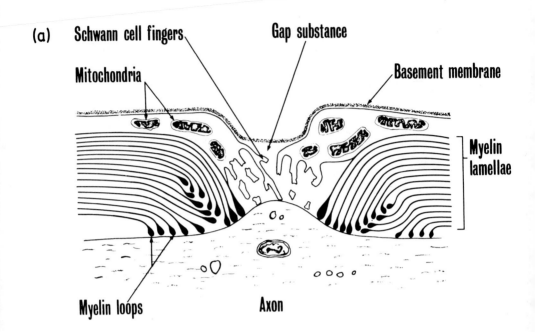

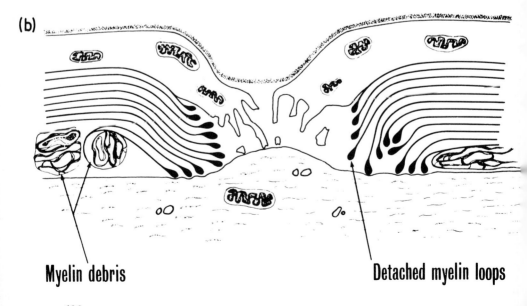

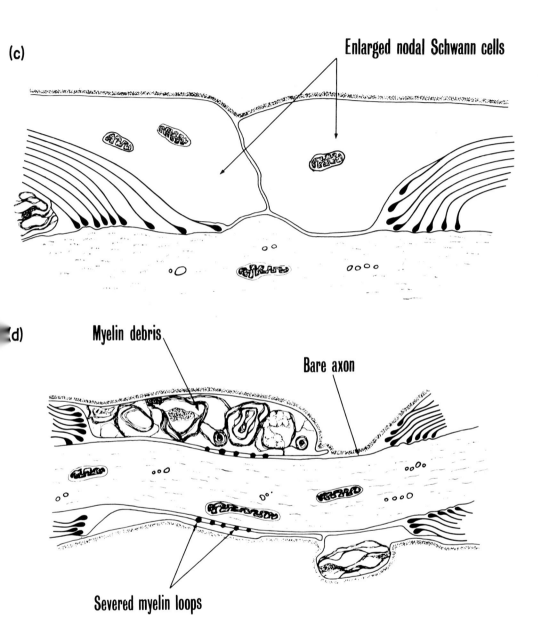

(c)

Enlarged nodal Schwann cells

(d)

Myelin debris

Bare axon

Severed myelin loops

Fig. 13.7 Diagram of changes at the node of Ranvier after intraneural injection of diphtheria toxin: (a) normal node of Ranvier of a large myelinated fibre; (b) 3 days – Schwann cell processes normal. Last-formed (outer) myelin loops detached from axolemma; (c) 7 days – Schwann cell fingers and gap substance replaced by swollen cytoplasm. Outer myelin loops detached from axolemma; (d) 10 days – marked nodal widening. Schwann cell fingers and gap substance absent. Much myelin debris. Severed myelin loops still present on the nodal axolemma. Axon may be bare of Schwann cell covering. Diagram based on 102 nodal profiles. (Reproduced from Allt and Cavanagh, (1969), by courtesy of *Brain*.)

689

the major dense line. In EAN the authors related the selective lysis at the intraperiod line to the possible distribution of 'neuritogenic' basic protein. Electron microscopy confirms that myelin loss in diphtheritic neuropathy progresses from the early formation of myelin ovoids to a complete separation of myelin debris and axon, such that they may occupy opposite sides of the Schwann cell in transverse profile (Webster *et al.*, 1961; Weller, 1965; Allt, 1968). The myelin debris normally retains its lamellate form in the early phase of its degradation. Webster (1964) has demonstrated putative myelin breakdown products within endothelial cells of endoneurial blood vessels.

In attempting to assess the extent of changes in the myelin sheath resulting from mechanical, toxic, or other agents it is necessary to appreciate that there are some 'normal' variations in the contour of the sheath. Webster and Spiro (1960) have described infoldings and protrusions of the myelin sheath, particularly in the paranodal region, as 'normal' features of the guinea-pig sciatic nerve. Whilst many of their illustrations may be explained by the paranodal crenation of the myelin sheath (Williams and Landon, 1963) others represent atypical modifications.

We (1969) considered unmyelinated axons and their associated Schwann (Remak) cells to be uninvolved in the changes of diphtheritic neuropathy, but Webster *et al.* (1961) however described focal fragmentation of Schwann (Remak) cell and axon membranes, and the dissolution of the axon filaments of some unmyelinated fibres.

Concerning the question of axonal involvement in myelinated fibres Webster *et al.* (1961) described the degeneration of a few axons of myelinated fibres in diphtheritic neuropathy in the guinea-pig. Weller and Mellick (1966) and ourselves (1969) failed to observe similar changes in the chicken or the rat respectively, although we found an increase in electron density of the axoplasm at widened nodes. Hughes, Narang and Kelso (1972) in an *in vitro* study reported that whilst the major effect of diphtheria toxin was upon the myelin sheaths, nerve cell bodies and axons also showed extensive degenerative changes. However, as the authors point out, their chick dorsal root ganglia cultures were exposed to a much higher and longer sustained concentration of toxin than could be achieved *in vivo*.

We (1969) described the ultrastructure of the changes leading to nodal widening (Fig. 13.7) in diphtheritic neuropathy in the rat. Our findings were largely in agreement with those of Ballin and Thomas (1968) for the same process in EAN. In addition to the detachment of terminal myelin loops from the paranodal axolemma (Fig. 13.7b) as described by Ballin and Thomas, we also observed severance of myelin lamellae at their junction with the myelin loops (Fig. 13.7d). We emphasized the early loss of nodal gap substance during the nodal widening process, and the absence of membrane-delimited dense bodies in the paranodal Schwann cytoplasm, although multivesicular bodies were occasionally observed at this site and within the nodal axoplasm. We drew attention to markedly widened nodal gaps of 10–50 μm at which terminal myelin loops were nevertheless still present at the terminations of most of the myelin lamellae. Such appearances were explained by either slipping of myelin loops over the axolemma surface, or the synthesis of new loops at the end of the intact region of myelin.

Since, according to the theory of saltatory conduction (Huxley and Stämpfli, 1949) the myelin sheath is considered to have an insulatory function, it can be anticipated that nodal widening and segmental demyelination will have detrimental effects on the electrophysiological properties of a nerve fibre. The possible functional significance of the morphological changes at the node of Ranvier is discussed below.

In diphtheritic neuropathy, we found ultrastructural evidence of a dysfunction of Schwann cell metabolism, both before and during the process of nodal widening. The Schwann cell was characterized by a paucity of cytoplasmic organelles, the swollen cytoplasm containing scattered 'membrane whorls'. It is probable therefore that the changes in the myelin sheath, including nodal widening, do not represent a direct effect of the toxin but an indirect effect, reflecting a general disturbance of the Schwann cell's metabolism; the biochemical basis for this effect of diphtheria toxin is discussed below. The importance of nodal widening therefore is not that it represents a primary effect of the diphtheria toxin but that it is probably the first visible evidence of diphtheritic neuropathy which has an important functional significance.

It is evident that diphtheritic neuropathy is quite different from EAN in that the breakdown of myelin in the former appears to be a consequence of a disturbance of Schwann cell metabolism, and the Schwann cell appears to play an active role in myelin lysis, with small numbers of macrophages playing a lesser role. In contrast, in EAN the primary event is an attack upon the myelin by invading mononuclear cells, and possibly humoral antibodies, involvement of the Schwann cell itself in the process of myelin degradation being secondary and minimal. In this situation the Schwann cell can be considered to play an essentially passive role in the demyelination process. This contrast between the two neuropathies helps to explain a prominent difference in the cytopathology of the two conditions. In diphtheritic neuropathy nodal widening generally precedes segmental demyelination since in a metabolically disturbed Schwann cell the nodal region becomes the most vulnerable part of the myelin sheath. In EAN however invading mononuclear cells attack the myelin sheath either at the node of Ranvier, or internodally and segmental demyelination can thus begin internodally. A generalized response by the Schwann cell to immune attack may also occur in EAN and this may contribute to the nodal widening which undoubtedly does occur in many instances. The role of humoral antibodies in these processes is unknown.

The temporary nature of the cytoplasmic disturbance of the Schwann cell in diphtheritic neuropathy was demonstrated by Allt and Cavanagh (1969). Ten days after the administration of the toxin most of the intracytoplasmic 'membrane whorls' had disappeared and Schwann cell organelles reappeared, notably numerous polysomes and granular endoplasmic reticulum. Such evidence of synthetic activity is likely to be related to (a) remyelination, (b) Schwann cell repair and proliferation and (c) the digestion of myelin debris.

Weller (1965), Weller and Mellick (1966), and Hallpike (1972) studied the role of lysosomes and hydrolases in myelin breakdown following diphtheritic intoxication in the hen and the rat by light and electron cytochemistry, and biochemical assay. Acid phosphatase activity was found to be significantly increased one day after inoculation with diphtheria toxin, and continued to rise steadily to the eighth day and beyond. At the fifth day activity was found to be three times normal yet no functional disability and no significant myelin degradation had occurred. Axons showed no evidence of acid phosphatase reaction, but acid protease showed a significant increase in the first two weeks after injection. Its coincident increase with acid phosphatase suggested that these enzymes have a common lysosomal origin. Neutral protease however is normally present in myelin fractions of peripheral nerve, and release of this protease was invoked to account for an increase in neutral protease activity in established diphtheritic neuropathy. Dense bodies (identified cytochemically as lysosomes) were found in the inner (juxta-axonal) and outer Schwann cell cytoplasm, and these were observed to increase in number up to six days after inoculation. Subsequently there was a marked decrease in lysosomes coincident with the onset of myelin breakdown, and dense bodies (primary lysosomes) were replaced by secondary lysosomes containing myelin debris. The authors therefore considered that hydrolytic enzymes may well play a role in initiating the disintegration of the myelin sheath in diphtheritic neuropathy. Hallpike went further to suggest that a common mechanism underlies other peripheral nerve disorders characterized by segmental myelin loss: activation of the Schwann cell lysosomal apparatus leading to local release of acid protease, which in turn attacks the myelin basic protein to cause disruption of the sheath.

Allt and Cavanagh (1969) found little evidence of the involvement of lysosomes in myelin breakdown in the young rat. We explained the findings of Weller in terms of two possibilities. Firstly, the mechanisms of early myelin disruption may differ in large and small fibres, since Weller was concerned largely with fibres of less than 5 μm in diameter, and Cavanagh and Jacobs (1964) had shown that such small fibres undergo rapid breakdown of whole internodes as a consequence of diphtheritic intoxication, while in large fibres damage may be restricted to the paranode or extended only gradually to the remainder of the internode. Our alternative suggestion was that the discrepancy between our observations and those of Weller may be related to the enormous differences in the susceptibilty of different species to diphtheria toxin, as noted by Jacobs (1967), the rat being much less sensitive than the hen.

Weller and Nester (1972) have recently investigated the problem by studying the histochemistry of single teased fibres and have demonstrated that while demyelination in small diameter fibres appears to be initiated by lysosomal enzymes, such enzymes are not involved in the primary disruption of the myelin sheath in the paranodal regions of large fibres. With reference to the relationship between lysosomes and diphtheria toxin, Weller and Mellick (1966) came to the conclusion that 'while it is possible that diphtheria toxin directly induces lysosome formation, it is more probable that this is a non-specific end result of a general disturbance to the metabolism of the cell'.

Brief descriptions of the fine structure of remyelination following diphtheritic neuropathy have been given by Webster et al. (1961), and Webster (1964) for the guinea-pig, and by Wiśniewski and Raine (1971) for the cat and rabbit. More detailed studies in the rat were reported by Allt (1969b, 1972b).

Remyelination following diphtheritic neuropathy is characterized, as in normal development, by the formation of a spiral of loose Schwann cell membranes which subsequently become compacted, with the elimination of intervening Schwann cell cytoplasm, to produce myelin lamellae with a regular repeat period, and the presence of active Schwann cell cytoplasm rich in granular endoplasmic reticulum and free ribosomes. As in EAN, however, I observed (1972b) several differences between remyelination in diphtheritic neuropathy and normal myelination during ontogeny. Whilst 88% of demyelinated axons were initially invaginated each within one Schwann cell (Fig. 13.6a), 12% of axons were enveloped by more than one Schwann cell process (Fig. 13.6b), but myelination by 'tunication', as described for EAN, was not observed in conjunction with this latter cellular relationship. As in EAN additional loosely associated Schwann cell processes were present with the confines of the old basement membrane of the fibre (Fig. 13.6e) although only for 36% of the axons; 'onion bulb' configurations (Fig. 13.6f) were only occasionally encountered. As in EAN the appearance of multiple Schwann cell processes is probably related to the Schwann cell proliferation which occurs in diphtheritic neuropathy (Jacobs, Cavanagh and Mellick, 1966). As in EAN, the thin myelin sheaths of early remyelination possessed Schmidt—Lanterman clefts, 'redundant' myelin and desmosome-like thickenings along the uncompacted myelin lamellae.

I described (1969b) regeneration of the node of Ranvier following diphtheritic neuropathy. Twenty-two days after inoculation the regenerating node of Ranvier (Fig. 13.8) had the simple structure of the developing node of the immature rat (Allt, 1969a). Paranodal bulbs of the axon and nodal constriction of the axon were slight or absent, so that there was little deviation from the cylindrical shape of the internode. All myelin loops reached the axolemma presenting a longitudinal series in profile and Schwann cell cytoplasm within the myelin loops, as in the immature node, was abundant. The adjacent Schwann cells simply abutted or overlapped one another at the node (Fig. 13.8) or terminated as branching processes projecting into the nodal gap. All of these appearances are very similar to those which I described (1969a) in normal development. The branching Schwann cell processes at the node had a diameter of 50—70 nm and sometimes contained a substructure of longitudinal filaments 10 nm in diameter causing them to closely resemble the finger-like processes of the normal adult node (Landon and Williams, 1963 and Chapter 1). However,

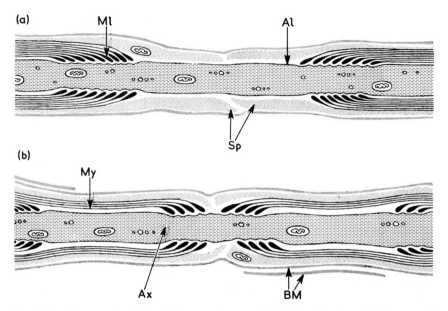

Fig. 13.8 Diagram to illustrate the two forms of nodal regeneration after intraneural injection of diphtheria toxin (Ax, axon; Al, axolemma; Ml, myelin loops; My, myelin lamellae; Sp, Schwann cell process; BM, basement membrane duplicated): (a) Nodal reconstitution associated with the formation of a whole new internode, where nodal widening is >15 μm. (b) Nodal repair by the pre-existing Schwann cell, where nodal widening is <15 μm. Diagram based on 14 nodal profiles. (Modified from Allt, (1969b), by courtesy of *Brain*.)

the processes of the regenerating node did not yet have the intimate and orderly relationship with the nodal axolemma found in the large mature node.

I described (1969b) two kinds of nodal regeneration (Fig. 13.8), the above description being applicable to both types. The first (Fig. 13.8), occurred in the majority of nodes and was associated with extensive myelin loss. It was interpreted to be the consequence of the establishment of a whole new internodal segment, by a Schwann cell laying down myelin *de novo* around a denuded axon. In these circumstances, the formation and appearance of the internodal myelin, and the development of the nodal apparatus, closely paralleled the processes of normal development.

The second type of nodal regeneration (Fig. 13.8) occurred when a nodal gap had been only moderately widened, usually to no more than 15 μm. Under these circumstances the repair mechanism was considered to involve either the extension of adjacent Schwann cells to meet each other at the original nodal site, and the laying down of new lamellae along the whole internode over the outer surface of the retracted sheath, or alternatively the reconstitution of the pre-existing, but broken, outer lamellae and their extension to cover the denuded axon. In either case the original internodal length was restored without the involvement of a new Schwann cell.

It is however necessary to exclude the possibility that the nodes of Ranvier I have described do not represent regenerated nodes but merely pre-existing undamaged nodes. It is also necessary to distinguish between nodal repair mechanisms involving paranodal deposition of new myelin lamellae, and partial demyelination producing thin paranodal myelin as described by Harrison, McDonald, Ochoa and Ohlrich (1972) in the cat spinal cord within only 6 hours of the injection of diphtheria toxin.

I showed (1969b) that at 10 days after injection of toxin (high dose level) all of the nodes of Ranvier examined by light microscopy (teased fibres) were widened to more than 10 μm, indicating that any nodes of Ranvier of normal appearance observed at 22 days had been reconstituted. At 22 days there was no evidence of continuing myelin breakdown or of disorganization of Schwann cell organelles, but there was however widespread evidence of remyelination, thin myelin sheaths, of both compacted and uncompacted lamellae, and 'active' Schwann cell cytoplasm, and the new paranodal myelin usually consisted of uncompacted lamellae at this time. Such appearances of the paranode were not seen during the active phase of demyelination, supporting the view that the paranodal thin myelin represents evidence of remyelination.

13.11 Effects of diphtheria toxin on cellular metabolism

Several authors have demonstrated that an effect of diphtheria toxin is to inhibit protein synthesis. For example, Strauss and Hendee (1959), in a study of the effect of diphtheria toxin on the metabolism of HeLa cells, found that on addition of saturating doses of toxin at 37°C protein synthesis, as indicated by methionine uptake, had ceased completely after 2 hours.

Collier and Pappenheimer (1964a and b) employing cell free extracts of HeLa cells and rabbit reticulocytes found that the presence of the cofactor NAD (nicotinamide adenine dinucleotide) was a *sine qua non* for toxin to exert its inhibitory effect in cell-free systems. They proposed that toxin specifically inhibits the transfer of amino acids from soluble RNA to the growing polypeptide chain. More recent studies (Honjo, Nishizuka, Hayaishi and Kato, 1968; Gill, Pappenheimer, Brown and Kurnick, 1969) have confirmed this view and demonstrated that toxin causes the reversible hydrolysis of NAD with the liberation of free nicotinamide. The ADP-ribose portion of NAD is linked to transferase II (one of the highly labile soluble enzymes involved in the assembly of amino acids into the polypeptide chain on the ribosome) inactivating the enzyme.

Matheson (1968a) demonstrated that the inhibition of protein synthesis by diphtheria toxin, as indicated by glycine uptake, occurs in rat sciatic nerve. Progressively less glycine was incorporated into the protein of an adult sciatic nerve with increasing concentrations of toxin. Similarly, Pleasure, Feldmann and Prockop (1973) using chick embryo sciatic nerves *in vitro*, found that diphtheria toxin did not increase the degradation of preformed myelin lipids or proteins, but that the toxin inhibited the synthesis of myelin proteolipid and basic proteins, and caused a secondary delayed reduction in the rate of incorporation of sulphatide into myelin. The authors put forward the interesting hypothesis that the synthesis of proteolipid and basic proteins is preferentially inhibited because these proteins are probably synthesized by ribosomes associated with the plasma membrane. The delay period of at least one hour before the effect of toxin is evident in cell systems (compared with the immediate effect in the cell-free systems) is accounted for by the time taken for the intact toxin (a protein of molecular weight of 62 000 daltons) to penetrate into the cell.

Jacobs (1967) attributed the greater susceptibility of Schwann cells of a young animal to toxin, as indicated histopathologically, to the relatively greater protein requirements of an immature Schwann cell. The Schwann cells of a young animal synthesize large quantities of protein during myelinogenesis for incorporation into new myelin lamellae, whereas in the adult, once myelination has ceased, protein is required only for replacement within the sheath. In support of this view Matheson and Cavanagh (1967) and Matheson (1968b) found that the rate of amino-acid incorporation in peripheral nerve was considerably greater in immature animals than in the adult, being about fourfold in the hen and more than tenfold in the rat. The authors proposed that the more rapid onset of damage in young animals due to diphtheria toxin can also be satisfactorily explained in terms of relative rates of protein synthesis. Jacobs ascribed the greater vulnerability of small fibres to diphtheria toxin compared with large fibres in terms of their relative surface areas, a relatively greater surface area of Schwann cell being available for the uptake of toxin in small fibres.

Majno, Waksman and Karnovsky (1960) in a study of diphtheritic intoxication in guinea-pig peripheral nerve observed a slow decrease in the total nerve lipid content from the fifth day after inoculation, and the incorporation of acetate into total lipids was profoundly and persistently depressed from 24 hours after inoculation. These changes were interpreted to be a manifestation of an early and persistent depression of the function of myelin maintenance. However it seems likely that the changes represent a secondary effect, the inhibition of protein synthesis probably preceding any dysfunction of lipid metabolism.

The breakdown of myelin and the formation of 'membrane whorls' in diphtheritic neuropathy, perhaps from intracytoplasmic membrane systems (Allt and Cavanagh, 1969), may be the direct result of an inhibition of protein synthesis. There is evidence that proteins have the property of stabilizing membrane systems (Kavanau, 1965): in discussing the role of proteins in mechanical stability of membranes, Kavanau describes the very effective way in which proteins stabilize emulsions, and how the proteins of mitochondria bind lipids to form a highly stable complex. The reported replacement rates for the protein moiety of myelin (i.e. protein 'turnover') vary (Davison and Peters, 1970; D'Monte, Mela and Marks, 1971; Smith, 1972; Fischer and Morrell,

1974): half-lives given for myelin basic protein and myelin proteolipid protein range from 12–95 days. Whatever the precise half-lives are, the amount of protein turnover could represent a critical aspect of the stability of the myelin sheath. It is likely that if replacement of protein in membranes is prevented by an inhibition of protein synthesis, as in diphtheria intoxication, the membrane systems will eventually become unstable and break down. The time necessary for this to occur probably explains the latent period of several days which elapses before myelin breakdown begins.

It is therefore becoming increasingly apparent that diphtheria toxin does not produce demyelination by acting directly on the membranes, as proposed by Webster *et al.* (1961) but instead interferes with the synthesis of one or more essential myelin components (Pleasure, Feldmann and Prockop, 1973). However, the mechanism by which demyelination is initiated in the central nervous system of cats within a few hours of localized injection of toxin, as reported by McDonald and co-workers (Harrison, McDonald and Ochoa, 1972; Harrison, McDonald, Ochoa and Ohlrich, 1972) remains unclear. McDonald and Sears (1970a) suggest the possibility that local oedema induced by the toxin may be involved in the pathogenesis of the lesion.

Waksman, Adams and Mansmann (1957) demonstrated that the immune mechanism was not involved in the pathogenesis of diphtheritic neuropathy, nor were the lesions inflammatory (as in EAN). There was no correlation between the development of the neuropathy and the production of circulating antibody (antitoxin) to diphtheria toxin, and no antibodies were produced against rabbit spinal cord or sciatic nerve as they are in EAE and EAN. Rabbits given whole body irradiation with 400 rads showed a drastic reduction in circulating lymphocytes, polymorphonuclear leucocytes and circulating antibodies but an unaffected disease process. It was concluded therefore that diphtheritic neuropathy is produced by a non-immune mechanism, (unlike EAN). It is evident therefore that the role of the immune response, if it is involved at all, is protective, serving to neutralize the diphtheria toxin. Whether or not the immune response is involved is determined by dose levels of toxin injected, as small doses of toxin, insufficient to induce antitoxin formation, nevertheless produced paralysis.

Several investigations have reported the effects of administering antitoxin (antibody) at varying times before and after injection of toxin (see Waksman, Adams and Mansmann, 1957). For example Cavanagh and Jacobs (1964) and Jacobs, Cavanagh and Mellick (1966) found that toxin was unavailable for inactivation by antitoxin one hour after injection of toxin, whereas no signs of functional disturbance developed when antitoxin was given 10 min before intraneural injection of toxin.

13.12 Electrophysiological changes in EAN and diphtheritic neuropathy

The effects of segmental demyelination and nodal widening on nerve conduction have been investigated in EAN (Kaeser and Lambert, 1962; Cragg and Thomas,

1964a; Hall, 1967b; Davis and Jacobson, 1971; Davis 1972) and diphtheritic neuropathy (Kaeser and Lambert, 1962; McDonald, 1963b; Morgan-Hughes, 1965, 1968; McDonald and Gilman, 1968; Koles and Rasminsky, 1972; Rasminsky and Sears, 1972). Some of the findings will be briefly discussed. The principal pathophysiological changes evident following demyelination are (a) a reduction in conduction velocity or a conduction block, and (b) an impaired response to repetitive stimulation.

Rasminsky and Sears (1972) have recently described a technique for recording from single undissected nerve fibres in the lumber ventral roots of the rat. By local application of diphtheria toxin they were able to demonstrate that conduction remains saltatory up to the stage of conduction block in demyelinating fibres, and does not become continuous as in normal unmyelinated fibres as had been previously suggested (Cragg and Thomas, 1964a). Slowing of conduction was attributed to changes in the passive electrical cable properties of the internode. There was an apparent increase in internodal capacitance and a decrease in internodal transverse resistance at internodes of demyelinating fibres, changes considered to have the effect of delaying excitation at the nodes. These changes in passive electrical properties appeared to occur primarily in the paranodal region, thus correlating with the pathology of nodal widening as described above. A more than twenty-five fold increase of internodal conduction time was tolerated before conduction block occurred in demyelinating fibres.

As in nerve fibres of the central nervous system (McDonald and Sears, 1970b), repetitive activation of demyelinated fibres was found by Rasminsky and Sears to cause a progressive increase in internodal conduction time culminating in intermittent or total conduction block. These changes were considered to be due to an accumulation of intracellular sodium with a consequent progressive decrease in the amplitude of the action potential. The authors postulated that the internal accumulation of sodium could result from deficient sodium pumping and related this to the breakdown of the nodal-paranodal complex in nodal widening as discussed above (Ballin and Thomas, 1968; Allt and Cavanagh, 1969). As Williams and Landon (1963) have suggested, the paranodal accumulations of mitochondria might be the energy source of the sodium pump, as the cytoplasm in which they lie is continuous with the nodal Schwann cell processes which abut upon the nodal axolemma (2 nm interspace: Anderson—Cedergren and Karlsson, 1966). Rasminsky and Sears point out that changes in internal sodium concentration which would have very little effect on conduction in normal fibres could be expected to have a considerable effect on conduction along internodes with a low safety factor (see below) such as those of a demyelinated fibre. The effect, in nodal widening, of the loss of nodal gap substance, which Langley and Landon (1968) have shown to contain a sulphated mucopolysaccharide with ion exchange properties, has yet to be elucidated.

Davis (1972) has described an impairment of repetitive impulse conduction in demyelinated nerves in EAN. Normal guinea-pig sciatic-peroneal nerves maintained at 37°C conducted compound action potentials with only a minor decrease in amplitude at stimulus frequencies up to 200 per second. In contrast demyelinating nerves maintained at 37°C demonstrated a rapid decrease in action potential amplitude when stimulated at rates as slow as 10–25 per second. McDonald and Sears (1970b) and Davis (1972) have proposed that this phenomenon may have clinical significance in the segmental demyelinating neuropathies as well as in CNS demyelinating disorders. Thus the failure of demyelinated axons to properly sustain repetitive activity could account for such symptoms in multiple sclerosis as the rapid increase of muscle weakness during exercise, and the 'fading out' of vision, while looking at an object continuously for several seconds, in those patients who have optic nerve lesions. Hall (1967b) had previously proposed that the neurological signs of EAN may result from a focal demyelination affecting the ability of fibres to transmit the rapid series of impulses which arise from muscle stretch receptors. He suggested that symmetrical ataxia of gait and instability of posture following displacement was due to interference with normal proprioceptive inflow to the central nervous system, provided largely by impulses from muscle stretch receptors.

Davis and Jacobson (1971) investigated the effect of both an increase and a decrease in temperature on conduction through demyelinating lesions in EAN in the guinea-pig. With normal nerves conduction can be blocked by an elevation of temperature of 34–36°C. For demyelinated, EAN nerves the same effect can be produced by a smaller increase in temperature, in some cases at temperatures of 15°C lower than for normal controls. Rasminsky (1973) found that in rat ventral roots demyelinated with diphtheria toxin, conduction block could occur in single fibres with an increase in temperature of only 0.5°C. The hypothesis proposed to account for this increased susceptibility to thermally-induced conduction blockade rests on the following premises: (a) the ratio of the action current generated by a nerve impulse to the minimum amount of current needed to maintain conduction is known as the safety factor, and is found to have a value of 5–7 in myelinated toad axons (Tasaki, 1953); (b) this ratio reflects the net effect of several variables which are involved in the maintenance of axonal conduction. The hypothesis proposes that if the safety factor is decreased by injury or disease to a very low level so that conduction only just occurs, then any additional detrimental factor such as a small increase in temperature might produce a conduction block, even though it would have little effect on normal nerves. Whilst the mechanism of the temperature effect is not known (see Rasminsky), the hypothesis accounts for the observation that only a small increase in temperature will produce a conduction block in demyelinating nerves. Conversely a small decrease in temperature would permit such a blocked nerve to conduct, or, in the case of a nerve conducting with a small safety factor, the effect would be to increase that safety factor.

This hypothesis would account for the well known effect of temperature on human demyelinating diseases such as multiple sclerosis where signs and symptoms are ameliorated by a small decrease in body temperature and exacerbated by similarly small increases in temperature (Guthrie, 1951).

Koles and Rasminsky (1972) constructed a computer model of a myelinated nerve fibre and simulated demyelination by increasing the capacitance and conductance of the myelin sheath of individual internodes or parts of internodes. The model consisted of 21 nodes and 20 internodes. Each internode had a myelin sheath represented by nine elements of parallel capacitance and conductance, and each element could be independently changed. The model showed that internodal conduction time increased as myelin thickness was decreased. Propagation continued through a single internode until myelin thickness was uniformly reduced to less than 2.7% of its normal value. Conduction failed earlier however if adjacent internodes were also demyelinating. Paranodal demyelination, as in nodal widening, was found to be especially effective in slowing impulse conduction. Propagation across a severely demyelinated internode was blocked by an increase in internal sodium concentration or an increase in temperature, insufficient to prevent conduction in a normal fibre. The authors emphasized the close correspondence between the results derived from the computer model and data derived experimentally.

Electrophysiological data are sparse for animals which have recovered from EAN. As Cragg and Thomas (1964a) explain, the reason is that severely affected animals do not survive and abnormalities are difficult to detect in the action potentials of nerves containing only a small proportion of affected fibres. Hall (1967b) obtained results from one animal (44 days after antigen injection) which still showed a marked conduction defect and persistent pathological changes despite the fact that it had made a complete symptomatic recovery from EAN. Hall was uncertain how to explain this paradox, but postulated a hypothetical 'central mechanism' which might compensate for the abnormal proprioceptive inflow. Cragg and Thomas found no abnormalities in electrical recordings from one guinea-pig injected 91 days previously and were able to demonstrate histological evidence of remyelination in the form of short internodes. Data from other experimental demyelinating conditions indicate that conduction velocity returns to approximately normal only after a long period. Morgan-Hughes (1965) found that in diphtheritic neuropathy in the guinea-pig the conduction velocity had returned to about half of its original value by the tenth week after injection. Subsequently the increase in conduction velocity progressed more slowly, and in some cases values at the lower limit of the normal range were not obtained until 7–8 months after injection.

Gilliatt (1966) considered that the slow improvement of conduction velocity is related to the gradually increasing myelin thickness of the affected segments. It has long been known that conduction velocity increases with myelin thickness (Sanders and Whitteridge, 1946) and fibre diameter (Gasser and Grundfest, 1939; Rushton, 1951). The role of nodal regeneration in EAN (Ballin and Thomas, 1969a) and in diphtheritic neuropathy (Allt, 1969b) in the reconstitution of normal conduction patterns has yet to be elucidated.

In regeneration, following segmental demyelination and Wallerian degeneration, the new internodes are usually short, due to the absence of the elongating effect of growth. It is therefore of interest to examine what effect the increased frequency of the nodes of Ranvier has upon conduction velocity. Sanders and Whitteridge (1946) came to the conclusion that conduction velocity is independent of internodal distance since they found a regenerated nerve (after crush) with short internodes conducted at a similar rate to a normal nerve of a corresponding diameter. Similarly Gilliatt (1966) argues that internodal length can vary within wide limits without velocity being affected, since fibre diameter and conduction velocity reach adult values early in man, probably by the eighth year, but by contrast internodal length continues to increase for as long as body growth continues. Morgan-Hughes (1965) observed short internodes on recovery from diphtheritic intoxication and yet obtained approximately normal values for conduction velocity.

Huxley and Stämpfli (1949) and Rushton (1951) provide *a priori* explanations for these observations. They determined that for a given size of fibre there will be an optimum internodal length for maximum conduction velocity. Lengths somewhat greater or smaller than this optimum will give nearly the same velocity but the energy losses in propagation will be proportional to the number of nodes in the stretch of nerve. Hence it will be most economical if the normal nerve has an internode somewhat greater than the optimum, since this will appreciably reduce the energy necessary for conduction without much change in speed. It follows that the reduction of the internode to a length somewhat below the optimum (as occurs after regeneration) will not change the velocity but will increase the energy required for impulse propagation, that is there will be a greater energy expenditure.

13.13 Wallerian degeneration and subsequent regeneration — introduction

The salient feature of Wallerian degeneration is that the primary lesion affects the axon with only secondary involvement of the Schwann cell and loss of myelin. It therefore affords an instructive contrast to segmental demyelination in which the lesion occurs in the Schwann cell, usually exclusively. Augustus Waller gave his name to this primary axonal degeneration, although he was not the first investigator to have examined the effects on nerve structure of a ligature or nerve section. Waller (1850) described the microscopical appearance of the hypoglossal and glossopharyngeal nerves of the frog following section. Whilst his terminology is necessarily archaic his precise account remains an impressive example of careful observation:

> During the four first days, after section of the hypoglossal nerve, no change is observed in its structure. On the fifth day the tubes appear more varicose than usual, and the medulla (*myelin sheath*) more irregular. About the tenth day the medulla forms disorganized fusiform masses at intervals.
> About the twentieth day the medullary particles are completely reduced to a granular state . . . where we find the presence of the nervous element merely indicated by numerous black granules, generally arranged in a row like the

beads of a necklace. In their arrangement it is easy to detect the wavy direction characteristic of the nerves. They are still contained in the tubular membrane, which is but faintly distinguished, probably from the loss of the medulla and from atrophy of its tissue.

Many studies since 1850 have further explored the changes occurring distal to a nerve section and the similar changes produced by nerve crush. Regeneration after nerve section, and the more orderly and reproducible regeneration after nerve crush, have also been the subject of many investigations. In this chapter it will be possible to consider only a selection from the vast literature which has accrued, and emphasis will be placed on the more recent light and electron microscope studies. This is justified, since it is in the nature of science that earlier work becomes assimilated, modified or is rendered obsolete by more recent studies.

The term 'Wallerian degeneration' will be used to describe degeneration distal to a cut or crush. It should not be used to describe changes proximal to the lesion nor, as is unfortunately widespread in the writings on neuropathology, any primary axonal degeneration induced by any means, be they mechanical, toxic or diseased states. If 'Wallerian' must be used in a wider sense than defined above, then the term 'Wallerian-type' is to be preferred.

Seddon (1943) proposed a clinical classification of nerve injury by mechanical trauma as follows:

(a) *Neurotmesis* ('cutting of the nerve'): injury in which all essential structures, including axons, have been severed. There is not necessarily a visible anatomical gap in the nerve, since the epineurial sheath may remain in continuity, but the effect on degeneration and regeneration is the same as after complete anatomical discontinuity.

(b) *Axonotmesis:* a lesion to the axon of sufficient severity to cause degeneration of the axon distal to the lesion; there is no interruption of the continuity of the endoneurium.

(c) *Neurapraxia:* ('non-acting nerve') injury in which paralysis occurs in the absence of peripheral degeneration.

The appeal of Seddon's classification is that not only does it distinguish between the types of degeneration, but also implicit within it are differences in the morphology of regeneration, functional loss and recovery, and hence clinical prognosis. The effects in experimental studies of endoneurial continuity (after crush) or discontinuity (after section) on subsequent nerve regerneration will be discussed in this chapter, as will neurotmesis and axonotmesis involving Wallerian degeneration of nerve fibres distal to the lesion. Neurapraxia will not be discussed.

The term 'neurilemma' has fortunately fallen into disuse with progress in electron microscopy, though even some electron microscopists have used the name (e.g. Satinsky, Pepe and Liu, 1964; Olsson and Sjöstrand, 1969), and any attempts to revive the term should be resisted. Young in 1942 wrote 'The term "neurilemma" has thus become hopelessly confused', and he tells us that Key and Retzius suggested that it should be abandoned as long ago as 1873. It has been used variously to mean the inner endoneurial sheath (sheath of Plenk and Laidlaw) the outer Schwann cell cytoplasm, the Schwann cell plasma membrane, the Schwann cell basement membrane, and combinations of these, and even in the nineteenth century the whole connective tissue of the nerve consisting of epi-, peri-, and endoneuria (see Young, 1942)! This historical confusion together with ultrastructural identification of the various structural components of the peripheral nerve have now rendered the term obsolete.

13.14 Histology of Wallerian degeneration

13.14.1 *Light microscopy*

The light microscopic descriptions of Wallerian degeneration and subsequent regeneration have been reviewed by Young (1942), Guth (1956) and Causey (1960). A brief summary of the earlier findings will be given followed by a more detailed consideration of some recent investigations.

Distal to a cut or crush the axon becomes irregular in shape and fragments. This process is accompanied by a retraction of the myelin sheath from the axon at the nodes of Ranvier, creating increased nodal gaps (Fig. 13.9a). The myelin sheath then breaks down into 'digestive chambers' or 'ellipsoids' (Fig. 13.9b) within which are contained axonal material which becomes degraded. The ellipsoids are progressively broken down into rows of spherical lipid droplets which are further degraded, together with axonal remains by Schwann cells and macrophages (Fig. 13.9c). The similar processes *in vitro*, produced by nerve crush in long-term cultures of dorsal root ganglia, have been described by Peterson and Murray (1965).

Degradation of the myelin debris and axonal remains is accompanied by proliferation of the Schwann cells which form, within the distal stump, the columns or 'bands of Büngner', and it is these columns which serve to guide the regenerating axons to their terminations. In a severed nerve proliferating cells migrate into the gap between the severed ends during the first few days after section. Migration occurs from both the proximal and distal ends, but chiefly from the distal, until the gap is bridged. The nature of the cell population that bridges this gap and the origin of macrophages in the degenerating nerve are considered below. Increased protein synthesis is apparent in the proliferating Schwann cells histochemically, and the significance of this feature is also considered later. Retrograde changes in the cell body, including chromatolysis, following axonal section are discussed elsewhere in this book (see Chapter 12).

Axonal outgrowths arise from the proximal side of the zone of trauma and traverse the gap in a severed nerve, guided by bands of Schwann cells within the gap. This is followed by reinnervation of the distal stump along the 'bands of Büngner', Initially the axons lie on the surface of the Schwann cells, but they later become embedded in the Schwann cell cytoplasm. Increase in axonal diameter occurs rapidly, e.g. 1.2 μm at 15 days, 2.3 μm at 25 days and 7.0 μm at 100 days. In addition to the outgrowth occurring from the cut ends of the axon, regeneration may also involve sprouting of new collateral branches, but as the regenerating nerve fibre increases in diameter such collaterals degenerate. Myelin sheaths are evident around the proximal ends of the regenerated axons within the first week after their outgrowth, but increase in thickness of the sheath is a slow process, requiring about a year for completion.

Axons arising from the proximal stump innervate the distal stump randomly, as can be shown when axons from one half of the proximal stump are allowed to reinnervate the whole of the distal stump and fail to follow their original pathways. Regenerating axons show no preference for degenerating as opposed to normal peripheral nerves, and removal of the muscle supplied has no effect on the extent of sprouting. However, the nature of their eventual peripheral connections greatly influences the final maturation of the regenerated fibres.

The rates of regeneration of nerves, i.e. distance traversed per unit time, for various nerves, in different species, and following different types of lesion, were reviewed by Guth (1956). Two examples will suffice: the average velocity of motor fibre regeneration in the rabbit is 2.0 mm per day after sectioning and 3.0 mm per day after crushing, the rate curve being linear (i.e. velocity is constant). As an example of regeneration of sensory nerves in man an overall average velocity of 4.6 mm per day was obtained, though in man the rate curve is curvilinear with a gradual deceleration, e.g. 8.5 mm per day in the upper arm decreasing to 2 mm per day at the wrist.

Certain characteristics of the fibre population of a regenerated nerve are influenced by the nature of the initial lesion. Following the crush of a nerve supplying a limb muscle in the rabbit, the regenerated fibres ultimately assume a fibre size spectrum which is bimodal, as in the normal animal. In contrast the fibre spectrum remains permanently unimodal after nerve section. 150–200 days after a crush, the number of fibres in the distal stump equals the number in the proximal stump, but after nerve section the number of fibres in the distal stump is permanently reduced. After both crush and cut the myelinated fibres of the proximal stump show a decreased diameter for 130 days, and only after a crush is there a subsequent restoration to approximately normal size.

Recent studies have clarified and extended these earlier findings. Williams and Hall (1971a and b) used a new incident light technique to examine the light microscope appearance of fibre degeneration *in vivo* induced by a crush. An important finding was that marked changes occurred in fibres during the first hour following crush (Fig. 13.9a). Earlier studies employing conventional histological techniques (Causey and Palmer, 1952) had described the earliest changes as occurring 24 hours after crush (except for widening of the nodal gap at the first nodes proximal and distal to the site of crush). Williams and Hall observed that whilst normal fibres examined for up to 6 hours show no change, a crush produced nodal widening and dilation of Schmidt–Lanterman incisures in all fibres, up to 5 mm from the site of crush, within 2 min. The same changes occurred in small fibres up to 2 cm distal to the crush within 10 min, and in some larger fibres over the next 60 min. During the next 36 hours the remaining large fibres between 2 and 4 cm from the crush became affected.

Williams and Hall have also described the progressive dissolution of the myelin sheath. The formation of ellipsoids, composed of axonal material surrounded by myelin, occurred by means of constrictions, in general at Schmidt—Lanterman incisures (Fig. 13.9b). The ellipsoids were progressively shortened by the formation of transverse partitions, producing irregular spheres and ovoids, such that by the fourth post-operative day few primary ellipsoids remained. By the fifth day myelin debris assumed two forms (still confined within the cylindrical territories of the degenerating fibres): the first consisted of relatively large spheres and ovoids, up to 10 μm in diameter, which displayed a periphery of optical density similar to the original myelin sheath, and the second of small spheres 1—2 μm in diameter, which were packed in the spaces between the larger debris. The small globules were seen to be formed by a process of 'pinching-off' from ends of the larger spheres and ovoids.

Between the fifth and thirtieth days after a crush, cells containing many small globules appeared in the endoneurial spaces and increased in number. The cells were flattened and elongated with irregular margins; they were observed to migrate outward until they came to lie beneath the perineurium, and by 20 days formed an almost continuous subperineurial cellular layer along the entire distal extent of the crushed nerves. Between 30 and 60 days following the crush this population of cells decreased until by 60 days only a few remained between the remyelinating fibres. Dissection of the perineurium and the fibre fascicles, and their examination *in vitro*, revealed that the globule laden cells remained in the endoneurial space without entering the perineurium.

Causey and Palmer (1953) were of the opinion that Wallerian degeneration, as indicated by nodal widening, progressed centrifugally, beginning at the site of the lesion and spreading towards the periphery but Donat and Wiśniewski (1973) were unable to find any differences in the nodal changes along the length of the nerve.

Webster (1965) described an increase in the number of Schmidt—Lanterman incisures distal to a crush as a prelude to myelin breakdown. The increase was apparent 12—48 hours after crush and was especially evident paranodally. Whilst this finding has now been generally accepted, Williams and Hall (1971a) consider it most likely that the apparent increase in number was in fact due to a sudden dilatation of previously closed, and therefore not readily apparent, incisures. In support of this contention the authors described dilatation of incisures as an early response to nerve crush, using their technique of continuous observation of degenerating fibres *in vivo*. Hall and Williams (1970) demonstrated a similar dilatation, which was reversible, under conditions of hypotonicity. On *a priori* grounds an increase in the number of incisures in Wallerian degeneration is not to be expected. Schmidt—Lanterman incisures are highly elaborate structures (Robertson, 1958a; Hall and Williams, 1970) which do exist *in vivo* (Hall and Williams, 1970) and in these two respects are comparable to the node of Ranvier (Robertson, 1959; Williams and Landon, 1963; Landon and Williams, 1963;

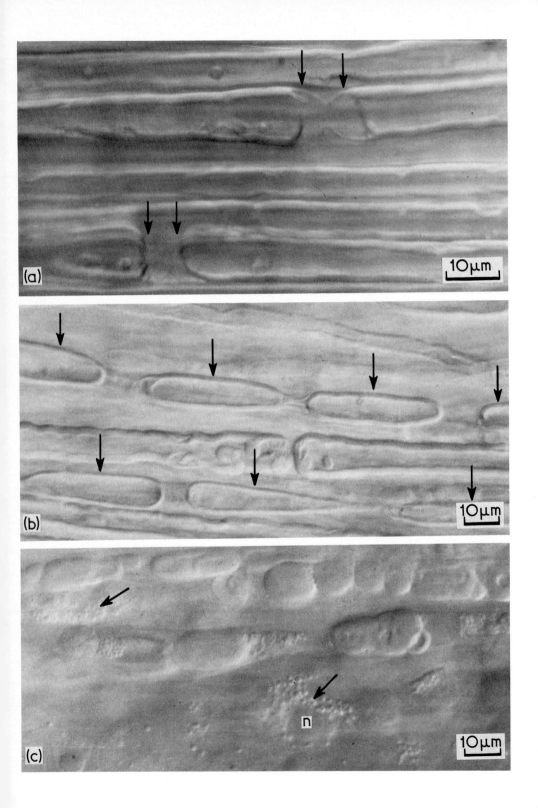

Williams and Hall, 1971a). That an essentially degradative process such as Wallerian degeneration should produce *de novo* such orderly and complex structures seems unlikely. This is not however to deny a role for the incisures in Wallerian degeneration: Webster observed that incisures were located at the regions of axonal narrowing and at the margins of myelin segments.

Williams and Hall (1971a and b) confirmed the importance of incisures in degeneration. Extreme dilatation of most incisures was followed by a progressive collapse and subsequently a severance and rounding-off of axon and myelin at incisures resulting in the formation of ellipsoids (Fig. 13.9b). Some ellipsoids initially contained incisures which were closed or in the early stages of dilatation. These incisures in turn showed dilatation and constriction, contributing to a shortening of the ellipsoids and their transformation into spherical and oval profiles. It is evident therefore that Schmidt—Lanterman incisures act as foci for the disruption of the myelin sheath.

The literature describing the histochemical changes occurring in Wallerian degeneration has recently been reviewed by Hallpike (1972 and Chapter 12). In summary, Hallpike describes two phases of myelin breakdown during Wallerian degeneration: in the first post-operative week the lipid staining properties of the degenerating fibres remains unchanged, while in the second week there is the onset of lipid degradation with the appearance of cholesterol ester. The loss of lipids is considered to be secondary to the breakdown of myelin protein by proteolytic enzymes (see Chapter 12).

Increased acid and neutral protease activity has been detected as early as 24 hours after nerve injury. In the first week both proteases show a two- to threefold increase in activity, with a further marked rise occurring in the second week. Free amino acids liberated from protein substrates within the nerve can be detected as a result of this enzymatic activity. The early released neutral protease is considered to be of axonal rather than myelin origin, whilst acid protease is probably lysosomal, being derived from axons, Schwann cells and macrophages.

Acid phosphatase showed a two- to threefold increase in activity in the first week after nerve section. The close similarities between the distribution and release of both acid phosphatase and acid protease supports the view that both enzymes are of lysosomal origin, and lysosomal activation in axons or Schwann cells thus appears to be an early event in Wallerian degeneration.

In diphtheritic nerves acid protease activity showed a significant increase in the first 2 weeks but neutral protease, probably derived from myelin, only showed increased activity in established diphtheritic lesions. In Wallerian degeneration however both proteases showed an early increase in activity, the release of neutral protease probably resulting from axonal damage.

Fig. 13.9 Adult mouse sciatic nerves distal to crush as observed *in vivo* using oblique incident illumination: (a) retraction and disappearance of paranodal myelin involving both heminodes (arrows) at 1 hour after crush; (b) during the acute phase the internodal myelin sheath rounds off at Schmidt—Lanterman incisures to form typical primary ovoids (arrows), which therefore correspond to cylindrico-conical segments (72 hours after crush); (c) typical debris-containing cells (arrows); nucleus (n) devoid of globules (7 days after crush). (Reproduced by courtesy of Susan M. Hall.)

The extensive literature describing biochemical studies in Wallerian degeneration is beyond the scope of this chapter and has been recently reviewed by Domonkos (1972), and Porcellati (1972).

As Williams and Hall (1971a) point out, theories which attempt to account for the underlying mechanism of fibre degeneration and ellipsoid formation are generally of two kinds, involving either the collapse of a long cylinder of fluid under surface tension after the loss of the turgor pressure normally supplied by the neuron (Young, 1945), or the activity of hydrolytic enzymes. However, these two explanations are not necessarily mutually exclusive. A combined mechanical and enzymatic process may well in fact occur in Wallerian degeneration, as Williams and Hall (1971a) and Weller and Mellick (1966) have suggested.

Olsson (1966) and Mellick and Cavanagh (1967, 1968a and b) have described an increased permeability of endoneurial blood vessels to labelled albumin in the region of trauma after section, crush and ligature. They showed that there is a proximal and distal movement of albumin within the nerve from the site of maximum concentration, and that the greater part moves in a distal direction if the endoneurial spaces are patent. Mellick and Cavanagh accounted for this movement in terms of a more rapid removal of protein by the perineurium (*vide infra*) distally than proximally. Olsson (1967) demonstrated an early mast cell degranulation in the region of nerve crush and nerve section but not distal to the lesion site. Mast cells in the epineurium, perineurium and endoneurium were all affected. He considered that the biogenic amines, heparin, histamine, and 5-hydroxytryptamine, liberated by the mast cells contributed to the increased vascular permeability induced by the mechanical trauma.

The perineurium is now well recognized to be a metabolically active diffusion barrier (Shantha and Bourne, 1968) and in this context can be considered to have an important homeostatic function, contributing to the maintenance of the constant composition of the endoneurial matrix. Mellick and Cavanagh (1968b) have proposed that following a crush, when blood-derived proteins leak into the endoneurial space, the perineurium may act to restore the composition of the endoneurial matrix, and they point out the possible importance of such changes in the *internal milieu* of the nerve on nerve function.

In Wallerian degeneration there is a marked increase in the cell population distal to the site of injury (Abercrombie and Johnson, 1946; Joseph, 1947, 1948, 1950; Thomas, 1948; Abercrombie, Evans and Murray, 1959). The increase is largely attributable to cells of local origin, and principally to Schwann cell proliferation. The greatest increase occurs in nerves containing many large myelinated fibres and the least increase in unmyelinated nerves. Abercrombie and Johnson (1946) investigated the cell population of the rabbit sciatic nerve following section. They found that the total cell population reached a peak at 25 days after section when it was 8.4 times the value of the normal nerve population, and that the period of steepest rise of the sigmoid growth curve occurred at 10–15 days. The population thereafter declined, e.g. at 225 days it was reduced to about 60% of the peak value, the greater part of the decrease occurring between 25 and 45 days. The Schwann cell ('tubal') population was 13 times greater than normal 25 days after section. At 225 days it was reduced to 55% of the Schwann cell population at 25 days, most of this reduction also occurring between 25 and 45 days.

Abercrombie, Evans and Murray (1959) investigated cell population changes in the rabbit abdominal vagus, a largely unmyelinated nerve. After 5 days of degeneration only a 60% increase in cell population was apparent, and no further change occurred between 5 and 10 days. The increase was therefore much less than for a nerve containing many myelinated fibres. After 10 days the cell population was observed to fall, and at both 25 days and 100 days did not depart significantly from the normal, thus again differing from myelinated nerves in which an increase in the population persists at these times. The authors demonstrated that the diminution in the numbers of macrophages present was insufficient to account for the decline in the total cell population.

The reason for the much more extensive proliferation of Schwann cells in myelinated nerve compared with unmyelinated nerves has not yet been elucidated. Thomas (1948) and Joseph (1947, 1948, 1950) found a correlation between fibre diameter and population increase; Abercrombie and Santler (1957) considered the initial density of cell population to be unimportant, and that the total mass of nerve fibre destroyed was the major determinant; Joseph (1948, 1950) considered the vacant space created by fibre degeneration to be important; whilst Abercrombie and Johnson (1946) postulated a chemical stimulus to cell division provided by the degenerating fibres. Similarly a satisfactory explanation for the decline in cell population has yet to be given. As Abercrombie and Johnson point out, the major decline occurs soon after the 25 day population peak, even when reinnervation is excluded as a complicating factor at this time by removal of a segment of nerve. Other factors, as yet undefined, must therefore be operating.

The changes induced in Schwann cells and fibroblasts by section of the sciatic nerve of the rabbit were investigated by Abercrombie and Johnson (1942) using tissue culture techniques. Portions of the proximal and distal stumps were explanted at varying times after section and the 'activity' of each explant was expressed as the amount of outwandering of Schwann cells and fibroblasts that occurred in vitro. Explants of normal nerve rarely showed any activity. In the distal stump Schwann cell activity began on the second day after section rising rapidly to a peak at 19–25 days, falling equally rapidly to 60 days and thereafter more slowly. In the proximal stump the maximum activity was never more than 10% of the maximum activity of the distal stump and was reached between 5 and 10 days after cutting the nerve. By contrast the Schwann cells from the distal stump of a largely unmyelinated nerve (rabbit abdominal vagus) showed a peak of activity at 5–10 days after section (Abercrombie, Evans and Murray, 1959).

The migratory activity of Schwann cells in vitro therefore closely parallels their proliferation *in vivo* in response to nerve section. The time of maximum activity corresponds to that of maximum proliferation, and the same diparity is found between myelinated and unmyelinated nerves in both the time at which maximum cell populations are reached, and their activity *in vitro*. As Abercrombie and co-workers point out, the stimulus to proliferation and migration may therefore be related. Lubińska (1961a) observed that, in the life-history of Schwann cells, phases of migratory and proliferative activity usually occur either before the formation or after the destruction of myelin, whereas the presence of myelin coincides with the sedentary and non-dividing condition of the cell. This, she suggests, implies that the maintenance of myelin is incompatible with the mobilized state of the Schwann cell.

It is during interphase that the synthesis of DNA, necessary for the doubling of genetic material, occurs in a dividing cell population and this part of interphase is termed the synthesis phase (S). Bradley and Asbury (1970) measured the length of the synthesis phase of Schwann cells in mouse sciatic nerve during Wallerian degeneration. Its duration was found to be 8.6–10.3 hours, and similar values were also obtained for 2 day old mouse sciatic nerve. Its duration was the same at 3 days after nerve section when the peak of mitotic activity occurred as indicated by autoradiographic labelling (15.5% of cells labelled) as at 9 days when only 0.8% of cells were labelled. The rapid onset of Schwann cell proliferation was indicated by the finding of labelled cells (1.9%) 19 hours after nerve transection. The authors show their data to be compatible with those of other studies in which indices of proliferation have been (a) counts of nuclei, (b) mitotic cells or (c) autoradiographic labelling.

Abercrombie, Evans and Murray (1959) assessed the proportion of mono-nuclear cells (chiefly macrophages) present in a degenerating nerve. In normal nerves they represented 2% of all cells, at 5 days after section 19%, at 10 days 15%, at 25 days 11% and at 100 days 5%. The population analysis was carried out on degenerating rabbit abdominal vagus nerve which contains few myelinated fibres. Nerves containing many myelinated fibres were found to contain markedly fewer macrophages on degeneration. The percentages obtained for the abdominal vagus nerve therefore probably represent maximal values.

In view of the difficulty of identification of cell types without the use of electron microscopy, it is necessary to interpret with some caution the precise percentage changes for each cell population as determined in light microscopic studies of Wallerian degeneration.

13.14.2 *Electron microscopy*

In early ultrastructural studies of Wallerian degeneration, Vial (1958) and Hönjïn, Nakamura and Imura (1959) described the initial axoplasmic changes distal to nerve section in the rat and mouse. The earliest changes were evident in the endoplasmic reticulum, which became fragmented into rows of vesicles, so that it was exceptional to find normal endoplasmic reticulum more than 24 hours after nerve section. Between 24 and 48 hours, neurofilaments lost their longitudinal orientation, and then underwent dissolution and were replaced by a finely granular material which subsequently became clumped, lying within a clear matrix. With the better techniques now available, it is clear that microtubules undergo the same changes as neurofilaments (Ballin and Thomas, 1969c; Donat and Wiśniewski, 1973). Concomitant with neurofilament disorganization, axonal mitochondria underwent a pronounced swelling. Vial emphasized the variation from one animal to another and even between different fibres in the same nerve in the rate at which these changes occurred, though the changes were always complete at 48 hours after section. At this time, some myelin sheaths were observed to have assumed complex infoldings, but as Webster and Spiro (1960) pointed out, some of these appearances could be accounted for by atypical configurations of the sheath which are occasionally seen in 'normal' nerve. In some cases they may also represent paranodal crenations of the sheath, typical of the normal paranode (Williams and Landon, 1963).

Schlaepfer (1974a) has proposed that the immediate cause of axonal microtubule and neurofilament disintegration is an influx of calcium ions into the axon at the point of the injury. By incubating segments of rat saphenous nerve in calcium-free media he was able to prevent the breakdown of axonal microtubules and neurofilaments; after the addition of calcium ions to the media, changes characteristic of early Wallerian degeneration occurred. Conversely, under conditions of energy deprivation the degenerative changes occurred more rapidly: after the addition of inhibitors of high-energy phosphate metabolism to the medium, degenerative changes began after two hours whilst under nutrient conditions they did not occur for 24–36 hours (Schlaepfer, 1974b). Schlaepfer proposes that a block of energy-dependent calcium-excluding mechanisms, followed by an influx of calcium ions into the axoplasm could initiate axoplasmic degeneration. *In vivo*, regions of the nerve proximal and distal to the site of the crush with intact axolemma and yet impaired vascular supply, due to crush or section, would be vulnerable to energy-deprivation which could contribute to the degenerative changes in these regions.

Several investigations (Hönjin, Nakamura and Imura, 1959; Ohmi, 1961; Webster, 1962; Lee, 1963; Holtzman and Novikoff, 1965; Zelena, Lubińska and Gutman, 1968; Ballin and Thomas, 1969c; Morris, Hudson and Weddell, 1972b; Donat and Wiśniewski, 1973; Schlaepfer, 1973) have variously described early axonal changes as involving focal accumulations of mitochondria, mitochondrial fragments, multivesicular bodies, lamellar bodies, dense bodies and vesicular profiles, occurring immediately proximal and distal to the cut or crush lesion (Fig. 13.10).

Donat and Wiśniewski recognized three distinct zones distal to the point of section on the basis of the distribution of accumulations of axonal organelles: zone 1 (the traumatic zone) consisted of the first 1–2 mm containing dense accumulations of organelles often arranged peripherally around centrally

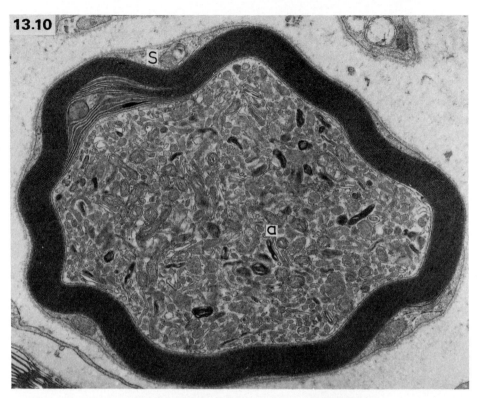

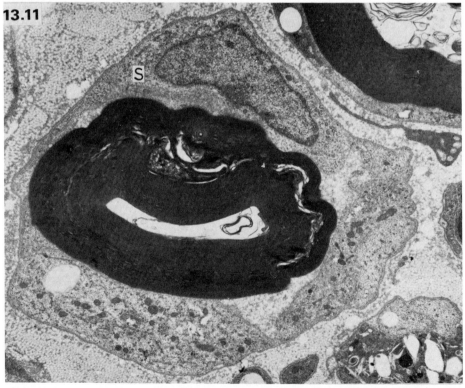

displaced filaments; zone 2 (the peritraumatic zone) occupied the next 2–3 cm and was characterized by paranodal accumulations of organelles; and zone 3 consisted of the rest of the nerve in which accumulations of organelles were rare. The cause of these accumulations is not understood, but several suggestions have been proposed e.g. block of retrograde flow (see Donat and Wiśniewski).

Martinez and Friede (1970) showed that the swelling of nerve fibres in the proximal stumps of transected nerves was quantitatively related to the increase in the concentration of axonal organelles. The findings accorded best with an active, selective redistribution of organelles operating with sufficient force to dilate the axon and myelin sheath. The phenomenon of myelin sheath expansion was therefore viewed as only incidental to a primary axonal alteration.

Thus in the proximal stump, close to the point of section the axon undergoes a transient reactive swelling, whilst distal to the transection there is a reduction in the volume of axoplasm during the initial phase of Wallerian degeneration. Friede and Martinez (1970a and b) showed that the myelin sheath accomodated these changes by distension and thinning, and by constriction and thickening of the sheath, at these two sites respectively. There was a corresponding decrease or increase in the number of myelin lamellae present, but the periodicity remained constant. These data were considered to provide proof of slippage of adjacent myelin lamellae resulting in rapid local changes in sheath size. In Wallerian degeneration two phases were recognized: (a) sheath adaptation (constriction) and (b) sheath disintegration. 'Myelin forms' consisting of a very thick myelin sheath enclosing little or no axoplasm (Fig.13.12) were considered to represent end stages of sheath constriction, while disintegration was characterized by bio-chemical degradation. Small fibres were observed to undergo sheath constriction faster than large fibres contrary to the conventional view that large fibres are the first to degenerate (e.g. Hönjin, Nakamura and Imura, 1959). Friede and Martinez considered that this view represents a misinterpretation of the data.

The early changes occurring in the myelin sheath during Wallerian degeneration were described by Williams and Hall (1971b). During the first 4 days after crush a progressive disruption of the myelin sheath was apparent, beginning at the incisures and nodes. At the incisures there was a widening of the incisural intraperiod line gap together with a splitting of the intraperiod line in the myelin adjacent to the incisure, to form a continuous intermembranous space. Subsequently myelin-derived material with a 4 nm repeat period collapsed into these spaces, and later became fused transversely across the fibre at sites of axonal constriction. This process resulted in the formation of islands of

---

Fig. 13.10   Early Wallerian degeneration showing accummulation of axonal organelles; myelin sheath still intact, 36 hours after section of rabbit cervical vagus nerve; within 0.5 cm of cut end. Schwann cell (S); axon (a). (x 24 000: Reproduced by courtesy of Dr R. H. M. King.)

Fig. 13.11   Later Wallerian degeneration demonstrating loss of axon; myelin sheath collapsed and showing some disorganization. 7 days after section of rabbit cervical vagus nerve; within 0.5 cm of cut end. Schwann cell (S). (x 8000: Reproduced by courtesy of Dr R. H. M. King.)

axoplasm enclosed within myelin-bound ellipsoids, the rounded ends being composed of the 4 nm repeat material. By the fourth day small lipid globules appeared at the ends of the ellipsoids, and these subsequently completely filled the spaces between the ellipsoids (correlating with the authors' *in vivo* observations). The Schwann cell cytoplasm contained aggregations of lamellar material often assuming oval or spherical profiles.

Accounts of myelin breakdown have been given by many workers e.g. Terry and Harkin (1959), Glimstedt and Wohlfart (1960), Barton (1962), Nathaniel and Pease (1963a), Satinsky, Pepe and Liu (1964), Thomas (1964a), Morris, Hudson and Weddell (1972a). Nathaniel and Pease, and Satinsky, Pepe and Liu have emphasized that the disappearance of myelin takes several months, and many Schwann cells retain myelin debris even whilst forming new myelin around regenerated axons. Thomas noted that in the spaces between myelin ovoids along the degenerating fibre, the Schwann tube usually showed a collapsed appearance with folding of the basement membrane, which nevertheless persisted intact.

Most electron microscope studies have recognized both Schwann cells and macrophages as being involved in myelin digestion (Terry and Harkin, 1959; Ohmi, 1961; Lee, 1963; Thomas, 1964a, 1966; O'Daly and Imaeda, 1967; Williams and Hall, 1971b) although Causey and Barton (1961), Nathaniel and Pease (1963a) and Morris, Hudson and Weddell (1972a) were able to obtain no evidence for macrophage involvement in myelin breakdown. Between 6 and 28 days after nerve section Thomas frequently observed macrophages containing myelin remains and multiple vacuoles lying within the Schwann cell tubes. In some cases macrophages were observed which were apparently in the process of leaving the Schwann tube, with part of the cell extending outside the tube through a discontinuity in the tube basement membrane. Macrophages were also observed lying free in the endoneurial space between Schwann tubes, particularly in perivascular locations.

The origin of the macrophages found in both the central and peripheral nervous systems following injury has been a matter of lengthy controversy, the details of which will not be discussed here. Thomas (1966), and Williams and Hall (1971b) considered it likely that the macrophages appearing in peripheral nerves during Wallerian degeneration were of haematogenous origin, as Cajal (1928) had proposed. Autoradiographic studies (Olsson and Sjöstrand, 1969) have lent further support to this view, without indicating what proportion of cells are exogenously derived. Thomas identified cells intermediate in character between mononuclear leucocytes and macrophages in the cellular outgrowth from the distal stump of transected nerves and discussed the possibility of there being a transitional series between the two cell types in traumatized peripheral nerves. Berner, Torvik and Stenwig (1973), on the basis of experimental labelling of blood monocytes with carbon particles considered that the digestion of cellular debris in Wallerian degeneration was performed by cells of endogenous origin only and excluded the involvement of blood monocytes. However, they considered that in the region of the crush (the traumatic region) haematogenous monocytes did have a phagocytic role. A similar view was taken by Liu (1974) in an autoradiographic and ultrastructural study, and the endogenous phagocytes were considered to be derived from vascular pericytes.

Electron microscope studies provide little evidence in favour of Schwann cells transforming into macrophages *in vivo*, as Weiss and Wang (1945) inferred from tissue culture studies. However, Morris, Hudson and Weddell (1972a) considered that Schwann cells containing myelin debris had the capacity to transform into cells lying 'free' in the endoneurial space, but were not able to act as phagocytes for any myelin other than their own.

Williams and Hall (1971b) identified three main cell populations within the endoneurial space distal to a crush performed one week earlier: these were the original Schwann cells containing myelin ellipsoids, small electron-dense globules and axonal remnants; the cells identified as newly differentiated Schwann cells containing 'active' cytoplasm and a few small dense globules; and globule-containing macrophages. Occasionally, other cell types were identified including large mononuclear cells devoid of debris, eosinophils, degranulating mast cells and endoneurial fibroblasts. Macrophages were not implicated in the initial lysis of myelin, however, unlike the situation seen in EAN. Myelin degradation was considered to occur initially within the Schwann cells, with lipid globules subsequently being extruded and taken up by macrophages. However, large masses of debris with a lamellar structure were not extruded.

Following nerve crush Williams and Hall (1971b) observed the appearance of lipid globules both within and between perineurial cells, associated with the disappearance of subperineurial globule-laden macrophages. A similar observation of globules within perineurial cells was made by Morris, Hudson and Weddell (1972c) in divided rat sciatic nerves but this was interpreted to indicate a transformation of Schwann cells (containing myelin breakdown products) into perineurial cells. By contrast O'Daly and Imaeda (1967) have described macrophages laden with myelin debris traversing gaps in the perineurium in Wallerian degeneration.

It is clear from the above descriptions that the macrophages in Wallerian degeneration do not initiate myelin lysis, and indeed are late arrivals on the scene, when myelin breakdown is already microscopically evident. Similarly in diphtheritic neuropathy, the macrophages (such as are present) are not implicated in the early myelin changes. In both neuropathies however there is evidence for an active role for the Schwann cell and an early and important role for hydrolytic enzymes in myelin breakdown. In EAN, in contrast 'macrophages' are specifically involved in splitting myelin lamellae and in their subsequent dissolution, the Schwann cell appearing to play a relatively passive role. Hydrolytic enzymes, which are likely to be macrophage-associated, are also important in the pathogenesis of EAN. As an exception to these generalizations Spencer and Thomas (1970) inferred that active splitting of myelin lamellae by macrophages occurred immediately proximal to the site of nerve section.

The process of nodal widening following nerve crush was examined in the rat by Ballin and Thomas (1969b and c). Myelin loops were observed to become separated from the axolemma by retraction, and by the insinuation of Schwann cell processes growing backwards from the node. The Schwann cell cytoplasm at the node increased in amount and the Schwann cell microvilli at the node, while remaining intact in the early stages, subsequently became separated from the axolemma by Schwann cell cytoplasm. Later, with loss of continuity of the axon at the nodes the myelin loops came together from opposite sides of the axon to form the end of an ovoid, or alternatively remained separated from one another, not now by the axon but by Schwann cell cytoplasm. Hall and Williams (1971a and b) have described similar findings in mice. As Ballin and Thomas point out, nodal widening in Wallerian degeneration differs in two notable respects from the same process in EAN and in diphtheritic neuropathy: the Schwann cell microvilli remain intact until a late stage in Wallerian degeneration, and complete denudation of the paranodal and nodal axon does not occur.

Earlier electron microscope studies of the responses of unmyelinated fibres to nerve crush or section have been reviewed by Thomas (1973). As he points out, these studies failed to make adequate distinction between unmyelinated axons and Schwann cell processes, resulting in contradictory reports which confused the degenerative and regenerative phases of the response to injury. More recent studies (Bray, Peyronnard and Aguayo, 1972; Dyck and Hopkins, 1972; Aguayo, Peyronnard and Bray, 1973; Matthews, 1973; Thomas and King, 1974) emphasize that the axonal changes are essentially the same as those observed in myelinated fibres. Thomas and King found that in the rabbit vagus nerve degeneration began in some unmyelinated axons as early as 24 hours after section, but axons of normal appearance were present for up to 5—6 days after section, while after 7 days no normal axons were observed. Both macrophages and Schwann cells were observed to take up axonal debris. Axonal swelling and organelle accumulation proximal and distal to the site of injury, similar to those seen in myelinated fibres have been described by Kappeler and Mayor (1969a,b), Bray, Peyronnard and Aguayo (1972) and Matthews (1973).

Holtzman and Novikoff (1965) have morphologically and histochemically characterized the various types of lysosomes present in both the axon and the Schwann cell following crush of rat sciatic nerves. They have also emphasized the very rapid histochemical appearance of acid phosphatase activity, i.e. within 2 hours of crushing. Weller and Mellick (1966) examined hen sciatic nerves after section for histochemical evidence of lysosomes and acid phosphatase activity. At 4 and 6 days after section no acid phosphatase could be detected in the Schwann cells, but was present at 6 days in endoneurial macrophages. At 10 days the majority of enzyme activity was found in Schwann cells, being most evident where myelin was in an advanced state of digestion.

13.15 Regeneration

13.15.1 *Light microscopy*

In normal peripheral nerve fibres internodal length increases with fibre diameter (Fig. 13.12a) since the largest fibres are the first to myelinate, and are thus subject to the greatest elongation during growth, as described earlier. However in regeneration following nerve crush in an adult animal remyelination occurs without subsequent internodal elongation, since no growth in length is occurring in the part of the body in which the nerve lies. As a consequence such regenerated internodes do not regain the normal relationship between internodal length and fibre diameter (Fig. 13.12b), and are relatively short (Hiscoe, 1947; Vizoso and Young, 1948; Cragg and Thomas, 1964b; Fullerton et al., 1965). Hiscoe reported an average length of approximately 300 μm in regenerated rat tibial nerves studied 30 days to 17 weeks after crush. There was only slight increase in average internodal length with fibre diameter e.g. fibres with an average diameter of 5.5 μm had an average internodal length of 288 μm whilst fibres of 9.5 μm average diameter had average internodal lengths of 298 μm.

The significance of the slight increase of internodal length with fibre diameter in regenerated nerves, described by both Hiscoe and Vizoso and Young, is not clear, but a small increase in limb length over the post-operative period (more than one year) could account for it. The authors provide no evidence to support this interpretation, although Vizoso and Young speak of '*little* or no growth' taking place. (By contrast one animal in which regeneration was observed following a crush at 11 days after birth demonstrated the elongating effect of growth upon internodal length). Hiscoe, on the other hand, considered that a secondary elongation of internodes had occurred on a minor scale, due to the presence of some fibres undergoing myelination before reaching the periphery. Whatever the true explanation, it may shed light on the results of experiments by Jacobs and Cavanagh (1969). They reported that in the hen, unlike the rat, rabbit and guinea-pig, a linear relationship between fibre diameter and internodal length is re-established in regeneration (Fig. 13.12f and g) after nerve crush (similar results were obtained in hen nerves following remyelination after segmental demyelination with diphtheria toxin. See Section 13.10.1). However, the slope of the regression line (regression coefficient) at 150 days after crush was less than one third that of the normal nerve i.e. internodal length increased much less with fibre diameter in a regenerated nerve than in normal nerve. Thus whilst the normal spectrum of axonal diameters had been re-established, the internodal lengths of the largest axons reached only about 1000 μm compared with over 2000 μm in unoperated nerves. Jacobs and Cavanagh suggested that the explanation for these surprising results should be looked for in the mechanism of selection of certain Schwann cells for remyelination and the elimination of others. Differences between species in the mechanism of selection could account for differences in the initial spacing of the myelinating Schwann cells and hence of internodal length. The details of the mechanism by which a linear increase of internodal length with axon diameter is achieved in regenerated hen nerves have yet to be elucidated.

Lubińska (1959) examined the last preserved internode proximal to the site of a crush in regenerating nerve fibres in cat and rabbit tibial and peroneal nerves. Such internodes varied from a half to a full normal internodal length. The nuclei of the associated Schwann cells appeared to be displaced distally,

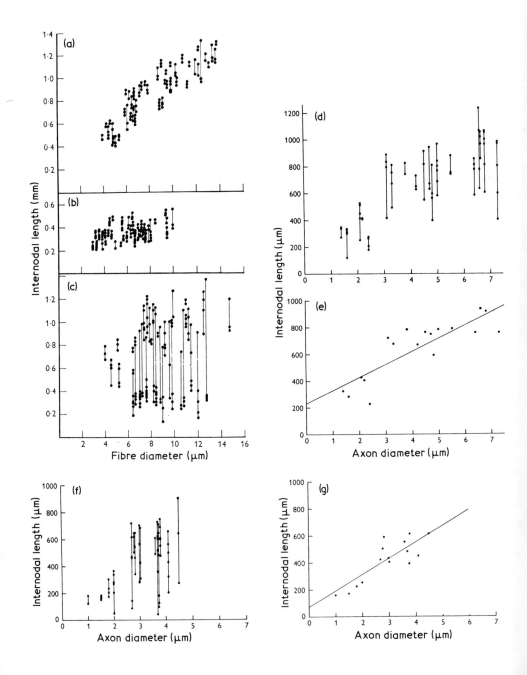

instead of being situated approximately centrally as in normal fibres, with the displacement in excess of the variation found within normal fibres. Her results demonstrated that when an internode is damaged by crush distal to the nucleus, the internode survives, albeit in shortened form. If however the crush occurred proximal to the nucleus the whole internode of myelin degenerated, emphasizing the importance of the integrity of the nuclear region. In some fibres proximal to a crush (Lubińska, 1961b), or a cut (Spencer and Thomas, 1970), a different response has been reported. The proximal portions of one to several internodes immediately above the lesion showed a loss of myelin, with preservation of the axons. These denuded regions subsequently remyelinated forming short intercalated internodes, as in segmental demyelinating diseases such as diphtheritic neuropathy and EAN. In the major (distal) part of the internode the myelin was retained but was grossly distorted. This region of the internode has been further examined by electron microscopy (Spencer and Thomas, 1970; Spencer and Lieberman, 1971), revealing macrophages and oedema fluid within spaces in the myelin sheaths.

Hiscoe (1947) investigated the distribution of Schmidt–Lanterman incisures in internodes of the tibial nerve of young and normal adult rats, and in adult rats in which the sciatic nerve had been crushed 30 days to 17 weeks previously. She found that the number of incisures per internode in all three groups of fibres increased in direct proportion to the size of the fibre. For any given fibre diameter however, young and regenerated nerves had somewhat more incisures per internode than in the adult. Hiscoe attributed this last finding to 'a slight precosity in the intercalation of additional incisures' during the growth of the fibres (the principle of intercalation of incisures being implicit in the increase of incisures with fibre size in development). It is evident therefore that whilst the developmental history of the nerve usually has a direct influence on the internodal length, e.g. the occurrence of short internodes following regeneration, it has little effect on the frequency of incisures. As Hiscoe points out, whilst a causal relationship does not always obtain between internodal length and fibre diameter, since the two may be changed independently, a more definite relationship between the number of incisures and fibre diameter can be inferred.

Fig. 13.12 Graphs of internodal lengths and fibre (or axon) diameters for remyelinating and regenerating fibres. (a)(b) and (c), guinea-pig lateral popliteal nerves; (a) normal nerves; (b) nerves after crush; (c) nerves after segmental demyelination (diphtheritic neuropathy or lead intoxication neuropathy). (d) (e) (f) and (g), hen sciatic nerve; (d) and (e) nerves injected with diptheria toxin 307 days previously; (f) and (g) nerves 85 days after crush. Vertical lines indicate individual nerve fibres and solid circles each internodal length (a, b, c, d, f). Regression lines calculated from the mean values of internodal lengths for each axon diameter (e, g). (e) and (g) show relationship between *mean* internodal lengths and axon diameters of the same fibres. (Fig. 13.12 (a), (b) and (c) reproduced from Fullerton *et al.* (1965), by courtesy of Dr P. M. Le Quesne and *The Journal of Physiology*; and Fig. 13.12 (d) – (g) from Jacobs and Cavanagh, (1969), by courtesy of Dr J. M. Jacobs and the *Journal of Anatomy*.)

The increase of frequency of incisures with increasing fibre size is sufficiently great to produce shorter segments between incisures in large normal fibres than in small normal fibres. The decrease in this segmental length between incisures that occurs with an increase in fibre size is in contrast with internodal length, which normally increases with fibre size. The relationship between segmental length and fibre size is retained in regenerated fibres, the average length decreasing from smaller to larger fibres, although the average length is far shorter than in normal adult fibres. This relationship again differs from that between fibre diameter and internodal length which does not normally retain its relationship with fibre diameter on regeneration. Hiscoe interpreted her findings to indicate an upper limit to the amount of myelin that the Schwann cell can maintain in a single segmental unit. Even with the increase in number of incisures with fibre size however, the relative volume of myelin per segment increases quite sharply. The relationship between incisure frequency and fibre diameter in remyelination after axon-sparing segmental demyelination e.g. diphtheritic neuropathy, appears not to have been investigated.

Peyronnard, Aguayo and Bray (1973) investigated Schwann cell internuclear distances in normal and regenerated unmyelinated nerve fibres from rat cervical sympathetic trunks. Median internuclear distances for normal nerves were 90–100 μm and for regenerated nerves 50–60 μm. The reduction of internuclear distance to a half of normal was related by the authors to the twofold increase in Schwann cell population present in the regenerated nerve and interpreted in terms of a reduced Schwann cell length (see Chapter 2).

It is not possible here to discuss the many studies of peripheral nerve regeneration which have demonstrated that the ultimate diameter of regenerated fibres is greatly influenced by the nature of the terminal ending (for a review see Guth, 1956). Suffice it to say that fibres unconnected with the periphery remain of small diameter, whilst motor fibres connected to a sensory terminal are larger than those without any peripheral connection, but are not as large as those that reinnervate a muscle. The removal of a large part of a muscle has no effect on nerve regeneration, and maturation is more complete when nerves grow into a denervated muscle than into a normal muscle. The results of experimental cross-union of different nerves are also reviewed by Guth. The essence of these findings is that the degree of myelination is determined by the parent axon and not by the nature of the degenerating distal stump (of whatever origin). However, a reduced myelin sheath thickness was observed after a cross-union of somatic and visceral nerves when large axons were directed along small connective tissue pathways.

Schröder (1972) measured myelin sheath thickness and axon size 6–24 months after a crush or nerve graft. The regenerated fibres showed a reduction of sheath thickness in the largest fibres compared with uninjured nerves and the largest regenerated fibres were smaller than those of normal nerves. As a consequence the regression line expressing the relationship between axon diameter and myelin sheath thickness showed a reduced slope when compared to that for normal nerves.

Thomas (1970) described two different and distinct appearances associated with Schwann cell proliferation in chronic neuropathies in man. In one type, Schwann cells formed a concentric array around central myelinated fibres ('onion bulbs' see Fig. 13.6f), an appearance he considers to be associated with a segmental demyelinating neuropathy. In the second type, large irregular clusters of Schwann cells were associated with several myelinated and unmyelinated axons. Thomas has demonstrated that the second appearance can be produced experimentally by repeated crush injury, and appears to be the consequence of repeated episodes of degeneration and regeneration.

13.15.2 *Electron microscopy*

Young (1942) attributed an important role to the endoneurial connective tissue sheaths in providing pathways for regenerating axons on the basis of his light microscopic observations. Thomas (1964a) subsequently investigated the problem with the electron microscope and observed the fate of these connective tissue sheaths in Wallerian degeneration. He found that at 7 and 10 days after nerve section the endoneurial sheaths were less clearly defined than in the normal nerve. The endoneurium was oedematous, and the collagen fibres were more widely separated than in the normal nerve. However, in the larger fibres it was still possible to identify, as in the normal nerve, an inner endoneurial sheath of irregularly arranged fibres (the sheath of Plenk and Laidlaw) and outside this, (and around smaller tubes) collagen fibres usually arranged parallel to the longitudinal axis of the 'Schwann tubes' (the sheath of Key and Retzius). The term Schwann tube refers to the space enclosed by the basement membrane previously containing the Schwann cell and axon (1964a). Thomas noted that in situations where the Schwann tubes had collapsed, so also had the endoneurial collagen sheaths, confirming the light microscope observations of Glees (1943).

An increase in the amount of endoneurial collagen was evident at later stages of degeneration, especially in material examined 28 and 35 days after nerve section. At this stage an additonal zone of closely packed collagen fibres, longitudinally orientated, was present between the Schwann tube basement membrane and the inner endoneurial sheath. The larger Schwann tubes were therefore surrounded by three separate layers of endoneurial collagen instead of the normal two layers (inner and outer). Whilst the limits of the Schwann tubes and 'bands of Büngner' are defined by the basement membrane, the endoneurial sheaths appear to provide the main structural support, reinforced as they are by the deposition of an additional dense layer of collagen fibres immediately adjacent to the basement membrane.

Thomas (1966) noted that the connective tissue situated peripherally at the base of the outgrowth from the distal stump was in direct continuity with the epineurial connective tissue of the stump. It therefore contained elastin fibres and collagen fibres of a larger diameter than more centrally located collagen typical of the endoneurium. Thomas (1963) had previously described these differences between epineurial and endoneurial connective tissue (see Chapter 3).

Thomas observed Schwann cell processes within the Schwann tubes at 7 and 10 days after nerve section, and by 21 days there was evidence of Schwann cell proliferation within the Schwann tubes to form the 'bands of Büngner'. Thomas (1964a), and Nathaniel and Pease (1963b) have attributed an important role to the persistent basement membrane in maintaining the structural integrity of the Schwann tube during degeneration. The basement membrane provides a tube which encloses proliferating Schwann cells such that they form a longitudinally continuous band, and such 'bands of Büngner' in turn provide pathways which guide regenerating axons to their terminations. Nathaniel and Pease (1963b) and Thomas (1964b) described the formation of new basement membranes by some of the proliferated Schwann cells, within the confines of the original basement membrane. The importance of the basement membrane is emphasized by the situation in nerve roots (Gamble, 1964; Thomas, 1964a) where little collagen is normally present but where nevertheless regeneration can occur as in nerve trunks (Nathaniel and Pease, 1963b; Gamble, 1964). It is unlikely therefore that the tubular endoneurial collagen sheaths have the function of delimiting the 'bands of Büngner', a function which can more readily be ascribed to the basement membrane. Even in nerve roots however Gamble described a great increase in the amount of collagen in association with regeneration 6 months after section but an orderly arrangement into tubular sheaths was not apparent. Haftek and Thomas (1968) observed that the basement membranes remained intact at the site of crush, and again considered them to be important as pathways for regenerating axons.

Regenerating axons are first found alongside of the 'band of Büngner' between the basement membrane and Schwann cells (Nathaniel and Pease, 1963b). Subsequently gutters form in the Schwann cells in which the axons become embedded. A mesaxon is thus formed and remyelination begins. Nathaniel and Pease observed remyelination as early as 7 days after crush, whilst remyelination following nerve section was not apparent until 21 days later (Terry and Harkin, 1957, 1959).

Several authors have noted that Schwann cells in Wallerian degeneration are typically rich in free ribosomes and granular endoplasmic reticulum (Vial, 1958; Glimstedt and Wohlfart, 1960; Nathaniel and Pease, 1963a; Satinsky, Pepe and Liu, 1964; Holtzman and Novikoff, 1965; Thomas, 1966). This 'active' appearance has been interpreted to be evidence of the synthetic activity typical of an actively dividing cell, or of the production of enzymes for myelin digestion.

After nerve section and separation of the cut ends, cellular outgrowths occur from both stumps. The outgrowth from the distal stump occurs at a greater rate and plays an important role in the re-establishment of continuity between the two segments. The identity of this outgrowth was disputed by light microscopists (see Thomas, 1966) and was variously ascribed to Schwann cells or fibroblasts (of various origins) together with, in some descriptions, capillaries, erythrocytes, leucocytes and macrophages. Concerned with the importance of this process in nerve regeneration Thomas investigated the problem using the greater resolution of electron microscopy. He was able to demonstrate that cords of Schwann cells, several cells thick and enclosed by a common basement membrane, extended from the distal stump, the cords being enclosed by a connective tissue framework (outgrowths of perineurium and endoneurium) containing fibroblasts, blood vessels, collagen fibres, granular and agranular leucocytes, macrophages, and erythrocytes. The columns of Schwann cells in the outgrowth were considered to be extensions of the 'bands of Büngner' in the distal stump, as described by Nathaniel and Pease (1963b) and Thomas (1964a). Liu (1973), on the basis of a light and electron microscopic and autoradiographic study, has put forward the heterodox view that the Schwann cells which unite proximal and distal stumps are derived from 'primitive reticuloendothelial cells around blood vessels' (pericytes) in the epineurium and endoneurium.

Thomas (1966) found no evidence to support earlier suggestions that endoneurial fibroblasts may be derived from blood-borne monocytes or from transformed Schwann cells. Since the connective tissue of the outgrowth was continuous with that of the distal stump he considered it likely that fibroblasts present in the outgrowth were derived by migration and proliferation from fibroblasts in the epineurium, perineurium and endoneurium.

Unmyelinated fibres appear to have the capacity to regenerate more rapidly than myelinated fibres (Bray, Peyronnard and Aguayo, 1972; Dyck and Hopkins, 1972; Aguayo, Peyronnard and Bray, 1973). For example, regeneration was evident in the rabbit anterior mesenteric nerve as early as two days after transection: numerous small axons (0.4 μm diameter) were present distal to the site of injury. Initially up to 200 axons were associated with one Schwann cell, but this number declined as axon groups were divided up into progressively smaller numbers by Schwann cells, though even by 13 weeks the axon–Schwann cell ratio was several times normal. Bray and Aguayo (1974) demonstrated a gradual loss of redundant axonal sprouts: the total axonal population, distal to crush, declined from four times normal at one month after nerve crush to within normal range 6 months after injury. Although distally, median axonal diameters remained at approximately half normal values throughout the six month period, there was a gradual increase in the proportion of axons with larger diameters. Proximal to the level of injury median axonal diameters were reduced one month after injury (attributable to retrograde atrophy), and the proportion of proximal axons of larger diameter also increased. Maturation of some unmyelinated axons, both proximally and distally, had occurred therefore.

In a light microscope study Evans and Murray (1954) demonstrated that, following crush of the rabbit vagus nerve, few regenerating unmyelinated axons reached the abdominal vagus nerve, but that these were instead diverted into the recurrent laryngeal nerve, normally consisting almost entirely of myelinated fibres. Since the regenerating axons had been diverted from a nerve (the abdominal vagus) which contains few myelinated fibres to one rich in myelinated fibres, it was possible that the presence of the myelinated fibres themselves might have had an important effect on the regeneration of unmyelinated axons. King and Thomas (1971) therefore examined the axon/ Schwann cell relationships in the regenerated recurrent laryngeal nerve. They found that the unmyelinated axons were usually immediately juxtaposed to a myelinated fibre, being arranged circumferentially or crescentically around the central myelinated fibre. Other groups of axons were however found lying free within the endoneurium. In both cases the unmyelinated axons were surrounded by their own Schwann cells and were never seen in close association with a Schwann cell which already contained a myelinated axon. The Schwann cells associated with unmyelinated axons were considered by King and Thomas to be derived from the proliferation of Schwann cells previously associated with myelinated axons. Such results indicate the plasticity of Schwann cells with regard to their potential to form myelin, and substantiate the view that factors intrinsic to the axon are the main determinants as to whether or not a particular Schwann cell forms a myelin sheath (see Chapters 1 and 2).

King and Thomas considered the possible reasons to account for the diversion of unmyelinated axons from the vagus nerve to the recurrent laryngeal nerve. Since the proliferation of Schwann cells in Wallerian degeneration in unmyelinated fibres is much less than in myelinated fibres (see above), they suggested that the process of formation of 'bands of Büngner' may be less effective than in myelinated fibres, and that the columns of Schwann cells formed may be discontinuous. Since continuous columns of proliferated Schwann cells appear to be necessary to guide the regenerating axons to their terminations, it is possible that the regenerating unmyelinated axons follow the continuous columns of cells formed by the degenerating myelinated fibres into the recurrent laryngeal nerve.

Thomas and Jones (1967) examined the regeneration of the perineurium in a region of nerve where a short segment had been removed. Regenerated axons and associated Schwann cells which had traversed the gap became surrounded by cells identified as fibroblasts which gradually acquired the characteristics of perineurial cells. The gap region thus acquired a multiple fascicle structure, with each small fascicle surrounded by perineurium. Morris, Hudson and Weddell (1972c) described the same changes immediately proximal to nerve section, but considered Schwann cells as well as fibroblasts to be transformed into perineurial cells. In both investigations the results were discussed with reference to the disputed mesodermal/neural crest origin of perineurium. The perineurium further proximal and distal to a crush was shown by Shanthaveerappa and

Bourne (1964) to undergo little or no change, either histologically or histochemically. The intact perineurial tube was therefore considered to be the primary guide enabling the regenerating axons to follow the Schwann cell tubes, and reach their proper destinations. Haftek and Thomas (1968) observed that in the region of a crush the perineurial cells were reconstituted at 3 days after trauma whilst at 1–2 hours no perineurial cells had remained and only their basement membranes persisted. Olsson and Kristensson (1973) found that at the site of crush the perineurium lost its normal properties as a diffusion barrier to labelled albumin which was then able to diffuse across the perineurium into the endoneurial spaces. They considered the deficient barrier function to be caused by the destruction of perineurial cells as described by Haftek and Thomas.

13.16 Electrophysiological changes in Wallerian degeneration and subsequent regeneration

Kaeser and Lambert (1962) examined the effect of section of the sciatic nerve of the guinea-pig on nerve function. Response of the foot muscle to stimulation of the distal stump could be elicited for a period of 40–45 hours. During this time the conduction velocity decreased only slightly i.e. to 80–90% of the normal value. The amplitude of the muscle action potential however fell sharply to 10% of the mean normal value after 40 hours, confirming the results of other investigations. Kaeser and Lambert proposed that the slight slowing of conduction occurring during the early stages of Wallerian degeneration was due to the larger and more rapidly conducting fibres degenerating before the slower fibres. In summary therefore, in Wallerian degeneration the amplitude of the action potential decreases until it disappears and nerve conduction is blocked, whilst the conduction velocity decreases little; whereas in segmental demyelinating conditions the conduction velocity decreases until conduction ceases, this decrease being accompanied by a fall in the amplitude of the action potential.

In view of conflicting evidence from earlier studies, Cragg and Thomas (1964b) re-examined the recovery of conduction velocity in regeneration following a nerve crush. It had previously been demonstrated that during the early stages of regeneration conduction velocity was reduced, and it was known that the fibres present had small axons, thin myelin sheaths and short internodes compared with the normal fibres. It was also recognized that in regeneration after nerve section, where normal fibre diameters are never restored, conduction velocity remained permanently reduced. In the circumstances of regeneration after nerve crush however, the question of the ultimate restoration of normal conduction velocity was a matter of some dispute. Cragg and Thomas's observations confirmed those earlier studies which had described a permanently reduced conduction velocity in regeneration following crush. The peroneal nerve of the rabbit showed a permanent 25% reduction in conduction velocity, there being no significant increase between 12 and 16 months after crush. A distal reduction in fibre diameter was observed, but it was considered to be insufficient to account for all of the slowing of conduction velocity, whilst the reduced internodal length (approximately 50% of normal) was not thought to have any effect. The magnitude of the permanent reduction in conduction velocity therefore remained unexplained.

Jacobson and Guth (1965) examined nerve regeneration in the sciatic nerve of the rat after crush. Recordings of action potentials could not be obtained in the immediate post-operative period further distally than 2 mm proximal to the lesion. At 4 days potentials were evident up to 2 mm distal to the lesion. The rate of regeneration increased exponentially from an initial rate of 0.3 mm per day immediately after the crush to 3.0 mm per day by 18 days. The amplitude of the action potential was 20% of normal by 56 days, while the conduction velocity was 75% of normal by 28 days and did not increase during the next 28 days.

Hopkins and Lambert (1972) found that regeneration of unmyelinated nerves, as indicated by the appearance of an action potential, was a rapid process compared with that occurring in myelinated fibres, thus confirming the histological results discussed above. Also in contrast to the findings in myelinated fibres, was their observation that conduction velocity had returned to the lower limit of normal by 30–40 days after the crush. Earlier studies on the restoration of conduction in regenerating nerves and the concomitant recovery of sensory and motor function are reviewed by Guth (1956).

13.17 Conclusion

A comparison of Wallerian degeneration and segmental demyelination serves to clarify the nature of the cellular relationship between axon and Schwann cell. It is apparent that the axon has the capacity to tolerate major, though transient, changes in its associated Schwann cells. A profound change in Schwann cells such as the loss of the myelin sheath has little or no effect on the morphological integrity of the axon. In segmental demyelinating diseases not only is the myelin sheath lost but the underlying cause of the disease may also have a deleterious effect on other Schwann cell functions, and in diphtheritic neuropathy, for example, it is evident that there is an inhibition of protein synthesis by the Schwann cells. Nevertheless, such a major disturbance of Schwann cell metabolism appears to produce no detectable morphological changes in the associated axons. Furthermore, in segmental demyelination the disease process may result in limited areas of axon becoming temporarily devoid of Schwann cells, again without apparent effect upon the axon.

Despite some suggestions to the contrary, there is so far no convincing evidence that the Schwann cell supports the axon in its trophic, ionic or energy requirements. A study of experimental peripheral nerve pathology affords no evidence for such roles and suggests that the Schwann cell either does not perform these functions or that they occur at a level which is not of critical importance to the survival of the axon. All that can be said with any certainty about the role of the Schwann cell in myelinated fibres is that it produces the myelin sheath which has insulatory properties and thus has an important function in saltatory conduction. The specific functions of the Schwann (Remak) cell in unmyelinated fibres have yet to be determined.

The Schwann cell is however clearly susceptible to changes in its associated axon. Following the axonal changes of Wallerian degeneration, the relationship of one Schwann cell to another is radically altered, and the cells temporarily lose their capacity to support a myelin sheath. It is possible to interpret these changes in the Schwann cell in Wallerian degeneration, including the loss of the myelin sheath, as being regenerative, in that it is part of a process of de-differentiation in preparation for the arrival of new axon sprouts. According to this view, Schwann cell proliferation can be seen as an essential but subordinate part of the process of de-differentiation. Hence the production by degenerating myelinated fibres of large numbers of Schwann cells, in excess of those for which there is an apparent functional role, may be related to the greater degree of differentiation of the Schwann cells of myelinated fibres when compared with those of unmyelinated fibres. However, whether the changes in the Schwann cell induced by nerve crush or section are viewed as being degenerative or regenerative, it is evident that the Schwann cell responds radically to axonal degeneration. While the survival of the Schwann cell is not dependent on the maintenance of the morphological integrity of the axon, the existence of a Schwann cell in its typically differentiated form depends upon its contact with an intact axon. By contrast the axon does not apparently respond to changes in the Schwann cells and is only affected by severance from the nerve cell body.

The preceding descriptions of EAN, diphtheritic neuropathy and Wallerian degeneration illustrate how well adapted the peripheral nervous system is to repair either the loss of the myelin sheath alone or complete fibre degeneration. Such studies of experimental peripheral nerve pathology also help to explain the relative incapacity of the central nervous system for self-repair. It is evident for example that the different kinds of cellular relationships existing between the Schwann cell and axon, and the oligodendrocyte and axon in the peripheral and central nervous system respectively, are in part responsible for differences in their capacity for remyelination.

The study of experimentally induced peripheral nerve pathology, as exemplified by the three systems described in this chapter, has made it possible to accumulate a detailed body of knowledge which it would have been impossible to have obtained from the study of human neuropathology alone. The potential value of such studies is well illustrated by those on experimental diphtheritic neuropathy in which the disease process has been minutely dissected in terms of its biochemistry, electrophysiology and histopathology. Whilst human diphtheritic neuropathy is, with few exceptions, no longer a medical problem, the value of obtaining a detailed understanding of such a model system is that, by analogy, it may further our understanding of other demyelinating diseases which are less amenable to direct investigation, and which remain major medical problems, an example being multiple sclerosis.

EAN is a different kind of experimental system since it provides a putative model for a specific human disease, the Guillain–Barré syndrome, and its validity as a model depends upon the degree of similarity between the two diseases. While this has not yet been completely determined, it is already apparent that EAN is a better model for the Guillain–Barré syndrome than EAE is for multiple sclerosis, a proposal which has been widely investigated. A good model showing many similarities between the experimental system and the human disease process has the obvious advantage of facilitating a detailed understanding of the human disease while allowing liberal experimentation in treatment.

The study of experimental Wallerian degeneration is again clearly of more than academic value. In an age in which mechanical injury to the nervous system is common e.g. in the motor car accident, a detailed knowledge of Wallerian degeneration and regeneration can greatly assist in the prognosis and treatment of nerve injury in man. Despite more than a hundred years of investigation some aspects of Wallerian change still remain to be elucidated such as, for example, those features of degeneration and regeneration which are specific to unmyelinated fibres.

Experimental neuropathology remains a most rewarding field for investigation, raising many fundamental questions of cell biology, but also promising an understanding, and thus a chance of treatment, of some of the most intractable and debilitating of human diseases.

Acknowledgements

I am indebted to several colleagues for helpful discussions, especially to Dr R. H. M. King.

References

Abercrombie, M. and Johnson, M. L. (1942) The outwandering of cells in tissue culture of nerves undergoing Wallerian degeneration. *Journal of Experimental Biology,* **19,** 266–283.

Abercrombie, M. and Johnson, M. L. (1946) Quantitative histology of Wallerian degeneration, I. Nuclear population in rabbit sciatic nerve. *Journal of Anatomy,* **80,** 37–50.

Abercrombie, M. and Santler, J. E. (1957) An analysis of growth in nuclear population during Wallerian degeneration. *Journal of Cellular and Comparative Physiology,* **50,** 429–450.

Abercrombie, M., Evans, D. H. L. and Murray, J. G. (1959) Nuclear multiplication and cell migration in degenerating unmyelinated nerves. *Journal of Anatomy,* **93,** 9–14.

Aguayo, A. J., Peyronnard, J. M. and Bray, G. M. (1973) A quantitative ultrastructural study of regeneration from isolated proximal stumps of transected unmyelinated nerves. *Journal of Neuropathology and Experimental Neurology,* **32,** 256–270.

Allt, G. (1968) *An Experimental Study of the Ultrastructural Relationships at the Node of Ranvier.* M.Phil. Thesis: University of London.

Allt, G. (1969a) Ultrastructural features of the immature peripheral nerve. *Journal of Anatomy,* **105**, 283–293.

Allt, G. (1969b) Repair of segmental demyelination in peripheral nerves: an electron microscope study. *Brain,* **92**, 639–646.

Allt, G. (1972a) Involvement of the perineurium in experimental allergic neuritis: electron microscopic observations. *Acta neuropathologica, (Berlin),* **20**, 139–149.

Allt, G. (1972b) An ultrastructural analysis of remyelination following segmental demyelination. *Acta neuropathologica, (Berlin),* **22**, 333–344.

Allt, G. (1975) The node of Ranvier in experimental allergic neuritis: an electron microscope study. *Journal of Neurocytology,* **4**, 63–76.

Allt, G. and Cavanagh, J. B. (1969) Ultrastructural changes in the region of the node of Ranvier in the rat caused by diphtheria toxin. *Brain,* **92**, 459–468.

Allt, G., Evans, E. M. and Evans, D. H. L. (1971a) The vulnerability of immature rabbits to experimental allergic neuritis: a light and electron microscope study. *Brain Research,* **29**, 271–291.

Allt, G., Evans, E. M. and Evans, D. H. L. (1971b) Experimental allergic neuritis: an assessment of the role of a serum factor in its aetiology. *Brain Research,* **32**, 255–257.

Allt, G., Evans, E. M., Evans, D. H. L. and Targett, G. A. T. (1971) Effect of injection of trypanosomes on the development of experimental allergic neuritis in rabbits. *Nature, (London),* **233**, 197–199.

Andersson-Cedergren, E. and Karlsson, U. (1966) Demyelination regions of nerve fibres in frog muscle spindle as studied by serial sections for electron microscopy. *Journal of Ultrastructure Research,* **14**, 212–239.

Arnason, B. G., Asbury, A. K., Åström, K. E. and Adams, R. D. (1968) EAN as a model for idiopathic polyneuritis. *Transactions of the American Neurological Association,* **93**, 133–136.

Arnason, B. G. W., Winkler, G. F. and Hadler, N. M. (1969) Cell-mediated demyelination of peripheral nerve in tissue culture. *Laboratory Investigation,* **21**, 1–10.

Arnason, B. G. W. and Chelmicka-Szorc, E. (1972) Passive transfer of experimental allergic neuritis in Lewis rats by direct injection of sensitized lymphocytes into sciatic nerve. *Acta neuropathologica, (Berlin),* **22**, 1–6.

Asbury, A. K. and Arnason, B. G. (1968) Experimental allergic neuritis: a radioautographic study. *Journal of Neuropathology and Experimental Neurology,* **27**, 581–590.

Åström, K. E. and Waksman, B. H. (1962) The passive transfer of experimental allergic encephalomyelitis and neuritis with living lymphoid cells. *Journal of Pathology and Bacteriology,* **83**, 89–106.

Åström, K. E., Webster, H. deF. and Arnason, B. G. (1968) The initial lesion of experimental allergic neuritis. A phase and electron microscopic study. *Journal of Experimental Medicine,* **128**, 469–495.

Ballin, R. H. M. and Thomas, P. K. (1968) Electron microscope observations on demyelination and remyelination in experimental allergic neuritis. Part I. Demyelination. *Journal of the Neurological Sciences,* **8**, 1–18.

Ballin, R. H. M. and Thomas, P. K. (1969a) Electron microscope observations on demyelination and remyelination in experimental allergic neuritis. Part 2. Remyelination. *Journal of the Neurological Sciences,* **8**, 225–237.

Ballin, R. H. M. and Thomas, P. K. (1969b) Electron microscope observations on nodal changes during Wallerian degeneration. *Journal of Anatomy,* **104**, 184–185.

Ballin, R. H. M. and Thomas, P. K. (1969c) Changes at the nodes of Ranvier during Wallerian degeneration: an electron microscope study. *Acta neuropathologica, (Berlin),* **14**, 237–249.

Barton, A. A. (1962) An electron microscope study of degeneration and regeneration of nerve. *Brain,* **85**, 799–808.

Berner, A., Torvik, A. and Stenwig, A. E. (1973) Origin of macrophages in traumatic lesions and Wallerian degeneration in peripheral nerves. *Acta neuropathologica, (Berlin),* **25**, 228–236.

Bradley, W. G. and Asbury, A. K. (1970) Duration of synthesis phase in neurilemma cells in mouse sciatic nerve during degeneration. *Experimental Neurology,* **26**, 275–282.

Bradley, W. G. and Jennekens, F. G. I. (1971) Axonal degeneration in diphtheritic neuropathy. *Journal of the Neurological Sciences,* **13**, 415–430.

Brandriss, M. W. (1963) Methotrexate: suppression of experimental allergic encephalo-myelitis by cytotoxic drugs. *Science,* **140**, 186—187.

Bray, G. M. and Aguayo, A. H. (1974) Regeneration of peripheral unmyelineated nerves. Fate of the axonal sprouts which develop after injury. *Journal of Anatomy,* **117**, 517—529.

Bray, G. M., Peyronnard, J. M. and Aguayo, A. J. (1972) Reactions of unmyelinated nerve fibres to injury. An ultrastructural study. *Brain Research,* **42**, 297—309.

Brostoff, S., Burnett, P., Lampert, P. and Eylar, E. H. (1972) Isolation and characterization of a protein from sciatic nerve myelin responsible for experimental allergic neuritis. *Nature, (London New Biology),* **235**, 210—212.

Cajal, R. Y. (1928) *Degeneration and Regeneration of the Nervous System.* Vol. I, pp. 92—98. Oxford University Press: London.

Calne, D. B. and Leibowitz, S. (1963) Suppression of experimental allergic encephalo-myelitis by cytotoxic drugs. *Nature, (London),* **197**, 1309—1310.

Carnegie, P. R., McPherson, T. A. and Robson, G. S. M. (1970) Experimental autoimmune encephalomyelitis. Digestion of basic protein of human myelin with cyanogen bromide and trypsin. *Immunology,* **19**, 55—63.

Causey, G. (1960) *The Cell of Schwann,* Ch. VII. E. & S. Livingstone Ltd: Edinburgh and London.

Causey, G. and Palmer, E. (1952) Early changes in degenerating mammalian nerves. *Proceedings of the Royal Society, London (Series B),* **139**, 597—609.

Causey, G. and Palmer, E. (1953) The centrifugal spread of structural change at the nodes in degenerating mammalian nerves. *Journal of Anatomy,* **87**, 185—191.

Causey, G. and Barton, A. A. (1961) An electron microscopic examination of degenerating and regenerating peripheral nerve. In *Cytology of Nervous Tissue,* Proceedings of the Anatomical Society of Great Britain and Ireland. pp. 75—77.

Cavanagh, J. B. and Jacobs, J. M. (1964) Some quantitative aspects of diphtheritic neuropathy. *British Journal of Experimental Pathology,* **45**, 309—322.

Chase, M. W. (1959) A critique of attempts at passive transfer of sensitivity to nervous tissue. In *Allergic Encephalomyelitis,* (ed.) Kies, M. W. and Alvord, E. C. pp. 348—374. Charles C. Thomas: Springfield, Illinois.

Collier, R. J. and Pappenheimer, A. M. (1964a) Studies on the mode of action of diphtheria toxin. *Journal of Experimental Medicine,* **120**, 1007—1018.

Collier, R. J. and Pappenheimer, A. M. (1964b) Studies on the mode of action of diphtheria toxin. *Journal of Experimental Medicine,* **120**, 1019—1039.

Cragg, B. G. and Thomas, P. K. (1964a) Changes in nerve conduction in experimental allergic neuritis. *Journal of Neurology, Neurosurgery and Psychiatry,* **27**, 106—115.

Cragg, B. G. and Thomas, P. K. (1964b) The conduction velocity of regenerated peripheral nerve fibres. *Journal of Physiology, London,* **171**, 164—175.

Davis, F. A. (1972) Impairment of repetitive impulse conduction in experimentally demyelinated and pressure-injured nerves. *Journal of Neurology, Neurosurgery and Psychiatry,* **35**, 537—544.

Davis, F. A. and Jacobson, S. (1971) Altered thermal sensitivity in injured and demyelinated nerve. A possible model of temperature effects in multiple sclerosis. *Journal of Neurology, Neurosurgery and Psychiatry,* **34**, 551—561.

Davison, A. N. and Peters, A. (1970) *Myelination.* pp. 138—140. C. C. Thomas: Springfield, Illinois.

D'Monte, B., Mela, P. and Marks, N. (1971) Metabolic instability of myelin protein and proteolipid fractions. *European Journal of Biochemistry,* **23**, 355—365.

Domonkos, J. (1972) Lipid metabolism in Wallerian degeneration. In *Handbook of Neurochemistry,* (ed.) Lajtha, A. Vol. 7, pp. 93—106. Plenum Press: New York and London.

Donat, J. R. and Wiśniewski, H. M. (1973) The spatio—temporal pattern of Wallerian degeneration in mammalian peripheral nerves. *Brain Research,* **53**, 41—53.

Dyck, P. J. and Hopkins, A. P. (1972) Electron microscopic observations on degeneration and regeneration of unmyelinated nerves. *Brain,* **95**, 223—234.

Dyck, P. J.., Thomas, P. K. and Lambert, E. H. (1975) *Peripheral Neuropathy.* W. B. Saunders: Philadelphia.

Elliot, G. A., Gibbons, A. J. and Greig, M. E. (1973) A comparison of the effects of melenestrol acetate with a combination of hydrocortisone acetate and medroxy-progesterone acetate and with other steroids in the treatment of experimental allergic encephalomyelitis in Wistar rats. *Acta neuropathologica, Berlin,* **23**, 95–104.

Evans, D. H. L. and Murray, J. G. (1954) Regeneration of nonmedullated nerve fibres. *Journal of Anatomy,* **88**, 465–480.

Eylar, E. H., Caccam, J., Jackson, J. J., Westall, F. C. and Robinson, A. B. (1970) EAE. Synthesis of disease inducing site of the basic protein. *Science,* **168**, 1220–1223.

Eylar, E. H., Jackson, J., Rothenberg, B. and Brostoff, S. W. (1972) Suppression of the immune response: reversal of the disease state with antigen in allergic encephalo-myelitis. *Nature (London),* **236**, 74–76.

Fischer, C. A. and Morrell, P. (1974) Turnover of proteins in myelin and myelin-like material of mouse brain. *Brain Research,* **74**, 51–65.

Fisher, C. M. and Adams, R. D. (1956) Diphtheritic polyneuritis. A pathological study. *Journal of Neuropathology and Experimental Neurology,* **15**, 243–268.

Freund, J. F. and McDermott, K. (1942) Sensitization to horse serum by means of adjuvants. *Proceedings of the Society for Experimental Biology and Medicine,* **49**, 548–553.

Freund, J. and Lipton, M. M. (1955) Experimental allergic encephalomyelitis after the excision of the injection site of antigen–adjuvant emulsion. *Journal of Immunology,* **75**, 454–459.

Friede, R. L. and Martinez, A. J. (1970a) Analysis of the process of sheath expansion in swollen nerve fibres. *Brain Research,* **19**, 165–182.

Friede, R. L. and Martinez, A. J. (1970b) Analysis of axon–sheath relations during early Wallerian degeneration. *Brain Research,* **19**, 199–212.

Fullerton, P. M. (1966) Chronic peripheral neuropathy produced by lead poisoning in guinea-pigs. *Journal of Neuropathology and Experimental Neurology,* **25**, 214–236.

Fullerton, P. M., Gilliatt, R. W., Lascelles, R. G. and Morgan-Hughes, J. A. (1965) The relation between fibre diameter and internodal length in chronic neuropathy. *Journal of Physiology, (London),* **178**, 26–28.

Gamble, H. J. (1964) Comparative electron microscopic observations on the connective tissues of a peripheral nerve and a spinal nerve root in the rat. *Journal of Anatomy,* **98**, 17–25.

Gasser, H. S. and Grundfest, H. (1939) Axon diameters in relation to the spike dimensions and the conduction velocity in mammalian fibres. *American Journal of Physiology,* **127**, 393–414.

Geren, B. B. (1954) The formation from the Schwann cell surface of myelin in the peripheral nerves of chick embryos. *Experimental Cell Research,* **7**, 558–562.

Gill, D. M., Pappenheimer, A. M., Brown, R. and Kurnick, J. T. (1969) Studies on the mode of action of diphtheria toxin VII. Toxin-stimulated hydrolysis of nicotinamide adenine dinucleotide in mammalian cell extracts. *Journal of Experimental Medicine,* **129**, 1–21.

Gilliatt, R. W. (1966) Nerve conduction in human and experimental neuropathies. *Proceedings of the Royal Society of Medicine,* **59**, 989–993.

Glees, P. (1943) Observations on the structure of the connective tissue sheaths of cutaneous nerves. *Journal of Anatomy,* **77**, 153–159.

Glimstedt, G. and Wohlrart, G. (1960) Electron microscope observations on Wallerian degeneration in peripheral nerves. *Acta morphologica neerlando-scandinavica,* **3**, 135–146.

Gombault, A. (1880–1881) Contribution à l'etude anatomique de la névrite parenchy-mateuse subaiguë ou chronique.- névrite segmentaire péri-axile. *Archives de neurologie (Paris),* **1**, 177–190.

Gregson, N. A., Kennedy, M. C. and Leibowitz, S. (1971) Immunological reactions with lysolecithin – solubilized myelin. *Immunology,* **20**, 501–512.

Guth, L. (1956) Regeneration in the mammalian peripheral nervous system. *Physiological Reviews,* **36**, 441–478.

Guthrie, T. C. (1951) Visual and motor changes in patients with multiple sclerosis. A result of induced changes in environmental temperature. *Archives of Neurology and Psychiatry, Chicago,* **65**, 437–451.

Haftek, J. and Thomas, P. K. (1968) Electron microscope observations on the effects of localized crush injuries on the connective tissues of peripheral nerve. *Journal of Anatomy,* **103**, 233–243.

Hall, J. I. (1967a) Studies on demyelinated peripheral nerves in guinea-pigs with experimental allergic neuritis. A histological and electrophysiological study. Part I. Symptomatology and histological observations. *Brain,* **90**, 297–312.

Hall, J. I. (1967b) Studies on demyelinated peripheral nerves in guinea-pigs with experimental allergic neuritis. A histological and electrophysiological study Part II. Electrophysiological observations. *Brain,* **90**, 313–332.

Hall, S. M. and Williams, P. L. (1970) Studies on the incisures of Schmidt and Lanterman. *Journal of Cell Science,* **6**, 767–791.

Hallpike, J. F. (1972) Enzyme and protein changes in myelin breakdown and multiple sclerosis. *Progress in Histochemistry and Cytochemistry,* **3** (No. 4), 1–215.

Harrison, B. M., McDonald, W. I. and Ochoa, J. (1972) Central demyelination produced by diphtheria toxin: an electron microscope study. *Journal of the Neurological Sciences,* **17**, 281–291.

Harrison, B. M., McDonald, W. I., Ochoa, J. and Ohlrich, G. D. (1972) Paranodal demyelination in the central nervous system. *Journal of the Neurological Sciences,* **16**, 489–494.

Heitman, R. and Mannweiler, K. (1957) Tierexperimentelle Untersuchungen über die 'allergische' Polyneuritis. *Deutsche Zeitschrift für Nervenheilkunde,* **177**, 28–47.

Hiscoe, H. B. (1947) Distribution of nodes and incisures in normal and regenerated nerve fibres. *Anatomical Record,* **99**, 447–475.

Holtzman, E. and Novikoff, A. B. (1965) Lysosomes in the rat sciatic nerve following crush. *Journal of Cell Biology,* **27**, 651–669.

Hönjin, R., Nakamura, T. and Imura, M. (1959) Electron microscopy of peripheral nerve fibres. III On the axoplasmic changes during Wallerian degeneration. *Okajimas Folia Anatomica Japonica,* **33**, 131–156.

Honjo, T., Nishizuka, Y., Hayaishi, O. and Kato, I. (1968) Diphtheria toxin-independent adenosine diphosphate ribosylation of aminoacyl transferase II and inhibition of protein synthesis. *Journal of Biological Chemistry,* **243**, 3553–3555.

Hopkins, A. P. and Morgan-Hughes, J. A. (1969) The effect of local pressure in diphtheritic neuropathy. *Journal of Neurology, Neurosurgery and Psychiatry,* **32**, 614–623.

Hopkins, A. P. and Lambert, E. H. (1972) Conduction in regenerating unmyelinated fibres. *Brain,* **95**, 213–222.

Hoyer, L. W., Good, R. A. and Condie, R. M. (1962) Experimental allergic encephalomyelitis: the effect of 6-mercaptopurine. *Journal of Experimental Medicine,* **116**, 311–327.

Hughes, D., Narang, H. K. and Kelso, W. (1972) The effects of diphtheria toxin on developing peripheral myelin in culture. *Journal of the Neurological Sciences,* **15**, 457–470.

Hurst, E. W. (1932) The effects of the injection of normal brain emulsion into rabbits, with special reference to the aetiology of the paralytic accidents of antirabic treatment. *Journal of Hygiene, Cambridge,* **32**, 33–44.

Hurst, E. W. (1955) The pathological effects produced by sera of animals immunized with foreign nervous or splenic tissue. Part II: Intra-arterial injection of serum. *Journal of Neurology, Neurosurgery and Psychiatry,* **18**, 260–265.

Huxley, A. F. and Stämpfli, R. (1949) Evidence for saltatory conduction in peripheral myelinated nerve fibres. *Journal of Physiology (London),* **108**, 315–339.

Jacobs, J. M. (1967) Experimental diphtheritic neuropathy in the rat. *British Journal of Experimental Pathology.* **48**, 204–216.

Jacobs, J. M., Cavanagh, J. B. and Mellick, R. S. (1966) Intraneural injection of diphtheria toxin. *British Journal of Experimental Pathology,* **47**, 507–517.

Jacobs, J. M. and Cavanagh, J. B. (1969) Species differences in internode formation following two types of peripheral nerve injury. *Journal of Anatomy,* **105**, 295–306.

Jacobson, S. and Guth, L. (1965) An electrophysiological study of the early stages of peripheral nerve regeneration. *Experimental Neurology,* **11**, 48–60.

Joseph, J. (1947) Absence of cell multiplication during degeneration of non-myelinated nerves. *Journal of Anatomy,* **81**, 135–139.

Joseph, J. (1948) Changes in nuclear population following twenty-one days degeneration in a nerve consisting of small myelinated fibres. *Journal of Anatomy,* 82, 146–152.

Joseph, J. (1950) Further studies in changes of nuclear population in degenerating non-myelinated and finely myelinated nerves. *Acta anatomica,* 9, 279–288.

Kabat, E. A., Wolf, A. and Bezer, A. E. (1948) Studies on acute disseminated encephalomyelitis produced experimentally in rhesus monkeys. *Journal of Experimental Medicine,* 88, 417–426.

Kaeser, H. E. and Lambert, E. H. (1962) Nerve function studies in experimental polyneuritis. *Electroencephalography and Clinical Neurophysiology,* Suppl. 22, 29–35.

Kapeller, K. and Mayor, D. (1969a) An electron microscopic study of the early changes proximal to a constriction in sympathetic nerves. *Proceedings of the Royal Society of London (Series B),* 172, 39–51.

Kapeller, K. and Mayor, D. (1969b) An electron microscopic study of the early changes distal to a constriction in sympathetic nerves. *Proceedings of the Royal Society of London (Series B),* 172, 53–63.

Kavanau, J. L. (1965) *Structure and Function in Biological Membranes.* Vols, I and II, pp. 39, 167 and 169. Holden-Day: San Francisco.

Kibler, R. F., Shapira, R., McKneally, S., Jenkins, J., Selden, P. and Chou, F. (1969) Encephalitogenic protein: structure. *Science,* 164, 577–580.

Khan, A. and Levine, S. (1974) Further studies on the inhibition of allergic encephalomyelitis by L-asparaginase. *Journal of Immunology,* 113, 367–370.

Kies, M. W., Murphy, J. B. and Alvord, E. C. (1960) Fractionation of guinea-pig brain proteins with encephalitogenic activity. *Federation Proceedings. Federation of American Societies for Experimental Biology,* 19, 207.

Kies, M. W., Thompson, E. B. and Ellsworth, C. A. (1965) The relationship of myelin proteins to experimental allergic encephalomyelitis. *Annals of New York Academy of Sciences,* 122, 148–160.

King, R. H. M. and Thomas, P. K. (1971) Electron microscope observations on aberrant regeneration of unmyelinated axons in the vagus nerve of the rabbit. *Acta neuropathologica (Berlin),* 18, 150–159.

Koles, Z. J. and Rasminsky, M. (1972) A computer simulation of conduction in demyelinated nerve fibres. *Journal of Physiology (London),* 227, 351–364.

Laatsch, R. H., Kies, M. W., Gordon, S. and Alvord, E. C. (1962) The encephalomyelitic activity of myelin isolated by ultracentrifugation. *Journal of Experimental Medicine,* 115, 777–788.

Lampert, P. W. (1969) Mechanism of demyelination in experimental allergic neuritis: electron microscope studies. *Laboratory Investigation,* 20, 127–138.

Landon, D. N. and Williams, P. L. (1963) Ultrastructure of the node of Ranvier. *Nature (London),* 199, 575–577.

Langley, O. K. and Landon, D. N. (1968) A light and electron histochemical approach to the node of Ranvier and myelin of peripheral nerve fibres. *Journal of Histochemistry and Cytochemistry,* 15, 722–731.

Lascelles, R. G. and Thomas, P. K. (1966) Changes due to age in internodal length in the sural nerve in man. *Journal of Neurology, Neurosurgery and Psychiatry,* 29, 40–44.

Lee, J. C. Y. (1963) Electron microscopy of Wallerian degeneration. *Journal of Comparative Neurology,* 120, 65–79.

Lehrich, J. R. and Arnason, B. G. (1971) Suppression of experimental allergic neuritis in rats by prior immunisation with nerve in saline. *Acta neuropathologica (Berlin),* 18, 144–149.

Leibowitz, S., Lessof, M. H. and Kennedy, L. A. (1968) The effect of antilymphocyte serum on experimental allergic encephalomyelitis in the guinea-pig. *Clinical and Experimental Immunology,* 3, 753–760.

Levine, S. and Hoenig, E. M. (1968) Induced localization of allergic adrenalitis and encephalomyelitis at sites of thermal injury. *Journal of Immunology,* 100, 1310–1318.

Levine, S., Sowinski, R. and Kies, M. (1972) Treatment of experimental allergic encephalomyelitis with encephalitogenic basic proteins. *Proceedings of the Society for Experimental Biology and Medicine,* 139, 506–510.

Lisak, R. P., Falk, G. A., Heinze, R. G., Kies, M. W. and Alvord, E. C. (1970) Dissociation of antibody production from disease suppression in the inhibition of allergic encephalomyelitis by myelin basic protein. *Journal of Immunology,* **104**, 1435–1446.

Liu, H. M. (1973) Schwann cell properties: I. Origin of Schwann cell during peripheral nerve regeneration. *Journal of Neuropathology and experimental Neurology,* **32**, 458–473.

Liu, H. M. (1974) Schwann cell properties: II. The identity of phagocytes in the degenerating nerve. *American Journal of Pathology,* **75**, 395–420.

Lubińska, L. (1958) Intercalated internodes in nerve fibres. *Nature (London),* **181**, 957–958.

Lubińska, L. (1959) Region of transition between preserved and regenerating parts of myelinated nerve fibres. *Journal of Comparative Neurology,* **113**, 315–335.

Lubińska, L. (1961a) Sedentary and migratory states of Schwann cells. *Experimental cell Research,* Suppl. 8, 74–90.

Lubińska, L. (1961b) Demyelination and remyelination in the proximal parts of regenerating nerve fibres. *Journal of Comparative Neurology,* **117**, 275–289.

Majno, G., Waksman, B. H. and Karnovsky, M. L. (1960) Experimental study of diphtheritic polyneuritis in the rabbit and guinea-pig. II. The effect of diphtheria toxin on lipide biosynthesis by guinea pig nerve. *Journal of Neuropathology and Experimental Neurology,* **19**, 7–24.

Martinez, A. J. and Friede, R. L. (1970) Accumulation of axoplasmic organelles in swollen nerve fibres. *Brain Research,* **19**, 183–198.

Matheson, D. F. (1968a) Incorporation of (C^{14}) glycine into protein of the adult rat peripheral nerve: effects of inhibitors. *Journal of Neurochemistry,* **15**, 179–185.

Matheson, D. F. (1968b) Influence of age in the incorporation of (C^{14}) glycine into isolated rat nerve segments *in vitro. Journal of Neurochemistry,* **15**, 187–194.

Matheson, D. F. and Cavanagh, J. B. (1967) Protein synthesis in peripheral nerve and susceptibility to diphtheritic neuropathy. *Nature (London),* **214**, 721–722.

Matthews, M. R. (1973) An ultrastructural study of axonal changes following constriction of post-ganglionic branches of the superior cervical ganglion in the rat. *Philosophical Transactions of the Royal Society,* **264**, 479–505.

McDonald, W. I. (1963a) The effects of experimental demyelination on conduction in peripheral nerve: a histological and electrophysiological study. I. Electrophysiological observations. *Brain,* **86**, 481–500.

McDonald, W. I. (1963b) The effects of experimental demyelination on conduction in peripheral nerve: a histological and electrophysiological study. II. Electrophysiological observations. *Brain,* **86**, 501–524.

McDonald, W. I. and Gilman, S. (1968) Demyelination and spindle function. Effect of diphtheritic polyneuritis on nerve conduction and muscle spindle function in the cat. *Archives of Neurology, Chicago,* **18**, 508–519.

McDonald, W. I. and Sears, T. A. (1970a) Focal experimental demyelination in the central nervous system. *Brain,* **93**, 575–582.

McDonald, W. I. and Sears, T. A. (1970b) The effects of experimental demyelination on conduction in the central nervous system. *Brain,* **93**, 583–598.

Mellick, R. (1969) The blood vessel permeability of peripheral nerve during primary demyelination and the effect of A.C.T.H. therapy on the permeability and on the functional disability. *Proceedings, Australian Association of Neurologists,* **6**, 133–138.

Mellick, R. and Cavanagh, J. B. (1967) Longitudinal movement of radioiodinated albumin within extravascular spaces of peripheral nerve following three systems of experimental trauma. *Journal of Neurology, Neurosurgery and Psychiatry,* **30**, 458–463.

Mellick, R. S. and Cavanagh, J. B. (1968a) Changes in blood vessel permeability during degeneration and regeneration in peripheral nerves. *Brain,* **91**, 141–160.

Mellick, R. S. and Cavanagh, J. B. (1968b) The function of the perineurium and its relation to the flow phenomenon within the endoneurial spaces. *Proceedings, Australian Association of Neurologists,* **5**, 521–525.

Morgan, I. (1947) Allergic encephalomyelitis in monkeys in response to injection of normal monkey nervous tissue. *Journal of Experimental Medicine,* **85**, 131–140.

Molnár, G. K., Riekkinen, P. J., Rinne, U. K. and Frey, H. J. (1974) Experimental allergic neuritis: a temporal correlation of the clinical signs, lymphocyte transformation and morphological findings to neurochemical phenomena in the peripheral nerves. Abstracts of the VIIth International Congress of Neuropathology, p. 211. Akadémiai Kiadó: Budapest.

Morgan-Hughes, J. A. (1965) Changes in motor nerve conduction velocity in diphtheritic polyneuritis. *Rivista di patologia nervosa e mentale*, 86, 253–260.

Morgan-Hughes, J. A. (1968) Experimental diphtheritic neuropathy: pathological and electrophysiological study. *Journal of the Neurological Sciences*, 7, 157–175.

Morris, J. H., Hudson, A. R. and Weddell, G. (1972a) A study of degeneration and regeneration in the divided rat sciatic nerve based on electron microscopy. I. The traumatic degeneration of myelin in the proximal stump of the divided nerve. *Zeitschrift für Zellforschung und mikroskopische Anatomie*, 124, 76–102.

Morris, J. H. Hudson, A. R. and Weddell, G. (1972b) A study of degeneration and regeneration in the divided rat sciatic nerve based on electron microscopy. III. Changes in the axons of the proximal stump. *Zeitschrift für Zellforschung und mikroskopische Anatomie*, 124, 131–164.

Morris, J. H., Hudson, A. R. and Weddell, G. (1972c) A study of degeneration and regeneration in the divided rat sciatic nerve based on electron microscopy. IV. Changes in fascicular microtopography, perineurium and endoneurial fibroblasts. *Zeitschrift für Zellforschung und mikroskopische Anatomie*, 124, 165–203.

Murray, P. K., Jennings, F. W., Murray, M. and Urquhart, G. M. (1974) The nature of immunosuppression in *Trypanosoma brucei* Infections in mice. II. The role of the T and B lymphocytes. *Immunology*, 27, 825–840.

Nathaniel, E. J. H. and Pease, D. C. (1963a) Degenerative changes in rat dorsal roots during Wallerian degeneration. *Journal of Ultrastructure Research*, 9, 511–532.

Nathaniel, E. J. H. and Pease, D. C. (1963b) Regenerative changes in rat dorsal roots following Wallerian degeneration. *Journal of Ultrastructure Research*, 9, 533–549.

O'Daly, J. A. and Imaeda, T. (1967) Electron microscopic study of Wallerian degeneration in cutaneous nerves caused by mechanical injury. *Laboratory Investigation*, 17, 744–766.

Ohmi, S. (1961) Electron microscope study on Wallerian degeneration of the peripheral nerve. *Zeitschrift für Zellforschung und mikroskopische Anatomie*, 54, 39–67.

Olsson, Y. (1966) Studies on vascular permeability in peripheral nerves I. Distribution of circulating fluorescent serum albumin in normal, crushed and sectioned rat sciatic nerve. *Acta neuropathologica (Berlin)*, 7, 1–15.

Olsson, Y. (1967) Degranulation of mast cells in peripheral nerve injuries. *Acta Neurologica Scandinavica*, 43, 365–374.

Olsson, Y. (1968) Topographical differences in the vascular permeability of the peripheral nervous system. *Acta neuropathologica (Berlin)*, 10, 26–33.

Olsson, Y. (1971) Studies on vascular permeability in peripheral nerves IV. Distribution of intravenously injected protein tracers in the peripheral nervous system of various species. *Acta neuropathologica (Berlin)*, 17, 114–126.

Olsson, Y. and Sjöstrand, J. (1969) Origin of macrophages in Wallerian degeneration of peripheral nerves demonstrated autoradiographically. *Experimental Neurology*, 23, 102–112.

Olsson, Y. and Kristensson, K. (1973) The perineurium as a diffusion barrier to protein tracers following trauma to nerves. *Acta neuropathologica (Berlin)*, 23, 105–111.

Paterson, P. Y. (1966) Experimental allergic encephalomyelitis and autoimmune disease. *Advances in Immunology*, 5, 131–208.

Paterson, P. Y. and Harwin, S. M. (1963) Suppression of allergic encephalomyelitis in rats by means of antibrain serum. *Journal of Experimental Medicine*, 117, 755–774.

Paterson P. Y. and Drobish, D. G. (1969) Cyclophosphamide: effect on experimental allergic encephalomyelitis in Lewis rats. *Science*, 165, 191–192.

Paterson, P. Y. and Hanson, M. A. (1969) Studies of cyclophosphamide suppression of experimental allergic encephalomyelitis in Wistar rats. *Journal of Immunology*, 103, 795–803.

Peterson, E. R. and Murray, M. R. (1965) Patterns of peripheral demyelination *in vitro*. *Annals of the New York Academy of Sciences*, 122, 39–50.

Peyronnard, J.-M., Aguayo, A. J. and Bray, G. M. (1973) Schwann cell internuclear distances in normal and regenerating unmyelinated nerve fibers. *Archives of Neurology, Chicago*. 29. 56–59.

Pleasure, D. E., Feldmann, B. and Prockop, D. J. (1973) Diphtheria toxin inhibits the synthesis of myelin proteolipid and basic proteins by peripheral nerve *in vitro*. *Journal of Neurochemistry*, **20**, 81–90.

Pollard, J. D., King, R. H. M. and Thomas, P. K. (1975) Recurrent experimental allergic neuritis: an electron microscope study. *Journal of the Neurological Sciences*, **24**, 365–383.

Porcellati, G. (1972) Amino acid and protein metabolism in Wallerian degeneration. In *Handbook of Neurochemistry*, (ed.) Lajtha, A. Vol. VII, pp. 191–219. Plenum Press: New York and London.

Raine, C. S., Wiśniewski, H. and Prineas, J. (1969) An ultrastructural study of experimental allergic encephalomyelitis in the peripheral nervous system. *Laboratory Investigation*, **21**, 316–327.

Rasminsky, M. (1973) The effects of temperature on conduction in demyelinated single nerve fibers. *Archives of Neurology, Chicago*, **28**, 287–292.

Rasminsky, M. and Sears, T. A. (1972) Internodal conduction in undissected demyelinated nerve fibres. *Journal of Physiology, London*, **227**, 323–350.

Rénaut, M. (1881) Recherches sur quelques points particuliers de l'histologie des nerfs. *Archives de Physiologie (Paris)*, **8**, 161–190.

Rivers, T. M., Sprunt, D. H. and Berry, G. B. (1933) Observations on attempts to produce acute disseminated encephalomyelitis in monkeys. *Journal of Experimental Medicine*, **58**, 39–53.

Robertson, J. D. (1958a) The ultrastructure of Schmidt–Lantermann clefts and related shearing defects of the myelin sheath. *Journal of Biophysical and Biochemical Cytology*, **4**, 39–46.

Robertson, J. D. (1958b) Structural alterations in nerve fibres produced by hypotonic and hypertonic solutions. *Journal of Biophysical and Biochemical Cytology*, **4**, 349–364.

Robertson, J. D. (1959) Preliminary observations on the ultrastructure of nodes of Ranvier. *Zeitschrift für Zellforschung und mikroskopische Anatomie*, **50**, 553–560.

Robinson, H. C., Allt, G. and Evans, D. H. L. (1972) A study of the capacity of myelinated and unmyelinated nerves to induce experimental allergic neuritis. *Acta neuropathologica, (Berlin)*, **21**, 99–108.

Rushton, W. A. H. (1951) A theory of the effects of fibre size in medullated nerve. *Journal of Physiology (London)*, **115**, 101–122.

Salvin, S. B. and Liauw, H. L. (1968) Immunologic unresponsiveness, immunity and enhancement in experimental allergic encephalomyelitis. *Journal of Immunology*, **101**, 33–42.

Sanders, F. K. and Whitteridge, D. (1946) Conduction velocity and myelin thickness in regenerating nerve fibres. *Journal of Physiology (London)*, **105**, 152–174.

Satinsky, D., Pepe, F. A. and Liu, C. N. (1964) The neurilemma cell in peripheral nerve degeneration and regeneration. *Experimental Neurology*, **9**, 441–451.

Scheinberg, L. C., Lee, J. M. and Taylor, J. M. (1967) Suppression of experimental allergic encephalomyelitis in mice by irradiation of the target organ. *Nature (London)*, **216**, 924–925.

Schlaeper, W. W. (1973) Effects of nerve constriction on oxygenated excised segments of rat peripheral nerve. *Journal of Neuropathology and experimental Neurology*, **32**, 203–217.

Schlaepfer, W. W. (1974a) Calcium-induced degeneration of axoplasm in isolated segments of rat peripheral nerve. *Brain Research*, **69**, 203–215.

Schlaepfer, W. W. (1974b) Effects of energy deprivation on Wallerian degeneration in isolated segments of rat peripheral nerve. *Brain Research*, **78**, 71–81.

Schröder, J. M. (1972) Altered ratio between axon diameter and myelin sheath thickness in regenerated nerve fibres. *Brain Research*, **45**, 49–65.

Schröder, J. M. and Krücke, W. (1970) Zur Feinstruktur der experimentell-allergischen Neuritis beim Kaninchen. *Acta neuropathologica (Berlin)*, **14**, 261–283.

Seddon, H. J. (1943) Three types of nerve injury. *Brain*, **66**, 237–288.

Shanthaveerappa, T. R. and Bourne, G. H. (1964) The effects of transection of the nerve trunk on the perineural epithelium with special reference to its role in nerve degeneration and regeneration. *Anatomical Record*, **150**, 35–50.

Shantha, T. R. and Bourne, G. H. (1968) The perineural epithelium – a new concept. In

The Structure and Function of Nervous Tissue, (ed.) Bourne, G. H. Vol. I, pp. 379–459. Academic Press: New York and London.

Sherwin, A. (1966) Chronic allergic neuropathy in the rabbit. *Archives of Neurology (Chicago)*, 15, 289–293.

Smith, M. E. (1972) The turnover of myelin proteins. *Neurobiology*, 2, 35–40.

Spencer, P. S. and Thomas, P. K. (1970) The examination of isolated nerve fibres by light and electron microscopy, with observations on demyelination proximal to neuromas. *Acta neuropathologica, Berlin*, 16, 177–186.

Spencer, P. S. and Lieberman, A. R. (1971) Scanning electron microscopy of isolated peripheral nerve fibres. Normal surface structure and alterations proximal to neuromas. *Zeitschrift für Zellforschung und mikroskopische Anatomie*, 119, 534–551.

Strauss, N. and Hendee, E. D. (1959) The effect of diphtheria toxin on the metabolism of HeLa cells. *Journal of Experimental Medicine*, 109, 145–163.

Tasaki, I. (1953) *Nervous Transmission*. p. 44. Charles C. Thomas: Springfield, Illinois.

Teitelbaum, D., Meshorer, A., Hirschfeld, T., Arnon, R. and Sela, M. (1971) Suppression of experimental allergic encephalomyelitis by a synthetic polypeptide. *European Journal of Immunology*, 1, 242–248.

Teitelbaum, D., Webb, C., Meshorer, A., Arnon, R. and Sela, M. (1972) Protection against experimental allergic encephalomyelitis. *Nature (London)*, 240, 564–566.

Terry, R. D. and Harkin, J. C. (1957) Regenerating peripheral nerve sheaths following Wallerian degeneration. *Experimental Cell Research*, 13, 193–197.

Terry, R. D. and Harkin, J. C. (1959) Wallerian degeneration and regeneration of peripheral nerves. In *The Biology of Myelin*, (ed.) Korey, S. A. pp. 303–320. Cassell: London.

Thomas, G. A. (1948) Quantitative histology of Wallerian degeneration II. Nuclear population in two nerves of different fibre spectrum. *Journal of Anatomy*, 82, 135–145.

Thomas, P. K. (1963) The connective tissue of peripheral nerve: an electron microscope study. *Journal of Anatomy*, 97, 35–44.

Thomas, P. K. (1964a) Changes in the endoneurial sheaths of peripheral myelinated nerve fibres during Wallerian degeneration. *Journal of Anatomy*, 98, 175–182.

Thomas, P. K. (1964b) The deposition of collagen in relation to Schwann cell basement membrane during peripheral nerve regeneration. *Journal of Cell Biology*, 23, 375–382.

Thomas, P. K. (1966) The cellular response to nerve injury. I. The cellular outgrowth from the distal stump of transected nerve. *Journal of Anatomy*, 100, 287–303.

Thomas, P. K. (1970) The cellular response to nerve injury. 3. The effect of repeated crush injuries. *Journal of Anatomy*, 106, 463–470.

Thomas, P. K. (1973) The ultrastructural pathology of unmyelinated nerve fibres. *New Developments in Electromyography and Clinical Neurophysiology*, 2, 227–239.

Thomas, P. K. and Jones, D. G. (1967) The cellular response to nerve injury. 2. Regeneration of the perineurium after nerve section. *Journal of Anatomy*, 101, 45–55.

Thomas, P. K. and King, R. H. M. (1974) The degeneration of unmyelinated axons following nerve section: an ultrastructural study. *Journal of Neurocytology*, 3, 497–512.

Thomas, P. K. and Lascelles, R. G. (1967) Hypertrophic neuropathy. *Quarterly Journal of Medicine*, 36, 223–238.

Turk, J. L. (1969) The cell-mediated immunological response. *Lectures on the Scientific Basis of Medicine*, 278–293.

Vial, J. D. (1958) The early changes in the axoplasm during Wallerian degeneration. *Journal of Biophysical and Biochemical Cytology*, 4, 551–556.

Vizoso, A. D. (1950) The relationship between internodal length and growth in human nerves. *Journal of Anatomy*, 84, 342–353.

Vizoso, A. D. and Young, J. Z. (1948) Internode length and fibre diameter in developing and regenerating nerves. *Journal of Anatomy*. 82, 110–134.

Waksman, B. H. (1959) Allergic encephalomyelitis in rats and rabbits pretreated with nervous tissue. *Journal of Neuropathology and Experimental Neurology*, 18, 397–417.

Waksman, B. H. (1961) Experimental study of diphtheritic polyneuritis in the rabbit and guinea pig. III. The blood-nerve barrier in the rabbit. *Journal of Neuropathology and Experimental Neurology*, 20, 35–77.

Waksman, B. H. and Morrison, L. R. (1951) Tuberculin type sensitivity to spinal cord antigen in rabbits with isoallergic encephalomyelitis. *Journal of Immunology*, **66**, 421–444.

Waksman, B. H. and Adams, R. D. (1955) Allergic neuritis: an experimental disease of rabbits induced by the injection of peripheral nervous tissue and adjuvants. *Journal of Experimental Medicine*, **102**, 213–236.

Waksman, B. H. and Adams, R. D. (1956) A comparative study of experimental allergic neuritis in the rabbit, guinea-pig and mouse. *Journal of Neuropathology and Experimental Neurology*, **15**, 293–333.

Waksman, B. H., Adams, R. D. and Mansmann, H. C. (1957) Experimental study of diphtheritic polyneuritis in the rabbit and guinea-pig. I. Immunologic and histopathologic observations. *Journal of Experimental Medicine*, **105**, 591–614.

Waller, A. V. (1850) Experiments on the section of the glossopharyngeal and hypoglossal nerves of the frog, and observations of the alterations produced thereby in the structure of their primitive fibres. *Philosophical Transactions of the Royal Society*, **140**, 423–429.

Webster, H. de F. (1962) Transient, focal accumulation of axonal mitochondria during the early stages of Wallerian degeneration. *Journal of Cell Biology*, **12**, 361–384.

Webster, H. de F. (1964) Some ultrastructural features of segmental demyelination and myelin regeneration in peripheral nerve. *Progress in Brain Research*, **13**, 151–174.

Webster, H. de F. (1965) The relationship between Schmidt–Lantermann incisures and myelin segmentation during Wallerian degeneration. *Annals of New York Academy of Sciences*, **122**, 29–38.

Webster, H. de F. and Spiro, D. (1960) Phase and electron microscopic studies of experimental demyelination I. Variations in myelin sheath contour in normal guinea-pig sciatic nerve. *Journal of Neuropathology and Experimental Neurology*, **19**, 42–69.

Webster, H. de F., Spiro, D., Waksman, B. and Adams, R. D. (1961) Phase and electron microscope studies of experimental demyelination II. Schwann cell changes in guinea-pig sciatic nerves during experimental diphtheritic neuritis. *Journal of Neuropathology and Experimental Neurology*, **20**, 5–34.

Weiss, P. and Wang, H. (1945) Transformation of adult Schwann cells into macrophages. *Proceedings of the Society for Experimental Biology and Medicine*, **58**, 273–275.

Weller, R. O. (1965) Diphtheric neuropathy in the chicken: an electron microscope study. *Journal of Pathology and Bacteriology*, **89**, 591–598.

Weller R. O. (1967) An electron microscopic study of hypertrophic neuropathy of Dejerine and Sottas. *Journal of Neurology, Neurosurgery and Psychiatry*, **30**, 111–125.

Weller, R. O. and Mellick, R. S. (1966) Acid phosphatase and lysosome activity in diphtheritic neuropathy and Wallerian degeneration. *British Journal of Experimental Pathology*, **47**, 425–434.

Weller, R. O. and Nester, B. (1972) Early changes at the node of Ranvier in segmental demyelination. Histochemical and electron microscope observations. *Brain*, **95**, 665–674.

Williams, P. L. and Landon, D. N. (1963) Paranodal apparatus of peripheral myelinated nerve fibres of mammals. *Nature (London)*, **198**, 670–673.

Williams, P. L. and Hall, S. M. (1971a) Prolonged *in vivo* observations of normal peripheral nerve fibres and their acute reactions to crush and deliberate trauma. *Journal of Anatomy*, **108**, 397–408.

Williams, P. L. and Hall, S. M. (1971b) Chronic Wallerian degeneration – an *in vivo* and ultrastructural study. *Journal of Anatomy*, **109**, 487–503.

Wiśniewski, H. M., Brostoff, S. W., Carter, H. and Eylar, E. H. (1974) Recurrent experimental allergic polyganglioradiculoneuritis. Multiple demyelinating episodes in rhesus monkey sensitized with rabbit sciatic nerve myelin. *Archives of Neurology*, **30**, 347–358.

Wiśniewski, H., Prineas, J. and Raine, C. S. (1969) An ultrastructural study of experimental demyelination and remyelination. I. Acute experimental allergic encephalomyelitis in the peripheral nervous system. *Laboratory Investigation*, **21**, 105–118.

Wiśniewski, H. and Raine, C. S. (1971) An ultrastructural study of experimental demyelination and remyelination. V. Central and peripheral nervous system lesions caused by diphtheria toxin. *Laboratory Investigation*, **25**, 73–80.

Yonezawa, T. and Ishihara, Y. (1967) Experimental allergic peripheral neuritis studied *in vitro*. *Journal of Neuropathology and Experimental Neurology*, **26**, 177.

Yonezawa, T., Ishihara, Y. and Matsuyama, H. (1968) Studies on experimental allergic peripheral neuritis. *Journal of Neuropathology and Experimental Neurology,* **27,** 453–463.

Young, J. Z. (1942) The functional repair of nervous tissue. *Physiological Reviews,* **22,** 318–374.

Young, J. Z. (1945) The history of the shape of a nerve fibre. In *Essays on Growth and Form,* (ed.) Le Gros Clark, W. E. and Medawar, P. B. pp. 41–94. Clarendon Press: Oxford.

Young, J. Z. (1950) The determination of the specific characteristics of nerve fibers. In *Genetic Neurology,* (ed.) Weiss, P. pp. 92–127. University of Chicago Press: Chicago.

Zelena, J., Lubińska, L. and Gutmann, E. (1968) Accumulation of organelles at the ends of interrupted axons. *Zeitschrift für Zellforschung und mikroskopische Anatomie,* **91,** 200–219.

14 ELECTROPHYSIOLOGICAL PROPERTIES OF PERIPHERAL NERVE

J.J.B. Jack

This chapter discusses present understanding of the best known function of peripheral nerve fibres, their ability to generate and conduct electrical signals.

Since the signal, or action potential, is a transient change in the potential recordable between the inside and the outside of a nerve fibre, it is natural to consider first the way in which such potential changes are achieved. The conventional assumption is that the changes in potential occur across the cell membrane, with free diffusion of (most) ions both inside and outside the cell (the 'membrane concept'). Readers interested in a radically different hypothesis, in which the resting membrane potential is explained by the ordering of ion-binding intracellular constituents, are referred to the work of Ling (1962) as well as the critique by Katz (1966, pp. 42–66).

If the potential recorded between the inside and outside of excitable cells is explained by the 'membrane concept', then any potential represents a separation of (ionic) charge between the two sides of the cell membrane. This separation of charge can be produced because the membrane has substantial electrical capacitance (usually about 1 μF per square centimetre of membrane). The capacitance of a patch of membrane can be charged, or discharged, in two basic ways: either by movement of charge across that patch of membrane or by spread of charge from another patch of membrane.

14.1 Charge movements across the membrane

On both sides of the surface membrane there are dilute aqueous solutions, predominantly of electrolytes, with the concentration of particular electrolytes varying on the two sides. Charge movement within the internal or external solutions is therefore by way of the movement of ions; with potassium ion being the main charge carrier internally and sodium and chloride ions externally. There is also good reason to believe that most, if not all, of the charge movement across the membrane is by the transfer of ions and not electrons (Hodgkin, 1951; Keynes, 1951; Hodgkin and Huxley, 1953; Brinley and Mullins, 1965; Rojas and Canessa-Fischer, 1968; Atwater, Bezanilla and Rojas, 1969). The question naturally arises as to how the ions cross the membrane. A primary distinction is made, in the types of ion movement which occur, on the basis of whether or not the movement requires energy. In any system consisting of two compartments separated by a permeable membrane, ions tend to move from one compartment to the other as a result of electrical and/or concentration differences. It is possible to give a precise quantitative description of the magnitude of these two effects such that, for a given concentration difference, there is a single electrical potential difference (called the equilibrium potential) for which there will not be net movement of the ion species. (Similarly one can define a comparable concentration difference necessary to hold an ion species in equilibrium, for a given electrical potential difference). If a particular ion species is out of equilibrium, then a net movement will occur, and it turns out that several ion species, including sodium, potassium and calcium, are out of equilibrium across the cell membrane. There will therefore be a tendency for these ions to have a net movement across the membrane, the magnitude of the movement being influenced by the ease with which they can cross, as well as the degree to which they are out of equilibrium. As will be seen later, the membrane can alter its properties so that a particular ion species can cross the membrane more or less readily. Such a process may be energy-consuming or producing, but the basic tendency of the ions to move does not require any energy other than that involved in producing the initial electrochemical disequilibrium for that ion species. These non-energy requiring ion movements are called 'passive movements'. At a first level of description these movements alone are sufficient to provide a basis for the resting membrane potential and the action potential. The energy-requiring movements, commonly called 'active transport', are most readily defined under conditions in which there is a net movement of the ion species against its electrochemical gradient, and are of importance in the maintenance of the electrochemical disequilibria for the various ion species.

14.1.1 *Passive movements of ions*

There are two main ways in which ion movements may be observed experimentally. The first is by chemical methods, such as the use of radioactive tracers or the observation of changes in concentration of an ion species within the intracellular or extracellular compartments. The advantage of these techniques is that they can give a direct measure of the movement, but they are still insufficiently sensitive to follow the rapid translocation of the small quantities of ions which are responsible for the action potential. Radioactive tracers have the further disadvantage that it is usually only possible to follow ion movements in one direction at a time, so that the *net* movement of the particular ion species is uncertain unless there is specific information available about the proportion of ions moving in the two directions, for a given electrochemical gradient. The second method is electrical and involves the measurement of the amount of current crossing the membrane for a particular electrical potential difference. Although generally possessing adequate sensitivity, both with respect to time and to quantity of charge moving, the method suffers the major limitation of not discriminating between different ion species; the ion species acting as major charge translocators have to be inferred from a variety of other experimental manoeuvres.

It is not surprising, in the face of these limitations, that certain assumptions are commonly made about the mechanism of ion permeation, to allow the development of a quantitative theory that can be used to interpret experimental results.

The first theoretical assumption made, as mentioned above, is that ions are subject to electrical and diffusional (thermal agitation) forces only. Other possibilities, such as hydrostatic pressure, are thought to be small and have therefore been neglected. It is then a straightforward matter to derive an equation describing the condition for equilibrium of an ion species by calculating the circumstance in which the work required to move the ion against the electrical gradient is exactly equal to the work required to move the same ion, in the opposite direction, against the concentration gradient (see Katz (1966) for an informal development, and Hope (1971) for a more rigorous treatment). The electrical gradient (membrane potential) at which an ion species is in equilibrium across a membrane permeable to it, is given by

$$E_c = \frac{RT}{zF} \log_e \left\{ \frac{[C]_o}{[C]_i} \right\} \tag{14.1}$$

where R is the gas constant, T is the absolute temperature, F the Faraday and z the valency of the ion concerned. The square brackets denote concentrations (or more strictly 'activities', which, roughly speaking, express the proportion of the total concentration which is in 'ionized' form) and the subscripts 'o' and 'i' are for 'outside' and 'inside' respectively. Equation (14.1) is called the Nernst equation.

As mentioned above, several ions, including sodium, potassium and calcium, are out of equilibrium across biological membranes. There will therefore be a net movement of each of these ion species down its electrochemical gradient (sodium and calcium into the cell, potassium out of the cell). This net movement of an ion species is a current. In order to describe its magnitude and direction, the electrochemical form of Ohm's law may be used

$$i_c = G_c \cdot (E_m - E_c) \tag{14.2}$$

where i_c denotes the current for a particular ion specise, C; G_c denotes the conductance of the membrane to that ion; E_m is the membrane potential and E_c the equilibrium potential for that ion (given by the Nernst equation, above).

It is obvious that the term for membrane conductance serves to describe the ease with which ions can cross the membrane; in experimental circumstances it is defined from the electrochemical forms of Ohm's law by knowing the membrane potential, the equilibrium potential for the particular ion and measuring the magnitude of current flow. It does not, however, refer to the properties of the membrane alone. The example usually offered as an illustration of this point is a membrane which is permeable to only one ion species, but the measurement of conductance is performed when the relevant ion is not present on either side of the membrane. No current will then flow, so that the conductance is defined by Ohm's law as zero. Similarly, if very small concentrations of the ion are present on both sides the conductance to that ion will be estimated to be very small because the limit on the amount of current flowing will be set by the number of relevant ions available to cross the membrane. In other words, at very low concentrations, it is the availability of ions to cross the membrane rather than the inherent properties of the membrane which limit the magnitude of the conductance. Furthermore, if the concentration of ion is quite high on one side of the membrane but very low on the other, the same reasoning would lead us to expect a very different magnitude for the conductance depending on the direction of net movement of the ion. Thus, in general, one might expect the magnitude of the conductance term to reflect not only the membrane properties but also to be related to both ion concentrations and imposed voltage.

There have been several theoretical attempts to get round this difficulty. The principal aim of these theories is to obtain a description of the membrane conductance in terms of a membrane property (defined as the membrane permeability to a particular ion species), with ion concentrations and membrane potential as independent factors. In order to interpret the data obtained from studies using radioactive tracers, it is also necessary to be able to predict the ratio of fluxes in the two directions for a given net flux. These theoretical treatments have to include assumptions concerning the way in which ions pass into and across the membrane. One very general approach is to assume that there is one or more energy barriers which the ions have to overcome before they can cross the membrane; the physical process of translocation need not be specified. Woodbury (1971) and Noble (1972a; see also, Jack, Noble and Tsien, 1975) have adopted this approach. Theories which assume a particular type of translocation also involve assumptions about the nature of the membrane structure (see Eisenman, Sandblom and Walker, 1967). Considerable guidance to the theoretical development is therefore obtained by comparing theoretical predictions with the behaviour of various types of artificially prepared membrane, where the membrane structure is fairly well understood and, to some extent, under experimental control. The literature in this field is now considerable and for details the reader is referred to the excellent reviews by Haydon and Hladky (1972) and Eisenman, Szabo, Ciani, McLaughlin and Krasne (1973).

Four principal mechanisms for ion permeation have been postulated. In one, the membrane is assumed to be homogenous, and once in the membrane the ions are assumed to move in accordance with the Nernst-Planck equation for electro-diffusion. Different versions of the theory then add further assumptions concerning, for example, the distribution of the electrical field across the membrane (see Cole, 1965, 1968). Another possible mechanism is that ions are carried across the membrane by the translocation of vesicles (e.g. Bennett, 1956), but this has yet to be explored by a theoretical treatment. The two mechanisms which have recently been most actively considered are that ions either move across the membrane in association with a lipid-soluble molecule ('carrier' mechanism) or that they traverse some physical gap in the membrane ('pore' mechanism). Impetus to the study of the two last mentioned mechanisms has come from three sources.

Firstly, on very general energetic grounds, treating the membrane as a thin region of low dielectric constant, it has been concluded that mechanisms of this kind are required to lower the barrier to ion permeation sufficiently to account for the observed magnitude of ion movements (Parsegian, 1969).

Secondly, the preparation of artificial membrane from a variety of lipid materials (Goldup, Ohki and Danielli, 1970; Haydon, 1970) has given considerable insight into possible mechanisms of permeation across biological membranes. Without further modification, artificial membranes are extremely impermeable to ions; the specific membrane resistance (of the order of $10^8 \, \Omega \, cm^{-2}$) being up to one hundred thousand times greater than that of nerve membranes. It is, however, possible to lower the resistance of the membrane dramatically by adding to it small amounts of certain molecules. Although the existence of some free ion diffusion is implicit in the finite, if high, specific resistance of the artificial membrane, the substantial permeability which can be induced by the added molecules is believed to be the consequence of them either acting as 'carriers' or as 'pore-formers' (Krasne, Eisenman and Szabo, 1971; Haydon and Hladky, 1972).

Finally, the direct study of the properties of certain biological conductances has given circumstantial evidence that ion transport occurs at sparsely located sites (Hille, 1970), some of whose properties can be explained by postulating that they are pores (Armstrong, 1971; Armstrong and Hille, 1972; Bezanilla and Armstrong, 1972; Hille, 1971, 1972, 1973).

The present theoretical circumstance is very unsatisfactory. For each of the three mechanisms assumed (electro-diffusion, carriers or pores) a variety of predictions may be made about the dependence of ionic conductance on either ion concentrations or membrane potential (see Eisenman et al., 1973; Läuger, 1972, 1973; Andreoli and Watkins, 1973). Rather than take each theoretical treatment in turn, it may therefore be more helpful to consider each of the assumptions used in the interpretation of experimental data, and discuss them in the light of both the different theories and the relevant experimental data.

Before entering upon this discussion, it is important to emphasize a fundamental distinction between different aspects of biological conductances: i.e. that their voltage-dependence may display two separate modes of behaviour. When the membrane potential is changed abruptly to a new value the current flowing also changes abruptly to a new value and then may either remain steady at that value or gradually (with time constants no briefer than 50 μs and as long as seconds) alter its magnitude. There is considerable evidence that these two aspects of the behaviour of biological conductances are separate properties, which have been called by Noble (1972a) the 'ion tranfer' reaction and the 'gating' reaction respectively. In the following, only the 'ion transfer' reaction is discussed; 'gating' reactions will be described when considering the mechanism of the action potential, although occasional reference has to be made to them when there is difficulty in deciding whether an experimental result is solely a property of the 'ion transfer' reaction.

Independence of ion movements

There are many different species of ion present on both sides of a nerve membrane, and hence there is a strong possibility that more than one type of ion could be crossing the membrane at the same time. Studies of the electrical properties of nerves only measure the total current crossing the membrane so that it is necessary to have a method of separating the current into its various ionic components. The standard assumption made is that 'the chance that any individual ion will cross the membrane in a specified interval of time is independent of the other ions which are present' (Hodgkin and Huxley, 1952a). This means that the flux of any ion species in one direction will be independent of the concentration of all other ion species on the side of the membrane from which it is moving and also independent of the concentration of all ion species (including its own) on the other side of the membrane. Changing the concentration of one ion, say sodium, on one side of the membrane (e.g. replacing it by an impermeant ion) will affect the magnitude of the sodium current without changing the potassium current. This was an essential assumption made by Hodgkin and Huxley (1952a) in separating the total ionic current into its two main components. (In making the separation, they did not need to assume the magnitude of the change in sodium current, because they were able to rely on the further assumption that most of the very early current, in response to a step depolarization, was carried by sodium ions.) This separation technique has been justified for the squid axon, by using the alternative technique of selectively blocking either the potassium or sodium conductance (with tetraethylammonium or tetrodotoxin, respectively; see Hille, 1970) but such a method is not generally valid. For example, the impermeant ion selected by Hodgkin and Huxley was choline and in the frog myelinated node this substance has a blocking action on the potassium conductance (Hille, 1967), so that its substitution for sodium externally, leads to a reduction in both sodium and potassium currents. The partial blocking action, on one or other conductance, is also not restricted to ions which normally are not present; recently it has been reported that changes in internal sodium ions lead to such an effect on the potassium conductance (e.g. Hille, 1973).

A theoretical extension of the independence principle allowed Hodgkin and Huxley (1952a) to predict the magnitude of the change in sodium current, when the concentration of sodium ions had been altered. Their experimental and theoretical results did not agree, but a reasonably good fit could be obtained by using a simple scaling factor. Hodgkin and Huxley thought this was due to a separate effect, of a 'gating reaction', because the reduced sodium concentration led to an increase in the resting membrane potential. Hoyt (1965), however, showed that both Hodgkin and Huxley's data and the related results of Adelman and Taylor (1964) for the sodium conductance, could equally well fit the assumption that the conductance did not obey the independence principle but was in fact ohmic, i.e. the current-voltage relation always remained linear. In order to obtain such fits, Hoyt had to assume a scaling factor of less than one when external sodium ion concentration was reduced, whereas Hodgkin and Huxley had used scaling factors greater than one. Hodgkin and Huxley had given a plausible argument for choosing a scaling factor greater than one, in that the increase in the membrane potential would lead to an increase in the resting value of h (one of the sodium conductance 'gating reactions' responsible for the closing of channels with depolarization: see *The Mechanism of the Action Potential*), and hence to a greater increase in sodium conductance in response to the same membrane depolarization, but Hoyt's scaling factor incorporates the concentration dependence of the conductance, unlike that of Hodgkin and Huxley, giving a reason for expecting the scaling factor to be less than one. Hoyt did not extend her analysis to the amphibian node of Ranvier, where Dodge and Frankhaueser (1959) had shown that the data were in good agreement with the prediction of the independence principle.

Hoyt pointed out that her treatment could not be extended to the case where the concentration of an ion species on one side of the membrane was reduced to zero, and tentatively concluded that the Ohm's law treatment might be appropriate for high concentrations of an ion species and the independence principle for low concentrations.

Hodgkin and Huxley (1952b) attempted to avoid the difficulties of disentangling effects on the 'gating reactions' from those on the 'ion transfer reaction' by studying the 'instantaneous' current-voltage relation for the sodium conductance. They compared results for normal sodium concentration with those obtained when the external solution contained no sodium ion. A difficulty with this experiment, which they pointed out, is that the actual value of external sodium in the latter case will be finite and changing with time. They therefore fitted the early experimental points with a curve assuming a 10% external sodium concentration and the later ones assuming zero external sodium. Neither curve provided a particularly good fit to their experimental points. Their early points (1–6 in their figure 7) roughly lie on a straight line so that, following Hoyt, an ohmic behaviour might be assumed. The conductance estimated from these points is about one third that found in normal sodium concentrations. Is there any way in which such a magnitude of conductance change can be predicted theoretically? As described later (see *Concentration dependence of an ionic conductance*, p. 752), a very simple theory for pores predicts that the magnitude of the conductance (at zero current) will be proportional to the square root of the product of the ion concentrations on the two sides of the membrane. Following Hodgkin and Huxley (1952b), and taking the external concentration for the early points to be 10% of the normal value, this theory predicts that the ratio of the two conductances should be 0.32:1. Such close agreement with the experimental result may, of course, be fortuitous but it does reinforce Hoyt's conclusion that the independence principle is not the only explanation for Hodgkin and Huxley's observations.

Hoyt (1965) has also made a study of the data for the potassium conductance of toad and squid axons and here, too, showed that an ohmic behaviour was as compatible with the experimental results as were predictions based upon the independence principle.

Binstock and Goldman (1971) studied the potassium conductance in the giant axon of *Myxicola* and noted that although the independence principle could be used to fit their data, the size of the scaling factor required seemed to be a function of external potassium concentration. It is not clear how this result can be explained, but it is certainly a further indication of the danger of assuming that the independence principle adequately predicts changes in the magnitude of ionic current.

Århem, Frankenhaeuser and Moore (1973) made a careful study of the resting sodium and potassium conductances of the toad node of Ranvier; they found that when the membrane potential was held at its resting value, changes in ionic concentration led to changes in membrane current that were not in accord with the independence principle. They pointed out that an alternative explanation, that would avoid disagreement with the independence principle, might be the existence of another current carrier in the resting membrane; but they provided evidence that the two most likely candidates, chloride conductance or an electrogenic pump, did not in fact make a significant contribution to membrane current.

The independence principle can also be used to predict the ratio of the fluxes of an ion species in the two directions. The equation (Ussing, 1949; Hodgkin and Huxley, 1952a) is;

$$\frac{M_i}{M_o} = \exp\left\{\frac{(E - E_c)zF}{RT}\right\} \tag{14.3}$$

where M_i is inward flux, M_o is outward flux, E is the membrane potential, E_c the equilibrium potential for that ion species, and z, F, R and T have the same meaning as in equation (14.1).

This equation is not generally obeyed. Hodgkin and Keynes (1955b) reported that the ratio of unidirectional fluxes of potassium across the squid axon membrane varied with driving force $(E - E_K)$ much more steeply than equation (14.3) predicts. Instead of a ten-fold change in the ratio for every 58 mV of driving force, a ten-fold change occured in about 23 mV. The data could therefore be fitted by the equation

$$\frac{M_i}{M_o} = \exp\left\{\frac{(E_m - E_c)zFn}{RT}\right\}.$$

(14.4)

where $n \stackrel{\scriptscriptstyle\sim}{=} 2.5$. The obvious presumption was that an interaction occurred between the potassium ions moving in the two directions, with the dominant flow effectively impeding the flow in the opposite direction. The specific model suggested by Hodgkin and Keynes (1955b) was a long narrow pore, in which two or three potassium ions could be present in 'single file'.

This experimental result provided the first circumstantial evidence that ions may cross the membrane through a pore, since both the electro-diffusion mechanism (Schwartz, 1971; see however, Mackey and McNeel, 1971, for a theoretical counterexample) and the carrier mechanism (Haydon and Hladky, 1972; but see Horowicz, Gage and Eisenberg, 1968, for the case when the carrier transports more than one ion of the same kind) would be expected to obey the independence principle.

Although Hodgkin and Keynes (1955b) took care to exclude other mechanisms it may be worth noting that an essential assumption of such flux studies is that only a single type of ion movement is being studied. For example, there might be a single type of passive movement which obeyed independence and an additional, largely unidirectional, flux (i.e. that part not accounted for by the theory of independence) due to a transport mechanism. Although a sharp distinction has been made between these two forms of ion movement, there are difficulties in making such a separation experimentally. The best known example of active transport in nerve is the sodium-potassium coupled pump, which uses ATP as a source of energy. This pump is usually pictured as irreversible, moving sodium outward and potassium inward, and it has been assumed that metabolic poisons or cardiac glycosides eliminate this form of ion movement. Recent evidence, however, suggests that this mechanism can function reversibly (e.g. Garrahan and Glynn, 1967) and, as pointed out by Chapman (1973), it is still an open question whether the cardiac glycosides inhibit the coupled fluxes in one direction only, leaving the opposite fluxes (sodium in, potassium out) either unaffected, or only partially inhibited (Mullins and Brinley, 1969).

A quite different problem, with respect to the predictive ability of the independence principle, arises in the case of radioactive tracer studies of sodium flux, in which, for a net inward movement of sodium, the ratio of fluxes can be less than that expected. Keynes and Swan (1959) first reported this phenomenon in an excitable cell, and they suggested that it represented an example of Ussing's 'exchange diffusion'. No net transport of the ion occurs because it is a one-for-one exchange, implying that the mechanism is electrically neutral and does not alter the concentrations of the ion on either side of the membrane; it can only be detected by the use of radioactive tracers.

These results highlight the difficulties which may be experienced in distinguishing the various types of ion movements across the membrane; not only to distinguish between active and passive ion movements but also as to whether there is a single type of passive ion movement (Brinley and Mullins, 1968; Mullins and Brinley, 1969; Shapiro and Candia, 1971; Sjodin, 1971). The problem is most acute when studying resting membrane fluxes; during the action potential the quantitive increase in the fluxes is so great that there is little error inherent in treating them as being due to a single type of passive movement.

Bezanilla, Rojas and Taylor (1970a) studied the large increase in sodium influx (and the sodium current) accompanying a step depolarization of the membrane, in internally perfused squid giant axons. When internal sodium was increased there was a decrease in sodium current, as expected, but they did not check the change in magnitude with that predicted by the independence principle. On the other hand they found that the sodium influx increased and they reported that, in one of the two experiments, this increase was well above their estimated experimental error. It would be expected from the independence principle that the sodium influx should have remained constant while the sodium efflux increased (leading to a reduction in net influx, or current). The authors suggest their results are in keeping with the sodium conductance obeying the independence principle, since the sodium influx did not decrease; but in fact, neither an increase nor a decrease are compatible with predictions based upon this principle.

It will be clear from this section that many biological conductances do not obey some of the predictions that can be derived from the independence principle. This does not mean that experimental analyses using this principle are incorrect; the qualitative, and many of the quantitative, features of the mechanism of the action potential have much additional support (see, for example, Hille, 1970; Bezanilla, Rojas and Taylor, 1970a,b). The situation is far less satisfactory, however, when one considers the membrane conductances that set the value of the resting membrane potential (see p. 760). The difficulty with the predictions of the independence principle is also reflected in other properties of ion conductances.

Voltage dependence of ion conductances

When a voltage difference is imposed between the ends of a metal resistor, the current flowing obeys Ohm's law; the current is equal to the voltage difference divided by the magnitude of the resistance – or the product of the voltage difference and the conductance, since conductance is the reciprocal of resistance. A variation in the voltage difference produces a concomitant variation in the current, because the conductance remains constant. This simple, 'ohmic', behaviour would not be generally expected for ionic conductances when there are concentration differences on the two sides of the membrane. As indicated earlier (p. 743), current might be expected to flow more readily from the high concentration side to the low concentration side, because of the greater availability of the permeant ion species. One early, and well-known, theoretical treatment of biological conductances (Goldman, 1943; Hodgkin and Katz, 1949) made exactly this prediction. The theory falls into the category of an electrodiffusion model, with the additional assumption that the electric field across the membrane is constant at rest, and remains so when there is a net movement of ions. It is therefore called the Goldman constant field theory.* With this special assumption it is an elementary matter to integrate the Nernst-Planck diffusion equation, to obtain a result for the relationship between current and voltage:

$$i_c = \frac{P_c z F^2 V}{RT} \cdot \frac{[C]_o - [C]_i \cdot \exp(FzV/RT)}{1 - \exp(FzV/RT)} \qquad (14.5)$$

where i_c is the current of the ion species, c; P_c is the membrane permeability to this ion, V is the membrane potential and the other symbols have their usual connotation.

Three things may be noted about this equation: firstly, it not only incorporates the dependence on voltage, but also (necessarily) dependence on the two concentrations. Secondly, the relationship is not linear (except when $[C]_o = [C]_i$, in which case $i_c = P_c(zFV[C]/RT)$. Finally, the equation is one derived for the steady-state. The treatment of the transient behaviour of electrodiffusion models is very complicated (e.g. Cohen and Cooley, 1965), but Cole (1965) has pointed out that it is likely that the steady-state is reached in a time (of the order of 0.1 μs) which is very brief compared with the resolution obtained in most physiological experiments.

This theoretical treatment, including some further predictions which are considered on p. 751, is the only one commonly used for the explanation or analysis of experimental results. This may seem surprising, since it has been clear for some time that electrodiffusion models are unlikely to be realistic versions of the ion permeation mechanism. Its continued use is probably a result of two factors. Experimentally the behaviour of some, but not all, biological conductances are similar to the predictions of the constant field theory (Hodgkin and Horowicz, 1959; Dodge and Frankenhaeuser, 1959; Hutter and Noble, 1960; Frankenhaeuser, 1962), and secondly, work on the predicted properties of 'pores' and 'carriers' indicates that these more likely candidates for passive ion movements may, under some circumstances, obey the predictions of the constant field model (e.g. Sandblom, 1967; Andreoli and Watkins, 1973).

Nevertheless it is clear that not all ion conductances obey the predictions of the constant field model. A clear exception was reported by Hodgkin and Huxley (1952b) for the sodium and potassium conductances of squid nerve, in which, at normal concentrations, the conductances were 'ohmic'. Frankenhaeuser (1960) suggested that this linearity could be explained by the electrodiffusion model as a consequence of fixed charges, altering the membrane field in such a way that the ion concentration in the membrane, and hence the

*This form of theoretical treatment had, in fact, been presented earlier by Mott and Gurney (p. 183 In: *Electronic Processes in Ionic Crystals*, Clarendon Press: Oxford (1940)).

conductance, does not change with alteration in the membrane potential. The result can, of course, also be explained by quite different models of ion transfer (e.g. Woodbury, 1971; Hall, Mead and Szabo, 1973; Läuger, 1972, 1973). Since these theoretical treatments, for 'pore' and 'carrier' models, lead to the prediction of a wide variety of voltage sensitivities depending on the particular characteristics of the 'pore' or 'carrier', it is obvious that an experimental determination is the only sure way to gauge the effect of voltage on an ion conductance. This conclusion may be reinforced by considering the behaviour of one of the potassium conductances found in many excitable membranes – the 'anomalous' or 'ingoing' rectifier. This conductance displays a voltage-sensitivity exactly the opposite to that discussed earlier, i.e. it passes current more readily from the low to the high concentration side than in the opposite direction. A detailed discussion of this conductance will be found in Adrian (1969).

Concentration dependence of ion conductance

In explaining the distinction between the terms permeability and conductance it has already been pointed out that, on simple expectations, the availability of ions might be a rate-limiting step in setting the magnitude of a conductance, for a given permeability of the membrane. It is therefore necessary to know the form of the dependence of conductance on concentration. Since the magnitude of the conductance may also be voltage-dependent, it is conventional to estimate it for small displacements from the zero-current point (i.e. near to the equilibrium potential for the ion species).

The constant field theory predicts the following relationship

$$G_{c(1_c \to 0)} = \frac{F^3}{(RT)^2} E_c \cdot p_c \cdot \left\{ \frac{[C]_1 [C]_2}{[C]_1 - [C]_2} \right\} \qquad (14.6)$$

where $[C]_1$ and $[C]_2$ denote the concentrations on the two sides of the membrane ($[C]_1 > [C]_2$), E_c is the equilibrium potential for the ion, p_c the permeability and the other terms have their usual significance. If $[C]_1 \gg [C]_2$ this leads to the simplification

$$G_c \approx \frac{F^2}{RT} p_c [C]_2 \log_e \left(\frac{[C]_1}{[C]_2} \right) \qquad (14.7)$$

so that the conductance, for low values of $[C]_2$ is nearly directly proportional to the concentration on the side of the membrane where it is lower. When $[C]_1 \approx [C]_2$ the conductance is approximately described by

$$G_c \propto \sqrt{([C]_1 \cdot [C]_2)}. \qquad (14.8)$$

There is now an extensive theoretical literature on the concentration dependence of ion conductances produced by 'carrier' mechanisms (Haydon and Hladky, 1972; Läuger, 1972; Ciani, Laprade, Eisenman and Szabo, 1973; Ciani, Eisenman, Laprade and Szabo, 1973). The essence of these studies is that at

751

lower concentrations there is a proportionality (whose exact form depends on the model) between conductance and concentration, and at higher concentrations the conductance may 'saturate', i.e. it does not increase with further increases in concentration.

Noble (unpublished) has studied the behaviour of a simple pore model in which it is assumed that there is no step change in concentration, i.e. the concentration of ions is a continuous function with distance from the bulk solutions through the membrane. The zero-current conductance is then proportional to the square root of the product of the concentrations on the two sides of the membrane. A similar result has been obtained by Hall, Mead and Szabo (1973) for an energy barrier model of ion permeation. With a single, symmetrical triangular energy barrier the zero-current conductance obeys a square root relation and, in addition, the current-voltage relation will be linear for small deviations from the zero-current point. Energy barrier models are independent of the exact mechanism of ion transfer, so this theory could apply to either a 'carrier' or to a 'pore' model. Hall *et al.* (1973) also point out that both the concentration dependence and the current-voltage relation will be very dependent on the exact form of the energy barrier, and in a slightly more general model, having a trapezoidal energy barrier, they showed that the concentration dependence of the zero-current conductance would take the form

$$g_c \propto ([C]_1)^n ([C]_2)^{1-n} \tag{14.9}$$

where $0 < n < \frac{1}{2}$ and $[C]_1 > [C]_2$.

A further expectation of a 'pore' model is that at high concentrations the conductance will saturate because an upper limit to the conductance will be reached when the rate limiting step is the rate at which they can move through the pore rather than the rate at which they could enter from solution (Hladky and Haydon, 1972).

Experimental work on the concentration dependence of ion conductances in excitable membranes is limited, and the results available are difficult to interpret. In the first place, when the concentration of an ion species is changed on one side of the membrane it is desirable to increase or decrease the concentration of another ion or solute to maintain the same tonicity — otherwise there may be water movement across the membrane with a consequent change in internal ion concentrations. Even if tonicity is maintained there may still be water movement, depending on the differential permeability of the membrane to the different ion species (e.g. Hodgkin and Horowicz, 1959). If tonicity is maintained by an uncharged solution there are effects on the voltage sensitivity of the 'gating reactions' of some ion conductances which greatly complicate the analysis (e.g. Chandler, Hodgkin and Meves, 1965; Mozhaeva and Naumov, 1972; Brismar, 1973). Finally, as mentioned earlier, if the ion species is replaced by another ion which is believed to be impermeant (e.g. choline) there may be an effect on the magnitude of the conductance because the independence principle is disobeyed.

There are a few studies where these difficulties appear to have been avoided. Hodgkin and Horowicz (1959) studied the resting potassium and chloride conductances of frog skeletal muscle. They found that the concentration dependence of the chloride conductance was in reasonable agreement with the expectations of constant field theory, and in keeping with its voltage dependence which also matches the predictions of this theory. It may be worth noting, however, that the results for concentration dependence were too scattered to decide whether constant field predictions or the square root relation mentioned above provided the better fit. In contrast, the results for the potassium conductance were unequivocal, in the sense that they definitely did not fit constant field theory (this conductance is the 'ingoing rectifier', mentioned earlier).

Århem, Frankenhaeuser and Moore (1973) studied the concentration dependence of the resting sodium and potassium conductances of the toad node of Ranvier under voltage clamp conditions. The node was clamped at the resting potential (about -70 mV) and the concentration of either sodium or potassium ions in the external solution was changed, without changing the concentration of the other ion (while this meant that there were changes in the osmolarity of the external solution, independent experiments suggested that in the time scale of the experiments water movements were negligible). It was therefore assumed that the observed current flow was of the ion species whose concentration had been changed. The constant field theory predicts that the change in the magnitude of the current flow, when voltage is held constant, will be directly proportional to the size of the concentration change (see equation (14.5)). Århem et al. (1973) found that for both potassium and sodium concentration changes the current was *not* linearly related to concentration, being less than expected when the external concentration of the ion was high. Such behaviour could be expected if the conductance obeyed the square root relation described above, and Århem et al.'s results have been plotted accordingly in Fig. 14.1. Note that the experimental measurement is of a *change* in the sodium or potassium current from its resting level and is not therefore the total current crossing the membrane. But, since

$$i_c = g_c \, (E_m - E_c),$$

and, on the assumption that

$$g_c \propto \sqrt{([C]_0 . [C]_i)}$$

and $[C]_i$ remains constant

$$i_c = K\sqrt{[C]_0} \, . \, (E_m - E_c).$$

Let i_{c_r} be the resting current, then

$$\Delta i_c = K\sqrt{[C]_0} . (E_m - E_c) - i_{c_r} \qquad (14.10)$$

so that, by plotting Δi_c against $\sqrt{[C]_0} \, (E_m - E_c)$ a straight line should be

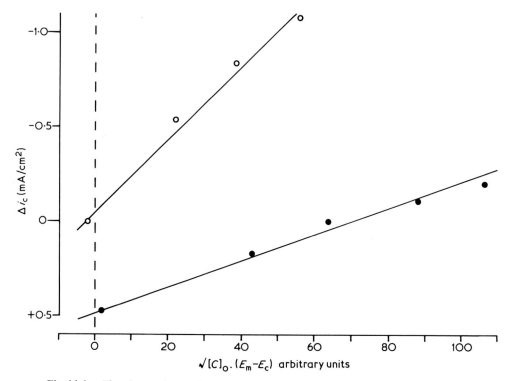

Fig. 14.1 The changes in membrane current, at constant membrane potential, (E_m), are shown for external solutions of different concentration $([C]_o)$. The abscissa plots the value of $\sqrt{[C]_o} \cdot (E_m - E_c)$, where the terms $\sqrt{[C]_o}$ and E_o both change with $[C]_o$. The ordinate gives the current in the test solution minus the current in ordinary Ringer solution. $(\circ — \circ)$ – potassium ion; $(\bullet — \bullet)$ – sodium ion. (Data measured from Fig. 3 of Arhem, Frankenhaeuser and Moore, (1973).)

obtained. The figure shows that the experimental results are in fair accordance with this prediction. The agreement may be fortuitous since it should be remembered that the square root relation was derived for the zero-current conductance whereas these measurements have been made at a fixed potential and hence away from the zero-current point. The concentration and voltage dependence of the conductances cannot therefore be separated but the results are compatible with a combination of a linear current voltage relation (i.e. conductance not voltage-dependent) and the square root concentration dependence predicted by Hall *et al.*'s (1973) triangular energy barrier model.

If this description is correct it is possible to deduce the total currents for sodium and potassium and hence the magnitude of the resting conductances. From equation (14.10) it may be noted that $i_{c_r} = -\Delta i_c$ when $E_m - E_c = 0$; this leads to $i_{K_r} = +0.05$ mA/cm^2 and $i_{Na_r} = -0.49$ mA/cm^2 and hence $g_{K_r} = 1.82 \times 10^{-3}$ S cm^{-2} and $g_{Na_r} = 4.05 \times 10^{-3}$ S cm^{-2}. The significance of this will be discussed further in the section on the resting membrane potential.

It has already been mentioned that the 'ingoing rectifier', a potassium conductance found in many membranes, does not obey the prediction of the constant field equation for voltage and concentration dependence. Hagiwara and Takahashi (1974) have made a careful study of this conductance in the starfish egg — a particularly favourable preparation in which the 'ingoing rectifier' is the predominant membrane conductance. They concluded that the conductance could be described by an equation of the form

$$g_K = A \cdot f(V - V_K) \cdot ([K^+]_0)^{\frac{1}{2}} \tag{14.11}$$

They did not study the effects of changes in $[K^+]_i$. Note that the 'voltage' dependence is a function of electrochemical gradient rather than absolute value of the membrane potential. The data given by Hodgkin and Horowicz (1959) for the same conductance in frog skeletal muscle are also in fair agreement with this equation. Hagiwara and Takahashi (1974) also noted that this conductance disobeyed the prediction of the independence principle; for example, the addition of some rubidium or calcium ion to the external solution leads to a reduction in the potassium conductance (the 'blocking' action of such ions had also been reported earlier for frog skeletal muscle by Adrian (1964)), and the membrane conductance displayed the phenomenon of 'anomalous mole fraction dependence' in an external medium containing tellurium and potassium, i.e. the conductance was at a minimum when both ions were present in substantial concentration and increased when either tellurium largely replaced potassium, or vice versa.

Ionic selectivity of conductances

Ions pass through the nerve membrane at sparsely located sites. Furthermore, individual sites have different properties so that the membrane can be regarded as possessing more than one population of 'ion transfer' sites or channels. In the case of squid giant axon there are two main populations, the so-called 'sodium' and 'potassium' channels. Although the names given to these channels imply a perfect selectivity for a single ionic species, it has become evident that the selectivity is not perfect; the 'sodium' channel for example, can transfer lithium, ammonium, potassium and calcium ions, although potassium and calcium move through it with much less ease.

The basis for this selectivity is still uncertain; reviews of the best developed theoretical account, the Eisenman—Williams electrostatic theory, will be found in Diamond and Wright (1969) and Chapter 8 of Jack, Noble and Tsien (1975).

Apart from requiring an explanation, this selectivity needs to be measured quantitatively. The present convention is to express the ease of transfer for a particular ion species as a ratio of its permeability to that of the ion species 'normally' transferred. Thus, the ease with which potassium moves through the 'sodium' channel of squid has been expressed as p_K/p_{Na} and given a value of about 0.08 (Chandler and Meves, 1965; Adelman, 1971). The exact values quoted in the literature are suspect, because they rely on assumptions such as the independence principle to derive the permeability ratio. Hille (1973) has pointed out that the estimated value of the ratio depends on the method by which it is derived; he suggests that the most suitable method is to measure the zero-current potential for the channel at two different concentrations of the relevant ion species and derive the permeability ratio using the Goldman-Hodgkin-Katz equation for zero-current potential. Since this equation is also of fundamental importance in the standard account of the membrane potential it needs to be discussed in some detail.

Equations for the zero-current potential

Hodgkin and Katz (1949) derived their equation for the zero-current potential using the assumptions of the Goldman constant field theory. The equation will be familiar to most readers since it is widely accepted as a quantitative description of the resting membrane potential. Assuming that only sodium and potassium have a significant net flux, it takes the form

$$E_o = \frac{RT}{F} \log_e \left\{ \frac{p_K.[K^+]_o + p_{Na} \cdot [Na^+]_o}{p_K.[K^+]_i + p_{Na} \cdot [Na^+]_i} \right\} \tag{14.12}$$

It was subsequently realized that the same type of equation could be derived for a much wider class of ion permeation mechanisms (e.g. Patlak, 1960; Sandblom and Eisenman, 1967; MacGillivray and Hare, 1969; Jacquez, 1971; Läuger, 1973; Szabo, Eisenman, Laprade, Ciani and Krasne, 1973; Coster, 1973; Førland and Østvold, 1974). It may not be obvious how this equation expresses the fundamental condition that the algebraic sum of the sodium and potassium currents is zero. This can be shown in the following way:

$$e^{E_o F/RT} = \frac{p_K.[K^+]_o + p_{Na} \cdot [Na^+]_o}{p_K.[K]_i + p_{Na} \cdot [Na^+]_i} \tag{14.13}$$

$$p_K([K^+]_o - [K^+]_i e^{E_o F/RT}) + p_{Na}([Na^+]_o - [Na^+]_i e^{E_o F/RT}) = 0$$

The first expression on the left hand side of equation (14.13) can be regarded as proportional to the potassium current, and the second expression to the sodium current. It can be seen that any ion permeation mechanism in which *each* of the current terms obeys the expression

$$i_c = p_c \cdot f(V) \cdot \{[C]_o - [C]_i e^{EF/RT}\} \tag{14.14}$$

will lead to a Goldman-Hodgkin-Katz description of the zero-current potential. $f(V)$ can be any function of voltage which is common to each of the current terms (as long as that function has the dimension of charge/mole), but can not be a function of ion concentrations if the independence principle is to be obeyed. In the case of constant field assumption

$$f(V) = \frac{F^2 E}{RT(1 - e^{EF/RT})} \tag{14.15}$$

As mentioned earlier this assumption means that the conductances, as defined by the electrochemical form of Ohm's law, are voltage dependent. But it was also pointed out that the sodium and potassium conductances of the squid axon have linear current-voltage relations (for the 'ion transfer reaction'). Can conductances with such a property still yield the same equation (14.12) for the zero-current potential? Frankenhaeuser (1960) suggested a modification to the Goldman constant field theory in which the electric field in the membrane was changed by the presence of fixed charges on one side of the membrane. Thus, for i_{Na}, assuming fixed negative charge on the inner surface of the membrane the current-voltage relation becomes linear when

$$f(V) = \frac{F^2 (E - E_{Na})}{RT(1 - e^{(E - E_{Na})F/RT})}$$

so that

$$i_{Na} = \frac{p_{Na} \cdot F^2 [Na]_o}{RT} \cdot (E - E_{Na}).$$

As Frankenhaeuser points out, in order to obtain a linear current voltage relation for the potassium conductance the nature of the fixed charge would have to be opposite (i.e. a positive charge on the inner surface, or a negative charge on the outer surface), so that the two values for $f(V)$ (in the description of i_{Na} and i_K respectively) would not be identical. In other words, this modification to the constant field theory description will not lead to the Goldman-Hodgkin-Katz equation.

A similar difficulty arises for the Goldman-Hodgkin-Katz equation in describing the zero-current potential for a membrane in which one of the conductances is the 'ingoing' rectifier (e.g. skeletal and cardiac muscle fibres, and some types of nerve cell). As described earlier the voltage-dependence of this conductance is quite unusual (see equation (14.11)) and it would not be expected to be obeyed by any other ion species (since the voltage dependence is a function of the electrochemical driving force on the potassium ion). This means that it is most unlikely that an explicit expression for the zero-current potential can be obtained when this conductance is one of the membrane components which needs to be included. An example of the effect of the 'ingoing' rectifier on the behaviour of the zero-current potential (resting membrane potential) is given by Noble (1965).

Setting aside the case discussed in the previous paragraph, is it possible to offer an alternative account of the zero-current potential that avoids the difficulty mentioned above when the conductances are not voltage-dependent? Since there is evidence that some conductances are not voltage-dependent, and their concentration dependence obeys a square root relationship rather than that predicted by the constant field theory, an obvious alternative is to assume that such a relationship will hold for all the conductances involved. In other words:

$$g_c = \frac{p_c \cdot F^2}{RT} \cdot \sqrt{([C]_o \cdot [C]_i)} \tag{14.16}$$

If sodium and potassium conductances are the only two involved, the zero-current equation becomes

$$E_o = \frac{(p_{Na}\sqrt{([Na^+]_o[Na^+]_i)} \cdot E_{Na}) + (p_K\sqrt{([K^+]_o[K^+]_i)} \cdot E_K)}{(p_{Na}\sqrt{([Na^+]_o[Na^+]_i)}) + (p_K\sqrt{([K^+]_i[K^+]_o)})} \tag{14.17}$$

Fig. 14.2 compares the predictions of equations (14.12) and (14.17) for the circumstance when $p_K \gg p_{Na}$. The method adopted was to first calculate the prediction of equation (14.12) taking a value of p_K/p_{Na} of 40 and concentrations of $[Na^+]_o = 120mM/l$, $[Na^+]_i = 10mM/l$, $[K^+]_i = 150mM/l$ and $[K^+]_o = 2.5mM/l$. The value of the zero-current potential is -83.3 mV, compared with the value of E_K of -103.1 mV. Next the value of the ratio p_K/p_{Na} was calculated, to obtain the *same* value of E_o, from equation (14.17). The required value is 13.2. Using these two values of p_K/p_{Na} in their respective equations, the behaviour of E_o for various values of $[K^+]_o$ (leaving other concentrations the same) was determined. The thin continuous line in Fig. 14.2 shows the predictions of equation (14.12) and the dashed line that of equation (14.17). The same general behaviour of the zero-current potential is displayed by the two accounts, so that it should be reasonably easy to fit a set of experimental points with both equations. The most notable difference between the two is the implication for the value of the permeability ratio – in this calculation, a three-fold difference.

As an example of the application of these two equations to experimental results, one can take the data of Chandler and Meves (1965) for the permeability ratio (p_{Na}/p_K) of the early 'sodium' channel in perfused squid giant axons. Chandler and Meves studied the zero-current potential for the channel when the internal concentration of sodium ion varied from 300 mM to 0 mM, with the external solution being K^+-free artificial sea-water. Strictly speaking equation (14.17) cannot be applied when $[K^+]_o$ and $[Na^+]_i$ are zero, but Chandler and Meves report that their KCl was contaminated with 0.33 mM sodium. No figure was given for the potassium contamination of 'K-free' artificial sea-water, but a value of 0.5 mM seems reasonable. These concentrations can then be converted into ion activities and the ratio of p_{Na}/p_K for the best fit to the data can be calculated. Using equation (14.12) a value of 11.7 is obtained, while equation (14.17) gives a value of 2.3. A distinction between the two accounts could have been made if there was experimental data for internal sodium activities between 35 and 5 m equiv./kg H_2O. In the absence of such results, it *might* be concluded, on the

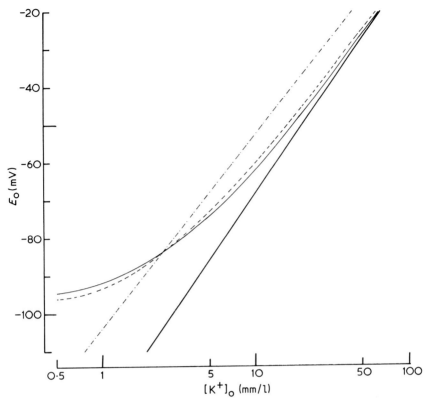

Fig. 14.2 Predictions of various equations for the zero-current potential. The abscissa shows the value of external potassium ion ($[K^+]$), on a logarithmic scale. The ordinate plots the value of the zero-current potential (E_o), with the usual convention that the sign reflects the excess charge on the internal surface. (———) – E_K. (———) – the values predicted by equation (14.12) (Goldman-Hodgkin-Katz equation). (– – – – –) – prediction of equation (14.17) (square root concentration dependence). (– · – · – ·) – the constant conductance description equation (14.18).

basis of the equally good fit provided by equation (14.17), that the selectivity ratio is less than 3 rather than the usually quoted figure of about 12. This example highlights the problem mentioned in the previous section (*Ion selectivity of conductances*)

Finally, it is worth noting that no single equation is likely to apply to all forms of biological conductance. The best-known example of a zero-current potential which could not be fitted by either equation (14.12) or (14.17) is the end-plate conductance of frog skeletal muscle (Takeuchi and Takeuchi, 1960; Takeuchi, 1963). Over a wide range of concentrations, the zero-current potential was found to fit the following description (with g_K and g_{Na} constant)

$$E_o = \frac{g_K \cdot E_K + g_{Na} \cdot E_{Na}}{g_K + g_{Na}}. \tag{14.18}$$

In other words the conductance appeared to lack any concentration or voltage dependence. For a further discussion of this interesting result the reader is referred to Bregestovski *et al.* (1972) and Rang (1974). The dotted line in Fig. 14.2 shows the behaviour of equation (14.18), when calculated in the same way as for (14.17). The g_K/g_{Na} ratio required is 7.4. Unlike the other two zero-current equations there is no marked curvature away from E_K at low potassium concentrations.

In conclusion, no single equation can give a general account of the zero-current potential for all individual conductances, or combinations of them. Only a few conductances have been examined carefully enough with respect to their concentration and voltage dependence, but since very few of them show the concentration dependence predicted by the constant field theory, and/or independence principle, it seems clear that the Goldman-Hodgkin-Katz equation is not a satisfactory general description of the zero-current potential. Much more complicated equations are certainly required to incorporate the ingoing potassium rectifier and conductances that disobey the independence principle in the sense that changing the concentration of one ion species affects the permeation process of another ion species.

The resting membrane potential

The standard account of the resting membrane potential holds that it is a diffusion potential in which potassium is the main ion involved (e.g. Hodgkin, 1958). In recent years this general account has been challenged in two ways.

First, it is evident that the active transport of ions can lead to the net transport of charge; for example, it appears to be generally true that in excitable cells the sodium-potassium pump generates a hyperpolarizing current (Ritchie, 1971; Thomas, 1972). This phenomenon is discussed on p. 774, but it may be helpful to point out that, in general, the direct contribution made by this pump in the steady-state will be of the order of only a few millivolts, and if the standard account is basically correct it only requires minor modification to accommodate this effect.

A more radical challenge to the basic hypothesis has recently been made by Århem, Frankenhaeuser and Moore (1973), based upon their study of the resting conductances of the toad node of Ranvier. The implications of their results is that some ion other than potassium (or chloride) is primarily responsible in setting the resting membrane potential. Before discussing this paper it may be useful to study two other peripheral nerve axons in which careful studies appear to give the conventional hypothesis some support.

Squid axon　　The Hodgkin-Huxley account of the membrane potential of the squid axon includes three conductances which are present in the resting state: a potassium conductance, a sodium conductance and a small 'leak' conductance. The potassium and sodium conductances are well-defined in their description because they represent those small fractions of the total conductances that are voltage-time-dependent (i.e. 'gated') and in which the 'gates' are open at the resting membrane potential. The 'leak' conductance is less well-defined: it is still uncertain which ion species is the main charge carrier, but the zero-current potential is usually described as being near the resting potential, and the current-voltage relation of the channel as being close to linear over the physiological range of resting potentials (Adelman and Taylor, 1961; Adelman, 1971).

The usual method of obtaining a quantitative description of the factors influencing the resting potential is to vary the ion concentrations on the external and (if technically possible) the internal side of the membrane. The experimental results so obtained, are then usually compared with the Goldman-Hodgkin-Katz equation, leaving the p_{Na}/p_K ratio as a free variable. Hodgkin and Katz (1949) treated the date of Curtis and Cole (1942) in this way, but found that they could not all be fitted by a single assumed value of p_{Na}/p_K (they also assumed a significant chloride permeability); when the axon was depolarized, in high $[K^+]_0$, the ratio appeared to decrease. This result was not surprising because a qualitative description of the voltage-dependent sodium and potassium permeabilities is that depolarization leads to a sustained increase in the potassium permeability but only a transient large increase in the sodium permeability.

Baker, Hodgkin and Shaw (1962) treated this possibility quantitatively by incorporating the Hodgkin-Huxley description of the steady-state voltage sensitivity of the sodium and potassium conductances. They also made the assumption that the sodium and potassium currents vary with concentration as predicted by the independence principle. Fig. 14.3 reproduces their illustration of the result of this approach. The open circles are the observations of Curtis and Cole and the continuous line the result of Baker et al.'s calculation. The theory predicts much less change in the membrane potential at low values of $[K^+]_0$ than is observed. Since it is uncertain whether the independence principle does apply to the sodium and potassium currents (i.e. that the change in current is directly proportional to the change in concentration) it is worth pointing out that a better match between theory and experiment would be obtained by assuming that the change in conductance scaled with the square root of the external concentration (c.f. Fig. 14.2).

Baker et al. (1962) also made an experimental study of the effects of changes in internal potassium concentration and fitted these results with a similar theoretical calculation. They found a good fit when external potassium concentration was low, but a much less satisfactory one for high external potassium concentrations. The good fit at low external concentrations may, in any case, be a coincidence since they assumed that the leakage current was carried by chloride ions; a dubious assumption as they themselves point out. Nevertheless correcting for this assumption may make only a minor change in the predicted potential (see Baker et al., 1962, p. 371), and it is difficult to escape the conclusion that, qualitatively, the membrane potential of the squid axon is the consequence of a relatively high potassium permeability. There is less

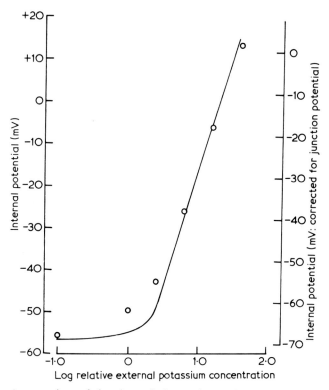

Fig. 14.3 A comparison of the observed changes in membrane potential of squid giant axons, when external potassium concentration is varied, with those predicted by the Hodgkin-Huxley model. The experimental data (open circles) is from Curtis and Cole (1942). The abscissa plots external potassium concentration logarithmically, in multiples of 13 mM. The axoplasmic concentration of potassium was taken as 369 mM/hg^{-1}. The line shows the theoretical prediction. a 12 mV junction potential was assumed to relate the curve (right hand ordinate) to the observations (left hand ordinate) (Reproduced from Baker, Hodgkin and Shaw (1962).)

certainty about the explanation provided for the deviation away from E_K, particularly at low values of $[K^+]_o/[K^+]_i$. If it were due to a 'sodium leak' one would expect a hyperpolarization on reducing external sodium concentration. Both Hodgkin and Katz (1949) and Hodgkin and Huxley (1952a) have reported a small effect of the expected kind, and it is generally assumed that the rest of the deviation is explained by the 'leak' conductance (which has a zero-current potential on the depolarizing side of the resting potential). Thus, the resting membrane potential in the squid axon seems to be adequately described, apart from the remaining uncertainties about the nature of the 'leak' conductance, and the appropriate equations needed to describe the concentration dependence of the sodium and potassium conductances.

Crayfish giant axon Strickholm and Wallin (1967) and Wallin (1967) studied the behaviour of the membrane potential in this preparation in response to changes in the external concentration of potassium, sodium and chloride ion. Qualitatively, the membrane potential changed with external potassium ion as expected, but there were some unexpected findings. First, reduction in the external sodium concentration did not produce a significant hyperpolarization. The tentative explanation offered for this observation was that the resting sodium permeability was relatively low by comparison with that in the squid (i.e. p_{Na}/p_K low) in keeping with Brinley's (1965) study of ion fluxes in the lobster axon. At normal potassium concentrations the effect of lowering external chloride was very small, so that, using the Goldman-Hodgkin-Katz equation, the p_{Cl}/p_K ratio was calculated to be 0.14. At high external potassium concentrations on the other hand, the membrane potential proved very sensitive to external chloride changes and a p_{Cl}/p_K ratio of nearly unity was estimated. Further experiments revealed that at low external potassium, chloride was out of equilibrium (E_{Cl} on the depolarizing side of E_m), but that as external potassium increased, internal chloride gradually came into equilibrium. A substantial volume increase accompanied the increased external potassium concentration due to the inward movement of both potassium and chloride ion. Strickholm and Wallin (1967) point out that such changes imply that at high potassium concentrations the membrane potential behaved like a potassium electrode (i.e. as for E_K), but that it was invalid to conclude on this basis that the membrane was predominantly permeable to potassium, because E_{Cl} was varying in the same way as E_K. Nevertheless their evidence for low (i.e. normal) values of external potassium suggest that in such circumstances the membrane is indeed predominantly permeable to potassium, with the deviation from E_K at least in part explained by leakage of both sodium and chloride ions since both are out of equilibrium. As there is insufficient evidence available to determine the concentration and voltage dependence of the resting conductances, it is not known what form of zero-current potential equation is appropriate.

Amphibian node of Ranvier. Huxley and Stämpfli (1951a,b) were the first workers to make direct measurements of the resting membrane potential of the frog node of Ranvier. Only changes in external sodium and potassium concentrations were made. Lowering the sodium concentration progressively caused a progressively larger hyperpolarization, whereas increase in external potassium produced a depolarization having the customary form, with the slope of the curve approaching that expected for E_K (slope of 51 mV for a ten-fold change, instead of the expected 58 mV slope).

Stämpfli (1959) extended this study and confirmed Huxley and Stämpfli's earlier observations for some axons. Other axons, which he believed to be in a more favourable physiological state because they had been particularly carefully and quickly dissected, showed a quite different response to small (up to 40 mM/l) increases in external potassium concentration. These depolarized to a much lesser extent, showing only a few millivolts change in resting potential. In some axons the resting potential in increased $[K]_0$ could be as much as 25 mV more hyperpolarized than E_K. At a critical value of membrane potential, usually about 5 mV more depolarized than the resting potential, these axons would regeneratively depolarize to a membrane potential just on the depolarized side of E_K. The nodal membrane resistance was much higher whilst the axon was in the state of being relatively insensitive to external potassium. These results were plausibly interpreted by Stämpfli (following a suggestion of Hodgkin) to indicate that in such axons the resting potassium conductance was low. The drop in membrane resistance and increased sensitivity to external potassium above a critical membrane potential was explained by Stämpfli to be due to activation of the voltage-dependent membrane potassium conductance. He therefore concluded that the resting potential in nodes in good condition was not set primarily by the diffusion potential for potassium.

Stämpfli (1959) considered the question of the major ion conductance that set the membrane potential. He suggested that it might be that of chloride ion, but found that increasing external chloride depolarized the membrane (when it was in the state of being insensitive to external potassium); clear evidence, when conventionally interpreted, that the conductance cannot be due to chloride. The evidence presented, that high external chloride tends to favour the state in which the node has a low potassium conductance, can be reinterpreted with hindsight as the effect either of changes of ionic strength shifting the voltage sensitivity of the potassium conductance (c.f. Brismar, 1973), or of choline blocking the potassium conductance (c.f. Hille, 1967). Stämpfli noted that raising external calcium ion had the same effect. Another piece of evidence indicating that chloride is not the main resting conductance is that estimates of the internal chloride concentration imply that E_{Cl} is about -40 mV (Hurlbut, 1963). The conclusion that can be drawn from this work, therefore, is that the resting potential is predominantly set by an unknown ion species (which is not potassium, sodium, chloride or calcium).

The observations of Århem, Frankenhaeuser and Moore (1973) gave further support to this conclusion. They voltage clamped a toad node of Ranvier at its resting level (-70 mV) and studied changes in the resting membrane current when the external concentrations of sodium, potassium and chloride were changed. They concluded that only a negligible fraction of the resting membrane current was due to chloride ion (<0.05 mA/cm^2) and, as indicated earlier, found that neither the sodium or the potassium current changed in accordance with the independence principle. An interpretation of the concentration dependence of these two conductances has been given earlier (see Fig. 14.1) and leads to the conclusion that the resting potassium current is $+0.05$ mA/cm^2 and the resting sodium current is -0.49 mA/cm^2. If we assign a maximal value of $+0.05$ mA/cm^2 (i.e. assuming that E_{Cl} is on the hyperpolarizing side of E_m) to a resting chloride current then it is clear that to obtain the zero current condition an outward current of about 0.4 mA/cm^2 is required. Århem et al. suggested that this could not be metabolically dependent ion current, because neither ouabain nor the metabolic inhibitor 2.4-dinitrophenol caused any detectable change in membrane current. Since the average total resting conductance of the node, as measured electrically, was about $28 \times 10^{-3}\,\mathrm{S\,cm^{-2}}$ whereas the total conductance contributed by potassium, sodium and chloride is of the order of $6 \times 10^{-3}\,\mathrm{S\,cm^{-2}}$ it is evident that a substantial conductance ($22 \times 10^{-3}\,\mathrm{S\,cm^{-2}}$) with a reversal potential of about $-90\,\mathrm{mV}$ is involved (providing that the interpretation, that the sodium and potassium conductances have a square root dependence on concentration, is correct). Bromm and Esslinger (1974) have also concluded that the resting potential is primarily set by an unknown ion species. It remains for further experiment to determine which one (or more) ion species is involved.

Therefore it is clear that the standard description that the resting membrane potential is primarily set by a potassium diffusion potential is not generally true, although it seems to hold for the giant axons of squid and crayfish. However, even in these cases, there is still considerable quantitative uncertainty attaching to the deviation of the resting membrane potential from E_K. In no case in which the concentration and voltage dependence of the resting conductances has been examined has any convincing evidence been obtained for the use of the Goldman-Hodgkin-Katz equation. It should therefore be abandoned as a general account and only used where there is clear evidence that *each* of the resting ion currents obeys equation (14.14). It remains to be seen whether an equation taking the form of equation (14.17) (but with additional ion species included) will prove to be more generally satisfactory, at least for those cases in which the ingoing potassium rectifier is not a large component of the resting conductance.

The mechanism of the action potential

The basic mechanism of the action potential is well known. Depolarization beyond a certain voltage leads initially to an increase in sodium conductance and, with a slightly greater delay, to an increased potassium conductance. Because the increased sodium conductance precedes the increase in the potassium conductance the membrane potential tends to go from its resting level towards E_{Na}. Repolarization occurs for two reasons. First, the increased sodium conductance is transient; even if a depolarization is maintained by experimental means the conductance decays back to near its resting level in a matter of milliseconds. Secondly, the delayed increase in the potassium conductance greatly speeds the process of repolarization.

The first analysis and quantitative description of this process was given for the squid giant axon over twenty years ago (Hodgkin, Huxley and Katz, 1952; Hodgkin and Huxley, 1952a,b,c,d). This work has been lucidly reviewed many times (e.g. Hodgkin, 1958, 1964; Woodbury and Patton, 1965; Noble, 1966; Katz, 1966; Cole, 1968; Hille, 1970) and it seems unnecessary to do any more than list the basic features of the description, including in the list further details that have emerged since the appearance of the original papers (e.g. Tsien and Noble, 1969; Hille, 1970; Noble. 1972a; Ehrenstein and Lecar, 1972; Keynes, 1972; Armstrong, 1974).

(1) The sodium and potassium conductances have a maximal value, per unit area of membrane; this is a reflection of the density of sparsely located sites, each with a relatively high value of maximal conductance.

(2) The sodium and potassium conductances are independent mechanisms that can be blocked selectively.

(3) The fundamental property of a single site is that it can exist only in an 'open' or a 'closed' state (i.e. conducting or not conducting).

(4) Usually several independent mechanisms ('gates') control whether the site is conducting. All of the 'gates' have to be in the favourable position of the two that they can occupy for the site to conduct. The sodium conductance possesses two qualitatively different types of 'gate'. One kind moves to the open position with depolarization (activation gate, m) and the other to the closed position (inactivation gate, h). For depolarizations of physiological duration, the behaviour of the potassium conductance can be explained by the behaviour of the activation gates (n) alone.

(5) If one examines the average behaviour of a population of similar 'gates', the proportion of them in the 'open' position, in the steady state, varies sigmoidally with voltage. Note that this description does not distinguish between two possibilities (not mutually exclusive): (1) that an individual gate jumps from the closed to the open position at a single value of membrane potential and the sigmoid curve reflects the distribution of that single 'threshold' value of potential for different gates in the population: and (2) that over a range of voltages the gates fluctuate back and forth between their open and closed positions so that the sigmoid curve describes the probability that the gates will be in the open position at any particular time.

The sigmoid curve has a very steep slope, implying that each 'gate' has more than one unit charge. For example the m (activation) gate of the squid sodium channel must have two unit charges, and if its movement from the closed to open positions only traverses part of the membrane, there must be more.

(6) If one studies the behaviour of a population of 'gates' with time, in response to a step change in voltage, the rate at which the gates move to their new steady state value can be described by a U-shaped curve (rate on the ordinate, potential on the abscissa). This measure of rate is not intended to represent the speed of a gating particle's movement, but rather the average frequency at which the population of gates makes a nearly instantaneous switch from the closed to the open position (or vice versa). In the detailed description, this U-shaped curve represented the sum of two rate coefficients, one for opening (α) and one for closing (β). These rate coefficients are instantaneous functions of voltage.

Some of the features listed above are interpretations of the physical mechanism that have been deduced since the original description. The Hodgkin-Huxley account can also be summarized mathematically: the total ionic current through the membrane is given by

$$i_i = i_{Na} + i_K + i_l \tag{14.19}$$

766

i_l is the leak current. Each ion current is in turn described by the electrochemical form of Ohm's law

$$i_c = g_c (E_m - E_c).$$

The dependence of each conductance on voltage and time are given by

$$g_{Na} = \bar{g}_{Na} \, m^3 h; \; g_K = \bar{g}_K n^4; g_1 = \text{constant}$$

where $\bar{g}_{Na}$ and $\bar{g}_K$ are the maximal values of the sodium and potassium conductances. The 'gating' variables m, h and n are functions of voltage and time. They take values between 0 and 1 according to the equation

$$\frac{dx}{dt} = \alpha_x \cdot (1 - x) - \beta_x \cdot x \tag{14.20}$$

where x represents m, h or n, and α_x and β_x are the opening and closing rate coefficients, which are instantaneous function of voltage. The dependence of α_x and β_x on voltage are described empirically and do not require any precise interpretation as to their mechanism.

This form of description has been remarkably successful in two ways. First, it has accurately predicted much of the observed behaviour of the squid giant axon, including the time course of the action potential, refractory period, anode break excitation and other threshold behaviour etc. Second, many other excitable cells have been similarly analyzed (amphibian node of Ranvier, see Frankenhaeuser and Huxley, 1964; lobster giant axon, see Julian, Moore and Goldman, 1962; frog skeletal muscle, see Adrian, Chandler and Hodgkin, 1970; sheep Purkinje fibre, see McAllister, Noble and Tsien, 1975; *Myxicola* giant axon, see Goldman and Schauf, 1973) and the description of the currents has been quite successful when taking the same general form. However there are several ways in which the original description has been found wanting. This finding has lead to suggestions of a variety of modifications; some of these are only minor additions while others represent quite substantial changes. These modifications will be summarized, but the list is restricted mainly to the studies of the squid and *Myxicola* giant axons.

(1) In the Hodgkin-Huxley description internal and external ion concentrations are assumed to be constant. Changes in internal concentration would be expected to occur only very slowly because of the large volume/surface ratio, so that the assumption is not an unreasonable one, although it would obviously need to be modified for small diameter axons. Changes in external concentration can occur readily in the squid axon however, because there is a restricted extracellular space having a diffusion barrier between it and the bulk of the external medium. A small number of action potentials can thus lead to a substantial rise in extracellular potassium concentration (Frankenhaeuser and Hodgkin, 1956). This situation leads to more complicated equations but it is still quite feasible to compute them (see Adelman and Fitzhugh, 1975). The exact modifications made should take account of the concentration dependence of the

maximal conductances, although, as discussed earlier, this is still an uncertain quantity.

(2) The voltage dependence of the 'gates' can be modified by a variety of agents. Frankenhaeuser and Hodgkin (1957) first described this effect for changes in external calcium ion. The major effect is a very simple one – the voltage dependence of both the steady-state curve and that of the rate coefficients are translated along the voltage axis, but not substantially modified in their absolute magnitude (Blaustein and Goldman, 1968; Hille, 1968; Gilbert and Ehrenstein, 1969; Brismar and Frankenhaeuser, 1972; Ehrenstein and Gilbert, 1973; Hille, Woodhull and Shapiro, 1975). Increase in calcium concentration shifts the voltage sensitivity in the depolarizing direction and vice versa for decreases in calcium concentration. Two possible explanations were discussed by Frankenhaeuser and Hodgkin (1957). Calcium ion could be acting by modifying the effect of fixed surface charge, thus affecting the local field acting on the 'gates', or alternatively calcium could be acting as 'blocking' molecule (requiring a large depolarization to displace it from the membrane). They favoured the former explanation. Although evidence has been presented recently that, in high concentrations, calcium can have a blocking action (Woodhull, 1973), the main effect on the conductances is most readily explained by the fixed charge hypothesis; the effect of the fixed charge is thought to be modified in two ways. First, the calcium ions, along with other cations, may 'screen' the surface charge by forming a diffuse double layer at the surface. Secondly, they may actually neutralize the charge by binding to it. Readers interested in the theoretical treatment of this effect are referred to the papers by Gilbert and Ehrenstein (1969), Brismar (1973), Brown (1974) and Hille, Woodhull and Shapiro (1975).

Various other cations, (including H^+ and Mg^{++}) and anions, and changes in total ion strength can produce similar effects (see Hille, Woodhull and Shapiro, 1975). These effects seem to apply to all the described gating mechanisms (i.e. m, h and n) but their magnitude varies. This has lead to deductions concerning both the physical position of the m and h gates across the membrane (see Woodhull, 1973) and the relative magnitudes of the local fields adjacent to the sodium and potassium channels.

There is also evidence for a fixed negative charge on the inner surface of the axon membrane, as Chandler, Hodgkin and Meves (1965) have found shifts in the h and m variables when the squid axon was perfused with solutions of low ionic strength. On the other hand Begenisich and Lynch (1974) did not find any substantial effects on the voltage dependence of the sodium and potassium conductances in squid axons when perfused with Ca^{++}, Co^{++}, Cd^{++} Ni^{++} and Zn^{++}, all of which are effective in screening external surface charge.

Once a complete empirical description of the effects of the concentration of various ion species on the fixed charges has been given, there should be no trouble in incorporating this into the Hodgkin-Huxley equations. In most physiological circumstances the concentrations will not change sufficiently for this to be a significant modification. The importance of the work described above lies rather in the insight it gives into the nature of the local mechanisms controlling the behaviour of the gates.

(3) The behaviour of the potassium gates does not always follow that predicted. Cole and Moore (1960) have reported that after a prolonged hyperpolarization the potassium conductance developed more slowly than expected (see also Frankenhaeuser and Hodgkin, 1957). Within the Hodgkin-Huxley description this required an equation of the form $g_K = \bar{g}_K \cdot n^{25}$, rather than $g_K \propto n^4$. It is not clear however whether this is the most appropriate modification (see Tsien and Noble, 1969; Hill and Chen, 1972; Roy, 1975).

Ehrenstein and Gilbert (1966) have reported a very slow inactivation of the potassium conductance of the squid axon. They suggest that this inactivation can be modelled by introducing a single parameter, similar to the h gate for the sodium conductance. The time constant near the resting potential for this process is of the order of 10 seconds so that it will only be of importance when considering phenomena like repetitive firing.

(4) The major difficulty faced by the Hodgkin-Huxley descriptions centres around recent descriptions of the process of inactivation of the sodium conductance. The main experimental discrepancies are as follows:

(a) The curve describing the steady-state voltage sensitivity of the h gate varies in its position along the voltage axis depending on the magnitude of the voltage test pulse that follows the conditioning pulse. This has been reported for both squid (Hoyt and Adelman, 1970; but see Jakobson and Scudiero, 1975) and *Myxicola* (Goldman and Schauf, 1972).

(b) The rate for inactivation can be measured in two ways: either from the time course of decay of the sodium conductance or from the time course of the effects of a conditioning pulse on a test pulse. In *Myxicola* the two measurements do not agree (Goldman and Schauf, 1973).

(c) In *Myxicola* there are small delays in the development of inactivation and in its recovery (Goldman and Schauf, 1972; Schauf, 1974).. A similar delay has been reported in the squid (Armstrong, 1970). On the basis of the Hodgkin-Huxley description inactivation should follow first order kinetics and thus be exponential, without a delay.

(d) Perhaps the most dramatic discrepancy can be seen in *Myxicola* axons in which a depolarizing conditioning pulse is followed by a larger test pulse. Providing the size of the conditioning pulse is chosen within a certain range, the sodium conductance will rise at the onset of the conditioning pulse and then decline to nearly zero. This finding can be interpreted from the Hodgkin-Huxley description to indicate that practically all of the inactivation gates have moved to the closed position, and hence it can be predicted that there will be a negligible rise in sodium conductance at the time of the test pulse; but in fact another large rise of sodium conductance is observed (see Goldman, 1975).

(e) Chandler and Meves (1970) have reported the occurrence of a complicated form of sodium inactivation in squid axons perfused with sodium fluoride solutions, in which the sodium conductance is not fully inactivated with long depolarizations. However, this would not be a significant effect within physiological durations of depolarization.

Two models have recently been proposed to explain some or all of these findings. Goldman (1975), following Hoyt (1963, 1968), has chosen a complex activation-inactivation mechanism that, when translated into a possible mechanism, implies five independent 'gates' each of which behave as follows:

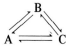

where A is the resting state, B the conducting state and C the 'inactivated' state. He has concluded that such a model gives a satisfactory description of the behaviour of the sodium conductance.

Jakobsson and Scudiero (1975) have offered a much less radical revision of the Hodgkin-Huxley description. They have left the behaviour of the h gate as in the original description and have postulated more complicated behaviour for the m gate:

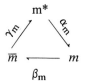

$\bar{m}$ represents the gate in the closed position, m^* is an intermediary position and m is the open position. α_m and β_m are instantaneous functions of voltage, as in the original description, but γ_m is a rate coefficient which is proportional to the rate of change of voltage, rather than to voltage *per se*. They point out that their model can explain the discrepancies listed under (a), (b) and (d). This model can also better describe certain features of repetitive firing (but see Adelman and Fitzhugh, 1975), and of accommodation observed in the squid axon, than can the original model.

It may be some time yet before appropriate experiments can be designed and performed to distinguish between these two proposals. One possible way of doing so has come from recent observations of a further current, named the 'gating' current, which must be added to the three currents listed earlier.

(5) In the summary of the Hodgkin-Huxley description given above the presumed 'gates' were postulated to have a charge and to move across the membrane in response to change in membrane potential; such a charge movement is a current and should therefore be detectable under suitable conditions. An essential feature of this current is that the total charge movement in response to the voltage step should be exactly balanced by an opposite charge movement following the return of the voltage to its original level, since the

'gates' are presumed to remain attached to the membrane. In this respect a 'gating' current is quite different from an ion current, and is formally equivalent to a capacitative current (see Keynes and Rojas, 1974).

Such a current has been recorded by several groups of experimenters (Armstrong and Bezanilla, 1974; Keynes and Rojas, 1974; Meves, 1974; Nonner, Rojas and Stämpfli, 1975a). It is evident that such measurements should provide an exquisitely sensitive test of the various proposals for the gating mechanism that have been offered. Unfortunately conflicting data have been described by the different groups. All workers do, however, agree that most of the gating current so far recorded is concerned with control of the magnitude of the sodium conductance. Armstrong and Bezanilla (see also Bezanilla and Armstrong, 1974, 1975; Armstrong, 1974) report two features of the current that are clearly at odds with the Hodgkin-Huxley description. The first of these is that gating current 'inactivates' in parallel with the sodium current. This is an unexpected effect if we assume that the major part of the gating current is explained by the rapid movement of the three m gates, since only the h gate movement should be involved in inactivation. These authors therefore suggest that a coupled activation-inactivation model of the gates, such as that due to Goldman, is appropriate. On the other hand both Keynes and Rojas (1974, Rojas and Keynes, 1975) and Meves (1974, 1975), deny that the gating current is inactivated in the potential range, and at the rate appropriate to the behaviour of h.

The second difference is that Bezanilla and Armstrong (1974, 1975) report that the time course of decline of the sodium conductance at the end of a depolarizing test pulse is not three times as fast as the decline in the gating current (as predicted by the Hodgkin-Huxley model) but is comparable in its time course. Keynes and Rojas (1974) drew attention to a similar result, but in a later paper (Rojas and Keynes, 1975) reported that there was indeed a difference in the time courses, and of the kind expected from the Hodgkin-Huxley model (Rojas and Keynes [1975] studied the rate coefficient for m, analyzed in the manner of Hodgkin and Huxley and found that their results failed to fit the original equations – there being a large discrepancy in the range −60 to −150 mV, which Hodgkin and Huxley had not examined experimentally. This means that if the Hodgkin-Huxley description is to be preserved a modification of the equation describing the voltage sensitivity of the rate coefficient is required.)

These discrepancies between experimental results will have to be resolved before any definite choice can be made concerning the most appropriate description of the factors governing the sodium conductance. Rojas and Keynes (1975) have presented a strongly argued case for the gating current reflecting the behaviour of the m gates. They have shown that their results are in accord with a theoretical treatment, with a Boltzmann distribution of charges between two states at different energy levels. Changes in membrane potential lead to a transition between these two states that can be described by first order kinetics. If they are correct they have provided a physical interpretation for the voltage sensitivity of the rate coefficients (in the Hodgkin-Huxley description).

If the movement of the m gates has indeed been detected, it is natural to ask whether there are comparable signs of the movement of the h and n gates. Keynes and Rojas (1974) and Rojas and Keynes (1975) have argued that even if present they will be much more difficult to detect; given the experimental discrepancies existing with respect to the main gating current it is, however, obviously premature to conclude that they do not exist (see also Bezanilla and Armstrong, 1975).

Given the existence of a gating current it is a fairly straightforward matter to incorporate it within the Hodgkin-Huxley description. If it represents the movement of the m gates then a term needs to be added

$$i_g = \bar{Q} \frac{dm}{dt} \tag{14.21}$$

where $\bar{Q}$ is the total charge associated with the gates in a unit area of membrane. Computations of the Hodgkin-Huxley equations with this modification have been reported by Adrian (1975).

(6) A further, small, current needs to be added to the Hodgkin-Huxley description. There is now good evidence for a voltage-time dependent conductance that predominantly selects calcium ions. Hodgkin and Keynes (1957) reported an increased calcium influx with each action potential of about 0.006 pmole cm^{-2} ($[Ca^{++}]_0 = 10.7$ mM). This may be compared with the net entry of sodium of about 4 pmole cm^{-2}, the calcium movement therefore contributing a negligible addition to the inward charge movement. Baker, Hodgkin and Ridgeway (1971) investigated this further and found that the calcium entry could be divided into two components: that entering via the 'sodium' channel and a late component entering by a separate channel, which was not the 'potassium' channel. Baker, Meves and Ridgeway (1973a,b) have described further properties of this calcium conductance. There are excellent reviews of these calcium movements and of their significance in excitation-contraction and excitation-secretion coupling (Baker, 1972; Reuter, 1973; Baker and Glitsch, 1975). One further possible significance for these inward calcium movements is that, in some tissues, at least, they can activate a prolonged conductance to potassium ions (Krnjevic and Lisiewicz, 1972; Jansen and Nicholls, 1973; Meech and Standen, 1974).

(7) In some respects the most radical challenge to the form of description adopted by Hodgkin and Huxley comes from experiments reported by Cohen and Landowne (1974; see also Landowne, 1972, 1973). They studied the net flux of sodium ions associated with impulses and found that they were very insensitive to changes in temperature (Q_{10} of about 1/1.2). The Hodgkin-Huxley theory predicts a much greater Q_{10}, of about 1/3.0, because the maximal conductances were thought to be fairly insensitive to temperature changes

whereas the gating variable have a large Q_{10} (≈ 3.0). Thus, on cooling the axon, the conductances would all have a much slower time course (but similar amplitude) to that observed at higher temperatures. The integral of the conductance, and hence the current, is therefore much larger at a lower temperature. The result reported by Cohen and Landowne is therefore very disconcerting for proponents of the conventional theory. If it cannot be explained within the usual theoretical framework, its discovery implies that the conversion of net fluxes into currents (and vice versa) is not valid; and as Cohen and Landowne point out, this conversion would not be valid if there was the possibility of the storage of charge (i.e. sodium ion) within the membrane. Such a storage implies a quite different mechanism for the ion permeation process to that usually assumed. A detailed presentation of a model with ion storage has been given by Offner (1972). Considerable experimental activity will doubtless be provoked by their observations. One possible explanation is that the previously measured estimates of the Q_{10} of the maximal sodium conductance are too low. Another factor which needs to be considered is the effect of K^+ accumulation and/or Na^+ depletion in the extracellular space.

(8) Another interesting challenge to the Hodgkin-Huxley description comes from the study of membrane 'noise'. Fishman (1973, 1975) has measured voltage noise in an isolated patch of squid axon membrane which is believed to be associated with the opening and closing of the potassium conductance. He analyzed his results with two possible interpretations in mind: the potassium conductance channel behaved either as a two-state conductance (open or closed) or as a multi-state conductance (having additional intermediary conductance values). Only the multi-state conductance model gave a good fit to his data.

His results have been criticized on the grounds that voltage noise will be affected by the complex impedance of the nerve membrane (Wanke, De Felice and Conti, 1974), and it has been claimed that only an analysis of current noise under voltage clamp will be informative about conductance changes in the membrane. Conti, De Felice and Wanke (1975) have provided a detailed analysis of this kind and have concluded that two of the components of the current noise are associated with the sodium and potassium currents respectively. Both components can be reasonably well fitted by a theory assuming only an open and closed state for the individual channels, but the data was too scattered to exclude the possibility of a multi-state model.

Further work on membrane noise should yield even greater insight into the molecular events underlying conductance changes (Verveen and De Felice, 1974). At the moment it appears that the simplest interpretation of the Hodgkin-Huxley equations, i.e. the two-state model, does not have to be modified. It will be interesting to see whether a component or components of the noise associated with gating movements can be detected; if it can it may be possible to decide whether an individual channel fluctuates spontaneously from the open to the closed position at a fixed voltage and to relate this to the voltage sensitivity of the rate coefficient.

14.1.2 *Active transport of ions*

The existence of any ion out of equilibrium and for which the membrane has a finite permeability, implies the presence of an active transport mechanism to maintain that disequilibrium. The best known example of such a mechanism in excitable cells is the 'sodium (-potassium) pump'.

The sodium pump

Since the major fluxes associated with the action potential are those of sodium and potassium, they are also the ion species with the greatest tendency to lose their electrochemical disequilibrium. Their concentration gradients must be maintained to retain a steady state, and thus it follows that the transport of sodium and potassium are the two largest fluxes attributed to active mechanisms. Studies in a variety of nerve tissues indicate that the major way this is achieved is by a coupled sodium-potassium transport mechanism that utilizes ATP as its immediate source of energy (Hodgkin and Keynes, 1955a; Caldwell, Hodgkin, Keynes and Shaw, 1960; Baker and Connelly, 1966; Brinley and Mullins, 1967, 1968; Mullins and Brinley, 1967, 1969; Rang and Ritchie, 1968a,b,c; Baker, Foster, Gilbert and Shaw, 1971). It is now generally accepted that the $(Na^+ - K^+)$-activated ATPase enzyme is intimately involved in effecting this transport (see Skou, 1975; Glynn and Karlish, 1975, for recent reviews). This is in keeping with the basic feature of this pump, that its activity is increased by increases in internal sodium concentration and/or of external potassium concentration. Some other factors which are known to influence the rate of pumping are: external sodium (a decrease increases the rate of pumping), temperature (at low temperatures the pump is inhibited), metabolic inhibitors (which inhibit it) and, of course, cardiac glycosides which, at least in high doses, inhibit it.

Several workers have studied the binding of radioactively labelled ouabain to membranes in order to estimate the density of sodium pumping sites (see Landowne and Ritchie, 1960). In mammalian non-myelinated nerve fibres the upper limit for the density of pump sites is about $750 \, \mu m^{-2}$. This is roughly thirty times the density of Hodgkin-Huxley sodium channels estimated for the same nerve (by studying the binding of tetrodotoxin, see Colquhoun, Henderson and Ritchie, 1972). The turnover rate for a single pump site (i.e. the maximum number of sodium ions extruded in unit time) is of the order of $40-100 \, s^{-1}$ at $37°C$. This rate is about 10^5 times slower than the rate of movement of Na^+ into the cell that has been calculated for the Hodgkin-Huxley sodium channel.

Electrical effects of the sodium pump

In the classical account of the sodium pump and its effect on the membrane potential, it was assumed that the transport of sodium and potassium was tightly linked, 1:1, so that the pump did not itself generate a current. The pump was necessary for the maintenance of the concentration gradients of the ion species, but did not make a direct contribution to the resting potential (see Katz, 1966). As Thomas (1972) has pointed out, there was already good evidence before 1960 that the pump could, at least in some circumstances, be electrogenic, and it is now clear that it is often, if not always, a current generator. One piece of evidence comes from the study of the ratio of the number of ions transported outwards by the pump to those transported inwards. In a variety of tissues the basic 'stoicheiometry' seems to be that for every molecule of ATP split, three sodium ions are pumped out and two potassium ions taken in (Hodgkin and Keynes, 1955a; Mullins and Brinley, 1969) — although the exact ratio of sodium to potassium is less certain. There is no good evidence for any other ion being involved (but see Moore, 1973, for a suggestion that H^+ may be transported out), but this is an unsatisfactory indication of the net charge transferred because of such a possibility. A more satisfactory procedure, therefore, is to measure the electrical effect of the pump directly. In order to find the proportion of extruded sodium (or other cation) that is not accompanied by an inward movement of potassium one needs to know both the total amount of sodium extruded, as well as the amount extruded uncoupled. Thomas (1969) was the first person to make such careful measurements, in a snail neurone, and he concluded that between one third and one quarter of the extruded sodium was uncoupled. Cooke, Leblanc and Tauc (1974) have also made such measurements in *Aplysia* neurones and have found between 40 and 65 per cent of the sodium extrusion was electrogenic. This discrepancy may reflect a variation in the coupling of sodium and potassium, a possibility that had been suggested earlier by various authors (see Mullins and Brinley, 1969; Cooke *et al.*, 1974). One important observation made in the squid axon is that the coupling ratio seemed to depend on the internal sodium concentration, more of the extruded sodium being uncoupled at high internal sodium concentrations. This may be helpful in interpreting observations that an increase in internal sodium may be followed by a marked hyperpolarization attributable to electrogenic pump activity, but there is less good evidence for it being electrogenic at resting levels of $[Na^+]_i$.

Once one has knowledge of the proportion of sodium that is extruded electrogenically it is a simple matter to calculate its effect on the membrane potential in the steady state. If c denotes the coupling ratio (proportion of potassium ions taken in to sodium pumped out) then the pump current is $(1-c)$ times the total amount of sodium extruded. But in the steady state the amount pumped out must be equal to the passive influx into the cell (in order to keep $[Na^+]_i$ constant). The algebraic sum of these two sodium currents is therefore $c \cdot g_{Na} \cdot (E_m - E_{Na})$. If the resting potential is a zero-current condition for sodium and potassium currents only, then it is given by:

$$g_K(E_R - E_K) + c \cdot g_{Na}(E_R - E_{Na}) = 0$$

or

$$E_R = \frac{g_K \cdot E_R + c \cdot g_{Na} \cdot E_{Na}}{g_K + c \cdot g_{Na}}. \qquad (14.22)$$

This formulation does not include any explicit dependence of the conductances on concentration and voltage. If these are known they can be readily included. For example if the Goldman-Hodgkin-Katz equation is applicable it becomes (Mullins and Noda, 1963):

$$E_R = \frac{RT}{F} \log_e \left\{ \frac{p_K [K^+]_i + c \cdot p_{Na} [Na^+]_i}{p_K [K^+]_o + c \cdot p_{Na} [Na^+]_o} \right\} \qquad (14.23)$$

whereas, if the conductances are not voltage-sensitive and have a square root dependence on concentrations, it becomes

$$E_R = \frac{p_K \sqrt{([K^+]_o \cdot [K^+]_i)} \cdot E_K + c \cdot p_{Na} \cdot \sqrt{([Na^+]_o [Na^+]_i)} \cdot E_{Na}}{p_K \sqrt{([K^+]_o [K^+]_i)} + c \cdot p_{Na} \sqrt{([Na^+]_o [Na^+]_i)}}.$$

$$(14.24)$$

If the conductances have no concentration or voltage dependence, equation (14.22) holds, with the conductance terms being constant. In all cases the only way in which the basic equations have been modified is that the 'effective' sodium permeability (or conductance) has been reduced by a factor equal to the coupling ratio.

It is a straightforward matter to show what contribution an electrogenic sodium pump makes to the resting potential, by calculating what the change in potential would be if the pump suddenly ceased to operate. The immediate effect (i.e. before ion concentration gradients ran down) can be calculated using each pair of equations (i.e. (14.12) and (14.23), (14.17) and (14.24) or (14.18) and (14.22)), assuming a particular p_K/p_{Na} (or g_K/g_{Na}) ratio. For example, taking the same values as those used for calculating Fig. 14.2, with $[K^+]_o = 2.5$ mM and a coupling ratio of $2/3$ the contribution made to the resting potential by the pump are -5.1 mV, -6 mV and -6 mV respectively.

It should be noted that these small effects on the resting membrane potential are a consequence of the assumption of a fairly large p_K/p_{Na} ratio. If the p_K/p_{Na} ratio is smaller, the membrane potential deviates further from E_K and the effect of the pump is relatively larger. A smaller coupling ratio will also lead to a larger contribution to the resting potential, but it can never be greater than the difference between the resting potential (without the pump working) and E_K because if $c = 0$ the resting potential predicted by equations (14.22), (14.23) and (14.24) is E_K. Note that the absolute magnitude of the resting membrane conductance ($g_m = g_K + g_{Na}$) does not affect the pump contribution. This is important to stress because the opposite has sometimes been implied (Hodgkin and Keynes, 1955a, Carpenter, 1973; Gorman and Marmor, 1974). This proposal is only valid if there is additional membrane conductance due to another ion (or if there are longitudinal gradients for intracellular sodium diffusion due, for example, to different surface/volume ratios of various regions of the cell).

One may therefore conclude that it is likely, for known coupling and p_K/p_{Na} ratios, that the electrogenic sodium pump has a small effect on the resting potential. This conclusion is in accord with careful experimental studies. Thomas (1969) reported values of -2.0 to -5 mV for a snail neurone, De Weer and Geduldig (1973) found the contribution was only -1.4 mV for the giant axon of squid and Gorman and Marmor (1974) obtained a value of just under -10 mV for a molluscan neurone.

In contrast, the transient effect of the pump can be considerable. The resting activity of the pump can be transiently increased by a variety of manoeuvres, the two main physiological ones begin an increase in internal sodium concentration and an increase of external potassium concentration. There is a large literature documenting these effects, and this is reviewed by Hurlbut (1970), Ritchie (1971) and Thomas (1972). Rather than repeat such a survey it may suffice to note that there are interpretive difficulties with many of the studies, particularly when the pump is activated by an increase in internal sodium.

(1) The activity of a neutral pump could be hyperpolarizing due to depletion of potassium in the immediate extracellular space.

(2) An increase in internal sodium may be accompanied by an increase in internal calcium, either because the sodium increase has been produced by a train of action potentials and hence also produced net calcium entry, or because of the postulated $Na^+ - Ca^{++}$ exchange mechanism (see p. 778). As mentioned earlier, an increase in internal calcium can increase a membrane potassium conductance such that, even if the pump were neutral, a hyperpolarization would be observed towards E_K (but not beyond it). On the other hand, if there is no calcium-activated potassium conductance, the increase in internal sodium would promote the inward movement of calcium by the $Na^+ - Ca^{++}$ exchange system. It is not known definitely whether this mechanism is a neutral exchange when it is operating in the direction sodium out, calcium in, but such a possibility should be borne in mind (when it is operating in the opposite direction the evidence, to be mentioned shortly, suggests it is not neutral).

There is insufficient suitable experimental evidence available to decide whether the coupling ratio (and hence the electrogenicity) is modified during the transient activation of the sodium pump, although there are hints that this may be so (e.g. Adrian and Slayman, 1966). Such an effect would help to explain the observation that while the sodium pump makes a negligible contribution to the resting membrane potential of the amphibian node of Ranvier (Århem, Frankenhaeuser and Moore, 1973), it can generate a very significant tetanic and post-tetanic hyperpolarization (Connelly, 1959; Schoepfle and Katholi, 1973). If the pump did vary its coupling ratio it might be expected that such a change would also be influenced by the level of the membrane potential. Several workers have sought such an effect, usually with negative results (e.g. Marmor,

1971), although it has been reported to occur in a snail neurone (Kostyuk, Kryshtal and Pidoplichko, 1972).

Only limited data is available on which one may make guesses about the functional significance of the electrogenicity of the sodium pump. The phenomenon has been implicated in the slow adaptation in repetitive firing of nerve cells and receptors (e.g. Sokolove and Cooke, 1971), and even in conduction block (e.g. Van Essen, 1973). These findings indicate that a possible function is to limit the firing of the cell so that large run-downs in the concentration gradient do not occur. On the other hand if the electrogenic response was not too vigorous it could serve to stabilize the membrane potential near the steady resting level in the face of an increased external potassium concentration (Gorman and Marmor, 1974), thus acting as a short-term 'buffer' and preventing depolarizing inactivation of the action potential mechanism. Quite apart from speculations about the electrical effects it may be noted that a net transfer of ions from the cell (particularly if the membrane has a significant anion conductance, leading to a passive following of that ion) will have a shrinking effect on the cell, because of the accompanying water movements. This may be important if the swelling which has been observed to follow a train of action potentials (Hill, 1950a,b) has any tendency to place the membrane under mechanical stress.

Calcium transport

In the squid axon there is roughly 400 μM/l present in the axoplasm, but 98 per cent of it is neither diffusible nor ionized; of the remainder most appears to be un-ionized leaving only about 0.3 μM of ionized calcium. There is therefore a very large electrochemical gradient to encourage calcium to move in across the membrane (normal concentration of sea water 11 mM), and there is evidence that the great bulk of the internal calcium is sequestered inside internal compartments, perhaps the mitochondria, probably by means of an ATP-dependent calcium pump. There is, however, no convincing evidence that a similar pump exists in the external membrane of nerve axons. The main mechanism of transport here seems to be a sodium-calcium exchange mechanism (for a review, see Baker, 1972). Although there are suggestions that ATP may be indirectly involved in this exchange process (Baker and Glitsch, 1973; DiPolo, 1974), it can proceed in the absence of internal ATP. Baker and his colleagues have presented evidence which is most simply interpreted in terms of a single reversible mechanism in which inward entry of sodium is coupled to an efflux of calcium (or vice versa). Although the stoichiometry of the reaction is not certain, it is probable that at least three sodium ions move in one direction for each calcium ion movement in the opposite direction. The predominant mode of operation normally is calcium efflux, sodium influx. On the above account it can be seen that the energy for the normally directed action is obtained from the run-down of the sodium concentration gradient and from the run-down of the membrane potential (since there is a net transfer of positive charge inwards). The mechanism can therefore be loosely regarded as 'parasitic' on the activity of the sodium pump. In keeping with the idea of a net transfer of charge, Mullins and Brinley (1975) have reported that calcium efflux is sensitive to changes in the membrane potential, hyperpolarization increasing and depolarization decreasing it. In electrical studies it will therefore appear to be a small conductance with a 'zero current' value somewhere on the depolarized side of E_R.

Other ion species

Amongst other ion species which are not distributed according to passive expectations are Mg^{++} (Baker and Glitsch, 1975), H^+ (e.g. Boron and de Weer, 1975), many amino acids (e.g. Schultz and Curran, 1970; Baker and Potashner, 1973), and, sometimes Cl^- (Keynes, 1953; Wallin, 1967; Lux, 1971). The Mg^{++} and some amino acids may be transported by means similar to the sodium-calcium exchange (Baker and Glitsch, 1975; Baker and Potashner, 1973), but the details of H^+ and Cl^- transport are still to be elucidated. The chloride pump mechanism is of special interest with respect to electrical behaviour. In some cells the net transport appears to be inward (Keynes, 1953; Wallin, 1967) but in others, such as the mammalian motor neuron, it is outward (Lux, 1971). Since there can be a significant chloride conductance, either at rest or induced by, for example, inhibitory synaptic action the nature of the chloride dis-equilibrium and the factors controlling it can be very important. Lux (1971) has presented evidence that the chloride pump can be blocked by ammonia and that this effect may be responsible for the generation and/or promotion of convulsions in certain pathological states.

14.2 The spread of charge

The axoplasm of nerve fibres is usually considered to have a fairly cylindrical structure. If the membrane surrounding it at one point is at a different value of potential from adjacent areas, there will be spread of current both inside and outside the axon acting to reduce this potential difference. Although radial spread of current (i.e. around the circumference of the fibre) can be important in special circumstances (see Eisenberg and Johnson, 1970), this account will be restricted to the longitudinal spread. This is the major form of current flow and considered in isolation it provides an adequate quantitative basis for studies of the excitation and propagation of the nerve impulse.

The basic equations for describing current flow along a cylindrical axon can be derived by simple application of Ohm's and Kirchoff's laws (see Taylor, 1963 and Jack, Noble and Tsien, 1975, for less cryptic accounts). The axoplasm is a simple resistance, so that, from Ohm's law (neglecting extracellular potential differences)

$$i_a = -\frac{(\partial V/\partial x)}{r_a} \qquad (14.25)$$

where i_a denotes axial current, r_a is axoplasmic resistance per unit length, V is the transmembrane voltage and x is distance. The minus sign occurs because of the convention that positive current flows in the direction of increasing x. From Kirchoff's law we can obtain an equation for the density of membrane current, since any change in axial current with distance must be due to membrane current flow:

$$\frac{\partial i_a}{\partial x} = -i_m \qquad (14.26)$$

The negative sign here is due to the convention that positive membrane current is outward. Differentiating equation (14.25) with respect to x

$$\frac{\partial i_a}{\partial x} = \frac{1}{r_a} \frac{\partial^2 V}{\partial x^2} \qquad (14.27)$$

one then obtains

$$i_m = \frac{1}{r_a} \frac{\partial^2 V}{\partial x^2} \qquad (14.28)$$

The membrane current is the sum of capacitative current (i.e. change in the charge distribution across the membrane capacitance) and total ionic current (i_i). If the membrane capacitance acts as a perfect capacitor (but see Cole, 1968; Jack, Noble and Tsien, 1975, Chapter 2; Fitzhugh and Cole, 1973)

$$i_c = c_m \frac{\partial V}{\partial t} \qquad (14.29)$$

where i_c is the capacitative current per unit length, c_m is the membrane capacitance per unit area and t denotes time. Hence

$$\frac{1}{r_a} \frac{\partial^2 V}{\partial x^2} = c_m \frac{\partial V}{\partial t} + i_i \qquad (14.30)$$

This is the standard equation for the description of current flow (and potential changes) in nerve. It only applies in this simple form to unmyelinated nerve in which there is no change in membrane structure at properties with distance.

Many solutions exist to this equation, depending on the exact electrical geometry considered, the nature of i_i and whether spatial or temporal variations in voltage can be neglected. Extensive discussion of these solutions will be found in Jack, Noble and Tsien (1975). For present purposes it is sufficient to concentrate on those that are relevant to the explanation of the excitation and propagation of the action potential. Unfortunately these are just the solutions that are most difficult to obtain because of the complicated, time-dependent non-linear dependence of i_i on V (see *Mechanism of the Action Potential*). When the Hodgkin-Huxley description of the ionic currents is incorporated into equation (14.30), it has not proved possible to obtain a solution without recourse to a digital or analogue computer. Nevertheless a guide to the behaviour of axons can be obtained by considering some simplifications to the full equation.

14.2.1 *Excitation*

One obvious simplification to try, is to neglect the time factor. In order to do this one needs to make certain assumptions about the nature of the ionic current. Excitation will not occur unless some of the voltage-dependent sodium conductance is activated, and an obvious approach is to consider the (artificial) case in which the sodium conductance is fully activated (i.e. m is allowed to go to its steady-state value, m_∞) without any activation (i.e. h remains at its initial value, h_0), and the potassium conductance remains at its resting value ($n = n_0$). This, and other possible simplifications to the Hodgkin-Huxley equations have been discussed extensively by Noble and his colleagues (Noble, 1966; Noble and Stein, 1966; Noble, 1972b; Jack, Noble and Tsien, 1975; Hunter, McNaughton and Noble, 1975).

Fig. 14.4 is a schematic representation of this simplification. The top part of the figure shows the change in the value of the sodium conductance with membrane potential. In the bottom half of the figure is the resultant current-voltage relation. Four relationships are shown. The dashed line represents the resting current-voltage relationship, with a zero-current voltage of -60 mV. The dashed–dot line is the relationship for the sodium current if the conductance were fully activated (i.e. $m = 1, h = 1$) for all voltages. The thin continuous line is the sodium current expected for the activation curve shown in the top part of the figure and the thick continuous line is the total membrane ionic current-voltage relation (sum of the resting current and the voltage-dependent sodium current). For about 30 mV on the depolarizing side of the resting potential the total ionic current is outward, but it then reverses and becomes inward. This cross-over point is the 'voltage threshold' for excitation of an action potential in a uniform patch of membrane. The argument for this is as follows: in a uniform patch of membrane, with no longitudinal spread of charge, the membrane current must be zero. The total membrane current is the sum of the applied current and the ionic and capacitative currents so that once the ionic current becomes net inward, the capacitative current will be outward even if the applied (inward) current ceases to pass. An outward capacitative current is equivalent to a reduction in the charge separated by the membrane capacity, so the membrane potential will tend to move further in the depolarizing direction. This in turn leads to a further increase in the net inward ionic current and a further movement of the membrane potential in the depolarizing direction. The rate of such movement at any moment in time is given by the ratio of the ionic current to the membrane capacitance. The depolarization will continue until the net ionic current becomes zero again, at about +35 mV. In the absence of any recovery process (sodium inactivation and the voltage-dependent increase in

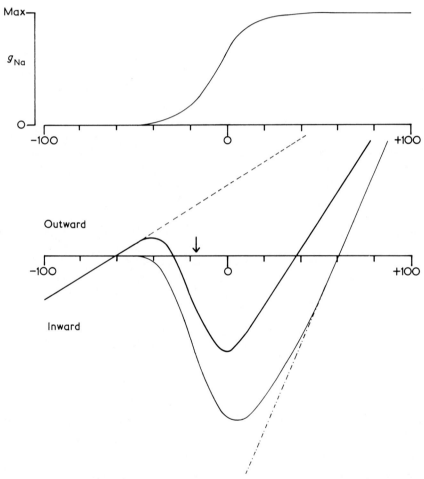

Fig. 14.4 The top half of the figure shows schematically the dependence of the sodium conductance (ordinate) on membrane potential (abscissa). The lower half of the curve plots four current-voltage relations, with voltage (abscissa) on the same scale as in the top half. (– – – – –) – is the assumed resting membrane conductance, (————) – plots the current-voltage relation for sodium ions due to the voltage dependence of the sodium conductance illustrated above, and (————) – shows the sum of these two currents. (– · – · – ·) – the current-voltage relation for sodium ions if the conductance always attained its maximal value.

potassium conductance) the membrane potential would be stable at this value. Noble (1966), and Jack, Noble and Tsien, (1975) Chapter 9) have discussed how these last processes alter the subsequent form of the total ionic current-voltage relationship and hence lead to repolarization.

Fig. 14.4 gives some insight into the factors setting the 'voltage threshold' in a uniform patch of membrane. The voltage threshold is the middle one of the three zero-current points along the voltage axis and is that potential at which the resting ionic current is equal and opposite to the voltage-dependent sodium current. Clearly this will be influenced by the ratio of the maximal sodium conductance to the resting membrane conductance and the form of voltage-dependence of the sodium conductance. For illustrative reasons the value of the resting membrane conductance has been chosen to be rather large (in relation to the maximal sodium conductance); in many nerve axons it is much smaller, so that the voltage threshold is nearer to the resting potential (for the same reason, the peak value of the action potential will then be nearer to the zero-current value for the sodium conductance).

In most physiological circumstances excitation is not achieved by uniform excitation, the depolarizing current being applied in one limited region. The extreme case is if all the applied current passes through the membrane at one point longitudinally (i.e. the applied current is passed equally around the circumference of the axon at one point). This form of excitation is called 'point polarization'. The conditions for excitation, with the above simplification, has been successfully analyzed (Noble, 1966, 1972). One way of summarizing the results, for an extended unmyelinated axon, is to say that the total ionic current, integrated with distance along the axon, must be inward (provided that the total ionic current-voltage relation is the same for all patches of membrane). The voltage-threshold now becomes the point on the uniform current-voltage relationship at which the *integral* of the net ionic current (taken from the resting potential, in the depolarizing direction) becomes inward. This point is marked with an arrow in Fig. 14.4. A recent exposition of this condition will be found in Jack, Noble and Tsien (1975, Chapters 9 and 12). Notice that in a point-polarized axon, at threshold, there will be a region on either side of the site of applied current where the membrane will be passing net inward ionic current. This is so because the voltage will decline, as a complicated function of distance, on either side of the point of applied current. At all distances where the voltage is above the 'voltage threshold' for the uniform patch of membrane there will be a net inward current as described in Fig. 14.4. Following Rushton, Noble (1972) has called the region the 'liminal length' for nerve excitation. It serves as an alternative description of the condition for excitation (with point polarization) i.e. that the membrane voltage be raised above uniform threshold over this length of the axon. The factors affecting the magnitude of the liminal length have been analyzed by Noble (1972).

This analysis may be extended to include a time factor for excitation. Noble (1972; see also Fozzard and Schoenberg, 1972) has discussed how the basic form of the strength-duration curve (see also, Noble and Stein, 1966; Cooley and Dodge, 1966) is related to the liminal length. The strength-duration curve gives the relationship between the strength of applied current and the time for which it must be passed, in order to achieve excitation.

The discussion above applies only to unmyelinated axons. There is as yet no comparable simplified treatment of myelinated nerve because of the mathematical difficulties in treating its complicated structure. The qualitative conclusions, however, would be expected to be similar. A digital computer solution for the initiation of an action potential in a myelinated nerve fibre has been given by Fitzhugh (1962).

14.2.2 *Propagation of the action potential*

In almost all peripheral nerve axons an action potential can be generated, and its propagation serves as the means of conducting the nervous 'message' (although see Bush and Roberts, 1968, for a well-documented exception). A quantitative account of the propagation of the action potential is based on the assumption that the spread of electrical charge by 'local circuits' is both necessary and sufficient. Although this was suggested at the turn of the century by Hermann, it was not until Hodgkin's study (Hodgkin, 1937a,b) that this assumption was justified. Goldman (1964) has reported some elegant experiments that put this assumption to a quantitative test; it survived.

The 'local circuit' theory accounts for impulse propagation in the following way. In an 'excited' patch of membrane the net ionic current is inward; part of this net inward current does not flow out across the local patch of membrane, but spreads along the longitudinal axis of the fibre to flow out across the membrane there. This outward flow of current reduces the membrane potential difference between the two regions by depolarizing it. There is an apparent paradox in this account because further depolarization in the 'just excited' region is explained by a net inward ionic current flow, whereas the depolarization ahead of the 'excited' region is accounted for by outward current flow. The paradox is resolved by considering the capacitative current flow − it is outward in both these regions, and it is this flow that indicates the *direction* of membrane potential movement. In the middle of the excited patch (just beyond the peak of the action potential) the capacitative current flow becomes inward as the direction of membrane potential change becomes repolarizing. Fig. 14.5 illustrates the currents flowing (for a detailed description, see Jack, Noble and Tsien, 1975, Chapter 9).

In this figure it will be noticed that the abscissa can be represented as either distance or time. This follows from the additional assumption that the axon properties and size are constant with distance. The action potential will then propagate at constant velocity, θ, so that

$$\theta = \frac{x}{t} \quad \text{i.e.} \quad x = \theta.t \tag{14.31}$$

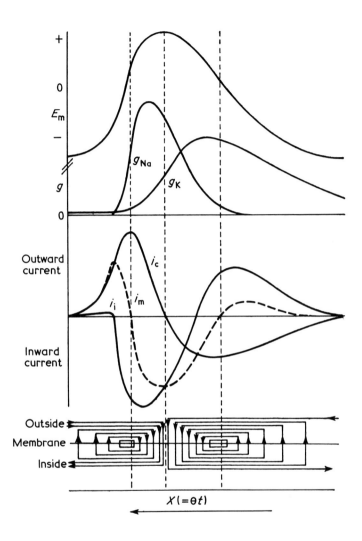

Fig. 14.5 Changes in conductance and currents flowing across the membrane during a propagated action potential. The abscissa is common to all the curves and represents either distance or time ($X = \theta t$). The vertical dashed lines join corresponding points on the figure. The uppermost curve shows the course of the membrane potential schematically, the one beneath the changes in sodium and potassium conductance, and the next the course of ionic and capacitative currents and of their algebraic sum, the membrane current (– – – –). The lowermost part of the figure shows the 'local circuit' currents. Note that the net axial current changes direction at the peak of the action potential (as does the capacitative current) whereas the ionic and membrane currents reverse their direction at other points. The membrane potential depolarizes substantially before there is any change in the value of g_{Na} or g_K because of 'local circuit' current flow. (Reproduced from Noble (1966).)

Substitution of equation (14.31) into equation (14.30) leads to

$$\frac{1}{r_a \theta^2} \cdot \frac{\partial^2 V}{\partial t^2} = c_m \frac{\partial V}{\partial t} + i_i$$

or

$$\frac{a}{2R_i \theta^2} \frac{\partial^2 V}{\partial t^2} = C_m \frac{\partial V}{\partial t} + I_i \tag{14.32}$$

where a is fibre radius, R_i intracellular resistivity ($= r_a/\pi a^2$), C_m membrane capacitance per unit area ($= c_m/2\pi a$) and I_i is membrane ionic current per unit area ($= i_i/2\pi a$).

This is a much less complicated equation to solve than the full partial differential equation (14.30) and it was solved by Hodgkin and Huxley (1952d) when their description of the voltage and time dependence of the ionic currents was incoporated. Unfortunately it is still quite a laborious computation, because a value of θ has to be guessed and then successive approximations made until the correct value of θ is obtained.

In myelinated nerve the 'local circuit' theory account is modified, to take account of the periodic structure of the nerve axon (see Huxley and Stämpfli, 1949; Tasaki, 1953; Stämpfli, 1954). There is good evidence that inward (i.e. sodium) currents are only generated at the nodes of Ranvier, while the internodes, covered with myelin, do not act as current generators. The local circuit current therefore has to spread along the internode in order to achieve excitation at the next node. The equations giving a complete description of propagation are accordingly much more complicated than for the unmyelinated axon (see Fitzhugh, 1962, 1969, 1973; Goldman and Albus, 1968; Hutchinson, Koles and Smith, 1970; Hardy, 1973b).

Simple models

In order to get some insight into the factors influencing the conduction velocity it is necessary, just as for excitation, to seek simplified models of the propagation process. Since the late 1930's there has been a profusion of such models whose features are reviewed in Fitzhugh (1969), Jack, Noble and Tsien (1975) and Hunter, McNaughton and Noble (1975). The most realistic, for unmyelinated axons, are those developed by Hunter *et al.* (1975), which assume that the recovery processes of the action potential (sodium inactivation and potassium activation) can be neglected. In terms of the Hodgkin-Huxley description this means

$$g_{Na} = \bar{g}_{Na} \cdot (m(t))^3 h_0, \qquad g_K = \text{constant}$$

where h_0 is a constant equal to the resting value of h. In one of their simplified models the rate constant (α) for change of m is not voltage-dependent, but, as

Hunter *et al.* discuss, this is not an unreasonable approximation over most of the range of the rising phase of the action potential. This model makes the following prediction

$$\theta \propto d^{1/2} R_i^{-1/2} C_m^{-5/8} \alpha_m^{3/8} \tilde{g}_{Na}^{1/8} \tag{14.33}$$

where d is fibre diameter, R_i is specific axoplasmic resistivity, C_m membrane capacitance per unit area, α_m the rate constant and $\tilde{g}_{Na}$ the maximal possible value of sodium conductance ($= \bar{g}_{Na} \cdot h_0$).

Hunter *et al.* have also presented models in which the rate constant can have a realistic (i.e. like the Hodgkin-Huxley description) dependence on voltage. From such models that have derived another equation of some experimental importance

$$\theta \propto (\dot{V}_{max} \cdot y)^{1/2} \tag{14.34}$$

where $\dot{V}_{max}$ is the maximum rate of rise of the action potential (i.e. the maximal value of dV/dt) and y is a 'shape factor' (shape referring to the particular time course of the rising phase). Thus, if the shape remains roughly constant, the conduction velocity is proportional to the square root of the maximum rate of rise. Combining equation (14.33) and the simpler form of equation 14.34 leads to (see Hunter *et al.*, equation (5.3))

$$\theta = K d^{1/2} R_i^{-1/2} C_m^{-5/8} \dot{V}_{max}^{1/2}. \tag{14.35}$$

Since R_i and C_m have been found to be roughly constant in unmyelinated axons of different sizes (e.g. Weidmann, 1951) this equation may assist experimentalists to estimate either fibre diameter or conduction velocity if only two measurements can be made on the axons. An alternative means of making such an estimate, from the time course of the rising phase of the action potential, has been given by Pickard (1969).

The models of Hunter *et al.* suffer from one major lack — recovery processes are not considered. This is most evident when dealing with the problem of the 'safety factor' for nerve conduction. Intuitively this term is intended to include some indication of the likelihood of conduction failure; but conduction does not fail in their models until the maximal value of the sodium conductance is reduced to such a level that the integral of the total current-voltage relation (integrated between the resting potential and the third zero-current point, see Fig. 14.4) is positive (i.e. net outward current) rather than negative (i.e. net inward current). This is also the condition in which the fibre is inexcitable (to 'point polarization'). In real axons the 'early' current-voltage relation can have an integral which is negative, but the recovery processes take place relatively too quickly for conduction to be possible. This is best exemplified by two examples: progressive reduction in the value of $\bar{g}_{Na}$ (for example, by blocking some of the sodium channels with tetrodotoxin, etc.) and the condition of 'heat block'. In the former case, computations for the standard Hodgkin-Huxley model of the squid axon, at 6.3°C, have shown that when the sodium conductance *alone* is reduced to less than one quarter of its usual value, conduction fails, but that if the sodium, potassium and leak conductances are all reduced together conduction does not fail until they are all about one twentieth of the usual value (see Colquhoun and Ritchie, 1972, Fig. 1). Similarly, the condition of 'heat block' occurs in the full model of the squid axon when the temperature is raised above about 45°C (in a real axon it occurs at about 36°C, see Chapman, 1967) because the prime effect of an increase in temperature is to increase the value of all rate constants (for m, h and n). At low temperatures the rate-limiting factor in the development of the recovery processes is their rate constant; but as they are increased the rate-limiting factor becomes the maximal rate of rise of the action potential (which is set by the value of the membrane capacitance and the maximal sodium conductance, neither of which are very temperature sensitive, as well as the rate constant for m). At some critical point the recovery processes 'catch up' sufficiently on the activation of the sodium conductance, so that the peak value of the action potential progressively falls and eventually is too small to sustain sufficient local circuit current for propagation to proceed.

This particular dissatisfaction with the simplified models can in part be rectified by a mathematical technique ('dimensional analysis') developed by Huxley (1959). He took equation (14.32) and considered the effects of modifying (1) the maximal value of *all* membrane conductances (by a factor, η,); (2) the membrane capacity (by a factor γ), and (3) *all* the rate constants (by a factor, ϕ). Equation (14.32) then becomes

$$\frac{a}{2R_i\theta^2\gamma C_m}\frac{d^2 V}{dt^2} = \frac{dV}{dt} + \frac{\eta I_i(\phi t)}{\gamma C_m}. \tag{14.36}$$

Letting $\tau = \phi t$ this equation changes to

$$\frac{\phi}{K}\frac{d^2 V}{d\tau^2} = \frac{dV}{d\tau} + \frac{\eta}{\gamma\phi}\frac{I_i(\tau)}{C_m} \tag{14.37}$$

where $K = 2R_i\theta^2\gamma C_m/a$

Thus for a value of $\eta/\gamma\phi$ for which conduction is possible there will be an appropriate value of ϕ/K. Let $\beta = \eta/\gamma\phi$, then

$$\frac{K}{\phi} = f(\beta)$$

where $f(\beta)$ needs to be determined. From the definition of K

$$\theta = \sqrt{\left(\frac{a}{2R_i\gamma C_m}\cdot\phi f(\beta)\right)}. \tag{14.38}$$

Huxley (1959) determined the value of $f(\beta)$, for various values of β, by numerical computation of equation (14.32). $f(\beta)$ monotonically increased as β increased.

The elegance of Huxley's analysis lies in the fact that once the relationship between β and $f(\beta)$ has been determined, the conduction velocity can be exactly predicted for any axon, as long as its difference from the squid axon can be characterized by the three modifications listed above. The following qualitative predictions also follow directly from his treatment:

(a) An increase in all ionic currents must lead to an increase in conduction velocity (and vice versa) since η is present only in the numerator of the argument of $f(\beta)$.

(b) Conduction velocity must always decrease as membrane capacity is increased (and vice versa) since γ appears, both times, in the denominator of equation (14.38).

(c) The effects of changing the rate constants will be complicated, since it appears in both the numerator and denominator of equation (14.38). Since $f(\beta)$ monotonically increases as β increases, one can predict that there will be an optimal value of ϕ at which conduction velocity is greatest. This prediction is important, since the main effect of an increase in temperature is to increase ϕ, so that there will be a temperature at which conduction velocity is maximal (see Huxley, 1959; Chapman, 1967).

Some simplified models of myelinated nerve fibres have been developed (e.g. Offner, Weinberg and Young, 1940; Landahl and Podolsky, 1949; Huxley and Stämpfli, 1949; Pickard, 1966; Namerow and Kappl, 1969; Deutsch, 1969), but the difficulties involved in making these realistic are immense. Reference to Hunter *et al.* will indicate that, at least for the unmyelinated axon, the conduction velocity can be very sensitive to the exact characteristics of the ionic current behaviour and it would be surprising if the same were not true for the myelinated axon (see Hardy, 1973b). Fortunately the myelinated axon is more amenable to 'dimensional analysis' (Rushton, 1951; Fitzhugh, 1973) but since the theories presented deal primarily with the effect of geometric factors, discussion of them will be deferred until later (see *Properties related to fibre size*).

To what extent do the simplified models or indeed the full Hodgkin-Huxley type of model, accurately predict conduction velocity? It was noted in the section on *The mechanism of the action potential* p. 770 that there was a quantitatively significant current, the 'gating current', that needed to be added to the Hodgkin-Huxley description. This will therefore be discussed, before considering the experimental observations and theoretical predictions of the effects of changes in external sodium concentration and temperature.

Effect of gating current

Hodgkin (1975) first drew attention to the fact that the gating current could have a significant effect on the conduction velocity, because it would act as an additional, non-linear, membrane capacitance: the larger the gating current, the larger the total effective membrane capacitance and hence the lower the conduction velocity. If it is correct to associate the gating current with the movement of m gates, then it follows that there will be an optimal number of sodium channels, because an increase in gating current would be associated with a larger value of $\bar{g}_{Na}$; this latter factor would, on it own, tend to increase conduction velocity. Hodgkin (1975) made a quantitative estimate of the optimal number of channels, both by the use of simple models (see also Hunter *et al.*, 1975) and also by using Huxley's (1959) 'dimensional' analysis, and he concluded that the optimal number was about 1000 channels/μm^2, the curve having a fairly flat maximum so that small deviations from this density would make little difference to the conduction velocity. As he pointed out, this figure was not completely secure since, in order to make the estimate, the gating mechanism had to be assumed to be equivalent to a fixed capacity (but, see Hunter *et al.*, 1975).

Adrian (1975) took up this problem and computed an equation of the form of (14.32) with the gating current modelled as indicated earlier. Hodgkin and Huxley (1952d) had already calculated the conduction velocity, without gating currents, and obtained a value of 18.8 ms^{-1} ($a = 238$ μm, $R_i = 35.4$ Ω cm, $C_m = 1$ μF cm^{-2}, $\bar{g}_{Na} = 120$ mS cm^{-2}, temperature = $18.5°$C). This was compared with the experimentally observed value of 21.2 m s^{-1}. Adrian repeated this calculation (with the resting potential set at -70 mV, instead of Hodgkin and Huxley's -62 mV, by a change in the zero-current potential for the leak conductance) and, for the same values listed above, found a value of 18.5 ms^{-1}. Adding the gating current (with C_m adjusted down to 0.88 μF cm^{-2} so that the total membrane capacity deduced from the time course of the foot of the action potential was 1.0 μF cm^{-2}) lead, in Adrian's calculation, to a conduction velocity of 14.7 ms^{-1}. This deviates significantly from the experimental value of 21.2 m s^{-1}.

Various forms of 'special pleading' might be proposed to resolve this apparent difficulty, but one at least of these can probably be ruled out. Since a precise description of the behaviour of the gating current is a subject of controversy, it might be thought that an alternative description would be of help. But any gating current, whatever its magnitude and kinetics, will tend to reduce the predicted conduction velocity and so exacerbate an already existing discrepancy (theory, 18.8 m s^{-1}; experiment, 21.2 m s^{-1}). In any case, this is not the only difficulty faced by Hodgkin-Huxley models in predicting conduction velocity.

Effect of change in $[Na^+]_0$

The Hodgkin-Huxley description of the squid axon can be used to predict the effects of changes in external sodium concentration on the conduction velocity of the nerve impulse. The qualitative result is that raising $[Na^+]_0$ should increase velocity, while lowering it should lead to a decrease in velocity. The magnitude of the changes will depend on the assumption made about the concentration dependence of the conductance, and on whether a change in $[Na^+]_0$ leads to any concomitant change in $[Na^+]_i$. Such a relationship could come about as a result of the effect on $[Na^+]_0$ on the rate of activity of the sodium pump – a decrease in $[Na^+]_0$ tending to increase the rate and hence, with a time course depending on the volume/surface ratio of the axon, lead to a decrease in $[Na^+]_i$. In the squid axon, having a diameter of about 500 μm, the volume/surface ratio is very large; the time course would be of the order of hours (Hodgkin and Keynes, 1955a) and can thus be neglected.

On the independence principle, a change in $[Na^+]_0$, with $[Na^+]_i$ constant, will lead to a different value for the sodium current, given by

$$i'_{Na} = i_{Na} \cdot \frac{[Na^+]'_0}{[Na^+]_0} \cdot \frac{1 - \exp[(E - E_{Na}')F/RT]}{1 - \exp[(E - E_{Na})F/RT]} \qquad (14.39)$$

where the stroke indicates the new values. Computations using this equation (and with $i_{Na} = m^3 h \bar{g}_{Na}$, etc.) have been performed by Colquhoun and Ritchie (1972). They found, for example, that halving the external sodium concentration leads to a decrease of conduction velocity to about 0.75 of its original value (see their Fig. 1B). This prediction seems to be in good accord with the observation of Hodgkin and Katz (1949) that the conduction velocity was reduced to 70 per cent in a squid axon bathed in half normal $[Na^+]_0$ (single experiment). The agreement may be spurious, however, because Colquhoun and Ritchie's computation was performed in the absence of the gating current. It is not possible, without further computation, to estimate the exact effect of the gating current in this circumstance because Huxley's dimensional analysis does not apply when the magnitude of only one of the conductances changes. An estimate in these circumstances might be much lower than 0.75 (or 0.7) since, as Huxley has shown, there is a much greater effect of an increased capacity when the values of the ion conductances are small.

Even if the result obtained for squid axon is roughly in accordance with that expected, the same is not true for either crab unmyelinated nerve or frog myelinated nerve fibres. Katz (1937) studied the effect of a reduction in external sodium ion on the conduction velocity of single crab nerve fibres, and found that halving the external concentration lowered the conduction velocity by only 4 per cent. This is a surprisingly small change since it would be predicted from equation (14.39) that the effect on the value of the maximal sodium conductance would be to halve it (i.e. assuming that E'_{Na} is not significantly different from E_{Na}). The minimal effect of this change of sodium conductance can in turn be estimated from the delayed activation model of Hunter et al., where

$$\theta \propto \tilde{g}_{Na}^{1/8}.$$

Assuming no change in membrane potential (i.e. h_0 remains constant), the minimal change in θ would be 8.3 per cent. Katz's result could be explained if the lowered sodium concentration led to a hyperpolarization and hence a significant increase in h_0, but it does raise the question of whether the independence principle is indeed applicable. If, instead, the sodium conductance was linear with a square root concentration dependence, the expected minimal change in θ(with no change in h_0) would be 4.2 per cent. These calculations ignore the effect of any gating current, and also of changes in external resistance, on conduction velocity; both of these factors would tend to decrease the velocity still further in the presence of a low external sodium concentration. It seems possible, therefore, that Katz's result can best be explained by assuming that lowered sodium *both* increases the value of h_0 and lowers maximal sodium conductance by an amount less than that predicted by the independence principle.

Colquhoun and Ritchie (1972) have presented similar results for mammalian unmyelinated nerve fibres, but in this case there is no difficulty in explaining their observations. A reduction of external sodium to 50 per cent produced, on average (see their Figs. 3, 4 and 6) a reduction in θ to 0.84, whereas 10 per cent $[Na^+]_0$ gave a mean value of 0.43. Since these fibres are small, there may have been adjustments in the value of $[Na^+]_i$ such that E_{Na} may have remained relatively constant. On the Hunter *et al.* model, the independence principle assumption would predict *minimal* reductions of θ to 0.92 (50 per cent $[Na]_0$ and 0.75 (10 per cent $[Na]_0$) because

$$\frac{\theta'}{\theta} \propto \left(\frac{[Na^+]'_0}{[Na^+]_0} \right)^{1/8}$$

whereas the square root assumption would lead to

$$\frac{\theta'}{\theta} = \left(\frac{[Na^+]'_0}{[Na^+]_0} \right)^{1/16}$$

and hence minimal reductions to 0.96 and 0.87 respectively. Since the observed reductions are greater than either of these sets of predictions they present no serious conflict: a greater reduction than predicted can, for example, be explained by assuming that the recovery processes intervene more effectively at lower sodium concentrations.

A careful study of the consequences of changes in external sodium on single fibres of frog myelinated merve has been made by Hardy (1973a,b). He found empirically that the following equation gave a good fit to his results

$$\frac{\theta'}{\theta} = \left(\frac{[Na^+]'_0}{[Na^+]_0} \right)^{0.524}$$

This is a much steeper dependence on external sodium than would have been predicted from either of the simple models for unmyelinated nerve but such models are unlikely to be applicable to this much more complicated structure.

Using the voltage-clamp description of the currents at the frog node of

Ranvier of Dodge and Hille, Hardy (1973b) compared the computed predictions for conduction velocity with those observed experimentally, His first difficulty was that, using the mean value reported earlier for myelin resistance and capacitance, and for nodal capacitance and 'leakage' and maximal sodium conductance, the predicted conduction velocity was only about half of the observed value and the time course of the action potential was also significantly different. Good agreement could be obtained, however, by selecting particular values of these parameters near to the previously observed range.

As reported earlier, it is usually accepted that the sodium conductance in amphibian node obeys the constant field/independence principle for concentration and voltage dependence. With this assumption, Hardy (1973b) found a large discrepancy between predicted and observed behaviour of the conduction velocity, when $[Na^+]_0$ was changed. The deviation was at low values of $[Na^+]_0$; the observed conduction velocity being about 50 per cent larger than predicted when $[Na^+]_0$ was one quarter of its normal value. As discussed earlier, this discrepancy would become larger if the computations had included the gating current that has been observed at the amphibian node (Nonner, Rojas and Stämpfli, 1975a). Hardy (1973b) considered some possible explanations for this phenomenon and favoured an explanation that the kinetic behaviour of the sodium conductance differs slightly from that described in Dodge's voltage clamp studies. Nevertheless, as he pointed out, the behaviour of the α_m rate constant would have to be sensitive to changes in $[Na^+]_0$. An alternative explanation, of course, is that the sodium conductance is less concentration dependent than the independence principle predicts. A quite different possibility, applicable to nerves conducting faster than predicted, is that sodium ion is not the only important inward charge carrier — another conductance, such as a calcium conductance, may have a significant effect, particularly in conditions of low sodium concentration.

Effect of temperature

The usual way of reporting the effect of temperature on biological variables is to quote a Q_{10}. This is defined as the factor by which a variable changes, for a temperature change of $10°C$. Thus, if conduction velocity doubles in value for a $10°C$ increase in temperature, the Q_{10} is 2.0. Extrapolation both within and outside the temperature range studied can be made on the assumption that a semi-logarithmic relationship exists between the change in the variable and the change in temperature. Taking the above example, if the temperature increases by $7.3°C$ then the conduction velocity will increase by a factor of $2^{7.3/10}$ $= 1.66$, whereas a $16°C$ increase will lead to an almost exact trebling of conduction velocity ($2^{16/10} = 3.03$). Extrapolation outside the measured temperature range is liable to be less accurate; for example, some nerve fibres show a fairly linear relationship between conduction velocity and temperature (Paintal, 1965); another way of describing this result is to say that the Q_{10}

varies systematically with the absolute level of temperature at which it is measured.

There are two types of nerve fibre in which the Hodgkin-Huxley type of description is available, as well as data about the temperature dependence of the relevant variables, including conduction velocity. For the squid giant axon the Q_{10} for all rate constants is roughly 3.0, the maximal conductances 1.5 and the axoplasmic conductivity 1.3 (see Huxley, 1959). Huxley pointed out that his dimensional analysis could then provide an indication of the Q_{10} for conduction velocity and he obtained a figure of 1.74 for the range 10–20°C. Chapman (1967) was the first to report careful measurements of the changes in conduction velocity associated with temperature variation for the squid giant axon. He found good agreement between predicted and observed changes in the range 5–25°C (where the Q_{10}'s for rate constants etc. had been measured earlier). The observed Q_{10} for the conduction velocity between 10° and 20°C was 1.7 ± 0.03 (S.D.). There thus seemed to be very satisfactory agreement between the Hodgkin-Huxley theory and observed behaviour.

The theoretical prediction did not, however, include the effects of 'gating current'. On the assumption that this current is associated with the movement of m gates, a Q_{10} of 3 would be expected for the rate of charge movement. This is, in fact, close to the observed average value of 2.5 ± 0.3 (Keynes and Rojas, 1974). Adrian (1975) computed the values for the Q_{10} of conduction velocity of the Hodgkin-Huxley model of the squid axon with and without gating currents. In the range 6.3–18.5°C he obtained a value of 1.49 with gating currents, as compared with 1.67 without (measured from his Fig. 3). The lower Q_{10} without gating current results from the fact that he did not include any effect of temperature on the maximal membrane conductance or axoplasmic conductivity. When this is allowed for, using Huxley's dimensional method, the figures are 1.62 and 1.77. The Q_{10} observed by Chapman for this temperature range is 1.73 (measured from his Fig. 1). Since there is very little scatter in Chapman's data in this range (S.D. of 0.03 for the temperature range 10–20°C), it is evident that there is a discrepancy between the prediction made by the Hodgkin-Huxley model, with gating, and the observed behaviour (the former being nearly four standard deviations away from the mean of the experimental range).

A much bigger discrepancy between theory and experiment turns up in Hardy's (1973a,b) study of frog myelinated nerve fibres. His observations, for variation in temperature around 15°C, gave a Q_{10} of 2.95. The predicted Q_{10} was 1.5. Hardy offered no explanation for this difference. If Hardy had included the effect of gating currents the predicted Q_{10} would have been even lower; this is a general expectation, whatever the exact kinetics of the gating current, because they add a component to the membrane capacitance that will tend to increase with temperature. As mentioned earlier, an increase in membrane capacitance must reduce conduction velocity and this will tend to cancel out the velocity increase caused by increases in the rate constants, the maximal membrane conductances and the axoplasmic conductivity.

One can summarize these last three sections very simply. The fit between experiment and theory for propagation of the action potential seemed to be reasonably good within the context of the original Hodgkin-Huxley description. Since the discovery of gating currents, and their incorporation into the model, the agreement is much less good. The observed value of the conduction velocity is too high, as is the Q_{10} for this process. At low external sodium the disagreement between predicted and observed velocity becomes even greater. All this evidence points to the need for a careful reassessment of the Hodgkin-Huxley model. The areas most obviously calling for careful experimental checking are the details of the kinetics of the voltage-time dependent conductances, their concentration dependence and, not least, a new study of the Q_{10} of the maximal value of the conductances. The last suggestion is of particular importance because, if it was found that this Q_{10} was substantially higher than 1.5 it would provide a simple explanation, not only of the Q_{10} of the velocity, but also of the smaller than predicted variation in net sodium influx with temperature, observed by Cohen and Landowne (1974). Another possibility is that at least some of the discrepancies may arise because the external 'series resistance' has not been incorporated into the computational modelling (see Hodgkin, 1975).

14.3 Properties related to fibre size

Nerve fibres vary widely in size, even within one animal, so it is naturally of interest to consider what the consequences of size are for their electrophysiological properties. As in the previous section, discussion will be largely confined to the effects on excitation and propagation of the action potential.

It is natural to start with the assumption that the only difference between nerve fibres of one type (i.e. myelinated or unmyelinated) is their size. It is then possible to predict their properties by the method of dimensional analysis (Rushton, 1951; Huxley, 1959; Fitzhugh, 1969). Providing this theory is correct, any observed deviation from such predictions then implies some failure of the initial assumption. A brief review following this line of argument has recently been published (Jack, 1975).

14.3.1 *Dimensional analysis*

The most complete discussion of nerve dimensional analysis in the literature is that given by Fitzhugh (1973); the prime concern of this section is to derive 'scaling relations' for fibre size, and readers interested in a more complete presentation are referred to Fitzhugh's paper.

Unmyelinated nerve fibres

The treatment of equation (14.32) in the previous section has already provided the expected 'scaling relation' for conduction velocity:

$$\theta \propto a^{1/2} \tag{14.40}$$

This prediction assumes that the external resistance can be neglected, and that the cross-section of the nerve fibre is circular. These factors can be readily allowed for, however (see Hodgkin, 1954; Fitzhugh, 1973):

$$\theta \propto \frac{1}{\sqrt{\left[S\left(\dfrac{R_i}{A} + r_e \right) \right]}} \propto \frac{1}{\sqrt{\left[S\left(\dfrac{R_i}{A} + \dfrac{R_e}{h} \right) \right]}} \tag{14.41}$$

where S is the membrane perimeter, A the cross-sectional area, r_e the external resistance per unit length, R_e the external resistivity and h the thickness of the 'shell' of external fluid. In experimental conditions the external resistance may be sufficiently high to lower conduction velocity (e.g. if the fibre is immersed in paraffin oil), but *in vivo* it is probably not a significant factor; so that, other things being equal, the conduction velocity will be proportional to the square root of the volume/surface ratio (= fibre radius or diameter, if circular).

The 'scaling relation' for excitation has been considered by Fitzhugh (1973) and Jack, Noble and Tsien (1975). Two possibilities need to be considered, depending on whether the current is applied by an intracellular microelectrode or by external electrodes. In the former case only the effects of fibre size on current distribution need to be considered. There are two effects:

(1) Distribution with axial distance: If the applied current is scaled so that the same voltage is achieved at the point of stimulation, the distribution of voltage with distance will scale with the square root of the fibre radius (see Noble and Stein, 1966), and hence the amount of current needed also tends to scale, with the square root of radius.

(2) Distribution radially: The larger the radius, the greater the circumference of the fibre. In order to keep current density per unit membrane area constant the current must scale, for this reason, with the fibre radius.

Combining these two considerations, one obtains the result that the current threshold for intracellular stimulation must scale as the 3/2 power of the fibre radius. If the fibre is not circular similar reasoning leads to the result

$$I_{th} \propto \sqrt{(AS)}. \tag{14.42}$$

In the above reasoning extracellular resistance has been neglected, but Fitzhugh (1973) has obtained the same result if h scales with a (or S).

If stimulation is brought about by external electrodes a simple result can be deduced when there is a large separation between the two electrodes; in such a situation the distribution of current between the different nerve fibres in a bundle will depend on fibre radius since the main resistance to current flow will be provided by the axial resistance, r_a (i.e. neglecting the contribution of membrane resistance). Since axial resistance is inversely proportional to the square of the radius, the scaling property for external stimulation between widely separated electrodes will be

$$I_{th} \propto a^{3/2} \cdot a^{-2} \propto a^{-1/2} \tag{14.43}$$

or, for non-circular fibres,

$$I_{th} \propto \sqrt{(AS)} \cdot A^{-1} \propto \sqrt{\frac{S}{A}} \tag{14.44}$$

Thus, in contrast to intracellular stimulation in which the current threshold is much greater in larger fibres, with extracellular stimulation of a nerve trunk the largest fibres have the lowest current threshold. (This conclusion differs from that reached by Fitzhugh [1973], but he does not appear to have considered the preferential distribution of extracellular current into larger fibres).

Myelinated nerve fibres

In myelinated fibres, analysis of the scaling relations is complicated by the many geometrical factors which have to be considered. Rushton (1951), Goldman and Albus (1968), Pickard (1969) and Fitzhugh (1969, 1973) have all discussed the problems, with Fitzhugh (1973) giving the most complete treatment. If we continue with the assumption that all myelinated fibres (in an animal species) are made of the same materials then scaling relations can be readily derived providing the following geometric conditions are satisfied (Fitzhugh, 1973)

$$l \propto D \left[\frac{\ln \partial}{R_i \partial^2 + R_e D/4h} \right]^{1/2} \tag{14.45}$$

and

$$\alpha \propto D[(R_i d^2 + R_e D/4h) \ln \partial]^{-1/2} \tag{14.46}$$

where l is internodal length, D external fibre diameter, $\delta(= D/d)$ is the ratio of external to axoplasmic diameter (d), α is nodal area and the other symbols have their usual meaning. If external resistance can be neglected these simplify to

$$l \propto d(\ln \delta)^{1/2} \tag{14.47}$$

$$\alpha \propto d(\ln \delta)^{-1/2} \tag{14.48}$$

There is evidence that real myelinated axons do obey equation (14.47) (Rushton, 1951; Coppin and Jack, unpublished), but it is less certain that equation (14.48) is obeyed (see Coppin, 1973).

On the assumption that both equations are indeed obeyed, Fitzhugh (1973) has given the scaling relation for conduction velocity

$$\theta \propto D \left[\frac{\ln \delta}{R_i \delta^2 + R_e D/4h} \right]^{1/2} \tag{14.49}$$

Neglecting extracellular resistance, this gives

$$\theta \propto D \left[\frac{\ln \delta}{R_i \delta^2} \right]^{1/2} \propto d \left[\frac{\ln \delta}{R_i} \right]^{1/2} \tag{14.50}$$

If the fibres are not circular in cross-section, equation (14.50) becomes

$$\theta \propto \left(\frac{A \ln \delta}{R_i} \right)^{1/2} \tag{14.51}$$

where A denotes the cross-sectional area of the axoplasm.

The scaling of current for excitation can be obtained by similar reasoning to that given for unmyelinated fibres. With an intracellular electrode inserted at a node of Ranvier it can be shown (Jack, unpublished) that the following proportionality relationship for the 'input conductance' (G_{in}) holds approximately

$$G_{in} \propto d(\ln \delta)^{-1/2} \tag{14.52}$$

and the current required to reach the same voltage at the point of current injection (in the steady state, at least) is thus

$$I_{th} \propto d(\ln \delta)^{-1/2}. \tag{14.53}$$

With extracellular electrodes widely spaced on a nerve trunk the threshold current for different sized fibres will therefore be

$$I_{th} \propto d^{-1} (\ln \delta)^{-1/2} \tag{14.54}$$

It is therefore possible to conclude that for both unmyelinated and myelinated fibres the threshold current for extracellular stimulation (when the fibres have identical membrane properties and extracellular resistance can be neglected) is inversely proportional to the predicted conduction velocity. Expressing the effects of extracellular stimulation by means of electrical excitability (reciprocal of current threshold) this means

$$E \propto \theta \tag{14.55}$$

for both myelinated and unmyelinated fibres (where E denotes excitability).

One further equation that is of value in interpreting experimental data is the relationship between the extracellularly recorded action potential, when recorded monophasically (V_e). This is given by (see Hodgkin and Rushton, 1946; Hodgkin, 1947b; Stein and Pearson, 1971)

$$V_e = V_m \cdot \frac{r_e}{r_a + r_e} \tag{14.56}$$

where V_m is the transmembrane potential. When the extracellular resistance is very low (and the amplitude of V_e hence small in comparison with V_m) this simplifies to

$$V_e \approx V_m \cdot \frac{r_e}{r_a} \approx \frac{V_m \cdot r_e \cdot A}{R_i} \tag{14.57}$$

$$\propto \frac{V_m \cdot r_e \cdot d^2}{R_i} \quad \text{(if the fibres are circular)} \tag{14.58}$$

14.3.2 Experimental results and their interpretation

As discussed in Jack (1975), there is clear evidence for both unmyelinated and myelinated fibres that their properties do not scale as predicted with fibre size. Although the evidence for any one fibre type in a single animal species is not always complete, the following generalizations seem to hold:

(1) In smaller fibres the conduction velocity is slower than predicted, so that the relationship between conduction velocity and fibre diameter tends to be a higher power than anticipated. For example, in insect unmyelinated fibres, Pearson, Stein and Malhotra (1970) found that

$$\theta \propto A^{0.35}$$

whereas the expected relationship would be

$$\theta \propto A^{0.25}$$

on the assumption that $A \propto S^2$ (i.e. constant fibre shape). Similarly in cat myelinated fibres, Coppin and Jack (1972) have deduced that

$$\theta \propto D^{1.5}$$

where D is the measurement of external fibre diameter made by Hursh (1939) and Lubinska (1960) in their studies of the relationship between fibre diameter and internodal length.

(2) In smaller fibres the time course of the action potential is slower. This was reported for insect unmyelinated fibres by Pearson, Stein and Malhotra (1970), and has also been observed in cat unmyelinated and myelinated fibres (Paintal, 1966, 1967). This finding would not be expected from dimensional theory because, if all fibres have the same membrane properties, the time course of the action potential should be constant (see Rushton, 1951; Jack, 1975).

(3) Although there does not seem to be any study of the electrical excitability of unmyelinated nerve fibres in a nerve trunk, the results for cat myelinated nerve fibres have been reported (see Coppin, C.M.L., Fig. 7.12 in Matthews, 1972). There is considerable scatter in the observations, but it is clear that the observed relationship between excitability and conduction velocity is not as predicted — the smaller the fibre the greater the deviation (towards a lower excitability than that expected).

There seems to be one exception to these generalizations: at least amongst larger amphibian myelinated nerve fibres the conduction velocity-fibre diameter relationship is in rough accord with dimensional expectations (see Tasaki, 1953; Hutchinson, Koles and Smith, 1970; Jack, 1975).

There are various possible explanations for these observed discrepancies. Table 14.1 gives a fairly exhaustive list of possible factors, with their effect on various measurable parameters; the predictions are based on dimensional considerations as discussed earlier (see also, Jack, 1975), when only that factor is varied systematically with fibre size. The point of this exercise is to see whether there is a single factor which, when changing with fibre size, could explain all the observed discrepancies. It will be evident from the list that there are four possibilities:

(1) membrane capacitance per unit area varies inversely with fibre size,

(2) maximal membrane conductances are reduced proportionally to fibre size,

(3) the rate constants for the voltage-time-dependent conductances become smaller as fibre size decreases,

(4) the concentration gradients (for sodium and potassium) become smaller as fibre size decreases.

Of these four, two can probably be rejected. According to the computations of Stein and Pearson (1971) based on the Hodgkin-Huxley model of the squid axon, increasing C_m has only a very small effect on the time course of the action potential. But in both unmyelinated (Pearson, Stein and Malhotra, 1970; Paintal, 1967) and myelinated (Paintal, 1966, 1967; Coppin, 1973 – see also, Jack, 1975) nerve fibres the changes in time course are considerable.

Decreasing the rate constants with decreasing size will tend to decrease θ, but increase V_m. Thus, V_e will not be proportional to A. But, in unmyelinated fibres Pearson, Stein and Malhotra (1970) found a good correlation between monophasic amplitude and cross-sectional area. Similarly, in myelinated fibres, Coppin and Jack (unpublished) have found that $V_e \propto \theta^2$ as would predicted as θ is approximately proportional to the square root of axoplasmic cross-sectional area (but, see later).

The only unitary explanations that remain, therefore, are that either the magnitude of the maximal membrane conductances or the concentration gradients decrease with fibre size*. As pointed out by Jack (1975), studies of tetrodotoxin binding in different nerves correlate well with the expectation that the maximal membrane conductances reduce with fibre size; unfortunately the available data is derived from different animal species having (unmyelinated) nerve fibres of different sizes so that some residual uncertainty persists.

There are teleological reasons for expecting that the maximal membrane conductances would decrease with fibre size, which relate to the problem created by the reduced volume/surface ratio of smaller fibres. If all fibres had

---

*An alternative explanation, applicable to myelinated nerve only, is that the nodal area is much larger in smaller fibres than required for dimensional scaling.

TABLE 14.1

Factor	Conduction velocity (θ)	Time course of action potential	Amplitude of action potential (V_m)	Electrical excitability in a nerve trunk (E)
Membrane capacitance (C_m)	Strong inverse effect i.e. increasing C_m decreases θ	Small effect: increasing C_m slows time course	Increasing C_m will tend to reduce V_m	Increasing C_m will reduce E
Axoplasmic resistance (R_i)	$\theta \propto (R_i)^{-1/2}$	No effect	No effect	$E \propto (R_i)^{-1/2}$
All maximal membrane conductances	Decreasing conductances decreases θ	Decreasing conductances slows the time course	Decreasing conductances will tend to reduce V_m	Decreasing conductances will reduce E
All rate constants	Decreasing rate constants will decrease θ	Decreasing rate constants greatly prolong time course	Decreasing rate constants will tend to increase V_m	Decreasing rate constants will tend to reduce E
Fibre shape	$\theta \propto \left(\dfrac{A}{S}\right)^{1/2}$	No effect	No effect	$E \propto \left(\dfrac{A}{S}\right)^{1/2}$ unmyelinated $E \propto \left(\dfrac{A}{S \ln \delta}\right)^{1/2}$ myelinated
Reduced concentration gradients	Decreasing gradients decreases θ	Decreasing gradients slows time course	Decreasing gradients reduces V_m	Decreasing gradients reduces E
External resistance	Increasing r_e decreases θ	No effect	No effect	——

similar membrane properties the same number of action potentials would exhaust the ion concentration gradients in smaller fibres much more quickly. A reduction in the maximal conductances would lead to a smaller sodium influx and potassium efflux per action potential for two reasons. Computations with the standard Hodgkin-Huxley model of the squid axon shows that reduction of all conductances leads to substantial reductions in the net sodium and potassium fluxes per action potential (S. B. Barton, unpublished). Furthermore, if gating current is included in the model, the saving is even greater, because a reduced number of channels means a smaller maximal gating current and hence a smaller effective capacitance (in the limiting case, with a maximally efficient action potential mechanism, the minimal sodium efflux will be directly proportional to the membrane capacitance, for a constant action potential size).

It seems likely therefore, that if a unitary explanation is appropriate the deviations from dimensional expectation observed for both myelinated and unmyelinated nerve fibres are due to a decrease in the density of ionic channels with fibre size. But is a unitary explanation appropriate? There are some slender hints that there may be other contributing factors. In the first place, a decrease in membrane conductances would tend to reduce V_m (and hence, V_e). In the Hodgkin-Huxley model of the squid axon a halving of the conduction velocity is accompanied by nearly a halving in V_m (see Jack, 1975). In cockroach nerve, Pearson, Stein and Malhotra (1970) report that conduction velocity in their smallest axon is less than one quarter of the expected value, so that by analogy with the squid axon model it would be thought that the value of V_m should be substantially reduced. But they also report that there is good agreement between V_e and the measured cross-sectional area of their fibres. On the face of it, there is therefore a substantial inconsistency in their account (they intepreted their results as due to a reduction in all membrane conductances with decreasing fibre size), but the inconsistency may perhaps be resolved by assuming that the recovery processes in these nerves were relatively very slow. This would tend to keep the action potential size constant, as its reduction in the squid axon model is a result of the increasing overlap in timing between sodium activation and the joint process of sodium inactivation and potassium activation, as the rising phase of the action potential tends to become the rate limiting step in changing the resting values of the various gating variables. It would be appropriate, therefore, to compare the results of Pearson *et al.* (1970) with a simple model of impulse propagation. In such models it can be shown that there is an exactly inverse relationship between rise time and maximum rate of rise of the action potential, so that

$$\theta \propto \frac{1}{(\text{Rise time})^{1/2}}.$$

A reduction in conduction velocity to one quarter should therefore be matched by a sixteen-fold increase in rise time. Pearson, Stein and Malhotra do not give values for the rise time, but for action potential duration. They reported that the deviations from predicted conduction velocities were directly proportional to the measured durations (i.e. slightly less than a four-fold difference in duration) and inspection of their records (their Fig. 3) indicates a similar range for the rise time. It therefore seems likely that changes in the maximal value of the conductances cannot provide the sole explanation for their observations.

In cat myelinated nerve fibres a similar study has been made of conduction velocity, rise time and extracellular action potential amplitude (see Coppin, 1973). Unfortunately there is no secure guidance as to the quantitative relationship existing between action potential time course and conduction velocity (for a given fibre size), although Hardy (1973b) has suggested from his computations that θ is roughly porportional to the square root of the maximum rate of rise. Inspection of his figure (Fig. 7) shows that this is a poor description, however, because the form taken is more like

$$\theta \propto \sqrt{(\dot{V}_{max} - \text{constant})}$$

which would, if the points were plotted on a log-log graph, be better described by a higher power than ½. There is another way of considering the experimental data, however. Coppin and Jack deduced that $\theta \propto D^{1.5}$, and since $V_e \propto \theta^2$, $V_e \propto D^3$. The observations were made over a four-fold range of D implying that V_m also varies over a four-fold range (r_e was found to be constant for the different sized fibres). Since the occurrence of a 30 mV action potential seems unlikely (assuming 120 mV for the largest fibres), because of the form of voltage dependence of the gates, either R_i systematically increases as D decreases, or there is a systematic change in fibre shape (with cross-sectional area being increasingly less than that predicted from the value of D^2, and hence d^2, as diameter decreases).

The value of R_i is usually presumed to be set by the ionic content of the axoplasm. Large changes in this value are unlikely since, if the ionic strength was low (without other molecules adjusting the tonicity) it would be expected that movement of water would occur out of the cell until, in the steady state, the ionic strength was the same in all fibres. The observations of Carpenter, Hovey and Bak (1973) are worth noting however. They found that R_i could be as much as twenty times the expected value, and they suggest that this might be due to an ordering of the intracellular water and/or ions. A systematic change in R_i is thus possible.

There is not much evidence for variation of fibre shape with size, but a hint comes from studies made of amphibian skeletal muscle. Håkansonn (1956) studied the relationship between conduction velocity and fibre diameter in isolated fibres and found a linear relationship, i.e. $\theta \propto d$. His method of measuring fibre diameter was to take the average of the major and minor 'diameters', since most fibres tend to be elliptical in cross-section, and such a measure gives a fairly accurate estimate of the circumference of a fibre. Hodgkin and Nakajima (1972b) did not measure diameter directly, but deduced it from the value of r_a. This measure of fibre diameter will be proportional to cross-sectional area. (Hodgkin and Nakajima, (1972a) had already showed, from measures of r_a and A in isolated fibres, that R_i was independent of fibre size.) The relationship found by Hodgkin and Nakajima (1972b) was that conduction velocity was proportional to the fourth root of cross-sectional area. Putting these two observations together leads to the suggestion that $A \propto S^4$ (instead of $A \propto S^2$). In other words, if all fibres are elliptical, the degree of eccentricity increases as fibre size decreases. It is unlikely that this is the whole explanation, since the average ratio of minor to major diameters was 0.8, it is possible that the value of r_e may have been significant in Hodgkin and Nakajima's experiment in which case the change in shape with size might be much smaller, if present at all.

In studies on nerve fibres there is no available evidence for variation in fibre shape, although it is notable that different workers using the same preparation have reached different conclusions about the relationship between conduction velocity and fibre diameter. For example, Hodes (1953) reported that $\theta \propto d$ in squid axons, whereas Young and his colleagues obtained, for the same diameter range, $\theta \propto d^{0.75}$ (Burrows, Campbell, Howe and Young, 1965). It is possible that the differences between these results reflect different techniques for 'diameter' measurement (e.g. whether perimeter or cross-sectional area were measured, and whether or not the fibres had been fixed, since the process of fixation and later preparative measures may produce differential swelling or shrinkage in fibres of different size. It is obvious that the resolution of these discrepancies for both unmyelinated and myelinated (c.f. Hursh, 1939; Boyd and Davey, 1968; Coppin and Jack, 1972) fibres will require attention to the measurement of both perimeter and cross-sectional area.

If it is correct that excitable cells are not circular in cross-section (see Keynes and Ritchie, 1965 and Chapter 2 for unmyelinated nerve fibres, and Berthold, 1968 and Chapter 1 for myelinated nerve fibres), and that the deviation from circularity is greater the smaller the fibre, it is tempting to speculate as to the reason for such an apparently disadvantageous arrangement. It is in fact disadvantageous for two reasons: first, for a given fibre perimeter the conduction velocity will be less than it would be if the fibre were circular, and secondly the volume/surface ratio is reduced even more than is implied by the value for fibre perimeter and thus an even smaller number of action potentials will exhaust the ion concentration gradients.

It has been suggested (Jack, 1975) that the explanation may lie in the fact that fibres tend to swell following a period of activity (Hill, 1950a, b; Lieberman, 1969; Cohen and Keynes, 1971). There are at least two possible causes for this swelling. First when sodium ions replace potassium ions internally they require more water of hydration, and second, if the membrane has a resting anion conductance with an equilibrium potential near to the resting potential, there will be a net flux of those anions (e.g. chloride) into the cell with each action potential, thus reducing the magnitude of the outward movement of potassium ion. Each action potential thus produces a net movement of salt and water into the cell, (and hence swelling) until the ion concentration gradients are restored by the action of the membrane pumps. The smaller the volume/surface ratio of the cell the greater the relative swelling, if each action potential produces the same net flux of ions. It has yet to be established whether such a possibility presents any serious threat to the mechanical integrity of excitable cells, but if if does two things become more intelligible. Smaller cells would tend to deviate further from circularity (which maximizes cross-sectional area for a given perimeter) in order to be better able to withstand the greater relative swelling following a period of activity. Secondly, the tentative conclusion that smaller cells may have smaller maximal conductances can be understood not only as a device to avoid run-down of their concentration gradients, but also as a means to reduce the amoung of swelling relative to that to be expected if they had the same maximal conductances per unit membrane area as larger fibres.

The same reasoning can also be used to explain an unusual feature of myelinated nerve structure – the paranodal folds (see Chapter 1). On the face of it, myelinated nerve fibres have a very large volume/surface ratio because the volume term includes the whole internodal region, whereas the effective surface for inward sodium movement is the nodal area. But there are two problems. Firstly diffusion into the internode is relatively slow and ions may take many minutes to move from the axoplasm adjacent to the node into the centre of the internode (see Hurlbut, 1963; Segal, 1970). Secondly, calculations on the Hodgkin-Huxley type model of myelinated nerve indicate that there is much more net inward flux of sodium ion than there is outward movement of charge (potassium and other cations out, anions in: see Hardy, 1973b, Fig. 2a). The nature of the main component of the resting conductance at the node is unknown, but if it is due to an anion, the net increase of electrolyte in the nodal axoplasm with each action potential would be substantial. Since water movements would also be expected to take place preferentially through the nodal membrane, there is the possibility of substantial local swelling following a burst of action potential activity. The increase in the perimeter of the myelin sheath on either side of the node (Williams and Landon, 1963) could therefore be interpreted as a means of allowing such swelling to occur without placing the sheath under too much mechanical strain.

The above speculations contain an underlying assumption which may be incorrect, viz. that fibres of different sizes are equally likely to undergo periods of intense activity. But the very fact that smaller fibres tend to have longer duration action potentials, and hence longer refractory periods (see Paintal, 1973, for a review), implies that there must be a lower value for their maximal firing frequency, and in any case, the firing frequency of nerve fibres will be set by the particular functional characteristics of the sensory receptor or nerve cell from which the impulses are normally generated. Any teleological speculations concerning the expected properties of different sized nerve fibres therefore need to include information about the normal functional role of the cell type discussed. Since very different functions may be subserved by, for example, receptors which have nerve fibres of similar diameter (see Boyd and Davey, 1968), the particular characteristics of nerve fibres may not be related simply to fibre size (see, for example, Bergman and Stämpfli, 1966).

Two features of the properties of peripheral nerve fibres, particularly in mammalian preparations, need further study. The first is the question of the safety factor for conduction in different types of nerve fibre, and hence their relative susceptibility to block by either 'pathological' (e.g. local anaesthetics, disease such as demyelination) or 'physiological' (e.g. prolonged, intense activity) phenomena. If the only change in nerve fibres of different size was a reduction in their maximal conductances with decreasing diameter, it would be expected that smaller nerve fibres would have a lower safety factor. But once a 'unitary' explanation for the various deviations from dimensional expectation has been abandoned, there is no reason why several factors should not all change together with fibre size. Thus, apart from maximal conductances and fibre shape (or the R_i value) it is also possible that the rate constants for the recovery processes become smaller, relative to that for sodium activation, as fibre size decreases, and this would tend to keep the safety factor fairly constant. Unfortunately it may be very difficult to obtain direct information about such possibilities, since voltage clamp studies on mammalian nerve fibres are unlikely to be easy, and so far, only one preliminary report of some successful experiments has appeared (Horackova, Nonner and Stämpfli, 1968).

A second problem is that of comparing myelinated and unmyelinated fibres. Both fibre types occur in vertebrate peripheral nerve and it is at present far from certain why this should be so. In a classical paper, Rushton (1951) suggested that the prime factor might be the tendency to maximize conduction velocity for a given fibre size. But Rushton's discussion was based on the belief that both myelinated and unmyelinated fibres obeyed dimensional expectations so far as conduction velocity was concerned. There is clear evidence for mammalian peripheral nerve that this assumption is incorrect (see Jack, 1975). The same kind of objection also applies to some of the discussion in Waxman and Bennett (1972), since neither of the conduction velocity–fibre diameter relationships they assumed ($\theta \propto d^{1/2}$, unmyelinated; $\theta \propto D$, myelinated) are likely to be appropriate. Further speculation seems premature until better methods are developed for studying the properties of very small nerve fibres.

14.4 Conclusion

In this chapter little attention has been given to the classification and description of the properties of peripheral nerve. These are admirably reviewed elsewhere (see Boyd and Davey, 1968; Paintal, 1973). Instead, attention has been focussed on the difficulties and uncertainties faced by present descriptions of the basic quantitative features of the resting potential and the action potential, including its excitation and propagation. Although the weight of evidence suggests that we are not likely to be given any major surprises about the qualitative aspects of such an account (unless more decisive for the storage of ions in the membrane (Offner, 1972) is obtained), it seems clear that the quantitative descriptions have a less secure basis.

It is argued that the standard equation for the resting membrane potential (the Goldman-Hodgkin-Katz equation) should be abandoned as this equation gives a misleading description of the relative ease with which various ion species can cross the membrane. It is unlikely that a single *explicit* equation will in fact prove adequate to describe all forms of zero-current potential in biological membranes, but whatever equation is used it requires to be justified by much more careful studies of the voltage and concentration dependence of each conductance component of the membrane.

It is a remarkable tribute to Hodgkin and Huxley that their careful description of the kinetics of the voltage-time-dependent conductances underlying the action potential mechanisms has survived largely intact, despite the profusion of further experimental tests. But it is now clear however that, at the very least, additions and minor modifications have to be made to their formulation. What is less certain is whether a radical reformulation of the kinetics of the gating variables is required. It is likely that there will be considerable problems of non-uniqueness in the predictions of alternative models, and it may therefore be some time before a single model is widely accepted.

This uncertainty has its implications when considering both excitation and propagation of the action potential. The quantitative account of the spread of electrical charge along nerve fibres appears to be correct; but when the theoretical model of the action potential process is married to 'local circuit theory', predictions based upon it do not always match the observations. Most of the discrepancies have emerged in relation to the velocity of propagation, probably because this has been the property most carefully studied. The absolute value of conduction velocity and its sensitivity to changes in temperature or external sodium concentration do not always conform to theoretical expectations, and any new model of the action potential mechanism will obviously have a greater chance of success if it can explain these experimental results.

There is quite good evidence that one or more of the specific membrane properties of peripheral nerve fibres change systematically with fibre size. Further studies are required before it is fruitful to explore the implications of this result in terms of a general theory of the relationship between function and nerve fibre structure.

Acknowledgements

I would like to thank Mr. D. Attwell, Dr I. Cohen, Professor A. L. Hodgkin and Dr D. Noble for their comments on the manuscript. Preparation of this chapter was begun while the author was visiting the Department of Biological Sciences,

Stanford University. I would like to thank Professor D. Kennedy, Dr D. Perkel and Professor N. Wessels for their kind hospitality.

References

Adelman, W. J. (1971) Electrical studies of internally perfused squid axons. In *Biophysics and Physiology of Excitable Membranes*, (ed.) Adelman, W. J., pp. 274–319. van Nostrand Reinhold Co.

Adelman, W. J. and Fitzhugh, R. (1975) Solutions of the Hodgkin-Huxley equations modified for potassium accumulation in a periaxonal space. *Federation Proceedings* **34**, 1322–1329.

Adelman, W. J. and Taylor, R. E. (1961) Leakage current rectification in the squid giant axon. *Nature (London)*, **190**, 883–885.

Adelman, W. J. and Taylor, R. E. (1964) Effects of replacement of external sodium chloride with sucrose on membrane currents of the squid giant axon. *Biophysics Journal*, **4**, 451–463.

Adrian, R. H. (1964) The rubidium and potassium permeability of frog muscle membrane. *Journal of Physiology*, **175**, 134–159.

Adrian, R. H. (1969) Rectification in muscle membrane. *Progress in Biophysics*, **19**, 341–369.

Adrian, R. H. (1975) Conduction velocity and gating current in the squid giant axon. *Proceedings of the Royal Society of London (Series B)*, **189**, 81–86.

Adrian, R. H., Chandler, W. K. and Hodgkin, A. L. (1970) Voltage clamp experiments in striated muscle fibres. *Journal of Physiology*, **208**, 607–644.

Adrian, R. H. and Slayman, C. L. (1966) Membrane potential and conductance during transport of sodium, potassium and rubidium in frog muscle. *Journal of Physiology*, **184**, 970–1014.

Andreoli, T. and Watkins, M. L. (1973) Chloride transport in porous lipid bilayer membrane. *Journal of General Physiology*, **61**, 809–830.

Århem, P., Frankenhaeuser, B. and Moore, L. E. (1973) Ionic currents at resting potential in nerve fibres from *Xenopus Laevis*. Potential clamp experiments. *Acta physiologica scandanavica*, **88**, 446–454.

Armstrong, C. M. (1970) Comparison of g_K inactivation caused by quaternary ammonium ion with g_{Na} inactivation. *Biophysical Society Abstracts*, **10**, 185a.

Armstrong C. M. (1971) Interaction of tetraethylammonium ion derivatives with the potassium channels of giant axons. *Journal of General Physiology*, **58**, 413–437.

Armstrong, C. M. (1974) Ionic pores, gates, and gating currents. *Quarterly Review Biophysics*, **7**, 179–209.

Armstrong, C. M. and Bezanilla, F. (1974) Charge movement associated with the opening and closing of the activation gates of the Na channels. *Journal of General Physiology*, **63**, 533–552.

Armstrong, C. M. and Hille, B. (1972) The inner quaternary ammonium ion receptor in potassium channels of the node of Ranvier. *Journal of General Physiology*, **59**, 388–400.

Atwater, I., Bezanilla, F. and Rojas, E. (1969) Sodium influxes in internally perfused squid giant axon during voltage clamp. *Journal of Physiology*, **201**, 657–664.

Baker, P. F. (1972) Transport and metabolism of calcium ions in nerve. *Progress in Biophysics*, **24**, 177–223.

Baker, P. F. and Connelly, C. M. (1966) Some properties of the external activation site of the sodium pump in crab nerve. *Journal of Physiology*, **185**, 270–297.

Baker, P. F., Foster, R. F., Gilbert, D. S. and Shaw, T. I. (1971) Sodium transport by perfused giant axons of *Loligo*. *Journal of Physiology*, **219**, 487–506.

Baker, P. F. and Glitsch, H. G. (1973) Does metabolic energy participate directly in the Na^+-dependent extrusion of Ca^{++} ions from squid giant axons? *Journal of Physiology*, **233**, 44–46P.

Baker, P. F. and Glitsch, H. E. (1975) Voltage-dependent changes in the permeability of nerve membranes to calcium and other divalent cations. *Philosophical Transactions of the Royal Society of London (Series B)*, **270**, 389–409.

Baker, P. F., Hodgkin, A. L. and Ridgway, E. B. (1971) Depolarization and calcium entry in squid giant axons. *Journal of Physiology*, **218**, 709–755.

Baker, P. F., Hodgkin, A. L. and Shaw, T. I. (1962) The effects of changes in internal ionic concentrations on the electrical properties of perfused giant axons. *Journal of Physiology*, **164**, 355–374.

Baker, P. F., Meves, H. and Ridgway, E. B. (1973a) Effects of manganese and other agents on the calcium uptake that follows depolarization of squid axons. *Journal of Physiology*, **231**, 511–526.

Baker, P. F., Meves, H. and Ridgway, E. B. (1973b) Calcium entry in response to maintained depolarization of squid axons. *Journal of Physiology*, **231**, 527–548.

Baker, P. F. and Potashner, S. J. (1973) The role of metabolic energy in the transport of glutamate by invertebrate nerve. *Biochimica et biophysica acta.*, **318**, 123–139.

Begenisich, T. and Lynch, C. (1974) Effects of internal divalent cations on voltage-clamped squid axons. *Journal of General Physiology*, **63**, 675–689.

Bennett, H. S. (1956) The concepts of membrane flow and membrane vesiculation as mechanisms for active transport and ion pumping. *Journal of Biophysical and Biochemical Cytology*, **2**, Supplement 99–103.

Bergman, C. and Ståmpfli, R. (1966) Différence de perméabilité des fibres nerveuses myelinisées sensorielle et motrices à l'ion potassium. *Helvetica physiologica et pharmacologica acta*, **24**, 247–298.

Berthold, C. H. (1968) A study on the fixation of large mature feline myelinated ventral lumbar spinal-root fibres. *Acta Societates Med. Upsal.*, **73**, Supplement 9, 1–36.

Bezanilla, F. and Armstrong, C. M. (1972) Negative conductance caused by entry of sodium and cesium ions into the potassium channels of squid axons. *Journal of General Physiology*, **60**, 588–608.

Bezanilla, F. and Armstrong, C. M. (1974) Gating currents of the sodium channels: three ways to block them. *Science*, **183**, 753–754.

Bezanilla, F. and Armstrong, C. M. (1975) Kinetic properties and inactivation of the gating currents of sodium channels in squid axon. *Philosophical Transactions of the Royal Society London (Series B)*, **270**, 449–458.

Bezanilla, F., Rojas, E. and Taylor, R. E. (1970a) Time course of the sodium influx in squid giant axon during a single voltage clamp pulse. *Journal of Physiology*, **207**, 151–164.

Bezanilla, F., Rojas, E. and Taylor, R. E. (1970b) Sodium and potassium conductance changes during a membrane action potential. *Journal of Physiology*, **211**, 729–751.

Binstock, L. and Goldman, L. (1971) Rectification in instantaneous potassium current-voltage relations in *Myxicola* giant axons. *Journal of Physiology*, **217**, 517–531.

Blaustein, M. P. and Goldman, D. E. (1968) The action of certain polyvalent cations on the voltage-clamped lobster axon. *Journal of General Physiology*, **51**, 279–291.

Boron, W. F. and de Weer, P. (1975) Studies on the intracellular pH of squid giant axons. *Biophysical Journal*, **15**, 42a.

Boyd, I. A. and Davey, M. R. (1968) *The Composition of Peripheral Nerves*, Edinburgh: Livingstone.

Bregestovski, P. D., Chailachjan, L. M., Dunin-Barkovski, V. L., Potapova, T. W. and Veprintsev, B. N. (1972) Effect of temperature on the equilibrium endplate potential. *Nature (London)*, **236**, 453–454.

Brinley, F. J. (1965) Sodium, potassium and chloride concentrations and fluxes in the isolated giant axon of *Homarus*. *Journal of Neurophysiology*, **28**, 742–772.

Brinley, F. J. and Mullins, L. J. (1965) Ion fluxes and transference number in squid axons. *Journal of Neurophysiology*, **28**, 526–544.

Brinley, F. J. and Mullins, L. J. (1967) Sodium extrusion by internally dialyzed squid axons. *Journal of General Physiology*, **50**, 2303–2331.

Brinley, F. J. and Mullins, L. J. (1968) Sodium fluxes in internally dialyzed squid axons. *Journal of General Physiology*, **52**, 181–211.

Brismar, T. (1973) Effects of ionic concentration on permeability properties of nodal membrane in myelinated nerve fibres of *Xenopus laevis*. Potential clamp experiments. *Acta physiologica scandinavica*, **87**, 474–484.

Brismar, T. and Frankenhaeuser, B. (1972) The effect of calcium on the potassium permeability in the myelinated nerve fibre of *Xenopus laevis*. *Acta physiologica scandinavica*, **85**, 237–241.

Bromm, B. and Esslinger, H. (1974) Ionic permeability at resting potential of Ranvier node. *Proceedings of the International Union of Physiological Sciences*, 26th Int. Congress **11**, 149.

Brown, R. H. (1974) Membrane surface charge: discrete and uniform modelling. *Progress in Biophysics*, **28**, 341–370.

Burrows, T. M. O., Campbell, I. A., Howe, E. J. and Young, J. Z. (1965) Conduction velocity and diameter of nerve fibres of cephalopods. *Journal of Physiology*, **179**, 39–40P.

Bush, B. M. H. and Roberts, A. (1968) Resistance reflexes from a crab muscle receptor without impulses. *Nature (London)*, **218**, 1171–1173.

Caldwell, P. C., Hodgkin, A. L., Keynes, R. D. and Shaw, T. I. (1960) The effects of injecting 'energy-rich' phosphate compounds on the active transport of ions in the giant axons of *Loligo*. *Journal of Physiology*, **152**, 561–590.

Carpenter, D. O. (1973) Electrogenic sodium pump and high specific resistance in nerve cell bodies of the squid. *Science*, **179**, 1336–1338.

Carpenter, D. O., Hovey, M. M. and Bak, A. F. (1973) Measurements of intracellular conductivity in *Aplysia* neurons: evidence for organization of water and ions. *Annals of the New York Academy of Sciences*, **204**, 502–530.

Chandler, W. K., Hodgkin, A. L. and Meves, H. (1965) The effect of changing the internal solution on sodium inactivation and related phenomena in giant axons. *Journal of Physiology*, **180**, 821–836.

Chandler, W. K. and Meves, H. (1965) Voltage clamp experiments on internally perfused giant axons. *Journal of Physiology*, **180**, 788–820.

Chandler, W. K. and Meves, H. (1970) Evidence for two types of sodium conductance in axons perfused with sodium fluoride solution. *Journal of Physiology*, **211**, 653–678.

Chapman, J. B. (1973) On the reversibility of the sodium pump in dialyzed squid axons. A method for determining the free energy of ATP breakdown? *Journal of General Physiology*, **62**, 643–646.

Chapman, R. A. (1967) Dependence on temperature of the conduction velocity of the action potential of the squid giant axon. *Nature (London)*, **213**, 1143–1144.

Ciani, S. M., Eisenman, G., Laprade, R. and Szabo, G. (1973) Theoretical analysis of carrier-mediated electrical properties of bilayer membranes. In *Membranes*, (ed.) Eisenman, G., Vol. 2, pp. 61–177. M. Dekker, Inc: New York.

Ciani, S., Laprade, R., Eisenman, C. and Szabo, G. (1973) Theory for carrier-mediated zero-current conductance of bilayers extended to allow for non-equilibrium of interfacial reactions, spatially dependent mobilities and barrier shape. *Journal of membrane Biology*, **11**, 255–292.

Cohen, H. and Cooley, J. W. (1965) The numerical solution of the time-dependent Nernst-Planck equations. *Biophysical Journal*, **5**, 145–162.

Cohen, L. B. and Keynes, R. D. (1971) Changes in light scattering associated with the action potential in crab nerves. *Journal of Physiology*, **212**, 259–275.

Cohen, L. B. and Landowne, D. (1974) The temperature dependence of the movement of sodium ions associated with nerve impulses. *Journal of Physiology*, **236**, 95–111.

Cole, K. S. (1965) Electrodiffusion models for the membrane of squid giant axon. *Physiology Review*, **45**, 340–379.

Cole, K. S. (1968) *Membranes, Ions and Impulses*. University of California Press: Berkeley.

Cole, K. S. and Moore, J. W. (1960) Potassium ion current in the squid giant axon: Dynamic characteristics. *Biophysical Journal*, **1**, 1–14.

Colquhoun, D., Henderson, R. and Ritchie, J. M. (1972) The binding of labelled tetrodotoxin to non-myelinated nerve fibres. *Journal of Physiology*, **227**, 95–126.

Colquhoun, D. and Ritchie, J. M. (1972) The interaction at equilibrium between tetrodotoxin and mammalian non-myelinated nerve fibres. *Journal of Physiology*, **221**, 533–553.

Connelly, C. M. (1959) Recovery processes and metabolism of nerve. *Review of Modern Physics*, **31**, 475–484.

Conti, F., de Felice, L. J. and Wanke, E. (1975) Potassium and sodium ion current noise in the membrane of the squid giant axon. *Journal of Physiology*, **248**, 45–82.

Cooke, I. M., Leblanc, G. and Tauc, L. (1974) Sodium pump stoichiometry in *Aplysia* neurones from simultaneous current and tracer measurements. *Nature (London)*, **251**, 254–256.

Cooley, J. W. and Dodge, F. A. (1966) Digital computer solutions for excitation and propagation of the nerve impulse. *Biophysical Journal*, **6**, 583–599.

Coppin, C. M. L. (1973) *A Study of the Properties of Mammalian Peripheral Nerve Fibres*. D.Phil. Thesis, University of Oxford.

Coppin, C. M. L. and Jack, J. J. B. (1972) Internodal length and conduction velocity of cat muscle afferent nerve fibres. *Journal of Physiology*, **222**, 91–93P.

Coster, H. G. L. (1973) The double fixed charge membrane. Solution-membrane ion partition effects and membrane potentials. *Biophysical Journal*, **13**, 133–142.

Curtis, H. J. and Cole, K. S. (1942) Membrane resting and action potentials from the squid giant axon. *Journal of Cellular and Comparative Physiology*, **19**, 135–144.

Deutsch, S. (1969) The maximization of nerve conduction velocity. *I.E.E.E. Trans. Systems Science and Cybernetics*, **5**, 86–91.

De Weer, P. and Geduldig, D. (1973) Electrogenic sodium pump in squid giant axon. *Science*, **179**, 1326–1328.

Diamond, J. M. and Wright, E. M. (1969) Biological membranes: The physical basis of ion and nonelectrolytes selectivity. *Annual Review of Physiology*, **31**, 581–646.

Dipolo, R. (1974) Effect of ATP on the calcium efflux in dialyzed squid giant axons. *Journal of General Physiology*, **64**, 503–517.

Dodge, F. A. and Frankenhaeuser, B. (1959) Sodium currents in the myelinated nerve fibre of *Xenopus laevis* investigated with the voltage clamp technique. *Journal of Physiology*, **148**, 188–200.

Ehrenstein, G. and Gilbert, D. L. (1966) Slow changes of potassium permeability in the squid giant axon. *Biophysical Journal*, **6**, 553–566.

Ehrenstein, G. and Gilbert, D. L. (1973) Evidence for membrane surface charge from measurement of potassium kinetics as a function of external divalent cation concentration. *Biophysical Journal*, **13**, 495–497.

Ehrenstein, G. and Lecar, H. (1972) The mechanism of signal transmission in nerve axons. *Annual Review of Biophysics and Bioengineering*, **1**, 347–368.

Eisenberg, R. S. and Johnson, E. A. (1970) Three-dimensional electrical field problems in physiology. *Progress Biophysics*, **20**, 1–65.

Eisenman, G., Sandblom, J. P. and Walker, J. L. (1967) Membrane structure and ion permeation. *Science*, **155**, 965–974.

Eisenman, G., Szabo, G., Ciani, S., McLaughlin, S. and Krasne, S. (1973) Ion binding and ion transport produced by neutral lipid-soluble molecules. *Progress in Surface and Membrane Science*, **6**, 139–241.

Fishman, H. M. (1973) Relaxation spectra of potassium channel noise from squid axon membranes. *Proceedings of the National Academy of Science*, **70**, 876–879.

Fishman, H. M. (1975) Noise measurement in axon membranes. *Federal Proceedings*, **34**, 1330–1337.

Fitzhugh, R. (1962) Computation of impulse initiation and saltatory conduction in a myelinated nerve fiber. *Biophysical Journal*, **2**, 11–21.

Fitzhugh, R. (1969) Mathematical models of excitation and propagation in nerve. In *Biological Engineering*, (ed.) Schwann, H. P., pp. 1–85. McGraw-Hill: New York.

Fitzhugh, R. (1973) Dimensional analysis of nerve models. *Journal of Theoretical Biology*, **40**, 517–541.

Fitzhugh, R. and Cole, K. S. (1973) Voltage and current clamp transients with membrane dielectric loss. *Biophysical Journal*, **13**, 1125–1140.

Førland, T. and Østvold, T. (1974) The biological membrane potential: a thermodynamic approach. *Journal of Membrane Biology*, **16**, 101–120.

Fozzard, H. A. and Schoenberg, M. (1972) Strength-duration curves in cardiac Purkinje fibres: effects of liminal length and charge distribution. *Journal of Physiology*, **226**, 593–618.

Frankenhaeuser, B. (1960) Sodium permeability in toad nerve and in squid nerve. *Journal of Physiology*, **152**, 159–166.

Frankenhaeuser, B. (1962) Potassium permeability in myelinated nerve fibres of *Xenopus laevis*. *Journal of Physiology*, **160**, 54–61.

Frankenhaeuser, B. and Hodgkin, A. L. (1956) The after-effects of impulses in the giant nerve fibres of *Loligo*. *Journal of Physiology*, **131**, 341–376.

Frankenhaeuser, B. and Hodgkin, A. L. (1957) The action of calcium on electrical properties of squid axon. *Journal of Physiology*, **137**, 218–244.

Frankenhaeuser, B. and Huxley, A. F. (1964) The action potential in the myelinated nerve fibre of *Xenopus Laevis* as computed on the basis of voltage clamp data. *Journal of Physiology*, **171**, 302–315.

Garrahan, P. J. and Glynn, I. M. (1967) The incorporation of inorganic phosphate into adenosine triphosphate by reversal of the sodium pump. *Journal of Physiology*, **192**, 237–256.

Gilbert, D. L. and Ehrenstein, G. (1969) Effect of divalent cations on potassium conductance of squid axons: determination of surface charge. *Biophysical Journal*, **9**, 447–463.

Glynn, I. M. and Karlish, S. J. D. (1975) The sodium pump. *Annual Review of Physiology*, **37**, 13–55.

Goldman, D. E. (1943) Potential, impedance, and rectification in membranes. *Journal of General Physiology*, **27**, 37–60.

Goldman, L. (1964) The effects of stretch on cable and spike parameters of single nerve fibres; some implications for the theory of impulse propagation. *Journal of Physiology*, **175**, 425–444.

Goldman, L. (1975) Quantitative description of the sodium conductance of the giant axon of *Myxicola* in terms of a generalized second-order variable. *Biophysical Journal*, **15**, 119–136.

Goldman, L. and Albus, J. S. (1968) Computation of impulse conduction in myelinated fibres; theoretical basis of the velocity-diameter relation. *Biophysical Journal*, **8**, 596–607.

Goldman, L. and Schauf, C. L. (1972) Inactivation of the sodium current in *Myxicola* giant axons. Evidence for coupling to the activation process. *Journal of General Physiology*, **59**, 659–675.

Goldman, L. and Schauf, C. L. (1973) Quantitative description of sodium and potassium currents and computed action potentials in *Myxicola* giant axons. *Journal of General Physiology*, **61**, 361–384.

Goldman, L. and Binstock, L. (1969) Leak current rectification in *Myxicola* giant axons. Constant field and constant conductance components. *Journal of General Physiology*, **54**, 755–764.

Goldup, A., Ohki, S+ and Danielli, J. F. (1970) Black lipid films. *Recent Progress in Surface and Membrane Science*, **3**, 193–260.

Gorman, A. L. F. and Marmor, M. F. (1974) Steady-state contribution of the sodium pump to the resting potential of a molluscan neurone. *Journal of Physiology*, **242**, 35–48.

Hagiwara, S. and Takahashi, K. (1974) The anomalous rectification and cation of selectivity of the membrane of a starfish egg cell. *Journal of Membrane Biology*, **18**, 61–80.

Håkansson, C. H. (1956) Conduction velocity and amplitude of the action potential as related to circumference in the isolated fibre of frog muscle. *Acta physiologica scandinavica*, **37**, 14–34.

Hall, J. E., Mead, C. A. and Szabo, G. (1973) A barrier model for current flow in lipid bilayer membranes. *Journal of Membrane Biology*, **11**, 75–97.

Hardy, W. L. (1973a) Propagation speed in myelinated nerve. I. Experimental dependence on external Na^+ and on temperature. *Biophysical Journal*, **13**, 1054–1070.

Hardy, W. L. (1973b) Propagation speed in myelinated nerve. II. Theoretical dependence on external Na^+ and on temperature. *Biophysical Journal*, **13**, 1071–1089.

Haydon, D. A. (1970) A critique of the black lipid film as a membrane model. In *Permeability and Function of Biological Membranes*, (eds.) Bolis, L., Katchalsky, A., Keynes, R. D., Loewenstein, W. R. and Pethica, B. A., pp. 185–194. North-Holland: Amsterdam.

Haydon, D. A. and Hladky, S. B. (1972) Ion transport across thin lipid membranes: a critical discussion of mechanisms in selected systems. *Quarterly Review of Biophysics*, **5**, 187–282.

Hill, D. K. (1950a) The effect of stimulation on the opacity of a crustacean nerve trunk and its relation to fibre diameter. *Journal of Physiology*, **111**, 283–303.

Hill, D. K. (1950b) The volume change resulting from stimulation of a giant nerve fibre. *Journal of Physiology*, 111, 304–327.

Hill, T. L. and Chen, Y. (1972) On the theory of ion transport across the nerve membrane. V. Two models for the Cole-Moore K⁺ hyperpolarization delay. *Biophysical Journal*, 12, 960–976.

Hille, B. (1967) Quaternary ammonium ions that block the potassium channels of nerves. *Biophysical Society Abstracts*, 11, 19a.

Hille, B. (1968) Charges and potentials at the nerve surface. Divalent ion and pH. *Journal of General Physiology*, 51, 221–236.

Hille, B. (1970) Ionic channels in nerve membranes. *Progress in Biophysics*, 21, 1–32.

Hille, B. (1971) The permeability of the sodium channel to organic cations in myelinated nerve. *Journal of General Physiology*, 58, 599–619.

Hille, B. (1972) The permeability of the sodium channel to metal cations in myelinated nerve. *Journal of General Physiology*, 59, 637–658.

Hille, B. (1973) Potassium channels in myelinated nerve. Selective permeability to small cations. *Journal of General Physiology*, 61, 669–686.

Hille, B., Woodhull, A. M. and Shapiro, B. I. (1975) Negative surface charge near sodium channels of nerve: divalent ions, monovalent ions, and pH. *Philosophical Transactions of the Royal Society of London (Series B)*, 270, 301–318.

Hladky, S. B. and Haydon, D. A. (1972) Ion transfer across lipid membranes in the presence of gramicidin A. I. Studies of the unit conductance channel. *Biochimica et biophysica acta*, 274, 294–312.

Hodes, R. (1953) Linear relationship between fibre diameter and velocity of conduction in giant axon of squid. *Journal of Neurophysiology*, 16, 145–154.

Hodgkin, A. L. (1937a) Evidence for electrical transmission in nerve. Part I. *Journal of Physiology*, 90, 183–210.

Hodgkin, A. L. (1937b) Evidence for electrical transmission in nerve. Part II. *Journal of Physiology*, 90, 211–232.

Hodgkin, A. L. (1947a) The membrane resistance of a non-medullated nerve fibre. *Journal of Physiology*, 106, 305–318.

Hodgkin, A. L. (1947b) The effect of potassium on the surface membrane of an isolated axon. *Journal of Physiology*, 106, 319–340.

Hodgkin, A. L. (1951) The ionic basis of electrical activity in nerve and muscle. *Biological Reviews*, 26, 339–409.

Hodgkin, A. L. (1954) A note on conduction velocity. *Journal of Physiology*, 125, 221–224.

Hodgkin, A. L. (1958) Ionic movements and electrical activity in giant nerve fibres. *Proceedings of the Royal Society of London (Series B)*, 148, 1–37.

Hodgkin, A. L. (1964) *The Conduction of the Nervous Impulse*, pp. 108. Liverpool University Press.

Hodgkin, A. L. (1975) The optimum density of sodium channels in an unmyelinated nerve. *Philosophical Transactions of the Royal Society of London (Series B)*, 270, 297–300.

Hodgkin, A. L. and Horowicz, P. (1959) The influence of potassium and chloride ions on the membrane potential of single muscle fibres. *Journal of Physiology*, 148, 127–160.

Hodgkin, A. L. and Huxley, A. F. (1952a) Currents carried by sodium and potassium ions through the membrane of the giant axon of *Loligo*. *Journal of Physiology*, 116, 449–472.

Hodgkin, A. L. and Huxley, A. F. (1952b) The components of membrane conductance in the giant axon of *Loligo*. *Journal of Physiology*, 116, 473–496.

Hodgkin, A. L. and Huxley, A. F. (1952c) The dual effect of membrane potential on sodium conductance in the giant axon of *Loligo*. *Journal of Physiology*, 116, 497–506.

Hodgkin, A. L. and Huxley, A. F. (1952d) A quantitative description of membrane current and its application to conduction and excitation in nerve. *Journal of Physiology*, 117, 500–544.

Hodgkin, A. L. and Huxley, A. F. (1953) Movement of radioactive potassium and membrane current in a giant axon. *Journal of Physiology*, 121, 403–414.

Hodgkin, A. L., Huxley, A. F. and Katz, B. (1952) Measurement of current-voltage relations in the membrane of the giant axon of *Loligo*. *Journal of Physiology*, 116, 424–448.

Hodgkin, A. L. and Katz, B. (1949) The effect of sodium ions on the electrical activity of the giant axon of the squid. *Journal of Physiology*, **108**, 37–77.

Hodgkin, A. L. and Keynes, R. D. (1955a) Active transport of cations in giant axons from *Sepia* and *Loligo*. *Journal of Physiology*, **128**, 28–60.

Hodgkin, A. L. and Keynes, R. D. (1955b) The potassium permeability of a giant nerve fibre. *Journal of Physiology*, **128**, 61–88.

Hodgkin, A. L. and Keynes, R. D. (1957) Movements of labelled calcium in squid giant axon. *Journal of Physiology*, **138**, 253–281.

Hodgkin, A. L. and Nakajima, S. (1972a) The effect of diameter on the electrical constants of frog skeletal muscle fibres. *Journal of Physiology*, **221**, 105–120.

Hodgkin, A. L. and Nakajima, S. (1972b) Analysis of the membrane capacity in frog muscle. *Journal of Physiology*, **221**, 121–136.

Hodgkin, A. L. and Rushton, W. A. H. (1946) The electrical constants of a crustacean nerve fibre. *Proceedings of the Royal Society of London (Series B)*, **133**, 444–479.

Hope, A. B. (1971) *Ion Transport and Membranes*. Butterworths: London.

Horackova, M., Nonner, W. and Stämpfli, R. (1968) Action potentials and voltage clamp currents of single rat Ranvier nodes. *Proceedings of the 24th International Physiological Congress*, **7**, 198.

Horowicz, P., Gage, P. W. and Eisenberg, R. S. (1968) The role of electrochemical gradient in determining potassium fluxes in frog striated muscle. *Journal of General Physiology*, **51**, 193–203s.

Hoyt, R. C. (1963) The squid giant axon. Mathematical models. *Biophysical Journal*, **3**, 399–431.

Hoyt, R. C. (1965) Non-linear membrane currents with ohmic channels. *Journal of Cellular and Comparative Physiology*, **66**, Supplement, 119–125.

Hoyt, R. C. (1968) Sodium inactivation in nerve fibers. *Biophysical Journal*, **8**, 1074–1097.

Hoyt, R. C. and Adelman, W. J. (1970) Sodium inactivation. Experimental test of two models. *Biophysical Journal*, **10**, 610–617.

Hunter, P. J., McNaughton, P. A. and Noble, D. (1975) Analytical models of propagation in excitable cells. *Progress in Biophysics*, **30**, (in press).

Hurlbut, W. P. (1963a) Sodium fluxes in desheathed frog sciatic nerve. *Journal of General Physiology*, **46**, 1191–1222.

Hurlbut, W. P. (1970) Ion movements in nerve. In *Membranes and Ion Transport*, Vol. 2, chapter 4, (ed.) Bittar, E. E., pp. 95–143. Wiley-Interscience: New York.

Hursh, J. B. (1939) Conduction velocity and diameter of nerve fibres. *American Journal of Physiology*, **127**, 131–139.

Hutchinson, N. A., Koles, Z. J. and Smith, R. S. (1970) Conduction velocity in myelinated nerve fibres of *Xenopus laevis*. *Journal of Physiology*, **208**, 279–289.

Hutter, O. F. and Noble, D. (1960) The chloride conductance of frog skeletal muscle. *Journal of Physiology*, **151**, 89–102.

Huxley, A. F. (1959) Ion movements during nerve activity. *Annals of the New York Academy of Sciences*, **81**, 221–246.

Huxley, A. F. and Stämpfli, R. (1949) Evidence for saltatory conduction in peripheral myelinated nerve fibres. *Journal of Physiology*, **108**, 315–339.

Huxley, A. F. and Stämpfli, R. (1951a) Direct determination of membrane resting potential and action potential in single myelinated nerve fibres. *Journal of Physiology*, **112**, 476–495.

Huxley, A. F. and Stämpfli, R. (1951b) Effect of potassium and sodium on resting and action potentials of single myelinated nerve fibres. *Journal of Physiology*, **112**, 496–508.

Jacquez, J. A. (1971) A generalization of the Goldman equation, including the effects of electrogenic pumps. *Mathematical Biosciences*, **12**, 185–196.

Jack, J. J. B. (1975) Physiology of peripheral nerve fibres in relation to their size. *British Journal of Anaesthesia*, **47**, 173–182.

Jack, J. J. B., Noble, D. and Tsien, R. W. (1975) *The Spread of Current in Excitable Cells*. Clarendon Press: Oxford.

Jakobsson, E. and Scudiero, C. (1975) A transient excited state model for sodium permeability changes in excitable membranes. *Biophysical Journal*, **15**, 577–590.

Jansen, J. K. S. and Nicholls, J. G. (1973) Conductance changes, an electrogenic pump and the hyperpolarization of leech neurones following impulses. *Journal of Physiology*, **229**, 635–655.

Julian, F. J., Moore, J. W. and Goldman, D. E. (1962) Current-voltage relations in the lobster giant axon membrane under voltage clamp conditions. *Journal of General Physiology*, **45**, 1217–1238.

Katz, B. (1947) The effect of electrolyte deficiency on the rate of conduction in a single nerve fibre. *Journal of Physiology*, **106**, 411–417.

Katz, B. (1966) *Nerve, Muscle and Synapse*. McGraw Hill: London.

Keynes, R. D. (1951) The ionic movements during nervous activity. *Journal of Physiology*, **114**, 119–150.

Keynes, R. D. (1963) Chloride in the squid giant axon. *Journal of Physiology*, **169**, 690–705.

Keynes, R. D. (1972) Excitable membranes. *Nature (London)*, **239**, 29–50.

Keynes, R. D. and Ritchie, J. M. (1965) The movements of labelled ions in mammalian non-myelinated nerve fibres. *Journal of Physiology*, **179**, 333–367.

Keynes, R. D. and Rojas, E. (1974) Kinetics and steady-state properties of the charged system controlling sodium conductance in the squid giant axon. *Journal of Physiology*, **239**, 393–434.

Keynes, R. D. and Swan, R. C. (1959) The effect of external sodium concentration on the sodium fluxes in frog skeletal muscle. *Journal of Physiology*, **147**, 591–625.

Kostyuk, P. G., Kryshtal, O. A. and Pidoplichko, V. I. (1972) Electrogenic sodium pump and the associated changes in conductivity of the surface membrane of neurones. *Biofizika*, **17**, 1048–1054.

Krasne, S., Eisenman, G. and Szabo, G. (1971) Freezing and melting of lipid bilayers and the mode of action of nonactin, valinomycin and gramicidin. *Science*, **174**, 412–415.

Krnjević, K. and Lisiewicz, A. (1972) Injections of calcium ions into spinal motoneurones. *Journal of Physiology*, **225**, 363–390.

Landahl, H. D. and Podolsky, R. J. (1949) On the velocity of conduction in nerve fibers with saltatory transmission. *Bulletin of Mathematical Biophysics*, **11**, 19–27.

Landowne, D. (1972) A new explanation of the ionic currents which flow during the nerve impulse. *Journal of Physiology*, **222**, 46–47P.

Landowne, D. (1973) Movement of sodium ions associated with the nerve impulse. *Nature (London)*, **242**, 457–459.

Landowne, D. and Ritchie, J. M. (1970) The binding of triated ouabain to mammalian non-myelinated nerve fibres. *Journal of Physiology*, **207**, 529–537.

Läuger, P. (1972) Carrier-mediated ion transport. *Science*, **178**, 24–30.

Läuger, P. (1973) Ion transport through pores: a rate-theory analysis. *Biochimica et biophysica acta*, **311**, 423–441.

Lieberman, E. M. (1969) Transient transmembrane water movements in crayfish axons detected by transmitted light interference microscopy. *Acta physiologica scandinavica*, **75**, 513–517.

Ling, G. N. (1962) *A Physical Theory of the Living State*. Blaisdell Publishing Company: New York.

Lubinska, L. (1960) Method of isolation of peripheral nerve fibres for quantitative morphological purposes. *Bulletin de l'Académie polonaise des sciences*, Ch. 2 Serie des Sciences biologiques, 8, 117–120.

Lux, H. D. (1971) Ammonium and chloride extrusion: Hyperpolarizing synaptic inhibition in spinal motoneurones. *Science*, **173**, 555–557.

McAllister, R,E., Noble, D. and Tsien, R. W. (1975) Reconstruction of the electrical activity of cardiac Purkinje fibres. *Journal of Physiology*, **251**, 1–59.

MacGillivray, A. D. and Hare, D. (1969) Applicability of Goldman's constant field assumption to biological systems. *Journal of Theoretical Biology*, **25**, 113–126.

Mackey, M. C. and McNeel, M. L. (1971) The independence principle. A reconsideration. *Biophysical Journal*, **11**, 675–680.

Marmor, M. F. (1971) The effects of temperature and ions on the current-voltage relation and electrical characteristics of a molluscan neurone. *Journal of Physiology*, **218**, 573–598.

Matthews, P. B. C. (1972) *Mammalian Muscle Receptors and their Central Actions*. Edward Arnold: London.

Meech, R. W. and Standen, N. B. (1974) Calcium-mediated potassium activation in *Helix* neurones. *Journal of Physiology*, **237**, 43P.

Meves, H. (1974) The effect of holding potential on the asymmetry currents in squid giant axons. *Journal of Physiology*, **243**, 847–867.

Meves, H. (1975) Asymmetry currents in intracellularly perfused squid giant axons. *Philosophical Transactions of the Royal Society of London (Series B)*, **270**, 493–500.

Moore, R. D. (1973) Effects of insulin upon the sodium pump in frog skeletal muscle. *Journal of Physiology*, **232**, 23–45.

Mozhaeva, G. N. and Naumov, A. P. (1972) Effect of surface charge on stationary potassium conductance of the Ranvier node membrane. 2 Changes in ionic strength of external solution. *Biophysics*, **17**, 644–649.

Mullins, L. J. and Brinley, F. J. (1967) Some factors influencing sodium extrusion by internally dialyzed squid axons. *Journal of General Physiology*, **50**, 2333–2355.

Mullins, L. J. and Brinley, F. J. (1969) Potassium fluxes in dialyzed squid axons. *Journal of General Physiology*, **53**, 704–740.

Mullins, L. J. and Brinley, F. J. (1975) Sensitivity of calcium efflux from squid axons to changes in membrane potential. *Journal of General Physiology*, **65**, 135–152.

Mullins, L. J. and Noda, K. (1963) The influence of sodium-free solutions on the membrane potential of frog muscle fibers. *Journal of General Physiology*, **47**, 117–132.

Namerow, N. S. and Kappl, J. J. (1969) Conduction in demyelinated axons – a simplified model. *Bulletin of Mathematical Biophysics*, **31**, 9.23.

Noble, D. (1965) Electrical properties of cardiac muscle attributable to inward going (anomalous) rectification. *Journal of Cellular and Comparative Physiology*, **66**, 127–135.

Noble, D. (1966) Applications of Hodgkin-Huxley equations to excitable tissues. *Physiological Reviews*, **46**, 1–50.

Noble, D. (1972a) Conductance mechanisms in excitable cells. In *Biomembranes*, Vol. 3, (eds.) Kreuzer, F.and Slegers, J. F. G. pp. 427–447. Plenum: New York.

Noble, D. (1972b) The relation of Rushton's 'liminal length' for excitation to the resting and active conductances of excitable cells. *Journal of Physiology*, **226**, 573–591.

Noble, D. and Stein, R. B. (1966) The threshold conditions for initiation of action potentials by excitable cells. *Journal of Physiology*, **187**, 129–162.

Nonner, W., Rojas, E. and Stämpfli, R. (1975a) Displacement currents in the node of Ranvier: voltage and time dependence. *Pflügers Archiv*, **354**, 1–18.

Nonner, W., Rojas, E. and Stämpfli, R. (1975b) Gating currents in the node of Ranvier: voltage and time dependence. *Philosophical Transactions of the Royal Society of London (Series B)*, **270**, 483–492.

Offner, F. F. (1972) The excitable membrane. A physiochemical model. *Biophysical Journal*, `12**, 1583–1629.

Offner, F., Weinberg, A. and Young, G. (1940) Nerve conduction theory: some mathematical consequences of Bernstein's model. *Bulletin of Mathematics and Biophysics*, **2**, 89–103.

Paintal, A. S. (1965) Effects of temperature on conduction in single vagal and saphenous myelinated nerve fibres of the cat. *Journal of Physiology*, **180**, 20–49.

Paintal, A. S. (1966) The influence of diameter of medulled nerve fibres of cats on the rising and falling phases of the spike and its recovery. *Journal of Physiology*, **184**, 791–811.

Paintal, A. S. (1967) A comparison of the nerve impulses of mammalian non-medullated nerve fibres with those of the smallest diameter medullated fibres. *Journal of Physiology*, **193**, 523–533.

Paintal, A. S. (1973) Conduction in mammalian nerve fibres. In *New Developments in Electromyography and Clinical Neurophysiology*, (ed.) Desmedt, J. E. Vol. 2, pp. 19–41.

Parsegian, A. (1969) Energy of an ion crossing a low dielectric membrane: solutions to four relevant electrostatic problems. *Nature (London)*, **221**, 844–846.

Patlak, C. S. (1960) Derivation of an equation for the diffusion potential. *Nature (London)*, **188**, 944–945.

Pearson, K. G., Stein, R. B. and Malhotra, S. K. (1970) Properties of action potentials from insect motor nerve fibres. *Journal of Experimental Biology*, **53**, 299–316.

Pickard, W. F. (1969) Estimating the velocity of propagation along myelinated and unmyelinated fibers. *Mathematical Biosciences*, **5**, 305–319.

Rang, H. P. (1974) Acetylcholine receptors. *Quarterly Review of Biophysics*, **7**, 283–399.

Rang, H. P.nd Ritchie, J. M. (1968a) The dependence on external cations of the oxygen consumption of mammalian non-myelinated fibres at rest and during activity. *Journal of Physiology*, **196**, 163–181.

Rang, H. P. and Ritchie, J. M. (1968b) On the electrogenic sodium pump in mammalian non-myelinated nerve fibres and its activation by various external cations. *Journal of Physiology*, **196**, 183–221.

Rang, H. P. and Ritchie, J. M. (1968c) The ionic content of mammalian non-myelinated nerve fibres and its alteration as a result of electrical activity. *Journal of Physiology*, **196**, 223–236.

Reuter, H. (1973) Divalent cations as charge carriers in excitable membranes. *Progress in Biophysics*, **26**, 1–43.

Ritchie, J. M. (1971) Electrogenic ion pumping in nervous tissue. *Current topics in Bioenergetics* **4** 327–356.

Rojas, E. and Canessa-Fischer, M. (1968) Sodium movements in perfused squid giant axons. Passive fluxes. *Journal of General Physiology*, **52**, 240–257.

Rojas, E. and Keynes, R. D. (1975) On the relation between displacement currents and activation of the sodium conductance in the squid giant axon. *Philosophical Transactions of the Royal Society London (Series B)*, **270**, 459–482.

Roy, G. (1975) Models of ionic currents for excitable membranes. *Progress in Biophysics*, **29**, 57–104.

Rushton, W. A. H. (1951) A theory of the effects of fibre size on medullated nerve. *Journal of Physiology*, **115**, 101–122.

Sandblom, J. P. (1967) A method to relate steady-state ionic currents, conductances, and membrane potential in ion exchange membranes with unknown thermodynamic properties. *Biophysical Journal*, **7**, 243–265.

Sandblom, J. P. and Eisenman, G. (1967) Membrane potentials at zero-current. The significance of a constant ionic permeability ratio. *Biophysical Journal*, **7**, 217–242.

Schauf, C. L. (1974) Sodium currents in *Myxicola* axons. Nonexponential recovery from the inactive state. *Biophysical Journal*, **14**, 151–154.

Schoepfle, G. M. and Katholi, C. R. (1973) Post-tetanic changes in membrane potential of single medullated nerve fibers. *American Journal of Physiology*, **225**, 1501–1507.

Schultz, S. G. and Curran, P. F. (1970) Coupled transport of sodium and organic solutes. *Physiological Reviews*, **50**, 637–718.

Schwartz, T. L. (1971) The validity of the Ussing flux ratio equation in a three-dimensionally unhomogeneous membrane. *Biophysical Journal*, **11**, 596–602.

Segal, J. R. (1970) Metabolic dependence of resting and action potentials of frog nerve. *American Journal of Physiology*, **219**, 1216–1225.

Shapiro, M. P. and Candia, O. A. (1971) Analysis of the components of ionic flux across a membrane. *Biophysical Journal*, **11**, 28–46.

Sjodin, R. A. (1971) Ion transport across excitable cell membranes. In *Biophysics and Physiology of Excitable Membranes*, (ed.) Adelman, W. J., pp. 96–124. van Nostrand Reinhold Co.

Skou, J. C. (1975) The $(Na^+ + K^+)$ activated enzyme system and its relationship to transport of sodium and potassium. *Quarterly Review of Biophysics*, **7**, 401–434.

Sokolove, P. G. and Cooke, I. M. (1971) Inhibition of impulse activity in a sensory neuron by an electrogenic pump. *Journal of General Physiology*, **57**, 125–163.

Stämpfli, R. (1954) Saltatory conduction in nerve. *Physiological Review*, **34**, 101–112.

Stämpfli, R. (1959) Is the resting potential of Ranvier nodes a potassium potential? *Annals of the New York Academy of Sciences*, **81**, 265–284.

Stein, R. B. and Pearson, K. G. (1971) Predicted amplitude and form of action potentials recorded from unmyelinated nerve fibres. *Journal of Theoretical Biology*, **32**, 539–558.

Strickholm, A. and Wallin, B. G. (1967) Relative ion permeabilities in the crayfish giant axon determined from rapid external ion changes. *Journal of General Physiology*, **50**, 1929–1953.

Szabo, G., Eisenman, G., Laprade, R., Ciani, S. M. and Krasne, S. (1973) Experimentally observed effects of carriers on the electrical properties of bilayer membranes –

equilibrium domain. In *Membranes*, (ed.) Eisenman, G. Vol. 2, pp. 179–328. M. Dekker, Inc: New York.

Takeuchi, A. and Takeuchi, N. (1960) On the permeability of end-plate membrane during the action of transmitter. *Journal of Physiology*, **154**, 52–67.

Takeuchi, N. (1963) Some properties of conductance changes at the end-plate membrane during the action of acetylcholine. *Journal of Physiology*, **167**, 128–140.

Tasaki, I. (1953) *Nervous Transmission*. Charles C. Thomas: Springfield, Illinois.

Taylor, R. E. (1963) Cable theory. In *Physical Techniques in Biological Research*, Vol. 6, (ed.) Nastuk, W. L., pp. 219–262. Academic Press: London and New York.

Thomas, R. C. (1969) Membrane current and intracellular sodium changes in a snail neurone during extrusion of injected sodium. *Journal of Physiology*, **201**, 495–514.

Thomas, R. C. (1972) Electrogenic sodium pump in nerve and muscle cells. *Physiological Reviews*, **52**, 563–594.

Tsien, R. W. and Noble, D. (1969) A transition state theory approach to the kinetics of conductance changes in excitable membranes. *Journal of Membrane Biology*, **1**, 248–273.

Ussing, H. H. (1949) The distinction by means of tracers between active transport and diffusion. The transfer of iodide across the isolated frog skin. *Acta physiologica scandinavica*, **19**, 43–56.

Van Essen, D. C. (1973) The contribution of membrane hyperpolarization to adaptation and conduction block in sensory neurones of the leech. *Journal of Physiology*, **230**, 509–534.

Verveen, A. A. and DeFelice, L. J. (1974) Membrane noise. *Progress in Biophysics*, **28**, 189–265.

Wallin, B. G. (1967) The relation between external potassium concentration, membrane potential and internal ion concentrations in crayfish axons. *Acta physiologica scandinavica*, **70**, 431–448.

Wanke, E., DeFelice, L. J. and Conti, F. (1974) Voltage noise, current noise and impedance in space clamped squid giant axon. *Pflügers Archiv*, **347**, 63–74.

Waxman, S. G. and Bennett, M. V. L. (1972) Relative conduction velocities of small myelinated and non-myelinated fibres in the central nervous system. *Nature New Biology*, **238**, 217–219.

Weidmann, S. (1951) Electrical characteristics of *Sepia* axons. *Journal of Physiology*, **114**, 372–381.

Williams, P. L. and Landon, D. N. (1963) Paranodal apparatus of peripheral myelinated nerve fibres of mammals. *Nature (London)*, **198**, 670–673.

Woodbury, J. W. (1971) Eyring rate theory model of the current-voltage relationships of ion channels in excitable membranes. In *Chemical Dynamics: Papers in honour of Henry Eyring*, (eds.) Hirschfelder, J. O. and Henderson, D., J. Wiley and Sons: New York.

Woodbury, J. W. and Patton, H. D. (1965) In *Physiology and Biophysics*, (eds.) Ruch, T. C. and Patton, H. D., chapters 1–3, W. B. Saunders: Philadelphia.

Woodhull, A. M. (1973) Ionic blockage of sodium channels. *Journal of General Physiology*, **61**, 687–708.

ADDENDA

Addendum to Chapter 2

A number of interesting studies on unmyelinated fibres have been published since this paper was submitted. The essential points made in some of those reports together with a reference are briefly summarized below.

1. *Fibrous proteins and axoplasmic transport in unmyelinated fibres.*
(a) Ochs, S. and Jersild, R. A. (1974) Fast axoplasmic transport in nonmyelinated mammalian nerve fibres shown by electron microscopic radioautography. *Journal of Neurobiology,* **5**, 373–377.
   In cat sciatic nerve, the same fast rate of axoplasmic transport is present in unmyelinated as was found earlier for myelinated fibres from a variety of animal species. The finding supports the concept that there is a common mechanism for fast transport in all nerve fibres.

(b) Banks, P., Mayor, D. and Owen, T. (1975) Effects of low temperatures on microtubules in the non-myelinated axons of postganglionic sympathetic nerves. *Brain Research,* **83**, 277–292.
   A rapid loss of microtubules in unmyelinated axons occurred on cooling nerves. Microtubules reappeared on rewarming and seemed to function normally with respect to their possible role in transport of storage vesicles along the axons.

2. *Regeneration of unmyelinated fibres.*
(a) Bray, G. M. and Aguayo, A. J. (1974) Regeneration of peripheral unmyelinated nerves. Fate of the axonal sprouts which develop after injury. *Journal of Anatomy,* **117**, 517–529.
   Early during regeneration of crushed cervical sympathetic nerves in rat, there is an absolute increase in the number of small axonal sprouts that invade the distal stump. This is accompanied by a uniform decrease in axonal diameters proximally. Eventually, there is a gradual decrease in the number of axonal sprouts, while the maximal axonal diameters increase on both sides of the injury.

(b) Weinberg, H. J. and Spencer, P. S. (1975) Studies on the control of myelinogenesis. I. Myelination of regenerating axons after entry into a foreign unmyelinated nerve. *Journal of Neurocytology,* **4**, 395–418.

Regenerating axons from a myelinated nerve become myelinated after entry into the distal stump of a previously unmyelinated nerve. This study confirms and extends the observation by Simpson and Young (cf. p. 141). However, the question of the origin of the myelinating cells remains open. That such cells are not carried distally by regenerating axons from the myelinated nerve has been elegantly demonstrated using radioisotope cell labelling, as described in the following two articles. (b1 and b2).

(b1) Aguayo, A. J., Epps, J., Charron, L. and Bray, G. M. (1976). Multi-potentiality of Schwann cells in cross-anastomosed and grafted myelinated and unmyelinated nerves. *Brain Research,* **105**, 1—20.

(b2) Aguayo, A. J., Charron, L. and Bray, G. M. (1975) Potential of Schwann cells from unmyelinated nerves to produce myelin. *Clin. Res.,* **23**, 641.

 (c) Wall, P. D. and Gutnick, M. (1974) Properties of afferent nerve impulses originating from a neuroma. *Nature,* **248**, 740—743.
Wall, P. D. and Gutnick, M. (1974) Ongoing activity in peripheral nerves: The physiology and pharmacology of impulses originating from a neuroma. *Experimental Neurology,* **43**, 580—593.

These electrophysiological studies provide evidence implicating immature regenerating nerve sprouts as the sources of abnormal impulses originating spontaneously in neuromas. On reaching cognitive levels such abnormal impulses may be interpreted as pain. Small myelinated and unmyelinated fibres would be involved.

3. *Observations on unmyelinated fibres in human nerves.*
(a) Carlsen, F., Knappeis, G. G. and Behse, F. (1974) Schwann cell length in unmyelinated fibres of human sural nerve. *Journal of Anatomy,* **117**, 463—467.

Using a procedure similar to that used by Ochoa and Mair (1969a) to assess mean internodal length of myelinated fibres, the authors have determined the length of Schwann cells from unmyelinated fibres in human sural nerve. From the length of the Schwann cell nucleus and the ratio of Schwann cells with and without nuclei encountered in cross sections, they reached a figure of 200—500 μm

(b) Buchthal, F., Behse, F., Dahl, K., Henriksen, X. and Sjö, O. (1974) Are there vasoconstrictors among unmyelinated fibres of nervous suralis in man? *Annual reports from the institute of Neurophysiology of the University of Copenhagen,* pp. 17—18.

Preliminary experiments measuring change in temperature and in blood flow in the cutaneous area innervated by the sural nerve following electrical nerve stimulation, indicate that some of the unmyelinated fibres of the sural nerve cause vasoconstriction in the skin of the dorsum pedis.

(c) Torebjörk, E. (1974) Single unit activity in afferent and sympathetic C fibres recorded from intact human skin nerves (Thesis). *Acta Universitatis Upsaliensis*, No. 211.

The report compiles five papers published between 1970 and 1974, providing comprehensive data on electrophysiological recordings of unmyelinated fibre activity related to sensory experience and autonomic phenomena in awake subjects: A most significant contribution to sensory physiology.

Addendum to Chapter 8

Since going to press, a number of important reviews have appeared. Among these is a detailed structural analysis of the carotid body of the rat, by McDonald and Mitchell (1975), which adds considerably to previous investigations. These authors have shown by degeneration experiments that the great majority of nerve terminals on glomus cells are sensory endings of glossopharyngeal nerve fibres, and that only a small proportion are efferent terminals, arising from preganglionic axons of the cervical sympathetic trunk. Reciprocal synapses, allowing two-way transmission, occur between afferent endings and glomus cells, and between individual glomus cells (of which two types can be distinguished structurally) so that these cells can be regarded as specialized interneurons. Parasympathetic and sympathetic ganglion cells also occur within the carotid body, with efferent processes terminating on arterioles supplying the organ. It is suggested that when the sensory endings are active they stimulate the related glomus cell to liberate catecholamines which in turn modify subsequent sensory activity. Efferent stimulation of only a few glomus cells would then be relayed to all those with synaptic interconnections, further modulating the release of catecholamines from glomus cells and so exerting central control on sensory responses. The autonomic innervation of the carotid blood supply serves as an additional means of altering carotid function by altering its vascular flow.

Three major reviews of muscle receptor structure, function and central actions have also recently appeared, as cited below (Barker; Hunt; McIntyre: all 1974).

Barker, D. (1974) Morphology of muscle receptors. In *Handbook of Sensory Physiology*, Vol. 3, Part 2, (ed.) Hunt, C. C., pp. 1–190. Springer: Berlin.

Hunt, C. C. (1974) The physiology of muscle receptors. In *Handbook of Sensory Physiology*, Vol. 3, Part 2, (ed.) Hunt, C. C., pp. 191–234. Springer: Berlin.

McDonald, D. and Mitchell, R. A. (1975) The innervation of glomus cells, ganglion cells and blood vessels in the rat carotid body: a quantitative ultrastructural study. *Journal of Neurocytology*, **4**, 177–230.

McIntyre, A. K. (1974) Central actions of impulses in muscle afferent fibres. In *Handbook of Sensory Physiology*, Vol. 3, Part 2 (ed.) Hunt, C. C., pp. 235–288. Springer: Berlin.

Addendum to Chapter 11

Since the completion of this review a number of original papers have been published containing additional pertinent information, particularly concerning the protein constituents of peripheral myelin. A selection of these papers is given below.

Brostoff, S. W., Kharkhanis, Y. D., Carlo, D. J., Reuter, W. and Eylar, E. H. (1975) Isolation and partial characterisation of the major proteins of rabbit sciatic nerve myelin. *Brain Research,* 86, 449–458.

Brostoff, S. W., Sacks, H., Dal Canto, M., Johnson, A. B., Raine, C. S. and Wisniewski, H. (1974) The P_2 protein of bovine root myelin: isolation and some chemical and immunological properties. *Journal of Neurochemistry,* 23, 1037–1044.

Brostoff, S. W., Sacks, H. and Di Paolo, C. (1975) The P_2 protein of bovine root myelin: partial chemical characterisation. *Journal of Neurochemistry,* 24, 289–294.

Butler, K. W. (1975) The effect of a myelin apoprotein on lipid structure: a spin probe study. *Canadian Journal of Biochemistry,* 53, 758–767.

Latovitzki, N. and Siberberg, D. H. (1975) Ceramide glycosyltransferase in cultured rat cerebellum: changes with age, with demyelination, and with inhibition of myelination by 5-bromo-2'-deoxyuridine or experimental allergic encephalomyelitis serum. *Journal of Neurochemistry,* 24, 1017–1022.

Martenson, R. E. and Deibler, Gladys E. (1975) Partial characterisation of basic proteins of chicken, turtle and frog central nervous system. *Journal of Neurochemistry,* 24, 79–88.

Nussbaum, J. L., Rouayrenc, J. F. and Mandell, P. (1974) Isolation and terminal sequence determination of the major rat brain myelin proteolipid P_7 apoprotein. *Biochemical and Biophysical Research Communications,* 57, 1240–1247.

Wood, J. G. and Dawson, R. M. C. (1974) Some properties of a major structural glycoprotein of sciatic nerve. *Journal of Neurochemistry,* 22, 627–630.

Wood, J. G. and Dawson, R. M. C. (1974) Lipid and protein changes in sciatic nerve during Wallerian degeneration. *Journal of Neurochemistry,* 22, 631–636.

Wood, J. G. and McLaughlin, Barbara J. (1975) The visualization of concanavalin-A binding sites in the interperiod line of rat sciatic nerve myelin. *Journal of Neurochemistry,* 24, 233–236.

INDEX

Abdominal plexus, 357
'Abnutzungpigment', 212
Acetylcholine (ACh), 615–6
  as transmitter substance, 498–9
  manufacture of, 499–500
  miniature end-plate potentials and,
    502–3
  receptor for, neuromuscular junction,
    477, 478
  release at synaptic cleft, effect,
    506–7
  release of, 500–6
  sensitivity of post synaptic membrane
    to, 501–2
Acetylcholinesterase (AChE), 221, 252,
    364, 365, 376, 377, 381
  activity of, 608–10, 615–6
Acetylthiodialine method, 609
Acid
  hydrolases, 607, 610
  phosphatase, 607, 610–11
    demyelination and, 645
  protease, 611, 625–6, 635, 637
Acridine orange fluorescence, 607
Acrylamide, effect of, 615, 631
Action potential
  conductance reduction and sodium
      and potassium flux reduction,
      802
  conduction velocity and, 740, 786–9,
      790, 791, 798, 799, 803, 806
    change with temperature increase,
      793
    excitation of, 781–4, 795, 796–8,
      807
    fibre diameter and, amphibian,
      803–4
    fibre size, 779–800
    sodium conductance and, 790–3
  mechanism of, 765–74, 807
  potassium concentration increase and,
    767
  propagation of, 781, 784–98, 807
  rise time and maximum rate of rise,
    802–3
  spread of, 779–81

Action potential (*cont.*)
  time course of, 799, 803
  'voltage threshold', 781, 783
Active transport, of ions, 741, 748, 760,
    774–9
Adhaerentes-like junction, 244, 248
Adrenaline, 366, 374
Alimentary canal, numbers of neurons in
    parts of, 384
Alkaline phosphatase, 611, 626
Amino peptidase activity, 625–6, 636
'Ampullar' dilatations, 193
Amyloid neuropathy, 652
Analgesic, path travelled to root sheath, 343
Aplysia, 775
Apparatus of Golgi-Rezzonico, 24, 30
Aryl sulphatases, 607, 651
Auditory nerve, 346, 348
Axon (*see also* Neuron)
  collaterals of Huber, 230
  flow, 608, 613–4, 631
  'reflex', 125
  section, 608, 631
  sprouts, 130
Axonotmesis, 703
Axotomy, 247, 262, 263

Baker's acid haematin, 618
Bands of Bünger, 140, 349, 704, 721, 722,
    723
  regenerating axons and, 722
Barrier
  blood-brain, 629, 679, 686
  blood-nerve, 194, 629–30
Basic myelin protein, 619, 621–5, 637,
    639, 642
Biliary cirrhosis neuropathy, 652
Bipolar neuroblast, 235
Black lipid membrane (BLM), 519, 520
Boltzman distribution of charges, 771
Boundary membrane, 163, 164, 165, 166,
    167, 174, 175, 177
  forerunner of extracellular connective
    tissue, 175
Bromine-Sudan Black technique, 617, 642
Butyrylcholinesterase, 609, 628

INDEX

C-fibres, 234
Capacitative current, 771
Carotid body, 442
Cathepsin, 607, 611
    D, 608, 611
Catecholamines, 114, 364, 366, 368, 613,
    614, 615, 632
Cauda equina, 330, 344
Cell
    anterior horn, 2, 279–329
    bipolar ganglion, 225
    capsule, 160, 172
    cerebellar, Purkiynjé, 260
    chromaffin, 365, 376
        amines of, 366
        shape of, 366
    cochlear, 1, 403
    death of, 199, 250
    dorsal root ganglion, 1, 2
    endothelial, 191, 197
        blood-brain barrier and, 194–5
        capillaries and, 194
        ion transporting functions, 215
    excitable, shape of, 804–5
    glial
        intramural ganglia, 387
        sympathetic ganglia, 358
    granule, 1, 225, 358, 365, 367, 439
        function, 366, 403
    HeLa, 696
    laminar, 172
    large pale (clear), 203
        characteristics, 219
        differences, small dark, prenatal rat,
          220
        divisions of, 219–20
        function, 221
    macrophage, 711, 715, 716
    Mast, 161, 191, 193, 339, 340, 358,
        434, 628, 629, 630, 643, 708
    Mauthner, 54, 608
    Merkel, 407, 408, 419
    mitral, 439
    nasal, 258
    Nissl substance of, 201–2
    oligodendrocytes, function, 344, 628
    perineurial, 165, 167, 168
        absorption of leaked protein by, 198
        tight junctions and, 165
    Purkinje, 1
    retinal amacrine, 1
    satellite (see also Neuron and
        Unmyelinated fibre), 13, 34, 56,
        58, 67, 70, 72, 75, 111, 136, 188,
        209, 231, 241, 358
        chromaffin cells and, 366
        ciliary ganglia and, 377
        cytoplasm of, 115, 242
        differentiation and mitotic
          capability, 253

Cell (cont.)
    function of, 247
    myelination of sensory ganglia and,
        249, 566
    nucleus of, 115, 200, 242
    outer surface of, 243
    peroxisomes, 217, 242
    relationship, other satellite cells, 243
    sensory ganglia and, 189
    shape of, 241, 242
    variation in, related to position on
        neuron, 244–5
  septal, 170
Schwann cell, 2, 4, 5, 6, 8, 9
    axon crush and, 704
    axon relationship and, 20, 41,
        58–59, 72, 137–8, 140, 168,
        231, 332, 333, 335, 336, 338,
        339
    axon regeneration and, 140, 141
    bands, devoid of axons, 134
    basement membrane of, 341, 346
    cholinesterase activity, 609
    'collagen pockets', 121
    critical axon diameter and, 14
    cytoplasm of, 18–21, 24, 30, 35, 36,
        37, 38, 40, 42, 46, 47, 48, 61,
        62, 73, 74, 75, 113, 116, 119,
        333, 348, 693, 696, 717
    cytoplasm and experimental
        allergic neuropathy (EAN),
        689
    collagen synthesis and, 177
    degeneration after crushing, 349
    dense bodies, 116
    derivation of, 13
    definition of, 16
    development of, 14, 34
    Diphtheria toxin and, 644
    diphtheritic neuropathy and, 689
    distribution in foetus, 14
    endoneurium and, 159, 161
    enzyme activity, 628–9
    experimental allergic neuritis (EAN)
        and, 670, 672, 676, 678
    EAN induction and, 681–2
    experimental diphtheritic neuritis
        (EDN), 686, 699
    EDN and cell disfunction, 692
    form of, 338
    function, 628–9
    golgi tendon organ and, 170
    ionic movements and, 53–54
    incisures of Schmidt-Lanterman
        and, 5
    in genital corpuscles, 171–2
    internode, cylindrico-conical
        segments, 5
    internuclear distances, unmyelinated
        fibres, 720

Cell (*cont.*)
    life history, 17
    lipid inclusions, 116
    lysosomes, 114
    material delivery to axon, 89
    material transfer in, 56
    Meissner's corpuscle and, 172
    Merkel disc and, 417
    microvilli, 717
    microvilli and ion movement, 52–53
    micropinocytosis, 121
    migratory activity following nerve
        crush, 710–11
    miniature end-plate potentials, 502
    'mosaic', 119
    myelin and, 27–28, 65, 68, 566, 623
    myelin degeneration and, 644
    myelin lamellae and, 40–41
    myelin removal in, 68–69
    myelination of peripheral system and
        Schwann cell length, 335
    myelinogenesis and, 14, 45, 59–60,
        63, 64, 69
    neuromuscular junction and, 477
    nucleus of, 21, 73, 200, 719
    paranodal apparatus of, 33–34, 48,
        53, 54
    'penicillate endings', 127
    peroxisome of, 242, 608
    'Pi' granules, 116
    processes, shape of, 129–30
    proliferation, chronic neuropathies in
        man, 721
    proliferation, following nerve section,
        710
    protein synthesis, 335
    recovery from EDN, 692–3
    regeneration following EDN, 694
    relation to node, 27–45, 46, 53
    response to injury, 583
    rippling movements at internode and,
        21
    sheath and, 28, 35
    suggested role of, 47, 73
    susceptibility to diphtheria toxin,
        697
    syncitial nature of, 111, 120
    synthesis activity following Wallerian
        Degeneration, 711
    teeth and, 452
    transformation to macrophages, 716
    unmyelinated fibre degeneration and,
        148, 150
    Wallerian Degeneration and, 630,
        632, 667, 715
sensory ganglion, 188–278
    action potentials and, 256
    'atypical' cell interpretation of,
        222–3
    axon hillock region of, 218, 227

Cell (*cont.*)
    axonal glomeruli of, 230–1, 233
    bimodal size distribution, 218, 219
    bipolar nature of, 225, 226
    classification of, by Nissl substance,
        203–4
    'dendro-axonal process' of, 226
    dense body lysosomes, 211–2
    dorsal root fibres and, 226
    electron dense vesicles, 215–6
    gamma amino butyric acid (GABA)
        and, 260–1
    GERL system of, 206, 208, 211,
        212, 220, 607–608
    glycogen membrane arrays of, 209
    Golgi apparatus of, 204–8, 211
    growth and differentiation in, 251–2
    initial portion of stem process, 227,
        229–30
    initial tract of axon, definition, 227
    lamellar bodies of, 208–9
    lipofuscin in, 212–3
    mesencephalic neurons, differences
        between, 255
    mitochondria of, 215
    molecule movement selection by, 237
    multipolar cells of, 222, 223
    myelination of, 248–9
    myelination of glomerular axons, 233
    nematosomes, 217
    neuromelanin in, 212–3
    neural crest and, 251
    nuclear inclusions, 200–1
    nucleolus, 201
    nucleus, characteristics of, 200
    numbers of, 199–200
        origin of, 249–50
        peripherally generated impulses and,
            257
        peroxidase containing bodies, 217
        physiological changes in, after injury,
            261–3
        pigment granules, shape of, 213
        regeneration after injury, 261–2
        satellite cell investment and, 252
        sizes of, 198–9
        somatotrophic organization of,
            258–60
        spontaneous discharge in, 257
        subsurface cisterns of, 209
        survival and satellite cell, 247–8
        unipolar nature of, 222, 225, 226
        volume of satellite cell sheath and,
            245
    sheath, 13, 109, 135
    small dark (obscure), 203
        characteristics, 219
        function, 221
    small intensely fluorescent (SIF), 225,
        365, 366

INDEX

Cell (*cont.*)
    spinal ganglion
        function, satellite cell absence, 247
        myelin of, 248
    sub-pial astrocyte, 345
    retinal bipolar, 1
    vestibular ganglion, 1
Cellules obscure, 219
Cementing disc, affinity for ions, 50, 52
Centrifugal inhibition, 403
Cerebroside, 617, 624, 630, 641
Cerebrospinal fluid, 342, 343
Charge
    spread of, 740, 779–95, 807
    storage of, 773, 807
Chemical transmitter, function of, 497, 498
Chemoreception, bacteria, 401
Chick
    extracellular connective tissue and, 175,
        176
    fibrillogenesis, 175–6
Cholesterol, 617, 618, 624, 625, 642
    esters, 618, 629, 630, 642, 652
Choline acetylase, 616
    acetyl transferase, 610
Chromatolysis, 254, 261, 263, 608
Colchicine, effect of, 614
Collagen pockets, 121
Complex paranode, 48
Conductance
    calcium, 772
        activated potassium, 777
    'leak', 760, 761, 762, 767, 788
    potassium, 760, 761, 765, 766, 783, 788
    sodium, 760, 761, 765, 766, 770, 771,
        776, 787, 788, 791
        charge with membrane potential,
            781–2
Conduction velocity, 3
    change in, effect of, 790–3
    'gating' current, effect of, 789–90, 795
    nerve impulses and, 784
    safety factor nerves, 787–8, 806
    simple models, 785–9
    temperature, effect of, 793–5
Connective tissue space, 162
    presence of, in body, 163–4
Corpuscles
    genital, 171
    Grandry, 408, 420
    Herbst, 408, 413, 415
    Meissner's, 171, 172, 415–6, 447, 454
    of Erzholz, 20
    of Vater-Pacini, 410
    Pacinian, 339, 400, 401, 402, 403, 404,
        405, 407, 408, 409, 410–3, 414,
        415, 447
    response from, 413–5
Corynbacterium diphtheriae, 683

Cranial nerve roots, definition of, 330
Crayfish, giant axon, 762–3
Creatine kinase, 607
Cresyl violet, 651
Cross of Ranvier, 28, 29, 33, 49
Curarine, effect of, 502, 505
Cutaneous endings, 171
Cyto centrum, 219

Da Fino silver technique, 208
Demyelination, 633, 635, 638, 642, 644–5,
    649
Dendritic glomerulus, 359
'Dense bodies', 211
Dentine, sensitivity of, 453
Dictyosomes, 204
Dimensional analysis, 788–9, 790, 795–9
Disease
    Fabry's, 651
    storage, 649–50
    Tangier, 652
    Tay-Sach's, 652
Doel, bulbous corpuscles of, 413
Dopamine, 366, 614–5, 632
Dorsal
    column nuclei, 448
    nerve roots, C fibre vulnerability, 343
    roots, 191, 209, 212, 220, 238, 258
Dura mater, 173

Earthworm, specialization of post junctional
    membrane, 469
Eighth cranial nerve, weakness of, 350
Eimer's organ, 417
Einerson's gallocyanin-chrome alum method,
    606
Eisenmann–Williams electrostatic theory,
    755
Elastic fibres, 189, 191
Endoneurium, 4, 49, 159
    appearance of, 339
    blood vessels and, 177–8, 339–40
    cellular populations in, 161–2
    diffusion barrier and, 165
    fibrils of, 161, 189, 190
    fibroblasts of, 339
    insulation from axon by, 5
    mast cells, lack of, 193
    motor end-plates and, 169–70
    muscle spindle and, 170
    nerve crush and, 708
    perineurial cells and, 165
    permeability of, 178
    protein leakage and endothelial cells, 197
    regenerating axon and, 721, 723
    Schwann tube and, 721
    subarachnoid space and, 173
End plate potential, 507–8
Enteric nervous system, 382

826

Epineurium, 4, 159, 194, 195, 197, 330, 343
  cellular populations in, 161
  dura mater and, 173
  fibrils of, 161
  motor endplates and, 169–70
  nerve crush and, 708
  sensory ganglia and, 189
  spinal nerve roots, 341
  sympathetic ganglia and, 357
Equilibrium potential, 741
'Espirocitos', 245
'Exchange diffusion', 748
Experimental allergic encephalomyelitis (EAE)
  antigens and, 680–2
  production of, 680
Experimental allergic neuritis (EAN)
  antigens and, 680–2
  characteristics of, 668–9
  electrophysiological changes and, 698–702
  histology of, 669–71
  immune response, 679–70
  lysis of intra period line, 688–9
  nodal widening, 689, 692
  permeability of spinal roots and, 676
  remyelination following, 676, 678
  suppression of, 682–3
Experimental diphtheric neuropathy (EDN)
  cellular metabolism and, 696–8
  characteristics of, 683–4
  differences of effect on myelin compared with EAN, 692
  electrophysiological changes and, 698–702
  enzyme activity and myelin breakdown, 693
  following remyelination, 694
  histology of, 684–96
  immune mechanism and, 698
  nodal widening and, 689, 692
  'short intercalary segments', 687

Familial Dyasautonomia (Riley–Day Syndrome), 137, 147
Fenestrated capillaries, 194, 195
Fetal human sciatic nerve, development of, 333
'Fibrae organicae', 107
Fibres
  C, 107
  nuclear bag, 423, 425, 426, 428
  nuclear chain, 423, 425, 428
  post-ganglionic, 370, 374, 379
  pre-ganglionic, 368, 379
  ratio between pre- and post-ganglionic, 369, 379
  varicose, 370

Fibrillary mechanism, 218
Fibrillenscheide of Key and Retzius, 159
Fibrils
  micro, 175
  primary, 175
Fixed surface charge, 768
Freund's adjuvant, 680
Fromman's lines, 33
Funiculi, 2, 14

'g', 9
'Gaine lamelleuse', 159
Gallus domesticus, 686
Ganglia
  autonomic nervous system of, 355–95
  boundary membrane, 357
  ciliary
    birds, 379–82
    histochemical reactions of, 377–8
    mammals, 376–9
  dendritic glomerulus, 359
  disposal of leaked protein, 198
  estimated numbers of, 358
  intramural, 382–8
    histochemistry of, 383, 384
  nucleus of cells of, 359
  paravertebral, 355, 361
    postganglionic fibres, 370, 372
  postganglionic fibres, myelination of, 379
  preganglionic fibres, acetylcholinesterase activity, 376
  prevertebral, 356, 361
  protein 'leakage' in, 195–8
  satellite cells and, 358–9, 374, 377
  sensory, 188–278
  superior cervical, nerve endings of, 363, 364
  sympathetic
    adrenalin and, 374
    amine distribution, 366
    Amphibia, 372
    capsule of, 357
    chromaffin cells of, 365–8
    classes of neurons, 359, 361
    classes of neurons, frog, 374
    dendrites, 359, 363
    divisions of, 355
    electron microscopy, 363, 366
    features of cells of, 361, 363
    fluorescence microscopy, 364, 374
    non-fluorescent neurons, function, 364
    number of neurons, 358
    paravertebral, 355
    preganglionic fibres, classification of, 368
    preganglion fibre/ganglion neuron ratio, 369, 370
    preganglionic fibres, origin and innervation, 368

Ganglia (*cont.*)
    preverterbral, 355, 357
    superior cervical, 358
    synapses and, 363, 372, 375
Ganglion cell-satellite cell complex, 191
Gap
    junction, 244, 252, 253, 255
    substance, 39, 40, 44, 45, 47, 243, 253,
       337, 609
'Gate'
    activation (m), 766, 768, 770, 771, 772,
       781, 788, 790
    activation–inactivation mechanism, 770
    current, 770–2, 789–90, 791, 793, 794,
       795, 796, 802
    potassium, 769
    voltage dependance, 768
'Gating reaction', 745, 746, 752, 766
Glial dome, 344, 346
Globoid cell leucodystrophy, 650–1
Glutamate, 237, 260
Glycogen, 209, 220, 242
Goldman constant field theory, 750, 751,
    753, 755, 756, 757
    modification of, 757
Goldman–Hodgkin–Katz equation, 756,
    757, 761, 763, 776, 807
Golgi apparatus
    enzymes of, 206
    form of, sensory ganglion cell, 204
    function of, 208
    GERL complex and acid hydrolase
       synthesis, 212
    outer stack face, form of, 206, 208
    receptor adaption, 403, 404
    tissue sheaths and, 170
Granular endoplasmic reticulum, 203, 204,
    206, 218, 219, 220, 242
Guillan–Barré syndrome, 667
Gustatory receptors
    central connections, 442
    responses of, 441–2
    structure of 440

'Haarschieben', 417
Hair follicles, lanceolate endings in, 416
Hair, receptor innervation, 447, 448
Hale colloidal iron technique, 44
Hairy skin, mechanoreceptive responses in,
    447
'Heat block', 787
Horseradish peroxidase, 194, 195, 197, 259
Hunter, unmyelinated axon models, 786–8
Hydraulic flow, theory of dental sensation,
    453
Hypertrophic neuropathy, 645

Incisures of Schmidt–Lanterman
    biological significance, 26

Incisures of Schmidt–Lanterman (*contd.*)
    dilation after nerve injury, 630
    diphtheritic neuropathy and, 688–9
    distribution following nerve crush,
       719–20
    EDN and, 684, 685
    motor neuron axon myelination and,
       296, 517
    myelin sheath of, 513
    nerve fibre crush and, 705, 706
    neuroplasmic flow and, 84– 85
    response to injury, mouse peripheral
       nerve, 582–3
    significance of, 26–27
    Wallerian degeneration and, 706, 707
Indoxyl acetate technique, 613
'Ingoing rectifier', 751, 753, 755, 757
Internode
    incisures of Schmidt–Lanterman and,
       5, 6, 7, 18
    length of, 4–5
    myelin sheath, passage of material
       through, 74
    node of Ranvier, 6, 7
Intraperiod line, 74, 625, 630
Ions
    active transport of, 741, 748, 760, 774–9
    conductance
       concentration dependance, 751–5,
          793
       selectivity of, 755–6 758
       voltage dependance, 749–51, 755
    movement
       independance of, 745–9, 752, 755,
          791, 792, 793
       methods of observation, 741
       passive, 741, 748
    permeation, mechanism for, 743
Isoniazid, effect of, 148, 631
Itch, humans, 445

'Jelly roll' hypothesis, 8

Karnovsky and Roots' technique, 609
Koelle and Friedenwald thiocholine
    method, 609
Krause, end bulbs of, 413

'Lamellated sheath of Ranvier', 159
Lamellar bodies, 208, 209
Lateral inhibition, process of, 402–3, 449
Lateral line mechanoreceptor, 400
Law
    Kirchoff, 779–80
    Ohm, 742, 743, 746, 749, 757, 767, 779
Lead, effect of, 644
Leucodystrophy
    Krabbe, 651
    Metachromatic, 650–1

'Liminal length', 783
Limulus, 401
Lipofuscin, 212, 213, 242, 608, 628
'Local currents', 784, 786
Lysosomes, 211, 212, 242, 607–8, 611,
    626, 631, 635, 644, 649

Marsupial, spinal ganglia of, 250–1
Mechanism
    'carrier', 744, 750, 751, 752
    'pore', 744, 750, 751, 752
Mechanoreceptors
    alimentary canal receptors, 430
    arterial chemoreceptors, 442–4
        sensitivity, 444
    classification, 409
    cutaneous endings of, 429–30
    cytology of, 406–7
    fibre routes to spinal cord, 448–9, 451
    golgi tendon organs, 422–3, 426
    gustatory receptors, 439–42
    in synovial joint, 430–2
    innervation of hair, 447, 448
    lanceolate endings, 416–7
    low threshold C-fibres, 429, 433, 447
    Merkel disc endings and, 417–9
    neuromuscular spindles, 423, 425,·
        426–9
        development of, 429
        efferent nerves and, 427
        responses from, 426–9
    nociceptors, 444–5
    nuclei of, 437
    olfactory receptors, 434, 437–9
    respiratory tract receptors, 430–1
    Ruffini terminals, 421
    supporting cells, 434–5
    thermoreceptors, 432–4
        effect of chemicals on, 434
    tissue relationship, 420–2
    type I, 402, 416, 417, 447, 448
    type II, 402, 422, 426, 447, 448
    urinary receptors, 430
    vascular baroreceptors, 431
Membrane
    artificially prepared, 743, 744
    charge movements across, 740
    concept, 740
    conductance and, 742, 743, 744, 746, 760
    current of, 781–2
    depolarization, 749
    ion
        concentration in, 750, 751, 752
        conductance, 'carrier' mechanism,
            751, 752, 764
        disequilibrium, 742
        independance of movement, 745–9
        movement across 740–1, 745, 755
        species and, 745

Membrane (*cont.*)
    Node of Ranvier resting potential, frog,
        763–5
    'noise', 773
    permeability of, 743, 744, 751
    potential 742, 784
    resting potential 749, 756, 760–5,
        776–7, 806
        alteration of, 761
    voltage threshold, 783
    zero current potential, 757, 763, 775,
        779, 781, 783, 787
'Membrane whorls', 692, 697
Mesencephalic nucleus, 253
Metachromasia, 629, 651–2
Metachromatic leucodystrophy (MLD),
    650–1
Mice, myelin abnormalities in, 579–82
Microfibrils, 191
Microtubules, 219, 229, 237, 242, 245
'Minimal membrane', 512
Motor end plate, 464–511
    barrier function and, 179
    chemical transmission and, 498
    en grappe configuration, 464, 473
    en plaque configuration, 464, 474
    formation of, 476
    function of, 495–6
    localization of, 478–9
    size of, 473
    tissue sheaths and, 169–70
Motor neuron
    axon
        hillock of, 295, 305, 315
        myelination of, 296
    cell bodies, 281
    changes in, after section, 283, 285,
        291–2
    cytoplasm of, 313
    dendritic tree of, 288–90
    detachment during development, 313
    distribution of M bouton types and,
        303–4
    dorsal root bouton of, 301
    electrical properties of, 286, 288
    embryology of, 313
    excitatory synapse, 312
    gamma type, 284
    growth of
        bouton and development, 318
        in kitten, 316
    importance of synapse removal during
        development, 319
    initial axon
        bouton loss after birth in kitten, 319
        presence of boutons on, in newborn
            kitten, 318
        segment of, 295, 315
    inhibitory synapse, 311

Motor neuron (*cont.*)
  models of, 287
  neuropil of, 291, 296, 313, 315
  nucleus of, 291, 313, 315
  phasic, 285–6, 302, 312
  proportions of bouton types on cell body
      and dendrites of, 304–5
  receptor field of, 288–9
  size of, 281, 283, 284, 315, 316
  synapses of, 298
    distribution, 309, 315
    types, 299–300
  tonic, 285–6, 302, 312
  tonic stretch reflex in kittens, 314
Muller, theory of specific nervous energy,
    396
Multiple sclerosis
  cerebroside loss and, 630
  demyelination disorders and, 700
  myelin sheath and, 583–5
  plaques, 638
  temperature effect on, 700
Muscle fibres
  contractile properties of, 486–7
  function of, 495
  miniature end plate potentials, 502
  motor nerve fibres to, 496–8
  newborn, sensitivity to ACh, 479
  slow fibres, 497, 498
  twitch, 497, 498
Muscle spindle
  atrophy of, 408
  generator potential, 400
  tissue sheaths and, 170
Myelin, 512–604
  abnormalities due to disease, 577,
      579–85
  birefringence of, 7, 8
  breakdown following EDN, 684, 686
  cerebroside dislocation from, 630
  classes of protein in, 637
  composition of, 520–2
  conduction velocity and, 515–6
  degredation, lysosomal enzymes and,
      672
  dissolution following nerve crush, 706
  enzyme association, 560–1
  enzymes of, 625–6, 628
  EAN and, 688–9
  fragmentation after nerve section, 630,
      635
  glycoprotein of, 561–2, 624
  growth of, 566–70
  inhibition by diphtheria toxin, 697–698
  intraperiod line, 24, 25, 625, 630
  isolation of, 522–4
  lipid composition of, 529, 531–2, 617,
      629–30, 641
  lipid turnover, 616–9
  lipoprotein complexes of, 526–3, 565

Myelin (*cont.*)
  loss of, 644–5, 649
  maturation of, 529
  membrane structure of, 586–8
  metabolism and synthesis, 570–7
  model of, 8
  multiple sclerosis and, 583–5
  myelinogenesis, manner of, 8
  phases of lipid breakdown during nerve
      degeneration, 641–3
  phospholipids of, 617–8, 642
  properties of isolated, 524–5
  protein
    composition, 525, 527–9, 549–50,
        553–5, 558–60
    histochemistry, 619–24
  PMR spectra of, 543, 544
  repeating lipid and protein layers, 7
  Schwann cell and, 720
  sheath, 5, 6, 616, 641
    accumulation of products of Schwann
        cell metabolism, 20–21
    amino acid transport across, 517
    axon regeneration and, 705
    changes during Wallerian degeneration,
        713, 715
    changes following axon crush, 704
    diphtheritic neuropathy, 689
    'discontinuities' in, 23
    form of, 18, 36, 38
    formation of, 8, 60–61
    formation by oligodendrocytes, 344
    function during saltatory conduction,
        692
    insulating properties, 518
    internodal axon and, 9
    lipid-protein nature of, 7–8, 624–5
    microtubules, function of, 41
    'normal' variations, 689
    oligodendrocytes, 344, 345
    properties of, 516–20
    role of, 513, 515–6
    Schwann cell and, 17, 18, 20, 78, 616
    sheath, 5, 6, 616, 641
    structure of, 533, 536–7, 539–41
    structure modification, techniques,
        544–8
Myelinated fibres, 1–105
  amphibian, conduction velocity and
      fibre diameter relationship, 800
  cat, conduction velocity and rise time,
      803
  degeneration in diphtheric neuropathy,
      689
  frog, Q_{10} value, 794
  models of, 789
  scaling relation, 797–9
  volume to surface ratio, 805
Myoneural end-plate, 168
'Myotactic unit', 428

Myxicola, 747, 767, 789

Naphthol AS–TR phosphatase, 607, 633
Nematosome, 217, 218
Nemiloff rings, 30
Nernst equation, 742
Nernst–Planck equation, 743, 750
Nerve
  crush
    incisures of Schmidt–Lanterman
      distribution following, 719–20
    recovery of conduction velocity
      following and, 725–6
    regeneration following, 718–25
  demyelination by EAN, 672
  injury, classification, 703
  splanchnic, 351
  endings
    calyciform, 380
    in intramural muscle, 384
    in sympathetic ganglia, 364
  fibre
    blocking, effect of, 745
    classification of fibre diameter, 3–4
    conductance of, 742, 743
    conduction velocities of, 3–4
    conduction velocities and
      temperature, 793–4
    connective tissue of, 4
    ion permeation, 742
    of Remak, 6
    peripheral, categorization of, 1–4
    regeneration following crush, 705
    safety factor for conduction, 806
    size and electrophysiological
      properties, 795–806
    swelling of, following activity,
      804–5
    to teeth, 452–4
    unmyelinated, Schwann cell
      internuclear distances, 720
  'growth factor', 136–7
  membrane (*see* Membrane)
  section, cellular outgrowths from, 723
  terminals, histochemistry, 615–6
  terminals, sensory, 396–463
  trunk, functional classification of fibres
    in, 2
Neural
  crest, embryological importance of,
    249–50, 251, 253, 330, 343,
    346, 408
  microtubules, 86–9
  processing, 399
  tube, cell derivation from 253, 330, 331
Neurofilaments, 12
Neurokeratin, 620–2, 624–5, 637, 639
Neuromuscular junction
  acetylcholine receptor site for, 477, 478,
    499
  basic features of, 465–73
  changes in after nerve section, 482
  development of, 476–7
  neuronal element of control, 482-3
  types of, 496–8
  ultrastructure of, 473–6, 485, 486
Neuromuscular spindle
  central control of, 428
  development of, 429
  reflex activities, 428
  responses of, 426–7
  structure of, 423–6
Neuron (*see also* Motor neuron)
  anaxonic, 1
  axon, 1, 2, 13
    ACh synthesis and, 499–500
    axonal transport along, 11
    axoplasm of, 10, 12
    Bands of Bünger and, 722
    bidirectional flow of material along,
      79–81
    changes following crush, 704
    composition of, 9–13
    concept of material flow along,
      77–78
    'critical diameter', 106
    current flow along, equations
      describing, 779–80
    dense cored vesicles of, 113
    depolarization and transmitter
      release, 504
    diameter of and conduction velocity,
      513
    diameter of and myelin sheath
      thickness, 63
    diameter of and sensory ganglion cell
      relationship, 199
    diameter to whole fibre diameter
      (d/D), 64, 65, 67, 68, 515–6,
      518
    dorsal root ganglion cell and, 239
    EDN and, 685
    fixed number of Schwann cells
      along, 67
    function of, 495
    'free endings', 445
    growth pattern, 14, 45–48
    guidance of, 136
    hillock of, 2, 218, 227, 295, 375
    initial segment of, 2, 254, 256, 295
    insulation from endoneurium, 5
    material flow along, 78–79, 81,
      82–83
    microtubules and material flow along,
      87–88
    myelination of, 59–70, 231, 238,
      296
    'nerve growth factor', 136
    neurofilaments and material flow
      along, 88–89

Neuron (*contd.*)
  neuroplasmic flow, physical
    mechanism mediating, 83–86
  oligodendrocytes, 345
  oxidative enzyme activity, 606–8
  periaxonal space, 5
  permeability of, 76
  paranodal bulb and, 34, 42
  'point polarized', 783
  protein synthesis in, 56–57
  protein synthesizing capacity, 608–15
  RNA of, 54–56
  synthesis of RNA, 55–56
  satellite cell and, 58–59, 69–70, 72,
    106, 107, 188, 245, 344
  satellite cell, spiralling around, 245
  Schwann cell and, 346, 348, 369,
    482, 516, 568, 676, 678, 724
  sodium flow into, during impulse
    passage along, 513, 515
  specialization of ending of, 467
  tight junctions and, 41, 75, 165,
    380, 517
  volume to surface ratio, 791, 796,
    800, 804, 805
 axonal glomerulus, 230–1
 axonal vesicle discharge and formation,
  483, 485
 bipolar, 1
 chromophyllic, 606
 classes of, 359, 361, 374
 cross union, effect of, 141
 dendritic tree of, 1
 'dendritic zone', 226
 description of, 1–2
 growth cones, 139, 140
 location of, 1–2
 mesencephalic, destination of, 254
 multipolar, 1, 346, 359
  course of, ventral horn and, 280–1
 neurites of, 1
 oligodendroglia, 2
 perikaryon, 1
 presence of, to stimulate neuromuscular
  junction, 476
 RNA distribution in, 54–56
 satellite cell complex and, 191, 243,
  244, 253
 size of, and satellite cell relationship, 245
 soma (perikaryon), 1
  function, 76–77
  material synthesis by, 89
 telodendroglia, 2
 ultrastructural differences in developing,
  236
 unipolar, 372
Neuron-glia unit, 58
Neuronal
 DNA, 606

Neuronal (*contd.*)
 RNA, 606
Neuropil, 291, 296, 315
 growth cones of, 313
Neurotmesis, 703
Neurotubule system, 86–9, 614–5
Neutral protease, 611, 625–6, 634–5
Nissl substance, 201, 203–4, 218, 252, 261,
 280, 291, 606, 608
Nociceptors
 categories of, 445
 definition of, 444
 mechanoreceptors, 445
 muscle, 445
 polymodal, 445
 teeth and, 453
 transduction in, 445
Node of Ranvier, 6, 7, 23, 27–28, 49, 54,
 60, 62, 73, 120, 346, 609, 612, 626,
 631, 635
 action potential and, 6, 9
 amphibian, sodium pump, 777
 axon crush and, 704
 axoplasm of, 44–45
 biconical expansion, 28
 changes induced by EAN, 674
 cholinesterase activity, 609
 conduction velocity and, 702
 development of, 45–48
 EDN and, 684
 frog, resting membrane potential,
  763–5, 767
 function of ions and, 52–53
 impulse conduction and, 48
 input conductance, 798
 ion exchange and, 50–52
 ionic environment of, 48–54
 microvilli of, 39–40, 47, 53
 morphogenesis, 46–47
 myelin sheath termination at, 513
 myelinated stem processes and,
  233–4
 oxide reductase activity, 612
 regeneration following EAN, 678
 regeneration following EDN, 694, 695
 role of, 29–30
 Schwann cell and, 345
 sodium current generation, 786, 793
 structure of
  electron microscopy, 34–45
  light microscopy, 28–34
 toad, conductance of, 760
 toad, ion conductance and, 747, 753
Nodose ganglion, 189, 221, 224, 225, 235,
 258
Noradrenergic neurons, 613
Nucleus of Edinger–Westphall, 379

'Occluding zonules', 166

Olfactory receptors
  central connections, 438–9
  responses of, 438
  structure of, 434–8
Olfactory roots, uniqueness of, 346
'Onion bulb', 129, 694, 721
Orthagociscus mola, 339
Orthophytes, 222
OTAN-method, 642
Oxidative enzyme activity
  axons, 612
  myelin, 626
  neuron, 606
  Schwann cell, 613

Pacinian corpuscle tissue sheaths and, 171,
    172
Paciniform ending, 413
'Paradoxical cold', 432
Paraganglia, 225
Paranodal apparatus, maturation of, 337–8
Paranodal bulb
  assymetry of, 33–34
  axon and, 42
  development of, 47–48
  myelin sheath and, 35–37, 48
  neurotubules, 42–43
Paranodal demyelination, 701
Paranodal folds, 805
Paraphytes, 222, 224, 230
PAS technique, 607, 619, 639, 652
  modification, 619
Passive movement of ions, 741
  experimental observation of, 741–2
Periaxonal space, 70–73, 75
  ion permeability in, 72
Perineurial sheath, 189, 193, 198
Perineurium, 189, 191, 194, 195, 197
  blood vessels and, 178
  capsule surrounding neuromuscular
    complex, 426
  cells of, 343
  cellular layers of, 165
  diffusion barrier and, 165–6
  distribution in nerves of, 160–1
  fibrils of, 161
  function of, 643
  golgi, tendon organ and, 170
  homeostatic function, 708
  motor endplates and, 169–70
  muscle spindle and, 170
  nerve fibre crush and, 706, 708, 716
  pacinian corpuscles and, 171
  peripheral termination of, 168–9
  pinocytosis, 179
  Schwann cell similarity and, 167, 241
  sensory ganglia and, 189
  subarachnoid angle and, 173–4

Perineurium (*contd.*)
  tight junctions and, 166–7, 174, 178,
    195
Peripheral nerve, multilamellar perineurial
    sheath of, 340–1, 343
  unmyelinated fibres, definition, 107
Perinodal gap, 49, 53
Peroxisome, 217, 242, 608
Phosphotungstic acid haematoxylin
    (PTAH), 622, 637
Pial envelope, 2, 167, 175, 348, 349
'Plasmastrassen', 213
Plexus
  Auerbach's, 382
  Meissner's, 382, 409
Point polarization, 783, 787
Pore theory, membrane conductance,
    746–7, 750
Potential
  generator, 400, 401, 402, 405
  resting, 399
Primitive band, 6
Protein, transport in central and peripheral
    axons compared, 236–7
Pump
  chloride, 779
  sodium
    activity rate, 791
    ATP, energy source for, 774
    as current generator, 775
    calcium transport and, 778–9
    electrical effects of, 774–8
    electrogenic function, 778
    Node of Ranvier, amphibian, 777
    tetanic nyperpolarization, 777
    transient effects, 777

'Quaking mouse', 579, 580, 582

Rabbit
  EAN, effect of, 669–70
  hair types of, 447
Rall, cable model of, 287, 288, 302
Ramus communicans
  grey, 357, 370, 374
  white, 355, 368
Rana, 230
  esculenta, 376
Ranvier (see node of)
Rat
  axon demyelination by EAN, 672
  axonal injury, 262–3
  axoplasmic changes distal to nerve
    section, 712
  diphtheritic neuropathy, 688–9
  dorsal root ganglia, EDN and, 684
  effect of diphtheria toxin, 645
  inhibition of protein synthesis, 696
  lysosomes and myelin breakdown, 693

Rat (*contd.*)
  neuromuscular junctions in diaphragm
    of, 474
  nodal widening following nerve crush,
    717
  remyelination following EDN, 687, 688
  sciatic nerve
    biochemical studies of, 335
    regeneration following crush, 726
  spinal roots, permeability to serum
    albumin, 676
  ventral root demyelination and
    conduction block, 700
Reaction
  'gating', 745, 746, 752
  'ion transfer', 744, 745, 746
Receptor
  cell–cell relationship, 407
  development of sensory cells, 407–9
  distribution of, 479, 481
  'field', 447
  synovial joint, central connections, 451
  transmitter substances and, 477–9
Receptor system
  action potential initiation, 401–2
  adaption of, 403–5
  classification of, 398
  initiation of conductance changes in,
    401
  neural processing, 402–3
  stimulus transmission, 398–9
Reich's π granules, 20, 613, 628–9, 632
Remak
  'cells', 115
  fibres, 106, 107, 115
Respiratory tract
  'irritant' terminals, 430
  'J' receptors, 431
  stretch receptors, 431
Reticular fibres, 161
Retinal rods, 400
Retrograde axonal flow, 613, 632
Root sheath, 174, 330, 341
Ruffini terminals, 400, 404, 421, 426

Saltatory conduction, 9, 29, 49, 73, 512,
    513, 516, 609, 610, 692
  diphtheria toxin, effect on, 699
  myelin sheath, function, 692
  requirements for theory of, 516–7
Schwann cell, *see* Cell
'Scaling relation', 796–9
Seddon's classification, 703
Segmental
  demyelination, 644, 651
  remyelination, 64–65
Senses, classification of, 346–7
Sensory endings, resting potential of, 399

Sensory ganglia (*see also* Cell)
  endoneurial vessels, permeability of,
    195, 196
  paraganglia of, 224–5
  vascularization of, 193–8
Sensory terminals, peripheral nerves of,
    396–463
Sheath (*see also* Epineurium, Endoneurium
    and Perineurium)
  Key and Retzius, 159, 339, 721
  Plenk and Laidlaw, 159, 161, 339, 704
Silver-gelatin autogram technique, 611, 625,
    634
Sodium-potassium coupled pump, 748, 760,
    774
  electrical effects, 774–5
Soleus muscle, alpha motor axons of, 285
Sphingomyelin, 618–9, 641
Spinal cord
  hemisection and terminal bouton
    degeneration, 310
  multipolar neurons of, 280
  paraventral ganglia of, 355
  white rami communicans, 355
Spinal nerve roots, 330–54
  analgesic and, 343
  blood vessels of, 339–40
  cellular sheaths of, 330, 341
  connective tissue of, 330
  degeneration of, 349–51
  development of, 331–2
  effect of crushing, 349
  endoneurial space, 343
  epineurium and, 341
  injuries and, 350
Spiny bracelet of Nageotte, 30, 31, 41, 65
Squid
  axon
    calcium transport and, 778–9
    conductances of, 760–2, 776, 768,
      769
    coupling ratio, 775
    Q_{10} ratio, 794
    sodium and potassium channels, 767
Starfish egg, conductance of, 755
Stem process, 226, 227, 231, 233
Stimulus
  accession, 398, 399
  transduction, 398, 399–401
Stratum internum perineurii, 166
Strength duration curve, 784
Subarachnoid
  angle, 173
  space, 173, 343, 350
'Sub-neural apparatus', 465
Substance P, 237, 260, 261
Substantia nigra, 218
Subsurface cisterns, 209

Sural nerve
  age changes in man, 148, 150
  d/D ratio, 516
Synapse (*see also* Terminal bouton)
  avian ciliary ganglion, 379–80
  excitatory on motor neuron, 312
  inhibitory on motor neuron, 311, 313
  intramural ganglia and, 384–5
  removal during growth, motor neurons, 319
  Renshaw, 311, 312
  types of, motor neurons, 299–300
Synaptic cleft, ACh and ion involvement, 505–6
Synaptic vesicle formation, 121
Synaptosomes, 615
Synovial joints, sensory receptors in, 450–2

Taste bud, 408, 440
Teeth, neural innervation of, 452–4
Terminal bouton
  C type, 209, 304, 309, 310, 312, 315, 317
    growth of, newborn kitten, 317
    inhibitory function, 311
  degeneration following spinal cord hemisection, 310
  determinants for classification, 300–1
  distribution, newborn kitten, 316–8
  F-type, 299, 300, 301, 304, 305, 309, 310, 312, 313, 315, 317, 319
    inhibitory function, 310–1
  M-type, 300, 301, 303, 310
    development of, kitten, 315, 316
    growth of, 317
  membrane covering, 305, 307, 317
  origin of, 309–10
  P-type, 300, 302, 303
  proportion of types on motor neurons 304–5
  S-type, 299, 301, 304, 305, 309, 315, 317, 319
  size of, newborn kitten, 316–8
  types of, motor neuron, 299–300
Thermoreceptive pathways, 449
Tight junctions, 195
Tongue, cells of, 440
Tonic stretch reflex, kitten, 314
Touch domes, 417
Trigeminal
  ganglion, permeability of vessels of, 195
  nerve root, 193, 195, 215, 217, 219, 221, 244, 258, 348
Triturus viridiscens, 477
Trophospongium, 244
Trypanosoma brucei, 682, 683
Tubuli primitivi, 106
Tylotrich hairs, 417, 447

Unit collagen fibrils, 161
Unmyelinated fibre, 106–158
  additional fibres and regeneration, 144
  axon
    composition of, 111–3
    contents of, 138
    diameter of, 132, 134
    growth of, 135–6, 139
    mechanism of growth guidance, 137
    numbers of in fibres, 131, 132
    patterns, 124–7
    Schwann cell cytoplasm and, 116, 119, 120, 124, 125, 126, 132, 135
    Schwann cell interface and, 120–1, 144
    separation from Schwann cell, 115–6
    shape of, 129–30
  axonal sprouts, 144, 146
  axoplasmic transport in, 114
  branching in, 125–6
  changes with age, 148–50
  collagen fibrils and, 121, 124
  conduction velocity, 138
  cross excitation, 124
  degeneration due to severance, 147–50
  discovery, 106, 108
  impulse conduction in, 146–7
  intranuclear distances, 120
  isoniazid and, 148
  misdirection during regeneration, 141–3
  models of, 786–9
  nuclei of, 120
  numbers of, 132
  'onion bulb' formation and, 129
  origin of, 108
  regenerative capacity, 111, 723
  regeneration in cut, 140–7, 177
  reinnervation of grafts, 143
  satellite cells and, 115
  scaling relation, 795–7
  Schwann cell length estimation, 120
  spatial relationship, myelinated fibres, 127, 129
  total ionic current, 783
Ussing's 'exchange diffusion', 748

Vagus nerve, 224, 250
Varicosities, 370
Vascular baroreceptor, 431
Ventral horn
  connections of, 356
  dendritic tree of horn cells, 289
  gamma motor neurons of, 284
  motor neurons
    newborn kitten, 314–5
    pools of, 290
  multipolar neurons of, 280–1

Ventral horn (*contd.*)
  neuron cell bodies, sizes of, 281, 283, 286
  neuropil ultrastructure, 296, 298
  Polio, effect on large motor neurons, 286, 293
  spinal border cells, 284
Vibrissal follicles, lanceolate endings, 417
Visual system, neural organization, 402
Voltage
  clamp, 753
  threshold, 781, 783
Vomeronasal organ of Jacobson, 434

Wallerian degeneration, 5, 84, 349, 582, 611, 613, 626, 644, 667, 674, 688, 701
  acetylcholinesterase activity, 631
  acid phosphatase, 633–4
  alkaline phosphatase, 633
  axon degeneration, 629
  axonal disintegration, 712
  axoplasm volume reduction, 713
  butylcholinesterase, 632
  cell population increase distal to injury, 708, 710
  demyelination and, differences, 645

Wallerian degeneration (*contd.*)
  electrophysiological changes, 725–6
  enzymes and, 631–6
  features of, 702–3
  histology of, 704–8, 710–3, 715–8
  incisures of Schmidt–Lanterman and, 706
  lipid changes and, 630
  macrophage population during, 711
  Marchi reaction to, 642
  myelin breakdown, phases of, 707
  'myelin forms', 713
  myelin fragmentation, 630, 637
  neurotoxic substances causing, 631
  oxidative enzyme activity, 631–2
  phospholipase activity, 633
  protein loss and, 637–9, 641
  Schwann cells and, 630, 632, 667, 715
  synthesis phase of Schwann cell during, 711
Weber–Fechner rule, 405
Weddell, 'pattern' theory of cutaneous sensation, 397, 398

Xenopus, 236

Zonal rotor, myelin isolation and, 523